Fundamentals of Nursing

CONTENT REVIEW PLUS PRACTICE QUESTIONS

PATRICIA M. NUGENT, RN, EdD
Professor Emeritus
Adjunct Professor
Nassau Community College
Garden City, New York
Private Practice—President of Nugent Books, Inc.

BARBARA A. VITALE, RN, MA
Professor Emeritus
Nassau Community College
Garden City, New York
Private Practice—Professional Resources for Nursing

F.A. Davis Company • Philadelphia

F. A. Davis Company
1915 Arch Street
Philadelphia, PA 19103
www.fadavis.com

Printed in the United States of America

Last digit indicates print number: 10 9 8 7 6 5 4 3 2 1

Publisher, Nursing: Robert G. Martone
Director of Content Development: Darlene D. Pedersen
Project Editor: Jacalyn C. Clay
Electronic Project Editor: Tyler R. Baber
Illustration and Design Manager: Carolyn O'Brien

Library of Congress Cataloging-in-Publication Data

Nugent, Patricia Mary, 1944- author.
  Fundamentals of nursing : content review plus practice questions /
Patricia M. Nugent, Barbara A. Vitale.
    p. ; cm.
  Includes bibliographical references and index.
  ISBN-13: 978-0-8036-3706-1
  ISBN-10: 0-8036-3706-3
  I. Vitale, Barbara Ann, 1944- author. II. Title.
  [DNLM: 1. Nursing Care—Examination Questions. 2. Nursing
Care—Outlines. WY 18.2]
  RT55
  610.73076—dc23
                          2013023818

*Dedicated to our
awesome grandchildren,
who inspire us,
who share their lives
and aspirations with us,
who communicate their energy to us,
and who give us their unconditional love!*

*Aiden, Alexander, Andie, Andrew,
Ava, Cade, Elle, James, Joseph, Nathan,
Ronan, Sean, William, and Carleigh,
our angel in heaven*

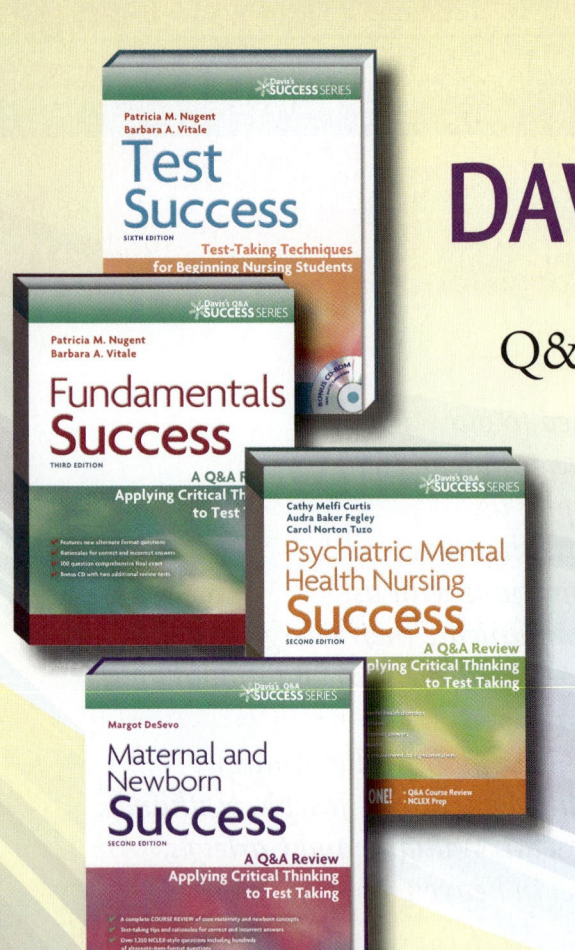
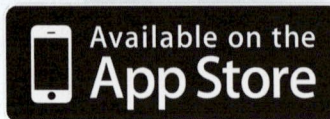
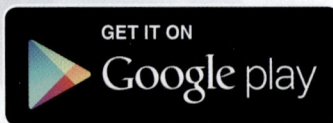
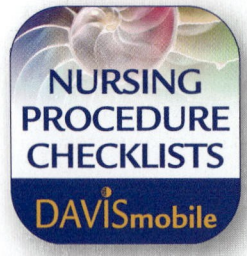
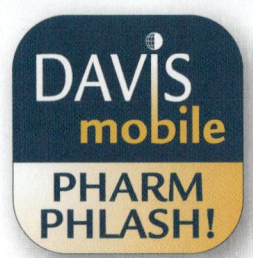
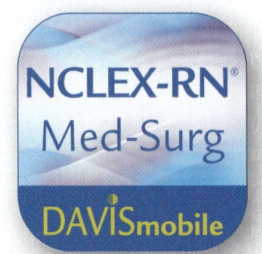
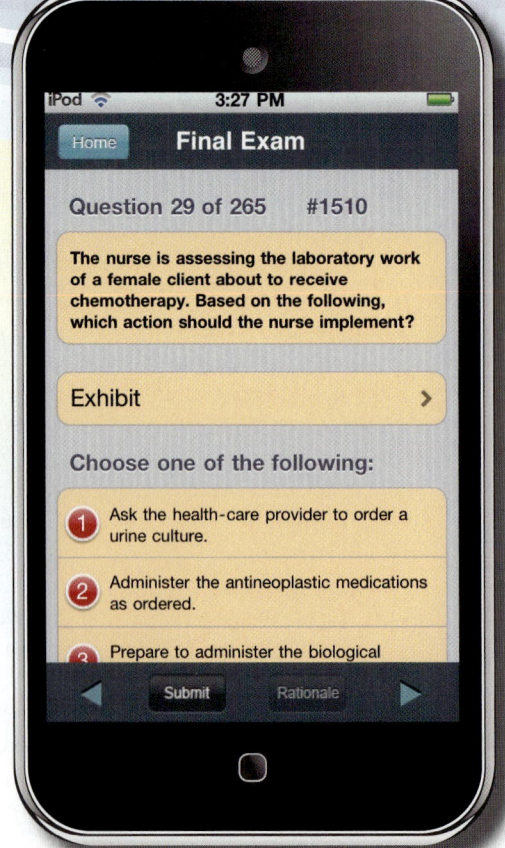
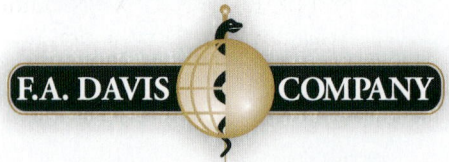

Why This Book Is Necessary

Most beginning nursing students have information overload. They must possess knowledge about a variety of subjects, including anatomy and physiology, psychology, sociology, medical terminology, diagnostic and laboratory tests, and growth and development, to mention a few. In addition, with the expanding roles and responsibilities of the nursing profession, the nursing information that beginning nursing students must learn is growing in depth and breadth exponentially. Fundamentals of nursing textbooks 20 years ago were approximately 300 to 400 pages in length. Today, they average 1,500 to 2,000 pages in length. This is more information than any beginning nursing student can possibly explore, remember, and apply in a stressful clinical situation without additional educational support. *Fundamentals of Nursing: Content Review Plus Practice Questions* provides that additional educational support!

Who Should Use This Book

Fundamentals of Nursing: Content Review Plus Practice Questions provides beginning nursing students with need-to-know information as well as questions to practice their ability to apply the information in a simulated clinical situation. This textbook is designed to:

- Be required by a nursing program as the sole fundamentals nursing textbook for a fundamentals of nursing course to be used in conjunction with reliable primary Internet sources for nursing information.
- Be required or recommended by a nursing program to be used in conjunction with a traditional fundamentals nursing textbook.
- Be used by beginning nursing students who want to focus on essential information contained in a fundamentals-of-nursing course.
- Be used by nursing students to learn how to be more successful when answering National Council Licensure Examination (NCLEX)–type multiple-choice and alternate-item format nursing questions early in their nursing education.
- Be used by nursing students preparing for the NCLEX-RN or NCLEX-PN examination to review basic nursing theory and practice.

What Information Is Presented in This Textbook

This textbook begins with a "Message to Test-Takers of Nursing Examinations," which includes information to help students maximize their ability to study effectively and achieve success when taking nursing examinations. General study strategies, specific study strategies, test-taking tips for answering multiple-choice questions and alternate-format questions, and the test plan categories for the NCLEX examinations are discussed.

The content is divided into five units. The first four units contain chapters that reflect the common, nucleus information contained in a fundamentals-of-nursing course. The fifth unit contains an integrated fundamentals of nursing examination.

- Unit I: Nursing Within the Context of Contemporary Health Care—This unit reviews nursing theories, legal and ethical issues, leadership and management, health-care delivery, and community-based nursing care.
- Unit II: Psychosociocultural Nursing Care—This unit reviews nursing care across the life span, communication and documentation, psychosocial and cultural nursing, and teaching and learning.
- Unit III: Essential Components of Nursing Care—This unit reviews the nursing process, physical assessment, infection control and wound care, safety, medication administration, and pharmacology.
- Unit IV: Basic Human Needs and Related Nursing Care—This unit reviews hygiene; mobility; nutrition; oxygenation; urinary elimination; fluid and electrolyte balance; gastrointestinal system; pain, comfort, rest, and sleep; and perioperative nursing.
- Unit V: Comprehensive Final Exam—This unit contains a 100-item fundamentals of nursing examination that integrates questions spanning content throughout the textbook. Each question contains rationales for correct and incorrect answers and the NCLEX test plan categories.

Each chapter presents need-to-know information in an outline format, eliminating nice-to-know, extraneous information. Just essential information is included, limiting the challenge of wading through excessive material. This approach assists students to focus on what is most important. The chapters include definitions of keywords and practice questions specific to their content. Multiple-choice questions as well as all the alternate-type questions included on NCLEX examinations are incorporated. Each question is coded according to the NCLEX test plan categories: Integrated Processes, including the Nursing Process, Client Need, and Cognitive Level. In addition, every question has the rationales for correct and incorrect answers. Studying rationales for the right and wrong answers to practice questions helps students learn new information or solidify previously learned information.

All questions in the textbook are included on line at davisplus.fadavis.com to provide the opportunity to practice taking NCLEX-type questions on a computer. In addition to these questions, two additional comprehensive tests are also posted online at davisplus.fadavis.com. Like the practice questions in the book, each question includes rationales for correct and incorrect answers and coding for the NCLEX test plan categories.

The textbook also presents a glossary of English words commonly encountered on nursing examinations. Familiarity with these words reduces the challenge of a test question because the student can focus on the theoretical content in the question.

Students should use every resource available to facilitate the learning process. We believe that this textbook will meet the needs of beginning nursing students who experience information overload!

Item Writers

MARY ANN HELLMER SAUL, PhD, RN, CNE
Professor
Nassau Community College
Garden City, New York

MICHAEL W. MANGINO, JR., RN, NP-PSYCHIATRY
Associate Professor
Suffolk Community College
Selden, New York

Medical Consultant

JOANNE M. VITALE, RPA-C
Coordinator of Bariatric Surgery
North Shore LIJ at Huntington Hospital
Huntington, New York

Reviewers

TINA K. ALLEN, BSN, MSN, EdD, RN
Associate Professor
School of Nursing/College of Health and Human
  Services
Troy University
Montgomery, Alabama

PAT FAHEY BACON, DNP, RN, FNP-BC
Coordinator Nursing Program and Nursing Faculty
Presentation College
Fairmont, Minnesota

CAROL BLAKEMAN, ARNP, MSN
Professor
College of Central Florida
Ocala, Florida

PEG BROADIE, MSN, CNE
Assistant Professor
Allen College
Waterloo, Iowa

REMYLIN BRUDER, DNP, RN
Associate Professor
Rochester College
Rochester Hills, Michigan

GLORIA BRUMMER, MS, RN, CNE, CEN
Assistant Professor
Department of Nursing
St. John's College
Springfield, Illinois

MARSHA CANNON, MSN, RN
Chairperson
University of West Alabama
Livingston, Alabama

EILEEN O. COSTELLO, MSN, RN
Dean, Health Sciences and Community Service Programs
Mount Wachusett Community College
Gardner, Massachusetts

MARNEE L. CRAWFORD, MSN, RN, CNE
Nursing Faculty
Northwest College
Powell, Wyoming

LEIGH ANN CREEL, RN, BSN, MSN
ADN Faculty/Nursing Instructor
Copiah Lincoln Community College
Wesson, Mississippi

CLAIRE CYRIAX, RN, MSN, LNC, CAPA
Nursing Faculty
Bergen Community College
Paramus, New Jersey

BONNIE DAVIS, PhD, RN
Director of Nursing
University of New England
Portland, Maine

KELLI DAVIS, RN, MSN
Nursing Instructor/ Faculty
Gadsden State Community College
Gadsden, Alabama

DEBORAH K. DRUMMONDS, RN, MN, CCRN, CEN
Assistant Professor
Abraham Baldwin Agricultural College
Tifton, Georgia

VICTOR DUARTE, MSN, RN, CCRN
Nursing Instructor
Front Range Community College, Larimer Campus
Fort Collins, Colorado

JACQUELINE FROCK, MSN, RN
Professor of Nursing
Oklahoma City Community College
Oklahoma City, Oklahoma

BELINDA FULLER, RN, MSN
Level 1 Coordinator
Gadsden State Community College
Gadsden, Alabama

NORENE GACHIGNARD, RN, MSN
Professor
North Shore Community College
Danvers, Massachusetts

WENDY GREENSPAN, RN, MSN, CCRN, CNE
Assistant Professor of Nursing
Rockland Community College
Suffern, New York

RENEE HARRISON, RN, MS
Nursing Outreach Coordinator
Tulsa Community College
Tulsa, Oklahoma

MICHELLE HORNACK, RN, MSN
Assistant Professor of Nursing
Graceland University
Independence, Missouri

SUSAN A. HUMENIK-SCHMIDT, MSN, RN
Assistant Professor of Nursing
Joliet Junior College
Joliet, Illinois

SHIRLEY JEANDRON, MSN, MBA
Nursing Instructor
Charity School of Nursing
Delgado Community College
New Orleans, Louisiana

CAROL JELFO, MSN, APRN-BC
Instructor, Associate Degree Nursing Program
West Georgia Technical College
Waco, Georgia

MARY ANN JOHNSTON, RN, MSN
Lecturer/Clinical Instructor
California State University, Stanislaus
Turlock, California

ANNE-MARIE JONES, MSN, RN, CNE
Assistant Professor of Nursing
Western Carolina University
Cullowhee, North Carolina

ELIZABETH KEENE, MSN/ED, RN, CNE
Assistant Professor, Nursing Program
Montgomery County Community College
Blue Bell, Pennsylvania

ANGIE KOONTZ, MSN, RN
Nursing Instructor
Caldwell Community College and Technical Institute
Hudson, North Carolina

RAEANN G. LEBLANC, DNP, GNP-BC, ANP-BC
Assistant Clinical Professor
University of Massachusetts
Amherst, Massachusetts

DIANE LITTEN, ARNP, MSN
Instructor, Chair—Nursing Department
Lake Sumter Community College
Clermont, Florida

KAREN LOCASCIO, MS, RN-BC
Assistant Professor of Nursing
Southern Maine Community College
South Portland, Maine

KATRINA LUTHER, RN, MSN
Nursing Instructor
Miles Community College
Miles City, Montana

BUFFI BEASLEY MCCAMBRIDGE, RN, MSN, BSN, BS
Faculty—Instructor and PreNursing Advisor
College of Nursing
Valdosta State University
Valdosta, Georgia

MAGDA SANDRA MCCARTHY, MSN, RN, CNE
Professor
Houston Community College
Houston, Texas

CATHY MCCAUGHEY, MSN, RN
Nursing Faculty/Adjunct
Los Medanos College
Pittsburg, California

AMY HILBURN MILLS, RN, MSN, CRNP
Assistant Professor
Troy University
Troy, Alabama

HEATHER PAULSEN, RN, BSN
Level 2 Team Leader and ASN Coordinator
Salish Kootenai College
Pablo, Montana

GLENDA REEDY, MSN, RN
Nursing Faculty
Caldwell Community College
Boone, North Carolina

LAURA SAUCER, RN, MSN
Program Director of Nursing
South University
Montgomery, Alabama

BARBARA A. SPRACKLIN, RN, MSN
Associate Professor
Bunker Hill Community College
Boston, Massachusetts

GERALDINE M. TYRELL, MSN, RN
Assistant Professor of Nursing
Bethel College
North Newton, Kansas

GRACE WAY, MSN, RN-C
Professor of Nursing
Seminole State College
Altamonte Springs, Florida

JANNA WICKHAM, RN, MSN
Nursing Faculty—Simulation
Lake Sumter Community College
Clermont, Florida

LICIA W. WILLIAMSON, RN, MSN
Instructor/Level 1 Coordinator
Lawson State Community College
Birmingham, Alabama

We want to thank Bob Martone, Publisher for Nursing, who has championed, guided, and supported us these last 19 years. He has worked with us to identify innovative and creative projects to meet the learning needs of nursing students and then entrusted us to accomplish the goals set forth in these publishing ventures. Bob is more than our publisher, he is a respected and valued friend and we treasure our collaborative relationship.

We also want to thank the talented and hardworking editorial team at F. A. Davis Company; their dedication, attention to detail, and perseverance to ensure excellence is greatly appreciated. While it is impossible to thank every person associated with the production of this textbook, we would like to identify a few individuals. Jaime Buss, our Content Editor, ensured that the textbook was well organized, accurate, complete, and well presented in outline format. She worked through hurricane Sandy with no electric power for two weeks and hardly missed a beat! Jacalyn Clay, our Project Editor at F. A. Davis Co., was always available for consultation, supported us enthusiastically which kept us motivated, and expertly kept the project on track. Linda Van Pelt, our Production Manager, skillfully transformed our manuscript into a book. We value her expertise and efforts. Thanks to Christine Becker, Project Manager, Progressive Publishing, and her team of copy editors and indexer for their detailed editing. Christine was extremely patient and supportive throughout the editing process and her efforts were greatly appreciated. Thank you to Rose Boul, Senior Art Coordinator of Graphic World, Inc., for the fabulous art work that supports visual learning. Keeping the art work organized was a tremendous task considering the large number of photographs, illustrations, and last minute changes. We would also like to thank the F. A. Davis Co. marketing department that provided creative and interest provoking marketing strategies. A special thanks to sales representatives, especially Don Weiss, for their student feedback and hardworking sales efforts.

We want to thank the reviewers for their knowledge, constructive criticism, and suggestions. We appreciate the feedback that added to the quality of the product. We are especially thankful to students, who constantly said that while standard fundamentals textbooks were rich resources of information, they felt overwhelmed when studying for nursing examinations. Students said that a textbook with just the need-to-know information would help them clearly focus on information essential to nursing theory and practice.

Finally, we want thank our husbands, Neil Nugent and Joseph Vitale, for tolerating the time that we dedicated to writing, editing, and proofing the manuscript. This textbook would not have been accomplished without their love and support. Special thanks to our children and their spouses Heather and James McCormack, Kelly and John Dall, Joseph and Nicole Vitale, John and JoAnne Vitale, and Christopher and Whitney Vitale, all of whom we are very proud. Love and kisses to our grandchildren, Joey, Andie, Andrew, Nathan, Alexander, William, and James Vitale; Sean, Ava, and Elle Dall; and Aiden, Cade, and Ronan McCormack, who all make our day with their smiles and accomplishments. A very special thanks to our grandsons Ronan McCormack and Joey Vitale for giving us permission to illustrate their surgical scars (badges of courage) in the physical assessment chapter.

PATRICIA M. NUGENT
BARBARA A. VITALE

Table of Contents

Message to Test-Takers of Nursing Examinations

To progress in a nursing program, you must achieve passing grades on course examinations. To pass nursing examinations you must know not only theory and principles of nursing but also theory and principles associated with other disciplines upon which nursing is based, such as anatomy, physiology, microbiology, psychology, sociology, mathematics, growth and development, and so on. Many factors influence your ability to learn all this information, such as genetic endowment, maturation level, past experience, self-image, mental attitude, motivation, and readiness to learn. You might not be able to change some of these factors; however, implementing study and test-taking strategies can enhance personal internal control, purposeful learning, and success on nursing examinations. The most important element in test success is to be over prepared. This text presents various learning strategies that can help you maximize your learning so that you are over prepared for examinations. In addition, it presents test-taking tips that will help you to understand what a test question is asking, how to examine options in a multiple-choice question, and how to eliminate incorrect options (distractors). For additional information on the strategies presented in this introduction, refer to *Test Success: Test-Taking Techniques for Beginning Nursing Students* published by the F. A. Davis Company.

Use General Study Strategies to Maximize Learning

1. Set short- and long-term learning goals because doing so promotes planned learning with a purpose.
2. Control internal and external distractors.
   - Select a study environment that allows you to focus on your learning and is free from external interruptions.
   - Limit internally generated distractions by challenging negative thoughts. For example, rather than saying to yourself, "This is going to be a hard test," say, "I can pass this test if I study hard."
   - Establish a positive internal locus of control. For example, say, "I can get an A on my next test if I study hard and I am over prepared," rather than blaming the instructor for designing "hard" tests.
   - Use controlled breathing techniques, progressive muscle relaxation, and guided imagery to control anxious feelings.

3. Review content before class because doing so supports mental organization and purposeful learning.
4. Take class notes.
   - Review class notes within 48 hours after class because doing so ensures that the information is still fresh in your mind.
   - Use one side of your notebook for notes and use the opposite page to identify additional information from the textbook or other sources.
   - Identify questions that you still have, and ask the instructor for clarification.
5. Balance personal sacrifice and time for relaxation. A rigorous course of study requires sacrifices in terms of postponing vacations, having less time to spend with family members and friends, and having less time to engage in personal leisure activities. However, you should find a balance that supports your need to meet course requirements and yet allows you time to rest and reenergize.
6. Treat yourself to a reward when you meet a goal because doing so supports motivation. Your long-term reward is to graduate and become a nurse. However, that reward is in the distance so, to stimulate motivation now, build in rewards when short-term goals are achieved.
   - An external reward might be watching a television program that you enjoy, having a 10-minute break with a snack, or calling a friend on the phone.
   - An internal reward might be saying to yourself, "Wow, I finished outlining that whole chapter; I am terrific" or "I feel great because I now understand the principles presented in this chapter."
7. Manage time effectively.
   - Examine your daily and weekly routine to identify and eliminate barriers to your productivity, such as attempting to do too much, lacking organization, or being obsessive-compulsive.
   - Learn to delegate household tasks.
   - Learn to say "no" to avoid overcommitting yourself to activities that take you away from what you need to do to meet your learning needs.
   - Get organized. Identify realistic daily, weekly, and monthly "to do" calendars. Work to achieve deadlines with self-determination and self-discipline.
   - Maintain a consistent study routine because doing so eliminates procrastination and establishes an internal readiness to learn.

- Recognize that you do not have to be perfect. If every waking moment is focused on achieving an "A," your relationship with family members and friends will suffer. The key is to find a balance and accept the fact that you do not have to have an "A" in every course to become a nurse.
- Capitalize on small moments of time to study by carrying flashcards, a vocabulary list, or a small study guide, such as one of the products in the *Notes* series by F. A. Davis Publishing Company.
8. Study in small groups. Sharing and listening increases understanding and allows for correction of misinformation.

Use Specific Study Strategies to Maximize Learning

1. Use acronyms, alphabet cues, acrostics, and mnemonics to help learn information that must be memorized for future recall.
2. When studying continually, ask yourself "how" and "why" because the nurse must comprehend the meaning of the "how" and "why" of information. For example, a nurse must know *how* much pressure compresses a capillary bed and *why* this level of compression will result in a pressure ulcer. Many questions on nursing examinations require the nurse to comprehend the how and why when identifying the correct option in a test question in terms of what the nurse should do first or next or what not to do.
3. Relate new information to something you already know to enhance learning. For example, if you are learning how to collect a sterile urine specimen from a urinary retention catheter, identify the principles that are common to those that you learned several weeks before about sterile technique when preparing a medication to be administered via a syringe.
4. Identify and study principles that are common among different nursing interventions because doing so maximizes the application of information in patient situations. For example, the principle of gravity applies when elevating a patient's legs on pillows to reduce edema, when holding an enema solution bag 12 inches above the level of the patient's anus to increase the flow of enema solution, and when raising the head of a patient's bed to lower abdominal pressure to facilitate ventilation.
5. Identify and study differences. For example, three patients may have an increase in blood pressure for three different reasons, such as obesity, acute pain stimulating the sympathetic nervous system, and decreased arterial compliance due to the aging process.

Use Test-Taking Tips to Maximize Success on Nursing Examinations

There is no substitute for being over prepared for a test. However, when you are uncertain of a correct answer, test-taking tips are strategies you can use to be test wise. By being test wise, you may be better able to identify what a question is asking and better able to eliminate one or more distractors. Your chances of selecting the correct answer increase when you are able to eliminate distractors from consideration. For example, when answering a traditional multiple-choice question that has four answer options, if you can eliminate one distractor from further consideration, you increase your chances of selecting the correct answer to 33 percent. If you are able to eliminate two distractors from further consideration, you increase your chances of selecting the correct answer to 50 percent.

Practice using the following test-taking tips to help you to understand what a question is asking and to eliminate distractors. Recognize that not all questions lend themselves to using test-taking tips. The practice questions in this textbook identify test-taking tips where applicable to help you learn how to apply them when answering a multiple-choice question.

Test-Taking Tips for Multiple-Choice (One Answer) Item

A traditional multiple-choice item typically presents a statement (stem) that asks a question. Usually, four statements that are potential answers follow the stem (options); one of which is the correct answer and three of which are incorrect answers (distractors). The test-taker must select the option that is the correct answer to receive credit for answering a traditional multiple-choice item correctly.

Test-taking tips describe strategies that can be used to analyze a traditional multiple-choice item and improve a test-taker's chances of selecting the correct answer.

Test-taking tip #1: Identify positive polarity of a stem.

- A stem with positive polarity is asking, "What should the nurse do when … ?"
- The correct answer may be based on understanding what is accurate or comprehending the principle underlying the correct answer.
- For example, a stem with positive polarity might say, "Which nursing action should a nurse implement when a patient who is being ambulated begins to fall?"
- **Study tip:** Change the stem so that it reflects a negative focus and then answer the question based on a stem with negative polarity. For example, "Which action should a nurse *not implement* when a patient who is being ambulated begins to fall?"

Test-taking tip #2: Identify key words in the stem that indicate negative polarity.

- A stem with negative polarity asks such questions as what the nurse should not do; what is contraindicated, unacceptable, or false; or what is the exception.
- Words in a stem that indicate negative polarity include *not, except, never, contraindicated, unacceptable, avoid, unrelated, violate,* and *least.*
- For example, a negatively worded stem might say, "Which action violates the principles of sterile technique when collecting a specimen from a surgical wound?"
- **Study tip:** Change the word that indicates negative polarity to a positive word and then answer the question based on a stem with positive polarity. For example, if a stem says, "Which action implemented by the nurse *violates* a principle of surgical asepsis?" change the word *violates* to *reflects.* You have just changed a stem with negative polarity to a stem with positive polarity.

Test-taking tip #3: Identify words in the stem that set a priority.

- The correct answer is something that the nurse should do first.
- Words in the stem that set a priority include *first, best, main, greatest, most, initial, primary,* and *priority.*
- For example, a stem that sets a priority might say, "What should a nurse do first when administering a tube feeding to a patient?"
- **Study tip:** After identifying the first step in the procedure for administering a tube feeding to a patient, place the remaining three steps in order of importance.

Test-taking tip #4: Identify options that are opposites.

- Options that are opposites generally reflect extremes on a continuum.
- More often than not, an option that is an opposite is the correct answer.
- If you are unable to identify the correct answer, select one of the opposite options.
- Some opposites are easy to identify, such as hypervolemia and hypovolemia or bradycardia and tachycardia, whereas others are obscure, such as bradycardia and rapid pulse rate or flat neck veins (indicating deficient fluid volume) and bounding pulse (indicating fluid volume excess).
- **Study tip:** Make flashcards that reflect the clinical indicator on one side and identify all situations than can cause that sign or symptom on the other side.

Test-taking tip #5: Identify patient-centered options.

- Patient-centered options focus on feelings, opportunities for patients to make choices, and actions that empower patients or support patient preferences.

- More often than not, a patient-centered option is the correct answer.
- For example, a patient-centered option might say, "What spices would you like me to sprinkle on your food?" or "Do you want to walk after your bath or after your lunch?" These example options give a patient an opportunity to make a choice, which supports independence. A nursing action that supports a patient's independence is an example of a patient-centered option.
- **Study tip:** Compose your own patient-centered options that would be a correct answer for the scenario presented in the question. "I would be mad, too, if my food were cold, but what can I do for you right now to make it better?," "How about if I write down the questions that you have for your doctor so that you don't forget to ask them when the doctor makes rounds today?," or "Losing a leg can be difficult."

Test-taking tip #6: Identify options that deny patients' feelings, needs, or concerns.

- Options that avoid patients' feelings, change the subject, offer false reassurance, or encourage optimism cut off communication.
- Options that deny patients' feelings, needs, or concerns are always distractors unless the stem has negative polarity.
- For example, an option that says, "You will feel better tomorrow," fails to recognize the patient's concerns about the pain that the patient is feeling today.
- If a stem with negative polarity says, "What should the nurse **avoid** saying when patients express concerns about the pain they are experiencing?" the option that says, "You will feel better tomorrow" is the correct answer. It is important to ensure that you identify the polarity of the stem.
- **Study tip:** Construct additional options that deny patients' feelings, needs, or concerns that relate to the scenario in the stem, such as, "Cheer up because things could be worse," "Don't worry; I promise that the pain will be less and less every passing day," or "The pain medication you are receiving should be adequate to relieve your pain."

Test-taking tip #7: Identify equally plausible options.

- Equally plausible options are options that are so similar that one option is no better than the other.
- Equally plausible options can both be deleted from further consideration.
- For example, one option says "Dyspnea" and another option says "Difficulty breathing." These two options are saying the same thing. One option is no better than the other; therefore, you can eliminate both from further consideration. Another example is if one option

states, "Encourage deep breathing exercises" and another option states, "Encourage the use of an incentive spirometer 10 times every hour." Both of these options present interventions that increase the depth of respirations. One option is no better than the other; therefore, you can eliminate both options from further consideration. By doing so, you increase your chances of selecting the correct answer to 50 percent.

- **Study tip:** Construct equally plausible options for the correct answer and identify equally plausible options for the options that are distractors.

Test-taking tip #8: Identify options with specific determiners (absolutes).

- A specific determiner is a word or phrase that indicates no exceptions.
- Words that are specific determiners place a limit on a statement that generally is considered correct.
- Words in options that are specific determiners include *all, none, only, always,* and *never.*
- For example, options with a specific determiner might say, "Use only water when bathing the perineal area" or "Patients should always be expected to provide their own care."
- Most of the time, options with specific determiners are distractors. However, there are some exceptions that focus on universal truths in nursing, such as interventions that focus on patients as individuals and the use of standard precautions. For example, "Always believe what patients report about their pain experience" and "Never leave a patient's room without implementing hand hygiene."
- **Study tip:** Construct examples of options with specific determiners so that you are able to recognize when an option has a specific determiner. Next, identify whether the option should be deleted or whether the option is an exception to the rule.

Test-taking tip #9: Identify the unique option.

- When one option is different from the other three options that are similar, examine the unique option carefully.
- More often than not, an option that is unique is the correct answer.
- For example, if a question is asking you to identify an expected patient response to a problem and three of the options identify an increase in something and one option identifies a decrease in something, examine the option that identifies the decrease in something because it is unique.
- **Study tip:** Construct options that are similar to the distractors and construct options that are similar to the unique option. Doing so can help you to distinguish among commonalities and differences.

Test-taking tip #10: Identify the global option.

- Global options are more broad and wide-ranging than specific options.
- One or more of the other options might be included under the umbrella of a global option.
- Examine global options carefully because they are often the correct answer.
- For example, a global option might say, "Keep patients clean and dry" versus a specific option, which might say, "Wash a patient's perineal area after toileting."
- **Study tip:** Construct as many specific options as possible that could be included under the umbrella of a global option. Construct as many global options as possible in relation to the content presented in the stem. Doing so will increase your ability to identify a global option.

Test-taking tip #11: Use Maslow's hierarchy of needs and the ABCs (Airway, Breathing, and Circulation) to identify the option that is the priority.

- This technique is best used when answering a question that asks what the nurse should do first or which action is most important.
- Examine each option and identify which level need according to Maslow is associated with each option. Identify whether any of the options are associated with maintaining a patent airway and, if not, examine each option from the perspective of maintaining breathing and so on.
- For example, in a question associated with postoperative care, an option that addresses the presence of an oral airway generally is the priority.
- **Study tip:** Start by identifying the action that is least important and work backward toward the option with the action that is most important. Then identify the reasoning behind the assigned order. This technique focuses on the how and why and helps you to clarify the reasoning underlying your critical thinking. This technique is often done best when working in a small study group.

Test-taking tip #12: Identify duplicate facts in options.

- Some options contain two or more facts. The more facts that are contained in an option, the greater your chances of selecting the correct answer.
- If you identify an incorrect fact, eliminate all options that contain the incorrect fact. After you eliminate options that you know are incorrect, move on and identify a fact(s) that you know is correct. Focus on the options that contain at least one fact that you know is correct.

- By eliminating options, you increase your chances of selecting the correct answer. By the process of elimination, you may even arrive at the correct answer even when unsure of all the facts in the correct answer.
- **Study tip:** Identify all the correct facts that you can that are associated with what the question is asking.

Test-taking tip #13: Practice test-taking tips.

- Practicing test taking is an effective way to achieve five outcomes.
  1. You can desensitize yourself to the discomfort or fear that you might feel in a testing situation.
  2. You can increase your stamina if you gradually increase the time that you spend practicing test taking to 2 to 3 hours. This practice will enable you to concentrate more effectively for a longer period of time.
  3. You will learn how to better manage your time during a test so that you have adequate time to answer all the questions.
  4. You will increase your learning when studying the rationales for the right and wrong answers. Also, by practicing the application of test-taking techniques and employing the study tips presented, you will learn how to maximize your learning associated with each test-taking tip.
  5. You will become more astute in determining what a question is asking and better able to identify when a test-taking tip might help you eliminate a distractor and focus on an option that might be the correct answer. Remember the old adage—practice makes perfect!!

Test-taking tip #14: Use multiple test-taking techniques when examining test questions and options.

- If using one test-taking technique to analyze a question is beneficial, think how much more beneficial it would be to use two or more test-taking techniques to analyze a question.
- Examine the stem first for a test-taking technique. For example, ask yourself, "Does the stem have negative polarity?" or "Is the stem setting a priority?"
- Next, examine the options. For example, ask yourself, "Do any of the options contain a specific determiner?" or "Is there a global option?" or "Is there a patient-centered option?"
- By using more than one test-taking tip, you can usually increase your success in selecting the correct answer.

Test-Taking Tips for Alternate-Format Items

Alternate-format items are purported by the National Council of State Boards of Nursing to evaluate some nursing knowledge more readily and authentically than possible with traditional multiple-choice items. To accomplish this, an alternate-format item does not construct a question with the same organization as a multiple-choice item. Each type of alternate-format item presents information along with a question using a distinctive format and requires the test-taker to answer the item in a unique manner. Some alternate format items use multimedia approaches, such as charts, tables, graphics, sound, and video. Understanding the composition of alternate-format items and strategies to analyze these items can increase your chances of selecting the correct answer.

1. *Multiple-Response Item*
   - A multiple-response item presents a stem that asks a question.
   - It presents five or six options as potential answers.
   - The test-taker must identify all (2 or more) correct answers to the question posed in the stem.
   - When answering a multiple-response item on a computer each option is preceded by a circle. The test-taker must place the cursor in the circle and click the mouse to select the desired answers.
   - **Test-taking tip:** Before looking at the options, quickly review information you know about the topic. Then compare what you know against the options presented. Another approach is to eliminate one or two options that you know are wrong; identify one option you know is correct; then eliminate another one or two options that you know are wrong. Finally, you should identify all the options you believe are correct. To do this, you can use some of the test-taking tips that apply to traditional multiple-choice questions, such as identifying options that are opposites; identifying patient-centered options; identifying options that deny patients' feelings, needs, or concerns; and identifying options with specific determiners (absolutes) to either eliminate options or to focus on potential correct answers.

2. *Drag-and-Drop (Ordered Response) Item*
   - A drag and drop item makes a statement or presents a situation and then asks the test-taker to prioritize five or six options.
   - The item may ask the test-taker to indicate the order in which nursing interventions should be performed, the order of importance of concerns, or actual steps in a procedure.
   - To be considered a correct answer, the test-taker must place all of the options in the correct order.
   - When answering a drag and drop item on a computer, the test-taker may highlight and click on the option or actually drag the option from the left side of the screen to a box on the right side of the screen. When practicing a drag and drop item in a textbook the text-taker can only indicate the priority order by listing the options in order by number.

- **Test-taking tip:** Use the ABCs (Airway, Breathing, and Circulation), Maslow's hierarchy of needs, and the nursing process to help focus your ordering of options. Identify the option that you consider to be the priority option; identify the option that you consider to be the least important option; then, from the remaining options, select the next priority option and the least priority option. Keep progressing along this same line of thinking until all the options have received a placement on the priority list.

3. *Fill-in-the-Blank Calculation Item*
   - A fill-in-the-blank calculation item presents information and then asks the test-taker a question that requires the manipulation or interpretation of numbers.
   - Computing a medication dosage, intake and output, or the amount of IV fluid to be administered are examples of fill-in-the-blank calculation items.
   - The test-taker must answer the item with either a whole number or within a specified number of decimal points as requested by the item.
   - **Test-taking tip:** Before answering a question, recall the memorized equivalents or formula that is required to answer the item; then perform a calculation to answer the item.

4. *Hot-Spot Item*
   - A hot-spot item presents an illustration or photograph and asks a question.
   - The test-taker must identify a location on the visual image presented to answer the question.
   - The answer must mirror the correct answer exactly to be considered a correct answer.
   - When answering a hot-spot item on a computer the test-taker uses a mouse, places the cursor on the desired location, and left clicks the mouse. These actions place an X on the desired location to answer the question. When answering a hot-spot item in a text book the test-taker is asked to either place an X on the desired location or identify an option indicated by an a, b, c, or d label presented in the illustration or photograph.
   - **Test-taking tip:** Read and reread the item to ensure that you understand what the item is asking. When attempting to answer a question that involves anatomy and physiology, close your eyes and picture in your mind the significant structures and recall their functions before answering the item.

5. *Exhibit Item*
   - An exhibit item presents a scenario, usually a patient situation.
   - The test-taker is then presented with a statement that asks a question.

- The test-taker must access information from a variety of sources. The information must be analyzed to determine its significance in relation to the question being asked to arrive at an answer.
- These items require the highest level of critical thinking (analysis and synthesis).
- When answering an exhibit item on a computer each option is preceded by a circle. The test-taker must place the cursor in the circle and click the mouse to select the desired answers.
- **Test-taking tip:** Identify exactly what the item is asking. Access the collected data and dissect, analyze, and compare and contrast the data collected in relation to what you know and understand in relation to what the item is asking.

6. *Graphic Item*
   - A graphic item presents a question with several options that are illustrations, pictures, photographs, charts, or graphs rather than text.
   - The test-taker must select the option with the illustration that answers the question.
   - When answering a graphic item on a computer each option is preceded by a circle. The test-taker must place the cursor in the circle and click the mouse to select the desired answer. When answering a graphic item in a textbook the test-taker is presented with an illustration and must select one answer from among several options or the test-taker is asked a question and must select one answer from among several options, each having an illustration.
   - **Test-taking tip:** When reading your textbook or other resource material visual images are presented to support written content. "A picture is worth a thousand words." Examine these images in relation to the content presented to reinforce your learning. Often times similar illustrations may be used in either hot-spot or graphic alternate test items.

7. *Audio Item*
   - An audio item presents an audio clip that must be accessed through a head set. After listening to the audio clip the test-taker must select the answer from among the options presented.
   - When answering an audio item on a computer each option is preceded by a circle. The test-taker must place the cursor in the circle and click the mouse to select the desired answer.
   - **Test-taking tip:** Listen to educational resources that provide audio clips of sounds that the nurse must be able to identify such as breath, heart, and bowel sounds. Engage in learning experiences using simulation manikins available in the on-campus nursing laboratory. When in the

clinical area use every opportunity to assess these sounds when completing a physical assessment of assigned patients. For additional resources access audio clips at wwwDavisPlus.com.

NCLEX-RN Test Plan and Classification of Questions

The National Council Licensure Examinations for Registered Nurses (NCLEX-RN) and for Licensed Practical/Vocational Nurses (NCLEX-PN) Test Plans (2013) primarily were designed to facilitate the classification of examination items and guide candidates preparing for the these examinations. These test plans were developed to ensure the formation of tests that measure the competencies required to perform safe, effective nursing care as newly licensed, entry-level registered nurses or licensed practical/vocational nurses. They are revised every 3 years after an analysis of the activities of practicing nurses, input from experts on the NCLEX Examination Committees, and National Council of State Board of Nursing's content staff and member boards of nursing to ensure that the test plans are relevant and consistent with state nurse practice acts. The detailed test plans for the NCLEX-RN and NCLEX-PN differ due to differences in the scope of practice for these professions. Each of these test plans can be found on the National Council of State Board of Nursing's Web site at www.ncsbn.org/nclex.htm.

Fundamentals of Nursing: Content Review Plus Practice Questions utilizes the NCLEX-RN Test Plan categories to analyze every question. This book contains more than 1,000 questions. The majority of the questions appear in the chapters that reflect the content in the question. In addition, there is a final examination in Unit 5 and two comprehensive examinations on davisplus.fadavis.com. Each question has the rationales for the correct and incorrect answers; offers a test-taking tip, if applicable; and is classified according to the following categories.

Integrated Processes Categories

Integrated processes are the basic factors essential to the practice of nursing, which are the nursing process, caring, communication and documentation, and teaching and learning. Because the nursing process provides a format for critical thinking, it is included for each question. Caring, communication and documentation, and teaching and learning are included when the intent of the question addresses one or more of these factors.

Nursing Process

- *Assessment:* Nursing care that collects objective and subjective data from primary and secondary sources.
- *Analysis:* Nursing care that groups significant data, interprets data, and comes to conclusions.

- *Planning:* Nursing care that sets goals, objectives, and outcomes; prioritizes interventions; and performs calculations.
- *Implementation:* Nursing care that follows a regimen of care prescribed by a primary health-care provider, such as administration of fluids, medications, and procedures, as well as performs nursing care within the legal scope of the nursing profession.
- *Evaluation:* Nursing care that identifies a patient's responses to medical and nursing interventions.

Caring

Nursing care that provides support, encouragement, empathy, concern, hope, and compassion to patients and significant others.

Communication and Documentation

Nursing care that reflects verbal and nonverbal interactions between the nurse and the patient, significant others, and members of the health team as well as documentation on a patient's clinical record that adheres to legal and ethical standards.

Teaching and Learning

Nursing actions that facilitate the acquisition of knowledge, skills, or attitudes by patients, family members, significant others, or staff members. The outcome of these interventions should promote a change in behavior.

Client Need Categories

Client needs reflect activities most commonly performed by entry-level nurses.

Safe and Effective Care Environment

- *Management of Care:* Nursing care that provides or directs the delivery of nursing activities to clients, significant others, and other health-care personnel. Management of care items account for 17 to 23 percent of the items on the NCLEX-RN examination.
- *Safety and Infection Control:* Nursing care that protects patients, significant others, and health-care personnel from health and environmental hazards. Safety and infection control items account for 9 to 15 percent of the items on the NCLEX-RN examination.

Health Promotion and Maintenance

Nursing care to assist patients and significant others to prevent or detect health problems and achieve optimum health, particularly in relation to their developmental level. Health promotion and maintenance items account for 6 to 12 percent of the items on the NCLEX-RN examination.

Psychosocial Integrity

Nursing care that supports and promotes the emotional, mental, and social well-being of patients and significant others as well as those with acute or chronic mental health problems. Psychosocial integrity items account for 6 to 12 percent of the items on the NCLEX-RN examination.

Physiological Integrity

- *Basic Care and Comfort:* Nursing care that provides support during the performance of the activities of daily living, such as hygiene, rest, sleep, mobility, elimination, hydration, and nutrition. Basic care and comfort items account for 6 to 12 percent of the items on the NCLEX-RN examination.
- *Pharmacological and Parenteral Therapies:* Nursing care related to the administration of medication, intravenous fluids, and blood and blood products. Pharmacological and parenteral therapies items account for 12 to 18 percent of the items on the NCLEX-RN examination.
- *Reduction of Risk Potential:* Nursing care that limits the development of complications associated with health problems, treatments, or procedures. Reduction of risk potential items account for 9 to15 percent of the items on the NCLEX-RN examination.
- *Physiological Adaptation:* Nursing care that meets the needs of patients with acute, chronic, or life-threatening physical health problems. Physiological adaptation items account for 11 to 17 percent of the items on the NCLEX-RN examination.

Cognitive Level Categories

This category reflects the thinking processes necessary to answer a question.

Knowledge

Information must be recalled from memory, such as facts, terminology, principles, and generalizations.

Comprehension

Information, as well as the implications and potential consequences of information identified, must be understood, interpreted, and paraphrased or summarized.

Application

Information must be identified, manipulated, or used in a situation, including mathematical calculations.

Analysis

A variety of information must be interpreted, requiring the identification of commonalities, differences, and interrelationship among the data.

Content Area Categories

Content area categories are not part of the NCLEX-RN Test Plan. These categories were added to indicate the name of the chapter in which the content being tested in the question can be found in this textbook.

Nursing Within the Context of Contemporary Health Care

Theory-Based Nursing Care

I. Definitions Related to Theory-Based Nursing Care

Nursing practice is based on a foundation of information that is viewed, organized, and utilized based on professional and personal influences. A nurse's knowledge base includes theories, models, frameworks, and a philosophy of nursing. Personal influences impact on both the patient and nurse and include such components as values, health beliefs, stress, and the ability to respond to stress.

A. Theory
1. Organized set of ideas and concepts that assists one to find meaning in experiences, organize thinking around a concept or idea, and develop new insight.
2. Way of viewing, describing, predicting, and controlling phenomena.

B. Model
1. Symbolic representation of a concept or framework.
2. Can be described in words or an illustration.

C. Framework
1. Broad, philosophical approach to a concept or idea.
2. Usually presented in an outline format.

D. Value
1. Something that a person holds in high regard.
2. Influenced by family, religion, school, and governmental traditions.
3. Influences the formation of beliefs and attitudes.

E. Health Belief
1. Concept about health that a person considers or accepts as accurate.
2. Influenced by social, cultural, and spiritual values.

F. **Philosophy**
1. Culturally determined system of beliefs, concepts, theories, or convictions.
2. Influences one's health practices (e.g., Jehovah's Witnesses do not accept blood transfusions, and Catholics do not accept abortion).

G. **Stress/Stressor**
1. Any physical, physiological, or psychological agent or condition that can cause imbalance in the body.
2. Can be internal (e.g., disease, anxiety, fear) or external (e.g., heat or cold, death of a loved one, an accident).
3. Can be positive (e.g., wedding ceremony, promotion at work) or negative (e.g., loss of a job, death of a loved one).
4. Types of stressors.
   a. Situational: Illness, accident, natural disaster.
   b. Developmental: Puberty, retirement, menopause.
   c. Physiologic: Genetic errors, vitamin deficiencies.
   d. Chemical: Medications, acids, bases.
   e. Physical: Incision, noise, extremes of environmental temperature, blunt trauma.
   f. Microbiological: Bacteria, viruses, fungi.
   g. Psychosociocultural: Excessive expectations regarding work, financial status, family dynamics.

H. **Adaptation**
1. Change that occurs in response to a stimulus (stressor).
2. Results from an ongoing effort to sustain internal and external balance.
3. Involves activation of voluntary and involuntary coping mechanisms to manage a stressor.

I. **Adaptive Capacity**
1. Physiological capability of a person to reestablish or sustain equilibrium.
2. Psychological capability of a person to reestablish or sustain equilibrium.

II. Theories of Nursing

Nursing theories identify and describe interrelated concepts that influence the practice of nursing. They provide a knowledge base that is broadly applicable to the variety of situations confronted by nurses. Each theory is unique, but they all include the patient as the focus of the theory.

A. **Care Deficit Theory of Nursing**—Dorothea Orem
1. Self-care is a purposeful learned behavior in response to a need.
2. Four concepts.
   a. Self-care: Self-initiated activities that a person performs to maintain life, health, and well-being.
   b. Self-care agency: An individual's ability to engage in self-care based on developmental level, experiences, and available resources.

   c. Therapeutic self-care demand: Comprehensive self-care actions required to meet personal self-care requisites.
   d. Self-care requisites: Actions directed to meeting universal needs common to all people, such as air, water, food, elimination, activity, rest, solitude/social interactions, safety, and promotion of human function.
3. Nursing implications.
   a. Promotes nursing care, such as acting, doing for, guiding, teaching, supporting, and providing a supportive milieu that increases patients' self-care abilities.
   b. Increases patients' self-care activities to maintain life, health, and well-being.

B. **Cultural Care Diversity and Universality Theory**—Madeleine Leininger
1. Transcultural care is a central and uniting feature of nursing.
2. Focuses on cultural care that addresses
   a. Preservation: Activities that help a patient maintain health.
   b. Accommodation: Activities that promote ways a patient adapts to and negotiates adjustments to health.
   c. Repatterning: Activities that help a patient reconstruct life patterns to promote health.
3. Nursing implications.
   a. Requires nurses to view nursing as a transcultural care profession.
   b. Requires nurses to provide culture-specific care that assists patients to achieve and maintain health.

C. **Human Caring Theory**—Jean Watson
1. Care should be based on values of concern, kindness, love of self and others, and respect for the spiritual domain.
2. Explains that nursing is an interpersonal process.
3. Ten factors: The first three factors relate to the science of caring, and the rest relate to a focus of nursing practice.
   a. Forming values.
   b. Instilling faith and hope.
   c. Cultivating sensitivity to self and others.
   d. Developing a helping-trusting relationship.
   e. Promoting and accepting expression of positive and negative feelings.
   f. Using problem-solving for caring processes.
   g. Promoting transpersonal teaching and learning.
   h. Providing supportive, protective, or corrective mental, physical, sociocultural, and spiritual environments.
   i. Assisting with meeting needs while preserving dignity and wholeness.

      j. Being open to dimensions of caring and healing that cannot be scientifically explained.

    4. Nursing implications.

      a. Supports caring as the basis of all nursing interventions and differentiates nursing from medicine, which is more concerned with curing.

      b. Encourages nurses to treat patients with care, respect, and dignity so that patients feel accepted, supported, and protected.

D. Adaptation Model—Sister Callista Roy

  1. A biopsychosocial adaptive system.

  2. Involves a feedback cycle of input and output of stimuli.

  3. Pronounces that a person modifies and integrates human and environmental components to achieve adaptation that supports survival, continuity, and growth.

  4. Holds that people respond in four modes.

    a. Physiologic: Relates to basic physiological issues (e.g., oxygenation, exercise, nutrition, elimination, fluid and electrolyte balance, and temperature regulation).

    b. Self-concept: Relates to the physical self (e.g., threats to bodily functions) or personal self (e.g., anxiety, guilt, and distress responses to physical or emotional stressors).

    c. Role function: Relates to a patient's ability to adapt to physical and emotional stressors to maintain personal life roles.

    d. Interdependence: Relates to issues that interrupt a patient's ability to maintain significant relationships.

  5. Nursing implications.

    a. Promotes patient adaptations in each of the four modes.

    b. Supports teaching about ways to alter internal and external environments to facilitate adaptations.

    c. Supports specific nursing care when adaptations are ineffective.

E. Functional Health Patterns—Marjory Gordon

  1. Framework for organizing data.

  2. Eleven health patterns.

    a. Health perception-health management.

    b. Nutritional-metabolic.

    c. Elimination.

    d. Activity-exercise.

    e. Sleep-rest.

    f. Cognitive-perceptual.

    g. Self-perception.

    h. Role-relationship.

    i. Sexuality-reproductive.

    j. Coping-stress tolerance.

    k. Value-belief.

  3. Nursing implications.

    a. Facilitates the collection and organization of data.

    b. Promotes identification of interrelated information that assists nurses to determine patients' health needs and appropriate nursing care.

F. Science of Unitary Human Beings—Martha Rogers

  1. Abstract theory focusing on a person as a cohesive whole, with a dynamic energy field that constantly interacts with environmental energy fields.

  2. Fields are characterized by a pattern, universe of open systems, and dimensionality.

  3. Nursing implications.

    a. Encourages nurses to focus on a person's wholeness.

    b. Promotes interventions based on interaction between human and environmental energy fields, such as therapeutic touch and direct/redirect patterns of interaction to increase achievement of health.

    c. Attempts to maintain an environment free from negative energy.

III. Theoretical Foundations Related to Concepts of Health, Wellness, and Illness

Health, wellness, and *illness* are terms used by people to reflect how they feel physically and/or emotionally. These terms, although used universally, are highly individualized, subjective, and influenced by a variety of factors. Theories have been developed to facilitate an understanding of the concepts and relationships between health, wellness, and illness.

A. Definition of Health

  1. Is highly personal and subjective and is based on one's individual perception.

  2. "A state of complete physical, mental, and social well-being and not merely the absence of disease or infirmity," according to the World Health Organization.

  3. "A dynamic state of being in which the developmental and behavioral potential of an individual is realized to the fullest extent possible," according to the American Nurses Association (1980).

  4. "An experience that is often expressed in terms of wellness and illness, and may occur in the presence or absence of disease or injury," according to the American Nurses Association (2004).

B. Definition of Wellness

  1. "A way of life oriented toward optimal health and well-being in which body, mind, and spirit are integrated by the individual to live more fully within the human and natural community," according to Myers, Sweeney, and Witmer (2000).

C. Definition of Illness
1. A state in which a person's status (e.g., physical, emotional, spiritual, developmental, intellectual, social) is diminished or impaired.
2. Not a disease but rather a response to a disease.

D. Health-Illness Continuum (Fig. 1.1)
1. Health is viewed along a continuum, with no distinct boundaries, that ranges from an excellent level of health to serious illness.
2. Placement on the continuum is determined by a person's self-perception and the perceptions of others; perceptions are influenced by many factors.
3. Placement on the continuum is dynamic and may change daily.
4. Nursing implications.
   a. Requires nurses to explore their own perceptions about health and illness and not impose them on patients.
   b. Assists nurses to identify where patients place themselves on the health-illness continuum because patients' health beliefs influence nursing care.

E. High-Level Wellness Grid—H. L. Dunn (Fig. 1.2)
1. Allows a patient's status to be plotted along an axis from peak wellness to death and against an intersecting axis from a very favorable environment to a very unfavorable environment.
2. Based on the intersection of the two axes, four quadrants of health and wellness are formed.
   a. Protected poor health (very favorable environment).
   b. Poor health (very unfavorable environment).

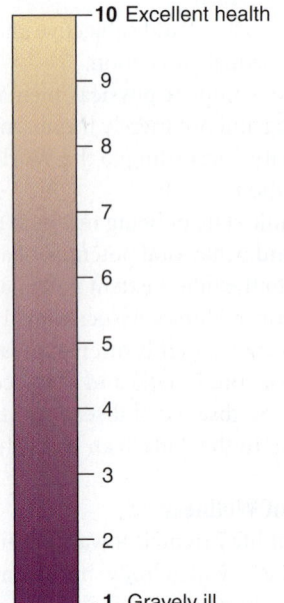

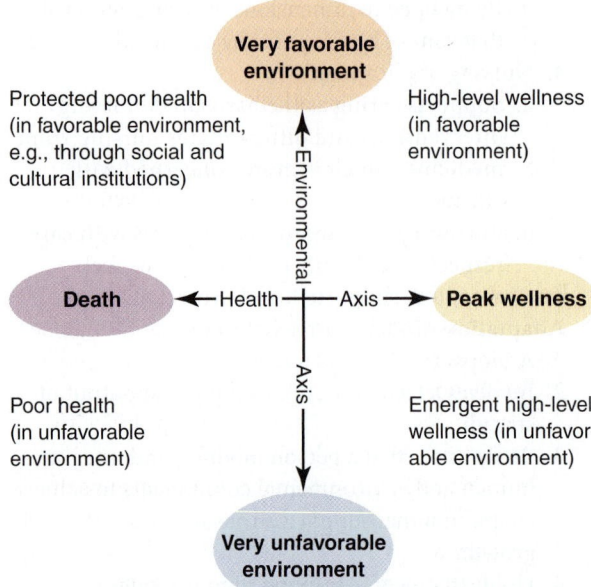

Fig 1.2 High-level wellness grid. (From U.S. Department of Health, Education, and Welfare. Public Health Service. National Office of Vital Statistics.)

   c. High-level wellness (very favorable environment).
   d. Emergent high-level wellness (very unfavorable environment).
3. Examples of environments.
   a. Favorable: Health insurance to pay for health services; supportive, caring family members; clean, uncrowded home environment.
   b. Unfavorable: Indigence or poverty; role responsibilities that interfere with health-seeking behaviors; lack of family; dirty, crowded home environment.
4. Nursing implications.
   a. Allows nurses to identify environmental factors that influence a patient's level of wellness.
   b. Facilitates prediction of whether patients' health will likely improve or decline on the basis of support or lack of support within the environment.

F. Wellness Model—Anspaugh, Hamrick, and Rosato
1. To achieve health and wellness, a patient must deal with features and dynamics within each of seven components of wellness.
   a. Physical.
   b. Social.
   c. Emotional.
   d. Intellectual.
   e. Spiritual.
   f. Occupational.
   g. Environmental.

2. Wellness requires working on all components of the model.
3. Nursing implications.
   a. Requires nurses to assess patients from seven perspectives.
   b. Facilitates a holistic approach to caring for patients because all components of wellness must be addressed.

G. Health Belief Model—Becker and Maiman; Rosenstock
1. Addresses the relationship between an individual's beliefs and behaviors.
2. Three components.
   a. Individual's perception of susceptibility to illness.
   b. Individual's perception of the seriousness of the illness.
   c. Individual's potential for action, which depends on benefits and barriers to taking action.
3. Nursing implications.
   a. Facilitates an understanding of patient behaviors.
   b. Provides a prediction of how patients might behave.
   c. Provides a basis for patient teaching.

H. Role Performance Model
1. Recognizes that all people generally fulfill a number of societal roles, such as parent, daughter or son, friend, and employee.
2. People who are able to fulfill their roles are considered healthy even though they may have an illness or disability.
3. Implies that people are unhealthy if they are unable to fulfill their roles.
4. Nursing implications.
   a. Requires nurses to explore patient perceptions about role performance versus the sick role to help plan and implement nursing care.
   b. Obligates nurses to foster independence when caring for patients who define their level of health by their ability to provide self-care.

I. Clinical or Medical Model
1. Interpretation of health is based on the presence or absence of signs and symptoms of illness, disease, or injury; a narrow interpretation of health.
2. A person is considered either healthy or sick; there is no continuum.
3. The model is based on the perception that a person is a physiological system with associated functions.
4. Nursing implications.
   a. Focuses on making nursing assessments in the physiological realm.
   b. Requires nurses to explore domains other than the physiological realm because this theory has a narrow interpretation of health.

IV. Theoretical Foundations of Nursing Practice

Nursing practice is an art and science that bases nursing care on information from a variety of disciplines (such as physical, social, and natural sciences) and related conceptual frameworks. A conceptual framework presents related ideas, statements, and concepts that address their significant interrelationships, providing an organized perspective to complex situations and problems. Theories that influence the discipline of nursing include those that present a framework reflective of growth and development, psychosocial issues, human needs, and death and dying.

A. Hierarchy of Basic Human Needs Model—Abraham Maslow (Fig. 1.3)
1. Human needs are arranged in a hierarchy of importance.
   a. Physiologic: Includes basic needs essential to maintain life (e.g., air, water, food, elimination, rest, sleep, sex, and activity).
   b. Safety and security: Includes the need to be physically and emotionally protected from injury (e.g., performing hand hygiene, sterile technique, effective mobility, and activities that promote trust; ensuring that the call bell is within the patient's reach, wheels are locked on equipment, and the bed is maintained in the lowest position; and explaining care before initiation).
   c. Love and belonging: Includes the need to give and receive love and acceptance and have a

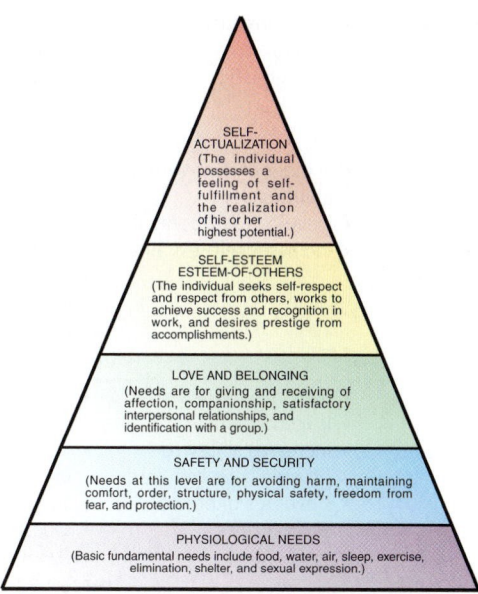

Fig 1.3 Maslow's hierarchy of basic human needs.

significant connection to family members, friends, and the community (e.g., treating patients with respect, ensuring privacy, and involving family members in care when appropriate).

    d. Self-esteem: Includes the need to have a positive self-regard, feel appreciated, and be independent and confident (e.g., encouraging independence, facilitating attainment of realistic goals, supporting roles, and accepting patients' values and beliefs).

    e. Self-actualization: Includes the need to achieve the highest potential within abilities (e.g., accepting patients as unique individuals, focusing on strengths, supporting hope, and teaching patients to be proactive in reaching their own potential).

  2. Human needs motivate behavior.

  3. Lower level needs must be met to some degree before higher levels needs are met.

B. **Theory of Psychosocial Development**—Erik Erikson

  1. Theory based on interrelationships between emotional and physical variables rather than psychosexual stages.

  2. Individuals at various stages of development cope with conflicts that may have a favorable or unfavorable outcome.

  3. Extent of resolution of preceding stage influences subsequent stages.

  4. Eight stages (Table 1.1).

MAKING THE CONNECTION

Maslow's Hierarchy and Nursing Implications

According to Maslow, human needs are arranged in a hierarchy of importance. Basic needs must be met to maintain life; then other needs emerge as previous needs begin to be met. Nurses can use this hierarchy to help identify patient needs and prioritize care. Patient needs must be considered within the context of a patient's developmental level (related to theories by researchers such as Erikson, Piaget, and Havighurst) because certain needs become more dominant at different stages of development (e.g., adolescents concerned about peer acceptance may place a higher importance on self-esteem needs). A patient's unique status (related to theories by researchers such as Roy; Gordon; and Anspaugh, Hamrick, and Rosato) must also be considered because personal factors can become more dominant when people are coping with illness (e.g., a woman who had a mastectomy might be more concerned about love and belonging needs or self-esteem needs than physiological needs).

  5. Nursing implications.

    a. Helps nurses understand human behavior.

    b. Helps nurses identify patients' stages of development and extent of task achievement.

    c. Helps nurses assist patients to develop coping skills associated with each task.

Table 1.1 Erikson's Stages of Psychosocial Development

Stage	Signs of Successful Achievement	Behaviors That Support Achievement	Signs of Unsuccessful Achievement	Behaviors That Precipitate Unsuccessful Achievement
Trust versus mistrust *Birth to 18 months*	• Develops trust in others • Is optimistic	• Basic needs are met consistently. • Supportive and affectionate care is received.	• Mistrusts others • Withdraws • Is estranged from others	• Basic needs are not met. • Impersonal and detached care is provided.
Autonomy versus shame and doubt *18 months to 3 years*	• Is independent within abilities • Develops self-control • Increases self-restraint	• Choices are allowed. • Ability to succeed or safely fail through experiences is allowed. • Appropriate praise and encouragement are provided.	• Has unnecessary dependence • Exhibits compulsive self-restraint • Has feelings of inadequacy • Is willful • Is defiant	• Overprotection occurs. • Limited choices are offered. • Shaming or insulting occurs. • Excessive criticism is received. • Harsh punishment is imposed.
Initiative versus guilt *3 to 5 years*	• Seeks new experiences • Is resourceful • Increases ability to provide basic self-care • Develops direction and purpose	• Accomplishments are recognized. • Creative activities are encouraged and supported. • Questions are answered.	• Is frustrated • Is hesitant to attempt new or challenging skills • Lacks self-confidence • Is pessimistic • Fears doing wrong • Blames self or feels guilty	• Creativity is limited. • Experimentation with new roles is discouraged. • Imagination and fantasy are stifled. • Behavior is consistently labeled as "bad."

Table 1.1 Erikson's Stages of Psychosocial Development—cont'd

Stage	Signs of Successful Achievement	Behaviors That Support Achievement	Signs of Unsuccessful Achievement	Behaviors That Precipitate Unsuccessful Achievement
Industry versus inferiority *6 to 12 years*	• Is eager to learn new skills • Thrives on realistic praise for accomplishments • Develops a sense of competency • Develops social skills	• Participation in activities that can be attained successfully within abilities is allowed. • Realistic recognition for accomplishments is given.	• Has feelings of inadequacy • Withdraws from peers and school	• Unrealistic expectations of the child are imposed by others. • Unwarranted or harsh punishments are imposed.
Identity versus role confusion *12 to 20 years*	• Explores various roles • Plans activities based on abilities • Integrates childhood experiences into a coherent sense of self or personal identity • Develops devotion and fidelity to others, especially peers	• Assistance is provided with decision making. • Encouragement to participate in family, school, and community endeavors is given. • Socially responsible behavior is supported.	• Has feelings of uncertainty about self • Is indecisive • Has difficulty making realistic plans	• Limited opportunities for decision making are offered. • Lack of interest or criticism by significant others in adolescent's activities or plans for the future.
Intimacy versus isolation *18 to 25 years*	• Develops meaningful relationships with friends • Develops an intimate relationship with another person • Develops a commitment to work or career goal	• Relationships with others are supported. • Exploration of career goals are encouraged and supported.	• Has impersonal relationships • Is unable to develop an intimate relationship with another person • Fears commitment to work or career goals • Feels isolated and rejected	• Relationships are criticized. • Disinterest in career goals by significant others.
Generativity versus stagnation *25 to 65 years*	• Becomes a productive member of society • Performs activities that promote the growth of others, particularly those in the next generation • Establishes a family • Engages satisfactorily in an occupation	• Emotional support is provided. • Activities, such as volunteerism, are supported.	• Is self-indulgent • Lacks interests • Is unable to promote the growth of others, particularly those in the next generation • Regresses to an earlier level of coping	• Emotional support is lacking. • Recognition and praise for accomplishments is lacking.
Integrity versus despair *65 years to death*	• Views life as meaningful • Feels respected by others • Respects self	• Review of life experiences is encouraged and supported. • Acceptance, appreciation, and respect are given by others.	• Has sense of loss and regret • Views life as meaningless • Has inability to adjust to changes associated with aging (e.g., physical changes, retirement)	• Achievement of goals does not occur. • Loss of a relationship with significant others occurs through isolation or death. • Multiple physical and/or emotional problems occur.

C. Theory of Cognitive Development—Jean Piaget
1. Thinking and reasoning develop through exposure to new experiences.
2. Four phases.
   a. Sensorimotor: Birth to 24 months; characterized by cognition, primarily through the senses and ability to process information on the physiological or emotional level.
   b. Preoperational: 2 to 7 years of age; characterized by an increasing ability to connect cognitively through language and actions.

    c. Concrete operations: 7 to 11 years of age; characterized by an increasing ability to organize information and use logical thought, ability to solve concrete problems, and less egocentricity.

    d. Formal operations: 11 to 15 years of age; characterized by use of abstract thinking and deductive reasoning and ability to examine alternatives.

3. Movement through phases is based on inherited intellect and environmental impact.

4. Each phase developed through
    a. Adaptation: Ability to adjust to and interact with the environment.
    b. Assimilation: Inclusion of new experiences and information within one's knowledge.
    c. Accommodation: Change in one's knowledge as a result of processing new experiences and information.

5. Nursing implications.
    a. Allows nurses to design nursing care, teaching plans, and activities that are appropriate for a child's developmental level.
    b. Helps nurses identify a child's developmental level and determine how far ahead to prepare the child for a procedure.

D. Developmental Stages and Tasks—Robert Havighurst

1. Each stage has a task requiring mastery.
2. Mastery of preceding tasks is essential for mastery of future tasks.
3. Six stages.
    a. Infancy and early childhood: Birth to 6 years of age.
    b. Middle childhood: 6 to 13 years of age.
    c. Adolescence: 13 to 18 years of age.
    d. Early adulthood: 19 to 30 years of age.
    e. Middle adulthood: 30 to 60 years of age.
    f. Later maturity: 60 years of age and older.
4. Nursing implications.
    a. Provides guidelines for supporting and evaluating task achievement.
    b. Facilitates identification of lack of task achievement, which requires interventions.

E. Psychoanalytic Theory—Sigmund Freud

1. Childhood experiences form unconscious motivation for behavior.
2. The basis of the theory is the development of balance between pleasure-seeking instincts and the standards of society.
3. Sexual energy is centered in body parts at different ages.
    a. Oral: Birth to 12–18 months.
    b. Anal: 12–18 months to 3 years.
    c. Phallic or oedipal: 3 to 6 years.
    d. Latency: 6 to 12 years.
    e. Genital: Puberty through adulthood.

4. The personality has three parts.
    a. Id (sexual energy): Represents instinctual urges, pleasures, and gratification; dominant in infants and children.
    b. Ego (realistic part of self): Balances what is wanted (id) and what is possible in light of societal limitations; begins to develop at 4 to 6 months of age.
    c. Superego (conscience): Regulates and restrains behavior by balancing the demands of the id and pressures of society; begins to develop at 5 to 6 years of age.

5. Nursing implications.
    a. Helps nurses to understand human behavior.
    b. Allows nurses to develop a plan of care based on a patient's psychosexual development and personality needs.

F. Theory of Stages of Moral Development—Lawrence Kohlberg

1. Theory helps to explain the development of moral code.
2. Each stage builds on the previous stage and develops over time.
3. Based on the ability to think at a higher level as one matures.
4. Based on the study of boys; validity of application to females is criticized.
5. Six stages.
    a. Obedience and punishment: Motivation for behavior is fear of negative consequences (e.g., punishment, disapproval).
    b. Individualism and exchange: Motivation for behavior is the desire for a positive consequence (e.g., good result, reward).
    c. Interpersonal relationships: Motivation for behavior is based on pleasing others because it is what others expect.
    d. Maintaining social order: Motivation for behavior is based on following rules.
    e. Social contract and individual rights: Motivation for behavior is based on differing values, beliefs, and opinions but adheres to standards agreed upon by society.
    f. Universal principles: Motivation for behavior is based on abstract reasoning, universal ethical principles (e.g., the "Golden Rule"), and principles of justice.
6. Nursing implications.
    a. Increases nurses' understanding that patient decision making is influenced by one's moral code.
    b. Helps nurses examine their own moral code and not impose their moral orientation onto patients and their family members.

G. Faith Development—James Fowler
1. Faith is a force of knowing that gives meaning to life.
2. It develops from interaction between a person and the environment.
3. New patterns of values, beliefs, and ways of thinking are added with each stage.
4. Six stages.
   a. Intuitive-projective: 3- to 7-year-old children imitate parental behaviors without thorough understanding.
   b. Mythic-literal: School-aged children may accept the concept of God and appreciate the perception of others.
   c. Synthetic-conventional: Adolescents begin to examine life-guiding beliefs, values, and personal religious practices.
   d. Individuative-reflective: Older adolescents and young adults assume responsibility for their own commitments, beliefs, and attitudes about faith.
   e. Conjunctive: Individuals integrate other viewpoints into their own understanding and identify personal conceptual realities in the context of faith development in others.
   f. Universalizing: Individuals achieve a universal perspective with absolute love and justice for humankind regardless of the religion or faith involved; this stage rarely is achieved.
5. Nursing implications.
   a. Increases nurses' understanding that spirituality is essential to providing holistic nursing care.
   b. Helps nurses to examine their own faith and not impose their own commitments, beliefs, and attitudes about faith onto patients and their family members.

H. Death and Dying Model—Elizabeth Kübler-Ross

DID YOU KNOW?
Patients have similar responses when coping with the diagnosis of a terminal illness or death and dying. Progression might not be linear; patients might not go through every stage or might experience several stages at the same time. In addition, some patients never reach the stage of acceptance.

1. Five stages.
   a. Denial.
   b. Anger.
   c. Bargaining.
   d. Depression.
   e. Acceptance.
2. Nursing implications.
   a. Assists nurses to assess patient behaviors associated with various stages of coping with death and dying.
   b. Promotes development of a plan of care appropriate to a specific stage of coping.
   c. Increases nurses' sensitivity to the needs of patients who are dying.

See also the section "Death, Dying, Loss, and Grief" in Chapter 8, "Psychological Support," p. 166.

CASE STUDY: Putting It All Together

Subjective Data

A 66-year-old woman is brought to a clinic by her female partner because of increasing shortness of breath and fatigue. The patient was reluctant to come to the clinic, but her partner insisted. The patient reports being diagnosed with emphysema 10 years ago and states, "I've been smoking since I was 15 years old, but I can't stop. The smoking finally got the best of me. I guess I should have stopped smoking when I was diagnosed with emphysema. If I had to do it over I would do a lot of things differently. I have so much phlegm; I cough all the time. I can hardly breathe, and I'm exhausted all the time. My partner hates that I always smell like smoke, and my fingers and teeth have turned yellow."

Objective Data

Vital Signs	
Temperature:	100.2°F, orally
Pulse:	88 beats/minute, regular
Respirations:	26 breaths/minute
Blood pressure:	138/84 mm Hg

Case Study Questions

A. Which of the following concerns identified by the nurse is the patient's primary problem and why. And why are the other concerns not the priority?

1. Impaired oxygenation due to retained secretions
2. Potential for falls because of overwhelming fatigue
3. Diminished self-esteem related to an inability to stop smoking
4. Impaired relationship with partner associated with changes in appearance

1. _____
2. _____
3. _____
4. _____

B. What additional objective data should the nurse collect in relation to the patient's respiratory status? Explain why each abnormal clinical indicator may have occurred by exploring its relationship to the patient's respiratory problem.

1. _____
2. _____
3. _____
4. _____
5. _____
6. _____
7. _____
8. _____

C. What statement indicates that the patient is struggling with one of the age-related tasks associated with Erikson's and Havighurst's developmental theories and why?

_____

D. Considering the concepts of the health belief model, what factors in the scenario indicate that the patient may be ready to make behavioral changes and why?

_____

REVIEW QUESTIONS

1. Which action is associated with a second-level need according to Maslow's hierarchy of needs?
   1. Taking deep breaths after exercising
   2. Hanging a self-made painting in a senior center
   3. Receiving weekly phone calls from adult children
   4. Removing scatter rugs after experiencing a fall in the home

2. A nurse identifies that a patient is experiencing a developmental stress. Which information about the patient supports this conclusion?
   1. Going through menopause
   2. Taking multiple medications
   3. Displaying signs of a vitamin deficiency
   4. Engaging in altercations with family members

3. Which statement by a nurse meets a second-level need according to Maslow's hierarchy of needs?
   1. "I see that you have applied makeup today for the first time since your surgery."
   2. "I am your nurse for the next 12 hours. You can use your call bell to page me."
   3. "Your wife can visit every day between 10 in the morning and 8 at night."
   4. "A physical therapist will be in today to complete an evaluation."

4. A middle-aged adult fell in the driveway at home and came to the emergency department to ensure that he had not sustained a bone fracture. Which statement made by the patient to the emergency department nurse indicates the developmental task of this age group?
   1. "If I get a cast, my fiancé will be furious because we're getting married next month and this will ruin the pictures."
   2. "I don't want you to call my place of employment about my health insurance coverage."
   3. "I must be out of here in a few hours because I have to coach my son's baseball team."
   4. "If my arm is broken, my friends will get another guy to complete our golf foursome."

5. Which nursing interventions meet a patient's physiological needs according to Maslow's hierarchy of needs? **Select all that apply.**
   1. _____ Closing the door to a patient's room to reduce noise
   2. _____ Wearing sterile gloves when changing a patient's dressing
   3. _____ Lowering the height of a patient's bed to the lowest position
   4. _____ Encouraging a parent to stay with a hospitalized child overnight
   5. _____ Providing assistive utensils so that a patient can eat independently

6. Dorothea Orem identified a theory of nursing. Which statement is associated with Orem's theory?
   1. Promotes nursing care that increases a patient's self-care abilities
   2. Helps nurses provide culture-specific care that assists patients to achieve and maintain health
   3. Assists nurses to identify behaviors associated with various stages of coping with death and dying
   4. Facilitates identification of a child's stage of development so that appropriate nursing care is planned

7. Which statement is accurate in relation to the concepts of health and wellness indicated in the presented theoretical framework?

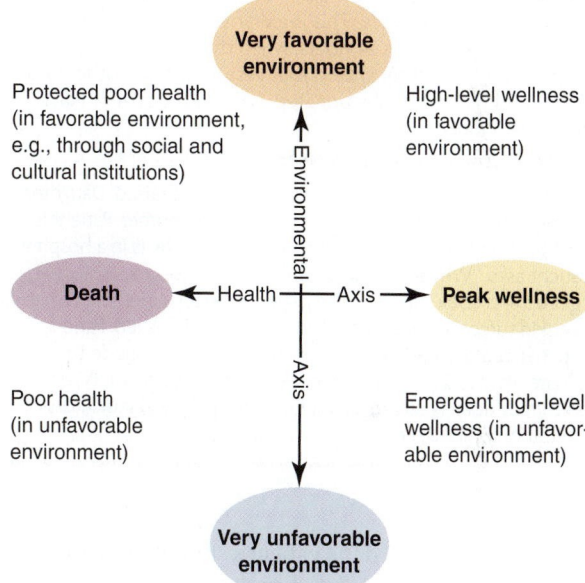

   1. Implies that people are unhealthy if they are unable to fulfill their roles in society
   2. Promotes meeting basic-level needs first and then progressing to higher level needs
   3. Supports teaching about how to alter internal and external factors to facilitate adaptations
   4. Facilitates prediction of whether patients will likely improve in health or experience a decline based on level of support

8. A nurse is caring for a patient newly admitted to the hospital because of altered mental state and to rule out a urinary tract infection (UTI) and brain attack.

Patient's Clinical Record

Vital Signs

Temperature: 102°F, rectally
Pulse: 120 beats/minute, irregular rhythm
Respirations: 26 breaths/minute
Blood pressure: 150/88 mm Hg

Emergency Department Nurse's Progress Note

Patient is a 75-year-old woman brought to the emergency department by her daughter, who found the patient wandering in the neighborhood without a winter coat or shoes. Patient recognizes the daughter and can state her name but is not oriented to time or place. This is a dramatic change in mentation since the previous 24 hours, when the patient was alert and oriented. Daughter shared that yesterday her mother said she felt burning when she urinated. IVF 1,000 mL 0.45% NaCl at 125 mL/hour.

Nurse's Admission Progress Note

Patient in semi-Fowler position. Upper side rails raised. Daughter sitting at bedside and quietly talking with her mother. Patient is unable to verbalize the time or recognize that she is in a hospital. Patient asks, "Why are these people in my house, and why can't I get up and cook supper?" The patient's mucous membranes are dry, skin turgor is inadequate, skin is warm and flushed. Patient experienced dyspnea when transferred to the commode to urinate. Voided 200 mL of urine, cloudy with sediment. IV set at 125 mL/hour. IV site dry, intact, free from clinical indicators of infiltration or inflammation.

The nurse reviewed the patient's clinical record and assessed the patient. Based on the collected data, which nursing action addresses a second-level need according to Maslow's hierarchy of needs?
1. Encourage the patient to increase oral fluid intake.
2. Seek an order for oxygen via a nasal cannula.
3. Activate the bed alarm on the patient's bed.
4. Take vital signs every four hours.

9. A nurse is caring for an older adult. Which statement by the patient indicates the conflict of ego integrity versus despair according to Erik Erikson's theory of development?
1. "I really don't trust any of my doctors and their treatment plan."
2. "I don't care what the doctor says, I will do it my way or no way."
3. "I hope that in my next lifetime I get the chance to become a doctor."
4. "I feel that I will never get better because nothing ever goes well for me."

10. A nurse is caring for an older adult male newly admitted to the hospital. The nurse understands the importance of organizing data and then prioritizing needs based on Maslow's hierarchy of needs. Place the following data collected by the nurse in order following Maslow's hierarchy of needs, progressing from first-level needs up to fifth-level needs.
1. Reported that he has difficulty taking a deep breath
2. Requested help with the telephone so that he can call his son
3. Informed the nurse that he feels dizzy when he moves to a standing position
4. Asked about his condition so that he can make realistic health-care decisions
5. Stated that he feels foolish when he can't find the right words to express himself
Answer: _____

11. A nurse identifies that a patient is experiencing a middle-adulthood developmental crisis. Which information supports the nurse's conclusion?
1. Failure to develop friendships with peers
2. Demotion to a lesser position at work
3. Powerless to postpone gratification
4. Inability to discuss eventual death

12. Which nursing action supports a patient's basic need for safety and security? **Select all that apply.**
1. _____ Positioning a commode next to a patient's bed at night
2. _____ Teaching a patient how to transfer from the bed to a chair
3. _____ Placing a patient's dentures in a labeled denture cup in the bedside table
4. _____ Assessing a patient's abdomen for clinical indicators of urinary retention
5. _____ Ensuring that a patient with neutropenic precautions is provided a mask when being transported for an x-ray

13. An older adult is living in a nursing home because of multiple chronic health problems. Which nursing action is **most** appropriate to assist the older adult to achieve the task associated with Erikson's stage of integrity versus despair?
1. Engage the patient in social activities.
2. Encourage the patient to reminiscence.
3. Provide the patient with opportunities to make choices.
4. Teach the patient the importance of balancing exercise, rest, and sleep.

14. Which statement is **most** associated with Sigmund Freud's psychoanalytic theory of personality development?
    1. Childhood experiences form unconscious motivation for behavior.
    2. People integrate various components to achieve adaptation, survival, and growth.
    3. Interrelationships between emotional and physical variables are more important than psychosexual stages.
    4. A person's energy field is characterized by a pattern, open systems, and dimensionality interacting with the environment.

15. Which nursing action is associated with Maslow's hierarchy of basic human needs model?
    1. The nurse identifies that although the patient has a serious chronic illness, the patient states that he feels healthy because he can meet the responsibilities required of him as husband and father.
    2. The nurse collects data about a patient and organizes it into eleven categories to determine the patient's health needs.
    3. The nurse plots a patient's health status in the quadrant of poor health with a very unfavorable environment.
    4. The nurse determines that the patient's need for oxygen is the priority.

1. **ANSWER: 4.**
   Rationales:
   1. Taking deep breaths after exercising is an example of a first-level need: meeting a physiological need.
   2. Hanging a self-made painting in a senior center is an example of a fourth-level need: need for self-esteem.
   3. Receiving weekly phone calls from adult children is an example of a third-level need: need for love and belonging.
   4. Removing scatter rugs after experiencing a fall in the home is an example of a second-level need: need for safety and security.
   Content Area: Theory-Based Nursing Care
   Integrated Processes: Nursing Process: Implementation
   Client Need: Safe and Effective Care Environment; Safety and Infection Control
   Cognitive Level: Analysis

2. **ANSWER: 1.**
   Rationales:
   1. Menopause is a developmental stress associated with a woman who no longer menstruates. Menopause generally occurs at approximately age 50.
   2. Medications are chemical, not developmental, stresses.
   3. A vitamin deficiency is a physiological, not a developmental, stress.
   4. Impaired family dynamics is a psychosociocultural, not a developmental, stress.
   Content Area: Nursing Care Across the Life Span
   Integrated Processes: Nursing Process: Analysis
   Client Need: Health Promotion and Maintenance
   Cognitive Level: Application

3. **ANSWER: 2.**
   Rationales:
   1. Supporting a patient's need for self-esteem is a fourth-level need according to Maslow.
   2. Providing information to a patient about who is providing care and who and how to call for help when necessary supports the need to feel secure and safe. This is a second-level need according to Maslow.
   3. Explaining when a spouse can visit helps meet love and belonging needs, a third-level need according to Maslow.
   4. Meeting a physiologic need, such as activity, nutrition, elimination, or oxygenation, is a first-level need according to Maslow.
   Content Area: Theory-Based Nursing Care
   Integrated Processes: Communication/Documentation; Nursing Process: Implementation
   Client Need: Safe and Effective Care Environment; Safety and Infection Control
   Cognitive Level: Application

4. **ANSWER: 3.**
   Rationales:
   1. This statement is unrelated to the task of generativity versus self-absorption associated with middle adulthood.
   2. This statement is unrelated to the task of generativity versus self-absorption associated with middle adulthood.

3. This statement is related to the task of generativity versus self-absorption associated with middle adulthood. This task is associated with giving back to the community.
   4. This statement is unrelated to the task of generativity versus self-absorption associated with middle adulthood.
   Content Area: Theory-Based Nursing Care
   Integrated Processes: Communication/Documentation; Nursing Process: Analysis
   Client Need: Health Promotion and Maintenance
   Cognitive Level: Analysis

5. **ANSWER: 1, 5.**
   Rationales:
   1. Closing the door to a patient's room to reduce noise supports the physiological needs of rest and sleep.
   2. Wearing sterile gloves when changing a patient's dressing protects against exposure to infectious microorganisms, which meets a patient's safety and security needs.
   3. Lowering a patient's bed to the lowest position helps to prevent a fall, which provides for the safety needs of the patient.
   4. Encouraging a parent to stay with a hospitalized child overnight supports the child's need to feel safe and secure as well as loved; it does not meet a patient's physiological needs.
   5. Providing assistive utensils helps a patient meet nutritional needs. In addition, it should support self-esteem needs because a patient may feel more independent.
   Content Area: Theory-Based Nursing Care
   Integrated Processes: Nursing Process: Analysis
   Client Need: Physiological Integrity; Basic Care and Comfort
   Cognitive Level: Analysis

6. **ANSWER: 1.**
   Rationales:
   1. This statement is related to Dorothea Orem's care deficit theory of nursing. Orem stated that self-care is a purposeful learned behavior in response to a need.
   2. This statement is related to Madeleine Leininger's culture care diversity and universality theory. She believed that transcultural care is a central and uniting feature of nursing.
   3. This statement is related to Elizabeth Kübler-Ross's theory on death and dying. She believed that patients have commonalities of responses when coping with the diagnosis of a terminal illness.
   4. This statement is related to Jean Piaget's cognitive development theory. She believed that thinking and reasoning developed through exposure to new experiences.
   Content Area: Theory-Based Nursing Care
   Integrated Processes: Nursing Process: Analysis
   Client Need: Health Promotion and Maintenance
   Cognitive Level: Knowledge

7. **ANSWER: 4.**
   Rationales:
   1. This statement is associated with the role performance model of health and wellness.
   2. This statement is associated with Abraham Maslow's hierarchy of basic human needs model of health and wellness.
   3. This statement is associated with Sister Callista Roy's adaptation model of health and wellness.
   4. This statement describes the purpose of H. L. Dunn's high-level wellness grid theory of health and wellness.

Content Area: Theory-Based Nursing Care
Integrated Processes: Nursing Process: Analysis
Client Need: Safe and Effective Care Environment;
Management of Care
Cognitive Level: Analysis

8. **ANSWER: 3.**
   Rationales:
   1. Oral fluid intake is associated with a physiological need, which is a first-level need, according to Maslow's hierarchy of needs.
   2. Seeking an oxygen order is associated with a physiological need, which is a first-level need, according to Maslow's hierarchy of needs. In addition, seeking an order for oxygen is premature. The nurse should collect additional data, such as a decreased oxygen saturation level, before arriving at the conclusion that the patient has an oxygen problem.
   3. **Meeting a patient's safety and security needs is a second-level need according to Maslow's hierarchy of needs. The patient is not oriented to time or place and may not understand the instruction to call for assistance when getting out of bed. A bed alarm will alert the nurse that the patient is attempting to get out of bed, and a caregiver can assist the patient immediately.**
   4. Taking the patient's vital signs every four hours is associated with assessing a person's physiological status, which is a first-level need, according to Maslow's hierarchy of needs.
   TEST-TAKING TIP: Identify the equally plausible options. Options 1, 2, and 4 are related to physiological needs and are equally plausible. Option 3 is related to a need other than meeting a physiological need.
   Content Area: Theory-Based Nursing Care
   Integrated Processes: Nursing Process: Implementation
   Client Need: Safe and Effective Care Environment; Management of Care
   Cognitive Level: Analysis

9. **ANSWER: 3.**
   Rationales:
   1. This response indicates mistrust of others, which may be associated with unsuccessful achievement of the task of trust versus mistrust related to Erik Erikson's theory of development.
   2. This response indicates willfulness, which may be associated with unsuccessful achievement of the task of autonomy versus shame and doubt.
   3. **Integrity versus despair is the task of the older adult. The person reviews life experiences and is either encouraged and views life as meaningful or has a sense of loss and regret. Nonachievement of a goal, such as becoming a doctor, may leave a person with a sense of loss or regret.**
   4. This response indicates pessimism, which may be associated with unsuccessful resolution of the task of initiative versus guilt.
   Content Area: Theory-Based Nursing Care
   Integrated Processes: Communication/Documentation;
   Nursing Process: Analysis
   Client Need: Health Promotion and Maintenance
   Cognitive Level: Analysis

10. **ANSWER: 1, 3, 2, 5, 4.**
    Rationales:
    1. The need for oxygen is a physiological need. Physiological needs are first-level needs according to Maslow's hierarchy of needs.
    3. A patient who reports feeling dizzy when moving to a standing position is experiencing hypotension, which increases the risk of a fall. A risk of falls is a safety issue and is a second-level need according to Maslow's hierarchy of needs.
    2. Wanting to talk to his son is related to love and belonging needs. The need to belong and feel loved is a third-level need according to Maslow's hierarchy of needs.
    5. When a person verbalizes feeling foolish, it indicates a loss of self-esteem. The need for self-esteem is a fourth-level need according to Maslow's hierarchy of needs.
    4. Making an informed and realistic health-care decision is characteristic of a self-actualized person. Self-actualization is a fifth-level need according to Maslow's hierarchy of needs.
    Content Area: Theory-Based Nursing Care
    Integrated Processes: Nursing Process: Planning
    Client Need: Safe and Effective Care Environment;
    Management of Care
    Cognitive Level: Analysis

11. **ANSWER: 2.**
    Rationales:
    1. Development of peer relationships is associated with the developmental tasks of 6- to 12-year-old children, not middle-aged adults.
    2. **Successfully fulfilling lifelong goals involving family, parenthood, employment, and role in society is associated with the developmental task of middle adulthood.**
    3. Inability to postpone gratification is associated with the developmental task of an 18-month-old to 3-year-old child, not a middle-aged adult.
    4. Confronting eventual death is associated with the developmental task of an adult 65 years of age or older, not a person in middle adulthood.
    Content Area: Theory-Based Nursing Care
    Integrated Processes: Nursing Process: Analysis
    Client Need: Health Promotion and Maintenance
    Cognitive Level: Analysis

12. **ANSWER: 1, 2, 3, 5.**
    Rationales:
    1. Positioning a commode next to a patient's bed provides for safety and security. The patient can easily transfer from the bed to the commode and avoid walking to the bathroom at night, which may precipitate a fall.
    2. Teaching a patient how to transfer from the bed to a chair includes actions that provide for safety. For example, teaching a patient to sit on the side of the bed until the blood pressure adjusts to the change in position will minimize dizziness and the potential for a fall that may occur if the person stands up too quickly.
    3. This action supports a patient's safety and security needs. Placing a patient's dentures in a labeled denture cup in the bedside table secures the dentures in a safe place with the patient's name.

4. Assessing and implementing nursing actions to address urinary retention is associated with the basic physiological need of urinary elimination, not a safety and security need.

5. This action meets the safety and security needs of a patient who has a low white blood cell count and is at risk for an infection. A mask will protect the patient from exposure to microorganisms while being transported for an x-ray.

Content Area: Safety
Integrated Processes: Nursing Process: Analysis
Client Need: Safe and Effective Care Environment; Safety and Infection Control
Cognitive Level: Analysis

13. **ANSWER: 2.**

Rationales:

1. Although engaging the patient in social activities is important, it is not the intervention that will help the patient achieve the major task associated with the older adult.

2. **Acceptance of one's worth and viewing one's life as meaningful is the task of the older adult. Engaging the older adult in reminiscing enables the patient to discuss one's past life and develop a sense of satisfaction with the life that was lived. Additional tasks of this age group include adjusting to physical decline and losses, establishing new roles, and preparing for death.**

3. Although providing the patient with opportunities to make choices is important because it supports self-esteem, it is not the intervention that will help the patient achieve the major task associated with the older adult.

4. Although teaching the patient about balancing exercise, rest, and sleep is important, it is not the intervention that will help the patient achieve the major task associated with the older adult.

TEST-TAKING TIP: Identify the word in the stem that sets a priority. The word *most* in the stem sets a priority.

Content Area: Nursing Care Across the Life Span
Integrated Processes: Caring; Communication/ Documentation; Nursing Process: Implementation
Client Need: Health Promotion and Maintenance
Cognitive Level: Application

14. **ANSWER: 1.**

Rationales:

1. This statement is associated with Sigmund Freud's psychoanalytic theory of personality development. Freud believed that all behavior has meaning and is unconsciously motivated by childhood experiences.

2. This statement is associated with Sister Callista Roy's adaptation model. Roy's model focuses on people as adaptive systems responding in the physiological, self-concept, role function, and interdependence modes.

3. This statement is related to Erik Erikson's theory of psychosocial development. Erikson's theory focuses on achievement of tasks viewed as crises throughout the life span.

4. This statement is associated with Martha Roger's science of unitary human beings. Roger's theory focuses on a person as a cohesive whole, with a dynamic energy field that constantly interacts with environmental energy fields.

TEST-TAKING TIP: Identify the word in the stem that sets a priority. The word *most* in the stem sets a priority.

Content Area: Theory-Based Nursing Care
Integrated Processes: Nursing Process: Analysis
Client Need: Psychosocial Integrity
Cognitive Level: Knowledge

15. **ANSWER: 4.**

Rationales:

1. This action is associated with the role performance model of wellness. Nurses should promote independence when caring for patients who define their level of health by their ability to meet role responsibilities.

2. This action is related to Marjory Gordon's functional health patterns. It is a framework for organizing data. The framework promotes identification of interrelated information that assists nurses to determine patients' health needs and appropriate nursing care.

3. This action is associated with Dunn's high-level wellness grid. It is based on the intersection of 2 axes forming 4 quadrants of health and wellness. The 4 quadrants include protected poor health (very favorable environment), poor health (very unfavorable environment), high-level wellness (very favorable environment), and emergent high-level wellness (very unfavorable environment).

4. **This action is associated with Maslow's hierarchy of basic human needs model, in which human needs are arranged in order of importance. The model promotes meeting basic level needs first, starting with physiologic and on to safety and security, love and belonging, self-esteem and, last, self-actualization.**

Content Area: Theory-Based Nursing Care
Integrated Processes: Nursing Process: Analysis
Client Need: Safe and Effective Care Environment; Management of Care
Cognitive Level: Application

Chapter 2

Legal and Ethical Issues

KEY TERMS

Administrative law (regulatory)—Rules and regulations developed by governmental administrative agencies to enforce laws passed by legislative bodies.

Assisted suicide—A competent person legally ends one's own life with medication prescribed by a primary health-care provider.

Attitude—Point of view that lasts over time and guides or influences behavior.

Autonomy—Right of people to have individual liberty and self-determination.

Belief—Opinion about something that people accept as true.

Beneficence—Refers to an action that benefits others or supports a positive outcome.

Common law—Laws based on judges' interpretation and application of constitutional and statutory laws to a set of facts presented in a court case.

Constitutional law—A group of laws that establish the powers and limits of the three branches of government (executive, legislative, and judicial).

Contract law—Laws based on a legally enforceable agreement (a contract) between individuals.

Criminal law—Laws that seek to punish a person for an offense against society.

Ethical dilemma—A situation in which a decision must be made between two or more actions and the best action is unclear.

Ethics—A structure of moral principles or standards that govern behavior.

Euthanasia—Premeditated termination of the life of a person suffering from an incurable or terminal illness.

Fidelity—Refers to making only promises or commitments that can be kept.

Justice—Refers to fairness and equality.

Morals—Personal or societal standards of what is right or wrong and good or bad.

Nonmaleficence—Refers to preventing or removing a patient from harm.

Nursing ethics—The study of ethical issues that occur in nursing and an attempt to provide standards or principles as a way to guide professional behavior.

Personal values—Beliefs that are internalized into one's own life to help guide personal behavior.

Professional values—Beliefs that help to guide professional behavior.

Proxy—A person identified to make health-care decisions for another individual (as in health-care proxy) when the individual is no longer able to make decisions.

Statutory law (legislative)—Laws enacted by federal and state legislative bodies, which are made up of elected individuals who represent the interests of voters.

Surrogate—Individual who legally is permitted to make health-care decisions for an incapacitated individual who does not have a health-care proxy.

Tort—A civil wrong inflicted or imposed on another person or their belongings.

Value—Belief about the worth of something; a belief, ideal, or action respected by an individual, group, or society.

Values clarification—Process by which individuals recognize, explore, and shape personal values.

Veracity—Truthfulness.

Vicarious liability—When accountability for a wrong is assigned to a person or entity that did not directly cause an injury, but has a contractual relationship with the person who did cause the wrong.

Whistle-blowing—Act of reporting workplace incompetence or unethical or illegal situations to someone who has the power to discontinue the wrongdoing.

I. Sources of Law

Nursing practice is influenced by many legal concepts. Therefore, nurses must understand the sources of law established and enforced by the government.

A. Constitutional Law
1. Based on the U.S. Constitution, a group of laws that establish the powers and limits of each of the three branches of government (executive, legislative, and judicial).
2. Grants broad individual rights and responsibilities.
3. Is the foundation of the U.S. justice system.
4. States can pass their own constitutions, but the laws and regulations contained within them must act in accordance with the principle precepts of the U.S. Constitution.

B. Statutory Law (Legislative)
1. Based on the laws enacted by federal and state legislative bodies, which are made up of elected individuals who represent the interests of voters.
2. Federal laws supersede state laws, and state laws supersede local laws.
3. Examples of federal and state laws are presented in the section "Specific Laws and Regulations that Guide Nursing Practice," page 24.

C. Administrative Law (Regulatory)
1. Based on rules and regulations designed to enforce the laws passed by legislative bodies.
2. Developed by governmental administrative agencies.
3. Example: Statutory law establishes nurse practice acts and authority for administrative functions of the state boards of nursing. The state board of nursing in each state is entrusted with the task of creating the rules and regulations detailing how the profession of nursing is practiced in the state.

DID YOU KNOW?

Although none of the standards published by professional organizations are statuary laws, their guidelines factor into what is considered reasonable and prudent nursing care.

D. Common Law
1. Evolves from court decisions, not through legislation.
2. Based on judges' interpretation and application of constitutional and statutory laws to a set of facts presented in a court case.
3. Generally follow precedent, meaning that judges apply the same rules and principles relevant in previous similar cases (doctrine of *stare decisis*— "let the decision stand").

E. Criminal Law
1. Seeks to punish a person for an offense against society; usually involves actions that jeopardize the safety and welfare of the public.
2. Must have a verdict based on guilt beyond a reasonable doubt.
3. Punishment for a minor crime (misdemeanor) generally is a fine or imprisonment for less than 1 year.
4. Punishment for a major crime (felony) is imprisonment for more than 1 year or possibly even execution, depending on the severity of the crime.

II. Civil Law

Civil law seeks to resolve a disagreement between a private individual and another individual or group. Verdicts are based on a preponderance of the evidence and punishment may include payment of money by the person being sued (defendant) to the person bringing the suit (plaintiff). Two types of civil law that influence standards for nursing practice are contract law and tort law.

A. Contract Law
1. Based on legally enforceable agreements (**contracts**) between individuals.
2. Requires.
   a. An agreement between legally competent individuals that indicates the responsibilities of each party.
   b. Understanding of provisions and responsibilities by each party.
   c. Payment for contracted actions performed.
3. Includes employment contracts, for example, in which:
   a. A nurse is expected to follow an employer's policies and standards consistent with federal and state law, satisfy the terms of agreed upon tasks and responsibilities, and respect the tasks and responsibilities of other health team members.
   b. In return, the nurse can expect sufficient and competent support in the delivery of care, reasonable treatment by providers of care and patients, payment for services, a safe working environment, and adequate resources to complete the contracted service.
4. Liability for a wrong may be assigned to a person or entity that did not directly cause an injury but has a contractual relationship with the person who did cause the wrong (**vicarious liability**). Examples include:
   a. *Respondeat superior* ("let the master answer"): When a hospital hires a nurse, the nurse functions as a representative of the institution and must perform within its policies and procedures; the hospital is responsible for the actions of the nurse.
   b. *Captain of the ship*: A health-care provider may be held liable for a nurse who is working under the direction of the health-care provider;

however, the nurse is also still liable for his or her own actions.

   c. *Borrowed servant:* When an employer directs a nurse to work for a second employer, the second employer is held accountable for the nurse's actions (e.g., agency nurse); however, the nurse is also still liable for his or her own actions.

B. Tort Law

   1. A **tort** is a civil wrong inflicted or imposed on another person or their belongings.

   2. Types of torts (Table 2.1).

     a. **Intentional tort:** Commission of a deliberate improper act (actual or threatened) that is beyond the legal limits of what is considered acceptable. It must be executed on purpose and with intent; however, no harm has to occur for liability to exist.

     b. **Quasi-intentional tort:** Making false statements, verbally (slander) or in writing (libel), about another person that harms the person's reputation, holds the person up to ridicule or contempt, or causes the person to be avoided.

     c. **Unintentional tort:** Commission or omission of an act that results in harm to another. However, there is no intent to do harm by the person committing or omitting the act. Negligence and malpractice are considered unintentional torts (see next section).

III. Negligence and Malpractice

The most common unintentional torts that affect nurses are negligence and malpractice. Both relate to failure to implement reasonable care according to standards that

Table 2.1 Types of Torts

Types and Definitions	Examples
Intentional Torts	
Assault Intentionally threatening to harm or touch a patient in an insulting, unjustifiable, or offensive manner.	• Stating, "Stop yelling or I will move you to the end of the hall." • Stating, "If you don't behave, you can't have your pain medication."
Battery Intentionally touching a patient's body or clothing or anything held by or attached to a patient in an angry, willful, negligent, or violent manner without consent.	• Performing a procedure without informed consent. • Forcefully undressing a patient. • Resuscitating a patient who has a do-not-attempt-resuscitation order. • Administering a medication refused by a patient.
Fraud Engaging in purposeful misrepresentation or reckless disregard of the truth to produce unlawful gain.	• Stating, "You should not feel any pain with this procedure," when it is commonly know that the procedure is painful. • Engaging in dishonesty when obtaining a nursing license. • Altering a medical record for the purpose of concealing the truth.
False imprisonment Intentionally and unjustifiably preventing movement or retaining a patient without consent or authority to do so.	• Refusing to discharge a patient from the hospital until he or she pays the bill. • Applying a restraint when doing so does not comply with the policies and procedures for restraint application.
Invasion of privacy Disclosing confidential information about a patient to an inappropriate person, sharing unnecessary information or gossip about a patient, or not honoring a patient's right to be left alone.	• Discussing confidential information on an elevator used by visitors. • Releasing information about a patient without consent. • Unnecessarily physically exposing a patient. • Asking unnecessary probing questions.
Quasi-Intentional Torts	
Defamation Communicating false derogatory information that harms a person's reputation, holds the person up to ridicule or contempt, or causes the person to be avoided. **1. Slander** Occurs when false derogatory information is stated orally. **2. Libel** Occurs when false derogatory information is stated in writing.	**1. Slander** • Maliciously stating that another nurse is incompetent without supportive data. • Commenting to another nurse that a patient is a child molester after hearing gossip from another caregiver. **2. Libel** • Documenting false information about the patient's sexual orientation in the patient's clinical record. • Documenting false derogatory information about a patient in an incident report.
Unintentional Tort	
See section III, "Negligence and Malpractice."	

results in injury to another. The differentiating factor is that malpractice is considered "professional negligence."

A. Negligence and Malpractice

1. **Negligence.**
   a. Occurs when a nurse fails to implement reasonable care as dictated by standards of care by omission or commission of an act and/or fails to act how a reasonable and prudent *layperson* would in similar circumstances.
   b. Must result in physical, emotional, or financial harm.

2. **Malpractice.**
   a. Professional form of negligence.
   b. Occurs when a nurse fails to provide an expected level of care consistent with professional standards of practice and/or fails to act how *another nurse* would in similar circumstances.
   c. Must result in physical, emotional, or financial harm.
   d. Litigation occurs when a patient (the plaintiff) initiates a civil suit in court against a provider of health care (the defendant). To prove malpractice, the plaintiff must establish by a preponderance of the evidence four elements of liability.
      (1) **Duty:** The nurse-patient relationship establishes that the nurse has a legal obligation to the patient when the patient seeks nursing care.
      (2) **Breach of duty:** The nurse's actions by omission or commission of an act failed to meet standards of care established by a job description, agency policy or procedures, the state nurse practice act, standards established by professional organizations, and/or a text deemed to be authoritative.
      (3) **Causation:** Involves two elements that must be proven by the plaintiff.
         (a) A nurse's action or inaction was the immediate cause of the plaintiff's injury (proximate cause).
         (b) A nurse should have known that the breach of the nursing standard could result in harm or injury (foreseeability).
      (4) **Damages:** A plaintiff must prove that physical, emotional, or financial harm or injury was the result of the breach of duty, such as pain, suffering, disfigurement, disability, medical expenses, or lost wages.

B. Common Malpractice Claims Related to Nursing Practice

1. Failure to assess the patient and make appropriate nursing diagnoses.
   a. Includes:
      (1) Failure to complete an admission assessment or assignment.
      (2) Failure to make ongoing assessments.
      (3) Failure to recognize a cluster of data that indicates a problem.
      (4) Failure to identify safety needs, such as a risk of falls or pressure ulcers.
      (5) Failure to listen to patient concerns or requests.
   b. To minimize the risk of litigation, the nurse must:
      (1) Make a complete assessment.
      (2) Have a strong knowledge base of the science of nursing, anatomy and physiology, sociology, psychology, chemistry, and so forth; collect, analyze, and recognize the significance of data; and have the ability to identify a patient's needs.
      (3) Make ongoing assessments until a patient is stable.
      (4) Listen to a patient's concerns or requests and respond appropriately.

2. Failure to plan appropriate nursing care.
   a. Includes:
      (1) Failure to design a plan of care according to facility policy and procedures.
      (2) Failure to include appropriate nursing interventions in the plan of care, such as failure to plan for assistance when a debilitated patient moves from a bed to a chair and subsequently falls or failure to plan to assist a patient with meals who is at risk for aspiration and who subsequently aspirates.
   b. To minimize the risk of litigation, the nurse must:
      (1) Formulate a plan of care for every patient, including problems/needs, goals/outcomes, and planned interventions.
      (2) Document the plan of care according to agency policy and procedures.
      (3) Include all appropriate nursing interventions in the plan of care to achieve the patient's goals/outcomes based on professional standards of care.

3. Failure to implement a plan of care appropriately.
   a. Includes:
      (1) Failure to follow standards of practice and agency policy and procedures, such as unsafe use of equipment, improper application of restraints, medication error, or disregard for do-not-attempt-resuscitation (DNAR) orders.
      (2) Failure to follow state laws or regulations concerning the prescription of medications and performance of medical/surgical interventions.
      (3) Failure to function as an advocate, such as failure to protect a patient's physical safety, report an impaired nurse, or report suspected abuse or neglect.

(4) Failure to respond to a patient's needs or requests in a timely manner, such as not proving pain medication or answering a call light.

(5) Failure to document critical information about a patient or a patient response to care, such as drug allergies, falls, untoward reaction to treatment or nursing care, patient status and progress, medication administration, response to interventions, and information provided by family members.

(6) Failure to communicate with other members of the health-care team, such as failure to notify the primary health-care provider of a change in a patient's condition or providing incomplete information at the change of shift report.

b. To minimize the risk of litigation, the nurse must:

(1) Know and understand acceptable legal limits of one's words or actions.

(2) Know who has a prescriptive license in the state and accept and implement prescriptions and orders only from these professionals.

🛑 (3) Accept assignments only for which one is qualified to provide safe and appropriate nursing care.

DID YOU KNOW?

A nurse has the right to refuse to be temporarily reassigned (floated) to an area in which he or she is unqualified to work. Staff members on the unit accepting a reassigned nurse have a responsibility for orienting the nurse to the unit and supporting the nurse in the performance of nursing care.

(4) Participate in continuing education to ensure competence in light of new technology and progress in nursing practice (e.g., know how to operate equipment before using it with a patient).

(5) Follow standards of care identified in the nurse practice act in the state in which the nurse works.

(6) Follow professional standards of care and agency policy and procedures (e.g., keep a bed in the lowest position, provide education and counseling, follow controlled drug policies and procedures, maintain confidentiality and privacy, ensure that informed consent is obtained for procedures).

(7) Employ the nursing process when identifying patient needs and providing patient care.
   (a) Assessment.
   (b) Analysis.
   (c) Planning.
   (d) Implementation.
   (e) Evaluation.

(8) Properly assign, delegate, and supervise subordinates, including only assigning tasks and responsibilities that are within the legal parameters of a person's role (e.g., only nurses are responsible for ongoing assessment, patient education, and completion of tasks that require sterile technique; nurse aides can take vital signs and assist patients with uncomplicated activities of daily living).

(9) Treat a patient with respect and dignity (e.g., address a patient by name, pull a curtain, provide draping, support patients' rights, explain what you are going to do and why).

(10) Involve a patient in the planning and implementation of care.

(11) Always function as a patient advocate (e.g., help a patient communicate wishes to other health-care providers and family members, question inappropriate medication and treatment orders, follow an agency policy to report impaired coworkers, intervene on the behalf of patients when patients are unable to protect themselves).

(12) Always respond to patient requests (e.g., assess the need for pain medication, answer call lights in a timely manner, order an alternate meal if requested).

(13) Always follow the rights of medication administration and question incomplete or inappropriate orders.

(14) Document all important information about a patient, nursing care planned for and provided, patient responses, and all events in the patient's medical record (e.g., progress notes, medication administration record, flow sheets, admission assessment form, discharge form).

(15) Report a change in a patient's condition that requires immediate action to the primary health-care provider.

(16) Employ the rapid response team when a patient's condition deteriorates.

(17) Provide a thorough report at the end of a shift to the nurse responsible for the continued care of the patient.

4. Failure to evaluate patient responses to interventions.
   a. Includes:
      (1) Failure to observe for nontherapeutic and therapeutic responses.
      (2) Failure to recognize significance of responses.
      (3) Failure to respond appropriately to nontherapeutic responses.

(4) Failure to notify the primary health-care provider of a patient's nontherapeutic responses.

(5) Failure to document the patient's therapeutic or nontherapeutic responses.

b. To minimize the risk of litigation, the nurse must:

(1) Always assess for therapeutic and nontherapeutic responses to an intervention (e.g., chills, fever, low back pain, dyspnea, and facial flushing indicating a hemolytic reaction to a blood transfusion).

(2) Respond appropriately to a nontherapeutic response (e.g., immediately stopping a blood transfusion and replacing it with normal saline solution if a hemolytic reaction occurs).

(3) Notify the primary health-care provider of nontherapeutic responses to interventions (e.g., immediately notifying the primary health-care provider if a patient has a hemolytic reaction to a blood transfusion and then waiting for treatment orders).

(4) Document all therapeutic and nontherapeutic patient responses to interventions (e.g., documenting medications given before a blood transfusion is initiated, patient evaluation afterward, therapeutic and nontherapeutic responses, immediate notification of the primary health-care provider in the event of a negative reaction, and follow-up care provided along with ongoing assessments and patient responses).

(5) Complete an incident report and follow facility policies and procedures when negative events occur (e.g., medication error, fall or injury involving a patient, visitor, or staff member).

IV. Informed Consent

When a patient agrees to be admitted to a hospital, the patient gives approval for routine care. However, each specialized procedure requires written informed consent specific for the stated procedure signed by the patient or the patient's surrogate.

A. **Elements That Must Be Met for a Patient to Give Informed Consent**

1. **Disclosure:** The patient must be provided with a thorough explanation of the risks, benefits, costs, and alternatives. It is the responsibility of the primary health-care provider to provide this information as well as answer all questions asked by the patient.

2. **Comprehension:** The patient must be able to repeat in his or her own words details about the procedure, including risks, benefits, costs, and alternatives.

3. **Voluntariness:** The patient must give his or her consent willingly.

4. **Competence:** The patient must be capable of understanding the information to make an informed decision.

a. Understanding is dependent upon the patient being alert, having intact cognition, and being a minimum of 18 years of age.

b. Minors younger than 18 years of age can sign a consent form if legally emancipated, a parent, or married.

B. **Nursing Care Related to Obtaining Informed Consent**

1. The nurse must ensure that all the criteria that relate to informed consent are met.

a. Disclosure: Ensure that the primary health-care provider has discussed details about the procedure, including risks, benefits, costs, and alternatives.

b. Comprehension: Instruct the patient, "State in your own words what you have been told about the procedure by your primary health-care provider." Determine if the information is consistent with details concerning the procedure.

c. Voluntariness: Ask the patient, "Are you signing this consent voluntarily without pressure from others?"

d. Competence: Ensure that the patient is at least 18 years of age or is an emancipated minor, a parent, or married and is alert with intact cognition. When a patient is incapable of participating in the decision-making process, an alternate decision-maker must be identified. Most states specify the order of priority, such as durable power of attorney, court-appointed guardian, parents, spouse, and adult children.

2. If a criterion is not met, it is the responsibility of the nurse to inform the primary health-care provider. The nurse should withhold signing the consent form until the deficiency is corrected.

3. A nurse's signature on the consent form indicates that the nurse was a witness to the patient's signature.

DID YOU KNOW?

Patients have the right to sign a form that states that they do not want to be informed of the details of a procedure.

V. Specific Laws and Regulations That Guide Nursing Practice

Federal and state laws have been established to protect individual rights and public interests. Nurses must have knowledge and understanding of these laws because of their impact on the profession of nursing and nursing practice.

A. Examples of Federal Laws
1. Bill of Rights.
   a. First 10 amendments to the U.S. Constitution.
   b. Examples of rights especially relevant to nursing practice are the rights of privacy, freedom of speech, and due process.
2. Americans With Disabilities Act.
   a. Established a mandate for eliminating discrimination against people with disabilities.
   b. Requires reasonable accommodation for individuals to perform their job and for patients (e.g., buildings must be wheelchair accessible, providers of care cannot discriminate against patients who have acquired immunodeficiency syndrome [AIDS]).
3. Comprehensive Drug Abuse Prevention and Control Act.
   a. Controls distribution and use of drugs that have a high potential for abuse or addiction, such as opioids, depressants, stimulants, and hallucinogens.
   b. Controlled drugs must be stored, handled, disposed of, and administered according to regulations established by the U.S. Drug Enforcement Administration (DEA).
4. Emergency Medical Treatment and Active Labor Act.
   a. Ensures access to emergency services despite an inability to pay for services.
   b. Forbids the transfer of indigent or uninsured individuals from a private to a public facility without adequate assessment and stabilization, except when:
      (1) The patient requests a transfer.
      (2) The facility does not have the capacity to stabilize the patient.
   c. Requires that, when transferred, a patient must be attended to by competent personnel and with appropriate equipment.
5. Occupational Safety and Health Act (OSHA).
   a. Established the Occupational Safety and Health Administration (an agency of the U.S. Department of Labor), which identifies and enforces regulations that protect individuals from work-related injury.
   b. Protects nurses, who have the potential for injury because of exposure to such hazards as radiation, chemotherapeutic agents, bloodborne pathogens, electrical equipment, sharps, and moving and lifting patients.
   c. Sets specific standards and requires the availability of certain equipment (e.g., mechanical lifts, personal protective equipment) to maintain a safe and healthful workplace for nurses.

DID YOU KNOW?
Occupational nurses have an essential role in helping maintain the health and safety of workers within the work setting.

6. Health Care Quality Improvement Act.
   a. Provides public identification of primary health-care providers who are disciplined or penalized for failure to meet legal standards of care.
   b. Established the National Practitioner Data Bank, which tabulates data about medical malpractice payments, unfavorable actions taken against clinical privileges, and measures taken by professional organizations that negatively affect membership.
7. National Labor Relations Act.
   a. Gives individuals the legal right to bargain with an employer as a group to improve working conditions and salaries (collective bargaining).
   b. The American Nurses Association (ANA) in 1944 stated that each state's nurses association can perform collective bargaining for nurses.
8. Newborns' and Mothers' Health Protection Act.
   a. Increased the length of stay in a hospital or birthing center for a mother and infant to no less than 48 hours after a vaginal birth and no less than 96 hours after a cesarean birth.
   b. Attempts to limit maternal and neonatal morbidity and mortality.
9. Health Insurance Portability and Accountability Act (HIPAA).
   a. Provides regulations that protect the confidentiality of health information and medical records.
   b. Sets standards for organizational identifiers, electronic transfer of patient information among organizations, uniform protection of all health information, and appropriate disclosure of protected health information.
   c. Requires nurses to:
      (1) Share patient information (e.g., verbally, electronically, or in writing) with only those members of the health-care team responsible for the patient. For example, nurses should:
         (a) Avoid posting signs that contain health-related information around patients' bed or on messages boards in a nursing station.
         (b) Avoid talking about patients in areas that can be overheard by others.
         (c) Avoid leaving patient documents (i.e., electronic or paper) unsupervised.

DID YOU KNOW?

Information about a patient's health-care status can be shared with people other than members of the health-care team when the patient gives written permission. In addition, student nurses are held to the same rules and regulations as licensed health-care providers.

(2) Inform patients verbally and in writing of their rights to privacy and confidentiality regarding their health information. For example, a nurse should not disclose that a person is a patient without expressed patient permission.

(3) Ensure that patients have the right to view and amend their own health records and obtain a copy of their clinical record upon written request. For example, a patient may want a copy of their medical records sent to another health-care provider for a second opinion.

10. Patient Self-Determination Act.
   a. Requires health-care agencies to provide patients written information about their rights when making decisions regarding health care.
   b. Requires all health-care providers who receive Medicare funds to explain advance directives to staff and patients (e.g., patient's wishes relative to health-care should incapacitation or an inability to make decisions occurs).
   c. Requires health-care providers to offer patients the opportunity to complete an advance directive.

B. Examples of State Laws
1. Mandatory reporting laws.
   a. Require reporting of communicable diseases and suspected abuse (e.g., physical, sexual, emotional, or verbal abuse; financial exploitation; neglect) of children, elders, and mentally disabled people by health-care providers or family members to authorities (e.g., Child Protective Services).
   b. Exist in most states.
   c. Vary by state, requiring nurses to know their own agency policy and state laws because, in some states, the employer is responsible for reporting suspected abuse or neglect.
   d. Provide for legal immunity from privacy laws if a nurse has made a report in good faith.
   e. Can charge nurses with a criminal or civil offence under the law if they do not report suspected abuse or neglect.
2. Good Samaritan laws.
   a. Offer immunity from liability in malpractice litigation to health-care professionals who provide assistance at the scene of an accident or in an emergency.

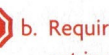 b. Require nurses to follow standards of practice and act in a prudent manner as would another nurse in similar circumstances.

   (1) Nurses should:
      (a) Only provide first aid, if possible.
      (b) Only employ actions that they are educated to do.
      (c) Instruct someone to get additional help.
      (d) Stay until the injured person leaves or is transferred by ambulance or until another qualified person assumes responsibility for the injured person.
      (e) Not accept compensation.
   c. Gross divergence from normal standards of care or recklessly or intentionally injuring a person can lead to litigation.
   d. Do not require nurses to render care to people outside of their contractual responsibilities to an entity.
3. Nurse practice acts.
   a. Safeguard the public by legally defining the nature and scope of nursing practice, describing how the nursing profession is governed, and defining criteria for nursing education.
   b. Are specific to each state; therefore, nurses should know and understand the nurse practice act of the state or states in which they work; this is critical for travel nurses and other nurses who work in more than one state.
   c. Generally give state boards of nursing the authority to regulate nursing practice and education within the state, including licensing, credentialing, and disciplinary procedures.
      (1) Licensing.
         (a) State boards of nursing have the authority to permit graduates of approved schools of nursing to take the National Council Licensure Examination (NCLEX-RN or NCLEX-PN).
         (b) After criteria for licensure are met (vary from state to state), the state board of nursing awards a nursing license that authorizes an individual the right to engage in the practice of nursing as a registered professional nurse or licensed practical nurse.
         (c) Certain states allow nurses to be licensed in one state and to practice in all states taking part in a multistate agreement (multistate compact).
      (2) Credentialing: Voluntary self-regulation that attempts to ensure proficiency of its

health-care providers and includes accreditation and certification.
  (a) Accreditation.
    - State boards of nursing examine and monitor a nursing program's ability to meet minimal expected standards for basic nursing education as well as evaluate ongoing efforts at continuous improvement of the program.
    - They generally require nursing programs to meet educational standards established by the National League for Nursing Accrediting Commission or the American Association of Colleges of Nursing.
    - Hospitals generally voluntarily seek accreditation by The Joint Commission, which ensures a minimum standard of quality of care is provided to patients.
  (b) Certification.
    - Professional organizations, such as the ANA, offer voluntary certification in specialty areas (e.g., oncology, geriatrics, pediatrics) when specific criteria are met, such as educational preparation, experience, evidence of continuing education, and a passing grade on an examination.
    - Some states permit a nurse to seek an advance practice license only if first certified by an approved specialty organization.
(3) Disciplinary procedures.
  (a) State boards of nursing generally are responsible for enforcing requirements by establishing disciplinary procedures.
  (b) Unprofessional conduct is reported to the state board of nursing, which follows a set procedure to determine whether the nurse has violated the state's nurse practice act. Punitive action (e.g., suspension, revocation of a license, attendance at a drug rehabilitation program) may result if proven guilty.

VI. Professional Guidelines for Nursing Practice

The role of the nurse has expanded dramatically because of the advent of new technology and changes in the delivery of health care within society. Patient and nurse rights, standards of nursing care, and specific policies and procedures within an entity are designed to protect both patients and nurses.

A. ANA Nurse's Bill of Rights
  1. Developed to "protect the dignity and autonomy of nurses in the workplace."
  2. Identifies seven conditions nurses should expect from the workplace that address issues related to the provision of safe, competent, and ethical nursing care as well as personal nurse-related issues.
    a. Right to practice nursing in a way that fulfills their obligations to society.
    b. Right to practice nursing within the legal scope of nursing practice and professional standards.
    c. Right to practice nursing in accordance with the Code of Ethics for Nurses.
    d. Right to advocate for patients and themselves without fear of retribution.
    e. Right to have fair compensation for their work.
    f. Right to work in a safe environment.
    g. Right to individually or collectively negotiate the conditions of their employment.

B. The Patient Care Partnership
  1. Asserts that patients have rights regarding their treatment when admitted to a health-care facility.
  2. Originally published as the Patient's Bill of Rights by the American Hospital Association; has evolved and now addresses patient expectations.
  3. Briefly identifies that patients should expect:
    a. High-quality care.
    b. A clean, safe environment.
    c. Freedom from abuse and neglect.
    d. To be involved in decisions.
    e. To receive information about the right to refuse care and resources available to help make decisions.
    f. Protection of privacy and confidentiality.
    g. Help with billing and insurance claims.
    h. Preparation and information on discharge from the facility.

C. Standards of Practice
  1. Are specific stipulations that guide the practice of nursing by outlining the scope, function, and role of nurses and nursing practice.
  2. May be general and relate to values within the profession or specific and relate to expectations of nursing care for an identified group of patients.
  3. Published by various states (e.g., nurse practice acts), professional organizations (e.g., ANA, Emergency Nurses Association), and federal organizations (e.g., The Joint Commission, Center for Medicare & Medicaid Services) to guide nursing practice.

D. Institutional Policies and Procedures
  1. Are not law.
  2. Are more specific than standards.

3. Include information specific to nursing practice that an employer expects a nurse to know and safely implement.

VII. Protection Against Litigation

By virtue of such factors as the complexity of nursing care, reengineering of health-care delivery, expanding role of the nurse, and expectations of patients and family members, as well as the litigiousness of society, nurses are at an increased risk for being accused of negligence or malpractice. Various safeguards exist that protect nurses from legal actions.

A. **Legal Safeguards for Nurses**
 1. Good Samaritan laws.
    a. Offer immunity from liability in malpractice litigation to health-care professionals who provide assistance at the scene of an accident or emergency.
    b. Require health-care professionals to act in a prudent manner consistent with standards of practice.
    c. Example: A nurse applies pressure with a shirt to a hemorrhaging wound that a patient sustained in an automobile collision. Later, the patient experiences a wound infection. The nurse is not libel for the patient's infection because the nurse acted in a prudent manner consistent to what another nurse would have done in a similar situation.
 2. Safe harbor.
    a. Provided for under state nurse practice acts.
    b. Protects a nurse from suspension, termination, disciplinary action, and discrimination if the nurse refuses to do or not do something because he or she believes that it is inappropriate and could be harmful.
    c. Example: A nurse working on a medical surgical unit who has no obstetrical nursing experience has a right to refuse to be floated to a birthing unit.
 3. Professional liability insurance.
    a. Contracts the nurse with an insurance company, who pays for legal fees and for judgment or settlement costs to the extent of the policy in the event of litigation.
    b. Provides some legal protection from malpractice litigation.
    c. Generally does not defend against claims of sexual abuse of a patient, damages caused while a nurse is under the effect of drugs or alcohol, unlawful actions, transmission of acquired immunodeficiency syndrome to a patient, or punitive damages.

4. Incident report.
    a. Clearly documents all the facts related to an incident, such as date, time, location, and a brief description of the incident in factual terms.
    b. In the event of litigation, helps to remind individuals involved what the facts were and avoids blurring of the facts over time.
    c. Should include quoted statements by the patient or individuals involved when possible; should not contain opinions, conclusions, or speculation and should not place blame.
    d. A nurse should document in the patient's medical record only how the injury occurred, the patient's response, and any actions taken; the nurse should not reference that an incident report was completed.

5. Informed consent.
    a. Protects a nurse from charges of battery if a patient claims that permission was not given for an invasive procedure.
    b. In the event a patient refuses to sign a consent form for a recommended intervention, the patient should be informed of the consequences of inaction and then be asked to sign a form that releases the health-care team and agency from responsibility.

6. Nurse practice acts.
    a. Protect a nurse by clearly defining the nature and scope of nursing practice and conditions under which a person can practice the profession of nursing.
    b. Requires nurses to work within the legal definition of their role to be protected.

7. Controlled substance laws.
    a. Protects a nurse from involvement in a situation of missing or misused controlled drugs.
    b. Requires nurses to follow all the rules and regulations established by the U.S. Drug Enforcement Administration related to storage, handling, administration, and disposal of controlled drugs to be protected by these laws.

8. Laws to protect "whistle-blowing."
    a. A **whistle-blower** is a person who unsuccessfully attempts to correct a quality-of-care issue within the normal channels of an organization and then resorts to going to an outside organization with the concern.
    b. Whistle-blowing should be a last resort when no action is taken in response to reported concerns, such as understaffing, reassignment, and excessive mandatory overtime.
    c. Some states have laws that protect whistle-blowers from reprisal.

B. **Nursing Actions to Protect Oneself From Litigation**

🛑 1. Know the legal parameters of the state nurse practice act in the state in which one works.

2. Follow laws that influence nursing practice.
3. Follow institutional policies and procedures.
4. Follow the ANA Standards of Nursing Practice.
5. Follow ethical parameters provided by the ANA Code of Ethics for Nurses.
6. Purchase professional liability insurance separate from what an employer provides to ensure that one's personal interests are protected.
7. Work only in a setting in which one is prepared to meet the challenges of delivering safe nursing care.
8. Keep current by attending educational and in-service programs.
9. Maintain competent nursing practice.
   a. Implement safe nursing care in the technical realm (e.g., perform skills safely and develop new skills in response to technological advances).
   b. Maintain cognitive competence (e.g., acquire new knowledge and apply it appropriately, especially in response to the results of evidence-based practice research).
   c. Ensure interpersonal competency (e.g., continue to develop communication skills to collaborate with patients and other members of the health-care team).
10. Be respectful of patients' rights and deliver nursing care in a compassionate manner.
11. Use the nursing process to plan and implement comprehensive nursing care.
12. Document all nursing activities and patient responses to interventions (see Chapter 7, "Communication and Documentation").

VIII. Ethical Nursing Practice

Nurses must perform self-examination to identify personal beliefs and values because these foundations drive the formation of one's character, morals, and ethics, ultimately influencing one's behavior in society. Then nurses must develop a professional ethical platform that does not impose their personal beliefs and values about what is acceptable and unacceptable onto patients and their family members. Incorporating the concepts of autonomy, beneficence, nonmaleficence, justice, and fidelity in conjunction with adhering to the laws and standards associated with the profession of nursing promotes the delivery of ethically competent nursing care. Nursing care becomes a challenge when decision-making conflicts occur among patients and their family members and even among health-care providers.

A. **Societal Factors That Contribute to Ethical Issues**

1. Advances in technology, such as:
   a. In vitro fertilization.
   b. Genetic engineering.
   c. Organ transplantation.
   d. Life support interventions.
   e. Procedures that reveal fetal impairment.
2. Multicultural population issues, such as:
   a. Multifaith society.
   b. Increased ethnic diversity.
   c. Groups with vastly different values and beliefs.
3. Increased consumer awareness, such as:
   a. Increased patient awareness of their rights.
   b. Internet availability of health information.
   c. Increased patient self-advocacy.
   d. Internet chat lines that facilitate discussion among people with the same disorder.
4. Cost-containment measures, such as:
   a. Nurses caring for increased numbers of more acutely ill patients, contributing to potentially unsafe situations.
   b. Decreased length of stay in health-care facilities, sending patients home while they still need skilled health-care services, which are not always readily available.

B. **Principles Related to Ethical Practice**

1. **Autonomy.**
   a. Refers to the right of people to have individual liberty and self-determination (i.e., patients have the right to make personal choices about treatment and care).
   b. Means that nurses should provide information so that patients can make personal choices regarding their care.
   c. Examples: Signing a consent form, continuing the intake of salt when a low-sodium diet is recommended, refusing blood products because of religious beliefs, signing one's self out of the hospital against medical advice.
2. **Beneficence.**
   a. Refers to the performance of an action that benefits others or supports a positive outcome.
   b. Examples: Irrigating a wound, administering a medication, turning and positioning an immobile patient.
3. **Nonmaleficence.**
   a. Refers to preventing harm, avoiding actions that can cause harm, and removing a patient from harm.
   b. The positive outcome of an action must be measured against the risk of potential harm.

   c. Example: Medicating a postoperative patient for pain and then ambulating the patient using a two-person assist addresses the need to improve circulation and to prevent harm while minimizing the risk of pain or a fall.

4. **Fidelity.**
   a. Refers to making only promises or commitments that can be kept.
   b. Means that a patient can expect that a nurse will honor agreements made verbally.
   c. Example: A nurse who promises to return immediately with pain medication is expected to honor that commitment.

5. **Justice.**
   a. Refers to fairness and equality (i.e., all patients should be treated fairly and equally regardless of individual factors, such as age, gender, skin color, ethnic origin, religious beliefs, sexual orientation, and medical diagnosis).
   b. Example: All people should have access to health care whether they have medical insurance or are indigent; just and fair policies and procedures should guide the allocation of organs for transplantation.

6. **Veracity.**
   a. Refers to being truthful, which is essential to a trusting nurse-patient relationship.
   b. Demonstrates respect for the patient.
   c. Necessary for a patient's right to make informed decisions.
   d. Examples: Providing truthful answers to patients who are asking questions about their prognosis; informing a patient when a procedure may be painful.

C. **Guides to Ethical Decision Making in Nursing**
  1. Nursing codes of ethics.
   a. Officially state ideals and values of the profession, provide a framework for making ethical decisions and are a standard for professional actions.
   b. Examples: The ANA Code of Ethics for Nurses (Box 2.1), International Council of Nurses' (ICN) Code of Ethics for Nurses.
  2. Institutional ethics committees.
   a. Generally consist of interdisciplinary health-care professionals, such as primary health-care providers, nurses, clergy, ethicists, and lay representatives.
   b. Establish guidelines, formulate policies and procedures, provide counseling and education, and conduct case reviews.
   c. Mediate in ethical dilemmas to facilitate resolution.
  3. Nursing ethics forums.
   a. May be unit-based or agency wide and are designed to provide opportunities for nurses

---

Box 2.1 Provisions of the American Nurses Association *Code of Ethics for Nurses*

1. The nurse, in all professional relationships, practices with compassion and respect for the inherent dignity, worth and uniqueness of every individual, unrestricted by considerations of social or economic status, personal attributes, or the nature of health problems.
2. The nurse's primary commitment is to the patient, whether an individual, family, group, or community.
3. The nurse promotes, advocates for, and strives to protect the health, safety, and rights of the patient.
4. The nurse is responsible and accountable for individual nursing practice and determines the appropriate delegation of tasks consistent with the nurse's obligation to provide optimum patient care.
5. The nurse owes the same duties to self as to others, including the responsibility to preserve integrity and safety, to maintain competence, and to continue personal and professional growth.
6. The nurse participates in establishing, maintaining, and improving health-care environments and conditions of employment conducive to the provision of quality health care and consistent with the values of the profession through individual and collective action.
7. The nurse participates in the advancement of the profession through contributions to practice, education, administration, and knowledge development.
8. The nurse collaborates with other health professionals and the public in promoting community, national, and international efforts to meet health needs.
9. The profession of nursing, as represented by associations and their members, is responsible for articulating nursing values, for maintaining the integrity of the profession and its practice, and for shaping social policy.

---

   to identify and discuss ethical issues associated with the provision of nursing care.
   b. Assist nurses in improving skills in ethical problem-solving and decision making.

D. **Development of a Personal Ethical Foundation**
  1. Nurses should identify and clarify their own values and beliefs.
  2. Nurses should form a personal ethical foundation.
  3. Nurses should integrate a personal ethical foundation with the ethics of the nursing profession (e.g., ANA Code of Ethics).
  4. Nurses should be aware of sensitive ethical issues.
  5. Nurses should continuously work at improving ethical decision-making abilities.

E. **Nursing Actions That Support Patients' Ethical Rights**
  1. Nurses should follow ethical codes provided by professional organizations.
  🛑 2. Nurses should support patient autonomy, especially when a patient's decision is not supported by family

members. The nurse must remember that the patient is the center of the health team and must be an advocate for the patient above all others.

3. Nurses should support patients and family members as they make decisions.
4. Nurses should accept patients' and family members' decisions, even if those decisions differ from the decisions a nurse would make for oneself; if unable to do so, nurses should remove themselves from responsibility for the care of the patient and family members.
5. Nurses should use an ethical decision model for guidance to identify the best response to a dilemma.
6. Nurses should use and participate in an institutional ethics committee.

IX. Legal Rights and Ethical Issues Related to End-of-Life Care

End-of-life issues have escalated dramatically due to advances in technology that prolong life, the increased number of older adults, and the desire of dying individuals to control their destinies with dignity. As a result, patients, family members, and health-care providers are faced with multiple ethical dilemmas, such as assisted suicide, euthanasia, withholding or termination of life-sustaining treatment, organ donation, and certification of death. Multiple legal instruments are available to address some of these issues, such as advanced health-care directives, health-care proxies, living wills, and do not attempt resuscitation (DNAR) orders.

A. Advance Health-Care Directives
1. Advance health-care directives are a set of instructions or directions stating a person's health-care requests if the person becomes incapacitated or unable to make decisions.
2. Health-care providers are required to offer patients the opportunity to complete an advance health-care directive.
3. Patients can cancel or make changes in advanced health-care directives at any time.
4. People should complete an advanced health-care directive before they become ill so that personal wishes are carried out when they become ill.
5. Health-care providers are protected from liability when they follow the instructions in an advance directive.
6. Advance health-care directives include health-care proxy (durable power of attorney for health care), living will, and DNAR orders.

B. Health-Care Proxy (Durable Power of Attorney for Health Care)
1. A health-care proxy is a document that identifies a person to make health-care decisions for a patient when the patient is no longer able to make decisions.
2. The contract may indicate certain conditions under which the proxy takes effect, such as irreversible coma or terminal illness.
3. It may include specific instructions about issues, such as withholding hydration, medication, parenteral nutrition, and mechanical ventilation.
4. It is a legal instrument signed by two witnesses.

C. Living Will
1. A living will is a document prepared by a competent person giving instructions associated with medical care to be delivered or not delivered if the person becomes unable to make decisions in the future.
2. A living will differs from a health-care proxy in that it does not identify a person as a proxy.

D. DNAR Orders
1. DNAR orders direct health-care providers not to attempt resuscitation in the event that a patient suffers cardiac or respiratory failure in a health-care facility or the home.
2. Health-care providers are not legally permitted to initiate DNAR orders without the consent of the patient, surrogate, or proxy.
3. Nurses and patients must know that a DNAR order does not mean do not treat.
4. DNAR orders may be suspended before surgery and reinstituted after surgery if the primary health-care provider has discussed this with and received consent from the patient or proxy.
5. Health-care professionals who initiate cardiopulmonary resuscitation in the presence of a DNAR order may be held accountable (i.e., sued by the family for pain and anguish; reported to the state board of nursing).

E. Assisted Suicide
1. Assisted suicide is the taking of one's own life after seeking and receiving a prescription from a primary health-care provider for a medication that will cause death.
2. Various criteria must be met determined by state law such as:
   a. State the intent to and be capable of self-administering medication that will end one's life.
   b. Be at least 18 years of age.
   c. Be terminally ill with fewer than six months to live as determined by two physicians.
   d. Meet certain psychiatric criteria and be counseled regarding other options including palliative and hospice care.
   e. Request a prescription from a physician for a medication that will cause death. Generally, there is a designated waiting period (e.g., 15 days) between the request for the prescription and the writing of the prescription by the physician.

3. The states of Oregon, Washington, and Vermont have passed laws that permit physicians to order medications that may be used by patients to cause their own death.
4. Physicians, nurses, and pharmacists are not required to participate in assisted suicide.
5. "The ANA (1994) believes that the nurse should not participate in active euthanasia [and assisted suicide] because such an act is in direct violation of the Code for Nurses with Interpretive Statements (Code for Nurses), the ethical traditions and goals of the profession, and its covenant with society. Nurses have an obligation to provide timely, humane, comprehensive and compassionate end-of-life care."

F. Euthanasia
1. Euthanasia is premeditated termination of the life of a person suffering from an incurable or terminal illness.
2. A person directly implements the cause of death.

3. The ANA believes that nurses should not participate in active euthanasia (see section IX, E, "Assisted Suicide").
4. No state in the United States currently allows euthanasia.

G. Withholding or Terminating Life-Sustaining Treatment, Food, and/or Fluid
1. People have the right to refuse recommended treatment as well as interventions that are life sustaining.
2. When patients are incapable of speaking for themselves, surrogates can make the decision to refuse or withdraw treatments for patients; states have specific protocols to determine the order of surrogacy.

H. Certification of Death, Organ Donation, and Postmortem Examination (See Chapter 8, "Psychosocial and Cultural Nursing," for information on these topics.)

CASE STUDY: Putting It All Together

A 17-year-old, accompanied by her mother, brings her one-week-old infant to the emergency department. The 17-year-old appears dazed, does not make eye contact, and rarely answers the nurse's questions. The grandmother tells the triage nurse that her daughter is a senior in high school, is unmarried, and lives at home. The nurse obtains the infant's vital signs, weighs the infant, and identifies that the infant is pale and lethargic. The grandmother, who is holding the infant, states, "The baby sleeps all the time and has difficulty sucking when given a bottle and stops a lot during a feeding." The triage nurse transports the infant and family members from the triage area to a room with a crib in the emergency department. When passing the main desk, the triage nurse says loud enough for other health team members to hear, "The baby's mother is on drugs. She had no business getting pregnant in the first place." Later, while the infant is waiting to be further assessed, the mother of the infant attempts to run out of the emergency department. A nurse grabs the mother's arm and pulls her back to the unit, saying firmly, "Where do you think you are going? Stay here. Your baby needs you!"

Case Study Questions

A. From whom should the informed consent be obtained to provide care to the infant? Why?

_____

B. During the intake interview, the triage nurse asks the following questions. Which questions are appropriate or inappropriate and why?

  1. "Why didn't you get married?"

  2. "Did you drink alcohol while you were pregnant?"

  3. "Where is the father of the baby now?"

  4. "Were you taking prescription or illegal drugs while you were pregnant?"

  5. "Did you experience any health problems during your pregnancy?"

  6. "Do you plan on going back to school or staying at home with your baby?"

  1. _____

  2. _____

  3. _____

  4. _____

  5. _____

  6. _____

C. Which nursing intervention is an example of an intentional tort, and why?

_____

D. Which nursing intervention is an example of a quasi-intentional tort, and why?

_____

REVIEW QUESTIONS

1. A home care nurse is visiting an older adult who experienced a brain attack 2 years ago and now has a sacral pressure ulcer. The nurse identifies that the patient and spouse both appear unkempt and the spouse appears tired and irritated. The patient is very quiet and avoids eye contact. Which nursing action is **most** appropriate?
   1. Explore with the patient and spouse their concerns.
   2. Assess the patient for signs of physical abuse and neglect.
   3. Discuss with the patient and spouse additional resources to help with the patient's care.
   4. Assess the patient's pressure ulcer and report findings to the primary health-care provider.

2. A patient is admitted to a home health-care program for palliative care. When completing the admission interview and nursing assessment the patient empathically states, "I want no intervention to extend my life other than keeping me comfortable." When talking with family members they want the patient to continue chemotherapy. What should the nurse do?
   1. Protect the patient's right to self-determination.
   2. Initiate a referral to a psychiatric nurse practitioner.
   3. Ask the patient to reconsider chemotherapy for the sake of the family.
   4. Refer family members to the primary health-care provider to resolve this issue.

3. A nurse is planning patient care based on moral and ethical principles. Which nursing statement demonstrates an effort to implement the principle of fidelity?
   1. "Let's talk about foods that are healthy and that you should include in your daily diet."
   2. "I know that you are out of work, so I have arranged for you to get follow-up care at our out-patient clinic."
   3. "You said that your son wants you to have this surgery. What is important is what you believe is best for you."
   4. "It's been half an hour and I am back as I promised to ensure that the pain medication I gave you is providing relief."

4. Which statements are associated with state nurse practice acts? **Select all that apply.**
   1. _____ Nurse practice acts identify what a nurse can and cannot do.
   2. _____ A purpose of state nurse practice acts is to regulate the practice of nursing.
   3. _____ The federal government is the regulating agency responsible for state nurse practice acts.
   4. _____ Student nurses are not obligated to meet the same standards of care as are licensed nurses.
   5. _____ If a student nurse is involved in a disciplinary action by the state board of nursing, the student may be prohibited from taking the National Council Licensure Examination.

5. A nurse is caring for an adult patient who is scheduled for surgery. Which action is not associated with the nurse ensuring a valid, legal consent?
   1. Observe the patient signing the consent form.
   2. Ensure that the patient is signing the consent form voluntarily.
   3. Assess if the patient has the capacity to make an informed consent.
   4. Review with the patient the risks and benefits of the surgery before the consent is signed.

6. Which situation should the nursing staff refer to the hospital ethics committee?
   1. The adult patient with renal insufficiency who refuses dialysis
   2. The wife who wants her unconscious husband to have a drug that is available in a phase-three trial
   3. The parents of a developmentally disabled adult who disagree with the health-care decisions of the court appointed guardian
   4. The adult patient recently diagnosed with metastatic cancer who wants hospice care but whose family wants chemotherapy to be given immediately

7. A nurse is implementing care based on moral and ethical principles. What should the nurse do **first** to accomplish a personal professional code of ethics consistent with the American Nurses Association *Code of Ethics for Nurses?*
   1. Deliver care that preserves and protects patient autonomy and self-determination.
   2. Explore personal values and beliefs because they affect nursing decisions.
   3. Implement culturally competent and sensitive nursing care to patients.
   4. Respect the inherent worth and uniqueness of each individual patient.

8. Which actions meet obligations regarding the Health Insurance Portability and Accountability Act (HIPAA) of 1996? **Select all that apply.**
   1. _____ Allowing patients the right to review and copy their clinical record
   2. _____ Providing access to a patient's clinical record to all members of the nursing team
   3. _____ Holding patient rounds in a hallway out of the hearing range of the patient being discussed
   4. _____ Explaining to a person inquiring about the condition of a patient that information about the patient is confidential
   5. _____ Giving medical information about an unconscious patient to a patient's daughter who is the person indicated in the patient's proxy directive

9. An older adult is diagnosed with atrial flutter with a 4-to-1 block. The atrial rate is 280 beats/minute and the ventricular rate is 70 beats/minute. The patient is admitted to the hospital and transferred to a medical unit. The patient is being treated with diltiazem (Cardizem), an antidysrhythmic, as well as continuous electrocardiogram monitoring. The primary health-care provider is contemplating performing cardioversion if the patient does not respond favorably to the antidysrhythmic. Later that evening, the patient reports feeling strange, so the nurse obtains the patient's vital signs and performs a physical assessment. The nurse concludes that the patient is stable and continues to follow the primary health-care provider's orders. During the night, the patient dies. Eventually, the patient's cause of death is determined to be a brain attack (cerebral vascular accident, stroke). The risk manager of the hospital reviews the patient's clinical record, specifically the vital signs, nurse progress notes, and electrocardiogram results.

Patient's Clinical Record

Vital Signs

Temperature: 99.2°F
Pulse: 90 beats/minute, irregular rhythm
Respirations: 26 breaths/minute
Blood pressure: 98/60 mm Hg

Electrocardiogram

Atrial fibrillation

Nurse Progress Notes

Patient reports feeling weak, tired, dizzy, and short of breath. States, "I feel very anxious and like my heart is pounding." Respirations are 26 breaths/minute but do not appear to be labored. Denies chest pain, nausea, and headache. Strength in both hands and feet are equal. Spoke with patient to provide reassurance.

The risk manager concludes that the nurse can be held accountable for which tort?
1. Assault
2. Battery
3. Negligence
4. Malpractice

10. A patient who has a history of schizophrenia and is hallucinating is brought to the emergency department of a community hospital. The primary health-care provider in charge refuses to admit the patient. The nurse attempts to educate the primary health-care provider regarding the law involving patients who are grossly disabled. The primary health-care provider still refuses to admit the patient. What is the nurse's **next** action?
    1. Admit the patient against the primary health-care provider's wishes.
    2. Refuse to discharge the patient as per the primary health-care provider's orders.
    3. Describe the primary health-care provider's behavior to the nursing supervisor and ask for guidance.
    4. Call the primary health-care provider's supervisor and explain that the health-care provider is acting inappropriately.

11. Which statements associated with a patient's clinical record are considered accurate? **Select all that apply.**
    1. _____ The clinical record belongs to the patient.
    2. _____ The Joint Commission examines patients' clinical records to substantiate compliance with standards of care.
    3. _____ Clinical records are used by a quality management committee to monitor quality of care provided by the facility.
    4. _____ Clinical records serve as a legal document that can be used in a court of law to prove that a standard of care was met or not met.
    5. _____ Parts of a clinical record can be copied and used only by student nurses if the patient's name and medical record number is removed.

12. A patient with paralyzed lower extremities (paraplegia) as a result of a spinal cord injury states that the employer said, "You cannot come back to work because the office is not set up for employees using wheelchairs." What nursing action is **most** supportive of this patient?
    1. Instruct a social worker to intercede on behalf of the patient.
    2. Report the patient's situation to the hospital's legal department to negotiate a compromise.
    3. Suggest that the patient seek employment where a wheelchair is able to maneuver about the work environment.
    4. Explain to the patient that employers must make reasonable accommodations to facilitate employment of disabled employees.

13. A nurse is caring for a patient receiving hospice care for terminal cancer. The patient has a transdermal opioid patch and a prescription for an oral opioid for breakthrough pain. The patient reports that the pain is excruciating. The nurse assesses the patient and identifies that the patient's pulse is 85 beats/minute, respirations are 10 breaths/minute and shallow, and the blood pressure is 98/68 mm Hg. What should the nurse do?
    1. Administer the prn opioid medication.
    2. Inform the primary health-care provider of the patient's respiratory rate.
    3. Call the nursing supervisor to ask for guidance in dealing with this situation.
    4. Hold the pain medication until the respirations increase to an acceptable rate.

14. Which statements accurately pertain to nursing licensure? **Select all that apply.**
    1. _____ A state board of nursing can never revoke a nursing license.
    2. _____ A nursing license can be refused as a result of unlawful actions.
    3. _____ A nursing license is not necessary when practicing nursing in the home setting.
    4. _____ A nursing license allows a nurse to practice in the state in which the license was issued.
    5. _____ A state board of nursing is responsible for ensuring that graduates of recognized schools of nursing take the NCLEX licensure examination.

15. A nurse is making every effort to implement nursing care based on moral concepts and principles of ethics. Which nursing statement demonstrates an effort to implement the principle of veracity?
    1. "Let's review the in-bed leg exercises that you need to perform after surgery."
    2. "Here is the pain medication that I promised I would get for you immediately."
    3. "After receiving this drug, you may feel bone pain, but it should subside in about a week."
    4. "I am going to move you to a room away from the nurses' station so that you sleep better at night."

16. Which term **best** describes the situation when a nurse says to a pediatric patient, "If you don't be quiet, I will not let your parents visit you today"?
    1. Battery
    2. Assault
    3. Negligence
    4. Abandonment

17. Which actions are a violation of the Health Insurance Portability and Accountability Act of 1996 (HIPAA)? **Select all that apply.**
    1. _____ Talking about a patient to another health professional in an elevator
    2. _____ Telling a neighbor about a famous person who currently is your patient
    3. _____ Documenting untrue information on purpose in a patient's clinical record
    4. _____ Leaving patient data on a computer screen in a hallway while administering medication
    5. _____ Completing an incident report about a patient situation and asking the nurse manager to review it

18. Which must be reported to legal authorities in some states in North America?
    1. Release against medical advice
    2. Communicable diseases
    3. Suspected child neglect
    4. Abuse of older adults

19. A primary nurse is caring for a 70-year-old adult who suffered a brain attack 10 days ago and is unresponsive. The patient did not sign a legal instrument identifying which adult child should make healthcare decisions in the event of incapacitation. Two of the adult children are adamant about not wanting a feeding tube inserted for nutritional support and two of the adult children are just as firm about wanting a feeding tube inserted. What should the nurse do to **best** help resolve this situation?
    1. Explain to the siblings all the advantages of inserting a feeding tube.
    2. Urge family members to discuss the matter of inserting a feeding tube with their spiritual advisor.
    3. Suggest that this issue about the feeding tube be presented to an ethics committee for consultation.
    4. Encourage the insertion of the feeding tube temporarily until the patient's status can be determined.

20. Which of the following is designed to protect the nurse?
    1. Americans with Disabilities Act
    2. Nurse practice acts
    3. Reporting of abuse
    4. Incident reports

21. A nurse accidentally administers a medication to the wrong patient and the patient experiences a serious untoward reaction. For which tort can the nurse be legally charged?
    1. Malpractice
    2. Assault
    3. Battery
    4. Fraud

22. Which are examples of violations of the Health Insurance Portability and Accountability Act (HIPAA)? **Select all that apply.**
    1. _____ Failure to fill out an incident report after a patient falls
    2. _____ Discussing a plan of care with other student nurses in a debriefing conference
    3. _____ Discussing test results with a patient in a populated sitting area in the unit lounge
    4. _____ Leaving a patient's vital signs sheet visible on a computer screen in the hallway while taking the patient's vital signs
    5. _____ Temporarily misplacing a form with the names of patients with their scheduled surgeries that is returned by a visitor

23. Which statement is accurate regarding a nurse practice act?
    1. Educational criteria that must be met by schools of nursing are legislated exclusively by a state's nurse practice act.
    2. Rules and regulations regarding the practice of nursing are identified in each state's nurse practice act.
    3. Nursing titles for a licensed nurse are regulated by the National League for Nursing.
    4. A nurse practice act provides federal oversight of what a nurse can and cannot do.

24. A patient who is staggering, slurring words, and is clearly incoherent is brought to the hospital via ambulance. A diagnostic evaluation reveals that the patient is grossly intoxicated but is in no medical distress. When called, the spouse says, "I've had it. I am done being an enabler. You handle it." The health-care provider refuses to admit the patient because the patient has no medical problem. What is the nurse's **most** appropriate action at this time?
    1. Request that the nursing supervisor talk with the primary health-care provider.
    2. Discharge the intoxicated patient as per the primary health-care provider's order.
    3. Have the primary health-care provider encourage the spouse to come to the emergency department.
    4. Inform the primary health-care provider that the patient is gravely disabled and should not be released.

25. A nurse is a defendant in a lawsuit. The plaintiff must provide evidence in the four elements of liability. Place the statements presented in the options related to meeting the elements of liability in the order of duty, breach of duty, causation, and damages.
    1. The patient experienced hypotension, fell, and fractured the head of the left femur as a result of receiving a diuretic that was not prescribed.
    2. The patient required surgery to repair the fractured femur and experienced a delay of chemotherapy for lung cancer.
    3. The nurse administered a diuretic to the wrong patient.
    4. The nurse is caring for a patient in the hospital.
    Answer: _____

1. ANSWER: 2.
Rationales:
1. If the patient is being neglected or abused by the spouse, the patient may not feel that this information can safely be conveyed to the nurse.
2. **Protecting the patient from neglect or abuse is the priority. The patient should be assessed further for signs of neglect or abuse. The patient's behavior may indicate fear. The spouse's appearance and behavior may indicate caregiver role strain. Inadequate turning and positioning, nutritional intake, and bathing and skin care can precipitate a pressure ulcer. Reporting suspected elder abuse or neglect to appropriate authorities is legally required by health-care professionals.**
3. This intervention is premature. Additional information is necessary for a comprehensive assessment. Respite care often is helpful in providing full-time caregivers an opportunity to experience a rest from providing 24/7 care to a family member.
4. Although assessing the pressure ulcer and reporting findings to the primary health-care provider should be done, it is not the priority.
TEST-TAKING TIP: Identify the word in the stem that sets a priority. The word *most* in the stem sets a priority. Identify the option that is most patient centered. Although all of the options are patient centered, option 2 is the only option that focuses on advocacy, which is an important role of the nurse.
Content Area: Legal and Ethical Issues
Integrated Processes: Caring; Nursing Process: Assessment
Client Need: Safe and Effective Care Environment; Management of Care
Cognitive Level: Application

2. ANSWER: 1.
Rationales:
1. **The patient has a right to refuse treatment and to be in charge of decisions regarding treatment and care. The nurse should support the decisions that are made by the patient.**
2. The patient's behavior does not indicate a need for a referral for psychological counseling.
3. This denies the patient's feelings. Asking the patient to reconsider chemotherapy for the sake of the family is not patient centered.
4. This action defers interventions that are within the legal role of nursing practice to another health-care professional.
TEST-TAKING TIP: Identify the option that is patient centered. Option 1 is the only option that focuses on the patient; it is a patient-centered intervention. Identify options that are opposites. Options 1 and 3 are opposites. Identify the option that denies the patient's feelings. Option 3 denies the patient's feelings.
Content Area: Legal and Ethical Issues
Integrated Processes: Caring; Communication/Documentation; Nursing Process: Implementation
Client Need: Safe and Effective Care Environment; Management of Care
Cognitive Level: Application

3. ANSWER: 4.
Rationales:
1. This is an example of the ethics principle of beneficence, not fidelity. Beneficence refers to the performance of an action that benefits others or supports a positive outcome.
2. This is an example of the ethics principle of justice, not fidelity. Ensuring that patients are treated equally, regardless of such factors as economics, age, gender, skin color, ethnic origin, religious beliefs, and sexual orientation, is associated with the principle of justice.
3. This is an example of the ethics principle of autonomy, not fidelity. Autonomy refers to the right to have individual liberty and self-determination. Patients have a right to make personal choices about treatment and care.
4. **This is an example of the ethics principle of fidelity. Fidelity is the duty to keep commitments. Patients need to know that nurses will honor verbal agreements.**
Content Area: Legal and Ethical Issues
Integrated Processes: Caring; Communication/Documentation; Nursing Process: Implementation
Client Need: Safe and Effective Care Environment; Management of Care
Cognitive Level: Analysis

4. ANSWER: 1, 2, 5.
Rationales:
1. **Each state has its own nurse practice act, which identifies the scope of nursing practice within the state; they identify what a nurse can legally do or not do.**
2. **Although state nurse practice acts regulate the practice of nursing, the main purpose is to safeguard the health, safety, and well-being of people in the community from maltreatment or injury related to nursing care.**
3. Each state, not the federal government, defines the nurse practice act in its own state.
4. Student nurses are held to the same standards of care as a licensed nurse.
5. **Since student nurses are held accountable for ensuring that standards of care are met, they are subject to disciplinary actions by the state board of nursing. A student nurse may be prohibited from taking the National Council Licensure Examination if it is determined that the student nurse failed to meet standards of care identified in the state nurse practice act.**
Content Area: Legal and Ethical Issues
Integrated Processes: Nursing Process: Analysis
Client Need: Safe and Effective Care Environment; Management of Care
Cognitive Level: Comprehension

5. ANSWER: 4.
Rationales:
1. It is the responsibility of the nurse to observe a patient signing an informed consent form.
2. It is the nurse's responsibility to ensure that the patient is agreeing freely and not being forced into having the surgery. Patients have the right to self-determination, which means they have the right to refuse treatment.
3. The patient has to be cognitively intact (have capacity) to understand the risks, benefits, and ramifications associated with the surgery for a consent to be legally valid.

4. Explaining the risks and benefits of surgery is the responsibility of the surgeon, not the nurse.
TEST-TAKING TIP: Identify the words in the stem that indicate negative polarity. The words *not associated* in the stem indicate negative polarity.
Content Area: *Legal and Ethical Issues*
Integrated Processes: *Nursing Process: Implementation*
Client Need: *Safe and Effective Care Environment; Management of Care*
Cognitive Level: *Application*

6. **ANSWER: 3.**
Rationales:
1. An adult patient who is cognitively intact has the right to self-determination; this means that the patient has a right to pursue or refuse medical treatment.
2. Requesting the use of an experimental drug by a person who has legal authority is not an ethical issue. However, to be accepted into a drug trial program, the patient must meet the criteria established by the individuals responsible for the program.
3. Although the legal guardian has the right to make medical decisions for this developmentally disabled adult, the involvement of the hospital's ethics committee may help to resolve the dispute between the parents and the guardian.
4. An adult patient who is cognitively intact has the right to self-determination; this means that the patient has a right to pursue or refuse medical treatment regardless of what family members want.
Content Area: *Legal and Ethical Issues*
Integrated Processes: *Communication/Documentation; Nursing Process: Implementation*
Client Need: *Safe and Effective Care Environment; Management of Care*
Cognitive Level: *Application*

7. **ANSWER: 2.**
Rationales:
1. Another step needs to be done before integrating ethical principles into one's nursing practice.
2. This is the first step in developing professional values. Professional values will develop and form as a student nurse expands knowledge and experience. First the nurse must identify personal values and beliefs before a conflict can be identified between personal values versus professional values. There may be times that personal values conflict with professional values, such as when a nurse who does not believe in abortion is asked to care for a patient scheduled for an abortion. Issues arise, such as can the nurse care for the patient in a nonjudgmental way?
3. Another step needs to be done before implementing culturally competent and sensitive nursing care to patients.
4. Another step needs to be done before integrating ethical principles, such as respecting the inherent worth and uniqueness of each individual patient.
TEST-TAKING TIP: Identify the word in the stem that sets a priority. The word *first* in the stem sets a priority. Identify the option that is unique. Option 2 is unique. It is the only option that is associated just with the nurse; options

1, 3, and 4 include the patient. Option 2 is the only option that presents a reason why the action is necessary, *because they affect nursing decisions.* For all these reasons, examine option 2 carefully.
Content Area: *Legal and Ethical Issues*
Integrated Processes: *Nursing Process: Analysis*
Client Need: *Safe and Effective Care Environment; Management of Care*
Cognitive Level: *Comprehension*

8. **ANSWER: 1, 4, 5.**
Rationales:
1. Patients have the right to examine, amend, and request a copy of their entire clinical record.
2. Only nursing team members directly responsible for caring for the patient have a right to access the patient's clinical record.
3. Rounds should be held in an area that is private so that only health team members can hear the conversation. If rounds are conducted in a hallway, visitors and other patients and nursing team members not responsible for the patient's care may overhear confidential information about the patient. Discussing patients in hallways, elevators, or dining areas violates HIPAA rules.
4. No information can be released to an inquiring individual without the permission of the patient. Health-care workers are not permitted to share the fact that the person is currently admitted or not admitted to the hospital.
5. If a patient is unable to participate in making personal health-care decisions, the patient's designated health-care proxy is responsible for making these decisions. An individual who is a health-care proxy must know all the risks and benefits of health-care interventions before making informed decisions for the patient.
TEST-TAKING TIP: Identify the option with a specific determiner. Option 2 contains the word *all,* which is a specific determiner. More often than not, an option with a specific determiner is a distractor.
Content Area: *Legal and Ethical Issues*
Integrated Processes: *Communication/Documentation; Nursing Process: Analysis*
Client Need: *Safe and Effective Care Environment; Management of Care*
Cognitive Level: *Application*

9. **ANSWER: 4.**
Rationales:
1. This scenario does not reflect an assault. An assault occurs when a person unjustifiably threatens to touch or harm another.
2. This scenario does not reflect battery. Battery is the intentional touching of a patient's body or clothing or anything held by or attached to a patient in an angry, willful, negligent, or violent manner without consent.
3. This scenario does not reflect negligence. Negligence occurs when a nurse fails to implement reasonable care as dictated by standards of care by omission or commission of an act and/or fails to act how a reasonable and prudent *layperson* would in similar circumstances.

4. The nurse had a professional relationship with and responsibility for the nursing care of the patient. The nurse failed to provide an expected level of care consistent with professional standards of practice and failed to act how *another nurse* would in similar circumstances. The patient's vital signs and physical assessment revealed that the patient was unstable, and the patient's electrocardiogram results converted from atrial flutter to atrial fibrillation. Atrial fibrillation can be a precursor to a brain attack (stroke). The rapid response team and the primary health-care provider should have been notified so that appropriate medical intervention could be performed.
Content Area: Legal and Ethical Issues
Integrated Processes: Nursing Process: Evaluation
Client Need: Safe and Effective Care Environment; Management of Care
Cognitive Level: Analysis

10. **ANSWER: 3.**
Rationales:
1. The nurse cannot admit a patient.
2. Although this is something that the nurse should do, there is another option that should be implemented first. A nurse should refuse to be involved in a discharge or any other action if it is known to be against policy or is unethical.
3. If a nurse believes an action by another professional is inappropriate, the nurse should seek guidance from the nurse's immediate supervisor.
4. It is inappropriate for a nurse to contact the primary health-care provider's supervisor. This does not follow the nurse's chain of command within a facility.
TEST-TAKING TIP: Identify the word in the stem that sets a priority. The word *next* in the stem sets a priority. Identify the options that are opposites. Option 1 and 2 are opposites. Examine options 1 and 2 carefully.
Content Area: Legal and Ethical Issues
Integrated Processes: Communication/Documentation; Nursing Process: Implementation
Client Need: Safe and Effective Care Environment; Management of Care
Cognitive Level: Application

11. **ANSWER: 2, 3, 4.**
Rationales:
1. The clinical record belongs to a facility or to a primary health-care provider if it is in a primary health-care provider's office; it does not belong to the patient. However, the information in the clinical record belongs to the patient.
2. The Joint Commission, in the process of accrediting a health-care facility, will audit patients' clinical records to ensure compliance with standards by which quality of health care is measured.
3. Quality management committees examine patients' clinical records to determine if there are any undesirable trends that indicate where improvement can be made in the delivery of care, such as success rates of procedures, frequency of agency acquired infections, occurrences of harmful events, and so on.

4. Comprehensive, detailed, and unambiguous documentation of the patient's status, nursing care provided, and the patient's response protect the nurse from false claims of negligence or malpractice.
5. A patient's clinical record cannot be copied and removed from the unit, even after the patient's name and medical record number are removed. This violates HIPAA regulations.
Content Area: Legal and Ethical Issues
Integrated Processes: Communication/Documentation; Nursing Process: Analysis
Client Need: Safe and Effective Care Environment; Management of Care
Cognitive Level: Knowledge

12. **ANSWER: 4.**
Rationales:
1. It is not the responsibility of a social worker to advocate for a patient in this situation.
2. It is not the responsibility of the legal department of a hospital to advocate for a patient in this situation.
3. It is not necessary for the patient to seek new employment.
4. The Americans with Disabilities Act, passed in 1990, requires employers to make reasonable accommodations (e.g., ramps, bathrooms, parking, elevators) to facilitate employment of people with disabilities. The patient should be made aware of one's rights indicated in the Americans with Disabilities Act and then be encouraged to seek compliance by the employer.
TEST-TAKING TIP: Identify the word in the stem that sets a priority. The word *most* in the stem sets a priority. Identify the options that are equally plausible. Options 1 and 2 are equally plausible. Identify opposite options. Options 3 and 4 are opposites.
Content Area: Legal and Ethical Issues
Integrated Processes: Caring; Communication/Documentation; Nursing Process: Implementation
Client Need: Safe and Effective Care Environment; Management of Care
Cognitive Level: Application

13. **ANSWER: 1.**
Rationales:
1. The American Nurses Association's *Code of Ethics* indicates that patients have the right to die in comfort. To be accepted into a hospice program, patients must complete a do-not-attempt-to-resuscitate form and understand that care is directed toward supporting comfort and dignity and not curative. Medicating a patient to achieve a comfortable and peaceful death is appropriate, even if by doing so it hastens death.
2. The health-care provider has already prescribed an intravenous opioid medication for the purpose of providing for a comfortable and peaceful death.
3. In a situation where a patient is receiving hospice care, pain medication may be administered, even it may hasten death. The intention of providing opioid medication is relief of pain and support for a comfortable and peaceful death.

4. Holding prescribed pain medication from a dying patient who has agreed to hospice care is cruel, unethical, and unacceptable.

TEST-TAKING TIP: Identify opposite options. Options 1 and 4 are opposites. Identify equally plausible options. Options 2 and 3 are equally plausible. They both seek direction in what to do next. Identify the most patient-centered option. Option 1 is the most patient-centered option.

Content Area: Legal and Ethical Issues
Integrated Processes: Caring; Nursing Process: Implementation
Client Need: Safe and Effective Care Environment; Management of Care
Cognitive Level: Application

14. **ANSWER: 2, 4, 5.**
Rationales:
1. A nursing license can be revoked or suspended for professional misconduct.
2. **This is an accurate statement. Candidates for licensure must self-report criminal convictions, chemical dependencies, and functional ability deficits.**
3. A nursing license is required to practice the profession of nursing in all settings.
4. **This is an accurate statement. Each state sets the criteria for the passing rate on the NCLEX examination. If you meet the criteria to practice nursing in one state, another state may grant a license to practice nursing in their state upon a person's application for this privilege (reciprocity).**
5. **Each state's board of nursing is responsible for ensuring that only graduates of recognized schools of nursing take the NCLEX examination. Administrators of schools of nursing inform state boards of nursing of the names of individuals who have successfully completed a nursing program. The graduate then completes an application to take the NCLEX examination, which is submitted to the state board of nursing.**

TEST-TAKING TIP: Identify options with a specific determiner. The word *never* in option 1 is a specific determiner. Generally, an option with a specific determiner can be eliminated from consideration.

Content Area: Legal and Ethical Issues
Integrated Processes: Nursing Process: Analysis
Client Need: Safe and Effective Care Environment; Management of Care
Cognitive Level: Knowledge

15. **ANSWER: 3.**
Rationales:
1. This is an example of the ethical principle of beneficence, not veracity. Performing an action that supports a positive outcome is an example of beneficence.
2. This is an example of the ethical principle of fidelity, not veracity. Fidelity refers to making only promises or commitments that can be kept. Promising to return immediately with pain medication and then immediately returning with the pain medication is an example of fidelity.
3. **This is an example of the ethical principle of veracity. Veracity refers to being truthful, which is essential to a**
trusting nurse-patient relationship. Informing a patient when a procedure may be painful is an example of veracity.
4. This is an example of the ethical principle of nonmaleficence, not veracity. Removing a patient from harm, preventing harm, and avoiding actions that may cause harm are associated with the principle of nonmaleficence. The positive outcome of an action must be measured against the risk of potential harm.

Content Area: Legal and Ethical Issues
Integrated Processes: Communication/Documentation; Nursing Process: Implementation
Client Need: Safe and Effective Care Environment; Management of Care
Cognitive Level: Analysis

16. **ANSWER: 2.**
Rationales:
1. Battery occurs when a person unlawfully touches another person without consent.
2. **Assault occurs when a person threatens harm to an individual. The patient does not have to be touched for the nurse to be charged with assault.**
3. Negligence occurs when a patient suffers an injury when a nurse fails to meet a standard of care.
4. Abandonment occurs when a nurse leaves a patient without an appropriate nursing replacement.

TEST-TAKING TIP: Identify the word in the stem that sets a priority. The word *best* in the stem sets a priority.

Content Area: Legal and Ethical Issues
Integrated Processes: Communication/Documentation; Nursing Process: Evaluation
Client Need: Safe and Effective Care Environment; Management of Care
Cognitive Level: Application

17. **ANSWER: 1, 2, 4.**
Rationales:
1. **This action violates HIPAA. Confidential information should be discussed only in an area where privacy is provided.**
2. **This action violates HIPAA. Information about a patient should be discussed only with appropriate members of the health-care team and individuals for whom the patient gives written consent.**
3. This action is fraud, not a violation of HIPAA.
4. **This action violates HIPAA. Information left on a computer screen that can be seen by people walking in a hallway violates confidentiality.**
5. Consulting with a nurse manager is an appropriate action and does not violate HIPAA.

TEST-TAKING TIP: Identify the word in the stem that indicates negative polarity. The word *violation* in the stem indicates negative polarity.

Content Area: Legal and Ethical Issues
Integrated Processes: Communication/Documentation; Nursing Process: Evaluation
Client Need: Safe and Effective Care Environment; Management of Care
Cognitive Level: Application

18. ANSWER: 4.
Rationales:
1. This event is not reportable to authorities in any state. A release against medical advice is a form that must be signed by a patient who wants to leave a hospital when the patient is advised not to do so by the primary health-care provider. It protects the health-care team members and the agency from legal liability in the event of negative consequences.
2. Notifying an agency, such as the health department, about the presence of a communicable disease is mandated in all states.
3. All states have laws that mandate that suspected child abuse or neglect be reported to appropriate authorities; for example, child protective services.
4. Not all states have mandatory reporting laws that protect adults over 60 years of age when abuse or neglect is suspected.
Content Area: Legal and Ethical Issues
Integrated Processes: Communication/Documentation; Nursing Process: Implementation
Client Need: Safe and Effective Care Environment; Management of Care
Cognitive Level: Knowledge

19. ANSWER: 3.
Rationales:
1. The issue is beyond solving at the primary nurse level. The adult children on both sides of the issue have a determined position.
2. Although this may be suggested to facilitate a different perspective of the issue that may help promote agreement, the spiritual advisor may have a limited focus that will not include the short- and long-term health-care issues.
3. This ensures that the two sides of this issue are explored in a nonconfrontational environment. The ethics committee will act as the patient's advocate and protect the rights of the patient, which is the focus of its activities.
4. The nurse should not give advice.
TEST-TAKING TIP: Identify the word in the stem that sets a priority. The word *best* in the stem sets a priority. Identify the option with a specific determiner. The word *all* in option 1 is a specific determiner. Rarely is an option with a specific determiner the correct answer.
Content Area: Legal and Ethical Issues
Integrated Processes: Communication/Documentation; Nursing Process: Implementation
Client Need: Safe and Effective Care Environment; Management of Care
Cognitive Level: Application

20. ANSWER: 1.
Rationales:
1. The Americans with Disabilities Act protects a person with a disability from discrimination by an employer. An employer is required by law to provide reasonable accommodation within the work setting to facilitate the job performance of a disabled person.
2. Nurse practice acts protect patients and society. They establish the minimum standards of care to be delivered by practicing nurses.

3. Mandatory reporting laws, such as the reporting of neglect or abuse of children, older adults, and people with mental illness or developmental impairments, are designed to protect those who are unable to protect themselves.
4. Incident reports are designed to identify problems and areas for quality improvement.
Content Area: Legal and Ethical Issues
Integrated Processes: Nursing Process: Analysis
Client Need: Safe and Effective Care Environment; Management of Care
Cognitive Level: Comprehension

21. ANSWER: 1.
Rationales:
1. The nurse can be charged with malpractice. Malpractice occurs when the nurse does not adhere to standards of nursing practice and it results in injury to the patient. Nurses are expected to act in a way a reasonably prudent person with the same education and experience would act in a similar circumstance.
2. Administering a medication to the wrong patient is not an example of assault. Assault occurs when a nurse intentionally threatens to harm or touch a patient in an insulting, unjustifiable, or offensive manner. An example is saying, "If you don't behave, you can't have your pain medication."
3. Administering a medication to the wrong patient is not an example of battery. Battery occurs when a nurse intentionally touches a patient's body or clothing or anything held by or attached to a patient in an angry, willful, negligent, or violent manner without consent. Examples include forcefully undressing a patient, resuscitating a patient who has a do-not-attempt-to-resuscitate order, and administering a medication refused by a patient.
4. Administering a medication to the wrong patient is not an example of fraud. Fraud occurs when there is purposeful misrepresentation intended to produce unlawful gain. Fraud is a reckless disregard of the truth. An example is stating, "You should not feel any pain with this procedure," when it is commonly known that the procedure is painful.
Content Area: Legal and Ethical Issues
Integrated Processes: Nursing Process: Analysis
Client Need: Safe and Effective Care Environment; Management of Care
Cognitive Level: Application

22. ANSWER: 3, 4, 5.
Rationales:
1. Failure to complete an incident report after a patient falls is not associated with HIPAA. This is related to failure to follow a policy or procedure of the agency.
2. Sharing clinical events and learning with other student nurses during a clinical post conference does not violate HIPAA as long as all members of the class maintain confidentiality of the patient's protected health information.
3. Any professional health caregiver who discusses protected personal health information within the hearing of unauthorized individuals is in violation of maintaining protected personal health information.

4. A computer screen with protected personal health information that is unattended or within the line of sight of an unauthorized person violates principles in HIPAA.

5. This is a violation of maintaining the confidentiality of protected health information. The information on the form was exposed to a visitor who is not a member of the health team.

TEST-TAKING TIP: Identify the word in the stem that reflects negative polarity. The word *violations* in the stem indicates negative polarity.

Content Area: Legal and Ethical Issues
Integrated Processes: Communication/Documentation; Nursing Process: Evaluation
Client Need: Safe and Effective Care Environment; Management of Care
Cognitive Level: Application

23. **ANSWER: 2.**
    Rationales:
    1. Educational criteria are established by the National League for Nursing Accrediting Commission (NLNAC) and the Commission on Collegiate Nursing Education (CCNE), which accredit schools of nursing.
    2. This is an accurate statement. Each state has a nurse practice act that safeguards the public by legally defining the nature and scope of nursing practice, describing how the nursing profession is governed, and defining criteria for nursing education.
    3. Each state's board of nursing determines the criteria for awarding licensure in their respective states based on satisfactory completion of a recognized school of nursing and achieving the passing rate determined by the state on the NCLEX-RN or NCLEX-PN examination.
    4. Nurse practice acts are legislated and enforced by each individual state, not the federal government.

    TEST-TAKING TIP: Identify the option with a specific determiner. The word *exclusively* in option 1 is a specific determiner. Generally, options with specific determiners are distractors.

    Content Area: Legal and Ethical Issues
    Integrated Processes: Nursing Process: Analysis
    Client Need: Safe and Effective Care Environment; Management of Care
    Cognitive Level: Knowledge

24. **ANSWER: 4.**
    Rationales:
    1. This is premature. The nurse needs to implement another option first.

2. This intervention may result in the patient causing self-harm or harm to others. The nurse should refuse to be involved in this patient's discharge.

3. The patient's spouse clearly has indicated no desire to help the patient at this time.

4. Patients who are visibly impaired are considered to be gravely disabled because they may cause self-harm or harm others; therefore, the person should not be released until sobriety is demonstrated. The nurse should explain this to the primary health-care provider.

TEST-TAKING TIP: Identify the word in the stem that sets a priority. The word *most* in the stem sets a priority.

Content Area: Legal and Ethical Issues
Integrated Processes: Caring; Communication/Documentation; Nursing Process: Implementation
Client Need: Safe and Effective Care Environment; Management of Care
Cognitive Level: Application

25. **ANSWER: 4, 3, 1, 2.**
    Rationales:
    4. This meets the requirement of *duty* associated with litigation. A nurse working as a representative of an agency has an implied contract with patients receiving care provided by a staff member of the agency.
    3. A nurse's actions by omission or commission that fails to meet standards of care meets the legal requirement of *breach of duty* associated with litigation.
    1. This statement indicates that the two elements of *causation* were met. The nurse administered a diuretic that was not prescribed by the primary health-care provider and the diuretic caused dehydration and subsequent hypotension that resulted in a fall.
    2. This statement addresses the damages suffered by the patient as a result of receiving the diuretic that was not prescribed by the primary health-care provider. Requiring surgery and the delay of the patient's chemotherapy treatment resulted in pain, suffering, and additional medical expenses. The patient experienced physical consequences of a longer hospitalization and recovery and the psychological consequences associated with the delay of cancer treatment.

    Content Area: Legal and Ethical Issues
    Integrated Processes: Nursing Process: Analysis
    Client Need: Safe and Effective Care Environment; Management of Care
    Cognitive Level: Analysis

Chapter 3

Leadership and Management

KEY TERMS

Accountability—Assumption of liability for the consequences of one's own actions and the actions of subordinates.

Authority—Power to direct the work of others.

Change—Process of transforming, modifying, or making something different.

Conflict—The disagreement of two or more people on an issue.

Delegation—Transfer of responsibility for the implementation of a task to another while retaining accountability for its outcome.

Leadership—Interpersonal process of motivating others in the accomplishment of a goal.

Management—Process of ensuring that tasks are accomplished to meet organizational goals.

Power—Authority to influence others or implement actions to achieve a goal.

Responsibility—Obligation to perform an assigned role.

I. Leadership

Leadership is an interpersonal process of motivating others in the accomplishment of a goal or to change. It involves *assisting* others to develop a sense of control and purpose, *developing* a commitment to accomplish a desired outcome, and *helping* others meet the challenges that arise in the fast-paced, technologically advanced, constantly changing health-care environment.

A. Behavioral Leadership Styles
 1. Behavioral leadership styles are associated with what a leader does.
 2. A nurse should know various leadership styles because each style lends itself to different settings and different situations. For example, an emergency might require a nurse to decide and act quickly, whereas a complex problem might require reflective thinking about and thorough discussion of the alternatives with others before making a decision.
 3. The most common behavioral leadership styles include the autocratic, democratic, and laissez-faire styles (Table 3.1).

MAKING THE CONNECTION

Autocratic Leadership Style and Clinical Practice

A nurse team leader identifies a small fire in a patient lounge. The nurse removes a patient who is in immediate danger and shuts the door to the dayroom. The nurse then instructs one employee to activate the fire alarm, two employees to close doors to all rooms on the unit as well as the fire cutoff doors, and two other employees to get ABC fire extinguishers. The nurse needed to use the autocratic behavioral leadership style in this situation because it required an immediate, efficient response. Therefore, the nurse team leader made decisions for the safety of patients and employees on the unit, gave direct orders to staff members, and assumed responsibility for the outcomes.

B. Transformational Leadership Theory
 1. Leaders motivate followers by communicating the importance of their vision (goal), inspiring commitment, and exciting others to participate in the

Table 3.1 Comparison of Behavioral Leadership Styles

Leadership Style	Control	Decision Making	Influence of the Leader	Responsibility	Efficiency
Autocratic	Retained by leader	By leader	High	Retained by leader	High
Democratic	Shared	By leader or shared	High	Shared	Moderate
Laissez-faire	Little or no control by anyone	Shared or by no one	Low	Relinquished by leader	Low

achievement of the vision. The vision is noble and for the good of humanity.

2. Transformational leaders often are characterized as being charismatic, energetic, optimistic, and courageous; having integrity; and being risk takers.

DID YOU KNOW?

Magnet certification is recognition given by the American Nurses Credentialing Center (ANCC), an affiliate of the American Nurses Association, to hospitals that meet criteria that indicate quality nursing care and support of professional nursing practice. Transformational leadership is essential to achieving Magnet certification because the criteria address the establishment of a collaborative culture that empowers nurses, promotes job satisfaction, advances nursing standards and practice, and provides quality patient care.

C. Situational Leadership Theories
1. Situational leadership theories propose that each circumstance may require a different leadership style because situations can be multifaceted and the individuals involved have different strengths and weaknesses.
2. The ability to acclimate to a situation is the central premise of situational theories.

D. Quantum Leadership Theory
1. *Quantum* is a "unit of radiant energy."
2. Quantum leadership theory is based on the concept that the fast growth of new information requires people to experience change, even as it is identified; this limits the thoughtful design and cautious implementation that other theories advocate.
3. It is based on the tenets of quantum physics.
   a. Leadership involves an interactive energy field between the leader and followers.
   b. Leadership cannot be estimated or structured.
   c. Leadership is not continuous.
   d. The impact depends on interaction (content and level) between the leader and followers.

II. Management

Management is the process of ensuring that tasks are accomplished to meet organizational goals. Managers are formally and authoritatively appointed to a position that inherently holds power and entitlement to implement and enforce decisions.

A. Management Activities
1. Identifying problems and implementing new initiatives.
   a. Determining the significance of collected data and identifying trends that indicate a problem.
   b. Implementing projects based on results of evidence-based practice research, new technology, and new ideas.
2. Planning: Developing goals and determining strategies that are most likely to achieve organizational goals.
3. Organizing: Obtaining and managing human and economic resources to meet desired clinical and financial goals.
4. Directing: Motivating, guiding, and leading staff members in meeting organizational goals.
5. Controlling: Using outcome criteria to measure effectiveness in goal achievement, ensuring ongoing evaluation, and implementing corrective actions when necessary.

B. Management Theories
1. Scientific management.
   a. Focuses on the task component of the management of subordinates.
   b. Based on the concept that when jobs are evaluated, tasks are planned so that they are more efficient and workers are provided with adequate incentives so that productivity increases.
2. Human relations–oriented management.
   a. Focuses on the interrelationship component of management.
   b. Includes two types of management styles.
      (1) *Theory X:* Managers believe that firm rules, continuous supervision, and fear of negative consequences produce effective, productive workers.
      (2) *Theory Y:* Managers believe that assistance, support, guidance, and rewards produce satisfied, inspired workers; managers work at addressing conflict and supporting mutual respect and understanding to ensure a setting in which individuals can be most effectual and productive (Table 3.2).

Table 3.2 Leadership Versus Management Traits

Leadership Traits	Management Traits
• Strive to influence and guide others (assisting, developing, helping)	• Strive to achieve organizational goals through influencing others (identifying, planning, organizing, directing, controlling)
• May or may not be a manager	• Must possess strong leadership skills to be effective
• Depend on a leadership style to generate power	• Use power for influence
• Communicate effectively verbally and in writing	• Have power and authority associated with their titles
• Collaborate effectively	• Are committed to achievement of organizational goals
• Think critically	• Are committed to excellence in nursing practice and ongoing quality improvement
• Are competent	• Understand power and organizational politics
• Are credible	• Understand economics, finances, and budgets
• Are respectful of others	• Have decision-making skills
• Are inspiring, motivating, and flexible	• Have delegation skills
• Use scientific problem-solving	• Are organized
• Think outside the box	• Are open to suggestions of subordinates
• Are self-aware and can assess their own effectiveness truthfully and openly	• Are fair and equitable in dealing with subordinates
	• Are sensitive to the needs of subordinates
	• Are responsible and accountable
	• Are experts in clinical practice

III. Nursing Management

Nurse managers are formally and authoritatively appointed to the position. Inherent in the position is the power and entitlement to implement and enforce organizational decisions. Actual responsibilities and activities depend on the specific position within the hierarchy of the organization in which a nurse manager works. To function in this role effectively, a nurse manager should have strong leadership traits.

A. Principles of Management Applicable to Nursing
  1. Authority.
     a. Managers have the authority to direct the work of others based on power associated with a title.
     b. Authority is expressed through leadership and management activities and is related to accountability and responsibility.
  2. Accountability.
     a. Managers assume liability for the consequences of their own actions and the actions of their subordinates.
     b. Accountability is reflected in one's personal ethical integrity, support of the philosophy and objectives of the organization, standards of nursing practice, and elements of the state nurse practice act.
  3. Responsibility.
     a. Managers assume the obligation to accomplish a task.
     b. Responsibility is assumed for the management and supervision of subordinates, utilization of financial resources, communication of information to and from subordinates, implementation of organizational policies and procedures, and achievement of organizational goals and objectives.

B. Examples of Activities of Nurse Managers
  1. Recruiting, hiring, and firing staff.
  2. Scheduling staff.
  3. Formulating and managing a budget.
  4. Establishing annual goals.
  5. Monitoring achievement of standards of practice.
  6. Supervising and counseling staff.
  7. Participating in and engaging staff in ongoing quality improvement activities.
  8. Providing for staff education.
  9. Providing a communication link among patients, upper management, and subordinates.
  10. Alerting administration to changing patient and subordinate needs.
  11. Problem-solving issues proactively or reactively.
  12. Conducting regular staff meetings.
  13. Making rounds with primary health-care providers and nursing team members.
  14. Encouraging staff to participate in interdisciplinary facility-wide committees.
  15. Encouraging staff to participate in nursing research.

C. Levels of Management in Nursing
  1. First-level managers.
     a. Are commonly responsible for managing daily activities associated with a specific group of people on a unit level, including delegating, supervising, and motivating staff to achieve organizational goals.
     b. Communicate staff and unit issues to unit-level managers, and communicate information from higher level managers back to staff on the unit.
     c. May have such titles as:
        (1) Primary nurse.
        (2) Team leader.
        (3) Charge nurse.
        (4) Case manager.
  2. Unit-level managers.
     a. Are commonly responsible for 24-hour operation of a nursing unit, including staffing schedules, budget management, supervision of staff, and ongoing quality improvement.
     b. Communicate information to middle-level managers and to first-level managers.
     c. May have such titles as:
        (1) Nurse manager.
        (2) Assistant nurse manager.

3. Middle-level managers.
   a. Are commonly responsible for supervising a number of unit-level managers and the overall functioning of areas, units, or departments for which they are responsible.
   b. Spend less time on day-to-day management issues and more time on departmental planning and interdisciplinary problem-solving.
   c. Function as liaisons between upper-level and unit-level managers.
   d. May have such titles as:
      (1) Nurse coordinator.
      (2) Supervisor.
      (3) Assistant director of nursing.
      (4) Associate director of nursing.
4. Upper-level (top-level) managers.
   a. Are commonly nurse executives who are responsible for determining organizational goals and developing strategic plans to achieve these goals.
   b. Are responsible for the overall management and practice of nursing within the organization.
   c. May have such titles as:
      (1) Director of nursing.
      (2) Vice-president for nursing.
      (3) Chief nurse.
      (4) Associate administrator.
      (5) Assistant administrator.
      (6) Vice-president for clinical care services (if also responsible for such areas as pharmacy and dietary).

IV. Power and Empowerment

Power relates to actions. It involves having the authority and ability to influence others to achieve a goal even in the presence of resistance. Empowerment relates to feelings. It involves personal feelings of competence and self-determination. Nurse managers must understand these concepts and integrate them into their practice.

A. Sources of Power
1. Power of authority: A person in a position of authority can mandate compliance as a result of the power of the position.
2. Power of reward: A manager can use incentives, such as pay increases or promotions, to influence others.
3. Power of coercion: A manager can use the threat of an undesirable performance evaluation or job termination to influence others; patients can return a less-than-satisfactory patient satisfaction survey or complain about a staff member to a charge nurse.
4. Power of expertise: A nurse can gain power by obtaining an advanced degree in nursing, such as nurse practitioner, or extensive experience in a

---

> ### MAKING THE CONNECTION
>
> #### Power Versus Empowerment
> Empowerment should not be confused with power. A person who has power might not *feel* empowered; to feel empowered, a person needs to feel confidence in his or her ability to do a good job, feel that individuals will listen, feel that the work is meaningful, and feel free to decide how work will get done. On the other hand, a person can feel empowered without having power. For example, nurses may feel empowered when they are treated with respect, receive recognition for a job well done, are given a reasonable work assignment, are included in organizational decisions, and have their contributions heard and valued.

specialty area, such as in pediatric, oncology, or emergency nursing.

B. Empowerment
1. Empowerment is a *feeling* of competence, a *feeling* of capability to influence another person, or a *feeling* of privilege or entitlement.
2. Nurse managers must support and nourish positive feelings of growth, accomplishment, and independence in subordinates that facilitate feelings of empowerment.

V. Delegation

The American Nurses Association (2009) defines *delegation* as the process of "transferring responsibility for the performance of an activity or task while retaining accountability for the outcome." Many changes in health-care delivery (e.g., reengineering of hospital organizations and downsizing the professional nursing workforce as a measure of cost containment) have resulted in the need for nurses to delegate tasks to unlicensed personnel, requiring nurses to spend more time in supervisory roles. The profession of nursing is working to ensure that unlicensed personnel are used only in supportive roles and not as substitutes for licensed nurses.

A. Five Rights of Delegation (must be met when a nurse delegates aspects of nursing care)
1. Right task: The task is appropriate for delegation.
2. Right circumstances: The nurse considers the appropriateness of the patient setting, available resources, and other relevant factors.
3. Right person: The task is delegated to a person who is competent to perform the task within his or her legal scope of practice.
4. Right direction/communication: The nurse provides a clear, concise description of the task, including what should be accomplished and how it should be accomplished.

5. Right supervision: The delegator is responsible for monitoring and evaluating the performance of the task and providing feedback to the person performing the task.

B. Policy Considerations Associated With Delegation
1. A registered nurse (RN) is responsible for delegating and supervising care provided by unlicensed individuals in health-care environments.
2. Each state has its own definitions, regulations, and directives regarding delegation.
3. The following general policy matters are common to all states regarding delegation.
   a. State nurse practice acts delineate the legal boundaries of nursing practice.
   b. There is a need for capable and properly supervised nursing assistive personnel in the delivery of cost effective, quality health care.
   c. An RN should assign or delegate tasks based on patients' needs and statuses, the risk of harm, constancy of a patient's condition, intricacy of the task, likelihood of the outcomes, capabilities of the staff member to whom the task is delegated, and the circumstances of other patient needs.
   d. All delegation decisions should be based on maintaining the safety and welfare of the public.
4. A nurse must understand the nurse practice act and the regulations and directives regarding delegation in the state in which the nurse works as well its application to the setting in which the nurse works.
5. Nurses are responsible for providing safe and effective nursing care over a range of care provided in various settings (e.g., hospital, nursing home, school, public health clinic, home-health agency).
6. In each setting, nurses are generally the coordinators of the health teams, which comprise a variety of licensed and unlicensed caregivers.

C. Nursing-Related Principles of Delegation
1. A nurse may delegate elements of care but retains responsibility to answer for personal actions associated with the nursing process.
2. Pervasive functions of assessment, planning, evaluation, and nursing judgment cannot be delegated.
3. A nurse must take into account the education and skills of the person to whom the nurse delegates components of care.
4. The decision to delegate should be based on the nurse's judgment regarding the condition of the patient, the abilities of nursing team members, and the amount of supervision that is necessary for the task delegated.
5. A nurse should delegate only those tasks permitted by the state nurse practice act and facility policies and procedures (Table 3.3).

Table 3.3 Care That May Be Performed by Unlicensed Assistive Personnel

Health-Related Functions (Illustrative and Not All Inclusive)	Non-Nursing Functions (Illustrative and Not All Inclusive)
• Making occupied and unoccupied beds • Obtaining routine vital signs, including temperature, pulse, respirations, and blood pressure • Bathing patients • Providing routine skin care • Promoting mobility, including ambulation and range of motion • Assisting with meeting routine urine and fecal elimination needs • Obtaining and reporting information at the direction of the registered nurse	**Housekeeping** • Cleaning unit surfaces, such as overbed and bedside tables • Disposing of trash • Changing linens on beds and stretchers • Stocking supplies **Clerical** • Recording routine data, such as temperature, pulse, respirations, blood pressure, and lab results • Checking clothing and valuables • Collating forms for new charts • Answering telephones **Transportation** • Transporting non-acute patients to tests off the unit, bodies to the morgue, and discharged patients to exits • Delivering medications, supplies, linens, specimens, and blood products **Dietary** • Delivering routine and isolation meal trays and nourishments • Recording food and oral fluid intake **Miscellaneous** • Assisting with visitors • Ordering stock medications and supplies

Adapted from New York State Nurses Association. (2004). *Position Statement: Registered Professional Nursing's Utilization of Unlicensed Assistive Personnel*. Retrieved October 25, 2012, from www.nysna.org/practice/positions/position1_04.htm, with permission.

6. A nurse must follow the Five Rights of Delegation and use professional judgment when delegating a task to another nursing team member.
7. A nurse must communicate effectively and ensure that communication is a two-way process between the delegator and the subordinate.
8. Nursing administrators are responsible for ensuring that assessment of policies and procedures and the evaluation of competence requirements associated with delegation are regularly conducted.

VI. Managing Change and Conflict

Change is the process of transforming, modifying, or making something different; it can also be defined as learning, growth, or progress. With the explosion of advances in technology and vast increases in knowledge, nurses must be able to incorporate new information into nursing practice to meet patients' needs. However, points of view and opinions about how something should be accomplished can cause conflict. Nurses must be willing to negotiate and compromise with other members of the health team to effect change.

A. Change Theory (Lewin)
1. Proposes a process to plan and implement change in organizations.
2. Purports that effective change entails three steps.
   a. *Unfreezing:* The need for change is identified, various supportive and resistive solutions are explored, and group members are motivated to change.
   b. *Moving:* Group members agree that the current status is unacceptable. Change is implemented after careful planning and with input from group members.
   c. *Refreezing:* Change is integrated, stabilized, and incorporated into practice.

B. Planned Change
1. A purposeful, intended, systematic effort by a person, group, or organization to alter its present state.
2. A nurse must identify factors relative to the change.
   a. What is the complexity of the change?
   b. What is the magnitude of the change (how many people/departments are involved)?
   c. Is there readiness for the change?
   d. What is the pace of the change (is it urgent or can it be implemented slowly)?
   e. What is the current stress level of participants?
   f. Are there forces of resistance within the organization?
3. A nurse should follow a process, such as the nursing process.
   a. Recognize the need for change.
   b. Identify the problem.
   c. Analyze possible solutions.

d. Choose a solution.
e. Plan for making the change (e.g., objectives, implementation steps, timetables, selection of individuals to implement the change, preparation to address resistance, and ways to stabilize the change).
f. Put the plan into effect.
g. Evaluate the outcomes of the change.
h. Stabilize the change (may be permanent).

C. Resistance to Change
1. Effective change requires the cooperation of all participants.
2. Individuals might resist change for four major reasons.
   a. Technical concerns, such as child-care needs.
   b. Psychosocial concerns, such as fear, anxiety, low tolerance to change, and impact on income.
   c. Threats to power, such as position or influence.
   d. Lack of knowledge or misunderstanding.
3. Nurse managers should identify and address issues that can contribute to resistance as early as possible.
4. Nurse managers need to identify and address resistive behaviors because they can undermine the effort to change.
   a. Obvious resistive behaviors include refusing to be involved in the process, writing negative memos, and organizing resistance.
   b. Passive-aggressive resistive behaviors include missing meetings and agreeing with the change but avoiding activities to implement the change.
5. Nurse managers should implement strategies for lowering resistance to change.
   a. Be prepared for resistance before change is introduced.
   b. Increase communication and information to overcome lack of knowledge and to correct misconceptions, which are often significant threats to change.
   c. Involve a resistive participant in developing and implementing the change, incorporating as many suggestions as feasible to ensure a vested interest in the success of the project.
   d. Reduce the anxiety and fears of participants by recognizing their competence, providing staff education programs that support new learning and personal growth, allowing time for learning and practice, providing a nonjudgmental climate where participants can verbalize feelings, and expressing appreciation for each participant's contributions.
   e. Assure participants, when possible, that no one will lose a job or position because of the change.

f. Make the organization's commitment to the project clear.

g. Identify the positive consequences of the change, including ways in which the change will benefit participants.

D. Conflict

1. Differing points of view and opinions about how something should be accomplished commonly result in conflict in the workplace.

2. Strategies for managing conflict.

   a. Recognize that health-care workers have differences (e.g., different ages, nationalities, cultures, income levels, genders, educational backgrounds, and lifestyles).

   b. Recognize that each person has personal values, beliefs, habits, and experiences.

   c. Understand that the clinical setting can be stressful, which can generate problems.

   d. Identify occurrences of conflict, which can occur between two individuals (e.g., two nurses, nurse and family member), workers of different shifts (workers on the day shift versus the night shift), or different departments (nursing and physical therapy, nursing and dietary).

   e. Address conflict in a constructive manner that leads to professional growth rather than rejection and anger.

   f. Handle conflict in a way that enables each party to gain insight into the other person's point of view; it can stimulate individuals to work together in more constructive ways, leading to increased productivity and improved relationships.

   🛑 g. Use a win-win approach to conflict resolution. For example, when possible, integrate a combination of suggestions from those offered from both sides of a conflict so that both sides gain some benefit.

   h. Engage in informal or formal negotiation if conflict cannot be managed through problem-solving.

CASE STUDY: Putting It All Together

A director of nursing at a local community hospital believes that nurses not only should be involved in the traditional roles of nursing (e.g., caregiver, teacher, advocate) but also should expand their roles into other areas associated with professional nursing. Based on this belief, the director of nursing invites all the nurse managers to a meeting to discuss future nursing initiatives. After a length of time with input from many of the nurse managers, the director of nursing makes the following statement: "We have discussed numerous interesting projects. However, I would like for us to begin with just one initiative. Since I firmly believe that nurses should be performing evidence-based practice, I really liked the suggestion that we conduct a small research project on each unit. What do you think?" Another discussion among the members of the meeting occurs, and the majority of nurse managers are in favor of instituting this initiative. The director of nursing then says, "I am sure that this is going to be an exciting new venture. Each unit can make its own determination on how to accomplish this goal. We have money in the budget, and we can hire a nurse researcher to assist you with your projects." After the meeting, one nurse manager of a medical unit says to another nurse manager, "I can't believe we are now going to have to do research projects. Don't you think we do enough already? Let's talk with the other nurse managers and see if we can reverse this decision." This nurse manager holds a unit meeting and tells the staff nurses, "We are going to be conducting a research project on our unit. I am not thrilled about having to do this, but we have no choice. Because we had three patients fall last month, I think we should attempt to reduce falls. I decided we should conduct a fall assessment for every patient, and for all patients at risk for falls, we should put a star over the bed and make them wear red socks. That way, the nursing staff will know who is at risk and hopefully ensure the safety of those patients. I expect you all to participate in this project, and if you don't, I will have to include that information in your next evaluation."

A month later, when the director of nursing calls another nurse manager meeting, three of the eight nurse managers did not attend, two said they were too busy, and the third took the day off to avoid the meeting.

Case Study Questions

A. What leadership style seems to be preferred by (1) the director of nursing and (2) the nurse manager of the medical unit, and why?

1. _____

2. _____

Continued

CASE STUDY: Putting It All Together   *cont'd*

_____ **Case Study Questions** _____

B. What management style seems to be preferred by (1) the director of nursing and (2) the nurse manager of the medical unit, and why?

   1. _____

   2. _____

C. What behaviors in the scenario reflect resistance, and why?

   1. _____

   2. _____

   3. _____

D. What types of power are exhibited in the scenario, and why?

   1. _____

   2. _____

   3. _____

REVIEW QUESTIONS

1. Which action is **most** appropriate for the nurse to delegate to an unlicensed assistive personnel (UAP)?
   1. Assisting a patient with a prosthetic leg to ambulate to the bathroom
   2. Teaching a patient with diabetes about the importance of eating an entire meal
   3. Helping a patient to drink contrast media that was poured into a cup by a nurse
   4. Asking a patient who recently had surgery about the intensity of pain being experienced

2. A nurse case manager is assessing an alert patient who is a candidate for a nursing home. Which is the **best** source of information about this patient?
   1. Primary health-care provider
   2. Family member
   3. Charge nurse
   4. Patient

3. A nurse is in charge of a team consisting of a registered nurse (RN), a licensed practical nurse (LPN), and a nursing assistant (NA). Which tasks should the nurse delegate to the LPN for the **most** effective use of the expertise of staff members? **Select all that apply.**
   1. _____ Take vital signs on a postoperative patient one day after surgery.
   2. _____ Perform a bed bath for a patient on contact precautions.
   3. _____ Obtain a blood glucose level on a patient with diabetes.
   4. _____ Provide patient education regarding a dressing change.
   5. _____ Discontinue tubing that was used to administer blood.

4. A nurse on the day shift is annoyed with the nurse on the night shift and reports concerns to the nurse manager. The day nurse states that the night nurse often does not complete patient assignments or provide for needed supplies, such as medication draws that are missing the next dose of medication, supplies that are not stocked for isolation rooms, and specimens that are not collected. What is the nurse manager's **best** response?
   1. "What do you think I should do to correct these problems?"
   2. "Which of these jobs can you assign to the nursing assistant on your team?"
   3. "Working nights is difficult, so do you think you can help the night shift staff when you can?"
   4. "When are you available so that I can arrange a meeting for the three of us to discuss these concerns?"

5. A nurse and a nursing assistant (unlicensed assistive personnel) are working together caring for a group of patients who recently had surgery. What action by the nursing assistant requires immediate intervention by the nurse?
   1. Reinforcing a dressing that is soiled with serosanguineous drainage
   2. Providing total assistance with a bed bath for a patient who is disoriented
   3. Giving a patient a cup of tea whose diet order was changed from NPO to clear liquid
   4. Assisting a patient to the bathroom on the second day after the patient had minor abdominal surgery

6. A charge nurse is delegating assignments to staff members working on a surgical unit. Which patient should be assigned to a recently registered nurse rather than an experienced registered nurse?
   1. A woman with an elevated temperature after surgery for an ectopic pregnancy
   2. A middle-aged patient who had elective surgery for repair of an abdominal hernia
   3. A young adult who had a fractured femur as well as multiple soft tissue injuries from an automobile collision
   4. An older adult male who had a transurethral resection of the prostate who has cherry red drainage from the continuous bladder irrigation

7. A nurse manager of an emergency department of a trauma center receives notification of a domestic terrorist attack in the community and that multiple casualties are en route to the hospital. What leadership style is **most** appropriate when the nurse manager responds to this event?
   1. Autocratic
   2. Democratic
   3. Laissez-faire
   4. Transformational

8. A nurse manager identifies that the nurse in charge on evenings needs additional in-service education about the legal roles of nursing staff members when the charge nurse assigns the:
   1. nursing assistant to monitor vital signs and determine those that are significant.
   2. registered nurse to teach a patient with a colostomy how to care for the stoma.
   3. licensed practical nurse to change several sterile dressings.
   4. nursing assistant to give a bath to a patient with dementia.

9. A nurse is seeking a position in nursing management. The nurse reads a classified ad that indicates that the hospital is seeking a person who will spend less time on day-to-day management issues and more time on departmental planning and interdisciplinary problem-solving. Which level manager is this agency seeking?
   1. Unit-level manager
   2. First-level manager
   3. Upper-level manager
   4. Middle-level manager

10. Which activity is appropriate for an unlicensed nursing assistant to implement?
    1. Collecting urine for a 24-hour creatinine clearance test
    2. Giving an obese patient a brochure on a 1,800-calorie diet
    3. Placing a tube feeding pump on hold while bathing a patient
    4. Helping with the insertion of a nasogastric tube by a primary health-care provider

11. Which is an example of an independent nursing intervention?
    1. Administering an enema
    2. Changing a soiled dressing
    3. Delegating the giving of a bath to a nursing assistant
    4. Assisting a patient with a transfer from a bed to a chair

12. A nurse manager of a patient care unit is determining if the nursing team members of the unit are meeting organizational goals. What should the nurse manager do **first**?
    1. Identify trends that indicate a problem.
    2. Plan approaches to meet patient needs.
    3. Develop strategies to achieve objectives.
    4. Share the purpose of the unit with colleagues.

13. A nurse manager believes in theory X human relations–oriented management. What behavior can a newly hired nurse expect the nurse manager to exhibit? **Select all that apply.**
    1. _____ Describing the continuous evaluation of nursing performance
    2. _____ Explaining the agency's policies regarding the use of sick days
    3. _____ Informing the nurse of the consequences for being late to work
    4. _____ Ensuring the nurse that an orientation program will provide guidance
    5. _____ Directing the nurse to seek assistance from another nurse when necessary

14. A nurse in charge of a patient care unit is considering staff member assignments. What criterion is **most** significant for the nurse to consider when delegating a task to another member of the nursing team?
    1. Who will ultimately be responsible for the patient's care?
    2. Is the activity within the person's job description?
    3. How much experience does the person have?
    4. What is the acuity level of the patient?

15. Which of the following is **most** related to the statement, "Managers have authority in the workplace"?
    1. Managers have the power to direct the work of others.
    2. Managers are expected to maintain personal ethical integrity.
    3. Managers assume the obligation to accomplish tasks associated with the job description.
    4. Managers assume liability for the consequences of ones' actions as well as those of subordinates.

16. Which statement by a nurse coordinator at a staff meeting exemplifies the major focus of leadership?
    1. "Every staff member will be scheduled to attend an in-service program on this new procedure."
    2. "A committee is being formed to develop a policy and procedure for the nursing manual regarding this new procedure."
    3. "I know from your past performance with other procedures that you have the expertise to implement this new procedure."
    4. "I expect that each unit will meet the criteria established by the state department of health regarding this new procedure."

17. A nurse manager of an emergency department identifies that a more efficient triage process is necessary. What should the nurse manager do to limit resistance to this change? **Select all that apply.**
    1. _____ Offer to transfer staff members to another unit if they do not support the new policies.
    2. _____ Allow adequate time for understanding the change before implementing the change.
    3. _____ Provide a nonjudgmental climate for people to voice their concerns.
    4. _____ Explain that the organization is committed to this change.
    5. _____ Assure participants that they will not lose their jobs.

18. A nurse manager is planning to implement a change in how administered medications are documented. What is **most** important for the nurse manager to do to avoid resistance to change?
    1. Incorporate incentives to promote a commitment.
    2. Establish multiple short-term goals to promote motivation.
    3. Convey to the staff that administration is committed to the new policy and procedure.
    4. Ensure that the new policy and procedure is consistent with the beliefs and ethics of staff members.

19. A staff nurse is counseled by the nurse manager regarding excessive time taken for lunch and breaks. The nurse manager indicates that if this behavior continues then the nurse will receive an undesirable performance evaluation. What type of power did the nurse manager exhibit?
    1. Reward
    2. Coercion
    3. Expertise
    4. Competence

20. An upper-level manager is assessing the qualities of several nurses who demonstrate leadership abilities for a promotion to a first-level management position. Which ability is required of a nurse manager that is not a necessity for a leader?
    1. Thinks critically
    2. Understands budgets
    3. Collaborates effectively
    4. Demonstrates competence

21. A nurse manager endorses the theory Y human relations–oriented management style. What intervention by the nurse manager reflects this style of leadership?
    1. Reviewing periodically the consequences for not adhering to steps listed in an activity in the procedure manual
    2. Explaining that an interim performance evaluation may be necessary if standards of care are not maintained
    3. Offering help when a nurse is overwhelmed with work at the end of a shift
    4. Ensuring that staff members adhere to policies established by the agency

22. Which situation involving a nurse is reportable to the state board of nursing?
    1. Omission of documentation of a medication that was administered intravenously
    2. Discussion of confidential information at a grand rounds meeting without the patient's consent
    3. Failure to monitor the blood glucose level of a patient with diabetes who became comatose and died
    4. Not placing a mouth guard in the mouth of a patient experiencing a tonic-clonic seizure who bites off the tip of the tongue

23. A charge nurse in a nursing home identifies that the weights of residents assigned to a particular nursing assistant are exactly the same as the week before. The nurse is concerned that the nursing assistant is not weighing residents and is falsifying the weights. What should the nurse do **first?**
    1. Confront the nursing assistant responsible for taking the weights.
    2. Report the problem regarding the nursing assistant to the nursing supervisor.
    3. Reweigh the residents assigned to the nursing assistant who had duplicate weights for both weeks.
    4. Assign the nursing assistant to take the weight of another resident and observe if the weight is actually taken.

24. A nurse manager identifies that the number of patients with hospital-acquired *Clostridium difficile* has increased on the unit during the past 3 months. The nurse manager recognizes that this issue must be addressed and involves the entire nursing team on the unit. Place the following interventions in the order in which they should be performed.
    1. Stabilize the change.
    2. Identify the expected outcomes of change.
    3. Evaluate the actual outcomes of the change.
    4. Explore and choose a solution to the problem.
    5. Identify why the *C. difficile* rate has increased.
    6. Put the plan into effect and deal with resistance.
    Answer: _____

25. A nurse coordinator is orienting a new manager to the responsibilities associated with scheduling staffing and managing a budget. Which type of power is **most** associated with a nurse coordinator functioning as a mentor?
    1. Reward
    2. Coercive
    3. Expertise
    4. Authority

26. When considering leadership styles, "democratic" leadership is to consultative as "autocratic" leadership is to:
    1. sharing.
    2. dictatorial.
    3. participative.
    4. collaborative.

27. A nurse manager implements a corrective action plan when a unit goal is not achieved. Which management function is being implemented by the nurse manager?
    1. Planning
    2. Directing
    3. Organizing
    4. Controlling

28. A nurse manager, in conjunction with the nursing team members on the unit, is instituting a new policy regarding criteria for assigning patients to specific rooms on the unit. After 3 weeks, the nurse in charge and a primary nurse engage in an intense discussion about how patients have been assigned. The nurse manager speaks with the two nurses and reviews the assignment of patients during the past week. Each nurse's perspective on the room assignments is as follows:

Charge Nurse's Perspective:
I have been following the criteria we identified at the beginning of this initiative. I reviewed every patient's physical and emotional status and compared it to the criteria we identified. I then considered if a private room was warranted and who the primary nurse was for the district in which the room was located. I think I have been consistent and fair to the nurses in my patient room assignments.

Primary Nurse's Perspective:
I do not think that the patient room assignments have been appropriate. It seems that I have been getting all of the patients who require the most work. At times, I feel that the charge nurse is favoring one of the other nurses and putting the less stressful patients in that district. Every day this week I have had a patient with a crisis on top of having to provide or supervise care for the rest of the patients in my district. It is not fair.

Nurse Manager's Perspective:
A review of the patients' assigned rooms indicated that the nurse in charge did follow the criteria identified at the beginning of the initiative. A review of the primary nurse's district and the assigned patients revealed that the nurse had an equal number of patients when compared to the other primary nurses. However, several of the patients did have more complex health problems. The primary nurse's district had three private rooms compared to the other districts, which have only one each.

What is the **best** intervention by the nurse manager?
1. Meet with the nurse in charge and agree that the criteria have been followed.
2. Remove one of the private rooms from the primary nurse's district and add it to another district.
3. Meet with the primary nurse and explain that they will continue with the initiative for another 6 weeks.
4. Arrange for a meeting of the nursing team and reconsider the criteria that were established for room assignments.

29. A nurse manager identifies that several medication errors occurred on the unit during the past month. What should the nurse manager do **next**?
1. Implement a plan of action.
2. Analyze factors involving the errors.
3. Choose a solution to address the issues.
4. Explore all possible strategies to prevent future errors.

30. A new float rotation schedule is to be implemented in the hospital. A staff nurse, in an exasperated tone, says to the nurse manager, "This new schedule is ridiculous." What is the nurse manager's **best** response?
1. "Do you really think that the schedule is unreasonable?"
2. "Share with me your concerns about this proposed new schedule."
3. "You need to work with the new schedule a little before being judgmental."
4. "I know that you are upset with the new schedule, but can you try to be more positive?"

REVIEW ANSWERS

1. ANSWER: 1.
Rationales:
1. Assisting patients with activities of daily living (e.g., bathing, dressing, ambulating) is within the legal role of UAP.
2. Patient teaching is within the legal scope of nursing practice because it requires in-depth knowledge about the content being presented and the principles of teaching/learning.
3. Contrast material is considered a diagnostic medication. Nursing care associated with medications is within the legal role of a licensed nurse, not UAP.
4. Patient assessment is within the legal scope of nursing practice because it requires in-depth knowledge and an assessment skill set.
TEST-TAKING TIP: Identify the word in the stem that sets a priority. The word *most* in the stem sets a priority.
Content Area: Leadership and Management
Integrated Processes: Communication/Documentation; Nursing Process: Planning
Client Need: Safe and Effective Care Environment; Management of Care
Cognitive Level: Application

2. ANSWER: 4.
Rationales:
1. The primary health-care provider is a secondary source.
2. The patient's family member is a secondary source.
3. The charge nurse is a secondary source.
4. The patient is the center of the health team and is the primary source for current objective and subjective data.
TEST-TAKING TIP: Identify the word in the stem that sets a priority. The word *best* in the stem sets a priority. Identify the option that is unique. Option 4 is unique because the other options identify people other than the patient.
Content Area: Physical Assessment
Integrated Processes: Communication/Documentation; Nursing Process: Assessment
Client Need: Safe and Effective Care Environment; Management of Care
Cognitive Level: Comprehension

3. ANSWER: 1, 3.
Rationales:
1. Delegating obtaining vital signs of this patient to an LPN, rather than an NA, is appropriate because the LPN has the knowledge to identify postoperative complications as they relate to the vital signs.
2. Delegating a bed bath for a patient on contact precautions to an LPN is inappropriate in this situation because an NA is capable of caring for patients on contact precautions.
3. Delegating blood glucose monitoring to an LPN, rather than an RN, is appropriate; the LPN has the knowledge and skill to perform this skill safely.
4. All patient education must be performed by an RN.
5. All interventions concerning the administration of blood should be performed only by an RN.
TEST-TAKING TIP: Identify the word in the stem that sets a priority. The word *most* in the stem sets a priority. Identify

the central person in the question. Although the question includes an RN, an LPN, and an NA, the LPN is the central person in the question.
Content Area: Leadership and Management
Integrated Processes: Communication/Documentation; Nursing Process: Planning
Client Need: Safe and Effective Care Environment; Management of Care
Cognitive Level: Analysis

4. ANSWER: 4.
Rationales:
1. The nurse manager is responsible for taking the initiative. The nurse manager should collect information, identify the problem, and implement an appropriate response. The night nurse's response to this statement may be an action that is inappropriate or impossible to implement.
2. This response suggests an intervention before collecting enough information to make an informed decision.
3. This response denies the night nurse's feelings and concerns.
4. Conflict resolution is best approached by having the individuals involved discuss the concerns. This approach allows each person to explain a personal point of view as well as gain insight into the other person's point of view. Suggestions from both perspectives will help achieve a win-win resolution.
TEST-TAKING TIP: Identify the word in the stem that sets a priority. The word *best* in the stem sets a priority. Identify the option that denies the day nurse's feelings and concerns. Option 3 denies the nurse's feelings and concerns. Identify the clang association. The word *night* in the stem and in option 3 is a clang association. Although options with clang associations often are the correct answer, the fact that this option denies the day nurse's feelings and concerns eliminates it from further consideration.
Content Area: Leadership and Management
Integrated Processes: Communication/Documentation; Nursing Process: Implementation
Client Need: Safe and Effective Care Environment; Management of Care
Cognitive Level: Analysis

5. ANSWER: 1.
Rationales:
1. This action requires the educational background and judgment of a licensed nurse. Additionally, the nurse must assess the patient further to ensure that the patient is not hemorrhaging.
2. Providing a bed bath is an activity that is within the scope of practice of a nursing assistant.
3. Assisting patients with prescribed diets is an activity that is within the scope of practice of a nursing assistant.
4. This is within the scope of practice of a nursing assistant. Generally, on the second day after minor abdominal surgery, a patient may need minimal assistance to ambulate safely. The nurse should assist a postoperative patient to ambulate for the first time after surgery and then evaluate the patient's response.

TEST-TAKING TIP: Identify the word in the stem that sets a priority. The word *immediate* in the stem sets a priority. Identify the central person in the question. Because the behavior of the nursing assistant is being evaluated, the nursing assistant is the central person in this question.
Content Area: Leadership and Management
Integrated Processes: Nursing Process: Evaluation
Client Need: Safe and Effective Care Environment; Management of Care
Cognitive Level: Analysis

6. **ANSWER: 2.**
Rationales:
1. An elevated temperature after an ectopic pregnancy may indicate peritonitis, which can be life-threatening. This patient should be cared for by a nurse more experienced than a new graduate.
2. **This patient is less likely to experience a life-threatening complication than the possible complications associated with the other patient situations. The other patients require more critical assessments that a more experienced nurse with a broader knowledge base and experiential background can draw upon when diagnosing, planning, and implementing nursing care.**
3. A patient who sustained multiple traumatic injuries may experience any number of serious life-threatening complications, which include hemorrhage, fat emboli, or neurovascular deficits, as a result of the fractured femur. This patient should be cared for by a nurse more experienced than a new graduate.
4. A patient who may be hemorrhaging should be cared for by a nurse more experienced than a new graduate. Also, the patient's continuous bladder irrigation flow rate should be managed so that clotting and tube obstruction are avoided.
TEST-TAKING TIP: Identify the central person in the question. The central person in this question is the newly licensed nurse.
Content Area: Leadership and Management
Integrated Processes: Communication/Documentation; Nursing Process: Planning
Client Need: Safe and Effective Care Environment; Management of Care
Cognitive Level: Analysis

7. **ANSWER: 1.**
Rationales:
1. **The autocratic leadership style is most appropriate in an emergency. Control and responsibility are retained by the leader and decisions are made by the leader. This style is highly efficient and appropriate in an emergency situation, where quick decisions are required.**
2. The democratic leadership style is not the most appropriate style in an emergency. The leader and subordinates share control and responsibility, and the democratic leadership style is only moderately efficient in emergency situations.
3. The laissez-faire is the least appropriate leadership style in an emergency situation because there is little or no control by anyone.
4. Transformational is a leadership theory, not a leadership style. Transformational leaders motivate followers by communicating the importance of their vision, inspiring commitment, and exciting others to participate in achievement of the goal.
TEST-TAKING TIP: Identify the word in the stem that sets a priority. The word *most* in the stem sets a priority.
Content Area: Leadership and Management
Integrated Processes: Nursing Process: Implementation
Client Need: Safe and Effective Care Environment; Management of Care
Cognitive Level: Application

8. **ANSWER: 1.**
Rationales:
1. **Determining the results of vital signs monitoring is not within the legal role of a nursing assistant. Although a nursing assistant may collect vital signs, determining the significance of vital signs is dependent on the educational preparation of a registered nurse.**
2. All teaching interventions require the expertise of a registered nurse.
3. A licensed practical nurse is educationally prepared to change sterile dressings.
4. A nursing assistant is educationally prepared to bathe a patient with dementia.
TEST-TAKING TIP: Identify the words in the stem that indicate negative polarity. The words *needs additional* indicate negative polarity. The question is asking, "Which action should not be implemented by the person delegated the task?"
Content Area: Leadership and Management
Integrated Processes: Nursing Process: Evaluation
Client Need: Safe and Effective Care Environment; Management of Care
Cognitive Level: Analysis

9. **ANSWER: 4.**
Rationales:
1. Unit-level managers are often responsible for 24-hour operation of a nursing unit, including scheduling staffing, budget management, supervision of staff, and ongoing quality improvement. Titles may be assistant nurse manager or nurse manager.
2. First-level managers are responsible for managing the work of daily activities of a specific group of people on a unit level. Titles may include primary nurse, team leader, or charge nurse.
3. Upper-level (top-level) managers often are nurse executives who are responsible for determining organizational goals and developing strategic plans to achieve the goals. They are responsible for the management and practice of nursing within the organization. Titles may include vice-president for nursing, associate administrator, or assistant administrator.
4. **Middle-level managers are responsible for supervising a number of unit-level managers and for the overall functioning of their assigned areas, units, or departments. They spend less time on day-to-day management issues and more time on departmental planning and interdisciplinary problem-solving. Titles may include nurse coordinator, supervisor, or assistant or associate director of nursing.**

Content Area: Leadership and Management
Integrated Processes: Nursing Process: Analysis
Client Need: Safe and Effective Care Environment; Management of Care
Cognitive Level: Comprehension

10. **ANSWER: 1.**
    Rationales:
    1. **This is an activity that an unlicensed nursing assistant is capable of performing safely. Collecting urine for a 24-hour creatinine clearance test does not require sterile technique. The collection container is set up by the nurse, and all staff members are instructed to add all of the urine voided by the patient during the 24-hour period to the collection container.**
    2. All activities related to patient teaching are the responsibility of a registered nurse. The registered nurse has the educational background regarding teaching principles and knowledge about the topic being taught and is therefore the qualified person to engage patients in teaching activities, not an unlicensed nursing assistant.
    3. Only a registered nurse or licensed practical nurse is permitted to place a feeding tube on hold.
    4. Only a registered nurse or licensed practical nurse is permitted to assist a primary health-care provider with an invasive procedure. An unlicensed nursing assistant does not have the educational foundation to assist other health-care providers with an invasive procedure.
    Content Area: Leadership and Management
    Integrated Processes: Nursing Process: Implementation
    Client Need: Safe and Effective Care Environment; Management of Care
    Cognitive Level: Application

11. **ANSWER: 3.**
    Rationales:
    1. An enema requires an order from a primary health-care provider and is a dependent function of a nurse.
    2. Changing a soiled dressing requires an order from a primary health-care provider and is a dependent function of a nurse.
    3. **Delegating responsibilities to nursing team members does not require an order from the primary health-care provider. Delegation activities are within the scope of practice of a registered nurse.**
    4. An order from a primary health-care provider is necessary before a nurse can transfer a patient out of bed to a chair.
    Content Area: Leadership and Management
    Integrated Processes: Nursing Process: Implementation
    Client Need: Safe and Effective Care Environment; Management of Care
    Cognitive Level: Application

12. **ANSWER: 1.**
    Rationales:
    1. **A nurse manager must engage in evaluation activities when determining if organizational goals are being met. Current outcomes must be compared to desired outcomes. When a problem occurs, it should be explored to determine if it is an isolated event or if it has occurred**

before. Problems that reoccur must be addressed to prevent continuation of the problem.
    2. Planning occurs earlier in the management process. Effective planning should result in the attainment of organizational goals.
    3. The development of strategies to achieve objectives occurs earlier in the management process. Effective strategies should result in the attainment of organizational goals.
    4. Although sharing this information with colleagues promotes collaboration, it does not evaluate whether organizational goals are being met.
    TEST-TAKING TIP: Identify the word in the stem that sets a priority. The word *first* in the stem sets a priority. Identify equally plausible options. Options 2 and 3 are equally plausible.
    Content Area: Leadership and Management
    Integrated Processes: Nursing Process: Evaluation
    Client Need: Safe and Effective Care Environment; Management of Care
    Cognitive Level: Application

13. **ANSWER: 1, 2, 3.**
    Rationales:
    1. **Managers who support theory X management principles believe that continuous supervision and evaluation produce productive workers.**
    2. **Managers who support theory X management principles believe that firm rules and regulations ensure that people will conform to the culture of the organization.**
    3. **Managers who support theory X management principles believe that the fear of negative consequences produces effective workers.**
    4. Managers who support theory Y management principles believe that guidance and support provide an atmosphere that produces effective workers.
    5. Managers who support theory Y management principles believe that assistance and mutual respect produce productive workers.
    Content Area: Leadership and Management
    Integrated Processes: Communication/Documentation; Nursing Process: Analysis
    Client Need: Safe and Effective Care Environment; Management of Care
    Cognitive Level: Analysis

14. **ANSWER: 2.**
    Rationales:
    1. The nurse who is delegating the task is ultimately responsible.
    2. **A nurse can delegate only those tasks permitted by the state nurse practice act and the policies and procedures within the agency. Legal parameters of practice are indicated in state nurse practice acts.**
    3. Although experience does broaden one's experiential background, each person within a job description must be minimally competent to perform required skills.
    4. Although a patient's acuity level is an important factor to consider, legal parameters of practice must be considered first.
    TEST-TAKING TIP: Identify the word in the stem that sets a priority. The word *most* in the stem sets a priority.

Content Area: Leadership and Management
Integrated Processes: Nursing Process: Planning
Client Need: Safe and Effective Care Environment; Management of Care
Cognitive Level: Application

15. **ANSWER: 1.**
    Rationales:
    1. This statement is associated with the concept of authority. Managers have the authority to direct the work of others based on the power associated with a title.
    2. This statement is associated with the concept of accountability.
    3. This statement is associated with the concept of responsibility.
    4. This statement is associated with the concept of accountability.
    TEST-TAKING TIP: Identify the word in the stem that sets a priority. The word *most* in the stem sets a priority. Identify the clang association. The word *work* in the stem and in option 1 is a clang association. Examine option 1 carefully.
    Content Area: Leadership and Management
    Integrated Processes: Nursing Process: Analysis
    Client Need: Safe and Effective Care Environment; Management of Care
    Cognitive Level: Comprehension

16. **ANSWER: 3.**
    Rationales:
    1. This statement reflects the use of the power of authority, which is related to management, not leadership.
    2. This statement is associated with producing a product, which is a function of a manager, not a leader.
    3. **This statement is associated with the transformational leadership style. Empowering and inspiring others by recognizing and respecting their knowledge and abilities supports cooperation when implementing change.**
    4. This statement reflects the use of the power of authority, which is related to management, not leadership.
    TEST-TAKING TIP: Identify the word in the stem that sets a priority. The word *major* in the stem sets a priority. Identify the option with a specific determiner. Option 1 contains the word *every*, which is a specific determiner.
    Content Area: Leadership and Management
    Integrated Processes: Communication/Documentation; Nursing Process: Implementation
    Client Need: Safe and Effective Care Environment; Management of Care
    Cognitive Level: Analysis

17. **ANSWER: 2, 3, 4, 5.**
    Rationales:
    1. This can be viewed by staff members as a threat.
    2. Communication, information, and participation are essential precursors to change. An increase in knowledge and time to process the information may promote a willingness to participate in the change with a positive attitude.
    3. Verbalization of concerns and feelings allows issues to be discussed with mutual respect. New information can

be provided and misinformation corrected. In addition, feelings can be validated.
    4. Organizational goals should be shared and clarified with the staff involved with the change. An organization committed to a change should provide the physical, emotional, and financial support necessary to successfully achieve the change.
    5. This fact provides a sense of security and may lower resistance to change.
    TEST-TAKING TIP: Identify opposites in options. Options 1 and 5, for all practical purposes, are opposites. People being transferred to another unit are in fact losing their present jobs. Identify options with a clang association. The word *change* in the stem and in options 2 and 4 are clang associations. More often than not an option with a clang association is a correct answer.
    Content Area: Leadership and Management
    Integrated Processes: Communication/Documentation; Nursing Process: Implementation
    Client Need: Safe and Effective Care Environment; Management of Care
    Cognitive Level: Application

18. **ANSWER: 4.**
    Rationales:
    1. Although this may be planned, it is not the priority. Incentives may motivate people with an external locus of control but not staff members with an internal locus of control.
    2. Although this may be planned because achievement of small steps is motivating, it is not the priority.
    3. This is the use of the power of authority and a veiled threat via the use of the power of coercion.
    4. **Change that is harmonious with beliefs and ethics is easier to implement than when not harmonious with beliefs and ethics. Change is difficult to implement when it is not consistent with the beliefs and ethics of staff members.**
    TEST-TAKING TIP: Identify the word in the stem that sets a priority. The word *most* in the stem sets a priority. Identify the equally plausible options. Options 1 and 2 are equally plausible. Both are interventions that a nurse manager may employ to motivate the nurses and therefore option 1 is no better than option 2.
    Content Area: Leadership and Management
    Integrated Processes: Nursing Process: Planning
    Client Need: Safe and Effective Care Environment; Management of Care
    Cognitive Level: Application

19. **ANSWER: 2.**
    Rationales:
    1. Offering an incentive, such as an increase in pay or a promotion, reflects the power of a reward.
    2. **The power of coercion is used when a negative consequence is used as a threat or an incentive to influence behavior.**
    3. The power of expertise results from knowledge and proficiency exhibited by a qualified, proficient individual.
    4. The power of competence is related to ability, capability, and proficiency; it does not involve identifying consequences or making threats.

TEST-TAKING TIP: Identify the options that are equally plausible. Options 3 and 4 both have to do with ability, proficiency, and capability. One is no better than the other.
Content Area: Leadership and Management
Integrated Processes: Nursing Process: Analysis
Client Need: Safe and Effective Care Environment; Management of Care
Cognitive Level: Analysis

20. **ANSWER: 2.**
Rationales:
1. Both leaders and managers must be able to think critically to function effectively in their respective positions.
2. Nurse managers usually are required to participate in the preparation of a budget or manage the finances of a unit within an agency.
3. Both leaders and managers must communicate and collaborate with other members of the health team.
4. Both leaders and managers must demonstrate competence to earn the respect of others; this is known as the power of expertise.
Content Area: Leadership and Management
Integrated Processes: Nursing Process: Analysis
Client Need: Safe and Effective Care Environment; Management of Care
Cognitive Level: Analysis

21. **ANSWER: 3.**
Rationales:
1. Focusing on negative consequences as a form of motivation to adhere to policies and procedures is a component of the theory X human relations–oriented management style.
2. Constant supervision of staff members is a component of the theory X human relations–oriented management style.
3. This intervention is associated with the theory Y human relations–oriented management style. This management style is concerned with support, guidance, and assistance as being integral to promoting effective, productive staff members.
4. This intervention is associated with the theory X human relations–oriented management style.
TEST-TAKING TIP: Identify the unique option. Option 3 is unique; it is the only option that is not autocratic.
Content Area: Leadership and Management
Integrated Processes: Caring; Nursing Process: Evaluation
Client Need: Safe and Effective Care Environment; Management of Care
Cognitive Level: Application

22. **ANSWER: 3.**
Rationales:
1. This is not a reportable incident to a state board of nursing. However, the nurse may be counseled and be required to attend an in-service program on medication administration.
2. Confidential information may be shared among a group of health-care professionals for educational purposes without the consent of the patient. In most cases the initials, not names, of patients are used to help maintain confidentiality. Also, health-care professionals understand that maintaining confidentiality of information shared at professional meetings is a standard of care protected by the *Patient Care Partnership: Understanding Expectations, Rights, and Responsibilities* and codes of ethics of various disciplines.
3. Monitoring a patient and protecting a patient from preventable complications are minimum standards of care and when violated can be reported to the state board of nursing. The nurse failed to meet these standards of care.
4. Placing a mouth guard in the mouth of a patient experiencing a tonic/clonic seizure is contraindicated because it may cause broken teeth. It is unfortunate that the patient bit off the tip of the tongue in this situation; however, the nurse's inaction was justified based on the nursing standard of care.
TEST-TAKING TIP: Identify the word in the stem that indicates negative polarity. The word *reportable* in the stem indicates negative polarity. The question is asking, "In what situation did a nurse *not* meet a nursing standard of care?"
Content Area: Legal and Ethical Issues
Integrated Processes: Communication/Documentation; Nursing Process: Evaluation
Client Need: Safe and Effective Care Environment; Management of Care
Cognitive Level: Application

23. **ANSWER: 3.**
Rationales:
1. The charge nurse does not have evidence to confront the nursing assistant.
2. The nurse should not follow through with this action until some evidence is provided that supports the alleged unethical behavior and the charge nurse counsels the nursing assistant.
3. If there is a substantial difference between the weights taken by the nursing assistant and the charge nurse, then there is some evidence to indicate that the nursing assistant was not following proper procedures. The next step is for the charge nurse to meet with and counsel the nursing assistant according to the policy and procedures of the facility.
4. This action will not confirm or disprove the previous behavior.
TEST-TAKING TIP: Identify the word in the stem that sets a priority. The word *first* in the stem sets a priority.
Content Area: Leadership and Management
Integrated Processes: Nursing Process: Implementation
Client Need: Safe and Effective Care Environment; Management of Care
Cognitive Level: Application

24. **ANSWER: 5, 4, 2, 6, 3, 1.**
Rationales:
5. The problem is that the incidence of *C. difficile* has increased. The next issue that must be addressed is why. What factors are causing the increase (e.g., health team members are not washing their hands adequately, lack of enough stations to perform hand hygiene, patients have high risk factors). A potential solution cannot be identified until the cause of the problem is identified.
4. A variety of solutions should be analyzed in relation to the problem. Pros and cons of each should be explored and then one should be selected as the method to prevent

the transmission of *C. difficile* on the unit. If too many interventions are included, it will be difficult to attribute a change to a specific intervention.

2. Expected outcomes provide specific, measurable criteria against which the actual outcomes can be compared. If the actual outcomes are the same as the expected outcomes, then the intervention is successful. This is the basis of evidence-based practice.

6. After everyone knows the direction of the planned change, then the plan can be put into effect. Resistance usually is more evident at this time because the health team members are expected to be actively involved in the change at this time.

3. When the timetable for the change is reached, then an evaluation of the plan must be conducted. Did the actual outcomes mirror the expected outcomes and why?

1. If the change is successful in reducing the incidence of *C. difficile* on the unit, then the change must be stabilized so that it is a permanent change. This involves ensuring that the factors and issues that supported the change continue into the future.

Content Area: Leadership and Management
Integrated Processes: Nursing Process: Planning
Client Need: Safe and Effective Care Environment; Management of Care
Cognitive Level: Analysis

25. **ANSWER: 3.**

Rationales:

1. The nurse coordinator is not using the power of reward. Power of reward is based on incentives to influence others, such as a pay increase.

2. The nurse coordinator is not using coercive power. Coercive power is based on retribution or the fear of punitive withholding of a reward.

3. The nurse coordinator is using the power of expertise, which is based on the respect one receives because of advanced education, ability, skills, knowledge, and experience. A nurse coordinator is a middle-level manager who has ascended the ranks from a staff nurse to first-level manager (e.g., team leader, charge nurse), to a unit-level manager (e.g., nurse manager), to a middle-level manager (e.g., supervisor, nurse coordinator).

4. Although the nurse coordinator has authority over the new nurse manager, the power of authority is not being used by the nurse coordinator when functioning as a mentor.

Content Area: Leadership and Management
Integrated Processes: Nursing Process: Analysis
Client Need: Safe and Effective Care Environment; Management of Care
Cognitive Level: Analysis

26. **ANSWER: 2.**

Rationales:

1. The word *sharing* is associated with the democratic, not autocratic, leadership style. The democratic leadership style fosters two-way communication and input from others and creates a spirit of teamwork that results in staff satisfaction.

2. The word *dictatorial* means domineering and is associated with the autocratic leadership style. Autocratic leaders use directive and controlling behavior and make decisions alone, without input from others.

3. The word *participative* is associated with the democratic, not autocratic, leadership style. The democratic leadership style fosters two-way communication and input from others and creates a spirit of teamwork that results in staff satisfaction.

4. The word *collaborative* is associated with the democratic, not autocratic, leadership style. The democratic leadership style fosters two-way communication and input from others and creates a spirit of teamwork that results in staff satisfaction.

TEST-TAKING TIP: Identify the unique option. Option 2 is unique because it is the only option that reflects the autocratic leader who makes decisions alone and independently. Options 1, 3, and 4 reflect involvement of others who contribute to a joint effort which is associated with the democratic leadership style.

Content Area: Leadership and Management
Integrated Processes: Nursing Process: Analysis
Client Need: Safe and Effective Care Environment; Management of Care
Cognitive Level: Comprehension

27. **ANSWER: 4.**

Rationales:

1. This is not an example of a management activity related to planning. Planning is associated with the development of goals, objectives, and/or outcomes and determining strategies that are most likely to achieve organizational goals.

2. This is not an example of a management activity related to directing. Directing is associated with motivating, guiding, and leading staff members in meeting organizational goals.

3. This is not an example of a management activity related to organizing. Organizing is associated with obtaining and managing human and economic resources to meet desired clinical and financial goals.

4. This is an example of a management activity related to controlling. Controlling is associated with using outcome criteria to measure effectiveness in goal achievement, ensuring ongoing evaluation, and implementing corrective actions when necessary.

Content Area: Leadership and Management
Integrated Processes: Nursing Process: Analysis
Client Need: Safe and Effective Care Environment; Management of Care
Cognitive Level: Comprehension

28. **ANSWER: 4.**

Rationales:

1. Individual meetings may lead the other members of the team to be suspicious about what was said. Lines of communication should be kept open among all members of the nursing team. Also, team members should be informed that the nurse in charge was following the criteria identified at the beginning of the initiative.

2. This is an authoritative approach and is premature. The private rooms may or may not be the cause of the perceived imbalance in patient room assignments.

3. This approach denies the primary nurse's concerns. This approach devalues the nurse at a time when the nurse should feel empowered. Six more weeks is unrealistic to wait.

4. The entire nursing team should be involved with new initiatives. When people are involved in the decision making, usually there is a vested interest in being successful.

TEST-TAKING TIP: Identify the word in the stem that sets a priority. The word *best* in the stem sets a priority.

Content Area: Leadership and Management
Integrated Processes: Communication/Documentation; Nursing Process: Implementation
Client Need: Safe and Effective Care Environment; Management of Care
Cognitive Level: Analysis

29. **ANSWER: 2.**
    Rationales:
    1. This action is premature.

    2. The occurrence of medication errors indicates a need for change. The next step involves identifying the problem: What factors are associated with the errors?

    3. A variety of strategies should be explored before deciding on a solution.

    4. The problem must be identified before potential strategies can be explored.

    TEST-TAKING TIP: Identify the word in the stem that sets a priority. The word *next* in the stem sets a priority. Identify the option with a specific determiner. The word *all* in option 4 is a specific determiner. More often than not, an option with a specific determiner is a distractor. Identify options with clang associations. The word *errors* in the stem and in options 2 and 4 are clang associations. Examine options 2 and 4 carefully because more often than not, an option with a clang association is the correct answer.

Content Area: Leadership and Management
Integrated Processes: Nursing Process: Assessment
Client Need: Safe and Effective Care Environment; Management of Care
Cognitive Level: Application

30. **ANSWER: 2.**
    Rationales:
    1. Although repeating the nurse's message is an invitation to respond, the nurse could respond with a yes or no answer that would close communication.

    2. This response encourages the nurse to elaborate on the statement, "This new schedule is ridiculous." It sends the message that the nurse manager is interested in the nurse's thoughts and feelings.

    3. This response is confrontational and accuses the nurse of being judgmental. This response will cut off communication.

    4. Although the first part of the statement is an attempt to validate feelings, the second part of the statement is confrontational because it implies that the nurse is being negative; this may shut off communication.

    TEST-TAKING TIP: Identify the word in the stem that sets a priority. The word *best* in the stem sets a priority. Identify the options that are equally plausible. Options 1, 3, and 4 are confrontational; one intervention is no better than the other. Identify the option that is unique. Option 2 is the only option that communicates to the nurse that the manager is interested in the nurse's concerns.

Content Area: Leadership and Management
Integrated Processes: Caring; Communication/Documentation; Nursing Process: Implementation
Client Need: Safe and Effective Care Environment; Management of Care
Cognitive Level: Analysis

Health-Care Delivery

Continuing education—Acquisition of information that keeps nurses abreast of new technology, theories, and clinical practice.

Nursing care delivery model—Organizational system that provides a framework for how nursing care is implemented and by which members of the nursing team.

Nursing certification—Voluntary endeavor to earn recognition for expertise in a specific area of nursing practice.

Primary health care—Care that focuses on maintaining an optimum level of wellness.

Role—Set of responsibilities and expected behaviors related to a position or status.

Secondary health care—Care that focuses on early detection of and intervention to cure disease and minimize further impairment.

Tertiary health care—Care that focuses on health restoration and palliation.

I. Settings for Health-Care Delivery

The health-care delivery system provides a variety of services across various settings to meet the health-related needs of the members of society. It is complex and continually changing based on such factors as federal and state legislation, reengineering of organizations, cost-containment issues, emergence of new health-care professions, and expectations of patients and their family members. Recent changes in health care, such as the increased emphasis on the provision of care within the community rather than in hospitals and the focus on health rather than illness, have influenced the settings in which health care is provided.

A. Classification of Health-Care Agencies
   1. Are classified in a number of respects.
      a. By state license when criteria are met.
      b. By ownership.
         (1) Public/official: Federal, state, or local governmental control.
         (2) Voluntary: Not-for-profit.
         (3) Proprietary: For profit.
      c. By focus of care or by mission, such as:
         (1) Orthopedic.
         (2) Pediatric.
         (3) Psychiatric.
         (4) Maternity.
         (5) General medicine and surgery.
         (6) Rehabilitation.
         (7) Hospice.

   d. Services offered generally are determined by the license, size, location, and mission of the agency.

B. Acute Care Hospitals
   1. Generally are involved with the diagnosis and treatment of acute and chronic illnesses.
   2. Services provided may include:
      a. Acute inpatient medical and surgical services.
      b. Outpatient care, such as ambulatory care services, diagnostic tests, day surgery, rehabilitative care, and emergency department administered care.
      c. Specialty services, such as a burn, spinal cord, or dialysis unit.

C. Outpatient Settings
   1. Include such settings as clinics, primary health-care provider's offices, ambulatory surgery centers, schools, occupational settings, and agencies that provide home-care services.
   2. Provide such services as minor surgical procedures, physical examinations, physical therapy, medical screenings, counseling, teaching, day care, and primary care.
   3. Examples of specific settings.
      a. Schools.
         (1) Provide health education, health promotion, and disease prevention interventions.
         (2) Coordinate with health-care professionals and implement assistance to ensure a meaningful learning experience within school settings for children with disabilities or health-care needs.

(3) Engage in case-finding activities, such as head lice and scoliosis screening, and make referrals to other health agencies as needed.

b. Occupational settings.
(1) Provide programs to support safety in the work environment.
(2) May provide annual employee health screenings.
(3) May provide health education on topics such as weight reduction and hypertension.
(4) May provide counseling services.
(5) May provide follow-up care after an injury.

DID YOU KNOW?

Increasing numbers of employers are providing health-care services and related benefits, such as exercise facilities, to their employees. The underlying reason is the belief that productivity is related to the health of a worker.

D. **Long-Term Care Settings**
1. Provide services on a continuum in a variety of inpatient and outpatient settings.
   a. Independent living setting.
   (1) Adults generally live in an independent apartment, care for themselves, and may have meals and housekeeping services provided.
   (2) Some facilities provide for leisure activities, banking hours, hair dresser services, rehabilitation services, and access to primary health-care providers at one's own expense within the building.
   b. Assisted living setting.
   (1) Adults receive some assistance with activities such as dressing and bathing, in addition to the provision of meals and housekeeping services.
   (2) Some facilities provide for leisure activities, banking hours, hair dresser services, rehabilitation services, and access to primary health-care providers at one's own expense within the building.
   c. Subacute unit in a skilled nursing home.
   (1) Provides comprehensive care for a person with an acute illness, injury, or exacerbation of a disease process in lieu of hospitalization.
   (2) Provides treatment interventions to avoid unnecessary and recurrent hospitalizations.
   d. Intermediate care setting.
   (1) Provides care for people who are disabled, older adults, and people who are not non-acutely ill but need less intensive care than services provided by a hospital or skilled nursing facility.
   (2) Care generally is provided by nonskilled and unlicensed personnel.
   (3) Usually provides custodial care.
   e. Skilled nursing care provided in a nursing home.
   (1) Facilities that are certified to participate in and receive remuneration from Medicare or Medicaid.
   (2) Requires people to meet specific criteria before admission, such as insurance, prescribed treatment, nursing services, and resources required.
   (3) Provides long-term care for people who need ongoing medical and nursing attention.
   (4) Provides short-term care for people discharged from a hospital who still require comprehensive medical and nursing care to facilitate recovery from an acute health event.
   (5) May specialize in services such as brain injury care or orthopedic rehabilitation.

E. **Hospice**
1. Provides care to patients with terminal illnesses as well as their family members and support persons.
2. Offers care in such settings as hospitals, skilled nursing homes, intermediate care settings, free-standing hospice settings, and private homes; locations vary depending on the patient's condition and the ability of family members to provide care at home.
3. Focuses on maintaining comfort and quality of life, not curative treatment.

F. **Home Care**
1. Associated with agencies that provide care in the home as well as outpatient services.
2. Examples include urgent care centers, day-care centers, use of hospital services and equipment on an outpatient basis, and residential treatment halfway houses where no treatment interventions are provided.

II. Types of Health-Care Services

Numerous types of health-care services are available to meet the complex needs of patients. These services can be categorized into primary, secondary, and tertiary care, each with its own unique focus. The complexity of care in each depends on a patient's individual needs, the primary health-care provider's knowledge and expertise, and the setting in which the health care is provided.

A. **Primary:** Health Promotion and Illness Prevention
1. Focuses on maintaining an optimum level of wellness.
2. Interventions decrease the risk of disease and disability.
3. Activities include sanitation, immunization, and lifestyle modifications, such as dietary counseling, smoking cessation, and exercise.

B. **Secondary:** Diagnosis and Treatment
1. Focuses on early detection and intervention to treat disease and minimize further impairment.

2. Involves acute medical care and surgical intervention.
3. Activities include regular dental exams, routine screenings (e.g., bone density testing and mammograms for women, human immunodeficiency virus testing, blood pressure and cholesterol testing), and x-rays.

C. Tertiary: Rehabilitation
1. Focuses on restoring function, maximizing results of treatment, and providing palliative care, such as supporting comfort and quality of life.
2. Focuses on maximizing abilities in light of chronic or irreversible conditions.
3. Activities include education and rehabilitation (e.g., learning how to use a wheelchair, learning to engage in activities of daily living to live independently, and making environmental modifications, such as installing grab bars and ramps and widening doorways in the home).

III. Health Team Members

Patient needs are multifaceted, complex, and require a multitude of people from a variety of health-care disciplines with specific expertise to assist patients to meet these needs. Because nurses have a unique relationship with patients, function as patient advocates, and, depending on the setting, provide care 24/7, they are commonly responsible for coordinating patient care. Nurses must know the members of the health team and the services they provide to perform the role of coordinator effectively. Although the nurse is the coordinator of the health team, the patient is the center of the health team.

A. The Patient
🛑 1. The patient is the center of the health team.

2. All members of the health team lend their expertise to assist the patient in meeting health-care goals.

B. Nursing Team Members
1. Nurse administrators.
   a. Establish and manage achievement of organizational goals, particularly those of the department of nursing and other related agency departments.
   b. Examples include vice-president for nursing, associate director of nursing, assistant director of nursing, nursing supervisor, nurse coordinator, and nurse manager.
2. Clinical nurse specialist (CNS).
   a. Functions as a resource to nurses caring for patients with complex nursing needs.
   b. Requires advanced education in a specific field.
   c. Examples include diabetic nurse educator, infection control nurse, and medical-surgical CNS.

3. Registered nurse (RN).
   a. Coordinates services provided by members of the health-care team.
   b. Provides direct nursing care.
   c. Supervises unlicensed nursing personnel.
4. Licensed vocational nurse (LVN) or licensed practical nurse (LPN).
   a. Provides uncomplicated bedside nursing care.
   b. Works in a structured setting under the supervision of an RN.
5. Unlicensed assistive personnel (UAP).
   a. Provides direct nursing care delegated by an RN.
   b. Performs activities generally related to assisting patients with activities of daily living and providing noncomplex tasks.
   c. Examples include nursing associate and nursing assistant.

C. Other Professional Team Members
1. Primary health-care provider: Person who has a prescriptive license, such as medical doctor (MD), physician's assistant (PA), and nurse practitioner (NP).
2. Pharmacist (RPh).
3. Dietitian (RD).
4. Respiratory therapist (RT).
5. Physical therapist (PT).
6. Occupational therapist (OT).
7. Social worker (SW).
8. Dentist (DDS).
9. Podiatrist (DPM).
10. Audiologist (Au.D).
11. Speech language pathologist (SLP).
12. Laboratory and radiology professionals (x-ray, ultrasound, and laboratory technicians).
13. Activity therapist (AT).
14. Certified child life specialist (CCLS).
15. Chaplain.

D. Supportive Team Members
1. Family members.
2. Unit secretary.
3. Transport staff.
4. Housekeeping personnel.
5. Security personnel.

IV. The Profession of Nursing

Nursing is considered both a profession and a discipline. As a profession, it is based on technical and scientific knowledge; has members who are knowledgeable, competent, and evaluated by peers; and has a code of ethics. As a discipline, nursing has its own scientifically based body of knowledge involving both a theoretical foundation and a practical aspect in the form of clinical skills. In addition, nursing integrates knowledge and principles associated with other disciplines, such as anatomy and physiology, psychology, sociology, communications, and mathematics. A variety of nursing education programs, from those providing entry into practice through the doctoral level, prepare nurses to practice as professional nurses on various levels of nursing practice and in various health-care settings. Nursing organizations support the practice of nursing by activities such as publishing position statements on important issues affecting nursing, encouraging and supporting nursing scholarship and research, and identifying standards of nursing practice and codes directing nursing practice. In addition they recognize expertise via certification of professional nurses who demonstrate proficiency in a specific area of nursing practice. Nurses should understand the educational programs available to continue personal growth and the services that nursing organizations provide to the profession of nursing.

A. Definitions of Nursing
1. According to the International Council of Nurses (INC), which represents nurses throughout the world, "Nursing encompasses autonomous and collaborative care of individuals of all ages, families, groups and communities, sick or well and in all settings. Nursing includes the promotion of health, prevention of illness, and the care of ill, disabled and dying people. Advocacy, promotion of a safe environment, research, participation in shaping health policy and inpatient and health systems management, and education are also key nursing roles."
2. According to the American Nurses Association (ANA), which represents nurses throughout the United States, "The protection, promotion, and optimization of health and abilities, prevention of illness and injury, alleviation of suffering through the diagnosis and treatment of human response, and advocacy in the care of individuals, families, communities, and populations."

B. Nursing Associations
1. American Nurses Association (ANA).
   a. Mission: "Nurses advancing our profession to improve health for all."
   b. National professional organization for nursing in the United States.
   c. Involved in such activities as publishing standards of nursing practice; lobbying for professional, political, and economic issues impacting health care and nursing; and certifying expert nurses who meet experiential and testing criteria.
   d. Online at *www.nursingworld.org.*
2. National League for Nursing (NLN).
   a. Mission: "Promote excellence in nursing education and build a strong and diverse nursing workforce to advance the nation's health."
   b. Organization of individuals such as nurses, non-nurses, and agencies.

c. Involved in such activities as providing a voice for nursing education and advocates for nurse educator interests in academic, professional, and political arenas.
   d. Online at *www.nln.org.*
3. National League for Nursing Accrediting Commission (NLNAC).
   a. Mission: "Supports the interests of nursing education, nursing practice, and the public by the functions of accreditation."
   b. Involved in such activities as accrediting nursing education programs, both postsecondary and higher degree, that offer either a certificate, diploma, or recognized professional degree.
   c. Online at *www.nlnac.org.*
4. International Council of Nurses (ICN).
   a. Mission: "To represent nursing worldwide, advancing the profession and influencing health policy."
   b. Involved in such activities as representing the profession of nursing worldwide via a federation of national nursing associations and collaborating with other organizations to provide access to focused information and research on major nursing and health topics (e.g., International Center for Nursing Human Resources).
   c. Online at *www.icn.ch.*
5. National Student Nurses' Association (NSNA).
   a. Mission: "To mentor students preparing for initial licensure as registered nurses, and to convey the standards, ethics, and skills that students will need as responsible and accountable leaders and members of the profession."
   b. Involved in such activities as representing student nurses; convening yearly conventions; and publishing *Image,* the official journal of the NSNA.
   c. Online at *www.nsna.org.*
6. Sigma Theta Tau International (STTI), the honor society of nursing.
   a. Mission: "To support the learning, knowledge and professional development of nurses committed to making a difference in health worldwide."
   b. Selects students in baccalaureate, masters, doctoral, and postdoctoral programs and practicing nurses for membership when they demonstrate excellence in nursing.
   c. Has a scholarly purpose rather than social purpose.
   d. Involved in such activities as providing awards and grants supporting nursing research; conducting biennial conventions to address organizational business and programs; and supporting a leadership institute, nursing research library, and global initiatives.
   e. Online at *www.nursingsociety.org.*

C. Nursing Education

1. Programs that prepare students to take the National Council Licensure Examination for Registered Nurses (NCLEX-RN).

    a. Diploma programs.

    (1) Were the most common nursing programs before the 1960s, when nursing education moved into community college and university settings; have dramatically declined in number.

    (2) Generally are under the sponsorship of a hospital and may provide college credit if associated with a community college.

    (3) Generally take 3 years to complete and focus on clinical experience.

    b. Associate degree programs, such as Associate Degree in Nursing (ADN), Associate of Arts (AA), Associate of Science (AS), or Associate in Applied Science (AAS).

    (1) Generally are 2-year programs offered by a community college or university; however, because many students are older with family and job responsibilities, may take 3 or more years of part-time study to complete.

    (2) Provide the basis for pursuing more advanced nursing education.

    c. Baccalaureate degree nursing programs, such as Bachelor of Science in Nursing (BSN). Offer two courses of study.

    (1) Generic: Generally are 3- to 4-year programs for students entering as freshman with a major in nursing.

    (2) General: Generally are 2-year programs for graduates of ADN programs or diploma programs with college credit; may offer a "fast track" option (12 to 18 months of continuous classes) for individuals with associate degrees in nursing.

    d. Master's entry program in nursing if the student earned a baccalaureate degree in another field.

    e. Doctoral entry program in nursing, which is similar to master's entry; has very limited enrollment.

2. Licensed practical nurse or vocational nurse programs that prepare students to take the National Council Licensure Examination for Practical Nurses (NCLEX-PN).

    a. Prepare graduates to provide uncomplicated bedside nursing care under the supervision of an RN.

    b. Generally are 1 to 1 1/2 years in length.

3. Programs that provide advanced degrees in nursing.

    a. Master's degree nursing programs, such as Master of Arts (MA), Master of Science (MS),
Master of Science in Nursing (MSN), and Master in Nursing (MN).

    (1) Prepare RNs with a BSN degree for advance practice.

    (2) Prepare nurses to assume advanced roles in clinical practice, education, research, and administration, such as Clinical Nurse Specialist (CNS), Certified Nurse Midwife (CNM), Certified Registered Nurse Anesthetist (CRNA), Nurse Practitioner (NP), nurse administrator, and professor of nursing education.

    (3) Generally take 1 1/2 to 2 or more years to complete.

    b. Doctoral programs in nursing, such as Doctor of Philosophy (PhD), Doctor of Nursing Science (DNS, DNSc), and Nursing Doctorate (ND).

    (1) Prepare nurses with master's degrees in nursing for advanced practice.

    (2) Focus of programs varies, such as clinical practice, administration, education, and theory development; however, all emphasize research.

D. Nursing Certification

1. Voluntary endeavor to earn recognition for expertise in a specific area of nursing practice.

2. Achieved in areas of practice, such as geriatrics, medical-surgical nursing, pediatrics, emergency nursing, nursing administration, nursing education, community health nursing, school nursing, and maternal-child nursing.

3. Provided by the ANA or specialty nursing organizations.

E. Evidenced-Based Practice

1. The use of research to prove the efficacy of a specific action. Evidenced-based practice in the context of nursing is the performance of nursing interventions based on rigorous scientific evidence and clinical effectiveness studies rather than tradition, intuition, or anecdotal information.

2. Research collects data that identifies which interventions will most likely produce expected patient outcomes.

3. Nursing practice based on evidence improves the quality of patient care, justifies nursing interventions, contains health-care costs, and expands the foundation of nursing as a profession.

F. Continuing Education

1. Many states require a certain number of hours of ongoing education (e.g., 15 to 30 hours every 2 years) or completion of classes on a specific topic (e.g., infection control, child abuse) for RN licensure renewal.

2. Classes ensure that nurses keep abreast of new technology, theories, and clinical practice.

3. Programs are offered by employers, colleges, professional nursing organizations, and professional journals.
G. In-Service Education
   1. Programs provided by employers.
   2. Generally focus on new equipment, introduction of new policies or procedures, or topics mandated by a state health department, such as infection control and cardiopulmonary resuscitation.

V. Delivery of Nursing Care

Nurses comprise the largest number of health-care professionals within most health-care settings. Utilization of their professional expertise requires a clear delineation of their roles and responsibilities as well as the use of a system that delivers nursing care that is safe, competent, and cost effective.

A. Roles of the Nurse (Table 4.1)
   1. A role is a set of responsibilities and expected behaviors related to a person's position or status.
   2. There are many common roles in the provision of nursing care regardless of the setting in which nurses work, and there are also differences in roles based on the unique services provided by particular health-care settings.

MAKING THE CONNECTION

In-Service Education and Job Performance

A nurse who works as a circulating and scrub nurse in a surgical unit in a hospital reads in a nursing journal about the development of a new device called the RF Assure Detection System. It is a mat that is placed on a surgical table under a patient and, prior to wound closure, can be used to scan a patient to identify retained surgical items. The nurse presents the technology to hospital administrators and convinces them to purchase the device. A nurse in the staff education department develops and presents an in-service education program for the nurses working in the surgical setting. This in-service education program about the new technology increases nurses' knowledge; promotes effective, efficient patient care; and helps to prevent patient complications.

 3. Nurses must have the knowledge and ability to assume appropriate roles when individualizing patient care and ensure that the roles are within the legal definition of the state nurse practice act within the state in which one works.

Table 4.1 Roles of the Nurse

Role	Examples of Nursing Care
Direct Caregiver Implements activities that address a patient's physical, psychosocial, developmental, sociocultural, and spiritual needs **Requires:** • Clinical proficiency • A supportive, empathetic, and caring bedside manner	• Assesses a patient • Performs technical skills, such as dressing changes, mechanical ventilation, and inserting and managing tubes and catheters • Administers medications • Provides emotional support • Evaluates outcomes of care
Patient Advocate Works with or on behalf of patients to meet their physical and emotional needs **Requires:** • Knowledge of human and legal rights • A nonjudgmental attitude • An assertive personality • Efficient communication skills	• Helps a patient explore options • Supports a patient's right to make decisions • Helps explain a patient's position to a health-care provider or family member • Helps patients to stand up for themselves • Protects the patient when the patient is unable to make decisions • Implements activities that protect the patient's human and legal rights, including the development of policies and procedures • Teaches patients how to prepare for office visits and how to prepare a list of questions for the primary health-care provider • Illustrates how to communicate with providers in new situations
Teacher Communicates clearly and accurately (verbally and in writing) with patients and their family members and people in the community to help them learn about their health and health care **Requires:** • Effective communication skills • Knowledge of teaching and learning principles	• Presents information about health-care procedures to maintain or restore health • Teaches patients how to access credible and reliable health-care information • Teaches healthy lifestyle behaviors, such as weight-loss strategies, smoking cessation, and a heart healthy diet • Teaches prenatal education classes • Provides preoperative teaching to prevent postoperative complications • Teaches self-administration of medications

Table 4.1 Roles of the Nurse—cont'd

Role	Examples of Nursing Care
Manager Influences others to achieve an identified goal **Requires:** • Knowledge of management theory • Knowledge of leadership theory • Effective communication skills • Ability to assume responsibility and accountability for the demands of the role	• Delegates and supervises nursing care activities of subordinate nursing team members • Evaluates outcomes of care delegated • Makes decisions regarding allocation of resources • Motivates staff members to achieve unit goals (See Chapter 3, "Leadership and Management," for additional information.)
Case Manager Oversees a patient's progress through the health-care system while ensuring that needs are identified and addressed **Requires:** • Organizational skills • Effective communication skills	• Oversees a patient's plan of care and functions as an advocate throughout the patient's hospitalization • Ensures that a patient's needs are met within the facility • Ensures continuity of a patient's health care within the community when preparing for discharge • Fulfills specific roles identified by the agency, such as discharge planning and managing referrals
Researcher Participates in planning and conducting evidence-based practice projects as well as implementing research results to the extent of one's educational preparation **Requires:** • Critical thinking ability • An inquisitive mind • Effective communication skills	• Participates as a member of a formal research committee • Assists in all phases of a research project • Incorporates findings into policy and procedure development • Facilitates the application of research results into practice (evidence-based practice) to improve patient care
Expert An individual who has specialized education, training, or experience in a particular field or activity and functions as a resource or in an expanded role **Requires:** • An advanced educational degree or certification in a specialty • Extensive experiential background in a particular field or activity	• Collaborates with other health team members regarding a plan of care for a patient with multiple or complex needs (e.g., clinical nurse specialist, diabetes nurse educator, enterostomal therapy nurse, infection control nurse, or dialysis nurse) • Provides primary care for a specific population, such as pregnant women, older adults, and children (e.g., nurse practitioner, psychiatric nurse practitioner) • Provides specialized services to patients (e.g., nurse anesthetist, certified registered nurse infusion)

B. Nursing Care Delivery Models

1. An organizational system that provides a framework for how nursing care is provided and by which members of the nursing team.
2. Continuously evolving because of societal health-care initiatives, organizational reengineering, increasing acuity of patients, and the need to address cost containment.
3. Types of nursing care delivery models.
   a. Primary nursing.
      (1) An RN is responsible for assigned patients throughout their hospitalization, 7 days a week, 24 hours a day (primary nurse).
      (2) The primary nurse does not deliver all care personally, but is responsible for ensuring that comprehensive and individualized care is delivered.
      (3) Primary nursing requires more registered nurses; however, it might not be more costly because it improves collaboration, avoids delays, and supports comprehensive care.
      (4) Communication is lateral; the primary nurse communicates directly with the nurses on the other shifts who are assigned to care for the patient.
      (5) Variations of primary nursing.
         (a) Total client-care: One nurse is responsible for the total care administered to a patient, but the nurse changes from shift to shift.
         (b) Modular nursing: Nurses are assigned to patients within a small segment of a nursing unit to ensure that patients receive care from the same personnel on a regular basis.
   b. Team nursing.
      (1) An RN team leader is responsible for a group of patients' plans of care and nursing care delivered and makes assignments based on the abilities of each team member,

such as RNs, LPNs, and unlicensed nursing personnel.

(2) Team members work together and share the work to be accomplished for a group of patients.

(3) The team leader is responsible for coordinating the team, planning care, and collaborating with professionals in other disciplines and often does not provide direct patient care.

(4) Although the focus is on patient assignments rather than tasks, tasks are assigned within the team.

(5) Communication occurs in a matrix (i.e., between the team leader and members and among team members).

c. Functional nursing.

(1) Functional nursing is a task-oriented approach whereby tasks are assigned based on a person's educational preparation.

(2) It is based on clearly defined job descriptions, policies, and procedures.

(3) The focus is efficiency and productivity, but can lead to fragmentation of care and failure to meet the emotional needs of patients.

(4) Communication occurs in a hierarchy from the head nurse to subordinates.

d. Case management (total care) model.

(1) An RN is responsible for planning, implementing, and evaluating care for a specific patient.

(2) The case manager is responsible for patient care across the continuum of practice settings to promote continuity of care and limit fragmentation and redundancy of care.

(3) This model commonly relies on critical pathways to ensure appropriate delivery of care and facilitate evaluation of the achievement of expected outcomes.

CASE STUDY: Putting It All Together

A nurse in a primary-care clinic administered immunizations to all the members of a family. The children received immunizations that were appropriate for their ages, the parents asked to be immunized against hepatitis B, and the older adult parent (grandmother) received a vaccine for shingles and a flu vaccine. All of the members of the family received complete physical examinations with routine blood work. The two adult women received bone density tests and mammograms. Eight months later, the grandmother's physical mobility became impaired because of osteoarthritis and the aging process. The primary health-care provider ordered physical therapy to help the grandmother learn how to use a walker. The family decided to make modifications to the house, adding grab bars in the bathroom and a ramp to the side door of the house so that the grandmother could walk out to the backyard independently. Two years later, the grandmother developed terminal stage IV ovarian cancer. The family was adamant about keeping her home to die.

Case Study Questions

A. Identify interventions associated with primary health care, and briefly discuss the focus of this type of health care.

_____

B. Identify interventions associated with secondary health care, and briefly discuss the focus of this type of health care.

_____

C. Identify interventions associated with tertiary health care, and briefly discuss the focus of this type of health care.

_____

D. What health-care service is available to assist the family with their goal of keeping the grandmother in the home to die and why?

_____

REVIEW QUESTIONS

1. Under which category is the agency Alcoholics Anonymous (AA) classified?
   1. Proprietary
   2. Voluntary
   3. Official
   4. Private

2. A nurse is caring for a patient who has shortness of breath because of chronic obstructive pulmonary disease and an upper respiratory infection. The patient reveals smoking several cigarettes a day. Which nursing intervention is associated with restoring this patient's health?
   1. Talking about managing work responsibilities while convalescing
   2. Suggesting attending a smoking cessation program
   3. Administering the prescribed antibiotic regimen
   4. Providing information about the ordered tests

3. Which interventions **most** likely are considered necessary by a company that provides health care insurance? **Select all that apply.**
   1. _____ Removal of an infected appendix.
   2. _____ Off-label use of a chemotherapeutic medication.
   3. _____ Bariatric surgery to promote weight loss of 100 lb.
   4. _____ Laser therapy for facial brown pigmentation due to sun damage.
   5. _____ Surgery to remove excess skin in the neck area after significant weight loss.

4. A patient is recovering from a brain attack (cerebrovascular accident) and experiencing dysphasia and aspiration. For which professional should the nurse seek a consultation referral from the primary health-care provider?
   1. Clinical nurse specialist
   2. Respiratory therapist
   3. Nurse practitioner
   4. Speech therapist

5. A patient experienced a brain attack (cerebrovascular accident) that resulted in a left hemiparesis. Which health-care professional is **most** appropriate to teach this patient how to recover and maintain abilities associated with activities of daily living?
   1. Occupational therapist
   2. Medical technician
   3. Physical therapist
   4. Primary nurse

6. An older adult who lives alone is recovering after surgery for a total hip replacement. Which is the **most** appropriate setting for this patient after discharge from the hospital?
   1. Home
   2. Hospice
   3. Skilled nursing facility
   4. Assistive living apartment

7. Patient needs are met in a variety of health-care settings. Place these settings in order, considering the progression from diagnosis to death.
   1. Hospice
   2. Outpatient clinic
   3. Acute care hospital
   4. Skilled nursing facility
   5. Intermediate care facility
   Answer: _____

8. Which setting has successfully reduced the overall cost of health care in the United States?
   1. Hospice
   2. Home care
   3. Rehabilitation facility
   4. Skilled nursing facility

9. An occupational nurse provides services related to primary prevention. Which action by the occupational nurse is an example of this type of service?
   1. Administering yearly flu vaccines to employees
   2. Measuring employee cholesterol levels twice a year
   3. Encouraging female employees to obtain routine mammograms
   4. Ensuring environmental accommodations for an employee who uses a wheelchair

10. Nurses working in acute care settings perform activities related to primary, secondary, and tertiary prevention. Which activity by a nurse in a hospital is related to secondary prevention?
    1. Teaching a patient's spouse how to administer an opioid injection
    2. Counseling a patient about a heart-healthy diet
    3. Instructing a patient how to use a walker
    4. Obtaining a patient's vital signs

11. A public health nurse is performing a variety of activities within the community. Which activities are examples of tertiary prevention? **Select all that apply.**

1. _____ Assessing the home environment of a patient with a spinal cord injury who is to be discharged

2. _____ Conducting a class at the local library about the importance of exercise

3. _____ Visiting a new mother who had a child with Down syndrome

4. _____ Teaching a patient how to perform a colostomy irrigation

5. _____ Screening school-aged children for scoliosis

12. A primary nurse is caring for an older adult who was admitted to the hospital for treatment of a new acute cardiac problem in addition to a history of chronic asthma, diabetes, and colitis. The patient is having difficulty coping with the additional self-care responsibilities associated with the new health problem. With whom should the primary nurse consult to **best** explore strategies to assist this patient with self-health care needs?

1. Nurse manager
2. Clinical nurse specialist
3. Licensed vocational nurse
4. Primary health-care provider

13. A 76-year-old man is hospitalized for pneumonia. His daughter has a meeting with her father's case manager to explore what should be done when her father is discharged. The nurse manager speaks with the patient's daughter, reviews the patient's medical history and present physical status, and identifies the community resources in the patient's community.

Additional Information

Patient's History

The patient experienced a brain attack (cerebral vascular accident, stroke) 3 years ago. He has right-sided hemiplegia and must use a wheelchair for ambulation. He wears a brace on his right leg and a splint on his right hand and forearm. The patient had periodic episodes of nighttime urine and fecal incontinence at home that have continued during the present hospitalization. He can perform some activities of daily living (ADLs) independently (e.g., brush teeth, comb hair, shave face, feed self, drink fluids), but needs assistance completing other tasks (e.g., complete bath, transfer from bed to wheelchair, toileting). He is mentally alert and is able to communicate effectively. The pneumonia is resolving, but he is weak and he has activity intolerance.

Interview With the Patient's Daughter

The patient's daughter is 52 years old, single, and works full time as an elementary school teacher. She states, "I love my dad very much and I like having him live with me. I have a wonderful home health aide who comes in from 8 a.m. to noon, Monday through Friday. She bathes my father, gives him breakfast and lunch, and cleans his bedroom. My dad has a medical alert button in case anything happens when I am not there. I am not getting any younger, and the job of caring for my dad is getting more demanding. It's nice to have someone in the house when I come home from school at 3:30, but I immediately get on another tread mill—taking my dad to the bathroom, making our dinner, washing our clothes, doing the food shopping, and all the chores around the house. The hardest part is cleaning him at night when he is incontinent. I don't mind caring for him, but 24/7 responsibility is tough. I refuse to put him in a nursing home."

Community Resources

Independent living apartment in an older adult development
Long-term care facility with skilled nursing
Older adult day-care center
Respite care center

What community resource should the nurse plan to explore with the patient and his daughter?

1. Independent living apartment in an older adult development
2. Long-term care facility providing skilled nursing care
3. Older adult day-care center
4. Respite care center

14. Which activity associated with the National League for Nursing Accrediting Commission has the greatest impact on the quality of care directly provided by a nurse?
    1. Approving nursing education programs
    2. Publishing standards of professional nursing practice
    3. Lobbying economic issues impacting on the profession of nursing
    4. Mentoring the professional development of future registered nurses

15. A nurse is promoted to the role of nurse manager. Which activities can the nurse expect to be included in this new job description that are not included in the role of case manager? **Select all that apply.**
    1. _____ Evaluating quality of nursing care delivered
    2. _____ Making decisions regarding allocation of resources
    3. _____ Ensuring continuity of care with community resources
    4. _____ Ensuring that patient needs are met in a timely manner
    5. _____ Overseeing a patient's progress through the health-care system

16. A nurse is interviewing for a position as head nurse for a medical-surgical unit. During the interview, the nurse manager mentions that primary nursing is the nursing care delivery model used in the agency. Which statement is associated with this nursing care delivery model?
    1. The delivery of nursing care is task oriented.
    2. Communication occurs in a hierarchy from head nurse to subordinate.
    3. The nurse is responsible for ensuring that comprehensive care is delivered.
    4. Responsibility for care is shared by nursing staff, but directed by a team leader.

17. Which nursing action reflects the caregiver role? **Select all that apply.**
    1. _____ Completes a dressing change ensuring that standards of care are met
    2. _____ Assesses a patient on return from the post-anesthesia care unit
    3. _____ Participates in developing policies that protect human rights
    4. _____ Supervises quality of care delegated to other team members
    5. _____ Helps a patient learn how to test a blood glucose level

18. A registered nurse graduated from an associate degree nursing program. The hospital in which the nurse works is requiring all registered nurses to attain a Bachelor of Science in Nursing (BSN) degree within 5 years. Which educational program should the college counselor suggest is the **most** appropriate for this nurse to attend?
    1. Masters in science nursing program
    2. Continuing education program
    3. In-service education program
    4. General nursing program

19. A patient who lives alone is scheduled to be discharged from the hospital with a large pressure ulcer that needs comprehensive nursing care. The service provided by which option is **most** appropriate for this patient?
    1. Assisted living facility
    2. Hospice care program
    3. Skilled nursing home
    4. Day-care center

20. Which activity associated with the American Nurses Association has the greatest impact on the quality of care provided by a nurse at a patient's bedside?
    1. Accrediting nursing education programs
    2. Publishing standards of professional nursing practice
    3. Lobbying economic issues impacting on the profession of nursing
    4. Mentoring the professional development of future registered nurses

REVIEW ANSWERS

1. ANSWER: 2.
Rationales:
1. Proprietary agencies are privately owned and operated to make a profit.
2. Alcoholics Anonymous (AA) is a voluntary organization. Voluntary agencies are not for profit and rely on professional and lay volunteers, in addition to a paid staff.
3. Official health agencies are supported by local, state, and/or national taxes.
4. Private agencies are privately owned and operated to make a profit.
TEST-TAKING TIP: Identify the equally plausible options. Option 1 and 4 are equally plausible. Agencies that make a profit are called *proprietary* or *private agencies*.
Content Area: Health-Care Delivery
Integrated Processes: Nursing Process: Analysis
Client Need: Safe and Effective Care Environment; Management of Care
Cognitive Level: Knowledge

2. ANSWER: 3.
Rationales:
1. Discussing concerns associated with responsibilities is related to facilitating coping, not restoring health.
2. Suggesting attending a smoking cessation program is related to preventing illness, not restoring health.
3. Antibiotics are curative and are given to restore health.
4. Explaining ordered tests is associated with promoting health, not restoring health.
Content Area: Health-Care Delivery
Integrated Processes: Nursing Process: Implementation
Client Need: Safe and Effective Care Environment; Management of Care
Cognitive Level: Application

3. ANSWER: 1, 3.
Rationales:
1. Surgery to remove an infected appendix is considered emergency surgery that is paid for by health-care insurance. Appendicitis can lead to perforation, peritonitis, and death if the appendix is not removed.
2. Off-label use of a medication generally is not covered by health-care insurance because efficacy has not been demonstrated.
3. Bariatric surgery to promote weight loss of 100 lb generally is covered by health-care insurance. Weight loss of less than 100 lb may be covered if the patient has a concurrent medical condition, such as diabetes or hypertension. It is believed that successful weight loss after bariatric surgery improves functioning; helps prevent complications, such as diabetes and hypertension; and improves quality of life. Although costly to provide initially, the person probably will have fewer health issues in the future.
4. Laser therapy to remove brown pigmentation of facial skin is not considered medically necessary to diagnose, treat, or improve functioning; this generally is not covered by health-care insurance.

5. Surgery to remove excess skin around the neck after significant weight loss is considered cosmetic and not medically necessary; this generally is not covered by health-care insurance. An exception to coverage for cosmetic surgery includes removal of pendulous abdominal skin that causes constant excoriation of touching skin surfaces, even with meticulous skin care. Reconstructive cosmetic surgery after a burn injury is covered by medical insurance.
Content Area: Health-Care Delivery
Integrated Processes: Nursing Process: Planning
Client Need: Safe and Effective Care Environment; Management of Care
Cognitive Level: Analysis

4. ANSWER: 4.
Rationales:
1. Although a clinical nurse specialist may provide care to a patient with impairment in swallowing, a clinical nurse specialist is not the professional educated to diagnose the specific mechanism that is impaired.
2. Respiratory therapists assess and treat patients with impairments of heart and lung functioning, not swallowing and speech.
3. A nurse practitioner is educationally prepared to diagnose illness and prescribe medications and treatments related to a patient's problems. However, nurse practitioners should consult with another health-care professional who can best determine the mechanism that is impaired when a swallowing problem exists.
4. Swallowing involves a complex mechanism that speech therapists are educated to diagnosis and treat; speech therapists assess, diagnose, and treat problems associated with speaking, language, articulation, vocal sound, and swallowing.
Content Area: Health-Care Delivery
Integrated Processes: Communication/Documentation; Nursing Process: Implementation
Client Need: Safe and Effective Care Environment; Management of Care
Cognitive Level: Application

5. ANSWER: 1.
Rationales:
1. An occupational therapist is the most appropriate professional to help this patient regain, acquire, improve, and maintain abilities related to activities of daily living, such as eating, dressing, bathing, grooming, cooking, and so on.
2. A medical technician works in a laboratory testing body fluid; activities may include evaluating blood levels of medication, crossmatching blood for blood transfusions, and examining tissues of the body.
3. A physical therapist is involved with preventing and limiting physical impairment and restoring function, strength, and coordination associated with mobility, not helping a patient cope with performing activities of daily living.
4. A primary nurse may be involved in coordinating the efforts of nursing team members with those of other health-care professionals involved in helping a patient recover

from an illness. A primary nurse provides nursing care and supports the plans of care established by professionals in other health-care disciplines.

TEST-TAKING TIP: Identify the word in the stem that sets a priority. The word *most* in the stem sets a priority.

Content Area: Health-Care Delivery

Integrated Processes: Nursing Process: Planning

Client Need: Safe and Effective Care Environment; Management of Care

Cognitive Level: Application

6. ANSWER: 3.

Rationales:

1. This patient lives alone and will not be capable of managing self-care.

2. There is no evidence in the stem that indicates that the patient has a probability of only 6 months to live, which is the central criterion for admission to a hospice program.

3. **Several weeks of rehabilitation services generally are ordered to promote strength, endurance, and mobility after a total hip replacement; the patient will require skilled nursing care and physical therapy.**

4. An assistive living arrangement may be an appropriate setting in the future if it is determined after rehabilitation that the patient can no longer live alone safely.

TEST-TAKING TIP: Identify the word in the stem that sets a priority. The word *most* in the stem sets a priority.

Content Area: Health-Care Delivery

Integrated Processes: Nursing Process: Planning

Client Need: Safe and Effective Care Environment; Management of Care

Cognitive Level: Analysis

7. ANSWER: 2, 3, 4, 5, 1.

Rationales:

2. **An outpatient clinic is a setting where secondary health care occurs (care that focuses on early detection and intervention to cure disease and minimize further impairment).**

3. **Acute care settings, such as hospitals, provide medical and surgical procedures to meet patients' immediate health needs.**

4. **After people have acute care needs met, they often are discharged earlier than in the past. As a result, these patients need skilled nursing care until, hopefully, they are capable of returning home.**

5. **Patients who are unable to return home after an experience in a skilled nursing facility usually are transferred to an intermediate care facility to meet their ongoing custodial needs.**

1. **As people reach the end of their lives, hospice care can provide supportive services for patients and their family members. Hospice provides palliative care so that patients can die with dignity and without pain.**

Content Area: Health-Care Delivery

Integrated Processes: Nursing Process: Analysis

Client Need: Safe and Effective Care Environment; Management of Care

Cognitive Level: Analysis

8. ANSWER: 2.

Rationales:

1. Although hospice care is less costly than a hospital in the provision of end-of-life care, it has not had as dramatic an impact as another setting in reducing overall costs of health care.

2. **Home care successfully provides a team approach to providing health care in the home, which is significantly less costly than providing the same care in a hospital or in a subacute unit in a long-term care facility.**

3. Although a rehabilitation facility can provide rehabilitation services less expensively than in the hospital setting, it is not the setting that has made the most impact in reducing overall costs of health care.

4. Although a skilled nursing facility provides skilled nursing care and subacute care for people in a less costly setting than a hospital, it is still more costly than another setting presented.

Content Area: Health-Care Delivery

Integrated Processes: Nursing Process: Analysis

Client Need: Safe and Effective Care Environment; Management of Care

Cognitive Level: Knowledge

9. ANSWER: 1.

Rationales:

1. **Primary prevention focuses on maintaining an optimum level of wellness and preventing disease or disability; it involves activities such as providing immunizations, promoting safety in the workplace, and counseling about life-style modifications (e.g., exercise, smoking cessation, and healthy diets).**

2. Secondary prevention involves early detection and intervention to cure disease and minimize impairment. An elevated cholesterol level alerts the employee to seek primary health-care supervision.

3. Secondary prevention involves early detection and intervention to cure disease and minimize impairment. Yearly physicals and routine dental care, mammograms, colonoscopies, and bone density tests are examples of secondary prevention.

4. Tertiary prevention includes activities such as making environmental modifications (e.g., ramps, widening doorways) for people recovering from physiological changes or rehabilitation and maximizing abilities.

TEST-TAKING TIP: Identify the options that are equally plausible. Options 2 and 3 are equally plausible because both involve health screening. Both tests are important; one is not more important than the other.

Content Area: Health-Care Delivery

Integrated Processes: Nursing Process: Implementation

Client Need: Health Promotion and Maintenance

Cognitive Level: Application

10. ANSWER: 4.

Rationales:

1. Education about palliative care that supports comfort is an example of tertiary care.

2. A heart-healthy diet will help maintain an optimum level of wellness; this is an example of primary prevention.

3. Teaching a patient how to use a walker is concerned with tertiary prevention; the nurse is providing information that will assist the patient to engage in the activities of daily living to live independently.

4. A patient's vital signs provide significant data and are integral to the diagnostic process; they assist with the identification of an illness, which is a part of secondary prevention.

TEST-TAKING TIP: Identify the unique option. Option 4 is unique; it is the only option that is obtaining, rather than providing, information.

Content Area: Health-Care Delivery
Integrated Processes: Nursing Process: Implementation
Client Need: Physiological Integrity; Reduction of Risk Potential
Cognitive Level: Application

11. ANSWER: 1, 3, 4.
   Rationales:
   1. This is an example of tertiary prevention; it is concerned with helping a patient to develop skills related to a chronic problem and become independent.
   2. This is an example of primary prevention; exercise is an activity that can promote wellness.
   3. This is an example of tertiary prevention. Down syndrome is a health problem caused by a genetic mutation. Life-long interventions are required to maximize the child's abilities and support the parents.
   4. This activity is an example of tertiary prevention. Colostomy irrigations may be a temporary or permanent requirement; regardless, it requires the learning of new skills to become independent for the length of time it exists.
   5. This is an example of secondary prevention; it involves the identification of a health problem so that appropriate interventions can be implemented as early as possible to promote a desirable outcome.
   Content Area: Health-Care Delivery
   Integrated Processes: Nursing Process: Planning
   Client Need: Physiological Integrity; Physiological Adaptation
   Cognitive Level: Analysis

12. ANSWER: 2.
   Rationales:
   1. The nurse manager is not the person with the most appropriate expertise to assist the primary nurse with this patient care situation.
   2. A clinical specialist has the most appropriate nursing education and experience to assist the primary nurse with this patient care situation. A clinical nurse specialist has the knowledge and ability to care for patients with complex nursing needs.
   3. A licensed vocational nurse does not have the educational or experiential background to best assist the primary nurse with this patient care situation.
   4. A primary health-care provider has a medical, not a nursing, educational, and experiential background.
   TEST-TAKING TIP: Identify the word in the stem that sets a priority. The word *best* in the stem sets a priority.
   Content Area: Health-Care Delivery
   Integrated Processes: Communication/Documentation; Nursing Process: Implementation

Client Need: Safe and Effective Care Environment; Management of Care
Cognitive Level: Application

13. ANSWER: 4.
   Rationales:
   1. The patient does not have the physical abilities to live in an independent care environment. The patient needs assistance with most of the activities of daily living.
   2. The patient does not need skilled nursing care. The patient needs assistance with the activities of daily living that can be provided by assistive nursing personnel.
   3. The patient is cared for in the morning by a home health aide and is competent to be alone for several hours until the daughter returns from work. An older adult day-care center will not meet the daughter's needs.
   4. A respite care center provides services that relieve family members from the caregiving role. In this situation, the daughter may be capable of keeping her father in the home if she has periodic opportunities to obtain adequate rest and relief from the daily responsibilities of caring for her father.
   Content Area: Health-Care Delivery
   Integrated Processes: Communication/Documentation; Nursing Process: Planning
   Client Need: Safe and Effective Care Environment; Management of Care
   Cognitive Level: Analysis

14. ANSWER: 1.
   Rationales:
   1. Approving nursing education programs, a role of the National League for Nursing Accrediting Commission, ensures that schools of nursing provide students with classroom and clinical experiences necessary to be prepared to take the National Council Licensing Examination.
   2. The American Nurses Association, not the National League for Nursing Accrediting Commission, establishes standards of nursing practice.
   3. Lobbying economic issues impacting the profession of nursing is one of the activities of the American Nurses Association, not the National League for Nursing Accrediting Commission.
   4. The National Student Nurses Association (NSNA), not the National League for Nursing Accrediting Commission, mentors the professional development of future registered nurses.
   TEST-TAKING TIP: Identify the word in the stem that sets a priority. The word *greatest* is the word in the stem that sets a priority.
   Content Area: Health-Care Delivery
   Integrated Processes: Nursing Process: Analysis
   Client Need: Safe and Effective Care Environment; Management of Care
   Cognitive Level: Comprehension

15. ANSWER: 1, 2.
   Rationales:
   1. A case manager is not responsible for evaluating the quality of nursing care delivered. A nurse manager is

responsible for the quality of care delivered by the members of the nursing team working in the areas assigned to the nurse manager.

2. A case manager is not responsible for making decisions regarding allocation of resources. A nurse manger is responsible for making decisions regarding allocation of resources within the assigned budget.

3. Case managers are responsible for ensuing continuity of care for patients transitioning back to the community setting with assistance from community resources.

4. Nurse managers and case managers both are responsible for ensuring that patient needs are met in a timely manner within their own area of responsibility.

5. Although a nurse manager ensures that the patient's needs are met within the acute care facility, it is the case manager's responsibility to ensure that a patient's needs are met through the entire health-care system.

TEST-TAKING TIP: Identify the words in the stem that indicates negative polarity. The words *not performed* in the stem indicate negative polarity. The question is asking, "What activity is not performed by a case manager?"

Content Area: Health-Care Delivery
Integrated Processes: Nursing Process: Analysis
Client Need: Safe and Effective Care Environment; Management of Care
Cognitive Level: Analysis

16. **ANSWER: 3.**

Rationales:

1. This statement is related to functional nursing. Functional nursing is a task oriented approach in which certain tasks are assigned to different people. It focuses on efficiency and productivity, but it can lead to fragmentation of care and failure to meet emotional needs of patients.

2. This statement is related to both functional nursing and team nursing, not primary nursing. In primary nursing the nurse communicates laterally with nurses on the other shifts who are assigned to care for the patient.

3. **This statement is related to primary nursing. A registered nurse is responsible for assigned patients throughout a patient's hospitalization, 7 days a week, 24 hours a day (primary nurse). The primary nurse does not deliver all care personally, but is responsible for ensuring that comprehensive and individualized care is delivered.**

4. This statement is related to team nursing. A registered nurse team leader makes assignments based on the abilities of each member of the team, such as registered nurses, licensed practical nurses, and unlicensed nursing assistants. Team members work together and share responsibility for the care of a group of patients. The team leader is responsible for coordinating the team, planning care, and collaborating with professionals in other disciplines and, therefore, often does not provide direct patient care.

Content Area: Health-Care Delivery
Integrated Processes: Nursing Process: Analysis
Client Need: Safe and Effective Care Environment; Management of Care
Cognitive Level: Knowledge

17. **ANSWER: 1, 2.**

Rationales:

1. In this scenario, the nurse is functioning in the role of caregiver. Direct care is given to a patient to meet physical, psychosocial, developmental, sociocultural, and spiritual needs.

2. In this scenario, the nurse is functioning in the role of caregiver.

3. In this scenario, the nurse is functioning in the role of advocate. An advocate protects the patient's personal and legal rights and supports and promotes the patient.

4. In this scenario, the nurse is functioning in the role of leader. A leader influences others to achieve goals.

5. In this scenario, the nurse is functioning in the role of teacher. A teacher presents information, assists with changes in behavior, and teaches skills related to learning self-care.

Content Area: Health-Care Delivery
Integrated Processes: Nursing Process: Implementation
Client Need: Safe and Effective Care Environment; Management of Care
Cognitive Level: Analysis

18. **ANSWER: 4.**

Rationales:

1. A master's degree nursing program prepares registered nurses with a baccalaureate degree in nursing for advanced practice, such as Clinical Nurse Specialist, Certified Nurse Midwife, Nurse Practitioner, nurse administrator, and nurse educator.

2. Continuing education programs generally offer credit hours applicable toward state requirements for renewal of a registered nurse license. These programs are offered by employers, colleges, professional nursing organizations, and professional journals. These programs ensure that nurses keep abreast of new technology, theory, and clinical practice.

3. In-service education programs are provided by employers and focus on such topics as new equipment, policies, or topics mandated by a state health department.

4. A general nursing program usually is a 2-year baccalaureate degree program for graduates of an associate degree nursing program. Generic programs are 3- to 4-year programs for students entering as freshman with a major in nursing.

TEST-TAKING TIP: Identify the word in the stem that sets a priority. The word *most* in the stem sets a priority.

Content Area: Health-Care Delivery
Integrated Processes: Communication/Documentation; Nursing Process: Planning
Client Need: Safe and Effective Care Environment; Management of Care
Cognitive Level: Application

19. **ANSWER: 3.**

Rationales:

1. An assisted living facility will not provide the level of skilled nursing care and medical attention needed by this patient at this time. Assisted living facilities help people with hygiene and dressing and provide meals and activities. Some limited nursing care may be provided, such as assistance with taking medications.

2. A hospice care program provides a medically directed nurse-coordinated program for terminally ill patients and their family members. Generally, this service is provided once the patient no longer seeks curative treatment and the patient is predicted to have less than 6 months to live. Comprehensive palliative care and emotional support for the patient and family members are provided. Grief support is also provided for family members and friends after the death of the patient.

3. **This setting provides skilled nursing and medical attention during the recovery phase of an illness. This setting provides skilled nursing care for a person who is not sick enough to require hospital care but is unable to provide for one's own needs at home (subacute care). In addition, subacute care services may help a patient prevent frequent hospitalization.**

4. A day-care center does not provide the level of skilled nursing care needed by this patient. A day-care center is designed to provide a safe environment for infants, children, and older adults who cannot be left alone at home. Interventions involving socialization, exercise and stimulation, and some noncomplex nursing care, such as help with medications, minor treatments, and counseling, may be provided.

TEST-TAKING TIP: Identify the word in the stem that sets a priority. The word *most* in the stem sets a priority.

Content Area: Health-Care Delivery
Integrated Processes: Nursing Process: Analysis
Client Need: Safe and Effective Care Environment; Management of Care
Cognitive Level: Application

20. ANSWER: 2.
Rationales:
1. The National League for Nursing Accrediting Commission (NLNAC) is responsible for accrediting nursing educational programs, not the American Nurses Association.

2. **The American Nurses Association establishes standards of nursing practice, which is the component of their responsibilities that has the greatest impact on a nurse's daily practice. Standards establish criteria that should be met when delivering nursing care.**

3. Although this is one of the activities of the American Nurses Association, another option has the greatest impact on the quality of nursing care delivered at the bedside.

4. The National Student Nurses Association (NSNA) mentors the professional development of future registered nurses, not the American Nurses Association.

TEST-TAKING TIP: Identify the word in the stem that sets a priority. The word *greatest* is the word in the stem that sets a priority.

Content Area: Health-Care Delivery
Integrated Processes: Communication/Documentation; Nursing Process: Analysis
Client Need: Safe and Effective Care Environment; Management of Care
Cognitive Level: Comprehension

Community-Based Nursing

I. Definitions Related to Community-Based Nursing

Community health-care terms are commonly confused and used interchangeably because they share similarities. However, these terms usually focus on different aspects of health-care delivery in the community. This section provides definitions that attempt to clarify the differences among common terms, such as community, population, community health nursing, community-based nursing care, and public health nursing.

A. Community
1. Group of individuals who share some characteristics, engage in multifaceted relationships, and have the capacity to act collectively.
2. Can include people living within a certain physical boundary (e.g., people living in New York City) or people who share a distinctive feature (e.g., Native Americans).

B. Population (Aggregate)
1. Cluster or group of people with at least one shared specific feature.
2. Examples include high-risk infants, adolescents, older adults, or a cultural group, such as Latino Americans.

C. Community Health Nursing
1. Concerned with protecting, promoting, maintaining, and improving health and quality of life.
2. Provides services to individuals, families, and groups within the context of a population.

D. Community-Based Health Care
1. Focuses on caring for individuals, families, or groups near where they live, work, and play.
2. Community settings include homes, health clinics, schools, assisted-living facilities, rehabilitation centers, nursing homes, and primary health-care providers' offices.

E. Public Health Nursing
1. Focuses on meeting the health needs of populations.
2. Provides services, such as prenatal care, immunizations for children, and screening for illnesses (e.g., tuberculosis, scoliosis), and helps to prevent individual disability and disease (e.g., correct use of automobile restraining devices for children, ways to reduce risk factors for cardiac disease).

II. Community-Based Settings

In addition to outpatient, occupational, extended care, school, and hospice care settings (see Chapter 4), health-care settings have evolved to meet the unique needs of certain populations within the community (e.g., some individuals reside in institutions, whereas others live in areas where health care is inaccessible). Creative initiatives and the use of technology (e.g., internet, fax machines) have increased the number of people who now have access to health care.

A. Mobile Health Clinics
1. Vans or buses with equipment and health-care professionals who provide primary and secondary health-care services at numerous places within a geographic area.
2. Bring health care to the people.
3. Help to service migrant workers, who pose a unique challenge to the provision of health-care services because they move about the country based on the timing of harvests.

B. Faith-Based Organizations
1. Religious organizations that provide health-care services to individuals.
2. Address patients' physical, emotional, and spiritual needs.
3. Activities associated with faith-based organizations.
   a. Coordination and training of volunteers who may provide such services as companionship visits and transportation to and from appointments.
   b. Development and facilitation of support groups.
   c. Referral services to community health-care facilities and programs.
   d. Presentation of programs involving health education, illness prevention, and health promotion.
   e. Discussion and education about health issues on an individual basis.
   f. Facilitation of assimilation of faith and health.

C. Correctional and Prison Environments
1. Provide routine examinations and screenings on a scheduled basis as well as acute care when needed.
2. Generally require nurses to meet certain physical criteria and complete special training to provide for their own safety, such as weapons training and security procedures.

D. Telehealth Care
1. Provides services to people who live in geographic areas where health care is not easily accessible.
2. Allows data to be transmitted via the internet, telephone, or fax machine to primary health-care providers and specialists for consultation.
3. Raises legal and ethical issues (e.g., who is responsible for the patient, how is patient confidentiality protected, and does the health-care provider have to be licensed in the state in which the patient lives?).

DID YOU KNOW?

The National Council of State Boards of Nursing's position on telehealth is that regulations associated with the state in which the patient lives are applicable.

III. Foundations of Community-Based Nursing

To work in the community, a nurse should understand the need for health care to be delivered in community settings and the ways in which health initiatives, such as Healthy People 2020, help a community and its population to achieve a healthier life. In addition, a nurse should understand the characteristics of a healthy community in order to be able to identify the characteristics of an unhealthy community. The following content provides information to help nurses better understand these issues.

A. Issues Promoting the Movement of Health Care Into the Community
1. Federal legislation identified a prospective payment system for Medicare based on illnesses and diseases. The introduction of diagnosis-related groups (DRGs) into the U.S. health-care system, in an effort to control costs, has resulted in patients being discharged sooner and sicker from the hospital to the community.
2. The aging of the U.S. population has resulted in a larger percentage of individuals in the community having chronic illnesses and disabilities, requiring supportive care for the patient and respite care for family members providing care.
3. The number of people who do not seek or cannot afford health care is increasing. Examples include vulnerable populations, such as people who are immigrants, homeless, living below the poverty level, uninsured, cognitively impaired, or abused.
4. The focus of health care is changing from treatment of diseases to health promotion and disease prevention, which emphasizes a nurse's teaching role and requires educating children before unhealthy habits become engrained.

5. More people prefer to die at home rather than in a health-care facility, necessitating the provision of both physical and emotional care for patients and family members.

B. Healthy People 2020 *(www.healthypeople.gov)*
1. A national initiative instituted in 1979, and updated every 10 years, that identifies health improvement goals and priorities and also includes new data on issues and progress achieved toward previous goals.
2. Provides objectives in a format that enables diverse groups to combine their efforts and work as a team.
3. Has a major impact on all health-care programs, but especially on activities and groups concerned with community health needs.
4. Has four overreaching goals, according to the U.S. Department of Health and Human Services (2012).
   a. "Attain high-quality, longer lives free of preventable disease, disability, injury, and premature death."
   b. "Achieve health equity, eliminate disparities, and improve the health of all groups."
   c. "Create social and physical environments that promote good health for all."
   d. "Promote quality of life, healthy development, and healthy behaviors across all life stages."

C. Characteristics of a Healthy Community
1. Has an awareness of its members, populations, and subgroups as being part of the community.
2. Provides opportunities for and encourages participation of individuals and groups in decision making related to issues affecting the community.
3. Ensures that communication remains open and information flows among all members and groups in every direction within the community.
4. Detects, investigates, and dissects problems and collaborates and coordinates a response among members and groups to meet their identified needs.
5. Ensures that community resources are available to all members and groups within the community.
6. Focuses on promoting a high level of wellness and health among all members and populations within the community.
7. Has a well-organized base of community resources available to meet needs and to intervene in a crisis or natural disaster.

IV. Components of a Community Assessment

The provision of nursing care in the community is based on the nursing process (assessment, analysis, planning, implementation, and evaluation). Assessment is the most significant step because it drives the rest of the nursing process. It must be comprehensive and accurate. When performing a community assessment, information must be collected about the physical environment and infrastructure of the community, characteristics of its population, available resources and services, and the economic and social systems within the community. This assessment may be conducted by a community health nurse or in collaboration with others, such as various members of the health-care team, members of community organizations, and government officials.

A. Physical Environment of the Community
1. Natural boundaries and size of the community.
2. Types of housing.
3. Average household income.
4. Location of agencies and resources.

B. Population of the Community
1. Characteristics of community members, such as age, gender, and educational level.
2. Growth trends.
3. Predominant ethnic and religious groups represented.
4. Population density.

C. Safety and Transportation Systems Available to the Population
1. Agencies and status of services provided regarding water and sanitation.
2. Air quality.
3. Telephone service.
4. Numbers of police and emergency services available.
5. Rail and bus systems.

D. Social Services Available to the Community
1. Schools, health-care agencies, and recreational facilities and the programs they provide.
2. Number of health-care providers and services available, such as sources of health-care information, extent of primary care, and home and long-term care services.
3. Number and types of spiritual institutions.
4. Recreational organizations and clubs, such as playgrounds, parks, beaches, and sports centers.

E. Status of the Members of the Community
1. Biological, emotional, and sociological nature of the community.
2. Biological statistics, including data on illness (morbidity) and death (mortality) rates and life expectancy of members of the community.
3. Emotional and sociological statistics, including data on indications of the general mental health of community members and satisfaction or dissatisfaction with characteristics or features of the community.

F. Economic Status of the Community
1. Industries, employers, and occupations within the community.
2. Economic level of the community, such as average household income.

3. Number of workplace health promotion and illness prevention programs.
4. Number of population receiving public assistance.

G. Social System of the Community
1. Statistics related to crime and drug abuse within the community.
2. Percentage of population attending school.
3. Ways communication flows.
4. Extent of interaction among members and groups within the community.
5. Kind of government that runs the community.
6. Extent of participation of members in health-care decision making within the community.
7. Availability of a welfare system to support the needy.
8. Types and extent of volunteer programs.

V. Specific Roles of Community-Based Nurses

Chapter 4, "Health-Care Delivery," explores traditional roles of the nurse and provides examples of nursing activities associated with each role. Here, some traditional roles of the nurse are discussed from the prospective of working within the community. In addition, a role specific to community health nursing—nurse epidemiologist—is presented.

A. Nurse Epidemiologist
1. Provides surveillance and monitoring activities to identify trends in health and risk factors that threaten the health of specific populations or the health of members of the general community.
2. Performs such activities as examining sources of information, case findings, field studies, surveys, and investigations; tracking illnesses, diseases, and death rates; and providing information and reports to appropriate local, state, or national officials.

B. Case Manager
1. Ensures that an appropriate plan of care is formulated and implemented to meet the needs of patients across a continuum of care within the community setting.
2. Coordinates and promotes continuity of care among health-care disciplines.

C. Advocate
1. Assists patients to work their way through the health-care system and obtain appropriate services.
2. Engages in political action at the local, state, or national level to advocate on behalf of the community.

D. Change Agent
1. Mediates within a family system or within the community, empowering people to effect change to better meet health-care needs.
2. Utilizes information related to facilitating change and managing resistance to change to be a more effective change agent.

E. Teacher
1. Focuses on health promotion and disease prevention with individuals and groups through educational activities.
2. Presents programs on such topics as prenatal classes, child safety, dental health, hypertension, and nutrition.
3. Targets groups in schools, community organizations, and businesses.

VI. Specific Competencies of Community-Based Nurses

All nurses should have a strong set of competencies to provide patient-centered, comprehensive, safe, and effective nursing care. However, community-based nurses commonly work autonomously and require in-depth expertise in specific areas of competency. They must be proficient in skills related to communication, collaboration, maintenance of continuity of care, and provision of care to individuals of different ages. In addition, community health nurses must be respectful of the varied values, beliefs, and cultural heritage of the populations within the community.

A. Collaborate With Others
1. Recognize that partnerships, networks, and coalitions are essential to effectively address the health-care needs of members and groups within a community.
2. Maintain collegial working relationships with other health team members to ensure consultation and cooperation in management of the delivery of care.
3. Collaborate with other health-care providers in identifying the need for change in social, political, economic, or health-care systems within the community.
4. Offer suggestions for changes compatible with the norms and values of the community.

B. Communicate With Others
1. Have excellent communication skills when working in a collaborative relationship with other health team members and when communicating with members and groups within a community.
2. Demonstrate respect verbally and nonverbally for the expertise that each professional brings to the team as well as for individual differences among members and groups within the community.

C. Maintain Continuity of Care
1. Coordinate delivery of health-care services between settings (e.g., hospital to home, rehabilitation center to assisted-living facility, or nursing home to hospital) and between and among providers of health care within the community.

⛔ 2. Be involved in discharge planning as soon as a patient is admitted to a hospital or extended-care facility when the person is expected to return to the community.

3. Know the resources, agencies, and services that are available in the community and make referrals on behalf of the patient to support continuity of care.

4. Ensure that, with the patient's consent, family members and significant others are included in the planning process because family members often are the main caregivers.

D. Provide Care Across the Life Span

1. Provide services to patients of all ages from the time they are born until they die.

2. Provide health-care services to special needs populations within different age groups, such as adolescents (e.g., pregnant teens who give birth to low-birth-weight and premature infants), pre-school and school-aged children (e.g., immunization programs, health screening, and nutrition services), and young adults (e.g., services for those who have sexually transmitted diseases or substance abuse problems).

3. Coordinate hospice care to assist terminally ill members of the community to die a peaceful, dignified death.

DID YOU KNOW?

Hospice is a concept, not a place to go to die. Hospice care provides interdisciplinary services that focus on maintaining comfort and quality of life of dying individuals and providing supportive care to grieving family members. Hospice care can be provided in extended-care facilities, freestanding hospices, or in the home. The location depends on the patient's physical and emotional needs and the ability of family members to provide care in the home. Although patients of all ages receive hospice care, a large percentage of these patients are older adults.

VII. Caring for Vulnerable Populations in the Community

A vulnerable population is a group of people who are at an increased risk for health problems because of multiple stressors, unhealthy behaviors, or lack of economic, social, and/or health-related resources. Examples of vulnerable populations include those who are homeless or indigent; immigrants; those who are severely mentally ill, abused, or neglected; older adults; infants and children; substance abusers; and those within a stigmatized population (see Box 5.1).

A. Commonalities of Nursing Care for Vulnerable Populations

1. Provide emotional and culturally sensitive care.

⛔ 2. Provide dignified, respectful, and nonjudgmental care.

Box 5.1 Traits of Vulnerable Populations

- Have a higher probability of developing illness and less favorable outcomes than other populations (because they have a combination of risk factors)
- Have a higher incidence of morbidity and mortality and a shorter life expectancy than the general population
- Have less access to health care
- Have greater difficulty managing reception of services because of a lack of personal and economic resources and dependency on others
- Experience a multiplicity of stressors that challenge delivery of appropriate and adequate health care
- Experience more positive outcomes when their needs are met early in a comprehensive manner before an issue becomes a crisis

---

3. Collaborate with other health-care professionals to ensure that comprehensive care is planned and implemented.

4. Engage patients in the planning process to ensure that they have input and a vested interest in goal achievement.

5. Involve family members in developing a plan of care to address patient needs if the patient gives consent or if the patient is a minor.

6. Establish priorities with the patient's input because what the nurse believes is most important might not be what is most important to the patient.

7. Promote and acknowledge patient abilities to foster independence and increase self-esteem.

8. Make referrals to appropriate community resources and services.

9. Arrange for transportation and child care to facilitate attendance at appointments.

10. Coordinate home-based care if the patient is unable to leave the home or if a vulnerable patient is at risk for not attending health-care services.

11. Arrange for participation in economic support programs, such as food stamps, Medicaid, and the Women, Infants, and Children (WIC) program.

12. Provide assistance for vocational counseling if the patient is able to maintain employment.

B. Individuals Who Are Infants (Birth to 1 Year) or Children

1. Infants and children are dependent on others to meet their physiological and emotional needs.

2. They have immature immune systems to protect themselves from infection.

3. They lack depth and breadth of physiological responses to stress.

4. They lack judgment, which may result in injury.

5. They may be born into a hostile environment (e.g., inadequate nutrition, parents who abuse substances, poverty).

6. Specific nursing care for infants and children.
   a. Ensure that infants and children receive immunizations.
   b. Ensure that they receive routine health care (e.g., initially monthly and then yearly) and dental care.
   c. Educate parents about positive health-care practices (e.g., nutrition, safety practices, and developmental expectations).

C. Individuals Who Are Older Adults

1. Includes a rising percentage of adults over age 85 because of an increase in life span; these frail older adults have multiple health problems, requiring comprehensive health care.
2. Also includes a rising percentage of adults over age 65 because of the aging of the large number of people born between 1946 and 1960 (baby boomer generation); these people have health promotion and illness prevention needs to maintain health and independence.
3. Demonstrate an increase in alcohol use in response to depression, lack of social support, and lack of companionship.
4. Experience socioeconomic stressors, such as retirement, inadequate income, social isolation, downsizing of home and lifestyle, and relocation, which can also cause psychological and physiological stress.
5. Generally live in their own homes, but may have impaired mobility or lack of transportation, which may require services to be provided in the home.

DID YOU KNOW?

Home-care services support independence and help avoid institutionalization of older adults.

6. Specific nursing care for older adults.
   a. Provide opportunities that support the developmental task associated with older adults (integrity versus despair).
   b. Assess patients for substance use (e.g., polypharmacy) and alcohol and prescription drug abuse.
   c. Encourage patients to engage in social activities available in the community.
   d. Arrange for home-care services so that older adults are able to remain in their own homes for as long as possible.
   e. Arrange for respite care that relieves family members from the caregiving role; varies in duration, from as short as a few hours so a family member can go to a movie or shop, to a week or more admission to a nursing home while a family attends an event or goes on vacation.

D. Individuals Who Are Homeless or Indigent

1. Generally live in substandard housing or in hazardous conditions, such as insect-or vermin-infested environments, or live outside in the elements.
2. Are less healthy because of such factors as inadequate nutrition, inaccessible facilities in which to bathe and wash clothes, inadequate rest, and absence of preventive health care, such as immunizations and health screenings.
3. Are at increased risk for accidental injury, assault, abuse, and infectious diseases, such as tuberculosis and skin and respiratory infections.
4. Have a higher incidence of severe mental illness, alcoholism, illegal drug use, and smoking than the general population.
5. Specific nursing care for homeless and indigent individuals and families.
   a. Help patients find mobile health clinics, soup kitchens, shelters, thrift shops, and housing.
   b. Teach the importance of and ways to maintain a clean, healthy environment.
   c. Teach homeless people ways to avoid violence.

E. Individuals Who Are Immigrants

1. Generally do not speak English well enough to communicate needs or find resources that support health and wellness and treat illness.
2. If in the country illegally, often do not seek health care until acutely ill because of a fear of being deported.
3. Often cannot afford health insurance or health-care services because of low paying jobs or dependence on day work.
4. Present with specific health problems, such as tuberculosis, intestinal parasites, dental decay, and hepatitis B.
5. May have experienced a traumatic event, such as war, natural disaster, lack of economic opportunity, or oppression, and are at risk for emotional distress.
6. Frequently engage in nontraditional healing practices that may or may not be helpful.
7. Specific nursing care for immigrant populations.
   a. Learn as much as possible about the patient's culture and its impact on the patient's health-care needs.
   b. Be sensitive to cultural values and beliefs and demonstrate respect for nontraditional healing practices unless they are harmful to the patient.
   c. Assess the patient for signs and symptoms of specific health problems unique to the patient's history, culture, and environment.
   d. Use a professional interpreter so that information can be correctly translated and confidentiality can be maintained; ensure that all questions are answered and understood to promote patient participation in the planning process.

F. Individuals Who Engage in Substance Abuse

1. Includes individuals who abuse illegal or prescription drugs and alcohol.
2. Often have economic and legal issues as well as health problems related to substance abuse, such as the expense of supporting the habit, arrest and conviction related to illegal activities acquiring drugs, and infectious disease as a result of sharing drug supplies.
3. Often experience a breakdown of the family and loss of support systems as the substance abuse becomes the focus of activities or because of abusive behavior.
4. Often present with complex medical problems (e.g., cocaine use can cause nasal, sinus, and cardiac problems; alcohol abuse can cause liver cirrhosis).
5. Specific nursing care for patients who engage in substance abuse.
   a. Observe for signs and symptoms of substance abuse, such as multiple missed appointments, chief complaint of insomnia or "bad nerves," multiple health-care providers, medication bottles with different provider names, requests for frequent refills of sedatives or analgesics, history of frequent sexually transmitted diseases, multiple abortions, gastrointestinal illnesses, chest pain or palpitations, and family history of addiction.
   b. Encourage patient participation in a substance abuse program.
   c. Refer the patient to appropriate legal services.

G. Individuals Who Are Mentally Ill

1. Are routinely cared for in the community rather than in psychiatric facilities.
2. Often refuse to take prescribed medications, which worsens their health status.
3. Often unable to self-perform activities of daily living.
4. Generally incapable of retaining a job, commonly resulting in their living below the poverty level and becoming homeless.
5. Often have many of the same needs as those of indigent and homeless people.
6. Specific nursing care for severely mentally ill individuals.
   a. Arrange for the patient to attend a day-care program for individuals with mental illness, if appropriate.
   🛑 b. Arrange for admission to a psychiatric facility if the patient becomes a danger to self or others.

H. Individuals Who Are Abused or Neglected

1. Includes those who are physically, emotionally, or sexually abused in addition to those who are neglected.

2. Most commonly are women, children, or older adults.
3. Have risk factors such as a relationship with another person who has a mental illness, an addiction (e.g., alcohol, drugs, gambling, sex), or a socioeconomic issue, such as excessive spending or lack of income.
4. Can receive help from community services in most communities, such as:
   a. The Victim Information Bureau that provides referrals to related services.
   b. Rape crisis centers that provide counseling and comprehensive services 24 hours a day.
   c. Emergency department companion programs that provide trained rape crisis counselors that meet children and adults in hospital emergency departments; the counselors provide nonjudgmental emotional support, information, referrals, and a change of clothes.
   d. Sexual assault nurse examiner (SANE) programs that provide special education to nurses so that they can care for rape victims in a SANE center (designated hospitals) by providing victim-centered care, medical evaluations, preventive medication for pregnancy and sexually transmitted diseases, evidence collection and storage, and a change of clothes.
   e. Multitude of programs that support children, adults, and family members individually and in groups when in crisis and when in need of continued support to resolve issues caused by an abusive event.
   f. Referral to an agency that provides an emergency safe haven or shelter.
   g. Access to counselors who provide support and advice as a victim and family members navigate the legal system.
5. Specific nursing care for abused individuals.
   a. Identify signs and symptoms of abuse or neglect (Box 5.2).
   b. Provide privacy when interviewing patients; ensure that interviews take place out of sight and hearing of suspected abusers (abused patients may fear retribution).
   🛑 c. Encourage patients who are currently unwilling to leave their abusive environments to have an exit plan, including a packed bag of clothes and toiletries, in the event a quick escape is necessary.
   d. Provide the telephone number of a domestic abuse hotline in the event immediate advice and emotional support is needed; instruct patients to memorize the phone number.
   e. Encourage patients to call 911 if personal safety is in immediate jeopardy.

Box 5.2 Signs of Abuse and Neglect

Child Sexual Abuse

- Vaginal or penile discharge
- Pain, itching, or trauma in the genital area
- Sexually transmitted disease
- Recurrent urinary tract infections
- Regressed behavior
- Fear of certain people or places
- Play that recreates sexual abuse
- Decreasing performance in school

Older Adult Abuse and Neglect

- Fractures or trauma inconsistent with stated cause
- Cigarette burns
- Scratches
- Bruising at different stages of recovery
- Chafing at ankles and wrists, indicating use of restraint
- Prolonged gap between injury and seeking of medical attention
- Dependence on caregiver
- Physical or cognitive impairment
- Combativeness

Domestic Abuse

- Fractures or trauma inconsistent with stated cause
- Multiple injuries involving face, head, breasts, and genitalia
- Ecchymotic areas around eyes, face, or neck
- Fractured nose or eye orbits
- Broken teeth
- Bruises at different stages of recovery
- X-ray evidence of old fractures
- Sense of helplessness, guilt, depression, or low self-esteem
- History of panic attacks, headaches, or anxiety

    f. When sexual abuse of a child is suspected, ensure that a child protective services counselor and a sexual assault nurse examiner or a primary health-care provider are present.
    g. For an adult who is sexually abused, ensure that a rape counselor and a primary health-care provider or sexual assault nurse examiner are present.
    h. Arrange for patients to be sheltered in a safe environment.
    i. Refer patients and family members to available community services.

 j. Report abuse or neglect when appropriate.

DID YOU KNOW?

All states mandate that nurses report suspected abuse or neglect of children to appropriate authorities, and most states mandate that nurses report suspected abuse or neglect of older adults and developmentally or cognitively impaired individuals to appropriate officials. Laws concerning reporting spousal abuse (i.e., intimate partner violence) and rape vary widely because some people believe that reporting violates the autonomy of the person being abused. Also, an adult patient who states that she or he is a victim of rape has to be the person who reports the rape to the authorities. However, a nurse should do everything possible to advocate for the patient.

I. **Individuals Who Are Within a Stigmatized Population**
  1. Often feel unaccepted and discriminated against and lack status and power.
  2. Includes individuals who have communicable diseases (e.g., human immunodeficiency virus [HIV], acquired immunodeficiency syndrome [AIDS], tuberculosis, hepatitis C), are mentally ill, or engage in behaviors that are denounced (e.g., substance abuse).
  3. Specific nursing care for stigmatized populations.
     a. Teach individuals who engage in high-risk behaviors ways to protect themselves from infection, such as using condoms and avoiding needle sharing.
     b. Refer patients who have HIV or AIDS to an HIV coordinator because these professionals have expertise to meet the needs of this vulnerable population.
     c. Provide patients with choices and opportunities to participate in planning care in an effort to empower them.

MAKING THE CONNECTION

Healthy People 2020 and Improved Health and Quality of Life

Healthy People 2020 sets objectives to improve the health and quality of life of people and communities and to reduce health disparities associated with vulnerable populations. The Healthy People Consortium & Partners, instituted by Healthy People 2020, is a rich resource for helping communities address health issues. In addition, The MAP-IT framework (Mobilize, Assess, Plan, Implement, Track) provides a foundation upon which to plan and evaluate community health initiatives. Nurses working in a community setting should have a thorough understanding of Healthy People 2020 and the resources available to assist them in addressing the needs of their community. For example, a public health nurse completes a community assessment and identifies that the health-care needs of homeless people are not being met. The nurse uses data provided by Healthy People 2020 to demonstrate the issues, networks with resources available through the Healthy People Consortium & Partners for advice and direction, and then uses the MAP-IT framework to design an initiative that addresses the needs of the homeless. Also, the nurse may use information from Healthy People 2020 to identify funding sources to underwrite the cost of implementing the program for the homeless in the community. Once the initiative is implemented, the nurse can track the outcomes of the initiative using the track guidelines in the MAP-IT framework.

CASE STUDY: Putting It All Together

A community health nurse working in the state of Florida in the United States performs a community assessment. Through surveillance and monitoring activities, the nurse identifies that at-risk populations within the community include older adults, immigrants, and homeless migrant workers. The nurse designs several initiatives to address the needs of these populations. Educational programs to address smoking cessation, nutrition, prenatal care, child safety, and ways to cope with the physiological changes of aging are presented throughout the community. The nurse works with a variety of community organizations, such as social organizations, to provide companions or drivers for older adults; the department of social services to obtain financial support for individuals and families; church groups to provide meals and places to sleep for the homeless; and governmental representatives to campaign for changes in immigration laws. Periodically, the nurse communicates with the members of the community and various agencies involved, keeping lines of communication open to collaboratively evaluate the effectiveness of initiatives and identify emerging needs.

Case Study Questions

A. What factors common to all of the at-risk populations make them at an increased risk for health problems?

1. _____
2. _____
3. _____
4. _____
5. _____

B. Identify and validate the roles the nurse assumed to meet the needs of vulnerable populations.

1. _____
2. _____
3. _____
4. _____

C. What specific competencies did the nurse exhibit in this scenario?

1. _____
2. _____
3. _____

D. What types of health-care services should be available to assist individuals who do not have access to health care?

1. _____
2. _____
3. _____
4. _____
5. _____
6. _____
7. _____
8. _____
9. _____
10. _____

REVIEW QUESTIONS

1. With what is community health nursing mainly associated?
   1. Delivering home health-care services
   2. Assisting economically disadvantaged high-risk groups
   3. Addressing the nursing needs of individuals or groups within the community
   4. Providing interventions that help people on the health end of the health–illness continuum

2. In what way is a home health-care nursing practice different from the acute care setting?
   1. The family is encouraged to provide emotional support.
   2. The patient is responsible for formulating outcomes.
   3. The nursing process is used as a framework for care.
   4. The nurse functions more autonomously.

3. The focus of the delivery of health care has changed from treatment to prevention. An increased emphasis on what aspect of nursing care will result?
   1. Community care
   2. Intensive care services
   3. Evidence-based practice
   4. Pathophysiology of illness

4. What focus is unique to community health practice when compared to acute health care?
   1. Family focused
   2. Individual focused
   3. Population focused
   4. Geographically focused

5. Which type of care is not designed to assist individuals and families with care in the home?
   1. Acute care
   2. Respite care
   3. Hospice care
   4. Restorative care

6. A nurse is preparing a health promotion class for individuals in the community. Which of the following topics should the nurse address because they are among the 10 indicators that are studied to determine if progress is made toward health goals identified in Healthy People 2020? **Select all that apply.**
   1. _____ Obesity
   2. _____ Tobacco use
   3. _____ Heart disease
   4. _____ Family planning
   5. _____ Physical activity

7. Which is **most** important when providing services to homeless individuals?
   1. Being aware of cultural beliefs
   2. Helping to find a source of food
   3. Teaching how to bathe in a public restroom
   4. Arranging for attendance at a day-care program

8. A nurse is caring for a patient who was brought to the emergency department by her husband who did not leave the wife's side and was overly solicitous. After a physical examination and an x-ray, the patient was diagnosed with a fractured arm. The patient stated that she is constantly clumsy. When the nurse assisted the patient into a hospital gown, the nurse identified multiple old bruises. The nurse suspects physical abuse. What should the nurse do **first**?
   1. Suggest preparation of an exit plan if the patient is reluctant to leave the abusive environment.
   2. Interview the patient outside the vision and hearing of the suspected husband.
   3. Report the suspected physical abuse of the patient to appropriate officials.
   4. Instruct the patient to call the police if personal safety is in jeopardy.

9. A school nurse, when performing scoliosis screening on a 12-year-old female student, identifies that the girl has multiple bruises on the arms and thighs. The school nurse talks with the student, reviews the student's school file, and interviews the student's classroom teacher.

▌ Additional Information

Student Interview

"My mom and I moved in with my mom's new boyfriend a couple of months ago. He has an 8-year-old girl and a 17-year-old boy. I have to go home right after school to babysit the girl. I hate living with them. The boy gives me a hard time and has beaten me up a couple of times. My mom doesn't believe me and tells me to stop making trouble. I can hear my mom crying at night after her boyfriend hits her. A couple of weeks ago, he hit me too. I am afraid he is going to start hitting me again."

Student's School File

Has had three different home addresses in the last year
   Grades have declined from a B average to a D+ average in the last 2 months
   Has been absent from school for a total of 15 days in the last 3 months
   Withdrew from participation in the marching band

Classroom Teacher Interview

"Over the past several months, I have noticed that she has become very quiet and has limited interaction with the boys in the class. Several times, I saw that she had some bruises. One time, she said she fell off her bike, and another time she said she fell down the front steps at home. I know her grades have declined, but she is not doing her homework. I try to support her the best that I can in class."

What is the **best** nursing intervention based on these assessments?
   1. Arrange for the mother to come to the school for a parent-nurse conference.
   2. Telephone the boyfriend to confirm the student's accusations.
   3. Call the public health nurse to make a home visit.
   4. Notify the authorities of suspected child abuse.

10. A nurse working in the community is functioning as a nurse epidemiologist. Which action implemented by the nurse is associated with this role?
    1. Monitors for risk factors that threaten the health of members of the community
    2. Engages in political action to represent health needs on behalf of members of the community
    3. Focuses on health promotion for groups of people as well as individuals within the community
    4. Ensures that plans of care meet patients' needs across the continuum of care within the community

11. A patient is diagnosed with pulmonary tuberculosis and must attend a clinic every week for treatment and follow-up health care. Which is **most** important to ensure that the patient is cured of tuberculosis when providing care in the community setting?
    1. Provide the patient with assistance regarding vocational counseling.
    2. Seek economic support for the patient, such as Medicaid, during recovery.
    3. Have the patient set the outcome criteria for the plan of care independently.
    4. Arrange home-based care if the patient is at risk for non-attendance at appointments.

12. A nurse is completing a community assessment to identify the status of the members of the community. Which information is **most** significant when identifying the health needs of the community in this area?
    1. Natural boundaries and size of the community
    2. Employers and occupations within the community
    3. Morbidity and mortality rates related to the community
    4. Crime rates and drug abuse associated with the community

13. Which setting for the provision of health-care services in the community is at the highest risk for potential legal and ethical issues?
    1. Migrant services
    2. Telehealth services
    3. Faith-based services
    4. Prison-based services

14. A public health nurse analyzes statistics about health issues in the community and identifies that domestic violence against women and their children is on the rise. Place the following interventions in the order in which they should be implemented to address this health-related problem.
    1. Design and implement outreach initiatives to access the targeted population.
    2. Identify the social system of the community and the social services available.
    3. Make referrals to appropriate community resources and arrange for transportation if needed.
    4. Collaborate with health-care professionals and women who personally have successfully dealt with this issue.
    5. Engage each individual in developing a personal plan for safety and acknowledge patient abilities to increase self-esteem.
    Answer: _____

15. A mother brings her 7-year-old daughter to the emergency department. The child has a high fever, reports cramping discomfort in the lower abdomen, and is sucking her thumb. The mother is concerned about possible sexual abuse because the daughter was cared for by an uncle while she and her husband were on vacation. What should the nurse do **first** before a physical examination of the child?
    1. Collect a urine specimen for a culture and sensitivity test.
    2. Interview the child to assess for clinical indicators of assault.
    3. Ask the mother to leave the bedside so that the child can be examined.
    4. Ensure that a sexual abuse health-care worker is present during the child's care.

1. **ANSWER: 3.**
Rationales:
1. The home setting traditionally was associated with the concept of community nursing. However, in the current health-care environment, the community includes such settings as schools, work environments, community centers, neighborhood clinics, and even mobile units that bring services directly to people in a neighborhood.
2. Community-based health activities are designed to help individuals and groups across all economic levels and low- as well as high-risk groups.
3. Community health nursing reaches out to people and groups outside of acute-care facilities. Services are provided in neighborhoods, which includes the home.
4. Community-based nursing assists individuals and groups from one end of the health–illness continuum to the other, not just the health end of the continuum.
TEST-TAKING TIP: Identify the word in the stem that sets a priority. The word *mainly* in the stem sets a priority. Identify the option with a clang association. The word *community* in the stem and in option 3 is a clang association.
Content Area: Community-Based Nursing
Integrated Processes: Nursing Process: Analysis
Client Need: Safe and Effective Care Environment; Management of Care
Cognitive Level: Comprehension

2. **ANSWER: 4.**
Rationales:
1. Family members are encouraged to provide emotional support to patients in all settings.
2. In all settings in which a nurse works, the nurse and the patient ideally formulate realistic, achievable, measurable, and acceptable goals together, not in isolation.
3. The nursing process is used in all settings in which the nurse works to identify and meet the actual and potential human responses to illness, disease, or injury.
4. The nurse functions more independently in the home setting, whereas in the acute setting, resources are immediately available for consultation and support.
TEST-TAKING TIP: Identify the central person in the question. The nurse in option 4 is the central person in the question.
Content Area: Community-Based Nursing
Integrated Processes: Nursing Process: Implementation
Client Need: Safe and Effective Care Environment; Management of Care
Cognitive Level: Knowledge

3. **ANSWER: 1.**
Rationales:
1. Health care is moving from the hospital to the community in response to an increased emphasis on health promotion and illness prevention. The words in the stem *changed from treatment to prevention* directs the nurse to the trend in health care whereby people are cared for more in the community rather than the acute-care environment. Also, because of prospective hospital reimbursement, lengths of stay are decreasing as patients are discharged more quickly than in the past and must rely on community resources to make the transition safely.
2. Intensive care areas are concerned with treatment, not prevention.
3. Evidence-based practice is associated with making decisions regarding nursing care based on some form of validation or demonstrated proof of superiority. Results of evidence-based practice research apply to all aspects of nursing care.
4. Primary health-care providers are more concerned about the pathophysiology of illness. Nursing practice, regardless of the setting, focuses on reacting to human responses.
Content Area: Community-Based Nursing
Integrated Processes: Nursing Process: Analysis
Client Need: Safe and Effective Care Environment; Management of Care
Cognitive Level: Comprehension

4. **ANSWER: 3.**
Rationales:
1. The family is included in both acute care and community health care.
2. Individuals are included in both acute care and community health care.
3. A characteristic of community health is that it focuses on the health status of people in an aggregate (people who, as a group, form a distinct population).
4. Neither acute care nor community health care is focused solely by geographic area. People who are served may come from different geographic areas, and groups can be identified by a variety of factors, such as common interests (e.g., citizens concerned about air pollution) or similar problems (e.g., homelessness, single-parent families).
TEST-TAKING TIP: Identify opposite options. Options 2 and 3 are opposites. In this situation, one of them is the correct answer.
Content Area: Community-Based Nursing
Integrated Processes: Nursing Process: Analysis
Client Need: Safe and Effective Care Environment; Management of Care
Cognitive Level: Knowledge

5. **ANSWER: 1.**
Rationales:
1. Acute care is provided by institutions with the highly skilled, intensive, specialized services that are provided by hospitals.
2. Respite care provides services so that caregivers can get relief from the stress of their responsibilities. Respite care can be provided in the home or nursing home setting.
3. Hospice care offers services that enable dying persons to stay at home with the support needed to die with dignity.
4. Restorative care, efforts that seek to reduce disability and reestablish function, is related to rehabilitation. Recovering lost functions or developing new compensating skills is commonly accomplished in the home setting.
TEST-TAKING TIP: Identify the word in the stem that indicates negative polarity. The word *not* in the stem indicates negative polarity.
Content Area: Community-Based Nursing
Integrated Processes: Nursing Process: Analysis
Client Need: Safe and Effective Care Environment; Management of Care
Cognitive Level: Knowledge

6. ANSWER: 1, 2, 5.

Rationales:

1. Obesity is one of the 10 leading health indicators identified in Healthy People 2020 that, when addressed, may motivate people to take action toward health promotion and illness prevention. Obesity increases the risks of many diseases, such as hypertension, cardiac disease, diabetes, osteoporosis, and so on.

2. Tobacco use is one of the 10 leading health indicators identified in Healthy People 2020 that, when addressed, may motivate people to take action toward health promotion and illness prevention. Smoking contributes to lung diseases, such as chronic obstructive pulmonary disease, emphysema, bronchitis, asthma, and lung cancer.

3. Heart disease is one of the 28 focus areas, not a health indicator, identified in Healthy People 2020.

4. Family planning is one of the 28 focus areas, not a health indicator, identified in Healthy People 2020.

5. Physical activity is one of the 10 leading health indicators identified in Healthy People 2020 that, when addressed, may motivate people to take action toward health promotion and illness prevention. People who engage in physical activity reduce the risks of heart disease, depression, colon cancer, and diabetes; activity increases muscle tone, muscle strength, and weight loss and contributes to psychological well-being.

Content Area: Community-Based Nursing
Integrated Processes: Teaching/Learning; Nursing Process: Planning
Client Need: Safe and Effective Care Environment; Management of Care
Cognitive Level: Analysis

7. ANSWER: 2.

Rationales:

1. Although this is important, it is associated with meeting a patient's need to feel accepted and to have self-esteem supported, third and fourth level needs respectively, according to Maslow's hierarchy of needs. Lower level needs must be met first before moving on to meeting higher level needs

2. Helping a homeless person find a source of food is the priority. Meeting nutrition needs is a first level need according to Maslow's hierarchy of needs.

3. Although this may be done, it is associated with preventing infection, which is related to safety and security, a second level need according to Maslow's hierarchy of needs. A first level need is the priority.

4. Day-care programs are not designed to care for homeless people. Day-care programs generally are designed to assist in meeting the needs of people who are mentally ill or older adults who need a sheltered environment during the day while family members are at work.

TEST-TAKING TIP: Identify the word in the stem that sets a priority. The word *most* in the stem sets a priority. Use Maslow's hierarchy of needs to help establish the priority.

Content Area: Community-Based Nursing
Integrated Processes: Caring; Nursing Process: Implementation
Client Need: Health Promotion and Maintenance
Cognitive Level: Application

8. ANSWER: 2.

Rationales:

1. Although this should be done if the nurse suspects physical abuse, it is not the priority.

2. This is the first thing the nurse should do if physical abuse is suspected. The patient is more likely to discuss physical abuse when not threatened by the presence of the suspected abuser.

3. This is premature. The nurse should first assess the patient in more detail. There is not enough evidence based on the data presented in the question to report suspected abuse to the appropriate officials.

4. Although this should be done if a nurse suspects physical abuse, it is not the priority.

TEST-TAKING TIP: Identify the word in the stem that sets a priority. The word *first* in the stem sets a priority. Identify the clang associations. The word *husband* in the stem and in option 2 is a clang association. The word *abuse* in the stem and the word *abusive* in option 1 is a clang association. The words *suspected physical abuse* in the stem and in option 3 is a clang association. Examine options 1, 2, and 3 carefully because they all contain clang associations.

Content Area: Community-Based Nursing
Integrated Processes: Caring; Communication/ Documentation; Nursing Process: Implementation
Client Need: Psychosocial Integrity
Cognitive Level: Application

9. ANSWER: 4.

Rationales:

1. The time it takes to arrange and conduct a parent-nurse conference may delay keeping the student safe. If confronted, the mother probably will deny the allegations. Also, this is not the role of a school nurse.

2. This is an unsafe intervention. Confronting the boyfriend to confirm the student's accusations will place the student in greater jeopardy. Also, this is not the role of a school nurse.

3. A school nurse does not have the authority to make a referral to a public health nurse. A person with a prescriptive license (e.g., physician, nurse practitioner, physician's assistant) has the authority to make a referral to a public health nurse.

4. Nurses have the responsibility and authority to report suspected cases of child abuse to the authorities. The nurse must be an advocate for the student to protect her from further harm. A home assessment will be made by the authorities and appropriate actions taken if necessary.

Content Area: Community-Based Nursing
Integrated Processes: Caring; Communication/ Documentation; Nursing Process: Implementation
Client Need: Safe and Effective Care Environment; Management of Care
Cognitive Level: Analysis

10. ANSWER: 1.

Rationales:

1. An epidemiologist implements surveillance monitoring activities to identify trends in health in addition to the presence of risk factors that have the potential to threaten the health of specific populations and the health of members of the general community.

2. This is the role of nurse advocate, not epidemiologist. In addition, the nurse working in the community functions as an advocate by assisting patients to work their way through the health-care system to obtain appropriate services.

3. This is the role of nurse educator, not epidemiologist.

4. This is the role of a nurse case manager, not epidemiologist.

Content Area: Community-Based Nursing
Integrated Processes: Nursing Process: Implementation
Client Need: Health Promotion and Maintenance
Cognitive Level: Comprehension

11. ANSWER: 4.

Rationales:

1. Although vocational counseling should be discussed, this will not cure the patient of tuberculosis.

2. Although the nurse may seek sources of financial assistance for the patient, this will not cure the patient of tuberculosis.

3. The patient should not be setting outcome criteria for the plan of care independently. The nurse and patient should identify outcomes and the plan to achieve the outcomes in a collaborative manner. Because tuberculosis is a communicable disease, outcomes have to be formulated that protect the public as well as the patient. For example, "The patient knows and implements at least 5 actions that will help reduce the risk of transmission of microorganisms to others or the environment." A patient acting independently may not be capable of identifying this as an essential outcome.

4. It is essential that patients with infections receive appropriate anti-infective medication according to the plan of care. Anti-infectives associated with any infection must be taken consistently, as ordered, to be effective. Since tuberculosis is a communicable disease and a public health risk, it is essential that a plan be placed in effect if a patient is at risk for not attending a treatment program. Home-care visits help to ensure that the treatment plan is being followed to meet the needs of the patient and protect people in the community.

Content Area: Community-Based Nursing
Integrated Processes:
Nursing Process: Implementation
Client Need: Safe and Effective Care Environment;
Management of Care
Cognitive Level: Application

12. ANSWER: 3.

Rationales:

1. This information reflects the physical environment of the community.

2. This information is associated with the economic status of the community.

3. Morbidity and mortality rates reflect the status of the members of the community.

4. This information is related to the social system of a community.

TEST-TAKING TIP: Identify the word in the stem that sets a priority. The word *most* in the stem sets a priority.

Content Area: Community-Based Nursing
Integrated Processes: Nursing Process: Implementation
Client Need: Health Promotion and Maintenance
Cognitive Level: Comprehension

13. ANSWER: 2.

Rationales:

1. This setting generally is at no greater risk for legal or ethical concerns than other traditional settings. Health-care services generally are provided in mobile clinics when meeting the health-care needs of migrant workers. However, these services present a unique challenge because workers and their family members move about the country based on the timing of harvests.

2. Telehealth services are at the highest risk for potential legal and ethical issues because they require data to be transmitted via the internet, telephone, or fax to primary health-care providers and specialists for consultation. Questions arise, such as: Who is responsible for the patient? How is confidentiality maintained? Does the primary health-care provider have to be licensed in the state in which the patient lives?

3. Faith-based settings generally are at no greater risk for legal or ethical concerns than other traditional settings. Faith-based settings generally offer services in regulated settings, such as hospitals, nursing homes, and clinics. Educational programs generally are provided by licensed health-care workers. In addition, volunteers usually provide supportive non-professional assistance, such as transportation and companionship, only after the volunteer meets training and educational criteria.

4. Prison-based settings generally are at no greater risk for legal or ethical concerns than other traditional settings. Prison-based care generally offers services in a regulated setting, such as a clinic or hospital-like unit within the prison. However, nurses working in a prison-based setting generally are required to meet special training to provide for their own safety.

TEST-TAKING TIP: Identify the word in the stem that sets a priority. The word *highest* in the stem sets a priority.

Content Area: Community-Based Nursing
Integrated Processes: Communication/Documentation;
Nursing Process: Analysis
Client Need: Safe and Effective Care Environment;
Management of Care
Cognitive Level: Analysis

14. ANSWER: 4, 2, 1, 5, 3.

Rationales:

4. Collaboration with health-care professionals involves people who have expertise in relation to the issue. Collaboration with women who personally have successfully dealt with this issue ensures that the discussion remains reality based.

2. Identification of the social system of the community and the social services available within the community are part of the assessment of the community. An assessment of the community also should include the physical environment and economic status of the community, the characteristics and status of its population, and the safety and transportation systems available.

1. After a problem is identified and explored with all significant people involved, then initiatives can be devised and carried out. The people in the target population must be reached before they can be helped.

5. Plans of care must be individualized. Women must be involved in the planning process to ensure that they have input and a vested interest in goal achievement. Women who are victims of domestic violence often feel overwhelmed, powerless, and helpless. Increasing self-esteem may be an initial step toward feeling empowered.
3. Once a plan is in place, then the appropriate community services should be made available to the woman, and every effort should be made to ensure that the woman is physically and emotionally supported.
Content Area: Community-Based Nursing
Integrated Processes: Caring; Communication/ Documentation; Nursing Process: Analysis
Client Need: Safe and Effective Care Environment; Management of Care
Cognitive Level: Analysis

15. **ANSWER: 4.**
    Rationales:
    1. This is not the priority at this time. However, this should be done before an antibiotic is initiated to treat an infection, such as a sexually transmitted infection or urinary tract infection.
    2. An interview with the child should be conducted by a trained sexual abuse health-care worker after the sexual abuse health-care worker has established a relationship with the child.
    3. The mother should remain with the daughter to provide emotional support at this time. If after further assessment there is a suspicion that the mother is the perpetrator of the sexual assault, the child should be interviewed out of the presence of the mother. This interview should be conducted by a sexual abuse health-care worker only after building a relationship with the child.
    4. This is the first thing that the nurse should do. A sexual abuse health-care worker is trained to meet the emotional and physical needs of a patient who has been sexually abused as well as meet the emotional needs of a nonabusive parent of a child who has been sexually abused.
    TEST-TAKING TIP: Identify the word in the stem that sets a priority. The word *first* in the stem sets a priority. Identify the clang association. The words *sexual abuse* in the stem and in option 4 are a clang association. Examine option 4 carefully.
    Content Area: Community-Based Nursing
    Integrated Processes: Caring; Nursing Process: Implementation
    Client Need: Safe and Effective Care Environment; Management of Care
    Cognitive Level: Application

Psychosocio-cultural Nursing Care

Chapter 6

Nursing Care Across the Life Span

KEY TERMS

Cooperative (associative) play—Child engaging in group play without rigid rules.

Egocentric—View of self as the center of the universe.

Male menopause (manopause, andropause)—Decreased production of androgens, such as testosterone, that results in decreased vigor and sexual desire; usually occurs between ages 45 and 55.

Menarche—Initiation of first menstruation.

Menopause—Permanent cessation of menstruation in women; usually occurs between ages 45 and 50.

Object permanence—Realization that objects moved out of sight still exist.

Parallel play—Child playing alongside, not with, other children.

Peer pressure—Intimidating, coercive behavior designed to persuade an individual to engage in activities in which the individual does not want to participate.

Puberty—Interval when secondary sex characteristics emerge and the ability to sexually reproduce occurs.

Role playing—Acting out of a character in a protective environment to practice a response that can be used when confronted with a similar situation in real life.

Separation anxiety—Child's infuriation, frustration, and fear precipitated by parental absence.

Stranger anxiety—Child's fear of people who are unfamiliar.

Therapeutic play—Use of toys, crafts, puppets, and other tools to assist a child to express feelings or concerns or to learn something new.

I. Infant

Infants are babies from 1 to 12 months of age. During this stage of development, babies experience dramatic physiological and psychosocial maturation as they begin to differentiate self from others.

A. Development
1. Physical.
   a. Weight triples.
   b. Chest measurement approaches head circumference.
   c. Has 6 to 8 teeth.
   d. Turns from abdomen to back by 5 months and back to abdomen by 6 months.
   e. Sits by 7 months.
   f. Crawls, pulls self up, and uses pincer grasp by 9 months.
   g. Walks holding on by 11 months.

2. Psychosocial.
   a. Oral phase of psychosexual development; infants obtain pleasure from oral gratification through stimulation of mouth, lips, and tongue.
   b. Is confronted with resolving the conflict of trust versus mistrust that leads to faith and optimism; if basic trust is not satisfied, the infant becomes insecure, fearful, and mistrusting.
   c. Is egocentric.
   d. Wants immediate gratification at 1 month; is able to tolerate some frustration and delay gratification at 8 months.
   e. Smiles and focuses on bright objects by 2 months.
   f. Laughs by 4 months.
   g. Has beginnings of separation anxiety at 4 to 8 months.
   h. Fears strangers by 6 to 8 months.

3. Cognitive.
   a. Sensorimotor phase; reflexes replaced by voluntary activity.
   b. Begins to understand cause and effect by 1 to 4 months.
   c. Realizes objects moved out of sight still exist (object permanence) by 9 to 10 months.
   d. Responds to own name and cries when reprimanded at 10 months.
   e. Uses and understands gestures, explores surroundings, throws kisses, gives hugs, may cling to security blanket or toy, and recognizes self as distinct from the environment by 12 months.
4. Language.
   a. Uses crying to signal displeasure during first 6 months.
   b. Babbles by 3 months.
   c. Imitates sounds by 6 months.
   d. Reacts to simple commands by 9 months.
   e. Says 1 word by 10 months; says 3 to 5 words and understands 100 words by 12 months.
5. Play.
   a. Plays alone (solitary play); revolves around own body.
   b. Play becomes more interactive and shows toy preferences by 3 to 6 months.
   c. Play involves sensorimotor skills by 6 to 12 months.
   d. Smiles at own image at 5 months.
   e. Enjoys peek-a-boo and bouncing in chairs at 7 months.
   f. Clutches soft objects at 8 months.
   g. Enjoys picture books at 10 months.
   h. Enjoys rough house play at 12 months.
6. Reaction to illness, hospitalization, and pain.
   a. Younger infant.
      (1) Recognizes pain, but is not emotionally traumatized by intrusive procedures.
      (2) Responses include high-pitched cry, irritability, tearing, stiff posture, fisting, brows lowered and drawn together, eyes tightly closed, mouth open, and difficulty sleeping and eating.
   b. Older infant.
      (1) Recognizes pain and may exhibit localized body response.
      (2) Responses include loud crying, facial expression of pain and anger, deliberate withdrawal of site affected by external stimulus, and pushing away of external stimulus.

B. Nursing Care
   1. Assess developmental level.
   2. Provide a consistent caregiver.
   3. Meet needs immediately to increase trust.

4. Provide a pacifier for comfort and to meet oral needs, especially if the infant is on nothing-by-mouth status; provide a nipple dipped in sucrose solution during painful procedures.
5. Foster parent bonding with the infant; encourage rooming-in, if possible.
6. Communicate with the infant through auditory (talking, singing), visual (eye-to-eye contact), and tactile (touching, holding) stimulation.
7. Support the mother's decision to breastfeed or bottle-feed.
8. Teach parents to provide appropriate nutrition.
   a. Provide adequate calories based on developmental needs.
   b. Introduce cereal and pureed foods around 5 to 6 months, progressing to chopped and then soft foods at 6 to 7 months, once dentition has begun.
   c. Provide finger foods to increase refinement of pincer grasp and hard crackers to provide pleasure and promote teeth eruption.
   d. Decrease volume of milk intake as more solid foods are ingested.
   e. Encourage weaning from bottle to cup progressively as readiness is demonstrated by improved hand-mouth coordination.
9. Teach parents to encourage age-appropriate play.
   a. Ensure play is interactive, recreational, and educational; rotate toys as developing skills progress.
   b. Encourage the infant to interact with self in mirror and with others to support social and creative growth.
   c. Provide a variety of toys because of short attention span to support cognitive growth.
   d. Provide black-and-white or brightly colored mobiles, stuffed animals, rattles, teething rings, push-pull toys, blocks, books with textures, and teething toys to support physical growth.
   e. Provide toys small enough to promote manipulation to develop fine motor skills, but larger than a fist to prevent aspiration.
10. Teach parents ways to prevent injury. (See the section "Age" under "Factors That Influence Patient Safety" in Chapter 13 for the reasons why infants are at risk for injury.)
   a. Suffocation and aspiration.
   🛑 **(1) Place in the supine position when sleeping.**
      (2) Avoid pillows, excessive bedding, tucked-in blankets, baby powder, bottle propping, latex balloons, buttons, plastic bags, and loose blind cords.
      (3) Avoid foods that can occlude the airway, such as nuts, grapes, hot dogs, hard candy, popcorn, and raisins.

(4) Ensure that the distance between crib slats is no more than $2\frac{3}{8}$ inches.

b. Motor vehicle injuries.

(1) Use a rear-facing car seat with five-point harness until the infant exceeds height and weight recommendations indicated by the manufacturer (usually 22–35 lb).

🛑 **(2) Do not leave an infant in a car unattended.**

c. Falls and head injuries.

(1) Supervise the infant on raised surfaces.

(2) Place gates at the tops and bottoms of stairs.

(3) Use restraints on infant seats, high chairs, walkers, and swings.

🛑 **(4) Never shake a baby because it can lead to head injury (shaken baby syndrome).**

d. Poisoning.

(1) Store agents in locked cabinets.

(2) Avoid secondhand smoke.

(3) Remove lead paint from surfaces in the home.

(4) Keep the poison control center number by the telephone.

e. Burns.

(1) Set the home's hot water heater at 120°F.

(2) Test water temperature before a bath and use a bathtub (not a sink) for baths.

(3) Avoid excessive exposure to the sun.

(4) Do not use a microwave to warm bottles.

(5) Put inserts in electric outlets.

(6) Install smoke detectors throughout the house.

f. Drowning.

(1) Supervise the infant when in or near water, such as a bathtub, toilet, bucket, pool, or lake.

(2) Keep bathroom doors closed and keep toilet lids down or use toilet seat guards.

II. Toddler

Toddlers are children 12 months to 36 months of age. Dramatic changes in growth and development during this stage promote the toddler's striving to differentiate self from others and attain independence.

A. Development

1. Physical.

a. Has a decrease in growth rate; birth weight quadruples by $2\frac{1}{2}$ years.

b. Anterior fontanel closes by 18 months.

c. Chest measurement is greater than head circumference.

d. Experiences a decrease in appetite (physiological anorexia), has 20 teeth, and has increased taste preferences.

e. Has a decrease in naps.

f. Achieves daytime bowel and bladder control at 2 to 3 years; nighttime control by 3 to 4 years.

g. Walks by 14 months; runs by 18 months.

h. Continues mastery of gross and fine motor movements.

2. Psychosocial.

a. Anal stage of psychosexual development; beginning development of independence with a focus on gaining control over excretory functions.

b. Is confronted with resolving the conflict of autonomy versus shame and doubt that leads to self-control; if unable to achieve autonomy, the child will have difficulty developing independence later in life.

c. Differentiates self from others; is able to separate from mother at $2\frac{1}{2}$ years for short periods.

d. Notes sex role differences and explores own body.

e. Withstands short periods of delayed gratification; negativistic.

f. May have a security object or may suck thumb for comfort.

g. Needs routines.

h. May fear sleep, engines, and animals.

i. May experience sibling rivalry with a newborn.

3. Cognitive.

a. Continuation of sensorimotor phase.

b. Preconceptional thought by 2 to 4 years; beginning of memory.

c. Has increased sense of time.

d. Begins asking "why" and "how" by 2 years.

e. Engages in magical thinking (i.e., considers personal thoughts are all powerful).

f. Is egocentric and has increased concept of ownership ("mine").

g. Begins to develop a conscience.

h. May begin to develop fears.

4. Language.

a. Increased comprehension: 4 to 6 words by 15 months; more than 10 words by 18 months; and more than 300 words and understands simple commands by 2 years.

b. Uses words "no" and "mine" constantly.

c. Talks incessantly; uses sentences by 2 years.

5. Play.

a. Interactions: alone and with peers and adults; can amuse self for brief periods.

b. Plays alongside, not with, other children (parallel play).

c. Types of play: recreational, imitative, and educational.

d. Activities: quiet, active, structured, and unstructured.

e. Environments: home, park, and preschool.

MAKING THE CONNECTION

Knowledge of Growth and Development and the Nursing Role

A nurse working in an emergency department is completing a comprehensive assessment of a toddler who was brought to the hospital by his father. The toddler is self-splinting his left arm and cries when the arm is touched. The nurse suspects that the toddler has sustained a left upper extremity fracture and keeps the arm immobilized until the boy can be seen by the primary care provider. The father states, "My son is always being defiant. He says no to everything and refuses to share toys with his sister, and is constantly saying, 'It's mine, its mine.' I can't get him to behave. I only tried to make him sit in a corner for 10 minutes to learn to behave and he kept getting up." The nurse concludes that the father does not understand normal growth and development of toddlers. The nurse explains that a toddler constantly saying "no" and "mine" is an expected part of growth and development. The nurse also explains that the toddler's behavior reflects egocentricity and striving for autonomy, which are associated with the developmental task of toddlers. The nurse suggests that the toddler be removed from a situation and told to sit quietly in "time-out" for a length of time no longer than his age (1 minute per year). A longer period of time is unrealistic, excessively punitive, and counterproductive. In this situation, the nurse functioned as a caregiver to and advocate for the child as well as a teacher, resource person, and counselor for the father.

Box 6.1 Phases of Separation Anxiety Associated With Separation From Parents Due to Hospitalization

Protest
- Lasts for a few hours to a few days
- Inconsolable crying
- Clinging to parents to prevent departure
- Rejection of others

Despair
- Follows protest phase
- Flat affect
- Sadness
- Passivity
- Unresponsiveness to stimuli
- Altered sleep
- Decreased appetite
- Moaning, rocking, thumb-sucking, and nose picking

Detachment and Denial
- Adjusts to the loss
- Lack of preference for parents
- Friendliness to all
- Interest in surroundings

---

6. Reaction to illness, hospitalization, and pain.
   a. Fears punishment, the unknown, and separation.
   b. Has increased stress in reaction to immobilization, isolation, and altered rituals.
   c. Expresses pain in a word ("ow").
   d. Clings to parent, cries, and regresses when in pain or anxious.
   e. Experiences separation anxiety (Box 6.1).

B. Nursing Care
1. Assess developmental level.
2. Provide a consistent caregiver.
3. Stay with the child.
4. Support routines.
5. Encourage rooming-in and family participation in child care.
6. Accept protest behaviors when toddler is separated from parents, and console the toddler when parents have to leave.
7. Provide familiar objects (e.g., teddy bear) from home.
8. Explain to the parents that the toddler's display of anger is healthy and expected.
9. Encourage independence.
10. Ignore regression, and praise appropriate behavior.
11. Provide massage, distraction, medications, and thermotherapy as ordered.
12. Use the services of a child life specialist who is educated to provide age-appropriate activities to assist a child to cope with illness or hospitalization.
13. Offer choices, avoid frustration, and provide for safety while ignoring tantrums.
14. Supervise interaction with infant siblings, give individual attention, include toddler in newborn care, and provide a doll for imitative play.
15. Teach parents to provide appropriate nutrition.
    a. Provide finger foods and support use of utensils to encourage self-feeding.
    b. Avoid the desire to feed the toddler to complete the task.
    c. Avoid using foods, such as sweets, for rewards or punishments.
16. Teach the parents to encourage age-appropriate play.
    a. Provide a variety of play experiences.
    b. Encourage play with banging toys and musical instruments to help the toddler release aggression through play.
    c. Provide push-pull, pounding board, and pedal-propelled riding toys and balls to support physical growth.

d. Provide telephones, dolls, safe kitchen utensils, dress-up toys, and trucks to support social and creative growth.

e. Provide crayons, nesting blocks, finger paints, and clay to support fine motor skills.

f. Provide simple puzzles, picture books, and appropriate television programs or videos to promote cognitive development.

17. Teach parents ways to prevent injury. (See the section "Age" under "Factors That Influence Patient Safety" in Chapter 13 for the reasons why toddlers are at risk for injury.)

a. Motor vehicles.

(1) Use a forward-facing seat with a five-point harness for all children 2 years and older and those who have exceeded height and weight recommendations for rear-facing seats.

(2) Use a belt-positioning booster seat when the child exceeds height and weight recommendations (usually 20–40 lb) for forward-facing seats.

🛑 (3) Do not leave the child in a car unattended.

b. Drowning.

(1) Supervise when in or near water.

(2) Fence or cover pools and hot tubs.

(3) Know cardiopulmonary resuscitation (CPR).

c. Burns.

(1) Turn handles of pots toward the back of the stove.

(2) Use front guards on radiators, space heaters, and fireplaces.

(3) Keep appliance cords, candles, and irons out of reach.

d. Suffocation and aspiration.

🛑 (1) Avoid foods that can occlude the airway, such as round and sticky foods (e.g., marshmallows, peanut butter) as well as nuts, grapes, hot dogs, hard candy, popcorn, and raisins.

DID YOU KNOW?

Children ages 1 to 3 years have the highest incidence of foreign body aspiration because the lumen of their airways is small. The right bronchus is the usual site of an obstruction because of its shorter length and straighter angle. Also, children of this age are just beginning to eat solid foods and their chewing and swallowing may not be effective. Hot dogs, round candy, nuts, and grapes account for approximately 40 percent of all aspirated foods. The severity of the obstruction depends on what was aspirated, the location of the obstruction, and the extent of the obstruction.

(2) Keep garage door openers inaccessible.

(3) Avoid toy boxes with heavy hinged lids, clothing with drawstrings, and appliances that cannot be opened from the inside.

e. Bodily damage.

(1) Do not permit the child to run with objects in the mouth or to run and jump near doors or furniture with glass.

(2) Teach the child to hold pointed objects downward.

(3) Keep tools and firearms in locked cabinets.

(4) Keep the child away from lawnmowers.

(5) Lock windows or use window guards on windows on second story or higher buildings.

(6) Teach the child never to go with a stranger or allow inappropriate touching.

f. Poisoning.

(1) Store agents in locked cabinets.

(2) Avoid secondhand smoke.

(3) Keep the poison control center number by the telephone.

III. Preschooler

Preschoolers are children between 3 and 5 years of age. Their growth and development supports their desire for direction and purpose and prepares them for entry into the school environment.

A. Development

1. Physical.

a. Average increase in weight of 5 lb/year and increase in height of 2.5 to 3 inches/year.

b. Increase in immune responses.

c. Increase in strength.

d. Refinement of gross and fine motor skills.

e. Dresses and washes self.

f. Goes up stairs with alternate footing at 3 years; skips and hops on one foot by 4 years; jumps rope and walks backward with heel to toe by 5 years.

g. Ties shoes, uses scissors, and prints a few letters by 5 years.

h. Achieves day and night bowel and bladder control usually by 3 to 4 years.

i. Eruption of permanent dentition possible during 5th year.

j. Visual acuity approaches 20/20 by 5 years; potential for amblyopia by 4 to 6 years.

k. Most body systems are mature and stable and can adjust to moderate stress.

2. Psychosocial.

a. Oedipal stage of psychosexual development; attaches to parent of opposite sex while identifying with same-sex parent, which encourages imitative and imaginative play.

b. Confronted with resolving the conflict of initiative versus guilt, leading to direction and purpose, which encourages endeavors; if initiative is not supported, the child may develop a sense of guilt that limits further initiative.

c. Is selfish and impatient and exaggerates.

d. Takes pride in accomplishments.

e. Is less defiant than a toddler and takes pride in manners and acting manly or womanly at 5 years.

f. Begins to differentiate between right and wrong (morality).

g. May have imaginary friend.

h. Develops personality by 5 years.

3. Cognitive.

a. Preoperational phase (two stages: preconceptual phase from 2–4 years and intuitive thought phase from 4–5 years), during which there is a shift from egocentricity to social awareness.

b. Has increased readiness for learning and curiosity about immediate world.

c. Considers others' views.

d. Understands past, present, and future by 5 years.

e. Begins to understand mathematical concepts.

f. Questions parental rules by 5 years.

4. Language.

a. Has totally intelligible speech.

b. Knows 900 words by 3 years; 1,500 words by 4 years; and 2,100 words by 5 years.

c. Language increases in complexity; uses all parts of speech and asks meaning of new words.

d. Asks "who," "what," "where," "when," and "why."

e. Stuttering and stammering common between 2 and 4 years.

5. Play.

a. Begins cooperative play; engages in group play without rigid rules (associative play).

b. Begins to notice group conformity; increases sharing by 5 years.

c. Engages in physical, manipulative, imitative, and imaginary play of acting like an adult.

d. Is at increased risk for pedestrian and motor vehicle accidents due to bicycle riding, running after balls into street, and crossing streets.

e. May cheat to win in games.

6. Reaction to illness, hospitalization, and pain.

a. Fears intrusive procedures, such as rectal temperature, injections, and ear examinations.

b. Fears pain, punishment, rejection, bodily harm, castration, mutilation, and darkness more than separation.

c. Is increasingly able to withstand temporary separation.

d. Views death as temporary.

e. Attempts to protect self from pain by crying, biting, hitting, and kicking.

B. **Nursing Care**

1. Explain interventions and reasons for them in language the child can understand.

 2. Engage the child in therapeutic play using visual aids and puppets; have the child handle appropriate equipment (e.g., stethoscope, syringe, bandages) on a doll; encourage a presurgical visit to the hospital, if applicable.

3. Engage the services of a child life specialist if available.

4. Encourage initiative, praise accomplished tasks, ignore regressive behaviors, and encourage choices.

5. Encourage self-care regarding activities of daily living, but provide supervision to maintain safety; allow the child to progress at own pace.

6. Balance activity and rest.

7. Teach the child how to dial 911 in case of an emergency and to give his or her full name and location.

8. Allow the child to explore own body without fear of punishment; ignore masturbation.

 9. Teach the child about stranger safety and recognition of unwanted touch; teach the child to report unwanted touch to a parent, school nurse, teacher, or other responsible adult.

10. Use distraction, thermotherapy, massage, and medications as ordered.

11. Assess for nonbinocular vision (strabismus).

12. Encourage parents to begin informal sex education.

13. Prepare the child for a painful procedure several minutes before it is to be performed; reward attempts to cooperate.

14. Teach parents to provide appropriate nutrition.

a. Encourage a variety of nutritious foods, capitalizing on color, flavor, and texture to expand the palate.

b. Encourage nutritious snacks, such as fruits and vegetables.

c. Encourage socialization during meals, including table manners.

d. Avoid threatening, bribing, or forcing a child to eat.

15. Teach parents to encourage age-appropriate play.

a. Arrange for preschoolers to play together.

b. Encourage safe playground play and use of sports equipment and bicycles to support physical growth.

c. Provide dress-up toys, puppets, and village sets to support social and creative growth.

d. Provide construction sets, musical instruments (e.g., drums, tambourines), and craft projects to develop fine motor skills.

e. Provide educational computer games (e.g., numbers, letters), simple board games, and activity books to support cognitive growth.

16. Teach parents ways to prevent injury. (See the section "Age" under "Factors That Influence Patient Safety" in Chapter 13 for the reasons why preschoolers are at risk for injury.)
    a. Bodily trauma.
       (1) Set examples for acceptable behavior by being a positive role model.
       (2) Teach the child to wear a helmet when riding a bicycle.
       (3) Encourage the child to recognize dangerous situations (e.g., pools, kitchen knives).
       (4) Teach the child to "stop, drop, and roll" if clothing is on fire.
       (5) Encourage the child to follow parenteral rules and provide positive or negative feedback based on the child's adherence or nonadherence to rules.
    b. Motor vehicles.
       (1) Use a forward-facing car seat until the child exceeds height and weight recommendations (usually 20–40 lb).
       (2) Use a belt-positioning booster seat when the child exceeds height and weight recommendations for forward-facing seats.

🛑 (3) **Do not leave the child in a car unattended.**

       (4) Teach the child to look both ways before crossing streets.
       (5) Encourage the child to play in yards or playgrounds instead of the street.

IV. School-Aged Child

School-aged children are 6 to 12 years of age. Their world enlarges dramatically during this phase, and growth and development support their increasing ability to perform complex social, cognitive, and motor behaviors.

A. Development
1. Physical.
   a. Average increase in weight of 4.5 to 6 lb/year and height of 2 inches/year; girls pass boys in height and weight by 12 years.
   b. Beginning of permanent teeth with front teeth.
   c. Puberty begins earlier in females (10 years) than in males (12 years).
   d. May be able to ride a bicycle and can print capital letters at 6 years.
   e. Develops good coordination and timing in motor activities by 9 years.
   f. Is skillful in most activities, such as skating, cycling, and skateboarding, and is able to use most tools skillfully and carefully by 10 years.
   g. Often appears awkward and lanky; may have difficulty coordinating muscle groups because of advancing bone growth at 11 years.
   h. Often overindulges in physical activity to point of exhaustion at 12 years.
2. Psychosocial.
   a. Latent stage of psychosexual development; tranquil stage between oedipal stage of early childhood and the genital stage of adolescence.
   b. Is confronted with resolving the conflict of industry versus inferiority, which leads to personal and interpersonal competence; if standards, whether internal or external, are not met, feelings of inferiority will develop.
   c. Identifies with peers of same gender by 6 to 10 years; begins to become interested in opposite gender by 10 to 12 years.
   d. Needs group approval and is highly competitive at 10 years.
   e. Develops intrinsic motivation (mastery, self-satisfaction).
   f. Behaves according to set norms; has decreased egocentricity.
   g. Develops self-image and body image; is increasingly concerned with physical appearance, hygiene, and need for privacy at 12 years.
   h. Begins to hero worship.
   i. Has many worries.
3. Cognitive.
   a. Develops concrete operations, inductive reasoning, and beginning logic by 7 to 11 years.
   b. Can count by multiples of 2, 4, 5, and 10 by 7 years.
   c. Classifies, serializes, tells time, and reads.
   d. Becomes more concerned about grades and failing at 9 years.
   e. Defines and understands abstract words, such as "peace" and "justice."
   f. Becomes more critical of own performance.
   g. Begins to think realistically about future and career by 11 years.
   h. Absorbs new information easily, shows interest in science and social studies, and is curious about people and places by 12 years.
4. Language.
   a. Vocabulary and comprehension expand; all sounds mastered by 12 years.
   b. Adult speech well established by 9 to 12 years.
5. Play.
   a. Has increased ego mastery, demands conformity in play, and is fanatic about rules.
   b. Is involved in peer relationships, such as team sports and clubs, and is highly competitive.
   c. Can play more complex board games.
   d. Is more selective about collections.

6. Reaction to illness, hospitalization, and pain.
   a. Fears the unknown, decreased control, dependency, disfigurement, and death.
   b. Personifies death as "boogyman" but has realistic concept by 9 to 10 years.
   c. Attempts to cooperate or stays rigid for procedures, but may cry, yell, or resist.
   d. Clenches fists, grits teeth, closes eyes, and wrinkles forehead in response to pain.
   e. Withstands some physical discomfort, but uses stall tactics to cope; self-image about reaction to pain is important.
   f. Desires more complete explanation of disease processes and scientific rationales for procedures.

B. **Nursing Care**
   1. Place with an age-appropriate roommate, and support visits from peers.
   2. Never belittle regression, resistance, or crying.
   3. Recognize accomplishments; avoid comparisons.
   4. Provide privacy; permit wearing underpants.
   5. Provide concrete details of procedures, emphasizing basic scientific aspects.
   6. Allow time for questions, and ask whether the child has any questions. Do not overwhelm the child with details, but provide honest, adequate answers. Reinforce that there is no such thing as a stupid question.
   7. Encourage expression of feelings, concerns, and fears; use puppets or visual aids for expression of feelings if appropriate. Explain that expressing feelings of sadness, anger, and love is acceptable.
   8. Allow manipulation of equipment, avoid procrastination, and praise attempts at cooperation.
   🛑 9. Provide choices, and allow the child to be involved in some decisions about care (e.g., how long parents should stay).
   10. Encourage diversional activities; seek assistance from a child life specialist, if available.
   11. Encourage completion of school work if the child is able; arrange for a tutor through the child's school.
   12. Support appreciation of worthwhile heroes.
   13. Help the child understand changes in body structure or appearance that make him or her different from peers.
   14. Use a pain scale, distraction, guided imagery, thought stopping, soothing music, massage, thermotherapy, and medications as ordered.
   15. Teach parents to provide appropriate nutrition.
       a. Teach principles of healthy nutrition (see the U.S. Department of Agriculture's MyPlate [*www.choosemyplate.gov*]).
       b. Encourage intake of foods high in vitamin D and calcium for bone growth.
       c. Encourage socialization during meals; avoid reprimands.
       d. Adjust caloric intake based on level of physical activity.
       e. Encourage intake of adequate breakfast at home or in a school nutrition program.
       f. Involve the child in meal planning and trips to the supermarket.

DID YOU KNOW?
According to the Centers for Disease Control and Prevention, the definition of childhood obesity is a body mass index at or above the 95th percentile for children of the same age and sex. Using that criterion, approximately 17 percent (12.5 million) of children and adolescents ages 2 to 19 years of age are obese in the United States. Since 1980, obesity prevalence among children and adolescents has almost tripled, and there are significant ethnic/racial and economic disparities. For example, Hispanic boys (2 to 19 years) are significantly more likely to be obese than non-Hispanic white boys, non-Hispanic black girls are significantly more likely to be obese than non-Hispanic white girls, and 1 in 7 low-income, preschool-aged children is obese.

16. Teach parents to encourage age-appropriate play.
    a. Encourage team sports and use of bicycles and skateboards to support physical growth.
    b. Encourage participation in groups, such as boy scouts or girl scouts, to support social and creative growth.
    c. Provide construction sets, musical instruments, and craft projects to support fine motor skills.
    d. Provide computer games and increasingly complex board games, such as Monopoly, to support cognitive growth.
17. Teach parents ways to prevent injury. (See the section "Age" under "Factors That Influence Patient Safety" in Chapter 13 for the reasons why school-aged children are at risk for injury.)
    a. Motor vehicles.
       (1) Teach the child pedestrian skills (e.g., cross streets in a crosswalk or at a corner with the light).
       (2) Encourage the child to play in a park rather than in the street.
       (3) Use a belt-positioning booster seat when the child exceeds weight and height recommendations for forward-facing seats; use a booster seat until the vehicle seat belt fits properly (usually 4 feet, 9 inches in height and between 8 and 12 years of age); then use the vehicle-provided lap and shoulder seat belts.
       (4) Seat all children under the age of 13 in the rear seat.

b. Physical and emotional harm.
   (1) Teach the child to wear eye, mouth, and ear protection with sports.
   (2) Avoid unsupervised gymnastics and climbing.
   (3) Reinforce previous teaching about playground safety, 911 notification in case of an emergency, and "stop, drop, and roll."
   🛑 (4) Teach the child to never go with a stranger or allow inappropriate touching; tell the child to report physical, verbal, emotional, or cyber bullying, sexual harassment, or abuse to a parent, school nurse, teacher, or other responsible adult.
c. Toxic substances: Practice role-playing to learn to say "no" to tobacco, drugs, and alcohol.

V. Adolescent

Adolescents are between 13 and 20 years of age. Adolescence is divided into multiple levels, depending on when profound physical, psychosocial, and cognitive changes occur. It is a transitional stage between childhood and young adulthood.

A. Stages of Adolescence
1. Early adolescence (as early as 11–14 years): transitions through puberty (Table 6.1).
2. Middle adolescence (15–17 years): transitions to peer group identification.
3. Late adolescence (18–19 years): transitions to adulthood.

B. Development
1. Physical.
   a. Uncoordinated, as linear exceeds muscular growth.
   b. Increased strength, especially in males.
   c. Slouching in early-maturing females to hide tallness.
   d. Overestimation of athletic ability in 16- to 18-year-olds, which increases the risk of accidents.

Table 6.1 Male Puberty Versus Female Puberty

Male Puberty	Female Puberty
• Generally occurs at 12 to 16 years	• Generally occurs at 10 to 14 years
• Enlargement of scrotum, testes, and penis	• Development of breasts and pubic and axillary hair
• Development of pubic, axillary, facial, and body hair	• Initiation of first menstruation (menarche)
• Initiation of nocturnal emissions and mature spermatozoa	• Initiation of ovulation about 12 months after menarche
• Deepening of voice	• Achievement of 95% of height by menarche
• Achievement of 95% of height by 15 to 16 years	

2. Psychosocial.
   a. Genital stage; abundance of libidinal drives as sexual maturity progresses.
   b. Is confronted with resolving the conflict of self-identity versus role confusion; strives to integrate self-concept and values with those of society; failure to achieve self-identity results in role confusion.
   c. Feels omnipotent.
   d. Engages in behaviors motivated by peer pressure; increases risky behavior.
   e. Is increasingly more confident and has increased interest in appearance.
   f. Desires independence, but may avoid responsibility and resists enforcement of discipline.
   g. Has increased interest in sex with experimentation; forms intimate relationships (opposite sex if heterosexual, same sex if homosexual).
   h. Is able to make sacrifices for long-range goals at 16 to 19 years.
   i. Is at increased risk for suicide and homicide (more frequently with males than females) related to economic deprivation, family dysfunction, and availability of firearms.
   j. May not seek medical care for sexually transmitted infections (STIs) due to lack of knowledge, guilt, shame, or fear.
3. Cognitive.
   a. Has formal operational thought; is capable of abstract, conceptual, and hypothetical thinking; and comprehends satire and double meanings.
   b. Has increased learning through inference versus repetition and imitation.
   c. Has difficulty accepting others' viewpoints; is idealistic.
   d. Is concerned with social, moral, and ethical issues.
   e. Develops a personal value system (value autonomy).
4. Language.
   a. Has increased vocabulary and reading comprehension.
   b. Experiments with language; uses jargon.
5. Play.
   a. Engages in individual and team sports for exercise; has increased social and personal development.
   b. Follows rules of complex games.
6. Reaction to illness, hospitalization, and pain.
   a. Similar to school-aged children, with increased need for independence, privacy, and body integrity.
   b. Has fear of disfigurement or decreased function.
   c. Has decreased need for parental visits, but separation from peers may be traumatic.

d. Has realistic concept of death, but emotionally may be unable to accept it.

e. Tolerates physical pain; stoicism important among males.

f. Clenches fist or teeth, self-splints, and has decreased interest and concentration in response to pain.

C. Nursing Care

1. Encourage visits by peers.

2. Talk to the adolescent directly, not through the parents, and show respect for level of knowledge.

3. Allow time for a relationship to develop; do not force self on adolescent.

4. Express an interest in the adolescent's life outside the hospital, especially hobbies, to aid communication.

5. Encourage questions and the expression of feelings and concerns.

6. Encourage participation in decision making, wearing own clothes, and performing own care.

7. Explain reasons for sexual characteristics that are developing; encourage discussion of changing body image.

8. Facilitate discussion about self-identify, role image, and goal direction.

9. Encourage positive role models.

10. Permit experience of competition, teamwork, and conflict resolution.

11. Use distraction, music, massage, and medications as ordered.

12. Teach parents to provide appropriate nutrition.

    a. Provide prescribed iron and B vitamins for increased muscle and tissue growth and red blood cell maturation, particularly in females following menarche.

    b. Teach the adolescent the importance of not following fad diets; encourage regular eating habits and avoidance of fast foods that are high in calories and salt.

    c. Provide nutritious between-meal snacks to meet increased caloric needs, physical growth, and emotional expenditure.

    d. Be alert for clinical indicators of anorexia nervosa, such as vomiting after meals, weight loss, cachexia, and tooth decay.

13. Teach parents to encourage age-appropriate play:

    a. Encourage participation in team sports and increasingly difficult sports, such as skiing and surfing, to support physical growth.

    b. Encourage participation in school activities, such as theater and chorus, to support social and creative growth.

    c. Provide musical instruments and advanced craft projects to support fine motor skills.

    d. Provide computer games and increasingly complex board games, such as chess, to support cognitive growth.

14. Teach parents ways to prevent injury. (See the section "Age" under "Factors That Influence Patient Safety" in Chapter 13 for the reasons why adolescents are at risk for injury.)

    a. Motor vehicles.

       (1) Assess the level of responsibility and ability to resist peer pressure.

       (2) Set limits on driving, and encourage wearing of lap and shoulder seat belts.

    b. Sports.

       (1) Encourage warming up and cooling down.

       (2) Encourage playing within abilities.

       (3) Encourage wearing protective gear.

    c. Violence, suicide, or homicide.

       (1) Assess risk due to frustration, deprivation, aggression, depression, and social isolation.

       (2) Keep firearms in locked closets.

       🛑 (3) **Teach the adolescent to report bullying, sexual harassment, or abuse to a parent, school nurse, teacher, or other responsible adult.**

       (4) Discourage membership in gangs.

    d. Sexually Transmitted Infections (STIs).

       🛑 (1) **Teach the adolescent sex education and STI prevention, such as engaging in abstinence, limiting number of partners, and using condoms.**

       (2) Engage the adolescent in role-playing to teach ways to resist peer pressure.

    e. High-risk behaviors.

       (1) Teach the adolescent to avoid body piercing, tanning beds, and tattoos.

       (2) Teach the adolescent to avoid drug abuse, tobacco use, and alcohol.

       (3) Teach the adolescent to check the depth of water before diving and to avoid swimming extended distances and in dangerous waters.

VI. Young Adult

Young adults are between ages 20 and 30 years. Young adulthood consists of multiple physical, psychosocial, and financial changes that involve decisions (e.g., intimate partner, career, high-risk behaviors) that can affect the quality and length of one's life.

A. Development

1. Physical.

   a. At height of bodily vigor; period of peak sexual capacity for males.

   b. Maximum level of strength, muscular development, height, and cardiac and respiratory capacity.

2. Psychosocial.
   a. Is confronted with resolving the conflict of intimacy versus isolation; development of friendships and an intimate love relationship are imperative; failure to achieve feelings of affiliation and love inherent in relationships causes one to feel isolated and alone.
   b. Has a vision of the future and imagines various possibilities for self; transfers an interest into an occupation.
   c. Defines and tests what can be accomplished.
   d. Seeks out a mentor to emulate as a guiding figure.
   e. Experiments with and chooses a lifestyle.
   f. Forms mature relationships with both males and females; may choose someone for a long-term relationship.
   g. Learns to understand masculine and feminine aspects of self as well as an adult concept of roles.
   h. Accepts responsibilities and pleasures of parenthood.
   i. May not seek medical care for STIs due to lack of information, guilt, shame, or fear.
   j. May continue to live with parents until financially solvent (increasing trend).
3. Cognitive.
   a. At close to peak of intelligence, memory, and abstract thought.
   b. Has maximum ability to solve problems and learn new skills.
4. Language: Has fully developed language.
5. Play.
   a. May participate in or enjoy watching sports activities.
   b. Engages in socialization with peers.
   c. Enjoys playing with own children or with children of others.
6. Reaction to illness, hospitalization, and pain.
   a. May feel dependence and/or a lack of autonomy.
   b. Chronic illness or prolonged hospitalization may interfere with establishment of intimacy and may result in isolation, loneliness, and withdrawal.
   c. Frustration and isolation may occur when goals related to choice of occupation, life partner, and procreation are not attained.

B. Nursing Care
1. Address by name, providing all necessary information.
🛑 2. Encourage participation in the plan of care and decision making; support independence and autonomy, especially when some aspect of physical, emotional, or financial dependence results.
3. Foster feeling of acceptance and belonging.

4. Encourage expression of feelings and concerns.
5. Praise accomplishments and encourage initiative.
6. Assist with coping with unexpected alterations in body image, lifestyle, or long-term goals.
7. Teach to maintain appropriate nutrition.
   a. Limit caloric intake if lifestyle is more sedentary than it was during adolescence.
   b. Encourage a heart-healthy, balanced diet; discourage intake of foods high in carbohydrates, cholesterol, saturated fats, sugar, preservatives, and additives.
   c. Seek guidance from a nutritionist regarding nutrition during pregnancy and lactation.
8. Teach ways to prevent injury. (See the section "Age" under "Factors That Influence Patient Safety" in Chapter 13 for the reasons why young adults are at risk for injury.)
   a. Sports.
      (1) Encourage warm-up and cool-down before and after activities.
      (2) Encourage play within abilities.
      (3) Encourage wearing of protective gear.
   b. STIs.
      (1) Engage in abstinence, limit number of partners, and/or use condoms.
      (2) Learn signs and symptoms of STIs and the need to seek health care if they occur.

VII. Adult

Adults are between the ages of 31 and 45 years. During this time, a realistic self-identify forms, concerns about career are paramount, and interest in mentoring the next generation emerges.

A. Development
1. Physical.
   a. Still near peak in late 30s, but has gradual decline in biologic functioning around 40 years.
   b. Peak sexual capacity for females occurs during mid-30s.
2. Psychosocial.
   a. Confronted with resolving the conflict of generativity versus self-absorption; inability to achieve generativity results in egocentricity and stagnation.
   b. Achieves a realistic self-identify.
   c. Accepts limitations while developing assets.
   d. Delays immediate gratification for future satisfaction.
   e. Struggles to establish a place in society; invests self in social structure, including work, family, and community.
   f. Has a stronger need to be responsible.
   g. Seeks advancement by becoming more creative and pursuing ambitions.

DID YOU KNOW?

Births to women ages 35 to 39 increased 47 percent from 1990 to 2008, and births to women ages 40 to 44 years increased 80 percent from 1990 to 2008. The main factor is related to women delaying marriage and/or motherhood as they seek attainment of higher education and establishment of a career. The advantages of delaying motherhood include financial security and less regrets. However, disadvantages include increased health risks for mother and baby, change in lifestyle, and fatigue associated with the physical care of a newborn due to the lower energy level associated with being older. The interesting impact is related to the delay of the developmental tasks of having and raising children, which is associated with the 20 to 30 age group. This, in turn, delays the achievement of the developmental task of generativity versus stagnation formerly associated with adulthood (31–45 years of age) as older first-time parents focus on family life and raising children.

3. Cognitive.
   a. Has perceptions based on reality.
   b. Takes longer to memorize, but still at peak in abstract thinking and problem-solving.
   c. Generates new levels of awareness; gives more meaning to complex tasks.
4. Language: Has fully developed language.
5. Play.
   a. May participate in or enjoy watching sports activities.
   b. Engages in socialization with peers.
   c. Enjoys playing with own children or with the children of others.
6. Reaction to illness, hospitalization, and pain.
   a. Illness can jeopardize job security, financial stability, and family cohesiveness, producing feelings of inadequacy.
   b. Illness heightens feelings associated with beginning bodily decline.
   c. Altered body image or function may interfere with solidification of a realistic self-identify.
   d. Chronic illness or prolonged hospitalization that stifles independence and creativity can lead to self-absorption and stagnation.
   e. Illness may interfere with sexual functioning.

B. Nursing Care
   1. Assess variables in the adult's environment that contribute to problems, such as economic, educational, health, and social variables.
   2. Assess knowledge of self and influence of current illness on self-image.
   3. Plan care so that the patient can maximize self-expression.

4. Assist to establish goals for long-term health maintenance.
5. Help to maintain judgment and initiative when external pressures of job and family interfere with internal comfort.
6. Encourage family discussion of needs and concerns; facilitate decision making and supportive relationships.
7. Teach to maintain appropriate nutrition.
   a. Encourage intake of a heart-healthy, balanced diet.
   b. Teach to eat in an unhurried, pleasant atmosphere.
   c. Encourage participation in a weight-reduction program, if necessary.
8. Teach ways to prevent sports-related injury. (See the section "Age" under "Factors That Influence Patient Safety" in Chapter 13 for the reasons why adults are at risk for injury.)
   a. Encourage warming up and cooling down before and after physical activity.
   b. Encourage play within abilities.
   c. Encourage wearing of protective gear.

VIII. Middle-Life Adult

Middle-life adults are between ages 46 and 64 years. The decline in physical abilities becomes more apparent, particularly the senses of hearing and vision. Concern for the next generation continues and may include grandchildren.

A. Development
   1. Physical.
      a. Has decreasing eye sight, especially close vision (may be one of the first signs of aging).
      b. Experiences gradual hearing loss; high-pitched sounds are impaired more readily than low-pitched sounds.
      c. Experiences gradual loss of taste buds in 50s and sense of smell in 60s.
      d. Has declining muscle strength because of decreased levels of estrogen and testosterone; takes longer to accomplish tasks.
      e. Experiences decreased lung capacity, which leads to decreased endurance.
      f. Skin begins to wrinkle due to decline in subcutaneous fat.
      g. Hair begins to turn gray.
      h. Experiences postural changes due to loss of calcium and reduced activity.
   2. Psychosocial.
      a. Continuation of resolving the conflict of generativity versus self-absorption.
      b. Middle years are rewarding if previous stages are fulfilled.

c. Responsibility of raising children declines; less financial strain once childbearing expenses are completed.

d. Often at height of career; may be leader in field.

e. Self-realization generally achieved as evidenced by more inner direction, no longer feeling the need to please everyone, being less likely to compare self with others, and approval of self without being dependent on standards of others.

3. Cognitive.

a. Begins to experience declining memory around 50 years.

b. Takes longer to learn new tasks and takes longer to perform old tasks.

c. Experiences increased practical judgment due to experiential background.

d. May tend to withdraw from mental activity or overcompensate by attempting the impossible.

4. Language: Has fully developed language.

5. Play.

a. May participate in or enjoy watching sports activities.

b. Engages in socialization with peers.

c. Enjoys playing with own children or grandchildren.

6. Reaction to illness, hospitalization, and pain.

a. Sensorimotor decline exaggerated by illness results in heightened feelings of aging.

b. Illness and recuperation may be prolonged due to reduced physiological and emotional adaptive capacity.

c. Illness occurring at this time of decreasing family responsibilities may lead to self-absorption and isolation.

d. Illness at height of one's career may promote denial and delay seeking medical attention; may produce resistance to hospitalization and curtail time necessary for recuperation.

B. Nursing Care

🛑 1. Allow discussion of frustrations of attempting to meet life's goals and voicing of concerns about the meaning and purpose of the rest of one's life.

2. Assist with goal setting that is realistic and attainable.

3. Focus on individual strengths rather than weaknesses; support ego strengths.

4. Encourage productive communication with mate and close friends.

5. Help to identify areas of meddling in their children's or close friend's lives; assist development of ways of coping with concerns for others in an objective and positive manner.

6. Encourage reaching out to others and giving assistance rather than isolating self.

7. Encourage expression of feelings about the empty-nest syndrome, if a concern.

8. Teach to maintain appropriate nutrition; same as in previous "Adult" category.

9. Teach ways to prevent injury. (See the section "Age" under "Factors That Influence Patient Safety" in Chapter 13 for the reasons why adults are at risk for injury.)

a. Sports: same as in previous "Adult" category.

b. Falls.

(1) Avoid turning and altering position quickly due to a decline in sensorium and balance.

(2) Eliminate cluttered environment.

IX. Older Adult (Early Late Years)

Older adults (early late years) are between 65 and 79 years of age. Their physical abilities continue to decline, and they are beginning to address the issues of satisfaction or dissatisfaction with their past and contentment or fear of the future.

A. Development

1. Physical.

a. Continued decrease in vigor and capacity; more frequent aches and pains.

b. Seventy percent rate themselves as healthy, but likely to have at least one major illness.

c. Changes in vision, hearing, sensation, posture, muscle strength, cardiovascular and neurologic functioning, and endurance as well as orthostatic hypotension may result in falls.

d. The ability to metabolize and excrete drugs decrease, increasing the risk of drug toxicity.

2. Psychosocial.

a. Confronted with resolving the conflict of ego integrity versus despair.

b. May be satisfied with life and able to accept personal strengths and weaknesses.

c. May be remorseful for what might have been, dissatisfied with the present, and fearful of the future, resulting in despair; reminisces.

d. Personality does not change, but may become more exaggerated.

e. May have intense feelings of aging and mortality when confronted with the reality of physical and mental changes.

f. Is adjusting to aging, decreased health, maintenance of quality of life, retirement, fixed income, death of spouse and friends, and change in residence.

g. May be more interested in utilizing own inner resources and less interested in obtaining rewards of society; feels a right to do what is important for self-satisfaction.

h. May become focused on bodily needs and comforts.

i. Feels sexual expression (e.g., love, touching, sharing, intercourse) are important and related to identity.

j. May provide moral support to grandchildren and be more tolerant of grandchildren than they were of own children.

k. Releases major authority of family to children while holding self in role of consultant.

l. Majority live in the community; increasingly more live in assisted living facilities; the percent of older adults over the age of 65 live in nursing homes are 1.1 percent for persons 65 to 74 years of age, 3.5 percent for persons 75 to 84 years of age, and 13.2 percent for persons 85 years of age and older.

3. Cognitive.
   a. IQ does not decrease, but mental acuity slows.
   b. Judgment and problem-solving remain intact, but processes may take longer.
   c. Long-term memory is better than short-term memory.

4. Language.
   a. Has fully developed language.
   b. May take longer to access words from memory.

5. Play.
   a. May engage in less physically demanding sports, such as golf, or watch sports activities.
   b. Engages in socialization with peers, although this declines as friends move away or die.
   c. May enjoy watching grandchildren play.

6. Reaction to illness, hospitalization, and pain.
   a. Has longer illness and recuperation secondary to decreased adaptive capacity.
   b. Has increased feelings of inadequacy and mortality.
   c. May experience frustration, anger, depression, and self-pity due to illness that limits or interferes with deserved goals of retirement or enjoyment of "golden years."
   d. May react to unfamiliar environments with confusion, anxiety, or fear.
   e. May feel dependence or hopelessness due to chronic illness, pain, or impending death.
   f. May have increased feelings of isolation and fear of death due to illness; may accept and prepare for death.

B. Nursing Care

1. Provide nursing care for older adults experiencing common problems associated with aging (Table 6.2).

2. Understand commonalities of aging, but approach each person as unique; avoid stereotyping because it denies uniqueness, decreases access to health care, and impacts negatively on the individual.

🛑 3. Encourage an older adult to discuss feelings about aging; facilitate feelings of pride in self-integrity.

4. Ensure access to health care and social services, especially in the home.

5. Encourage ongoing follow-up medical care and health promotion and illness prevention activities within the patient's abilities; provide aggressive treatment for critical illnesses, if desired.

6. Assess for digestive or intestinal disturbances, such as gastric acidity and constipation, that occur with aging.

7. Encourage engagement in self-satisfying endeavors.

8. Encourage the patient to seek harmony in relationships with significant others.

9. Encourage social involvement outside the home.

10. Accept an older adult's need for love and belonging and to have sexual needs met; provide for privacy, and encourage exploration of medications or devices to minimize dysfunction.

11. Help others to see that older adults deserve dignity and respect.

12. Teach to maintain appropriate nutrition.
    a. Have multiple small meals or between-meal snacks to ensure adequate intake of calories.
    b. Use spices other than salt to compensate for a decline in taste and smell.
    c. Reduce caloric intake because metabolic and activity levels decline.
    d. Encourage daily dental hygiene and to visit a dentist regularly.
    e. If experiencing difficulty with shopping or cooking, seek assistance of community agencies that can help shop, serve, or deliver meals to the home; if on a limited income, apply for food stamps or seek assistance from community food banks.
    f. Maintain adequate intake of fiber and fluid and reduce intake of high-fat foods to promote fecal elimination; discourage use of laxatives and enemas because they can become habitual.

13. Teach ways to prevent injury. (See the section "Age" under "Factors That Influence Patient Safety" in Chapter 13 for the reasons why older adults are at risk for injury.)
    a. Falls:
       (1) Follow safety precautions, such as using grab bars, railings, and walkers; rising slowly; and keeping feet apart for a wide base of support.
       (2) Use ambulation assistance devices, as indicated.

Table 6.2 Common Problems Associated With Aging and Related Nursing Care

Problem	Nursing Care
Bowel and Bladder Incontinence • Incontinence is not part of the aging process. • It may be aggravated by decreased muscle tone of anal and urinary sphincters and prostatic hyperplasia.	• Ensure screenings for urinary tract infection and bladder or prostate cancer. • Assist with hygiene and skin care. • Institute bowel and bladder retraining.
Adverse Drug Effects • Multiple health problems require an increase in prescriptions (polypharmacy), commonly with decreased coordination among health-care providers. • Decreased hepatic and renal function can result in accumulation, drug toxicity, and increased paradoxical effects.	• Coordinate care among health-care team members. • Identify unnecessary or excessive doses of medications; explore medications that may be discontinued, changed to a lower dose, or substituted by a less-toxic drug • Assess for adverse or toxic effects. • Teach the patient to read over-the-counter drug labels to avoid accidental overdose when taking multiple products.
Cognitive Impairment Not part of the aging process. • **Delirium:** Acute decrease in cognition; potentially reversible; associated with acute illness. **Clinical manifestations:** Lability; fear; delusions; increased pulse, respirations, and blood pressure; hallucinations; illusions; disorientation; dilated pupils; diaphoresis; sleep disturbance; tremors. • **Dementia:** Chronic, progressive, irreversible disorder; progresses from mild to severe; ultimately requires total care. **Clinical manifestations:** Intellectual decline, such as decreased short-term memory, language, insight, and judgment; self-preoccupation; can be passive, as evidenced by flat affect and decreased spontaneity, or irritable, as evidenced by sarcasm, decreased concern for others, and paranoia. • **Sundowning syndrome:** Thought to be associated with disturbance in circadian rhythms; associated with seasonal affective disorder and depression. **Clinical manifestations:** Agitation, confusion, and disorientation in late afternoon and evening.	• Provide a safe, nonstimulating, familiar environment with consistent routines and caregiver. • Use a calm, unhurried, nondemanding approach. • Consider the patient's mood and easy distractibility when planning care. • Reorient to time, place, and person; use simple language and visual clues. • Promote independence within ability; assist with activities of daily living. • Encourage reminiscing about earlier years. • Identify events that increase agitation, such as environmental stimuli, altered routines, strangers, increased expectations, and "lost" items. • Involve in simple, repetitive tasks and one-on-one activities. • Promote involvement in therapy, such as music and pet therapy, and current events. • Support primary caregivers and encourage periodic respite care.
Alcohol Abuse • Develops secondary to depression, loneliness, and lack of social support.	• Explore effective coping strategies. • Refer the patient to Alcoholics Anonymous.
Risk of Suicide • Occurs secondary to multiple losses, such as loss of loved ones and health, and lack of social support. • 20% of older adults experience depression, feelings of hopelessness, and isolation.	• Assess for suicide risk. • Provide reality orientation, validation therapy, and reminiscence. • Support body image. • Encourage psychological counseling. • Obtain an order for an antidepressant. • Refer the patient to social services for home-care services.
Decreased Sexual Response and Erectile Dysfunction • Sexual response takes longer due to decreased testosterone and estrogen, chronic health problems, and medications. • Can occur secondary to unavailable partner or cognitive impairment.	• Provide privacy, support dignity and nonjudgmental attitude. • Encourage verbalization of concerns. • Suggest lubricant, penile prostheses, or medication to promote erection, as applicable.
Sexually Transmitted Infections • Need for sexual expression continues. • Increased society recognition that sex is natural and acceptable, even if single by choice or after death of spouse.	• Maintain a nonjudgmental attitude. • Teach about sexually transmitted infection prevention.

(3) Remove scatter rugs from the home environment.

b. Motor vehicles.

(1) Assess ability to drive (e.g., vision, hearing, sensation in feet, reflexes, judgment).

 (2) Encourage the older adult to give up driving when impairment jeopardizes the safety of self or others; encourage family members to take away car keys if the individual is incompetent to drive.

X. Older Adults (Later Years)

Older adults (later years) are 80 years and older. Their physiological abilities continue to decline and may progress to the point that they are frail, their psychosocial environment narrows significantly, and they begin to address the inevitability of death.

A. Development

1. Physical.
   a. Experience additional sensory problems, including diminished sensation to touch and pain.
   b. Are at risk for falls due to diminished physical and sensorial abilities and orientation to space and sense of balance.
   c. Experience more acute and chronic health problems.
   d. May experience decreased control of urinary and anal sphincters, resulting in incontinence, due to illness.

2. Psychosocial.
   a. Continuation of the conflict of ego integrity versus despair; continues to reflect on past life and comes to terms with self.
   b. Few significant relationships remain; death of friends, family, and associates and an increased inability to leave the home cause isolation.
   c. Dependence, hopelessness, and helplessness may occur in response to significant impairment of adaptive responses and structural and functional alterations associated with aging.
   d. May be preoccupied with immediate bodily needs and personal comforts; gastrointestinal tract frequently becomes a major focus.
   e. May provide others with an example of wisdom and courage.
   f. May be concerned with own mortality; may cope with process of dying and prepare for own death.

3. Cognitive.
   a. Has better memory for past than present; repetition of memories occurs.
   b. May use confabulation to fill in memory gaps; forgetfulness may lead to safety problems.
   c. Increased arteriosclerosis may lead to mental illness, such as organic brain syndrome.

4. Language.
   a. Has fully developed language.
   b. May take longer to access words from memory.

5. Reaction to illness, hospitalization, and pain.
   a. May experience helplessness and despair because of multiple health problems and impairments causing dependence.
   b. May become egocentric due to a significant decline in physical and mental status, producing behavior that is demanding, inflexible, irritable, hostile, and suspicious.
   c. May experience confusion, disorientation, anxiety, and fear in response to hospitalization.
   d. May have feelings of relief that life is nearly over.

B. Nursing Care

1. Provide interventions to meet safety needs, such as bed or chair alarms, bed bolsters, or mattresses on floor next to bed, if necessary.
2. Assist with ambulation or teach use of a walker or cane; encourage wearing sturdy shoes and removing scatter rugs and other potential risk factors in the home.
3. Encourage independence with activities of daily living within abilities and assist as needed; praise accomplishments.
4. Provide constant supervision as needed.
5. Allow the patient to proceed at own pace; support personal-care rituals.
6. Assess physical status because the patient might not experience pain due to diminished sensitivity of nerve endings.
7. Follow bowel and bladder routine or training, if appropriate.
8. Orient to time, place, and person as needed; keep a clock and calendar in view.
9. Ask questions about the past to foster reminiscence; avoid becoming annoyed when the patient is repetitious.
10. Allow the patient to explore the meaning of life and listen to expressed feelings in a nonjudgmental manner.
11. Provide for dignity, such as pulling curtains and draping the patient when providing direct care.
12. Support dying individuals in accordance with desires, religious convictions, and beliefs.
13. Facilitate visits by a pastoral counselor of choice if desired by the patient.
14. Support family members so that they are capable of helping a dying relative. (See Chapter 8, "Psychological Support, Nursing Care for Family Members of a Patient Who is Dying.")
15. Teach ways to prevent injury. (See the section "Age" under "Factors That Influence Patient Safety" in Chapter 13 for the reasons why older adults are at risk for injury.)
    a. Falls.
       (1) Use hand rails, shower seats, and raised toilets to support safety.
       (2) Use grab bars, railings, and a cane or walker as needed for ambulation.

(3) Rise slowly.

(4) Keep feet apart for a wide base of support.

b. Polypharmacy.

  (1) Consult with the primary health-care provider before taking over-the-counter medications.

  (2) Ensure that the primary health-care provider is notified of all medications prescribed by other health-care providers.

(3) Take medications only for the length of time prescribed; discard unused medications.

(4) Encourage use of a pill box organizer to simplify taking medications and provide a visual cue when medications were not taken on time.

CASE STUDY: Putting It All Together

A public health nurse makes an initial home visit to assess the needs of a 75-year-old woman who was discharged after surgery for a fractured hip. She moved permanently into her daughter's home. The daughter has a 10-month-old infant who was born 6 weeks premature, a 3-year-old toddler, and a 5-year-old child. The daughter's husband works in another state and comes home every other weekend for 2 days. During the home visit, the public health nurse assesses all the children as well as the grandmother. The assessment findings are as follows:

Infant

• Turns from abdomen to back and from back to abdomen

• Is not sitting, crawling, or pulling self-up to a standing position

• Is not using a pincer grasp

• Holds on to mother and refuses to go to nurse

• Reacts to simple commands

• Enjoys peek-a-boo

Toddler

• Has 14 teeth

• Has made no progress with daytime bladder and bowel control

• Sucks thumb while holding a security blanket

• Is fearful of loud noises

• Is always saying "mine" and "no"

5-year-old

• Needs help with dressing and undressing

• Climbs stairs using the right foot first for each step

• Hops on two feet, but not on one

• Is unable to tie shoes

• Does not print letters

• Takes pride in accomplishments

• Is difficult to understand when speaking

• Has a limited vocabulary

• Fears temperature and ear examinations

75-year-old grandmother

• States that she is not as strong as she once was

• States that she is fearful of falling and is using a walker

• States that she has been depressed since her husband died 6 months ago and since losing her home

---

Case Study Questions

A. Which assessments of the 10-month-old indicate that the infant is meeting developmental norms? Which assessments indicate a developmental delay?

Assessments that meet developmental norms include:

1. _____

2. _____

3. _____

4. _____

Assessments that indicate a developmental delay include:

1. _____

2. _____

3. _____

Continued

CASE STUDY: Putting It All Together

cont'd

___ **Case Study Questions** ___

B. The nurse collects and analyzes the data related to the toddler. Which data are typically associated with toddlers and which are a cause for concern?

Data typically associated with toddlers include:

1. _____

2. _____

3. _____

Data that raise a cause for concern include:

1. _____

2. _____

C. Identify four clusters of data related to growth and development delays in the 5-year-old, and list nursing interventions planned to address each cluster.

1. _____

2. _____

3. _____

4. _____

D. Identify nursing interventions the nurse should implement to address the needs of the grandmother before leaving the home?

1. _____

2. _____

3. _____

4. _____

5. _____

6. _____

REVIEW QUESTIONS

1. What is the **best** site for the nurse to inject a newborn with vitamin K?
   1. Deltoid muscle
   2. Dorsogluteal muscle
   3. Ventrogluteal muscle
   4. Vastus lateralis muscle

2. A nurse is assessing several newborns who are all approximately 12 hours old. Which clinical manifestation should alert the nurse to notify the primary health-care provider?
   1. Apical rate of 130 beats/minute
   2. Respiratory rate of 74 breaths/minute
   3. Head circumference approximately equal to chest circumference
   4. Crown to rump length approximately equal to head circumference

3. Preoperative teaching was performed for a 4-year-old child regarding elective surgery. Which is the **least** appropriate method to assess if the teaching was effective?
   1. Ask the child to repeat what the nurse said.
   2. Have the child write down what was learned.
   3. Provide a coloring book for the child to draw what was taught.
   4. Use role playing so that the child can demonstrate what is going to be done.

4. A nurse is planning a health promotion program for a group of middle-aged adults. Which topic is **most** appropriate for this age group?
   1. Stress management
   2. Importance of exercise
   3. Adequate nutritional intake
   4. Maintenance of a safe home environment

5. The nurse is caring for a chronically ill freshman college student who is 21 years old. The patient experienced numerous hospital admissions over the years and long convalescent periods at home after each hospitalization, delaying educational goals. Which personal characteristics of the patient may interfere with the achievement of the developmental task associated with young adulthood? **Select all that apply.**
   1. _____ Accepts limitations
   2. _____ Delays gratification
   3. _____ Occupied with self-absorption
   4. _____ Concerned about an altered body image
   5. _____ Struggling to establish a place in society
   6. _____ Attempting to perform own activities of daily living

6. Which information should the nurse consider when planning and implementing nursing care for toddlers?
   1. Friends are important.
   2. Dependency is desired.
   3. Rituals are comforting.
   4. Organized group play is preferred.

7. Which educational intervention is **most** important when teaching older adults?
   1. Teaching about safety precautions in the home environment
   2. Providing suggestions about maintaining a healthy diet
   3. Presenting strategies to avoid the empty nest syndrome
   4. Exploring actions that support a healthy lifestyle

8. A nurse is caring for an adolescent admitted to the hospital for multiple fractures in a lower extremity requiring a large external fixation device. Which nursing intervention is **most** important when planning care for this adolescent?
   1. Encourage discussion of concerns about outcomes of the injury.
   2. Suggest playing a complex board game with another patient.
   3. Allow as much self-care as possible.
   4. Cover the leg with a bedspread.

9. A nurse is caring for a 20-year-old college student who is scheduled for outpatient surgery to revise an unattractive scar on the arm. During preoperative teaching, the patient shares having anxious feelings. From whom does the nurse anticipate the patient will benefit **most** when the person is providing emotional support?
   1. Professor
   2. Friends
   3. Parents
   4. Sibling

10. A nurse is assessing the developmental level of a toddler. Which activity does the nurse determine is beyond this child's ability?
    1. Riding a tricycle
    2. Completing multiple chores
    3. Beginning control of elimination
    4. Walking up steps without assistance

11. A nurse is assessing the developmental level of a preschool-aged child (4–5 years of age). Which behavior can the nurse expect to identify?
    1. Making change for small amounts of money
    2. Playing a game of catch with a small ball
    3. Using words within complete sentences
    4. Investing energy in having a collection

12. A nurse is assessing the developmental level of an adolescent (12–18 years). What developmental changes can the nurse generally expect? **Select all that apply.**

1. _____ Feeling independent from parents
2. _____ Demonstrating concern for personal appearance
3. _____ Exploring interests that may evolve into a career plan
4. _____ Beginning determination of one's own beliefs and values
5. _____ Working toward developing a mature relationship with another person

13. A nurse is assessing the reflexes of a 9-month-old child. Which reflex is a cause for concern in this child?
1. Present gag reflex
2. Negative Babinski reflex
3. Positive tonic neck reflex
4. Absent palmar grasp reflex

14. A nurse is presenting a class on infant development and care to a group of adolescents who are learning to be babysitters. Which statement by a participant indicates that further teaching is necessary?
1. "I should burp the baby frequently when feeding a bottle."
2. "I can rock the baby if crying occurs after being fed."
3. "I must place the baby on the back for sleeping."
4. "I may gently shake a baby to get its attention."

15. A nurse in the child health clinic obtains a health history from a parent of a 24-month-old child. Which physical activity should the nurse expect the parent to report was first evident during toddlerhood?
1. Running
2. Hopping
3. Skipping
4. Crawling

16. A nurse is caring for a group of children ranging in age from infancy to adolescence. The nurse considers the psychosocial task associated with each child's developmental level. Place the nursing intervention specifically associated with each developmental level progressing from infancy through adolescence.
1. Encourage independence.
2. Recognize accomplishments.
3. Support a positive self-concept.
4. Provide activities within abilities.
5. Meet physical needs immediately.
    Answer: _____

17. An older adult who was hospitalized has been experiencing sundowning syndrome. What interventions should the nurse include in the patient's plan of care? **Select all that apply.**

1. _____ Follow the preset daily routine.
2. _____ Hurry through direct patient care.
3. _____ Provide a nonstimulating environment.
4. _____ Explain in detail what care will be performed.
5. _____ Use a motion sensor device on the patient's bed.

18. A nurse is obtaining a health history and performing a physical assessment of an older adult. Which clinical manifestations associated with aging should the nurse expect? **Select all that apply.**

1. _____ Impaired balance
2. _____ Close vision impairment
3. _____ Diminished muscle strength
4. _____ Intermittent urinary incontinence
5. _____ Decreased hearing of low-pitched sounds

19. A nurse is assessing an older adult. Which clinical indicator should be communicated to the primary health-care provider because it is not associated with the aging process?
1. Tenting of skin on the back of the hand
2. Exaggerated premorbid personality
3. Delayed sexual response
4. Lability of mood

20. Which statement by an adult child about the child's 90-year-old father indicates ageism?
1. "My father was always egocentric, but it has gotten worse as he has gotten older."
2. "My father's physical status has progressively declined these last few years."
3. "I am so tired of him constantly talking about past experiences."
4. "I would rather die than reach the useless age of my father."

21. A nurse in the child health clinic is assessing a preschool-aged child. Which behaviors that may indicate a developmental delay should the nurse bring to the attention of the primary health-care provider? **Select all that apply.**

1. _____ Goes up and down stairs using both feet on each step
2. _____ Is unable to dress self without assistance
3. _____ Has imprecise fine motor skills
4. _____ Uses magical thinking
5. _____ Falls frequently

22. For which physical changes associated with aging should a nurse assess when assisting an older adult with a bath? **Select all that apply.**
1. _____ Increased sweat gland activity
2. _____ Decreased pigment cells in hair
3. _____ Decreased vascularity of the skin
4. _____ Increased sebaceous gland activity
5. _____ Increased collagen fibers in the dermis

23. A nurse identifies that a patient is experiencing a developmental crisis specifically associated with middle adulthood. Which assessment identified by the nurse supports this conclusion?
1. Inability to postpone satisfaction
2. Incapable of facing one's mortality
3. Problems maintaining peer relationships
4. Difficulty achieving a sense of fulfillment

24. What safety instruction addresses a major cause of accidental death among people from all developmental levels?
1. Resist pressure to engage in high-risk activities.
2. Rise slowly to a standing position.
3. Wear a seat belt when in a car.
4. Cut all food into small pieces.

25. A nurse is teaching a group of parents of school-aged children about motor vehicle accidents and child safety. Which information is **most** important for the nurse to include in this program?
1. Front passenger seats can be occupied by children when they weigh more than 110 lb.
2. Ensure that safety seats are appropriate for the height and weight of the child.
3. Children 14 years of age should ride in the back seat of a vehicle.
4. Children 4 to 10 years of age should use a booster seat.

26. A hospitalized older adult who is allergic to pollen has an allergy attack and the primary health-care provider prescribes diphenhydramine (Benadryl) 50 mg every 4 hours by mouth. The patient experiences extreme drowsiness and the nurse calls the primary health-care provider for instructions regarding the next dose. The primary health-care provider instructs the nurse to give one-half the present dose when the next dose is due. Since the diphenhydramine is in the form of a capsule that cannot be cut in half, the nurse acquires diphenhydramine elixir that states that there is 12.5 mg per 5 mL. How much solution should the nurse administer? Record your answer using a whole number.
Answer: _____ mL

27. A nurse is caring for an 18-month-old child. Which behavior is expected when assessing the child playing?
1. Playing interactively with another child
2. Being fanatical about rules in a game
3. Unwilling to share a favorite toy
4. Cheating to win a game

28. A nurse is planning a health promotion program for school-aged children. Which information is **most** important for the nurse to include in this program?
1. Encouraging nutritious snacks
2. Demonstrating how to care for teeth
3. Reporting bullying to a responsible adult
4. Seeking medical care for sexually transmitted infections

29. An 18-year-old male freshman in college comes to the local urgent care center on 4/8/2013. The student visited the center several times in the last year. The nurse reviews the student's clinic file, reviews the primary health-care provider's diagnosis and orders for the present clinic visit, and interviews the student.

Additional Information

Patient's Clinic File

9/10/2012: Greenish yellow penile discharge, swollen painful testes; gonorrhea; single dose ceftriaxone (Rocephin) 250 mg IM
11/2/2012: Thick yellow penile discharge, burning on urination; gonorrhea; single dose ceftriaxone (Rocephin) 250 mg IM

Primary Health-Care Provider: Diagnosis and Orders

Patient has chancre on shaft of penis; enlarged, nontender lymph node in right groin; primary syphilis; single dose of benzathine penicillin G 2.4 million units IM.

Patient Interview

Now that I am away from home, I can do what I want. I've been having a good time. I love girls; the more the merrier. Last time, the nurse said I could have complications from an infection, but I'm healthy and that is not going to happen to me. I don't know what the big deal is. If I get an infection, it can be cured with a shot.

Which statement by the nurse is **most** appropriate?
1. "If you are not worried about yourself, at least think about your partner."
2. "I will have to notify local health authorities about your infection."
3. "Let's talk about how you can protect yourself in the future."
4. "Consider what this is doing to your future health."

30. A public health nurse is visiting an 80-year-old widow who recently was discharged from a rehabilitation center after recovering from a fall. The woman shares that her three children and their families live several states away. The nurse identifies that the patient looks fatigued, uses a walker to get around the house, and lives independently in her own home. She receives a little help from the community in the way of supermarket deliveries and a cleaning person who comes every other week. Which should the nurse identify as the main concern?

1. Risk for falls
2. Potential for loneliness
3. Decline in distant memory
4. Hopelessness regarding the situation

1. ANSWER: 4.
Rationales:
1. The deltoid muscle is too small to be used in infants and children.
2. The dorsogluteal muscle is less well developed than the preferred muscle for an intramuscular injection in a newborn. The dorsogluteal muscle develops as the child begins to bear weight on the lower extremities.
3. The ventrogluteal muscle is less well developed than the preferred muscle for an intramuscular injection in a newborn. The ventrogluteal muscle develops as the child begins to bear weight on the lower extremities.
4. The vastus lateralis muscle is the best site for an intramuscular injection in a newborn because it is better developed than the gluteal muscles, which are poorly developed.
TEST-TAKING TIP: Identify the word in the stem that sets a priority. The word *best* in the stem sets a priority. Identify the unique option. Option 4 is unique because it has three words and option 1, 2, and 3 have only two words. Examine option 4 carefully.
Content Area: Nursing Care Across the Life Span
Integrated Processes: Nursing Process: Implementation
Client Need: Physiological Integrity; Pharmacological and Parenteral Therapies
Cognitive Level: Application

2. ANSWER: 2.
Rationales:
1. The expected apical rate of a newborn is 120 to 140 beats/minute. An apical rate less than 80 to 100 beats/minute (bradycardia) or more than 160 to 180 beats/minute (tachycardia) should be reported to the primary health-care provider.
2. The expected respiratory rate of a newborn is 30 to 60 breaths/minute. A respiratory rate more than 60 breaths/minute or periods of apnea lasting 20 seconds or longer should be reported to the primary health-care provider.
3. Head and chest circumference may be equal for the first 1 to 2 days of life because of molding. Approximately 2 days after birth, the head circumference, typically 13 to 14 inches (33–35 cm), is about 1 inch (2 to 3 cm) larger than the chest circumference.
4. The crown-to-rump length, typically 12.5 to 14 inches (31–35 cm), is approximately equal to head circumference in the newborn.
TEST-TAKING TIP: Identify the word in the stem that indicates negative polarity. The words *to notify* in the stem indicate negative polarity. It instructs the test-taker to identify the clinical manifestation that is unexpected. Use the concept of the ABCs (airway, breathing, and circulation) of assessment to answer this question. No option is related to airway. Option 2 is related to breathing. Examine option 2 carefully.
Content Area: Nursing Care Across the Life Span
Integrated Processes: Nursing Process: Implementation
Client Need: Safe and Effective Care Environment; Management of Care
Cognitive Level: Analysis

3. ANSWER: 2.
Rationales:
1. A 4-year-old child probably will be able to repeat what was taught. However, the nurse should assess the child further to determine understanding, not just recall.
2. A 4-year-old child does not have the manipulative or cognitive skills to write down what was learned.
3. Using a coloring book to assess knowledge is an appropriate intervention. A child of this age can manipulate a crayon and is probably familiar with this type activity.
4. Role playing is an appropriate intervention. A child of this age likes to imitate others.
TEST-TAKING TIP: Identify the word in the stem that indicates negative polarity. The word *least* in the stem indicates negative polarity.
Content Area: Nursing Care Across the Life Span
Integrated Processes: Teaching/Learning; Nursing Process: Evaluation
Client Need: Health Promotion and Maintenance
Cognitive Level: Application

4. ANSWER: 1.
Rationales:
1. Middle-aged adults are faced with many stresses, including earning a living, supporting a family, paying for children's educational expenses, saving for retirement and, for many middle-aged adults, caring for aging parents.
2. Although learning about exercise is important for middle-aged adults, another option is more appropriate.
3. Although learning about nutrition is important for middle-aged adults, another option is more appropriate.
4. Maintaining a safe home environment is more appropriate for families with young children and for older adults who are more prone to falls than middle-aged adults.
TEST-TAKING TIP: Identify the word in the stem that sets a priority. The word *most* in the stem sets a priority.
Content Area: Nursing Care Across the Life Span
Integrated Processes: Teaching/Learning; Nursing Process: Planning
Client Need: Health Promotion and Maintenance
Cognitive Level: Application

5. ANSWER: 3, 4.
Rationales:
1. Accepting limitations enables a person to be realistic about career choices. This should not interfere with the developmental tasks associated with young adulthood.
2. The ability to delay gratification is a responsible behavior and should not interfere with the resolution of the conflict of intimacy versus isolation, the conflict associated with young adulthood.
3. Self-absorption may interfere with establishing an intimate relationship with another person, which is one of the developmental tasks of this age group.
4. When patients have concerns about altered body image, they may believe that they are no longer desirable. If this belief is held by a young adult, the person may withdraw in an effort to protect the ego.
5. Struggling to establish a place in society is expected in this age group. It is part of the process of confronting the conflicts associated with young adulthood.

6. Attempting to perform personal activities of daily living is responsible behavior expected of a young adult. This will not interfere with resolving the conflict of intimacy versus isolation associated with young adulthood.
Content Area: Nursing Care Across the Life Span
Integrated Processes: Nursing Process: Analysis
Client Need: Health Promotion and Maintenance
Cognitive Level: Analysis

6. **ANSWER: 3.**
Rationales:
1. Socialization with peers is just beginning during the preschool years of 3 to 6. School-aged children 6 to 12 years of age learn to play in groups and develop special friendships, and adolescents 12 to 18 years of age are concerned with establishing close relationships with peers where they feel valued and accepted.
2. Toddlers struggle for autonomy and independence, not to be dependent.
3. **Toddlers feel most comfortable with structured routines that are expected (e.g., a bedtime routine that the toddler can anticipate: having a bath, putting on pajamas, brushing the teeth, listening to a story, singing a song, and giving and receiving hugs and kisses). Knowing what to expect reduces anxiety.**
4. Organized group play takes on significance for school-aged children 6 to 12 years of age.
Content Area: Nursing Care Across the Life Span
Integrated Processes: Caring; Nursing Process: Planning
Client Need: Health Promotion and Maintenance
Cognitive Level: Application

7. **ANSWER: 1.**
Rationales:
1. **As older adults physically decline, they are prone to falls and accidents in the home environment. Prevention of falls and a safe home environment are essential to explore when teaching older adults.**
2. Maintaining a healthy diet is not specific to older adults. A healthy diet should be an educational focus for all age groups.
3. Presenting strategies to avoid the empty nest syndrome generally is specific to the late-middle-adult age group as children leave home to pursue their educations or live independently. In addition, not everyone has children.
4. Exploring actions that support a healthy lifestyle is not specific to older adults. Leading a healthy lifestyle should be an educational focus for all age groups.
TEST-TAKING TIP: Identify the word in the stem that sets a priority. The word *most* is the word in the stem that sets a priority. Identify the equally plausible options. Options 2 and 4 are equally plausible. One is no better than the other because option 4 includes the concept in option 2.
Content Area: Nursing Care Across the Life Span
Integrated Processes: Teaching/Learning; Nursing Process: Planning
Client Need: Health Promotion and Maintenance
Cognitive Level: Application

8. **ANSWER: 1.**
Rationales:
1. **Encouraging ventilation of feelings is critical in this age group. Adolescents are concerned about body image and generally fear disfigurement or decreased function.**
2. Although engaging the patient in diversional activities is important, it is not the priority.
3. Although it is important to support independence, it is not as important as the action in another option.
4. A bedspread may be too heavy to rest on top of an external fixation device. If the patient feels self-conscious about the apparatus, the nurse can place a draw sheet over a bed cradle to provide for privacy.
TEST-TAKING TIP: Identify the word in the stem that sets a priority. The word *most* in the stem sets a priority. Identify the clang association. The word *injury* in the stem and in option 1 is a clang association. Examine option 1 carefully.
Content Area: Nursing Care Across the Life Span
Integrated Processes: Caring; Communication/Documentation; Nursing Process: Planning
Client Need: Health Promotion and Maintenance
Cognitive Level: Application

9. **ANSWER: 2.**
Rationales:
1. A professor is not the person who generally affords the most benefit when providing emotional support to a young adult. Professors are often placed in the same group as parents by young adults because they are seen as authority figures.
2. **Friends are most important to a young adult. Generally, a young adult will benefit most from the emotional support provided by peers.**
3. Young adults are beginning to separate from parents as they seek independence. Young adults are more likely to rely on a person identified in another option rather than parents.
4. More likely, the young adult will seek support from a person identified in another option rather than a sibling.
TEST-TAKING TIP: Identify the word in the stem that sets a priority. The word *most* in the stem sets a priority.
Content Area: Nursing Care Across the Life Span
Integrated Processes: Nursing Process: Analysis
Client Need: Health Promotion and Maintenance
Cognitive Level: Application

10. **ANSWER: 2.**
Rationales:
1. Riding a tricycle is within the expected range of motor development for a toddler 12 to 36 months of age.
2. **Completing multiple chores is beyond the developmental activities of a toddler. This behavior is associated with school-aged children 6 to 12 years of age.**
3. Beginning control of elimination is within the expected physiological development of a toddler.
4. Walking up steps without assistance is within the expected range of motor development of a toddler.

TEST-TAKING TIP: Identify the words in the stem that indicate negative polarity. The words *beyond this child's ability* in the stem indicate negative polarity. The question is asking, "What activity is a toddler unable to do?"
Content Area: Nursing Care Across the Life Span
Integrated Processes: Nursing Process: Assessment
Client Need: Health Promotion and Maintenance
Cognitive Level: Application

11. **ANSWER: 3.**
Rationales:
1. Making change for small amounts of money is within the expected psychosocial development of a school-aged, not preschool-aged, child.
2. Throwing and catching a small ball is within the expected motor development of a school-aged, not preschool-aged, child.
3. Increasing vocabulary and using words in complete sentences are within the range of expected psychosocial development for a 4- to 5-year-old child (preschooler).
4. Having a collection or hobby is within the expected psychosocial development of a school-aged, not preschool-aged, child.
Content Area: Nursing Care Across the Life Span
Integrated Processes: Communication/Documentation; Nursing Process: Assessment
Client Need: Health Promotion and Maintenance
Cognitive Level: Application

12. **ANSWER: 2, 3, 4.**
Rationales:
1. Feeling independent from parents occurs during young adulthood, not adolescence. Young adults demonstrate emotional, social, and economic responsibility for their own lives.
2. Adolescents generally are concerned about their personal appearance. Hair style, clothing, and skin care are important factors associated with adolescents as they search for self-identity.
3. Adolescents explore areas for their own learning as well as those that may interest them as a potential career.
4. Adolescents examine their values, beliefs, standards, and morals. They may discard those adopted from parents for those that they believe are more appropriate for themselves.
5. Developing a mature relationship with another person occurs during young adulthood, not adolescence. According to Erikson, the developmental task of young adulthood is intimacy versus isolation.
Content Area: Nursing Care Across the Life Span
Integrated Processes: Nursing Process: Assessment
Client Need: Health Promotion and Maintenance
Cognitive Level: Application

13. **ANSWER: 2.**
Rationales:
1. A gag reflex is present at birth and continues throughout life. This reflex helps to prevent aspiration of respiratory secretions, fluids, and food.

2. A positive Babinski reflex (the big toe dorsiflexes and the other toes hyperextend when the sole of the foot is stroked) is evident at birth and can be elicited until the infant is approximately 1 year of age. A negative Babinski reflex during the first year of life and a positive Babinski reflex after the first year of life indicate possible upper motor neuron damage.
3. A tonic neck reflex (fencing reflex) is elicited when an infant's head is turned to one side, the arm and leg on that side extend and the arm and leg on the opposite side flex. This is assessed with the infant in the supine position. This reflex disappears after 4 to 6 months of age.
4. A palmar grasp reflex occurs when a small object is placed in the palm of the hand, resulting in the hand curling around it. This reflex disappears at about 8 to 10 months of age.
TEST-TAKING TIP: Identify the word in the stem that indicates negative polarity. The words *cause for concern* indicate negative polarity. What reflex is not expected in a 9-month-old child?
Content Area: Nursing Care Across the Life Span
Integrated Processes: Nursing Process: Assessment
Client Need: Health Promotion and Maintenance
Cognitive Level: Analysis

14. **ANSWER: 4.**
Rationales:
1. An infant may swallow air when feeding, when sucking too quickly, or when having allergies. Frequent burping may help minimize associated abdominal/intestinal discomfort.
2. Cuddling and rocking will comfort a crying infant. Additional measures to comfort a crying infant include swaddling, finding the most comfortable position, and positioning the infant in a baby swing or vibrating chair.
3. Sleeping in the supine position is desirable. Research demonstrates that positioning an infant on the back, not prone, greatly decreases the risk of sudden infant death syndrome (SIDS).
4. An infant or young child should never be shaken, even gently, for any reason. Shaken baby syndrome (SBS) can cause a whiplash that may result in severe brain injury, especially in infants. Blindness, spinal cord damage, cerebral damage, subdural hematoma, and neurological impairments can occur.
TEST-TAKING TIP: Identify the words in the stem that indicate negative polarity. The words *further teaching* indicate negative polarity. The question is asking, "What should not be done when caring for an infant?"
Content Area: Nursing Care Across the Life Span
Integrated Processes: Teaching/Learning; Nursing Process: Evaluation
Client Need: Health Promotion and Maintenance
Cognitive Level: Application

15. **ANSWER: 1.**
Rationales:
1. Toddlers develop gross motor skills and usually are able to walk by 14 months of age and run by 18 months of age.

2. Preschoolers have increasing strength and the physical ability to hop.

3. Preschoolers have the coordination and physical ability to alternate legs to perform skipping.

4. Infants are capable of crawling, pulling self up, and using pincer grasp by 9 months of age.

Content Area: Nursing Care Across the Life Span
Integrated Processes: Nursing Process: Assessment
Client Need: Health Promotion and Maintenance
Cognitive Level: Application

16. **ANSWER: 5, 1, 4, 2, 3.**
Rationales:
5. The task of infancy is the development of trust. When basic physiological needs are met immediately, the infant feels safe and secure and develops trust.
1. The task of toddlerhood is the development of autonomy. Personal decision making and having independence (within parameters of safety) help to promote autonomy.
4. The task of preschoolers is the development of initiative. Successful completion of activities within one's abilities promotes motivation and initiative.
2. The task of school-aged children is industry. Learning new information and skills promotes being productive.
3. The task of adolescence is the development of a self-identity. Recognition from others and internal satisfaction with personal accomplishments help to promote a positive self-concept.

Content Area: Nursing Care Across the Life Span
Integrated Processes: Caring; Nursing Process: Analysis
Client Need: Safe and Effective Care Environment; Management of Care
Cognitive Level: Analysis

17. **ANSWER: 1, 3, 5.**
Rationales:
1. Daily routines provide structure and repetition that limit the unknown. Patients are more in control and less anxious if they know what to expect.
2. The opposite is true; an unhurried routine is less demanding and less likely to precipitate anxiety.
3. Less stimuli are better than a stimulating environment. Excessive stimuli precipitate confusion, increase anxiety, and exacerbate the sundowning syndrome.
4. Simple communication (e.g., declarative statements, short sentences with one noun and one verb) with just the essential information is less confusing.
5. A motion sensor will alarm if a patient attempts to get out of bed. The alarm will alert the nurse so that supervision can be provided.

Content Area: Nursing Care Across the Life Span
Integrated Processes: Communication/Development; Nursing Process: Planning
Client Need: Health Promotion and Maintenance
Cognitive Level: Application

18. **ANSWER: 1, 2, 3.**
Rationales:
1. Impaired balance is associated with aging because the spinal column begins to deteriorate and vertebral fractures and loss of cartilage between the vertebrae occur; these changes alter the center of gravity and body alignment, resulting in difficulty maintaining balance.
2. Close vision impairment (presbyopia) occurs because the lens becomes less elastic and is no longer able to accommodate to close objects.
3. Diminished muscle strength occurs because body and bone mass decrease. The effects of decreased joint mobility inhibit the ability to exercise to the extent possible when younger.
4. Urinary incontinence is not associated with aging; it is associated with urinary tract infections and decreased tone of the muscles in the pelvis. This can occur at any age, especially in women.
5. Decreased hearing of high-pitched sounds (presbycusis), not low-pitched sounds, occurs with aging because the hair cells in the cochlea deteriorate with aging.

Content Area: Nursing Care Across the Life Span
Integrated Processes: Nursing Process: Assessment
Client Need: Health Promotion and Maintenance
Cognitive Level: Application

19. **ANSWER: 4.**
Rationales:
1. Tenting on the back of the hand often occurs in older adults because of a decrease in subcutaneous fat. Tenting should be assessed over the sternum in older adults. Tenting is not a reliable indicator of dehydration in older adults. The nurse needs additional information before contacting the primary health-care provider.
2. A person's personality does not change as one ages, but the intensity of the personality may increase.
3. A delayed sexual response is experienced with aging because, in women, the vaginal mucosa becomes thinner and dry, erectile difficulties and lengthening time for ejaculation occur in men, and less intense orgasmic contractions occur in both men and women. These responses result from a decline in estrogen or testosterone.
4. An unstable or constantly changing mood (lability of mood) is unrelated to aging; it may be related to physical problems (e.g., brain attack) or emotional problems (e.g., bipolar disorder). Consistent feelings (e.g., sadness, anger, frustration) may occur with the loss of personal abilities, independence, and/or loved ones.

TEST-TAKING TIP: Identify the words in the stem that indicate negative polarity. The words *not associated* in the stem indicate negative polarity. The question is asking, "What physical characteristic is not related to aging?"

Content Area: Nursing Care Across the Life Span
Integrated Processes: Communication/Documentation; Nursing Process: Implementation
Client Need: Safe and Effective Care Environment
Cognitive Level: Application

20. **ANSWER: 4.**
Rationales:
1. This may occur as people age and is referred to as an exacerbation of a person's premorbid personality. This statement does not reflect ageism.
2. All systems of the body gradually decrease in size and function as one ages (e.g., decreased mass and strength in

both bones and muscles, decreased joint mobility, impaired balance and coordination). This statement does not reflect ageism.

3. The adult child may be frustrated by the father's behavior, but the adult child's statement is not a reflection of ageism.

4. This comment reflects ageism because it assumes older adults are useless. Ageism is negative attitudes and beliefs about older adults that include stereotyping, prejudice, or discrimination against people based on their age.

TEST-TAKING TIP: Identify the options that are equally plausible. Options 1 and 2 are equally plausible. One is no better than the other. Options 1 and 2 can be eliminated from consideration.

Content Area: Nursing Care Across the Life Span
Integrated Processes: Communication/Documentation; Nursing Process: Analysis
Client Need: Health Promotion and Maintenance
Cognitive Level: Application

21. **ANSWER: 1, 2, 5.**
    Rationales:
    1. Climbing up and down steps using alternate feet, not using two feet on each step, is expected by 3 years of age.
    2. A preschool-aged child should be able to don clothing without assistance, except for back closing garments.
    3. Imprecise fine motor skills are still obvious during the school-aged years of 6 to 12 years.
    4. Magical thinking is commonly associated with 3- to 5-year-old children.
    5. Falling frequently is expected by a toddler, not a preschool-aged child.

    TEST-TAKING TIP: Identify the words in the stem that indicate negative polarity. The words *behavior* and *developmental delay* are the key words in the stem that indicate negative polarity. The question is asking, "Which behaviors are not expected of a preschool-aged child?"

    Content Area: Nursing Care Across the Life Span
    Integrated Processes: Communication/Documentation; Nursing Process: Assessment
    Client Need: Safe and Effective Care Environment; Management of Care
    Cognitive Level: Analysis

22. **ANSWER: 2, 3.**
    Rationales:
    1. Sweat gland activity decreases, not increases, with aging.
    2. Hair turns white or gray because pigment cells in hair decrease as a person ages.
    3. Decreased vascularity of the skin occurs with aging, causing coolness and pallor.
    4. Sebaceous gland activity decreases, not increases, with aging.
    5. Collagen and elastin in the dermis deteriorate with aging, causing the skin to become wrinkled.

    TEST-TAKING TIP: Identify the equally plausible options. Options 1, 4, and 5 all refer to physiological processes that increase with aging. Options 2 and 3 refer to physiological processes that decrease with aging. Since aging is associated with a decline in many physiological processes give special consideration to options 2 and 3 when attempting to answer this question.

Content Area: Nursing Care Across the Life Span
Integrated Processes: Nursing Process: Assessment
Client Need: Health Promotion and Maintenance
Cognitive Level: Application

23. **ANSWER: 4.**
    Rationales:
    1. Children between the ages of 18 months and 3 years are concerned with learning how to delay satisfaction, not middle-aged adults.
    2. Coping with death is one of the developmental tasks of older adults, not middle-aged adults.
    3. Developing peer relationships is a developmental task of children who are 6 to 12 years of age as well as adolescents, not middle-aged adults.
    4. The most important developmental task of middle adulthood is successfully achieving goals that involve family, career, and society. A developmental crisis occurs when a middle-aged adult has difficulty achieving these goals.

    Content Area: Nursing Care Across the Life Span
    Integrated Processes: Nursing Process: Analysis
    Client Need: Health Promotion and Maintenance
    Cognitive Level: Analysis

24. **ANSWER: 3.**
    Rationales:
    1. Instructing a person to resist high-risk activities is most appropriate for adolescents who are vulnerable to peer pressure because they want to be accepted and belong.
    2. Instructing a person to rise slowly to a standing position is most appropriate for older adults because their voluntary and autonomic reflexes have declined and made them vulnerable to orthostatic hypotension and falls.
    3. The leading cause of accidental death in infants, toddlers, preschoolers, school-aged children, adolescents, and adults is motor vehicle accidents. Motor vehicle accidents are one of the leading causes of injuries in older adults after falls. Seat belts reduce the incidence of morbidity and mortality.
    4. Many foods are small or soft and do not need to be cut into small pieces. Although cutting food into small pieces is advisable for everyone, it is most significant in infants and toddlers. Risk for choking is the greatest between 6 months and 3 years of age.

    TEST-TAKING TIP: Identify the option with a specific determiner. Option 4 contains the word *all* which is a specific determiner. An option that contains a specific determiner rarely is the correct answer.

    Content Area: Safety
    Integrated Processes: Nursing Process: Implementation
    Client Need: Safe and Effective Care Environment; Safety and Infection Control
    Cognitive Level: Analysis

25. **ANSWER: 2.**
    Rationales:
    1. Children 12 years of age or younger, regardless of weight, should ride in the back seat of a vehicle. This action is associated with a 30 percent reduction in the risk of a fatal injury in a vehicular accident.

2. Age, height, and weight appropriate automobile safety seats are essential to protect infants and children when in a motor vehicle accident.

3. This option does not indicate the weight of the child. If the child is 14 years of age and weighs greater than 110 pounds, the child may sit in the front seat. Children 12 years of age or younger and children older than 12 years of age but weighing less than 110 pounds should ride in the back seat of a vehicle.

4. Booster seats are safer than a seat belt alone for average-size children 4 to 8 years of age, not 4 to 10 years of age. Children who are older than 4 years of age should not transition to a booster seat until they outgrow the criteria for using a five point harness safety seat.

TEST-TAKING TIP: Identify the word in the stem that sets a priority. The word *most* in the stem sets a priority. Identify the unique option. Option 2 is unique because it is the only option that does not have a number. Identify the global option. Option 2 is global in that it is broad and all encompassing. Examine global options carefully.

Content Area: Safety
Integrated Processes: Teaching/Learning; Nursing Process: Planning
Client Need: Safe and Effective Care Environment; Safety and Infection Control
Cognitive Level: Application

26. **ANSWER: 10.**
Rationale:
The ability to metabolize and excrete drugs decreases in older adults. Medications may require a reduction in the size of the dose to prevent toxicity. Solve the problem using ratio and proportion.

$$\frac{\text{Desire } 25 \text{ mg}}{\text{Have } 12.5 \text{ mg}} = \frac{x \text{ mL}}{5 \text{ mL}}$$

$$12.5\, x = 25 \times 5$$

$$12.5\, x = 125$$

$$x = 125 \div 12.5$$

$$x = 10 \text{ mL}$$

Content Area: Medication Administration
Integrated Processes: Nursing Process: Planning
Client Need: Physiological Integrity; Pharmacological and Parenteral Therapies
Cognitive Level: Application

27. **ANSWER: 3.**
Rationales:
1. Children between the ages of 12 and 36 months do not engage in interactive play. They play next to, not with, their peers.
2. Rigidity about rules of a game is associated with the play of children between the ages of 6 to 12 years of age.
3. Children 12 to 36 months of age (toddlers) are egocentric. They frequently use the word "mine" and are reluctant to share favorite toys without encouragement.

4. Cheating to win a game is associated with children 3 to 5 years of age when they engage in cooperative play (associative play).
Content Area: Nursing Care Across the Life Span
Integrated Processes: Nursing Process: Assessment
Client Need: Health Promotion and Maintenance
Cognitive Level: Application

28. **ANSWER: 3.**
Rationales:
1. Although teaching about nutritious snacks is important because of the increased incidence of obesity in children, it is not the priority for school-aged children.
2. Although teaching about care of the teeth is important, this is not as high a priority as another option.
3. This is the priority from among the options presented. Being the target of bullying is extremely damaging to the ego. Children who are bullied are known to commit suicide or may resort to extreme violence in retaliation.
4. Information about sexually transmitted infections should be explored in a health promotion program for adolescents, not school-aged children.
TEST-TAKING TIP: Identify the word in the stem that sets a priority. The word *most* in the stem sets a priority.
Content Area: Nursing Care Across the Life Span
Integrated Processes: Teaching/Learning; Nursing Process: Planning
Client Need: Health Promotion and Maintenance
Cognitive Level: Application

29. **ANSWER: 3.**
Rationales:
1. This is a judgmental response that may cut off communication.
2. Although this is a true statement, it may be perceived as a threat by the patient. It is a confrontational statement that may cut off further communication.
3. The patient does not perceive a benefit in changing his behavior because the consequence is insignificant to him. The patient stated, "I do not know what the big deal is. If I get an infection, it can be cured with a shot." The patient should be taught how to consistently use safe sex practices (e.g., condoms, uninfected sex partner) to prevent the acquisition and transmission of sexually transmitted infections.
4. This statement will have no impact on the patient. The patient has stated, "Last time the nurse said I could have complications from an infection, but I am healthy and that is not going to happen to me." This statement indicates that the patient does not perceive that he is at risk for complications; he is in denial.
TEST-TAKING TIP: Identify the word in the stem that sets a priority. The word *most* in the stem indicates a priority.
Content Area: Nursing Care Across the Life Span
Integrated Processes: Communication/Documentation; Teaching/Learning; Nursing Process: Implementation
Client Need: Health Promotion and Maintenance
Cognitive Level: Analysis

30. ANSWER: 1.

Rationales:

1. **Risk for falls is the priority. The patient is fatigued, uses a walker, lives alone, and has a history of a fall; these are risk factors for a future fall.**

2. Although this is a concern, it is not as important as another option.

3. Older adults generally experience a decline in recent, not distant, memory.

4. No data in the stem indicate that the patient feels hopeless.

TEST-TAKING TIP: Identify the word in the stem that sets a priority. The word *main* in the stem sets a priority. Identify the word in the stem that is clang association. The word *fall* in the stem and in option 1 is a clang association. Examine option 1 carefully.

Content Area: Nursing Care Across the Life Span
Integrated Processes: Nursing Process: Analysis
Client Need: Safe and Effective Care Environment; Management of Care
Cognitive Level: Application

Communication and Documentation

I. Communication

Communication is a dynamic, purposeful, reciprocal process of sending and/or receiving a message. The need to communicate is universal because it is the way people convey and fulfill needs.

A. Concepts About Communication
1. All verbal and nonverbal communication transmits meaning.
2. Communication is a learned process.
3. Communication can occur within the self (intrapersonal); between two people (interpersonal); or when sending a message to or communicating within a group, such as with public speaking, small self-help and social groups, and group therapy.
4. Recurring ideas and thoughts (themes) communicated during an interaction provide insight to a patient's feelings.
5. A trusting relationship is basic to effective communication.
6. A patient's degree of expression (emotional affect) reflects the patient's mood.
7. Humor is highly subjective; it can mean different things to different people.

8. Patients have a potential for growth as a result of verbal and nonverbal communication.
9. Previous patterns of communication can become inadequate when one is ill or under stress.
10. Communication is confidential information and should be shared only with health team members.

B. Elements of Communication
1. **Sender** (encoder/source): Person who conveys a message.
2. **Message:** Information communicated; includes language, words, voice intonation, and gestures.
3. **Channel** (mode): Vehicle used to convey a message; includes written, oral, and touch.
4. **Receiver** (decoder): Person who acquires a message.
5. **Feedback** (response): Response from the receiver to the sender.

C. Factors Affecting the Communication Process
1. Attitudes, values, beliefs, and experiences.
2. Culture, education, and language.
3. Developmental level.
   a. The very young are concrete thinkers and have little or no experience.
   b. Adults are more abstract thinkers.

c. Older adults may have vision and hearing loss that interferes with communication.

4. Gender.
   a. Males and females generally communicate differently from an early age.
   b. Females seek intimacy and validation and reduce differences; boys use language to negotiate status and establish independence.
   c. Differences are changing as gender roles become less distinct.

5. Authority one ascribes to a role (e.g., some see nurses as authority figures, whereas others see nurses as servants).

6. Ineffective perception or selective inattention: May distort a message.

D. Barriers to Communication

1. Unwillingness to listen to another point of view.
2. Physical factors, such as an uncomfortable environment (e.g., too hot or too cold), excessive noise, or distractions.
3. Adaptation to disease, such as impaired ability to communicate through speech, writing, or signs because of brain dysfunction (e.g., receptive or expressive aphasia); impaired ability to say words (dysarthria); impaired cognition (e.g., dementia or delirium); oral problems; fatigue; and pain.
4. Treatment related factors, such as laryngectomy, or artificial airways, such as tracheostomy or endotracheal tube.
5. Psychological factors, such as lack of privacy, anxiety, and fear.

E. Phases of the Communication Process

1. Preinteraction phase.
   a. This phase occurs before meeting the patient.
   b. The nurse gathers information about the patient.
2. Orientation phase.
   a. Initially, the nurse is in the stranger role.
   b. The nurse meets a patient and begins to establish a relationship of rapport and trust.
   c. Introductions and initial exchange of information occurs.
   d. The purpose of the visit is explained, roles are clarified, and an agreement or contract about the relationship may be formulated.
   e. The termination phase is initiated in this phase.
3. Working phase.
   a. Most communication occurs during this phase.
   b. This phase is the active part of the relationship.
   c. The nurse and patient work together to address patient needs, feelings are shared, caring is demonstrated, and mutual respect is maintained.
   d. The nurse may function as caregiver, counselor, teacher, resource person, and so on.
   e. The nurse motivates a patient by identifying progress and supporting movement toward independence.

f. Anxiety may increase during this phase as the patient may need to learn new adaptive behaviors.
g. Preparation for the termination phase continues.

4. Termination phase.
   a. Actual termination occurs at the conclusion of a relationship.
   b. Termination occurs at discharge, at the end of a shift, or when the goals of the relationship are achieved.
   c. Goals and objectives are summarized, adaptive behavior is reinforced, and additional resources available are arranged for the patient.
   d. Some patients become emotional during this phase because they feel angry, rejected, or fearful of leaving a safe environment; the nurse needs to address these feelings.

F. Modes of Communication

1. **Verbal communication:** Uses spoken or written words to communicate a message.
   a. Characteristics.
      (1) Clarity: Simple words and sentence structure are better understood.
      (2) Intonation: Reflects feeling behind words; loud or soft volume, cadence, and pitch can impart a message, such as anger, excitement, sarcasm, and fear.
      (3) Pacing: Speed, rhythm, and patterns of delivery can convey anxiety, indifference, and attention; pace must be fast enough to maintain interest, but slow enough for receiver to decode the message.
      (4) Relevance: Message needs to be conveyed when the receiver is ready and able to receive the message; information has to be important to the patient.
   b. Nursing care.
      (1) Build a therapeutic relationship.
         (a) Place oneself in the patient's place mentally and emotionally (empathy).
         (b) Acknowledge the patient's individuality; be flexible when meeting needs.
         (c) Address the patient by name; avoid using terms of endearment, such as "grandma" and "honey."
         (d) Respect values and beliefs.
         (e) Provide privacy.
         (f) Maintain credibility and genuineness; be truthful, respond to needs promptly, and follow through on promises.
      (2) Let the patient take the lead in the communication process.
      (3) Use simple words and sentence structures; keep messages brief.

(4) Ensure intonation and pace of words convey professional confidence, respect, interest, and acceptance of the patient.

(5) Ensure that message is relevant and a priority for the patient.

(6) Use humor carefully; although it may lighten the mood, it can be misunderstood and offend a patient.

🛑 (7) Validate congruence between verbal messages and nonverbal behavior.

2. **Nonverbal communication:** Message that is sent and received without use of spoken or written words; involves use of body language; may be more accurate than verbal communication because it is less consciously controlled.

a. Characteristics.

(1) Facial expression: Can convey meaning or mask emotions; some expressions are universal, such as a smile (happiness) or a frown (displeasure); can be subtle, such as raising the eyebrows.

(2) Gestures: Emphasize spoken word; some have same meaning regardless of culture, such as waving indicates hello or goodbye; different gestures may have similar meanings, such as shaking a fist versus cold, stillness when angry; shaking the head "yes" may indicate the message has been received even though message is not understood.

(3) Eye contact: In Western cultures, indicates interest and attention, whereas downcast eyes may indicate low self-esteem, powerlessness, and sadness; however, in some cultures, downcast eyes show respect.

(4) Posture and gait: Erect posture, head held up with a rapid gait indicates well-being and confidence; slumped, slow, shuffling gait with head held low indicates illness, depression, or impaired self-esteem; crossing legs and arms indicates a defensive posture.

(5) Touch: Generally conveys caring, concern, encouragement; some patients do not like to be touched, and touching is unacceptable in some cultures (e.g., only relatives can touch an orthodox Jewish man).

(6) Territoriality and space: People have a physical zone around the body that is culturally and individually defined.

(a) Intimate: 0 to 18 inches; used for providing nursing care or emotional support, such as hygiene and hand holding.

(b) Personal: 1.5 to 4 feet; used for therapeutic communication, such as nurse-patient conversation, counseling, and teaching.

(c) Social and public: 4 feet and beyond; used when performing more formal interventions, such as making rounds, teaching a class, or facilitating a group.

b. Nursing care.

(1) Be aware of a patient's culture and its impact on nonverbal communication.

(2) Demonstrate behavior that supports a therapeutic relationship, such as eye contact, caring facial expression, unhurried behavior, and open posture.

(3) Validate the meaning of body language to ensure messages are received as intended.

🛑 (4) Validate the meaning of body language that is not congruent with the spoken word.

(5) Use touch cautiously so as not offend the patient.

(6) Explain what is going to be done and why before entering a patient's personal space; entering personal space may be perceived as a violation of a patient's territory and the patient may feel uncomfortable, threatened, or anxious.

(7) Knock before entering a patient's room, and ask permission before entering a patient's closet or bedside drawer.

(8) Close the door, pull the curtain, or drape the patient when engaging in nursing care that requires privacy because doing so conveys respect.

II. Therapeutic Versus Nontherapeutic Communication

Therapeutic communication is interaction between a nurse and a patient in which the nurse focuses on the feelings, concerns, needs, and/or objectives of the patient. Nurses must develop a repertoire of verbal and nonverbal techniques that can be used to facilitate therapeutic communication as well as be aware of the various attitudes and approaches that can hinder communication. The therapeutic use of self is the most valuable tool that nurses have to facilitate therapeutic communication and ultimately develop an effective nurse-patient relationship.

A. Therapeutic Communication: See Table 7.1
B. Nontherapeutic Communication: See Table 7.2

III. Nursing Care for Patients With Special Communication Needs

A patient's physical, emotional, or cultural status may result in a diminished or absent ability to receive, process, or send a message. When impaired communication occurs between a patient and a nurse, it is the nurse's responsibility to identify what is interfering with the communication process.

Table 7.1 Therapeutic Communication Techniques and Related Nursing Care

Therapeutic Communication Technique	Related Nursing Care
Silence • Provides time for the patient to process what was said, reflect, and articulate a response. • Encourages the patient to initiate or continue a conversation.	• Maintain an open posture. • Maintain an unhurried manner.
Offering Self • Indicates a nurse's attention and interest without expectations.	• Maintain an open posture. • Maintain an unhurried manner. • Example: Say, "I will sit with you for a while."
Open-Ended Questions • Allows the patient to control the direction of the conversation to an area of concern.	• Ask questions that require more than one-word answers and invite a more detailed response. • Example: "Tell me about how you have been managing your illness."
Direct Questions • Facilitates collection of objective information. • May interfere with exploration of feelings because they may be too blunt and threatening.	• Keep questions short and simple. • Example: "Have you received the pneumococcal (PVC) vaccine?"
Paraphrasing • Encourages further discussion by repeating content in same or similar words. • Conveys that the message was understood. • Allows the patient to hear what he or she said.	• Listen attentively. • Focus on content. • Example: The patient says, "When I'm discharged, I might have a hard time because I live alone." The nurse responds, "You sound concerned about how you are going to manage."
Reflection • Encourages further discussion by focusing on emotional themes and feelings. • Indicates active listening. • Helps the patient to identify emotional themes and feelings.	• Listen attentively. • Focus on feelings rather than content. • Example: The patient says, "I don't understand how I had a heart attack. I don't smoke or eat fatty foods, and I exercise regularly." The nurse responds, "It must be frustrating to have a heart attack when you did everything right."
Clarifying • Encourages elaboration on unclear messages. • Ensures that the message is understood as intended; minimizes misunderstanding.	• Be nonjudgmental; do not place responsibility for lack of understanding on the patient. • Example: "I don't understand what you mean when you say that your pain feels like melting lava."
Focusing • Directs conversation to areas of concern; targets discussion to key points. • Encourages the patient to expand on an idea, thought, or feeling.	• Focus on the priority topic of concern. • Example: "Earlier you mentioned that you are having a problem with recurrent diarrhea."
Validating • Identifies and supports what the patient feels or believes. • Demonstrates respect for the patient. • Demonstrates empathy.	• Maintain a nonjudgmental, empathetic demeanor. • Example: "I can understand how difficult it must be to wait 5 days for a biopsy result."
Touch • Communicates caring, concern, and encouragement.	• Use touch cautiously because some patients prefer not to be touched, touch can be misunderstood, and touch invades a person's intimate space. • Examples: Hold a patient's hand or place an arm around a patient's shoulder.
Summarizing • Highlights important points in a conversation, such as progress made and tasks that may still need to be accomplished.	• Review just the most important points. • Provide a summary in writing when appropriate. • Example: "Let's review what we accomplished today."

Once the cause has been identified, the nurse can formulate an individualized plan to promote communication.

A. Commonalities of Nursing Care

1. Reduce noise and minimize distractions.
2. Stand in front of the patient while making eye contact.
3. Be alert to nonverbal cues and behavior.
4. Explain everything that is going to be done and the reasons why using simple words and sentence structures.
5. Give the patient adequate time to formulate a message and respond to a message.

Table 7.2 Nontherapeutic Communication and Preventive Nursing Care

Nontherapeutic Communication	Preventive Nursing Care
Being Judgmental • Imposes the nurse's opinions, values, beliefs, and standards on the patient. • Demonstrates lack of respect for the patient.	• Be aware of own values, beliefs, standards, and opinions and do not impose them on others. • Use words that demonstrate acceptance. • Maintain an empathetic demeanor.
Using Medical Jargon • Confuses patients. • Communicates that the nurse is not interested enough to make information understandable. • Demonstrates a demeanor of superiority and arrogance.	• Use words that can be understood; avoid use of medical jargon, such as medical terminology, acronyms, and slang. • Offer opportunities to ask questions; answer all questions to the patient's satisfaction. • Seek feedback to ensure understanding.
Using Ridicule or Sarcasm • Conveys a hostile attitude through words or tone of voice.	• Avoid cutting, caustic, and hostile remarks. • Avoid ridicule.
Using Probing Questions • Invades privacy because it attempts to obtain information to satisfy one's curiosity. • Pressures the patient to discuss topics before he or she is ready.	• Ask questions based on the patient's needs, not curiosity. • Use open-ended questions.
Focusing on Self • Demonstrates lack of interest in the patient. • Demonstrates an attitude of self-importance and egocentricity.	• Remember that the patient is the center of the health team. • Focus on the patient's needs and not self-needs.
Stereotyping • Devalues patient uniqueness and individuality. • Demonstrates opinions either blatantly or subtly, such as men who cry are not manly, and patients who are health-care professionals do not need health teaching.	• Assess own beliefs, such as stereotypes, biases, and prejudices, and ensure that they do not affect professional relationships. • Accept each patient as unique.
Changing the Subject • Indicates lack of interest in the patient's concerns or feelings. • Reflects that the nurse feels uncomfortable talking about the topic. • Cuts off communication when the patient may be ready to discuss an emotionally charged topic.	• Identify health-care topics that cause anxiety within one's self and seek education or counseling to become therapeutic in the health-care role. • Listen attentively. • Focus on the patient's concerns.
Providing False Reassurance • Minimizes the patient's concerns. • Violates trust.	• Answer questions truthfully; base reassurance on facts. • Address underlying concerns.
Minimizing Feelings • Devalues the validity of the patient's feelings.	• Use the communication technique of reflection. • Address feelings.
Giving Advise • Bases responses on one's own values and beliefs rather than on what is important to the patient. • Limits the patient's right to be a partner in problem-solving. • Supports dependence and is controlling.	• Assist the patient to explore his or her own feelings, concerns, opinions, and options. • Assist the patient to use critical thinking to arrive at a conclusion.
Using Clichés, Colloquialisms, and Slang • Trivializes the patient's concerns. • Causes misunderstanding.	• Use words that the patient can understand. • Avoid comments that may have ambiguous meanings or multiple interpretations.
Using Terms of Endearment • Demonstrates lack of respect. • Reflects an unprofessional demeanor.	• Call the patient by his or her name. • Avoid use of intimate names (e.g., honey, dear, sweetie, mom, or pop).
Responding Defensively by the Nurse • Demonstrates the nurse's attempt to protect the self rather than focus on the patient's concerns; defensive responses usually are precipitated by patients who are angry, demanding, or critical. • Minimizes the patient's concerns. • Focuses on content rather than feelings.	• Identify the underlying cause of the patient's behavior; patients' angry, demanding, or critical responses are attempts to protect the self; all behavior has meaning. • Focus on the patient's feelings. • Involve the patient in identifying a resolution, such as, "I am sorry that I did not meet your expectations. What can I do now to help you?"

Continued

Table 7.2 Nontherapeutic Communication and Preventive Nursing Care—cont'd

Nontherapeutic Communication	Preventive Nursing Care
Challenging the Patient • Requires the patient to defend his or her feelings or point of view. • Ignores the patient's feelings and rights. • Causes the patient to abandon a coping mechanism that may be temporarily therapeutic.	• Accept the patient's right to have his or her own feelings, beliefs, and point of view. • Support the patient's coping mechanisms, unless they are destructive to self or others; abandoning a coping mechanism can leave a patient defenseless.
Asking "How" or "Why" • Threatens or intimidates the patient. • May leave the patient unsure how to answer the question.	• Use open-ended questions. • Explore issues with the patient so that he or she can develop insight and come to own conclusions about "how" or "why."
Asking Too Many Questions • Overwhelms the patient emotionally and may invade the patient's privacy or precipitate feelings of "being interrogated." • Overwhelms the patient physically.	• Assess the patient's physical and emotional stamina to engage in data collection. • Use several shorter sessions to collect data.
Engaging in Nonprofessional Involvement • Oversteps boundaries of the therapeutic nurse-patient relationship. • Befriends the patient, but actually abandons the patient because the nurse is unable to fulfill professional role.	• Maintain a professional relationship with the patient as the center of the health team; avoid personal and social relationships. • Minimize self-disclosure; use it judiciously. • Explain the nurse-patient relationship, and set limits if necessary.

6. Seek feedback to ensure that the message is received as intended.
7. Repeat a message using different words if the message was not understood.

B. Patients Who Are Angry
1. Assess for the cause of anger because all behavior has meaning.
2. Assess for verbal and nonverbal signs of escalating aggression, such as a loud voice, clenched fist and jaw, narrowed eyes, and physical agitation.
3. Model acceptable behaviors, such as keeping a calm voice with a normal volume, tone, and pace.
4. Validate the patient's feelings.
5. Avoid touching the patient because it may be perceived as a threat.

🛑 6. Do not turn your back to an angry patient or avert your eyes away from the patient; position yourself between the patient and the door.

C. Patients Who Have Aphasia
1. Assess the patient's ability to communicate through speech, writing, or alternate means of communication, such as gestures, a picture board, and computer programs.
2. Promote communication when the patient has an inability to formulate and/or send a message (expressive aphasia).
   a. Use questions that require a one-word answer or a short response.
   b. Give the patient ample time to formulate a message; do not complete sentences for the patient.
   c. Use alternate means of communication, such as picture cards, blinking the eyes once for yes and twice for no, a computer, a puff-activated communication device, or a voice synthesizer.
3. Promote communication when the patient has an inability to understand communicated information (receptive aphasia).
   a. Use simple words and sentences; vary words when repeating a message.
   b. Augment verbal messages with gestures and facial expressions.
   c. Augment verbal communication with picture cards or objects, such as holding up a cup of water to encourage fluid intake.

D. Patients Who Are Confused
1. Use short sentences and convey concrete ideas.
2. Speak slowly.
3. Use questions that require a one-word answer or a short response.
4. Break down instructions into simple steps.
5. Augment verbal communication with picture cards or objects, such as holding up a comb to indicate the need for hair care.

E. Patients Who Are Hearing Impaired
1. Ensure that the patient is wearing a hearing aid, if available; ensure that a hearing aid is functioning, is inserted properly, and is cleaned and stored with a label.
2. Stand on the patient's side with more acute hearing; speak at a normal pace using a low tone because high-pitched sounds are harder

to hear; use a slightly louder volume, but do not yell.

3. Face the patient, enunciate words (without exaggeration), and to facilitate lip reading avoid chewing gum or holding a hand in front of the mouth when speaking.

4. Use gestures and facial expression to augment verbal communicate.

5. Determine whether the patient knows sign language, and seek the assistance of sign-language specialists if applicable.

6. Provide writing materials to support communication if the patient is able to write and is literate.

F. Patients Who Are Unresponsive

(!) 1. Assume that the patient's hearing is intact because hearing is believed to be the last sense lost before death. Never talk about a patient or others in front of the patient thinking that the patient cannot hear.

2. Talk to the patient in a normal volume, tone, and pace.

3. Explain what you are going to do and the reasons why before touching a patient.

G. Patients Who Are Visually Impaired

1. Provide adequate lighting.

2. Speak in a normal volume because the patient is not hearing impaired.

3. Explain what you are going to do if you have to touch the patient and seek permission first.

4. Orient the patient to surroundings, such as furniture in room and food on a plate using a clock as a format (e.g., meat is at 12, green beans at 3, potatoes at 6).

H. Patients Who Do Not Speak English

(!) 1. Seek the help of a professional interpreter fluent in the patient's language (e.g., use a telephone service that provides translation services); avoid the use of non-educated translators or family members because inaccuracies may occur (inadvertently or deliberately) as well as confidentiality may be jeopardized.

2. Use a translation book that presents common questions and answers in the nurse's and patient's language.

3. Use pictures, body language, and environmental cues to communicate until an interpreter is available.

I. Patients With a Physical Barrier (e.g., endotracheal tube, laryngectomy)

1. Encourage the patient to use eye blinks, hand squeeze, writing tools, such as a magic slate, flash cards or pictures, or a communication board to communicate.

2. Reinforce and praise efforts to communicate.

IV. Types of Interactions Between the Nurse and Other Health-Care Team Members

Information about patients must be communicated between nurses and among nurses and other members of the health team, including patients and their families. Whether the interaction is verbal or written, a systematic approach is preferred so that the message is clearly, concisely, and accurately transmitted and received.

A. Systematic Approach to Communication

1. Framework to facilitate thorough communication among health-care professionals to provide a culture of safety for the patient.

2. Current movement occurring in the health-care community toward setting standards related to interdisciplinary communication (e.g., the Joint Commission is requiring that a systematic approach be used during nursing change of shift reports and when a nurse seeks a telephone order from a primary health-care provider).

3. Example: SBAR.

a. Situation: Identify self, title, facility; identify patient, date of birth, gender; reason for collaboration.

b. Background: Patient's present issue, relevant medical history, summary of background.

c. Assessment: Vital signs and clinical indicators outside expected range, severity of patient issue, nurse's clinical impression.

d. Recommendation: Explain what is required and urgency of what is required; make suggestions.

MAKING THE CONNECTION

Systematic Approach to Communication and Clinical Practice:

A patient with no previous history of acute or chronic health problems is admitted to a hospital for surgical removal of a mass in the ascending colon. After an uneventful recovery in the postanesthesia care unit, the patient is transferred to a surgical unit. The patient is receiving a patient-controlled analgesia intravenous infusion containing morphine. In addition to the basal dose of 1 mg/hour, the patient is allowed a 0.2 mg on-demand dose with a lock-out interval of 10 minutes. The patient can self-administer six 0.2 mg doses per hour, for a total of 1.2 mg/hour, with a maximum dose of 8.8 mg in 4 hours. As the postoperative period progresses, the nurse identifies that the patient's personal pain rating scale has increased from a range of 2 to 3 to a range of 4 to 5 and the PCA pump history indicates that the patient has been pressing the button every 5 minutes in the last hour. The nurse

Continued

MAKING THE CONNECTION—cont'd

assesses the patient. The patient's vital signs are: T—99.6°F; P—92 beats/minute and regular; R—22 breaths/minute, regular, and shallow; BP—134/88 mm Hg. The patient states that the incisional pain is sharp and rates it as a 7 on a scale of 0 to 10. The patient is lying in one position, has clenched fists, and is exhibiting a facial grimace. The patient's oxygen saturation is 96 percent, the urinary catheter is draining an adequate amount of clear yellow urine, and the dressing is dry and intact. The nurse concludes that the patient's analgesic prescription is inadequate to relieve the patient's pain and places a phone call to the patient's primary health-care provider. The nurse uses the SBAR format to provide a systematic approach when communicating with the primary health-care provider.

Situation: Hello, this is Ms. Jones. I am a registered nurse from Longview Medical Center. I am caring for Mr. Smith, who was born April 5, 1939, and I am calling about his patient-controlled analgesia (PCA).

Background: Mr. Smith had no acute or chronic health problems prior to this admission. He had surgery at 0800 this morning for resection of a tumor in his ascending colon. His PCA prescription is morphine basal dose of 1 mg/hour and he is allowed a 0.2 mg on-demand dose with a lock-out interval of 10 minutes. The patient can self-administer six 0.2 mg doses per hour, for a total of 1.2 mg/hour, with a maximum dose of 8.8 mg in 4 hours. In the last hour, Mr. Smith has pushed the trigger of the PCA pump every 5 minutes.

Assessment: Mr. Smith states that his pain is a 7 on a scale of 0 to 10. His vital signs are T—99.6°F; P—92 beats/minute and regular; R—22 breaths/minute, regular, and shallow; BP—134/88 mm Hg. He is lying in one position, has clenched fists, and is exhibiting a facial grimace. The patient's oxygen saturation is 96 percent, the urinary catheter is draining an adequate amount of clear yellow urine, and the dressing is dry and intact. I think that Mr. Smith is in excessive pain and the prescribed dose of morphine is inadequate to control his pain.

Recommendation: Mr. Smith has been in excessive pain for an hour and it is important to adjust the morphine prescription. Could you please increase the basal dose, increase the on-demand dose, or shorten the lock-out time?

B. Change of Shift Report
1. Given by a nurse who is finishing a shift to a nurse who is responsible for continuing care of the patient.
2. May be verbal, written, or audiotaped; may include walking rounds where two or more nurses visit the patient as part of the report.
3. Includes basic data about the patient, current assessment of the patient's health status, recent interventions and patient responses, dependent and independent nursing interventions to be implemented, report of patients who are off the unit temporarily (includes purpose, when they are expected to return, and nursing care that is anticipated), and patients who have been admitted, transferred, or discharged.

C. Telephone Reports
1. Method by which critical information, such as laboratory test results, may be communicated to the unit.
2. Method by which nurses can report a change in a patient's condition to a primary health-care provider.
3. Require the nurse to identify self by name and title, state relationship with the patient, and concisely and accurately report the patient's condition, including vital signs, any clinical findings, and any intervention already performed for the patient.

D. Transfer and Discharge Reports
1. Concisely summarize all pertinent data about a patient that are needed to implement immediate care.
2. Include, but are not limited to, discharge from the postanesthesia care unit (PACU); discharge to another facility, such as a nursing home or rehabilitation center; discharge to another service within the facility; and discharge from the hospital to home.

E. Reports to Family Members
1. Provide a progress report to designated family members; the patient gives legal consent to disclose confidential information to a designated person.
2. A code word, functioning as a PIN number, is required from a caller before a nurse can give information over the telephone.

DID YOU KNOW?

Nurses legally are not permitted to acknowledge that a person is admitted to a facility. Acknowledging a patient's presence without the patient's consent violates the patient's right to confidentiality and Health Insurance Portability and Accountability Act (HIPAA) laws.

F. Nursing and Interdisciplinary Team Conferences
1. Nurses and other health team members meet to discuss a patient's needs and coordinate a patient's care.
2. Promote critical thinking from a multidisciplinary perspective.

G. Incident Reports
1. Are required in response to any occurrence out of the ordinary that results in or is likely to result in harm to a patient, employee, or visitor.

2. Used for quality improvement activities, not for disciplinary actions against a staff member.
3. Promote identification of high-risk trends, which promote the development of educational programs to address the prevention of the problem. (For more information, see Chapter 2, "Legal and Ethical Issues.")

V. Documentation

Documentation is the act of creating a written record. It involves the insertion of information about a patient onto paper forms kept in a chart or electronically in a paperless charting system. Documentation should include information about patient assessments, plans of care, interventions provided, and patient responses. The written record is a legal document that also is used to promote quality assurance, reimbursement to third-party payers, education, and research.

A. Admission Nursing Assessment
1. Initiates a database about the patient.
2. Provides information with which subsequent information can be compared.

B. Kardex
1. Communicates basic information about the patient for easy reference.
2. Generally includes the plan of care.
3. Is updated continuously.
4. Is not usually part of the legal clinical record.
5. Has been losing favor since the advent of electronic clinical records.

C. Plan of Care
1. Communicates the strategies identified to address patient needs.
2. May be a nursing care plan or an integrated health team plan.
3. Is part of the patient's permanent record.

D. Clinical Pathways
1. Collaborative case management plan for a patient with a specific diagnosis or procedure.
2. Includes expected outcomes, interventions to be implemented, and the sequence and timing of those interventions.

E. Flow Sheets
1. Document routine aspects of nursing care.
2. Include forms, such as for vital signs, weight, I&O, skin assessment, and activities of daily living.

F. Medication Administration Record (MAR)
1. Documents all the patient's prescribed and administered or omitted medications.
2. May contain a section to record why a drug was not administered or contain specific information relative to before or after administering a drug, such as blood pressure before an antihypertensive and objective pain scale results before and after pain medication is administered.

G. Progress Notes
1. Inform other members of the health-care team of the patient's progress.
2. May use various formats.
   a. Narrative.
      (1) Traditional method that provides a story about the patient's status, all care provided, and patient responses.
      (2) May make finding important information difficult because it includes documentation of all routine care.
   b. Charting by exception (PIE).
      (1) Includes:
         (a) **Problem** identification.
         (b) **Interventions** provided.
         (c) **Evaluation** of patient outcomes.
      (2) Documents information other than routine care (routine care is documented on a separate flow sheet).
      (3) Assigns a number to each identified problem, providing easy reference.
      (4) Simplifies and streamlines documentation.
   c. Problem-oriented charting (SOAP).
      (1) Includes:
         (a) **Subjective** data: What the patient or family members' state.
         (b) **Objective** data: Measurable data.
         (c) **Assessment:** Conclusions (may be presented as nursing diagnoses).
         (d) **Plan:** Actions designed to address the patient's problem.
      (2) Provides a structured logical format to charting.
   d. Focus charting.
      (1) Uses format of data, action, and response in a narrative note.
      (2) Ensures a focus on planning (action) and evaluation (response).
   e. Case management—critical pathway.
      (1) Includes key elements used by all disciplines to monitor and document interventions performed on a daily schedule so that outcomes are achieved when expected.
      (2) When a goal is not met when expected because of a complication or unexpected event (variance), the event and actions in response to the event are documented.
      (3) Promotes collaboration, communication, and teamwork.
      (4) Attempts to ensure that interventions are implemented as expected, increasing quality of care and discharge in a timely manner.

H. Nursing Responsibilities Related to Documentation
1. Documentation do's.
   a. Use only black ink.
   b. Ensure writing is legible and easy to read.
   c. Use only acceptable abbreviations.
   d. Use correct spelling and grammar.
   e. Sign each entry with a signature and title.
   f. Indicate the date and time of each entry, using a 24-hour clock (Fig. 7.1).
   g. Ensure that each page of the medical record contains patient identification at the top of the page; verify this information before charting.
   h. Record facts and observations.
   i. Quote what the patient says and/or describe the patient's behavior for ongoing quality management, for peer review, and in a court of law.
   j. Draw one line through a recorded mistake, indicate above or next to the entry that it is an error, and initial the mistake; the word to use usually is approved by the facility.
   k. Draw a single line though any blank spaces above your signature to ensure that no additional information can be added by another person.
   l. Record events chronologically and as close as possible to the time they occur.
   m. Record the patient's response to visits by health-care providers, consultants, and other caregivers, such as speech, respiratory, and physical therapists.
   n. Record all telephone calls concerning the patient.

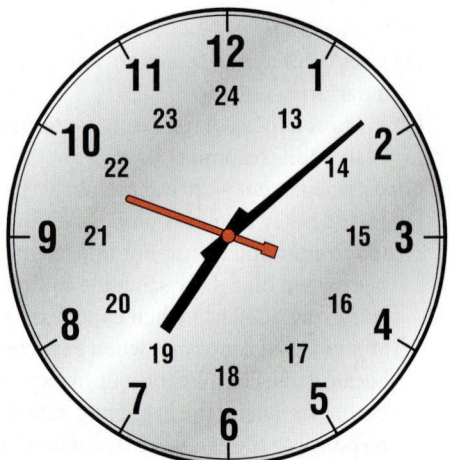

Fig 7.1 24-Hour Clock. (From Wilkinson and Treas [2011]. *Fundamentals of Nursing*, Vol. 1, 2nd ed. Philadelphia: F. A. Davis Company. With permission.)

   o. Record only pertinent and appropriate information as concisely as possible.
   p. When inserting a late entry, identify that the note is a late entry.
   q. Record all care implemented and the patient's response to care.

DID YOU KNOW?

If an intervention is not documented, it is considered not done. Charting should be thorough, clear, and concise. Entries in a medical record document the care provided and the status and progress of a patient.

2. Documentation dont's.
   a. Never leave a blank space above your signature in which someone could add something later.
   b. Never chart interventions before they are delivered.
   c. Do not use correction fluid or obliterate mistaken entries.
   d. Avoid charting opinions or terms that label a patient (e.g., "demanding," "uncooperative," and "unpleasant").
   e. Never chart for another nurse.
   f. Never alter a previously written entry.
   g. Never back date a note; instead, enter the current date and time with the word "addendum" and then add the note with the date and time it should have been documented.
   h. Avoid using the word "patient" because it is unnecessary.
   i. Avoid judgmental words that mean different things to different people (e.g., "good," "poor," "sufficient," "decreased," "bad," "normal," "abnormal").
   j. Avoid terms of generalization (e.g., "seems to be" or "appears").
   k. Do not use abbreviations that are not included in the facility's policy and procedure manual or abbreviations disallowed by the Joint Commission (Table 7.3).

DID YOU KNOW?

In 2002, the Joint Commission (formerly the Joint Commission on the Accreditation of Healthcare Organizations [JCAHO]) identified a national patient safety goal requiring accredited organizations to develop and implement a list of abbreviations not to use in their organization. In 2004, the Joint Commission identified a minimum list of dangerous abbreviations, acronyms, and symbols that must be included on an organization's do-not-use list of abbreviations as part of the requirement for meeting this goal.

Table 7.3 Abbreviations to Avoid in Documentation

Abbreviation	Meaning	Preferred Documentation
IU*	international unit	international unit
MS*	morphine sulfate	morphine sulfate
MSO_4, $MgSO_4$*	magnesium sulfate	magnesium sulfate
qd, q.d., QD, Q.D.*	every day	daily
qod, q.o.d., QOD, Q.O.D.*	every other day	every other day
u, U*	unit	unit
AS, AD, AU	left ear, right ear, both ears	left ear, right ear, each ear
cc	cubic centimeters	mL, milliliters
d/c, D/C, DC	discharge or discontinue	discharge, discontinue
hs, qhs	hour of sleep, bedtime	nightly, at bedtime
OS, OD, OU	left eye, right eye, each eye	left eye, right eye, each eye
sub q, SQ, SC	subcutaneous	subcutaneously
TIW	three times a week	three times weekly, 3 times weekly
µg, mcg	microgram	microgram
@	at	at
&	and	and
°	hour	hour, h, or hr

Use of "0" in a Medication Dose

Eliminate trailing zero after a decimal point dose* 1.0 mg can be mistaken for 10 if decimal is not seen.	1 mg
Insert a leading zero before a decimal point dose* .5 mg can be mistaken for 5 mg if decimal is not seen.	0.5 mg

*Included on the Joint Commission's Official "Do Not Use" List of dangerous abbreviations, acronyms, and symbols. The Joint Commission. (2004). Facts about the official "Do Not Use" list. Retrieved July 1, 2012, from www.jointcommission.org/assets/1/18/Do_Not_Use_List.pdf.

CASE STUDY: Putting It All Together

On a Saturday evening, a tractor trailer loses control, crosses the median of a roadway, and causes a ten-car pileup in the oncoming lanes of a highway. The hospital disaster plan is activated, and many health team members respond to the emergency department of the local hospital. The emergency department is filled to capacity and has a lot of noise and commotion because of the presence of patients, family members, and health team members.

A patient who reports severe pain in the hip as a result of the accident is placed on a stretcher in an alcove in the hallway until a room becomes available. The patient is accompanied by her adult daughter and 5-year-old grandson. The daughter and grandson were passengers in the car, but they did not sustain any injuries and were not admitted to the emergency department. The nurse positions a curtain around the patient's stretcher and stands near the head of the bed, facing the patient. The nurse cannot sit because a chair would block the hallway, creating an unsafe situation.

While making eye contact with the patient, the nurse introduces himself by name and title and states that he is going to conduct an interview and perform a physical assessment. The nurse asks whether the patient prefers that the daughter and grandson stay or step to the other end of the hall during the interview. The patient says that it is alright for the daughter and grandson to stay during the interview.

The grandson appears anxious and is pulling on the linen at the foot of the grandmother's bed. The nurse observes the patient grimacing and rubbing her right hip. Before the nurse can assess the patient's pain, the patient stated, "I am so angry. I was riding in the right lane, and I was on cruise control within the speed limit. Why did this have to happen?" The nurse responds, "It must be frustrating to know that you did everything right and still had something like this happen."

When beginning the pain assessment, the nurse asks, "What is the intensity of your pain on a scale of 0 to 10?" The nurse also says, "Tell me the location of the

Continued

CASE STUDY: Putting It All Together *cont'd*

pain and what it feels like." The patient is breathing in short, shallow breaths; shaking her head from side to side; and, with her eyes closed, states, "The pain in my right hip is crazy. It is unbearable." The nurse responds, "Can you explain in more detail what you mean by 'crazy'?"

After diagnostic tests have been completed, the primary health-care provider informs the patient that surgery to repair the right hip will be performed in the morning. The nurse then transports the patient to the orthopedic unit and reinforces the information about the patient being scheduled for an ORIF in the morning. After being transferred to a bed on the orthopedic unit, the patient begins to cry and says, "I am sorry I'm crying. I am such a big baby." The nurse touches the patient's arm and responds, "It's okay to cry. You had a lot happen to you today. Everything is going to be fine. Try to be strong and a good role model for your grandson."

Case Study Questions

A. Identify the nursing actions that facilitated communication and the rationales for why they are effective in promoting communication.

1. _____
2. _____
3. _____
4. _____
5. _____

B. Identify factors in this scenario that can be barriers to communication and explain why.

1. _____
2. _____
3. _____
4. _____
5. _____

C. Identify the interviewing skills the nurse used when communicating with the patient and explain why these skills are effective in promoting communication.

1. _____
2. _____
3. _____
4. _____
5. _____
6. _____

D. Identify the nursing responses that were nontherapeutic?

1. _____
2. _____
3. _____

REVIEW QUESTIONS

1. A nurse is caring for a patient who is unconscious. What is the sense that is **most** important to a person who appears to be unconscious?
   1. Taste
   2. Smell
   3. Touch
   4. Hearing

2. What is **most** effective when the nurse is developing a therapeutic relationship with a patient?
   1. Catharsis
   2. Confrontation
   3. Trustworthiness
   4. Recommendations

3. What is **most** important for the nurse to do when assessing a patient's nonverbal expressions?
   1. Increase the patient's self-awareness.
   2. Validate their meaning.
   3. Remain observant.
   4. Explore feelings.

4. A nurse is caring for a patient who is blind. What should the nurse do to facilitate communication? **Select all that apply.**
   1. _____ Overarticulate when speaking.
   2. _____ Speak slightly louder than usual.
   3. _____ Indicate when you are going to leave the room.
   4. _____ Announce your presence when entering the room.
   5. _____ Explain your intentions before touching the patient.

5. Which question asked by the nurse will elicit the **most** specific information?
   1. "How long ago did the pain in your left knee start?"
   2. "I think I heard you say that you have concerns about going home."
   3. "Tell me more about yourself before you were admitted to the hospital."
   4. "Could you tell me more about the dark feeling that you say you have been having?"

6. Which concept about communication is essential for the nurse to include in a foundation for nursing practice?
   1. Communication is an instinctive process.
   2. Communication through humor is highly objective in nature.
   3. Previous patterns of communication may be ineffective when one is ill.
   4. Verbal communication is more meaningful than nonverbal communication.

7. A nurse is interacting with a patient at a local mental health clinic. The nurse states, "So, you've come here today because you feel you cannot go on." What phase of the nurse-patient relationship does this interaction reflect?
   1. Working
   2. Termination
   3. Preinteraction
   4. Orientation phase

8. Which documentation regarding the administration of a medication is recorded accurately according the Joint Commission?
   1. Coumadin 5 mg QOD for 7 days
   2. Heparin 5,000 units Sub-Q daily
   3. $MgSO_4$ 1.0 g for hypertension
   4. Calcium 600 mg po qd

9. A nurse is working with a severely visually impaired patient. Which approaches will be **most** effective when communicating with this patient during a bed bath? **Select all that apply.**
   1. _____ Speak in a louder volume.
   2. _____ Enunciate every word slowly.
   3. _____ Stand directly in front of the patient.
   4. _____ Tell the patient exactly what will happen.
   5. _____ Use touch to emphasize what is being done.

10. A nurse is attempting to identify a patient's concerns. Which communication technique is **most** appropriate for the nurse to use?
    1. Silence
    2. Reflection
    3. Paraphrasing
    4. Open-ended question

11. A nurse is checking a patient's graphic sheet (shown here) to verify when the patient exhibited the lowest temperature. What time on May 6th was the patient's temperature the lowest?

GRAPHICS

DATE	5/6/2011						
HOSPITAL DAY	2						
POST OP DAY	2						
TIME	0400	0800	1200	1600	2000	2400	0400
C F							
40.0 104							
39.4 103							
38.8 102							
38.3 101							
37.7 100							
37.2 99							
36.6 98							
36.1 97							
35.5 96							
35.0 95							
PULSE		88	76	80	74		
RESPIRATIONS		16	14	18	16		
BLOOD PRESSURE		140/84	138/84	130/88	128/82		
HEIGHT 5'2"	WEIGHT 125						
TYPE OF DIET	Clear liquids						
%	B 80%		L 50%		S		

1. 0800
2. 1200
3. 2000
4. 2400

12. When talking with a patient, a nurse states, "Since speaking with you for a while, it seems that you are very worried about your upcoming surgery." In which phase of the nurse-patient relationship is this statement **most** appropriate?
1. Working
2. Orientation
3. Termination
4. Preinteraction

13. A patient who is about to have a mastectomy is wringing her hands, and her eyes are darting around the preoperative unit. Which statements by the nurse are **most** appropriate to explore the patient's potential concerns? **Select all that apply.**
1. _____ "It is alright to be a little nervous before having surgery."
2. _____ "Do you have any concerns regarding your surgery?"
3. _____ "Tell me about the surgery you are about to have."
4. _____ "Have you thought about alternatives to surgery?"
5. _____ "You will feel better after the surgery is over."

14. Which intervention by the nurse is **least** appropriate during the orientation phase of the nurse-patient relationship?
1. Discussing boundaries of the therapeutic alliance
2. Explaining the time frame of their interaction
3. Introducing themselves to each other
4. Exploring personal issues

15. Which information is **most** informative when giving a change-of-shift report?
1. A patient with dementia is confused.
2. A patient reports that incisional pain is now tolerable.
3. A patient's blood pressure is within the expected range.
4. A patient walked down the hall with no activity intolerance.

16. A nurse is using the SBAR communication technique during a crisis. Which nursing intervention reflects the R step of this technique?
1. Recording the reaction of the patient to the crisis
2. Reassessing the patient after medical intervention
3. Recommending a potential action to manage the crisis
4. Reporting the situation to the primary health-care provider

17. An 86-year-old man is admitted to an intermediate care facility after discharge from the hospital for treatment of left-sided weakness and an inability to verbally express himself clearly. He is being assessed to identify his physical, occupational, and speech therapy needs. The nurse reviews the patient's family history, performs a physical assessment, and interviews the patient.

Patient's Clinical Record

Family History

An 86-year-old man had a brain attack, resulting in left hemiparesis and expressive aphasia. The patient lives with his 78-year-old wife. The couple live alone, but are visited frequently by a daughter and a son, who both live approximately 30 minutes away.

Physical Assessment

The patient has left hemiparesis and wears a hand and forearm splint on the left arm to prevent contractures. The patient ambulates safely with the use of a tripod cane. The patient needs assistance with activities of daily living. The patient is continent of urine and feces. The ability to chew and swallow solid food safely is intact, but on infrequent occasions experiences dribbling from the corner of the mouth when drinking fluids.

Patient Interview

The patient was oriented to time, place, and person. He pointed to things for which he had difficulty finding the words such as "pen" or "bathroom." He became frustrated and banged on the table when he could not clearly communicate his thoughts. He had an angry facial expression and turned away from his wife when she was unable to understand what he was saying.

Which nursing action addresses this patient's **most** urgent need?
1. Thicken all beverages and soups.
2. Maintain the splint on the upper extremity.
3. Explore interventions to facilitate communication.
4. Encourage the children to participate in their father's rehabilitation.

18. A nurse asks a patient, "How are you feeling?" The patient responds, "I am doing fine" while looking toward the floor. The nurse identifies that the verbal and nonverbal communication are incongruent. What is the nurse's **most** appropriate response?
1. "What is bothering you?"
2. "Let's talk about your illness."
3. "I am glad you are doing fine."
4. "Are you sure nothing is bothering you?"

19. The nurse should anticipate that the patient with what condition will **most** likely have difficulty conveying needs verbally?
1. Receptive aphasia
2. Hearing impaired
3. Delirium
4. Blind

20. Which nursing actions are common to patients who have impaired hearing or impaired vision? **Select all that apply.**
1. _____ Repeating the message using different words if the message was not understood
2. _____ Being alert for nonverbal cues and behavior
3. _____ Using gestures to augment verbal language
4. _____ Using a clock to orient food on a plate
5. _____ Providing for adequate lighting

21. A nurse is talking with a patient about the patient's concerns. Which nursing action reflects the **most** important component of verbal communication in this situation?
1. Answering questions that the patient is asking
2. Taking the lead in the interaction
3. Using simple sentence structure
4. Speaking in a calm cadence

22. A nurse answers a patient's question while standing by the side of the patient's bed. The patient responds saying, "Oh well, I just know that I am going to be fine," and then begins to cry, using a head shaking gesture to indicate "no." What should the nurse do **first**?
1. Pat the patient's hand.
2. Sit in a chair near the head of the patient's bed.
3. Get a tissue from the bedside drawer for the patient.
4. Use an open-ended question to explore the patient's feelings.

23. A nurse is caring for a patient who is hearing impaired but refuses to wear hearing aids. What are the **most** appropriate ways to have a verbal interaction with this patient? **Select all that apply.**
1. _____ Speak in a normal volume.
2. _____ Speak in a very loud volume.
3. _____ Use a soft, higher pitched voice.
4. _____ Use a deep, slightly louder voice.
5. _____ Stand directly in front of the patient.
6. _____ Ensure that the patient knows that a conversation is to begin.

24. A patient in the emergency department says to a nurse, "I have been so sick for a while with pain in my stomach and nothing seems to work." Which statement by the nurse demonstrates the use of an open-ended question?
1. "Tell me what you have been doing to manage your illness."
2. "Would you like for me to sit down with you for a little while?"
3. "Can you tell me how long you have been experiencing this pain?"
4. "It must be frustrating when nothing works to make you feel better."

25. A patient says to a nurse, "I periodically get a weird feeling in my head. It is so frustrating not to have a specific diagnosis. I am not thrilled about having this test tomorrow, but maybe I will get some answers." Which statement by the nurse is an example of the interviewing technique of clarification?
   1. "You sound upset about the test that you are having tomorrow."
   2. "Can you describe what you mean by a strange feeling in your head?"
   3. "I can understand how frustrating it is not to have a definitive diagnosis."
   4. "Did your primary health-care provider say you would get the results of the test right away?"

26. An inservice educator is correcting a test taken by a newly hired nurse regarding the use of abbreviations. Which abbreviations specifically disallowed by the Joint Commission did the nurse identify correctly? **Select all that apply.**
   1. _____ qd
   2. _____ mL
   3. _____ OD
   4. _____ Sub-Q
   5. _____ MgSO$_4$

27. Which nursing action is considered acceptable nursing practice when documenting in a patient's clinical record?
   1. Only chart for another nurse in the event of an emergency.
   2. Always initial an entry when adding a comment to a previously written progress note.
   3. When documenting an opinion, such as "The patient is demanding," also include examples of the patient's behavior.
   4. For an addendum to a note, enter the current date, the word "addendum," and the date and time it should have been documented.

28. A nurse working on the day shift receives a telephone call from the night nurse who just left the unit. While in the parking lot, the night nurse remembered the need to document nursing care given to a patient. What is the **best** action by the day nurse?
   1. Leave room in the progress notes for the night nurse to enter the note on the nurse's return the next night.
   2. Enter the note dictated by the night nurse, note that it was dictated, and sign and date the note.
   3. Suggest that the night nurse enter an addendum note on the nurse's return the next night.
   4. Encourage the night nurse to return to the hospital to enter the progress note.

29. A nurse is providing preoperative teaching for a patient who is scheduled for a pacemaker insertion in 3 days. The patient tells the nurse, "I am so nervous. I never had surgery before." What is the nurse's **most** therapeutic response?
   1. "What is it that concerns you the most?"
   2. "Has anyone in your family had surgery before?"
   3. "Being anxious before surgery is a normal response."
   4. "Having a pacemaker inserted is a routine procedure."

30. A nurse is orienting a newly admitted patient to the patient's bedroom environment. The patient tells the nurse, "I have difficulty hearing. I left my hearing aids at home." What is the nurse's **most** important intervention?
   1. Facing the patient directly when speaking
   2. Speaking clearly when conversing with the patient
   3. Ensuring that communicated information is understood
   4. Eliminating excess background noise when having a conversation

31. A patient has an appointment in the department of ambulatory surgery to receive preoperative teaching from a nurse. Place the following interventions in the order that they should be performed by the nurse when communicating with the patient.
   1. Summarize the goals and objectives of the meeting.
   2. Read the patient's chart before meeting the patient.
   3. Explain the purpose of the visit to the clinic.
   4. Verify the patient's identification.
   5. Provide preoperative teaching.
   6. Introduce self.
   Answer: _____

32. A nurse is documenting in a patient's clinical record and realizes that it is the medical record of another patient. What should the nurse do?
   1. Draw a line through the entry, indicate that it is an error, and sign and date the entry.
   2. Ask the nurse in charge to countersign the entry, indicating that it was an error.
   3. Apply white-out to the entry so that it is not readable.
   4. Use a black magic marker to obliterate the entry.

33. A nurse is documenting a variance associated with an interdisciplinary plan of care, describing the event and actions in response to the event. What type of documenting format is the nurse using?
   1. Critical pathway
   2. Focused charting
   3. Charting by exception
   4. Problem-oriented charting

34. A nurse communicates the strategies identified to address the patient's needs. Which documentation format should the nurse use to **best** communicate this information?

1. Progress notes
2. Plan of care
3. Flow sheet
4. Kardex

35. Which statements by a nurse are examples of non-therapeutic communication? **Select all that apply.**

1. _____ "I can't believe that you didn't eat all of that beautiful dinner."
2. _____ "We are going to start an IV with a piggyback in a few minutes."
3. _____ "Let's review what we accomplished today learning about insulin."
4. _____ "Take a deep breath. You are getting excited over very simple surgery."
5. _____ "I know you're angry about the cold coffee, but occasionally these things happen."

1. **ANSWER: 4.**
   Rationales:
   1. Although being able to taste is important, it is not the most important sense to an unconscious patient.
   2. Although being able to smell is important, it is not the most important sense to an unconscious patient.
   3. Although touch is important, it is not the most important sense to an unconscious patient.
   4. Hearing is the most important sense to an unconscious patient because it is believed to be the last sense that is lost. The senses receive stimuli from the environment and hearing keeps one in contact with others.
   TEST-TAKING TIP: Identify the word in the stem that sets a priority. The word *most* in the stem sets a priority.
   Content Area: Communication and Documentation
   Integrated Processes: Communication/Documentation;
   Nursing Process: Analysis
   Client Need: Psychosocial Integrity
   Cognitive Level: Knowledge

2. **ANSWER: 3.**
   Rationales:
   1. Catharsis should not occur before trust is developed because the patient is vulnerable and must have faith that the nurse will be accepting and supportive.
   2. Confrontation should not occur before trust is developed because the patient is vulnerable and must have faith that the nurse will be accepting and supportive.
   3. Trustworthiness results from being responsible and dependable.
   4. Recommendations and advice promote dependence; the patient should be assisted to problem-solve.
   TEST-TAKING TIP: Identify the word in the stem that sets a priority. The word *most* in the stem sets a priority.
   Content Area: Communication and Documentation
   Integrated Processes: Caring; Communication/
   Documentation; Nursing Process: Implementation
   Client Need: Psychosocial Integrity
   Cognitive Level: Application

3. **ANSWER: 2.**
   Rationales:
   1. Self-awareness cannot be attained without first exploring the meaning of behavior.
   2. The meaning and significance of behavior must be declared or clarified by the patient; otherwise, they are just assumptions by the nurse.
   3. Just remaining observant is inadequate; the nurse must explore the meaning of behavior.
   4. Feelings may not be related to the nonverbal behavior.
   TEST-TAKING TIP: Identify the word in the stem that sets a priority. The word *most* in the stem sets a priority.
   Content Area: Communication and Documentation
   Integrated Processes: Communication/Documentation;
   Nursing Process: Assessment
   Client Need: Psychosocial Integrity
   Cognitive Level: Application

4. **ANSWER: 3, 4, 5.**
   Rationales:
   1. Some people overarticulate when speaking with a person who is deaf, not blind. However, this should be avoided because it is perceived as mumbling by people who are hearing impaired.
   2. Speaking slightly louder is unnecessary. The patient is blind, not deaf.
   3. This is common courtesy. A blind person may be unaware that you have left the room if not told.
   4. This is common courtesy. Also, it supports a sense of security. The person who is blind has a right to know who is in the room and why the person is there.
   5. Touching patients who are blind without first telling them what you are doing can be frightening and should be avoided.
   Content Area: Communication and Documentation
   Integrated Processes: Communication/Documentation;
   Nursing Process: Implementation
   Client Need: Psychosocial Integrity
   Cognitive Level: Application

5. **ANSWER: 1.**
   Rationales:
   1. The question in option 1 is a direct question and is seeking specific information about when the pain started. It can be answered with a short answer.
   2. The question in option 2 is used to validate whether what was heard was the message that was sent.
   3. The question in option 3 is an open-ended question and allows the patient to determine the direction and extent of the information shared.
   4. The question in option 4 is a clarifying question. It asks the patient to expand on information already shared and invites the patient to continue the discussion.
   TEST-TAKING TIP: Identify the word in the stem that sets a priority. The word *most* in the stem sets a priority. Identify the unique option. To obtain specific information, the nurse must ask questions that start with how, what, where, when, or why. Option 1 is the only option that asks a direct question; this option is unique.
   Content Area: Communication and Documentation
   Integrated Processes: Communication/Documentation;
   Nursing Process: Implementation
   Client Need: Psychosocial Integrity
   Cognitive Level: Analysis

6. **ANSWER: 3.**
   Rationales:
   1. Communication is learned; it is not instinctive.
   2. Humor is subjective, not objective, in nature. Humor may be interpreted as having many different meanings. What is "funny" to one person may be insulting to another.
   3. This is a true statement. The nurse should assess a patient's communication pattern and determine if the patient is able to express feelings and communicate needs effectively.
   4. What people verbalize really may not be what they believe or feel. Nonverbal language (e.g., behavior, gestures) often is more meaningful and emotionally charged than what is spoken.

TEST-TAKING TIP: Identify the word in the stem that indicates a priority. The word *essential* in the stem sets a priority.
Content Area: Communication and Documentation
Integrated Processes: Communication/Documentation;
Nursing Process: Analysis
Client Need: Psychosocial Integrity
Cognitive Level: Knowledge

7. **ANSWER: 4.**
   Rationales:
   1. The working phase involves attempts at problem-solving with the patient.
   2. The termination phase involves summarization of goals and objectives.
   3. The preinteraction phase occurs prior to the nurse meeting the patient.
   4. **The orientation phase involves gathering information from the patient and identifying patient needs.**
   TEST-TAKING TIP: Identify the option with a clang association. The word *phase* in the stem and in option 4 is a clang association.
   Content Area: Communication and Documentation
   Integrated Processes: Communication/Documentation;
   Nursing Process: Implementation
   Client Need: Psychosocial Integrity
   Cognitive Level: Analysis

8. **ANSWER: 2.**
   Rationales:
   1. The Joint Commission requires that QOD be spelled out as *every other day*.
   2. **The use of Sub-Q for subcutaneously is not disallowed by the Joint Commission.**
   3. The Joint Commission requires that magnesium sulphate be spelled out. It disallows the use of a trailing 0 after a decimal. In addition, the route and frequency are not included in this prescription.
   4. The Joint Commission requires that qd be spelled out as *daily*.
   Content Area: Communication and Documentation
   Integrated Processes: Communication/Documentation;
   Nursing Process: Implementation
   Client Need: Safe and Effective Care Environment;
   Management of Care
   Cognitive Level: Application

9. **ANSWER: 4, 5.**
   Rationales:
   1. Speaking louder to a visually impaired person will not help the person see better and may be interpreted by the patient as demeaning.
   2. Enunciating more clearly will not help the patient see better. This approach is appropriate for a patient who is hearing impaired.
   3. The nurse should be standing directly next to the patient while giving a bed bath. It is the close proximity to the patient rather than being in front of the patient that is important.
   4. **Telling the patient exactly what will happen before and during the bed bath provides both information and emotional support.**

5. **Using touch with a visually impaired person promotes communication because it engages another sense.**
   TEST-TAKING TIP: Identify the word in the stem that sets a priority. The word *most* in the stem sets a priority.
   Content Area: Communication and Documentation
   Integrated Processes: Caring; Communication/
   Documentation; Nursing Process: Implementation
   Client Need: Psychosocial Integrity
   Cognitive Level: Application

10. **ANSWER: 4.**
    Rationales:
    1. Silence is not the most appropriate technique to identify concerns. It provides no direction to gather information.
    2. Reflection is not the most appropriate technique to identify concerns. With this technique a feeling that the nurse identified in the patient's conversation is reflected back to the patient. This may not be an accurate interpretation by the nurse, and it is more directive than another communication technique.
    3. Paraphrasing is not the most appropriate technique to identify concerns. Paraphrasing restates the main idea of the patient's message in similar but different words. This may be too directed in that the nurse decides what part of the patient's message to rephrase.
    4. **Open-ended questions are the best way to identify a patient's concerns because this technique allows a patient to take the initiative and direct the conversation to any topic desired by the patient.**
    TEST-TAKING TIP: Identify the word in the stem that sets a priority. The word *most* in the stem sets a priority. Identify the option that is unique. Option 4 is unique because it is the only option with 3 words and a hyphen.
    Content Area: Communication and Documentation
    Integrated Processes: Caring; Communication/
    Documentation; Nursing Process: Implementation
    Client Need: Psychosocial Integrity
    Cognitive Level: Application

11. **ANSWER: 4.**
    Rationales:
    1. At 0800, the patient's temperature was at its highest at 100.2°F.
    2. The patient's temperature at 1200 was not at its lowest. At 1200, the patient's temperature was 99.2°F.
    3. The patient's temperature at 2000 was not at its lowest. At 2000, the patient's temperature was 99.2°F.
    4. **The patient's temperature at 2400 was at its lowest, at 98.4°F.**
    TEST-TAKING TIP: Identify the equally plausible options. Options 2 and 3 are equally plausible. They are both 99.2°F. One is no better than the other. Eliminate options 2 and 3 from further consideration.
    Content Area: Communication and Documentation
    Integrated Processes: Communication/Documentation;
    Nursing Process: Evaluation
    Client Need: Safe and Effective Care Environment;
    Management of Care
    Cognitive Level: Analysis

12. ANSWER: 1.

Rationales:

1. This statement is most appropriate during the working phase because, by this phase, the patient and nurse have talked for a while, which allows the nurse to verbalize the implied.

2. During the orientation phase, the nurse is just getting to know the patient and it is inappropriate to verbalize the implied.

3. This statement is inappropriate in the termination phase because, by the time the termination phase is reached, the patient's issues and concerns should have been addressed.

4. This statement does not apply to the preinteraction phase; this phase involves gathering information before meeting with the patient.

TEST-TAKING TIP: Identify the word in the stem that sets a priority. The word *most* in the stem sets a priority.

Content Area: Communication and Documentation
Integrated Processes: Communication/Documentation; Nursing Process: Implementation
Client Need: Psychosocial Integrity
Cognitive Level: Application

13. ANSWER: 1, 2.

Rationales:

1. This statement lets the patient know that it is alright to be nervous; it provides the patient with an opportunity to express feelings if desired.

2. This statement invites the patient to discuss her concerns about the surgery.

3. This statement assesses knowledge about the surgery, but does not explore the patent's anxiety or concerns.

4. This statement is inappropriate and may increase the patient's anxiety.

5. This statement invalidates the patient's anxiety. There is no way the nurse can predict that the patient will feel better after the surgery.

TEST-TAKING TIP: Identify the word in the stem that sets a priority. The word *most* in the stem sets a priority. Identify the option with a clang association. The word *concern* in the stem and option 2 is a clang association. Identify the option that denies the patient's concerns. Option 5 denies the patient's concerns.

Content Area: Communication and Documentation
Integrated Processes: Caring; Communication/Documentation; Nursing Process: Implementation
Client Need: Psychosocial Integrity
Cognitive Level: Analysis

14. ANSWER: 4.

Rationales:

1. Defining limits and parameters is part of the orientation phase of a nurse-patient relationship. It provides a guide for the future relationship.

2. Explaining the anticipated time frame of the relationship is part of the orientation phase of a nurse-patient relationship.

3. Introducing oneself is part of the orientation phase of a nurse-patient relationship. Patients have the right to know who is providing care.

4. Exploring personal issues is the least appropriate of the options presented during the orientation phase of a nurse-patient relationship. A therapeutic alliance must be established before exploring personal issues.

TEST-TAKING TIP: Identify the word in the stem that indicates negative polarity. The word *least* in the stem indicates negative polarity.

Content Area: Communication and Documentation
Integrated Processes: Communication/Documentation; Nursing Process: Planning
Client Need: Psychosocial Integrity
Cognitive Level: Application

15. ANSWER: 2.

Rationales:

1. Although it is important to know that a patient with dementia is confused and disoriented, these responses are commonly associated with a medical diagnosis of dementia.

2. Knowing that incisional pain is now tolerable is the evaluation step of the nursing process; ongoing evaluation of the effectiveness of the management of pain is most important of the options presented.

3. Although a patient's blood pressure being within the expected range is important to know, it is within a normal, not abnormal, range; this information is not as significant as information in another option.

4. Although knowing that a patient walked down the hall with no activity intolerance is important to know, it is a normal, not abnormal, expectation; this is not as significant as information in another option.

TEST-TAKING TIP: Identify the word in the stem that sets a priority. The word *most* in the stem sets a priority.

Content Area: Communication and Documentation
Integrated Processes: Communication/Documentation; Nursing Process: Evaluation
Client Need: Safe and Effective Care Environment; Management of Care
Cognitive Level: Application

16. ANSWER: 3.

Rationales:

1. The A step (Assessment) in the SBAR communication framework includes the patient's status in relation to the crisis.

2. There is no step in the SBAR communication framework that addresses a reassessment of the patient.

3. The R in the SBAR communication framework stands for suggested Recommendations. Once the nurse explains the Situation (e.g., identify self, title, facility; identify the patient's date of birth and gender; and reason for collaboration), provides Background information (e.g., patient's present issue, relevant medical history, and summary of background), and provides an Assessment (e.g., vital signs and clinical indicators outside expected range, severity of patient's issue, and nurse's clinical impression), then the nurse makes a Recommendation (e.g., explains what is

required, urgency of what is required, and makes suggestions).
4. The **R** in the SBAR communication framework does not denote reporting the crisis. The entire SBAR technique is a reporting format; each step reports a specific piece of information regarding the crisis.
Content Area: Communication and Documentation
Integrated Processes: Communication/Documentation;
Nursing Process: Implementation
Client Need: Safe and Effective Care Environment;
Management of Care
Cognitive Level: Analysis

17. **ANSWER: 3.**
Rationales:
1. Occasional difficulty with fluids is not the priority at this time. However, direct supervision should be provided to ensure that this occasional difficulty is not a serious problem. Patients should be encouraged to enjoy food and liquid until the difficulty progresses to a point where it presents a risk for aspiration.
2. Although use of the splint should be maintained, it is not the most serious concern at this time.
3. This is the priority at this time. The patient is exhibiting anger and frustration with his inability to express himself and communicate his feelings and needs.
4. Although the nurse may explore the son and daughter's interest in participating in their father's rehabilitation, this is not the priority.
TEST-TAKING TIP: Identify the word in the stem that sets a priority. The word *most* in the stem sets a priority. Identify the option with a specific determiner. Option 1 contains the word *all,* which is a specific determiner.
Content Area: Communication and Documentation
Integrated Processes: Caring; Communication/
Documentation; Nursing Process: Planning
Client Need: Psychosocial Integrity
Cognitive Level: Analysis

18. **ANSWER: 4.**
Rationales:
1. This statement is inappropriate because the nurse is making an assumption.
2. This response focuses on a topic that may not be the patient's concern.
3. Since the verbal and nonverbal communications are incongruent, the nurse should not assume the patient is doing fine.
4. This response seeks further information because the patient's verbal and nonverbal communications are incongruent.
TEST-TAKING TIP: Identify the word in the stem that sets a priority. The word *most* in the stem sets a priority. Identify the options that deny the patient's feelings. Options 2 and 3 ignore the patient's behavior and therefore deny the patient's feelings or concerns.
Content Area: Communication and Documentation
Integrated Processes: Caring; Communication/
Documentation; Nursing Process: Assessment
Client Need: Psychosocial Integrity
Cognitive Level: Application

19. **ANSWER: 3.**
Rationales:
1. The patient with expressive, not receptive, aphasia has an impaired ability to verbalize a message.
2. People who are hearing impaired generally are able to verbalize a message; they may have difficulty receiving a message.
3. Of the four options presented, the patient with delirium is the most likely person to have difficulty verbalizing needs effectively. Delirium is a temporary disturbance in cognition accompanied by incoherent speech and altered sensory perception. It may be caused by a variety of acute problems, such as hypoxia or a metabolic problem associated with such conditions as renal or liver impairment.
4. Most patients who are blind are able to encode and decode a verbal message.
TEST-TAKING TIP: Identify the word in the stem that sets a priority. The word *most* in the stem sets a priority.
Content Area: Communication and Documentation
Integrated Processes: Communication/Documentation;
Nursing Process: Analysis
Client Need: Psychosocial Integrity
Cognitive Level: Analysis

20. **ANSWER: 1, 2, 5.**
Rationales:
1. Repeating the message using different words if the message was not understood is common nursing care for patients who are either hearing or visually impaired. Additional or different words help to clarify a message.
2. Being alert to nonverbal cues and behavior is common nursing care for patients who are either hearing or visually impaired.
3. Although many gestures have universal meanings that can augment verbal language, gestures are not helpful when a patient is visually impaired. Using gestures in addition to the spoken word is most effective when communicating with patients who are hearing impaired.
4. Using a clock to orient food on a plate is helpful to the patient who is visually impaired. It is not necessary for the patient who is hearing impaired.
5. Providing for adequate lighting is common to caring for patients who are either hearing or visually impaired. Adequate lighting enables some patients who are considered legally blind, but who have some limited vision, to see shadows and outlines of people and objects in the environment. Patients who are hearing impaired may lip-read to facilitate reception of a message; adequate lighting promotes lip-reading.
Content Area: Communication and Documentation
Integrated Processes: Communication/Documentation;
Nursing Process: Analysis
Client Need: Psychosocial Integrity
Cognitive Level: Analysis

21. **ANSWER: 1.**
Rationales:
1. Answering questions posed by a patient is related to the concept of relevance. Although some of the other options are important to effective communication, providing answers to questions posed by the patient is the priority.

2. The nurse should not take the lead when discussing a patient's concerns. The nurse should use open-ended and other nondirect interviewing techniques that encourage the patient to lead the discussion to topics that concern the patient.

3. Although using simple words and sentence structure support clarity, another option is the priority.

4. Although speaking in a calm cadence is important because it conveys professional competence and respect for the patient, it is not the priority.

TEST-TAKING TIP: Identify the word in the stem that sets a priority. The word *most* in the stem sets a priority. Identify the clang association. The word *patient's* in the stem and *patient* in option 1 is a clang association. Examine option 1 carefully.

Content Area: Communication and Documentation
Integrated Processes: Communication/Documentation; Nursing Process: Implementation
Client Need: Psychosocial Integrity
Cognitive Level: Application

22. **ANSWER: 2.**
Rationales:

1. This intervention is inappropriate at this time. Touch should be used carefully because some patients believe that it is an invasion of their personal space.

2. **The first step is to sit at the head of the bed. This indicates to the patient that you are staying and interested.**

3. A nurse should not enter a patient's bedside drawer without permission. The bedside cabinet and overbed table are the patient's personal space.

4. This is premature. Silence is more appropriate.

TEST-TAKING TIP: Identify the word in the stem that sets a priority. The word *first* in the stem sets a priority.

Content Area: Communication and Documentation
Integrated Processes: Caring; Communication/Documentation; Nursing Process: Implementation
Client Need: Psychosocial Integrity
Cognitive Level: Application

23. **ANSWER: 4, 5, 6.**
Rationales:

1. If the nurse speaks in a normal volume, the patient probably will not hear the message.

2. A nurse should speak a little louder than usual, not very loud, to a patient who is hearing impaired but does not wear a hearing aid. Speaking too loud may be perceived by the patient as aggression.

3. This approach is inappropriate. As people age, they tend to lose the ability to hear higher pitched sounds.

4. **Older adults hear lower, rather than higher, pitched voices as a result of the aging process. Speaking slightly louder and deeper will aid the patient in hearing the message.**

5. **Standing in front of the patient will promote communication because the patient will be able to see the nurse's lips, which may aid in the reception and comprehension of the message.**

6. **Ensuring that the patient knows when a conversation is going to begin allows the patient to be prepared to listen.**

TEST-TAKING TIP: Identify the word in the stem that sets a priority. The word *most* in the stem sets a priority. Identify the option with a specific determiner. The word *very* in option 2 is a specific determiner. Option 2 can be deleted. Identify the opposite options. Options 3 and 4 are opposites. More often than not, one of the options that is an opposite is a correct answer.

Content Area: Communication and Documentation
Integrated Processes: Communication/Documentation; Nursing Process: Implementation
Client Need: Psychosocial Integrity
Cognitive Level: Application

24. **ANSWER: 1.**
Rationales:

1. **This is an open-ended question. It requires more than just a yes-or-no answer. Open-ended questions permit the patient to control the direction of the discussion.**

2. This is an example of offering of the self. It indicates the nurse's attention and interest without expectations. It is not an open-ended question.

3. This is an example of a direct question. Direct questions generally are used to collect objective data.

4. This is an example of reflection. It lets the patient know that the nurse has heard the message and is being empathetic.

Content Area: Communication and Documentation
Integrated Processes: Communication/Documentation; Nursing Process: Implementation
Client Need: Psychosocial Integrity
Cognitive Level: Analysis

25. **ANSWER: 2.**
Rationales:

1. This is an example of paraphrasing. It repeats content in the same or similar words used by the patient.

2. **This is a clarifying question. It asks the patient to elaborate on an unclear message, which helps to minimize misunderstanding.**

3. This is an example of reflection. It is a validating statement because it identifies and supports what the patient feels and demonstrates empathy.

4. This is a direct question that does not focus on the patient's feelings.

TEST-TAKING TIP: Identify the equally plausible options. Options 1 and 3 are equally plausible. They both address the patient's feelings—upset and frustrated.

Content Area: Communication and Documentation
Integrated Processes: Communication/Documentation; Nursing Process: Implementation
Client Need: Psychosocial Integrity
Cognitive Level: Analysis

26. **ANSWER: 1, 3, 5.**
Rationales:

1. **According to the Joint Commission, every day or daily must be written out. QD and qd are no longer acceptable abbreviations.**

2. According to the Joint Commission, milliliters or cubic centimeters (cc) may be abbreviated only as mL.

3. According to the Joint Commission, right eye must be written out. OD and od are no longer acceptable abbreviations.

4. The Joint Commission does not specifically address the use of an abbreviation for subcutaneous. According to the Institute for Safe Medication Practices, Sub-Q must be written out as subcutaneously.

5. According to the Joint Commission, magnesium sulphate must be written out. $MgSO_4$ is no longer an acceptable abbreviation.

TEST-TAKING TIP: Identify the word in the stem that indicates negative polarity. The word *disallowed* indicates negative polarity. The question is asking, "What abbreviations cannot be used as directed by the Joint Commission?"

Content Area: Communication and Documentation
Integrated Processes: Communication/Documentation; Nursing Process: Evaluation
Client Need: Safe and Effective Care Environment; Management of Care
Cognitive Level: Application

27. **ANSWER: 4.**
Rationales:
1. It is never acceptable to chart for another nurse. Nurses are responsible for only their own actions.

2. The nurse should never alter a previously written entry in the patient's clinical record. When the correct procedure for adding an addendum to a note is followed, no one can claim that an attempt was made to alter the previous note surreptitiously.

3. A nurse should describe a patient's behavior and avoid using judgmental words (e.g., demanding) to characterize behavior.

4. **This is the correct procedure for entering an addendum to a progress note. This avoids a claim by another that a previous note was altered surreptitiously.**

TEST-TAKING TIP: Identify options with specific determiners. The word *only* in option 1 and the word *always* in option 2 are specific determiners. Rarely are options with specific determiners the correct answer.

Content Area: Communication and Documentation
Integrated Processes: Communication/Documentation; Nursing Process: Implementation
Client Need: Safe and Effective Care Environment; Management of Care
Cognitive Level: Knowledge

28. **ANSWER: 4.**
Rationales:
1. Blank spaces between entries and between the end of a note and one's signature should be avoided. This prevents anyone from entering a note later, which is an unacceptable practice.

2. A nurse should never enter a note for another person. A nurse should only enter notes for patients for whom the nurse is responsible.

3. This action should be suggested if the night nurse refuses to implement an action presented in another option.

4. **This is the best advice the day nurse should give the night nurse. This avoids the need for the night nurse to add an "addendum" note the next night.**

TEST-TAKING TIP: Identify the word in the stem that sets a priority. The word *best* in the stem sets a priority.
Content Area: Communication and Documentation
Integrated Processes: Communication/Documentation; Nursing Process: Implementation
Client Need: Safe and Effective Care Environment; Management of Care
Cognitive Level: Application

29. **ANSWER: 1.**
Rationales:
1. **This response is open ended and allows the patient to talk about whatever the patient wants to discuss.**
2. This response takes the focus away from the patient.
3. This response minimizes the patient's feelings and may cut off further communication.
4. This statement invalidates the patient's concerns and may interfere with further communication.

TEST-TAKING TIP: Identify the word in the stem that sets a priority. The word *most* in the stem sets a priority. Identify the options that deny the patient's feelings. Options 3 and 4 minimize the patient's feelings and concerns. Identify the equally plausible options. Options 3 and 4 are equally plausible.
Content Area: Communication and Documentation
Integrated Processes: Caring; Communication/Documentation; Nursing Process: Assessment
Client Need: Psychosocial Integrity
Cognitive Level: Application

30. **ANSWER: 3.**
Rationales:
1. Although facing the patient may facilitate lip reading, it does not ensure that the patient will receive the message accurately.
2. Although speaking clearly may be done, it will not help the immediate situation.
3. **Feedback from the patient must be obtained to ensure that the instructions about the environment are understood. This is the primary outcome of any patient teaching, regardless of the physical status of the patient.**
4. Although eliminating background noise helps to eliminate competing stimuli, it does not ensure that the message will be received accurately.

TEST-TAKING TIP: Identify the word in the stem that sets a priority. The word *most* in the stem sets a priority. Identify equally plausible options. Options 1, 2, and 4 are equally plausible because they all address how to improve the transmission of a verbal message to a person who has impaired hearing. Identify the unique option. Option 3 is unique because it is the only option that involves an intervention that obtains feedback from the patient.
Content Area: Communication and Documentation
Integrated Processes: Communication/Documentation; Nursing Process: Implementation
Client Need: Psychosocial Integrity
Cognitive Level: Application

31. **ANSWER: 2, 6, 4, 3, 5, 1.**
Rationales:
2. This permits the nurse to gather significant information about the patient before actually meeting the patient.

6. Patients have a right to know who is providing care and the role that the person fulfills.

4. It is essential that the nurse verify the patient's name with at least two qualifiers. This ensures that the nurse is sharing confidential information with the correct person.

3. Explaining the goals and objectives provides an orientation for the patient regarding the remainder of the interaction. It provides an initial exchange of information.

5. Preoperative teaching is the working phase of this relationship. The nurse imparts information, provides teaching, explores patient concerns, and evaluates the patient's understanding.

1. At the completion of the session, it is essential that the nurse review what was achieved. This is best accomplished by briefly reviewing the desired outcomes of the preoperative teaching session.

Content Area: Communication and Documentation
Integrated Processes: Teaching/Learning; Nursing Process: Planning
Client Need: Safe and Effective Care Environment; Management of Care
Cognitive Level: Analysis

32. **ANSWER: 1.**
    Rationales:
    1. This is the correct procedure for indicating a documentation error. The word used to indicate that the entry is incorrect is determined by policy and procedure of an agency.
    2. It is not necessary to have a stricken entry counter-signed by the nurse in charge.
    3. Documentation that is in error should not be obliterated by white-out to avoid any concern that an attempt was made to fraudulently alter the clinical record.
    4. Documentation that is in error should not be obliterated by a black magic marker to avoid any concern that an attempt was made to fraudulently alter the clinical record.
    TEST-TAKING TIP: Identify the equally plausible options. Options 3 and 4 both indicate an action that obliterates the entry. One is no better than the other. Eliminate options 3 and 4 from further consideration.
    Content Area: Communication and Documentation
    Integrated Processes: Communication/Documentation; Nursing Process: Implementation
    Client Need: Safe and Effective Care Environment; Management of Care
    Cognitive Level: Application

33. **ANSWER: 1.**
    Rationales:
    1. A critical pathway includes key elements used by all disciplines to monitor and document interventions performed on a daily schedule so that outcomes are achieved when expected. When an outcome is not achieved as expected, the health-care professional is required to document the variance, including the event and the action in response to the event. This approach is designed to ensure that interventions are implemented as expected, increasing quality of care and discharge in a timely manner.

2. This is not an example of focused charting. Focused charting uses the format of data, action, and response in a narrative note. It focuses on planning and evaluation.

3. This is not an example of charting by exception. Charting by exception documents information other than routine care. Routine care is documented on a separate flow sheet. It assigns a number to each identified problem, providing for easy reference. It streamlines documentation following the format of problem identification, interventions provided, and evaluation of patient outcomes.

4. This is not an example of problem-oriented charting. Problem-oriented charting follows the SOAP format. Subjective data, Objective data, Assessment, and Plan. This approach provides a structured, logical format to charting.

Content Area: Communication and Documentation
Integrated Processes: Communication/Documentation; Nursing Process: Implementation
Client Need: Safe and Effective Care Environment; Management of Care
Cognitive Level: Comprehension

34. **ANSWER: 2.**
    Rationales:
    1. Progress notes inform other members of the health-care team of interventions and status of the patient in response to interventions.
    2. **This is the purpose of a plan of care. It may be a nursing plan of care or an integrated health team plan.**
    3. Flow sheets document routine aspects of nursing care and include forms such as weight, vital signs, I&O, and skin assessment.
    4. The Kardex is used to communicate basic information about the patient for easy reference. Although some Kardexes contain a section on the plan of care, it is a secondary source of information and usually it is not part of the legal clinical record. In addition, Kardexes are losing favor with the advent of electronic charting.
    Content Area: Communication and Documentation
    Integrated Processes: Communication/Documentation; Nursing Process: Implementation
    Client Need: Safe and Effective Care Environment; Management of Care
    Cognitive Level: Comprehension

35. **ANSWER: 1, 2, 4, 5.**
    Rationales:
    1. This is a judgmental statement and demonstrates a lack of respect for the patient. The better response is, **"I see that you did the best that you could with regard to eating your dinner." This is an empathetic response that demonstrates acceptance.**
    2. **The statement uses medical jargon which the patient may not understand. Medical jargon may confuse a patient and communicates that the nurse is not interested enough to make information understandable. The nurse should use language that the patient understands, offer opportunities for questions, and evaluate the patient's understanding.**
    3. This is the therapeutic communication skill of summarization. It highlights important points in a conversation or teaching session and may identify what still needs to be accomplished.

4. This statement minimizes the patient's concerns and violates trust. The better response is, "Let's talk about what concerns you have regarding the surgery so that you will feel more comfortable."

5. This is a defensive nontherapeutic response to a patient who is angry. The better response is, "I am sorry that your coffee was cold this morning. How about I get you a nice hot cup of coffee right now?"

TEST-TAKING TIP: Identify the word in the stem that indicates negative polarity. The word *nontherapeutic* in the stem indicates negative polarity. The question is asking, "Which statements are inappropriate or do not promote communication?"

Content Area: Communication and Documentation
Integrated Processes: Communication/Documentation; Nursing Process: Evaluation
Client Need: Psychosocial Integrity
Cognitive Level: Analysis

Chapter 8

Psychosocial and Cultural Nursing

KEY TERMS

Adaptation—Disturbance in the human system in response to an event or stimulus.

Affect—Observable, outward expression of mood.

Aggression—Hostile verbal, symbolic, or physical behavior that intimidates others.

Anger—Emotion precipitated by extreme displeasure.

Anxiety—Unpleasant emotional state that spans the range of mild to severe with accompanying escalation of uncomfortable physiological and motor responses.

Assimilation—Process of acquiring a new cultural identity by adapting to the norms of the dominant cultural group.

Behavior—Physical mannerisms that can be observed by others.

Bereavement—Mourning period following a loss.

Body image—Subjective mental image of one's physical appearance and functioning.

Cognition—Intellectual operations, such as the capacity to think, reflect, and reason.

Coping (adaptation)—Use of healthy and effective choices to reduce stress.

Culturally appropriate—Care based on knowledge of the cultures and ethnicities of individuals for whom care is provided.

Culturally competent—Care that addresses the overall context of the patient's condition in a culturally appropriate manner.

Culturally sensitive—Respect for the cultures and ethnicities of individuals for whom care is provided.

Culture—Nonphysical traits, beliefs, attitudes, values, and customs common to a group and handed down from one generation to the next.

Culture shock—Situation that occurs relative to transition from one culture to another, whereby previous coping is ineffective.

Defense mechanisms—Mainly unconscious mental processes used to protect the self from anxiety precipitated by external threats or internal tensions.

Delusion—Fixed false belief without an external stimulus.

Discrimination—Unequal treatment of people or groups based on race, ethnicity, gender, social class, sexual orientation, or other characteristics.

Ethnicity—Group within a social system that has common traits or characteristics, such as language or religion.

Ethnocentric—Belief that one's own culture is better than the cultures of others.

External locus of control—Motivation generated from outside the self.

General attitude—Manner of acting that demonstrates one's temperament.

Grief—Overall physical, emotional, cognitive, spiritual, and behavioral response to loss or bereavement.

Hallucination—False sensory perception without an external stimulus.

Insight—Ability to understand the causes and significance of one's attitudes, emotions, moods, and behaviors.

Internal locus of control—Motivation generated from within the self.

Judgment—Ability to formulate a rational opinion or make a conventional decision based on available information.

Continued

KEY TERMS—cont'd

Loss—Unwanted change, removal, or reduction of worth of a valued object, person, or situation; can be actual or perceived, physical, or psychological.

Maladaptive coping—Occurs when unhealthy and ineffective choices are used to reduce stress.

Mood—Continued emotion that has a significant impact on a person's view of the world.

Mourning—Social and cultural expressions that convey feelings of sadness and grief.

Perception—Recognition and interpretation of stimuli.

Personal identity—Person's view of the self as a unique, separate, and distinct individual.

Prejudice—Negative belief that is generalized to all members of a group; also called *racism*.

Race—Classification of individuals based on physical characteristics or genetic indicators, such as skin color, hair texture, features, and bone structure.

Religion—System of beliefs associated with the worship of a superior being and the nature and purpose of the universe.

Self-concept—Totality of a person's perception of the physical and psychological self.

Self-esteem—Degree to which a person believes others view him or her as well as how one views oneself.

Sensory status—Ability to receive, discern, and react to seeing, feeling, hearing, or sensing aromas.

Socialization—Process of being nurtured within a culture and assimilating the features and uniqueness of the group.

Stereotyping—Presuming that all people of a group are alike, commonly unrelated to reality and precipitated by racism or discrimination.

Suicidal ideation—Thoughts of suicide or self-injurious acts expressed verbally or symbolically.

Suicide—Self-inflicted death.

Suicide attempt—Self-directed act that may result in minor or major injury by a person who intended to die.

Suicide gesture—Self-directed act that results in minor injury.

Suicide threat—Expression of intent to commit suicide without action.

Thought processes—Processes associated with cognitive activities, including thinking, reasoning, reflecting, conceiving ideas, conceptualizing, and having opinions; attention, concentration, and expectation; orientation; level of consciousness; and memory are also involved.

Transcultural nursing—Learning and exploring different cultures in relation to cultural norms, health beliefs, and health practices with the objective of delivering health care within the framework and perspective of the patient's culture.

I. Psychosocial Health

Psychosocial health begins within the self in relation to self-concept ("Who am I?"). Self-concept is a complex construct composed of self-esteem, body image, personal identity, personal strengths, and role performance. It is constantly evolving as a result of gender, parental and social influences, growth and development, socioeconomic status, personal motivational resources, successes or failures, and health-related stressors (e.g., illness, disability, and aging). Nurses must understand the influence of this information, the theories that relate to the development of self-concept, and the general concepts related to stress and coping (adaptation) to be prepared to help patients maintain psychosocial health.

A. Self-Concept
  1. Overview.
     a. Totality of a person's perception of the physical and psychological self.
     b. Frame of reference from which an individual identifies and interrelates with the environment and others.
     c. Dynamic process that changes throughout life as one is exposed to different experiences and when one compares oneself to others.
     d. Characteristics of a person with positive self-concept.
        (1) Has a clear understanding of self and others.
        (2) Finds productive ways of finding meaning in life.
        (3) Relates to others in a fulfilling manner.
        (4) Can manage problems using effective coping strategies.
        (5) Is more willing and able to take action to improve health.
     e. Characteristics of a person with a negative self-concept.
        (1) Does not value oneself.
        (2) May become stalled in the ability to find meaning in life.
        (3) May have difficulty engaging in respectful relationships.
        (4) May resort to ineffective or destructive ways of coping.
        (5) May not have energy to engage in activities to improve health.
        (6) Is less willing or unable to take action to improve health.

f. Can be challenged or negatively impacted by health problems, such as illness, disability, or disfigurement.
  (1) Patients may not have personal strengths to manage change in a positive way.
  (2) Patients may react with ineffective coping, such as anger, depression, and even suicide. (See the section "Nursing Care to Support Psychosocial Health" later in this chapter for nursing interventions to support patients who are angry, depressed, or suicidal.)
g. Can be improved through nursing interventions that help a patient to view oneself more positively, use positive strategies to improve relationships with others, employ more effective and positive coping strategies, and accept a change or deterioration in health and quality of life.

2. Components of self-concept.
  a. **Self-esteem.**
    (1) Judgment of one's own worth.
    (2) May reflect personal admiration or respect for self in relation to the totality of the ideal self or a certain part of the self (e.g., appearance, intellect, accomplishments).
    (3) Based on one's view of the self in relation to personal standards or standards set by others; also influenced by how others view the person.
  b. **Body image.**
    (1) Subjective mental image of one's physical appearance and functioning.
    (2) Can be altered by a loss of a body part or function, disfigurement, or developmental changes.
    (3) Can change over time in response to alterations in one's physical appearance and functioning.
      (a) Change in the body can negatively affect a person's self-concept, health, and health-seeking behaviors.
      (b) Sudden change in the body, such as paraplegia or amputation of an extremity, generally is more traumatic than a gradual change in the body associated with aging.
      (c) Change in the body's appearance or function may precipitate denial, anger, despair, and depression.
  c. **Personal identity.**
    (1) Person's view of the self as a unique, separate, and distinct individual.
    (2) Influenced by culture and socialization, beginning in childhood when a person identifies with parents and extended family members and then by teachers, friends, and other people with whom the person comes in contact.
    (3) Remains relatively stable over time.
    (4) Characteristics of a person with a strong personal identity.
      (a) Values own viewpoints, perceptions, and contributions.
      (b) When faced with a crisis, is more likely to work hard to address the challenge.
    (5) Characteristics of a person with a weak personal identity.
      (a) May not value own viewpoints and perceptions or view contributions in a positive frame of reference.
      (b) Is more likely to compare self with others and be influenced by others.
      (c) When faced with a crisis, is more likely to limit activities or blame illness or disability on others.
  d. **Personal strengths.**
    (1) Components within a person that one draws upon to manage stressful situations in life, such as a positive mental attitude, talents, pride in life achievements, and positive coping skills.
    (2) Can be drawn upon by patients to manage stress.
  e. **Role performance.**
    (1) Throughout life, people are expected to engage in roles, such as child, parent, spouse, sibling, grandparent, employee, and so on.
    (2) People tend to view themselves in light of the roles that they are expected to fulfill and whether they can fulfill them successfully.
    (3) Health challenges and developmental changes due to aging can affect how successfully one is able to meet role expectations.
    (4) Role changes in life require transition.
      (a) Can be situational, such as death of a spouse or child, divorce, job termination, and relocation.
      (b) Can be developmental, such as commencement of a career, marriage, parenthood, retirement, and so on.
    (5) People with a strong self-concept are better able to draw upon personal strengths to adjust to changes in role than people with a weak self-concept.

3. Factors affecting self-concept.
  a. Developmental level.
    (1) As people age, self-concept is less affected by others.
    (2) Adults generally view inadequacies and faults less as confirmation of incompetence

and see them more as difficulties common to all people.

b. Gender.

(1) Women tend to place a higher value on teamwork and cooperation and have a higher self-concept for verbal and social competence than men do.

(2) Men tend to place a higher value on personal achievement and have a higher self-concept for mathematical and physical dimensions than women do.

c. Socioeconomic status.

(1) Socioeconomic status (social class) is related to one's level of income and ability to support oneself.

(2) The higher the social class, generally the stronger the self-concept.

d. Family and peer relationships.

(1) Social identity is facilitated by interactions between infants and parents and expands as the child ages through relationships with other family members, including siblings, grandparents, aunts, uncles, and cousins.

(2) As children age, they are less influenced by family and more influenced by peers and peer pressure.

e. Personal motivational resources.

(1) **Internal locus of control:** People are motivated from within and believe that their actions can exert control over their lives; they take responsibility for their actions and are more able to handle unanticipated adverse situations in a more optimistic light.

(2) **External locus of control:** People are motivated from outside of the self and believe that control of situations is attributable to external factors, other people, organizations, or a superior being; they are more likely to blame others for a situation or seek recognition from others for motivation.

f. History of success or failure.

(1) History of success contributes to a positive self-concept; multiple experiences resulting in success encourages a person to seek new challenges, especially if the person has a strong support system.

(2) History of failure contributes to a negative self-concept; multiple experiences resulting in defeat or failure may predispose a person to expect failure in the future or even to avoid opportunities for growth because of the fear of failure.

g. Illness, disability, and aging.

(1) The United States is a youth-oriented society in which physical attractiveness, vitality, health, and youth are valued.

(2) Body disfigurement; chronic illness; loss of a body part; and wrinkles, loss of hair, and other signs of aging may pose a serious threat to a person's self-concept.

B. Theories Related to the Development of Self (also see "Theoretical Foundations of Nursing Practice" in Chapter 1, "Theory-Based Nursing Care," p. 7)

1. **Erikson's theory of psychosocial development.**

a. Consists of eight developmental stages.

(1) Infant (trust versus mistrust): As an infant receives supportive behaviors and experiences the meeting of needs, the infant develops trust in self and others.

(2) Toddler (autonomy versus shame and doubt): As a toddler experiences self-control through exploration of the environment and independence, personal identity, body image, and self-esteem develop.

(3) Preschooler (initiative versus guilt): As a child relates with family members and through the development of sexual identity, the child begins to establish a role identity.

(4) School-aged child (industry versus inferiority): As a child experiences successful performances and recognition, self-confidence and continued growth of self-concept occurs.

(5) Adolescent (identity versus role confusion): As an adolescent integrates the tasks of earlier stages, the adolescent searches for a secure sense of self.

(6) Young adult (intimacy versus isolation): As a young adult develops intimate relationships with others, the sense of self progresses and the individual establishes new roles, such as partner, parent, occupational role, and so on.

(7) Middle-aged adult (generativity versus self-absorption): As an adult achieves goals and is concerned with the next generation, a new sense of identity develops along with a continued integration of roles and increasing self-concept.

(8) Older adult (integrity versus despair): As an older adult accepts personal accomplishments or feels a lack of personal worth and value, the individual develops positive, negative, or ambivalent feelings about the self.

b. Each stage requires achievement of specific tasks that cultivate and advance growth and development of a positive self-concept, self-esteem, personal identity, and role performance.

c. Inability to achieve or incomplete achievement of a task affects one's ability to satisfactorily achieve later tasks.

d. Understanding of Erickson's eight stages directs nursing interventions that support movement toward task achievement associated with each stage of development.

2. **Coopersmith's four components of self-esteem.**
   a. Identifies critical components in the development of positive self-esteem that occur during childhood and adolescence.
   b. Consists of four critical components.
      (1) Acceptance and worthiness: A person cultivates a sense of self based on the quality and quantity of care and concern received from others.
      (2) Power and control: Toddlers learn power and control of the environment through exploration and learning the cause and effect of behavior; initiative continues to develop, especially in school-aged children as they learn the difference between a leader and a follower in team sports and competitive activities.
      (3) Moral worth and virtue: Morals and values of parents and other important individuals in a child's life are internalized by preschool- and school-aged children and are integrated into behavior in an attempt to please significant others.
      (4) Competence and mastery: As developmental milestones are reached, a growth in abilities leads to task achievement and feelings of competence and mastery.
   c. Understanding of this theory helps direct nursing interventions that support growth and development associated with each component of self-esteem development.

C. Stress and Coping
   1. Stress.
      a. An external or internal event (stressor) precipitates a response in an individual; can be positive or negative, but is usually perceived as a threat to physical or psychological functioning.
      b. Sources of stressors.
         (1) From within a person (internal), such as infection and fear.
         (2) From outside a person (external), such as death of a spouse and relocation.
      c. Types of stressors.
         (1) **Situational stressors** are unpredictable and may occur anytime in the life span (e.g., divorce, illness, and death of a loved one).
         (2) **Psychological stressors** arise from events or in response to primary or secondary stressors (e.g., inconsistent care during childhood, violent environment, exposure to physical or emotional abuse, history of separation from parents, rejection by peers,

mental illness, problems at work, and impaired family dynamics).
         (3) **Developmental stressors** are associated with a predictable event that occurs at an expected time in a person's life (e.g., beginning school, puberty, marriage, parenthood, pregnancy, commencement of a career, midlife crisis, family responsibilities, menopause, caring for parents, physical changes of aging, and retirement).
         (4) **Microbiological stressors** include bacteria, viruses, and fungi. Some infections precipitate psychological stress associated with the stigma of a disease (e.g., sexually transmitted diseases) or isolation (e.g., methicillin-resistant *Staphylococcus aureus*, *Clostridium difficile*).
         (5) **Chemical stressors** are toxic substances that can precipitate physiological or psychological changes within an individual (e.g., smoking, drug or alcohol addiction, habitual use of prescribed or over-the-counter drugs).
         (6) **Physical and physiological stressors** are stimuli that change the structure or function within the body (e.g., pain, obesity, paralysis, loss of vision or hearing, incontinence, impaired function, disease, disfigurement, amputation, physical abuse or neglect, terminal illness) and that may precipitate an emotional response (e.g., impaired body image, feelings of loss).
   2. Coping (adaptation).
      a. A disturbance in the human system in response to a stimulus perceived as a threat to physical or psychological functioning.
      b. Adaptive coping occurs when healthy and effective choices are used to reduced stress.
      c. Maladaptive coping occurs when unhealthy and ineffective choices are used to reduce stress; multiple concurrent stressors, a high intensity of a stressor, and/or a prolonged exposure to a stressor can exhaust a person's ability to adapt.
      d. Personal factors that influence adaptation.
         (1) Perception of the stressor (e.g., the extent to which the person's view of it is realistic or exaggerated).
         (2) General health (e.g., chronic illness can decrease a person's ability to adapt effectively).
         (3) Extent of support system (e.g., family, friends, neighbors, and religious groups).
         (4) Other factors (e.g., age, success of previous coping, and life experience).
      e. Personal approaches to coping.
         (1) Actions that remove or change the stressor, such as resigning from an excessively demanding job.

(2) Defense mechanisms help people to adapt to stress. (Table 8.1).

    (a) Mainly unconscious mental processes used to protect the self from anxiety precipitated by external threats or internal tensions.

    (b) Are adaptive because they protect a person from anxiety through the release of tension; however, when extreme, they become maladaptive.

(3) Avoiding the stress, such as using stairs instead of an elevator if one is claustrophobic.

f. Psychological reactions to stress include feelings, thoughts, and behaviors that are expressed, such as anxiety, fear, anger, aggression, depression, embarrassment, guilt, paranoia, hopelessness, helplessness, powerlessness, forgetfulness, disorganization, resistance to authority, and use of defense mechanisms.

g. Physiological responses to stressors begin with generalized responses (see Table 11.1, "Stages of the General Adaptation Syndrome and Related Nursing Care," in Chapter 11, p. 242 and the section "Inflammatory Response: Local Adaptation Syndrome" in Chapter 12, p. 296). If adaptation is unsuccessful, then pathophysiological responses (diseases) occur.

II. Mental Health Assessment

A mental health assessment is an important component of a comprehensive health assessment. Various stressors, whether they are situational, physical, physiological, developmental, psychological, microbiological, or chemical, impact a person's mental and emotional functioning. Keep in mind that humans have a biopsychosocial connection as well as a holistic response to stressors. Therefore, adaptations to stressors may be reflected in a person's appearance, general attitude, behavior, activity, sensory and cognitive status, thought processes, judgment, insight, mood, affect, speech pattern, self-concept, self-esteem, body image, perception, ability to control one's impulses, potential for violence, level of anxiety, and use of defense mechanisms to protect the ego. Before the nurse can identify a plan of action to address a patient's mental and emotional needs, the nurse must first collect, cluster, and determine the significance of data reflective of the patient's mental and emotional status.

A. Components of a Nursing Mental Health Assessment

1. Stressors: Stimuli that precipitate a change in an individual.

    a. Assess for internal stressors.

    b. Assess for external stressors.

2. Appearance: Outward aspects of an individual.

    a. Note the patient's grooming and hygiene, posture, eye contact, and clothing.

Table 8.1 Defense Mechanisms

Defense Mechanism	Example
Compensation: Increased capabilities in one area to make up for deficiencies in another.	Nonathletic student joins the debate team.
Denial: Ego unable to accept painful reality.	Person assumes false cheerfulness or fails to seek medical help when needed.
Displacement: Directing anger toward less threatening substitute.	Patient yells at a significant other after being diagnosed with cancer.
Intellectualization: Situation dealt with on cognitive, not emotional, level.	Patient discusses all test results but avoids focusing on fears and feelings.
Projection: Attaching to others feelings that are unacceptable to self.	Preoperative patient says to wife, "Don't be scared."
Rationalization: Attempt to logically justify or excuse unacceptable behaviors.	Mother of a latchkey 10-yr-old says, "He needs to learn to be self-sufficient."
Reaction formation: Opposite reaction to the way one really feels.	A person does not like a neighbor but is overly friendly.
Regression: Retreat to an earlier, more comfortable developmental age.	Adolescent has a temper tantrum when told not to do something.
Repression: Unconscious blocking of unacceptable thoughts from the conscious mind.	A woman has no recollection of her father's sexual abuse.
Suppression: Conscious blocking of thoughts from the mind.	"I'll worry about that after my test tomorrow."
Undoing: Actions or words cancel previous actions or words to decrease guilt.	Husband gives wife a gift after abusing her.

From Vitale (2013). *NCLEX-RN Notes: Content Review and Exam Prep.* Philadelphia: F. A. Davis Company. With permission.

b. Determine whether the patient's appearance is congruent with his or her developmental stage and age.

3. General attitude: Manner of acting that demonstrates one's temperament.
   a. Assess whether the patient responds in a positive adaptive manner or in a maladaptive manner.
   b. Assess whether the patient is friendly or distant, hostile or aloof, open or defensive, passive or aggressive, guarded, suspicious, or resistive.

4. Behavior (physical mannerisms that can be observed by others) and activity (quality or quantity of behaviors).
   a. Note mannerisms, such as gestures.
   b. Identify whether the patient is rigid or relaxed and has tremors or tics.
   c. Determine whether the patient is restless, agitated, hyperactive, or calm.
   d. Identify whether activity and behavior are congruent with feelings.

5. Sensory status: Ability to receive, discern, and react to seeing, feeling, hearing or sensing aromas.
   a. Assess ability to receive visual stimuli.
   b. Assess ability to receive auditory stimuli.
   c. Assess ability to receive olfactory stimuli.
   d. Assess ability to receive tactile stimuli.

6. Cognition and thought processes: Processes associated with intellectual operations, such as the capacity to think, reflect, and reason; conceiving ideas, concepts, and opinions; attention, concentration, and expectation; orientation; level of consciousness; and memory.
   a. Assess whether thinking is organized, rapid, slow, or repetitious.
   b. Determine the length of the patient's attention span.
   c. Assess level of consciousness, such as level of alertness.
   d. Assess orientation to person, place, and time.
   e. Assess memory, such as recall, recent, and remote.
   f. Assess ability to concentrate.
   g. Assess content of cognition (e.g., delusional, suicidal, obsessive, paranoid, phobic, or expressing religiosity or magical thinking).

7. Judgment (ability to formulate a rational opinion or make a conventional decision based on available information) and insight (ability to understand the causes and significance of one's attitudes, emotions, moods, and behaviors).
   a. Assess decision-making, problem-solving, and coping abilities.
   b. Assess ability to understand cause and effect.

8. Mood: A continued emotion that has a significant impact on a person's view of the world.
   a. Assess whether the patient is emotionally labile, depressed, apathetic, sad, anxious, fearful, irritable, happy, elated, guilty, despairing, angry, ashamed, proud, content, or confident.
   b. Assess whether the patient's mood has the potential for precipitating harm to self or others.

9. Affect: Observable, outward expression of mood.
   a. Assess the patient's ability to vary emotional expression.
   b. Identify whether the patient's affect is congruent with mood or is flat, blunted, diminished, or inappropriate.

10. Speech pattern: Vocalization of sounds and words that reflect elements of speech.
    a. Assess verbal communication, such as tone, volume, rate of speech, fluency, and enunciation, and its congruency with the patient's feelings and behavior.
    b. Assess for rapid talking (pressured speech).
    c. Assess for impaired ability to communicate through speaking, writing, or behaviors (aphasia). Determine whether the patient is having difficulty receiving a message (receptive aphasia) or sending a message (expressive aphasia).
    d. Assess the fluency of speech, such as whether the patient is hesitant, is mute, or exhibits a latent response.

11. Self-concept: Totality of a person's perception of the physical and psychological self, including self-esteem and body-image.
    a. Assess the presence of negative or positive statements about self.
    b. Determine the extent of satisfaction with self-esteem and body image.

12. Perception: Recognition and interpretation of stimuli.
    a. Determine whether the patient has a history of hallucinations (command or auditory), delusions, or illusions.
    b. Determine whether the patient has a history of feeling detached or separated from oneself or feeling that one is being treated as an object rather than a person (depersonalization).

13. Impulse control: Ability to resist urges, drives, or temptations related to an action that may cause harm to self or others.
    a. Assess whether the patient exhibits disinhibition, aggression, hyperactivity, hypersexuality, or other inappropriate social behavior.
    b. Assess whether the patient has the potential for precipitating harm to self or others.

14. Potential for violence: Likelihood of the use of force or physical compulsion to abuse or cause injury to oneself or others.

🛑 a. Assess for progressive behaviors that indicate an increasing risk of violence toward others (e.g., increased muscle tension, pacing, use of profanity, verbal and physical aggression).

🛑 b. Assess for progressive behaviors that indicate an increasing risk of violence toward self (e.g., depression, suicidal ideation, suicide threat, suicide gesture, suicide attempt).

15. Family and social systems.
    a. Identify significant others and resources that influence the patient.
    b. Assess ability to attain and maintain interpersonal relationships.
    c. Assess the extent of the patient's support system.

16. Spiritual status: Belief in a relationship with a higher power, divine being, or infinite source of energy in an effort to discern meaning in life.
    a. Identify patient's level of comfort with beliefs, values, and spiritual/religious beliefs.
    b. Identify whether the patient has an affiliation with a religious organization.

17. Anxiety: An unpleasant emotional state that spans the range of mild to severe with accompanying escalation of uncomfortable physiological and motor responses; may promote or hinder function and learning depending on the level of anxiety.
    a. Assess the patient's level of anxiety (Table 8.2).

18. Defense mechanisms.
    a. Assess for use of defense mechanisms (see Table 8.1).
    b. Identify whether defense mechanisms being used are adaptive or maladaptive.

III. Nursing Care to Support Psychosocial Health

Stress is a part of everyday living from the moment people get up in the morning until they go to bed at night. However, stress can multiply when a person is confronted with additional consequences associated with illness and disease. Nurses should implement actions that address needs common to all people adapting to stress. In addition, nurses should know how to meet the specific needs of patients who are exhibiting maladaptive coping behaviors, such as patients who are anxious, depressed, suicidal, angry, aggressive, or hyperactive and those who are experiencing delusions or hallucinations. This section discusses these common and specific nursing interventions.

Table 8.2 Levels of Anxiety and Related Signs and Symptoms

Factor	Mild	Moderate	Severe	Panic
Perception	Broad, alert.	Narrowed, focused.	Greatly narrowed, selective attention.	Distorted, scattered.
Motor activity	Slight muscle tension.	Increased muscle tension, tremors.	Extreme muscle tension, increased motor activity.	Erratic behavior, combative or withdrawn.
Communication	Questioning.	Pitch changes, voice tremors.	Difficulty communicating.	Incoherent.
Mood	Relaxed, calm.	Energized, nervous.	Irritable, extremely upset.	Panicky, angry, terrified.
Physiological responses	Normal vital signs (VS).	Slight increase in pulse and respirations.	Fight or flight response: increased VS, dilated pupils, hyperventilation, headache, diaphoresis, nausea, diarrhea, urgency, frequency.	Continuation of fight or flight response; may exhibit dyspnea, pallor, hypotension.
Learning	Enhanced, uses learning to adapt.	Impaired, focuses on one issue, selective attention.	Greatly diminished, improbable, decreased concentration, increased distractibility.	Impossible, unable to learn.

From Vitale (2013). *NCLEX-RN Notes: Content Review and Exam Prep.* Philadelphia: F. A. Davis Company. Adapted with permission.

A. Common Nursing Care

1. Provide basic nursing care for all patients.

   a. Always introduce yourself and explain what you are going to do and why.

   b. Address the patient by name and always speak in a respectful manner.

   🛑 c. Recognize that all behavior has meaning.

   d. Actively listen to the patient's message.

   e. Maintain a safe, supportive, and nonjudgmental environment.

   f. Use interviewing techniques to encourage ventilation of feelings; do not deny or approve feelings.

   g. Maintain eye contact and use touch appropriately.

   h. Provide privacy when performing procedures or discussing something of a personal or sensitive nature.

   i. Accept and respect the patient as an individual; provide choices, when able, to promote independence.

   j. Do not talk about the patient to others in front of the patient.

   k. Set simple, fair, consistent expectations and limits about behavior; address inappropriate behavior immediately.

   l. Help the patient to test new interpersonal skills.

   m. Encourage activities that involve the patient in recovery.

   n. Include family members, with the patient's consent.

   o. Implement actions that support spiritual needs, such as supporting religious rituals and arranging for visits with a spiritual advisor.

   p. Recognize that sexual needs persist throughout life; maintain nonjudgmental acceptance of the patient's need to meet sexual needs and provide privacy when patient engages in meeting sexual needs.

   q. Discuss sexual concerns with the patient, especially when the patient has a physical illness or change in body image that impacts self-esteem and self-concept.

2. Provide nursing care to promote self-concept and self-esteem.

   a. Establish a therapeutic relationship, emphasizing honesty, consistency, and a nonjudgmental attitude.

   b. Help to develop and achieve realistic goals.

   c. Help to identify past achievements and personal strengths.

   d. Encourage the patient to be as independent as possible; include the patient in planning care and encourage performance of self-care.

   e. Discourage self-criticism and negative self-talk; teach the patient to substitute positive self-talk.

   f. Be supportive and use positive, affirming language.

   g. Support personal preferences and previous routines when able.

   h. Encourage involvement in activities that offer opportunities for success.

   i. Encourage the use of communication skills that promote interpersonal relationships.

   j. Help the patient to cope with dependency needs associated with illness or the aging process.

   k. Refer the patient to self-help groups as needed.

3. Provide nursing care to promote a positive body image.

   a. Ensure that one's body language and facial expressions do not reflect revulsion, fear, or rejection.

   b. Reinforce personal strengths.

   c. Encourage discussion of the illness, surgery, or trauma that caused the altered body image and explore options associated with living with the altered change in body image.

   d. Support the patient through the various stages of loss, and explain to the patient that anger, crying, and depression are expected responses.

   e. Urge the patient to be kind to oneself; point out when the patient is being unrealistically critical about his or her body and to try to look at strengths to support personal identity.

   f. Suggest that the patient identify what is liked about his or her body and refer to it when feeling down.

   g. Encourage acceptance of positive comments about appearance.

   h. Practice role playing, allowing the patient to respond to negative comments from others about his or her appearance.

   i. Encourage the patient to surround him- or herself with positive, upbeat people who are not critical.

   j. Provide for interaction with people who have comparable body changes.

   k. Help identify all available resources.

   l. Assess the response of family members and intervene if they are negatively affecting the patient.

4. Provide nursing care to promote role enhancement.

   a. Help the patient to differentiate between ideal and actual role performance; help the patient to recognize that it is acceptable not to be perfect.

   b. Help the patient to focus on positive and supportive change.

   c. Help the patient to identify current and future roles; encourage reminiscence by older adults.

    d. Discuss expectations and modification of roles in light of the patient's lifestyle, family, and specific health changes.

    e. Facilitate alteration in roles among family members, such as redistribution of responsibilities and behaviors in expanded roles as a result of the patient's health problem.

B. Caring for Patients Who Are Anxious

  1. Introduction.

    a. Anxiety is a feeling of uneasiness and apprehension that occurs in response to a nonspecific, vague threat to the patient's physical, emotional, or social integrity that activates the autonomic nervous system.

    b. Anxiety ranges from mild to severe.

    c. Mild to moderate anxiety supports motivation and may encourage a person to take positive action.

    d. Severe anxiety interferes with a person's ability to focus and communicate, causes one to be easily distracted, increases motor activity, and consumes energy because all behavior is directed toward seeking relief.

    e. Once a nurse understands the signs and symptoms distinguishing the various levels of anxiety, the nurse can assess the level of anxiety experienced by a patient.

  2. Nursing care.

    a. Assess level of anxiety.

    🛑 **b. Stay with the patient during a panic attack and provide for safety.**

    c. Provide a single room and decrease environmental stimuli.

    d. Validate somatic complaints, but do not call attention to them.

    e. Assist with relaxation techniques, such as deep breathing and muscle relaxation, to decrease anxiety.

    f. Help the patient identify and avoid anxiety-producing situations.

    g. Postpone teaching when anxiety reaches higher than a moderate level.

    🛑 **h. Intervene when acting-out impulses may harm self or others.**

C. Caring for Patients Who Are Depressed

  1. Introduction.

    a. Depression generally is described as feeling sad, powerless, or hopeless and is related to low self-esteem, anxiety, and various psychiatric disorders.

    b. Depressed people tend to retreat from people and reality.

    c. Depression theories include chemical imbalance due to hormonal, neurological, or genetic factors; loss and emotional detachment; negative thinking; ineffective family and interpersonal relationships; socioeconomic factors; and loss of function, illness, and disability.

    d. Clinical indicators include anger, anxiety, guilt, sadness, tearfulness, regression, restlessness, withdrawal, self-blame, blaming others, preoccupation with loss, anorexia or overeating, headache, backache, chest pain, constipation, hopelessness, and powerlessness.

      (1) Hopelessness is when a person lacks the psychic energy to seek or comprehend alternatives because of a distressed emotional state.

      (2) Powerlessness is described as verbalizing a lack of control or influence over a situation and is externally based; a person can feel powerless but still have hope.

    e. Failure to address a depressive episode early can lead to major depression, described by the American Psychiatric Association as a depressed mood or markedly diminished interest or pleasure in all or almost all activities for more than 2 weeks, plus four or more of the following:

      (1) Increased or decreased weight (5%); increased or decreased appetite.

      (2) Psychomotor changes (agitation or retardation).

      (3) Altered sleep (insomnia or hypersomnia).

      (4) Decreased concentration or indecisiveness.

      (5) Decreased energy or fatigue.

      (6) Feelings of worthlessness or inappropriate guilt.

      (7) Recurrent thoughts of death or suicide.

  2. Nursing care.

    a. Accept feelings of worthlessness, hopelessness, and powerlessness as real to the patient.

    🛑 **b. Monitor for risk of suicide, especially as depression lifts and energy increases.**

    c. Sit quietly next to the patient and then encourage one-to-one interaction.

    d. Spend time with the patient to support worthiness; provide realistic praise.

    e. Accept, but do not reward, dependence; provide simple choices.

    f. Encourage self-care.

    g. Minimize isolation; involve the patient in simple, repetitive activities.

    h. Assist the patient to identify and replace self-deprecating thoughts with positive thoughts through cognitive restructuring.

    i. Avoid false reassurance and excessive cheerfulness.

    j. Implement measures to support self-esteem.

D. Caring for Patients Who Are Suicidal
1. Introduction.
   a. Risk of suicide is associated with stress, loss, depression, hopelessness, helplessness, serious illness, substance abuse, social isolation, young adults and adolescents, single older adults (higher in men), mood disorders, sexual identity crisis, and history of previous attempts.
   b. Levels of suicidal behavior.
      (1) **Suicidal ideation:** Thoughts of suicide or self-injurious acts expressed verbally or symbolically.
      (2) **Suicide threat:** Expression of intent to commit suicide without action.
      (3) **Suicide gesture:** Self-directed act that results in minor injury.
      (4) **Suicide attempt:** Self-directed act that may result in minor or major injury by person who intended to die.
      (5) **Suicide:** Self-inflicted death.
2. Nursing care.
   a. Provide constant observation and a safe environment, such as no sharps, belts, and shoelaces and assignment to a two-bed room.
   b. Identify the patient's behaviors, involving giving away possessions or putting affairs in order, as precursors to a suicide attempt.
   c. Ask the patient whether he or she has a plan and means to carry out suicide.
   d. Encourage writing a no-suicide contract.

DID YOU KNOW?

A no-suicide contract is an agreement that outlines what a person should do if feelings of suicide occur. The contract should include:

- **A statement that the patient realizes that it is never okay to die by suicide.** This encourages the patient to internalize the concept that suicide is not an acceptable way to manage feelings.
- **Ways for the patient to get help if feeling suicidal.** This provides a list of things to do or people to call if the patient should feel suicidal; it eliminates the burden of having to decide who to call and how to initiate the call when emotionally distraught, confused, and unsure about what to do.
- **The patient's signature.** This is done after the terms of the contract are reviewed to ensure that there are no misunderstandings about the contract and that the patient understands that suicide cannot be attempted under any circumstance.
- **Identification of a place for the patient to keep the contract.** This is done so that if the patient feels suicidal, the patient can quickly find the contract.
   e. Focus on strengths rather than weaknesses.
   f. Identify factors that precipitated or contributed to the suicide crisis and address them.
   g. Encourage exploration of consequences, such as impact on others if successful, feelings about death, and reasons for living.
   h. Assist with problem-solving; prioritize problems and focus on one at a time.
   i. Help the patient write a list of sources of support and community resources and ways to ask for help.
   j. Ensure that family members are aware of the need to maintain safety because most suicides occur within 90 days after hospitalization.

E. Caring for Patients Who Are Angry or Aggressive
1. Introduction.
   a. Anger is an emotion precipitated by extreme displeasure; it can progress to acting out behavior, such as aggression.
   b. Aggression is hostile verbal, symbolic, or physical behavior that intimidates others.
   c. Anger and aggression are associated with delirium, dementia, substance abuse, mania, paranoid schizophrenia, and conduct disorders. They may be a response to a reality-based stimulus or associated with the defense mechanism of displacement.
   d. Clinical indicators include a clenched fist, furled brow, glaring eyes, tense mouth, clenched teeth, flushed face, and raised or lowered voice.
   e. Signs of anger escalation include disproportionate anger, pacing, agitation, suspiciousness, throwing objects, and verbal and physical threats.
2. Nursing care.
   a. Assign the patient to a single room.
   b. Use nonthreatening body language and a calm approach; respect the patient's personal space and do not touch.
   c. Monitor for frustration, irritation, increasing anxiety, or distorted thinking that may precede violence.
   d. Anticipate needs to decrease stress that can cause anger.
   e. Assist the patient to express anger in acceptable ways, such as using words, writing a list of grievances, engaging in physical exercise, and using assertiveness; provide positive reinforcement for acceptable behavior.
   f. Teach the patient to interrupt aggressive patterns, such as counting to 10 or removing self from the situation.

g. Always position oneself between the patient and the door to provide an escape route.

h. If behavior becomes aggressive, request assistance from other staff members and use short command sentences such as, "John, calm down."

🛑 i. Follow policies and procedures for progressively managing aggressive patients if verbal interaction is ineffective, such as removing the patient from the situation and vicinity of others, offering an as-needed medication, using seclusion, and applying restraints.

F. Caring for Patients Who Are Hyperactive
  1. Introduction.
     a. Hyperactivity is characterized by increased motor activity and speech, impulsivity, inattention, and an expansive or irritable mood.
     b. It is associated with attention deficit hyperactivity disorder or a manic episode associated with a psychiatric disorder, such as bipolar disorder.
  2. Nursing care.
     a. Provide a safe, nonstimulating environment.
     b. Approach the patient in a calm, nonargumentative manner.
     c. Channel hyperactivity into safe, controlled activities.

🛑 d. Use easy distractibility to redirect inappropriate behavior.

     e. Keep activities simple, repetitive, and of short duration.
     f. Use rewards, such as tokens or praise, to support appropriate behavior.
     g. Balance energy expenditure and rest.
     h. Provide high-protein and high-calorie handheld foods.

G. Caring for Patients Who Experience Delusions or Hallucinations
  1. Introduction.
     a. A **delusion** is a fixed, false belief without an external stimulus.
     b. A **hallucination** is a false sensory perception without an external stimulus.
  2. Nursing care.
     a. Recognize and accept that delusions and hallucinations are real to the patient; stay with the patient because delusions and hallucinations increase with isolation.

🛑 b. Identify commands that direct the patient to commit an act of violence that may harm the self or others.

     c. Distract from delusions by encouraging the patient to listen to music or walk and talk with the nurse.

d. Point out reality, but do not reason, argue, or challenge delusions or hallucinations.

e. Focus on meaning and feelings rather than content.

f. Praise reality-based perceptions.

g. Identify factors that can exacerbate sensory and perceptual disturbances, such as reflective glare, lights, and television and computer screens.

h. Teach self-coping for delusions, such as recreational activities and diversionary activities.

i. Teach self-coping for hallucinations, such as exercising; listening to music; saying, "Stop; go away!"; and engaging in structured activities.

IV. Death, Dying, Loss, and Grief

Although feelings of loss and grief can occur with any situation in which a person experiences a change or reduction in a valued object, situation, or ability, they are usually related to the death of a significant other or oneself. Death is inevitable because every human being will die. Although the provision of nursing care during the dying process addresses physical needs, the main focus of nursing care is on the patient's and family members' psychosociocultural needs. Models of grieving provide frameworks that reflect the ways in which people generally cope with dying and death. These models provide nurses with information that can help identify a patient's progression toward death, which allows the nurse to formulate a plan of care that addresses individualized needs during specific stages of dying. Although a patient's body is cared for respectfully after death, the major focus of care shifts to the needs of the family.

A. Introduction.
  1. Loss is an unwanted change, removal, or reduction of worth of a valued object, person, or situation.
     a. Can be actual, such as death of a spouse or amputation.
     b. Can be perceived, such as loss of stamina or feeling less womanly after a hysterectomy.
  2. Bereavement refers to the mourning period following a loss.
  3. Grief is the overall physical, emotional, cognitive, spiritual, and behavioral response to loss or bereavement.
     a. Factors affecting grief include the importance of the loss, amount of psychosocial support, unresolved conflict at the time of the loss, anticipated or unexpected loss, and number of losses experienced in a short period.
     b. Uncomplicated grieving is normal grieving.
     c. Complicated or dysfunctional grieving occurs over an extended length of time (more than 2 years) or involves excessive intensity of emotion or maladaptive responses, such as severe depression or addictive behaviors.

d. Anticipatory grieving is grief experienced before the actual loss; it generally occurs when a person is caring for another person with a chronic, deteriorating illness, such as Alzheimer's disease.

4. Mourning refers to the social and cultural expressions that convey feelings of sadness and grief, such as crying, religious rituals, burial practices, and expression of condolence.

5. Quantifying death by primary health care providers is guided by two sets of criteria.
   a. The President's Commission for the Study of Ethical Problems in Medicine and Biomedical and Behavioral Research (1981) defines death as: "Absence of respiration and circulation; irreversible absence of all brain functions, including the brain stem."
   b. The Harvard Medical School Criteria of Death consists of five components:
      (1) Unreceptive and unresponsive to stimuli.
      (2) No movements.
      (3) No breathing.
      (4) No reflexes.
      (5) Flat electroencephalogram.

B. Models of Grieving
1. **Engel's model of grief.**
   a. Consists of six phases.
      (1) Shock and disbelief: A person is in denial or intellectually accepts the loss, but not emotionally.
      (2) Developing awareness: Reality of the loss is internalized and psychological pain is experienced.
      (3) Restitution: Process of mourning that includes funeral, religious practices, and rituals.
      (4) Resolving the loss: Grieving person centers energy on thoughts and beliefs about the deceased.
      (5) Idealization: All negative thoughts and feelings about the deceased are initially repressed; as time passes, the person incorporates some unique characteristics of the deceased into one's own personality.
      (6) Outcome: Psychological dependence on the deceased lessens, the person begins to focus on moving forward, and the person begins to seek new relationships.
2. **Kübler-Ross's stages of grieving.**
   a. Classic theory for health-care professionals to help guide patient-centered care to those who are dying.
   b. Has five stages (Table 8.3).
   c. Not all people move through every stage; progression through stages is not contingent on completing the previous stage.

Table 8.3 Kübler-Ross's Stages of Grieving

Stage and Responses	Nursing Care
Denial: "Not me"; unable to believe loss; may exhibit cheerfulness.	• Explore own feelings about death and dying. • Accept, but do not strengthen, denial. • Encourage communication.
Anger: "Why me?"; questioning; resists loss with hostility and anger.	• Recognize anger is a form of coping. • Do not abandon the patient or become defensive. • Help others to understand the patient's anger.
Bargaining: "Yes, me, but . . ."; barters for time and may express guilt for past behavior.	• Assist with ventilation of feelings, such as guilt, fear, sadness. • Help with unfinished business, if appropriate.
Depression: "Yes, me"; realizes full impact; grieves future losses; may talk, withdraw, cry, or feel extremely lonely.	• Convey caring; use touch; sit quietly with the patient. • Acknowledge sad feelings. • Accept and support grieving.
Acceptance: "OK, me"; accepts loss; may have decreased interest in activities and people; may be quiet or peaceful.	• Support completion of personal affairs. • Support family participation in care. • Do not abandon the patient and family. • Help family members to understand and allow the patient's withdrawal.

   d. Movement through stages may be nonsystematic and may not be linear; the person may be in two stages at the same time; and, after completion of one stage, the patient may regress back to a previous stage.
   e. Nurses should encourage verbalization of feelings regarding the stage the patient is in and should not attempt to move patients to subsequent stages because doing so depends on the patient's readiness and coping abilities.

C. Hospice and Palliative Care
1. Hospice programs provide holistic care to patients with a terminal illness and their family members; hospice care can be provided at home or in hospitals, long-term care facilities, or free-standing hospice agencies.
2. Palliative care focuses on supporting comfort and quality of life.

D. Nursing Care for a Patient Who Is Dying
1. Answer questions honestly.
2. Meet spiritual needs expressed by the patient.

3. Encourage independence and offer choices, such as "Who do you want in the room with you now?" and "What can we do to help you go peacefully?" Acknowledge that the patient has control over the plan of care and goals.

4. Support social needs; recognize that the patient may want to mend a strained relationship or spend time with particular people or family members.

5. Assist with final arrangements, such as persons to notify, funeral arrangements, and completion of any last wishes when possible.

6. Balance activity and rest.

7. Implement measures to maintain hygiene, grooming, and skin integrity.

8. Provide for physical needs, such as elimination, nutrition, and oxygen.

9. Provide for adequate pain control. Also, accept an informed decision not to be medicated so that interaction with family members can be maintained.

10. Provide care for an unconscious patient.
    a. Continue to talk to as if hearing is intact.
    b. Wet the patient's lips and mouth.
    c. Use artificial tears to keep eyes moist.
    d. Turn the patient on his or her side and raise the head of the bed if respirations are congested and noisy (death rattle).

11. Understand that some patients wait for a specific date to die or until family members arrive; others wait until loved ones leave so as not to die in their presence.

E. Nursing Care for Family Members of a Patient Who Is Dying

1. Explain the stages of death and dying to family members so that they understand their loved one's behavior, and explain that dying patients may interact minimally with family members.

2. Involve family members in direct patient care if that is the patient's and their wishes.

3. Encourage family members to ensure their own needs are met (e.g., food and rest); provide chairs or recliners so that family members can stay near.

4. Keep family members informed about physical signs that indicate active dying, such as falling blood pressure, diaphoresis, and mottled, cold skin.

5. Explain that moaning and grunting are common behaviors when death is near and may not mean that the patient is uncomfortable.

6. Encourage family members to continue to occasionally talk to a dying unconscious patient.

7. Do not impose on family members at the moment of death; accept family members' behaviors, such as picture taking and lying next to or hugging the body; allow family members as much time as they need to be with the body; stay near and wait quietly until they are ready to move away from the body.

8. Remove any tubes or lines attached to the patient (unless an autopsy is required) according to policy and procedure; straighten bedcovers; and make patient look as natural as possible.

9. Take family members to view the body when they arrive, if they wish.

10. Transfer the body after family members have viewed the body or stated a preference not to view the body.

11. Offer support by saying, "I am sorry for your loss." Avoid efforts to minimize loss by saying, "She is in heaven now" or "You still have your children." Ask family members "How can I help?" or "What would you like me to do?"

F. Body Preparation and Postmortem Care

1. Be aware that death is generally pronounced by a primary health-care provider or coroner; however, some states grant advanced practice nurses and nurses working in long-term care facilities, home-health care, and hospice agencies the authority to pronounce death.

2. Consider any legal issues related to postmortem care (Box 8.1).

3. After a person is pronounced dead and family members have left, prepare the body or delegate the task to unlicensed assistive personnel, as appropriate.
   a. Respect cultural and spiritual preferences, noting that some cultures require family members to wash the body.
   b. Follow facility policies and procedures regarding hygiene, grooming, and dressing changes.
   c. Remove tubes and lines unless an autopsy is scheduled.
   d. Provide postmortem care per facility policy.
      (1) Secure a postmortem set, which contains items such as a plastic sheet called a *shroud*, identification tags, soft gauze, and padding.
      (2) Position the body in functional alignment.
      (3) Position a pillow under the head and shoulders to reduce the risk of settling blood, which can cause discoloration.
      (4) Place dentures in the mouth.
      (5) Close the eyes.
      (6) Tie soft gauze under the chin and around the head to keep the mouth set in a natural position.

Box 8.1 Legal Issues Related to Postmortem Care

Certification of Death

- U.S. laws mandate that a death certificate be completed and filed with the local health or other government office for every person who dies.
- Certificates of death are also necessary for legal matters and insurance purposes.

Organ Donation (Upon Death)

- All states have accepted the Uniform Anatomical Gift Act for organ donation.
- Generally, a person carries an organ or tissue donor card that stipulates all or specific organs and tissues that a person wishes to donate upon death; some states use a section of the driver's license as a donor card.
- Documents no longer require a witness to the person's signature or a family member's consent.
- An organ procurement team member may approach family members about organ donation in the absence of a donor card.

Postmortem Examination (Autopsy)

- An autopsy is an examination of a body to establish the cause of death.
- It is required in the event of an unexpected, suspicious, or violent death.
- Family member must give consent for an autopsy.
- The legal system may seek a court order for an autopsy in some situations.

    (7) Pad and tie the wrists together gently to hold the arms close to the body.
    (8) Place an identification tag on the patient's toe or ankle.
    (9) Enclose the body within a shroud and place an identification tag on the shroud.
  e. Arrange to have the body transported to the morgue or removed by funeral home personnel.
  f. Be aware that most facilities have a special stretcher to transport a body to the morgue; it looks like a regular stretcher, but the body is enclosed below so that it is not visible to visitors and other patients.

V. Cultural Nursing Care

Nurses are encountering increasing diversity among the populations for whom they provide care. To be culturally sensitive, appropriate, and competent, nurses must understand the characteristics, customs, and rituals common to various cultures. Even still, nurses must consider the fact that no two people within a culture are likely to have identical views. Therefore, nursing care must always be individualized for each patient.

A. Characteristics of Culture
1. Culture is values, beliefs, practices, and traditions that are shared by members of a group; it provides an identity.
2. Culture is complex and is reflected in many aspects of life and on many levels, such as art, literature, attire, language, customs, rituals, and practices.
3. Culture is taught and learned through life experiences, such as incidents, practices, traditions, and encounters with individuals within the culture.
4. Culture affects communication. For example:
  a. Different cultures may have different languages or dialects of the same language that pose a challenge for not only the patient, but also for care providers.
  b. American culture is associated with assertive, self-determined independence.
  c. Asian cultures value group harmony, show respect to elders and family leaders, consider direct eye contact disrespectful or aggressive, and engage in ambiguous communication, such as using incongruent agreeing statements rather than saying "no," which is considered disrespectful. The nurse needs to seek feedback to ensure that agreeing statements actually reflect understanding or consent.
5. Cultures are organized based on family relatedness and status within a family or society, such as gender, age, and education. For example:
  a. A Korean mother is subject to the authority of her husband and to the oldest son in the absence of the father.
  b. In many African cultures, the woman is the leader and decision-maker of the family.
  c. In some cultures, men have a higher status than women and receive care before women.
6. Culture influences physical placement when communicating with others and is related to personal space and territoriality. For example, North Americans tend to stand 18 inches apart when communicating with one another, whereas people from Arab cultures stand closer.
7. Culture influences time orientation regarding whether a person is past, present, or future oriented. For example, North Americans are future-oriented, whereas Latinos are more present-oriented.
8. Cultures observe life events with traditions and/or religious rituals.
  a. Beliefs and rituals associated with a variety of cultures.
    (1) Female circumcision is practiced in some African cultures.
    (2) Religious rites of passage may occur at puberty, such as a Bat or Bar Mitzvah in the Jewish faith or confirmation in Catholic and Protestant faiths.

    (3) Females must participate in a ritual bath after each menstruation and before resuming intimate relations with a spouse in the Orthodox Jewish, Islamic, and Hindu cultures.

    (4) Various cultures have specific attitudes and beliefs about cremation, organ donation, and autopsy because of the belief that the dead must face the creator with the body undesecrated.

  b. Beliefs and rituals associated with different cultural and religious groups (Table 8.4).

9. Culture affects health beliefs and practices:

  a. Some cultures have folk healers (e.g., shaman, herbalist, medicine man) and folk practices to help restore health, such as religious healing rituals, amulets or talismans worn to ward off evil, and energy (qi) to restore yin/yang balance.

  b. Asian Americans may tolerate pain stoically because they view pain as something that cannot be controlled.

MAKING THE CONNECTION

Patients' Religious Beliefs and Practices and the Provision of Nursing Care

Dying and death customs and rituals associated with the Jewish faith include having a family member or representative present while a patient is actively dying and remaining with a body until it is buried. This practice fulfills the desire to provide a constant presence for the person who is dying and for the body until burial. The body is washed with warm water by a member of the family or a member of the Chevra Kaddisha society, and then men are wrapped in a prayer shawl, while women are wrapped in a white burial shroud. The body is placed in a simple pine box and buried as soon as possible, often within 24 hours after death. Additional rituals include tearing an article of clothing to symbolize the loss, covering mirrors, and mourning for seven days (Shiva), when community members bring food to the family and reminisce about the deceased.

To support these customs and rituals, the nurse should provide privacy for the dying patient and significant others. A lounge chair or bed should be provided for the person staying with the patient who is dying. Discuss with the family if the body can be touched after death or if arrangements should be made for a member of the Chevra Kaddisha society to care for the body. Obtain from the family the name of a funeral establishment that conforms to Jewish customs and rituals and arrange for removal of the body.

B. Cultural Diversity

1. Trends in the United States.

  a. The United States is a multicultural society, consisting of people from dissimilar cultural and ethnic groups. The U.S. Census Bureau reported 127 nationalities indicated as "first ancestry reported" during the 2010 census.

  b. Racial and ethnic minorities accounted for 91.7 percent of all growth in the U.S. population from 2000 to 2010. Hispanics were responsible for 56 percent of the nation's population growth between 2000 and 2010.

  c. The U.S. Census Bureau predicts that, in 2050, the majority of the U.S. population will consist of what was referred to in 2007 as "minority groups" (Hispanic—30 percent, African American—15 percent, Asian—9 percent, and others—2 percent).

2. Inequalities in health, illness, and death rates correlate with racial and ethnic groups.

  a. People from minority groups are less healthy and experience higher rates of illness and death than white (non-Hispanic) individuals in the United States; for example:

    (1) Infant mortality among African Americans is 1.5 to 3 times more likely to occur than with people from other races/ethnicities.

    (2) People with HIV/AIDS are disproportionately higher within racial/ethnic minorities with the exception of Asian/Pacific Islanders than with whites.

    (3) Cardiovascular disease accounts for the largest proportion of inequality in life expectancy between whites and blacks.

    (4) Preventable hospitalization rates increase as economic level decreases. In addition, there are large disparities in preventable hospitalizations in racial/ethnic groups, with blacks reflecting a rate double that of whites.

    (5) Disparities in smoking and alcohol consumption exist among American Indians and Alaska Natives despite overall declines in other groups.

    (6) Eighty-three percent of individuals newly diagnosed with tuberculosis are reported to be individuals from racial or ethnic minority groups.

  b. *Healthy People 2020* identifies national health promotion guidelines.

    (1) Two overreaching goals include increasing quality and years of healthy life and eliminating health inequalities based on gender, ethnicity, education, income, disability, geographic location, and sexual orientation.

Table 8.4 **Common Beliefs of Different Cultural and Religious Groups**

Culture or Religion	Common Beliefs
African American/Black	• Are generally a matriarchal culture. • May have many family members at the bedside. • Are present-oriented. • May distrust others. • May consume a diet high in fat. • Generally believe in prayer, use of herbs, laying on of the hands, magic rituals, and Voodoo. • May believe illness is due to disharmony and that healing is spiritual. • May refuse advance directives.
Amish	• Prefer that birth and death occur in the home. • Need permission from the church to seek care in a hospital. • Accept anesthesia, surgery, blood transfusions, blood products, dental care, and organ transplantation other than the heart (heart transplantation is unacceptable because Amish believe that the heart is the soul of the body). • Avoid health insurance because it demonstrates lack of faith. • Limit end-of-life care so that assets are used for the living. • Generally are afraid of disability, but not death.
Arab, Muslim, Islamic	• Most Arabs are Muslims and are united by the Islam faith; there is no separation of church and state. • Believe in six terms of faith: one must follow Allah; one must follow the Qur'an, Torah, and Psalms; each person has two angels appointed to them; Muhammad (the greatest prophet) is used to deliver Allah's messages; life after death and hell; and Allah has power over everything. • Believe in five pillars of faith: following Allah and Muhammad, praying facing Mecca five times a day, helping poor and impoverished people, fasting between sun up and sundown during the month of Ramadan (unless ill), and making a pilgrimage to Mecca at least once during one's lifetime. • Do not eat pork. • Do not permit women to make autonomous health-care decisions; husbands are the decision makers. • If female, may prefer same-sex care givers, may wear a small leather bag around the neck containing a locket with religious writings, and may cover their body with clothing so that only the face or the eyes are exposed. • May not practice birth control (strict Muslims), but may allow abortions for health reasons. • May request that the body or head be positioned facing toward Mecca when dying. • May request that a family member or representative provide a ritual bath after death.
Asian American	• Generally include several generations in the nuclear family and may include extended family members. • Have respect for elders. • Are subordinate to authority. • Value self-respect and self-control. • Believe health is a state of balance of the physical and spiritual. • Believe illness is disharmony of yin and yang. • Have a rich history of Eastern medicine that includes herbs, diet, application of hot or cold, acumassage, acupressure, and acupuncture to reestablish balance. • May stoically cope with disability, discomfort, and pain.
Buddhist	• Admire Buddha (Enlightened One) as a way of life. • Believe in avoiding evil, being moral and pure, calming the mind so as to observe rather than react, and doing good by helping others. • Believe in multiple cycles of birth, life, death, and rebirth until a person is no longer involved with desire and the self; goal is to achieve eternal life without further reincarnation (nirvana) and achievement of liberty and freedom from distress and suffering. • Do not engage in formal ceremonies; however, observe the birthday of Buddha. • Accept modern medicine, surgery, and technology. • Consider illness part of life and therefore do not offer prayers for healing. • On the seventh day after death, read the Tibetan Book of the Dead to liberate the patient's soul from the nether worlds (Tibetan Buddhists).

Continued

Table 8.4 Common Beliefs of Different Cultural and Religious Groups—cont'd

Culture or Religion	Common Beliefs
Catholic	• Believe in the Father, Son, and Holy Spirit and that redemption comes through the blood of Jesus, the Son of God. • Believe that the pope and clergy have prominence over individuals. • Priests administer the sacraments, which include Baptism, Reconciliation, Eucharist, Anointing of the Sick, and Matrimony. A member of the faith can baptize in an emergency if a priest is unavailable. Bishops administer the sacraments of Holy Orders and Confirmation. • Participate as a congregation at a religious service called the Holy Sacrifice of the Mass, where bread and wine is transformed (transubstantiation) into the body and blood of Christ and then distributed in the form of bread wafers (Eucharist) and sips of wine. • Engage in penance and acts of good work during Advent (time period before Christmas) and Lent (time period before Easter Sunday) to prepare for the celebration of the birth of Christ and Christ's resurrection after death on the cross. • Do not ingest meat on certain days, such as Fridays during Lent. • Accept the rhythm method as the only acceptable form of birth control. • Prohibit sterilization, suicide, euthanasia, and abortion. • May desire baptism of a critically ill neonate or infant.
Christian Scientist	• Believe in a unique form of Christianity that teaches a dependence on God and not the medical establishment for health care. • Do not smoke tobacco or drink alcohol and may not drink coffee or tea. • Believe that illness is due to lack of knowledge, fear, or sin and that a person will recover when the circumstance is corrected. • Engage in Christian Science health-care remedies and prayer. • Denounce drug therapy and surgery, but do permit setting of a fracture. • May require the U.S. court system to intervene on behalf of infants and children when parents refuse life-saving treatments.
European American/ non-Hispanic White	• Believe in independence, individuality, and autonomy. • Believe that health is a balance in emotional and physical well-being. • Accept health care in a variety of settings and care based on the newest technologies and approaches. • Supplement traditional medical care with alternative therapies, such as acupuncture, spinal adjustment, massage, herbal therapy, aromatherapy, and naturopathy.
Jehovah's Witness	• Forbid blood transfusions and blood products, but may use artificial blood expanders (may require the U.S. court system to intervene on behalf of infants and children when parents refuse life-saving treatment). • Do not permit sterilization, abortion, and organ transplantation. • Allow birth control, autopsy, and cremation. • Do not permit use of tobacco and recreational drugs. • Do not eat food with blood (animals must be bled according to custom to be acceptable, and some members do not eat meat at all). • May drink alcohol but drunkenness is unacceptable.
Jewish	• Believe that there is only one God who is everywhere and that people have a free will and are responsible for their choices and actions. • Believe in the Torah and Old Testament to show them how to worship and treat others. • Consist of Orthodox, Conservative, and Reformed congregations; Orthodox congregations follow Jewish law more strictly than Conservative and Reformed congregations. • Observe the Sabbath on Saturday and holy days such as Yom Kippur, Rosh Hashanah, and Passover. • May only eat food that is permitted and that is slaughtered and prepared following strict laws of Kashrut (kosher diet), if Orthodox or Conservative Jew. • Prohibit pork, but permit meat from animals that are cloven footed and cud chewing; do not ingest dairy at the same meal as meat; require two separate sets of dishes, pots, and utensils to ensure that meat and dairy products are maintained separately; can eat fish with scales and nonpredatory birds. • May wear a head scarf or a wig and clothing that is modest and covers the arms and most of the legs to show respect to God (Orthodox Jewish women). • Practice sexual self-denial during menstruation and a ritual bath afterward (a husband cannot touch his wife until after the ritual bath). • Practice rituals, such as hand washing, scripture reading, using prayer beads, meditation, praying before and after meals, and lighting candles on the Sabbath.

Table 8.4	**Common Beliefs of Different Cultural and Religious Groups—cont'd**

Culture or Religion	Common Beliefs
Jewish (cont'd)	• Engage in a ceremony called a *bris* 8 days after birth, in which a Jewish male is circumcised by a *mohel* and named; infant females are named during a ceremony in the synagogue on the first Sabbath after the birth. • Engage in a religious rite of passage called a Bat or Bar Mitzvah at puberty. • Do not consider neonates to be human until birth of the head or after three-quarters of the body is born. • Cherish health and life to the degree that no intervention is permitted to alleviate pain and suffering if it hastens death. • Generally do not consider psychiatric care helpful. • Believe that a person should be with the patient when death occurs and with the body until burial, which should occur within 24 hours; burial society volunteers (Chevra Kaddisha) wash the body, close the eyes, wrap it in a linen shroud, and may lay it on the floor until burial. • After death of a loved one, observe a mourning period (sit Shiva) during which people gather to pay respect and focus on the memory of the deceased. • Prohibit tattoos, suicide, euthanasia, embalming, and cremation.
Hindu	• Believe in Brahman, the underlying universal life force. • Believe the aim in life is relief from the karmic cycle of death and reincarnation; leading a good life will lead to a higher status in the next life. • Believe illness may be caused by actions in a past life. • May revere several or more gods and goddesses. • May wear a religious thread around the wrist or body. • Observe Mahashivarathri, a celebration of Lord Shiva. • Believe family members are important to each other. • Believe that illness is due to supernatural causes that imbalance bile, phlegm, and wind (body humors). • Believe that pain is due to the anger of a higher power and therefore one must bear the condition and situation. • Believe in the tenets of astrology. • Pray and meditate after bathing; prefer to wash in water that is free flowing. • Do not accept abortion, circumcision, suicide, and euthanasia. • Use birth control, participate in organ donation, and receive blood transfusions. • Accept health care only from a person of the same gender. • If female, wear saris that cover the body except for the arms and feet. • Cremate the body within 24 hours because doing so is believed to release the body from connection with the earth. • Are vegetarians, eat sweets and yogurt at all meals, and use large amounts of spices. • Eat with only the right hand because the left hand is used for toileting activities.
Hispanic and Latino	• Generally have extended family members living together; emphasis is on the group. • Believe in faith and spirituality. • Believe health is a gift from God, a reward, or good luck. • Believe in prayer, miracles, wearing religious medals or amulets, herbs, rituals, and hot and cold therapy. • Believe illness is an imbalance in hot and wet, hot and dry, cold and dry, and/or cold and wet. • May consider illness to be a punishment.
Mormon (Church of Jesus Christ of Latter-day Saints)	• Believe in Jesus and one God and the sacred writing of the Book of Mormon (believed to be given to Joseph Smith by an angel). • Follow a strict health code that advises healthful living. • Forbid alcohol, coffee, cola, tea, and overeating, and observe monthly fasting. • Wear a sacred undergarment that is only removed for bathing and can be removed for surgery but must be treated with respect. • Permit circumcision, organ transplantation, and autopsy. • Permit cremation only if required by law. • Forbid abortion, sterilization, drug abuse, and smoking. • Provides a subsidized welfare system and financial assistance for congregants who are ill.
Native American	• Believe in a spiritual power, acceptance of nature, tradition, sharing, and respect of elders. • Treat the body with respect. • Engage in rituals, ceremonies, chanting, exorcisms, dancing, sand painting, meditation, use of herbs, and wearing amulets. • Believe health is living in harmony with nature. • Believe illness is a concern of the family, extended family, and tribe.

Continued

Table 8.4	Common Beliefs of Different Cultural and Religious Groups—cont'd

Culture or Religion	Common Beliefs
Protestant	• Believe that Jesus is the mediator between man and God and that Jesus' death redeems and with God's grace makes redemption possible. • Believe in the authority of the scriptures in the Holy Bible and Books of Doctrine particular to specific religions, such as Lutheran, Baptist, and Methodist. • Believe that individuals are prominent over the authority of a minister, priest, or pastor. • May attend services, receive Communion, and celebrate Easter Sunday and Christmas. • May fast in preparation for certain religious celebrations, such as Easter Sunday.
Seventh-day Adventist	• Hold the Sabbath on Saturday and spend the day worshiping and resting. • Forbid tattoos, body piercings, alcohol, opioids, stimulants, and caffeine. • Believe that healing is precipitated when a minister anoints a patient with oil. • Believe that prayers advance healing. • Accept birth control for married couples. • Allow abortion when medically necessary. • Prohibit euthanasia, but accept stopping medical support. • Consider death to be like sleep; believe that the body and soul remain together until Christ comes again. • Follow kosher dietary laws, and most are vegetarians.

(2) For more information about Healthy People 2020, see the section "Healthy People 2020" in Chapter 5, Community-Based Nursing, p. 83.

3. Nurses are challenged with meeting the needs of a culturally diverse population.
   a. The U.S. Department of Health and Human Services (2010) reports that 83.2 percent of nurses are white (non-Hispanic).
   b. Nurses will be caring for ever-increasing numbers of individuals with different cultural and ethnic backgrounds, educational preparation, financial status, disabilities, genders, and sexual orientation and come from different geographic locations.
   c. Conflicts in health-care delivery are commonly related to cultural misunderstandings.

C. **Providing Culturally Competent Nursing Care**
   1. To meet the needs of the culturally diverse population, nurses must be:
      a. **Culturally sensitive:** Have respect for the cultures and ethnicities of individuals for whom they are providing care.
      b. **Culturally appropriate:** Implement care based on knowledge of the cultures and ethnicities of individuals for whom they are providing care.
      c. **Culturally competent:** Implement care that addresses the overall context of the patient's condition in a culturally appropriate manner.
   2. To provide culturally competent nursing care, nurses should:
      a. Study and learn about cultures and religions that are different from their own.

   b. Explore their true feelings about various cultures and identify their own personal biases and prejudices, if any exist.

   🛑 c. Provide nonjudgmental nursing care that is accepting and respectful of a patient's culture, beliefs, and rituals.

   d. Explore a patient's spiritual beliefs and/or religious affiliation and steps that can be taken to better support spiritual and religious needs.
   e. Respectfully handle religious articles, such as the Bible, the Koran, rosary beads, prayer beads, religious jewelry, medals, amulets, icons, and totems, and nonjudgmentally accept tattoos that have a religious, spiritual, or special meaning to the patient.
   f. When a significant other has authority within the family, with the patient's consent, involve that person in decision making.
   g. Ensure modesty when providing nursing care; assign a caregiver of the same gender as a patient if requested; support a patient's desire to wear clothing that is more modest than a hospital gown.
   h. Arrange for a dietician to collaborate with a patient who has specific dietary preferences, such as people who follow a kosher diet, do not eat pork, eat only vegetables, or avoid meat on certain days of the week.
   i. Help patients explore their feelings if a health-care intervention that they desire is prohibited by their religion (e.g., a patient who wants a blood transfusion whose religion prohibits the administration of blood or blood products).

j. Explore and document refusal of care related to religious beliefs to ensure that it is the patient's desire and communicate the information to other health-care team members.

k. Arrange for a spiritual advisor or leader to visit or perform religious rituals.

l. Provide time and privacy for rituals, and provide extra seating for participants.

m. Avoid bathing the patient for several hours if a ritual involved anointing with oils.

CASE STUDY: Putting It All Together

A nurse is caring for a 42-year-old man who was admitted 7 days ago to the burn unit with partial-thickness burns on his neck, hands, and lower arms and patches of deep partial-thickness burns of his face, chest, and anterior upper arms. The nurse received report from the night nurse, completed a physical assessment, and interviewed the patient.

Night Nurse Report

Pt. admitted 7 days ago after sustaining partial-thickness burns of his neck, hands, and lower arms and patches of deep partial-thickness burns of his face, chest, and anterior upper arms. Vital signs are slightly elevated and experiencing dyspnea at times. Voiding straw-colored urine greater than 50 mL/hour.

Ringer's lactate, 100 mL/hour, running as ordered

Urinary retention catheter, hourly urine output

Nasal oxygen at 2 L/minute; oxygen saturation 95%

Electrolytes within expected range at this time; basic metabolic panel every a.m.

Intake and output in balance at this time

Tracheostomy set and suction apparatus on unit

Vitamin C 500 mg PO daily

Ancef 1 g IVPB every 8 hours

IPPB with normal saline solution qid

Protonix 40 mg IVPB q24 hours

PCA: Dilaudid 1 mg per hour with 0.2 mg/15 minute lockout, not to exceed 7.2 mg in 4 hours

Physical Assessment

Vital signs	
Respirations:	28 breaths/minute, dyspnea.
Pulse:	110 beats/minute, regular.
Temperature:	99.8°F, rectal.
Blood pressure:	146/88 mm Hg.

Partial-thickness burns (erythema and blanching with pressure) on the neck, hands, and lower arms, involving more than 12% of body and patches of deep partial-thickness burns (erythema, moist blebs, and blisters) on face, chest, and anterior upper arms, involving 5% of body.

Singed hair on the forehead and sides of the head, absence of eyebrows and eyelashes, singed nostril hair, and sooty sputum noted.

Patient demonstrating an increase in muscle tension, rapid talking when discussing the event, a hoarse voice with tremors when talking, and restless behavior, evidenced by nervously moving about in bed and shaking a lower leg.

Alert and oriented to time, place, and person.

Patient Interview

Patient is able to recall the accident. He explained that he was home alone when the fire started. His three children were in school. Patient stated that he cares for his three children alone: "It's just me and the kids now, with a little help from my neighbors, since my wife took off with another man a year ago. I'm a baggage handler at the airport at night and was doing a few chores before I went to sleep when the fire occurred. I tried to put the flames out myself, but they spread too quickly. The entire kitchen, ceiling, and bedroom over the kitchen were heavily damaged. My children are staying with neighbors temporarily so that they can go to their school until I can make other arrangements. I'm worried about money, but I have homeowner's insurance and health insurance with my job. I am not sure what will be covered or how many sick days I have. You just get a little bit ahead—a house, no big bills, and a little breathing room. This is really going to set me back, but I'm not going to worry about that now." Patient states that he has not seen his children since the accident, but spoke to them a few times on the phone. He said, "I'm worried that my face will scare the kids, and I don't know how my coworkers will react when they see me. People will be horrified because I look like a monster. I think I'll have to get another job that doesn't require me to leave the house so I don't scare others." He went on to say, "I have been able to deal with what life has tossed at me because I always want to do right by my kids, but this is more than I can handle. Maybe it would be better for the kids if I just killed myself." Patient is open and willing to share concerns and feelings while maintaining eye contact most of the time. Occasionally, he used hand gestures that were congruent with verbalized feelings, such as shaking his head, shrugging his shoulders, and drawing his hand across his neck, as if he were cutting his throat when talking about killing himself. He spoke in a sad tone,

Continued

CASE STUDY: Putting it All Together

cont'd

had a sad facial expression and slumped posture, and avoided eye contact when discussing the financial and emotional setback of this event. Patient's speech was hesitant at times when he became emotional. However, he put on a big smile and said, "I have great kids who give me no trouble. I told them that they had to 'be strong.'"

Case Study Questions

A. Identify specific examples of stressors that the patient is experiencing or is at risk for experiencing grouped in relation to the types of stressors.

1. Situational

a. _____

b. _____

c. _____

d. _____

2. Psychosocial

a. _____

b. _____

c. _____

d. _____

e. _____

f. _____

3. Developmental

a. _____

b. _____

4. Microbiological

a. _____

b. _____

5. Physiological

a. _____

b. _____

B. Identify data collected in the following areas when making a mental health assessment of the patient.

1. Stressors _____

2. Appearance _____

3. General attitude _____

4. Activity and behavior _____

5. Sensory and cognitive status _____

6. Thought processes _____

7. Judgment and insight _____

8. Mood _____

CASE STUDY: Putting It All Together   *cont'd*

_____ **Case Study Questions** _____

9. Affect _____

10. Speech _____

11. Self-concept and self-esteem _____

12. Perception _____

13. Impulse control _____

14. Potential for violence _____

15. Family and social systems _____

16. Spiritual status _____

17. Signs and symptoms of anxiety _____

18. Use of defense mechanisms _____

C. Which piece of data indicates the priority problem and why?

_____

D. Identify at least 10 specific nursing interventions that the nurse should implement to help the patient achieve the following nursing outcome: "The patient will remain safe from self-injury."

1. _____
2. _____
3. _____
4. _____
5. _____
6. _____
7. _____
8. _____
9. _____
10. _____
11. _____
12. _____
13. _____
14. _____
15. _____

REVIEW QUESTIONS

1. A nurse is assigned to care for a patient who is admitted for an abortion. Abortion is against the religious beliefs of the nurse. There is no other nurse to whom the patient can be assigned. What should the nurse do?
   1. Care for the patient in a nonjudgmental manner.
   2. Provide just basic physiological care for the patient.
   3. Arrange to have the patient moved to another unit within the hospital.
   4. Explore with the patient the reason for the procedure including alternatives.

2. A nurse is caring for a patient who was admitted to the hospital for cardiac bypass surgery. What patient statement indicates that the patient has an internal locus of control?
   1. "My future is in the hands of my health-care team."
   2. "Many people in my family have coronary artery disease."
   3. "I experienced the chest pain very suddenly out of nowhere."
   4. "I have decided to try cardiac rehabilitation after I am discharged."

3. Many people who are independent and perform all of their activities of daily living become dependent and demanding when physically ill and hospitalized. What defense mechanism should the nurse conclude they are exhibiting?
   1. Denial
   2. Regression
   3. Compensation
   4. Reaction formation

4. A 57-year-old woman who had a mastectomy, radiation, and chemotherapy 6 years ago for breast cancer is admitted to the hospital because of metastasis to the lung. The patient had no respiratory symptoms and the metastasis was identified on a chest x-ray during a routine physical. The nurse reviews the patient's diagnostic test results, obtains the patient's vital signs, and interviews the patient.

Patient's Clinical Record

Vital Signs

Temperature: 99.4°F orally
Pulse: 90 beats/minute, regular
Respirations: 24 breaths/minute, regular rhythm
Blood pressure: 138/84 mm Hg

Diagnostic Test Results

Oxygen saturation: 97%
Serum sodium: 142 mEq/L
Serum potassium: 4.2 mEq/L
Chest x-ray reveals a lesion in the left lower lobe
Dual x-ray absorptiometry test to measure bone density:
 T score +1

Patient Interview

Patient is crying and angrily states, "I can't believe it came back. I went through so much. I had surgery, radiation, and chemo and I've been taking medication ever since. My whole life changed 6 years ago. I gave up wine, I don't eat a lot of fatty foods, and I eat only vegetables that have antioxidants. By doing all this, I thought I had it beat."

Which nursing intervention is the priority based on this information?
   1. Maintaining a patent airway
   2. Providing emotional support
   3. Monitoring serum electrolytes
   4. Supporting the limbs when changing the patient's position

5. The spouse of a patient who is dying tells the nurse, "Even though I want to visit, I can come only once a week because I work and have a dog that I need to walk and feed." Which defense mechanism does the nurse identify the spouse is using?
   1. Projection
   2. Sublimation
   3. Compensation
   4. Rationalization

6. What is psychosocial development **most** influenced by?
   1. Food
   2. Society
   3. Alcohol
   4. Genetics

7. A patient stands 6 inches from the nurse and begins to talk to the nurse in a loud voice. The nurse feels uncomfortable with this behavior. What is the **most** appropriate response by the nurse?
   1. "I would like to talk to you, but you are standing too close to me."
   2. "If you come closer to me you will have to stay in your room."
   3. "You are much too close to me; you must step back."
   4. "Please step back because you are scaring me."

8. A patient with terminal cancer is projecting unwarranted and excessive anger onto a friend who is visiting. The friend approaches the nurse crying and states, "I do not know what is wrong with my friend." What is the **most** appropriate response by the nurse?
   1. "It is your friend's true personality coming out."
   2. "Do not take what your friend is saying personally."
   3. "Your friend is attempting to cope with a serious illness."
   4. "Although this anger is directed at you, it is not your fault."

9. A nurse is assisting a moderately cognitively impaired patient with morning care. What is the nurse's **most** appropriate verbal intervention to help the patient get dressed?
   1. "Would you like to put on brown pants or blue pants before you go to breakfast?"
   2. "Here are your clothes. Would you rather get dressed before or after you have breakfast?"
   3. "The brown pants look good on you. Put them on and go to the dining room for breakfast."
   4. "Pick the outfit you would like to wear today and then go to the dining room for your breakfast."

10. A nurse is caring for a patient with low self-esteem. What can the nurse do to promote the patient's self-esteem? **Select all that apply.**
    1. _____ Provide simple choices.
    2. _____ Assist with setting achievable goals.
    3. _____ Teach the patient relaxation techniques.
    4. _____ Point out the patient's past achievements.
    5. _____ Help the patient to identify personal strengths.

11. A nurse working in the emergency department of a hospital is interviewing an extremely agitated patient who keeps standing up, pacing, and sitting down. Which statement by the nurse is **most** appropriate?
    1. "Please sit down so that we can discuss your concerns."
    2. "Your behavior is inappropriate and you have to try to control it."
    3. "Let's go to a quiet room because your anxiety may be contagious."
    4. "Come with me for a walk and you can describe what is bothering you."

12. Parents bring a 3-month-old infant to the pediatrician because the infant has been crying on and off for hours at a time for several weeks. One parent states that, after a bottle, the baby repeatedly draws up the legs, arches the back, and cries for 4 to 5 hours. Both parents convey being frustrated and exhausted from lack of sleep. Which concern is **most** important that the nurse should include in a teaching program for these parents?
    1. Infant colic
    2. Failure to thrive
    3. Shaken baby syndrome
    4. Sudden infant death syndrome

13. A nurse working in the emergency department of a hospital is assessing a 3-year-old child with a burn injury. Which assessment should alert the nurse to collect additional information because of a concern regarding potential child abuse?
    1. Grease burn on the arm
    2. Evidence of a burned tongue
    3. Scalding burns on both hands
    4. Second degree sunburn on the back

14. Which interventions are examples of nursing actions designed to support psychosocial coping? **Select all that apply.**
    1. _____ Reviewing health-care options with parents of a mentally impaired child
    2. _____ Taking a patient's vital signs just before implementation of a procedure
    3. _____ Discussing strategies about how to live with a diagnosis of cancer
    4. _____ Providing names of resource agencies in the community
    5. _____ Changing a patient's dressing 3 days after surgery

15. A patient is scheduled to have an amputation of the left arm near the shoulder because of a crushing injury sustained during an accident. According to Maslow's hierarchy of needs, which human need does the nurse expect to be **most** affected?
    1. Safety
    2. Security
    3. Self-concept
    4. Self-actualization

16. A nurse is caring for a patient from a Hispanic culture who is dying. What might the nurse expect from the patient's family?
    1. Desire for time for reflection in a peaceful and quiet environment
    2. Request that a religious representative care for the body after death
    3. Expression of happy thoughts to facilitate the dying patient's journey
    4. Loud moaning and expressions of grief during the patient's last hours

17. A nurse is caring for a Native American patient admitted for cardiac care who believes in the benefit of a medicine man with healing powers (shaman). What should the nurse do when planning care for this patient?
    1. Ensure privacy for the performance of healing religious rituals.
    2. Check meal trays to verify that meat is not served with dairy products.
    3. Consult with a dietician to ensure that the patient receives a vegetarian diet.
    4. Accept the decision that a heart transplant violates the belief that the heart is the body's soul.

18. A nurse is planning care for a patient who is a Jehovah's Witness. What action is **most** appropriate?
    1. Ensure that a kosher menu is provided for meal selection.
    2. Verify with certainty that the patient does not want a blood transfusion.
    3. Assign a female nursing assistant to help the patient with activities of daily living.
    4. Consult with the dietician regarding avoidance of pork and milk during the same meal.

19. Which response by the nurse is **most** effective when attempting to reduce a patient's hostility about an event?
    1. "I am here to help you."
    2. "You need to calm down now."
    3. "What can I do now to help address this situation?"
    4. "Do you think that you can be objective at this time?"

20. A nurse is caring for an unconscious patient who sustained a brain injury. What should the nurse include in a stimulation program? **Select all that apply.**
    1. _____ Rub lotion on the extremities.
    2. _____ Perform range-of-motion exercises.
    3. _____ Explain thoroughly everything that is done.
    4. _____ Keep a radio on in the background at all times.
    5. _____ Provide mouth care using a mint-flavored agent.

21. A patient with a blood glucose level of 550 mg/dL is diagnosed with type 1 diabetes and is admitted to the hospital for further diagnostic testing and treatment. The next day the patient says to the nurse, "They told me I have diabetes and I will have to give myself shots of insulin and test my glucose several times a day. What is this all about?" What is the nurse's **best** initial response?
    1. "I will give you some pamphlets that explain everything you need to know about diabetes."
    2. "Although it sounds overwhelming at first, eventually you'll learn these skills."
    3. "It must be difficult for you to have a serious chronic disease."
    4. "Let's talk a little bit about what it means to have diabetes."

22. A nurse is caring for a patient who experienced numerous panic attacks. Place the following nursing interventions in the order that they should be performed when caring for this patient.
    1. Identify which nursing interventions reduce the patient's anxiety level.
    2. Maintain a nonjudgmental approach when caring for the patient.
    3. Stay with the patient when the patient is having a panic attack.
    4. Explore own feelings about people who have panic attacks.
    5. Assess the patient's level of anxiety.
    Answer: _____

23. An older adult shares, "I am a member of the Amish community and have been using herbs and receiving treatment from my community's practitioner for abdominal pain. After 6 months, the pain increased and my skin turned yellow. I received permission from my elders to come to the hospital." After multiple diagnostic tests, the patient is diagnosed with inoperable pancreatic cancer and the primary health-care provider indicates that the situation is terminal. Which statement by the nurse is **most** appropriate when discussing discharge plans with the patient?
    1. "When the time comes would you like to receive hospice care?"
    2. "What can we do for you that will help keep you in your own home?"
    3. "What do you plan to do since your community does not permit chemotherapy?"
    4. "Would you prefer to be discharged to a nursing home where you can receive skilled nursing care?"

24. A nurse notes on a male patient's medical record that the patient is Catholic. Which statement by the nurse shows sensitivity for the patient's religious practices?
    1. "Would you like me to give your name to the priest who is distributing the Eucharist?"
    2. "I will let the dietary department know not to send dairy on the same tray as meat."
    3. "I will assign a male nursing assistant to help you with your bath this morning."
    4. "Can I remove your sacred undergarment when I give you a bath?"

25. A nurse is caring for a woman who is a member of the Church of Jesus Christ of Latter-day Saints (Mormon). Which statement by the nurse demonstrates a lack of sensitivity for the patient's religious related practices?
    1. "I am assigning a male nursing assistant to help care for you tonight."
    2. "I have to remove your head covering so that I can wash your hair."
    3. "I will ensure that you get coffee with your dinner tonight."
    4. "I prayed last night for you that you would get well."

26. A nurse is attempting to meet the psychosocial needs of a patient. Place the following steps in the order in which they should be performed?
    1. Use interviewing techniques and do not deny feelings.
    2. Introduce yourself and explain what you are going to do.
    3. Identify patient needs and involve the patient in recovery.
    4. Address the patient by name and speak in a respectful manner.
    5. Listen to the patient and recognize that all behavior has meaning.
    Answer: _____

27. A nurse is assessing a patient's level of anxiety. Which level of anxiety is the patient exhibiting when the patient is irritable, displays increased motor activity, and exhibits selective attention?
    1. Mild
    2. Panic
    3. Severe
    4. Moderate

28. A nurse is caring for a patient who states, "I hear voices that keep telling me what to do." What is the nurse's **best** response?
    1. "Do you find them frightening?"
    2. "How often do you hear the voices?"
    3. "Is there anything I can do for you?"
    4. "What are the voices saying to you?"

29. Which nursing intervention is **most** specific to help a patient develop a positive body-image?
    1. Facilitate exploration of future roles.
    2. Help the patient identify past achievements.
    3. Support the patient through various stages of loss.
    4. Assist the patient to avoid anxiety producing situations.

30. A nurse is assessing a recently admitted patient's mental status, particularly thought processes. What should the nurse assess?
    1. Is the patient happy versus sad?
    2. The length of the patient's attention span.
    3. Are the patient's emotional expressions stable?
    4. The ability of the patient to exhibit disinhibition.

31. Three days after a stressful event, a person can no longer remember what there was to worry about. What defense mechanism should the nurse conclude that the person may be using?
    1. Repression
    2. Regression
    3. Displacement
    4. Intellectualization

32. A nurse is caring for a group of patients with a variety of psychosocial problems. Which interventions are appropriate regardless of a patient's problem? **Select all that apply.**
    1. _____ Sit quietly next to the patient.
    2. _____ Treat the patient with respect.
    3. _____ Encourage ventilations of feelings.
    4. _____ Maintain a nonjudgmental attitude.
    5. _____ Position self between the patient and the door.

33. A nurse is caring for a patient who is hyperactive. What is the **best** approach to use with this patient?
    1. Plan a variety of challenging activities.
    2. Provide a nonstimulating environment.
    3. Encourage the patient to rest several times a day.
    4. Suggest that the patient engage in a game of chess.

34. A nurse identifies that a patient who will have surgery in the morning is exhibiting mild anxiety. What behaviors exhibited by the patient supported this conclusion by the nurse?
    1. Patient appeared calm but was alert and was asking numerous questions.
    2. Patient had increased muscle tension and kept focusing on one topic.
    3. Patient was extremely upset and had difficulty concentrating.
    4. Patient had flight of ideas and exhibited erratic behavior.

35. A patient is exhibiting severe anxiety associated with a 3-year struggle with colon cancer. The primary health-care provider prescribes gabapentin (Neurontin) 100 mg three times a day for the anxiety. The primary health-care provider indicates that the oral solution form of the drug be dispensed because the patient has difficulty swallowing tablets. The gabapentin solution states that there are 250 mg/5 mL. How much solution should the nurse administer? Record your answer using a whole number.
    Answer: _____ mL

REVIEW ANSWERS

1. ANSWER: 1.
Rationales:
1. There are times when a nurse may have to care for a person whose personal values are different from one's own. In these instances, the nurse should care for the patient in a nonjudgmental manner based on the standards of nursing practice.
2. This care is inadequate; the patient has both physiological and emotional needs.
3. This is unrealistic and places the needs of the nurse before the needs of the patient.
4. The patient has made the decision to proceed with the abortion. The nurse's role is to support the patient's right to self-determination.
TEST-TAKING TIP: Identify the patient-centered option. Option 1 is patient centered.
Identify the option that contains a specific determiner. Option 2 contains the word *just* which is a specific determiner. Rarely options with a specific determiner are the correct answer.
Content Area: Psychosocial and Cultural Nursing
Integrated Processes: Caring; Nursing Process: Implementation
Client Need: Psychosocial Integrity
Cognitive Level: Application

2. ANSWER: 4.
Rationales:
1. The statement in option 1 assigns responsibility for future personal health to members of the health team. This statement reflects an external, not internal, locus of control.
2. The statement in option 2 is a statement of fact and is not assigning responsibility for future growth to others or to oneself (neither external nor internal locus of control).
3. The statement in option 3 is a statement of fact and is not assigning responsibility for future growth to others or to oneself (neither external nor internal locus of control).
4. The statement in option 4 accepts personal responsibility for one's future health status. This demonstrates an internal locus of control.
Content Area: Psychosocial and Cultural Nursing
Integrated Processes: Communication/Documentation; Nursing Process: Analysis
Client Need: Psychosocial Integrity
Cognitive Level: Analysis

3. ANSWER: 2.
Rationales:
1. Patients may use denial during an illness, but this generally will not make them dependent and demanding.
2. During a crisis, one may regress to a stage that provokes less anxiety in an attempt to cope with an unacceptable situation. Regression to a childlike, demanding stage can occur under stress.
3. Compensation is a mechanism that is used to make up for a lack in one area by emphasizing capabilities in another.

4. Reaction formation is used when a patient acts in a way opposite to internal feelings.
Content Area: Psychosocial and Cultural Nursing
Integrated Processes: Nursing Process: Analysis
Client Need: Psychosocial Integrity
Cognitive Level: Analysis

4. ANSWER: 2.
Rationales:
1. In this scenario, the patient is experiencing no respiratory symptoms and the patient's oxygen saturation is 97 percent. There are no data that indicate an inability to manage respiratory secretions or that the airway is compromised. Adequate oxygenation of cells occurs when the oxygen saturation is between 95 and 100 percent.
2. The patient is in Kübler-Ross's stage of grieving known as *anger*. The patient is asking, "Why me?" The nurse must encourage the patient to ventilate feelings and provide emotional support.
3. The patient's serum electrolytes are within the expected range. The expected range for serum sodium is 135 to 145 mEq/L and the expected range for serum potassium is 3.5 to 5.0 mEq/L.
4. A T score is measured in the number of standard deviations from the level expected in a young adult. The patient's bone density T score of +1 is within the acceptable range of +1 to –1 standard deviation from the expected young adult score. T scores between –1 and –2.5 standard deviations indicate osteopenia, and T scores of less than –2.5 standard deviations indicate osteoporosis.
Content Area: Psychosocial and Cultural Nursing
Integrated Processes: Nursing Process: Planning
Client Need: Psychosocial Integrity
Cognitive Level: Analysis

5. ANSWER: 4.
Rationales:
1. Projection is the denial of emotionally unacceptable feelings and the attribution of traits to another person.
2. Sublimation is the substitution of a socially acceptable behavior for an unacceptable feeling or drive.
3. Compensation is making up for a perceived deficiency by emphasizing another feature perceived as an asset.
4. Rationalization is offering a socially acceptable or logical explanation to justify an unacceptable feeling or behavior.
Content Area: Psychosocial and Cultural Nursing
Integrated Processes: Communication/Documentation; Nursing Process: Analysis
Client Need: Psychosocial Integrity
Cognitive Level: Analysis

6. ANSWER: 2.
Rationales:
1. Food is only one aspect of a society and its culture; the primary purpose of food is to meet physiologic needs.
2. A person's cultural environment, which includes the family and the community, has the greatest impact on psychosocial development.
3. Although alcohol meets some individuals' psychological needs and is served in social situations, it is not the factor that most influences psychosocial development.

4. Although some theorists identify genetics as a factor related to personality and behavior, it is not the most influential factor in psychosocial development.
TEST-TAKING TIP: Identify the word in the stem that sets a priority. The word *most* in the stem sets a priority. Identify the option with a clang association. The word *psychosocial* and the word *society* in option 2 is an obscure clang association. *Society* is closely related to *psychosocial*. Carefully consider option 2. More often than not, an option with a clang association is the correct answer.
Content Area: Psychosocial and Cultural Nursing
Integrated Processes: Nursing Process: Analysis
Client Need: Psychosocial Integrity
Cognitive Level: Comprehension

7. **ANSWER: 1.**
   Rationales:
   1. This statement demonstrates interest in the patient while setting limits on behavior.
   2. This statement is inappropriate and threatening.
   3. This statement sets limits, but does not validate the patient.
   4. This statement sets limits, but does not validate the patient. The nurse's statement about being scared may give the patient the message that the nurse cannot keep the situation safe.
   TEST-TAKING TIP: Identify the word in the stem that sets a priority. The word *most* in the stem sets a priority.
   Content Area: Psychosocial and Cultural Nursing
   Integrated Processes: Communication/Documentation; Nursing Process: Implementation
   Client Need: Psychosocial Integrity
   Cognitive Level: Application

8. **ANSWER: 4.**
   Rationales:
   1. This is an inaccurate and inappropriate response. The way people respond to stress is not necessarily their true personality.
   2. Although this response is somewhat helpful, it is not the best response to meet this visitor's needs.
   3. Although this statement reflects reality, it is not the best response in this situation.
   4. This statement is most appropriate because it validates the friend's concerns and supports the friend.
   TEST-TAKING TIP: Identify the word in the stem that sets a priority. The word *most* in the stem sets a priority. Identify the central person in the question. The friend is the central person in the question. The nurse's intervention should meet the friend's needs.
   Content Area: Psychosocial and Cultural Nursing
   Integrated Processes: Caring; Communication/Documentation; Nursing Process: Implementation
   Client Need: Psychosocial Integrity
   Cognitive Level: Analysis

9. **ANSWER: 1.**
   Rationales:
   1. This statement provides the patient with a simple choice and adequate direction.

2. This statement does not give the moderately cognitively impaired patient enough guidance. The concept of before versus after may not be understood.
3. This statement takes control away from the patient.
4. The patient may not have the cognitive ability to make this decision. Receiving two directions at once may be overwhelming.
TEST-TAKING TIP: Identify the word in the stem that sets a priority. The word *most* in the stem sets a priority.
Content Area: Psychosocial and Cultural Nursing
Integrated Processes: Communication/Documentation; Nursing Process: Implementation
Client Need: Psychosocial Integrity
Cognitive Level: Application

10. **ANSWER: 2, 4, 5.**
    Rationales:
    1. This approach is not necessary for a patient with low self-esteem. This approach is more appropriate for people who are depressed and do not have the emotional energy to make decisions.
    2. When goals are attained, it promotes motivation and positive feelings of achievement. This promotes a positive self-esteem.
    3. Learning relaxation techniques will not directly influence self-esteem. Learning relaxation techniques directly relates to reducing anxiety in people who are anxious or experiencing a panic attack.
    4. Past achievements are accomplishments that promote positive feelings. This promotes a positive self-esteem.
    5. Reviewing personal strengths accentuates the positive. Personal strengths provide a foundation on which to build future strengths.
    Content Area: Psychosocial and Cultural Nursing
    Integrated Processes: Caring; Nursing Process: Implementation
    Client Need: Psychosocial Integrity
    Cognitive Level: Application

11. **ANSWER: 4.**
    Rationales:
    1. This statement by the nurse, although courteous, may make the patient more agitated. This is an unrealistic request.
    2. Telling a patient to control behavior may make the patient more agitated. The patient may not be able to control the behavior.
    3. Stating that the patient's anxiety may be contagious is nontherapeutic and possibly may make the patient feel worse.
    4. Offering to walk with the patient during the interview allows the patient to expend energy while voicing concerns.
    TEST-TAKING TIP: Identify the word in the stem that sets a priority. The word *most* in the stem sets a priority. Identify the option that denies the patient's needs. Option 1 denies the patient's need to move around. Identify the options that are not patient-centered. Option 2 is confrontational and not patient-centered. The patient is unable to control the behavior. Option 3 is not patient centered because by saying that the patient's anxiety may be contagious implies

that the patient may harm others. Identify the patient-centered option. Option 4 is patient centered. It is the only option that allows the patient to continue moving about while the nurse addresses the patient's concerns.
Content Area: Psychosocial and Cultural Nursing
Integrated Processes: Caring; Communication/Documentation; Nursing Process: Implementation
Client Need: Psychosocial Integrity
Cognitive Level: Application

12. ANSWER: 3.
Rationales:
1. Although infant colic is a concern and should be addressed, it is not the priority in this situation.
2. There is no evidence to support the conclusion that the infant is not thriving. Failure to thrive is suspected when an infant falls below the fifth percentile for height and weight.
3. **When exhausted, frustrated, and overwhelmed, a person, out of desperation, may resort to shaking a child who is constantly crying. The parents should be taught appropriate comforting techniques and told what can happen to an infant if shaken. It is also important for the parents to have a respite from the crying child to sleep, rest, or relax.**
4. Although implementing measures to prevent sudden infant death syndrome, such as avoiding the prone position when sleeping, is important, it is not the priority in this situation.
TEST-TAKING TIP: Identify the word in the stem that sets a priority. The word *most* in the stem sets a priority. Identify the central person in the question. The parents are the central persons in the question.
Content Area: Psychosocial and Nursing
Integrated Processes: Teaching/Learning; Nursing Process: Implementation
Client Need: Safe and Effective Care Environmental; Safety and Infection Control
Cognitive Level: Application

13. ANSWER: 3.
Rationales:
1. A grease burn generally is not a *red flag* indicating potential child abuse. Hot water and grease burns are the most common cause of burns in children younger than 3 years of age.
2. A burned tongue indicates that the child most likely ingested food or fluid that was too hot. However, it could be considered child neglect if the caregiver provided the child with a nutrient that was hotter than intended and intentionally did not check its temperature first. This is often associated with heating food in a microwave, which should be avoided when heating food or liquids for infants and children. Intentional avoidance of providing physical or emotional care to another, such as a child or older adult, is considered neglect.
3. **Scalding burns on both hands or feet and cigarette burns are most often associated with child and elder abuse than with an accident. Further assessments should be made to determine if abuse is the cause when these signs are identified. Abuse is harm or injury**

(e.g., physical, emotional, or sexual) to a child, adult, or older adult.
4. A sunburn is not a *red flag* indicating potential child abuse. However, it could be considered child neglect if the caregiver intentionally did not apply suntan protection on a sunny day.
Content Area: Psychosocial and Cultural Nursing
Integrated Processes: Nursing Process: Assessment
Client Need: Psychosocial Integrity
Cognitive Level: Application

14. ANSWER: 1, 3, 4.
Rationales:
1. **This intervention assists parents in making decisions about a child. Coping is associated with restoring homeostasis (balance, equilibrium) and involves thinking processes and behaviors designed to deal with stressors. Nursing interventions can help patient's develop adaptive (effective) coping mechanisms or to recognize maladaptive (ineffective) coping as the first step in correcting unhealthy coping behaviors.**
2. Taking a patient's vital signs is physical assessment, not an intervention to support coping.
3. **Discussing strategies about how to live with a diagnosis of cancer is designed to help a patient effectively adapt (cope) to the devastating emotional toll of living with a life-threatening disease.**
4. **Providing this information can lead a patient and family members to agencies that can facilitate coping (physically and emotionally) with home-care health promotion and illness prevention.**
5. Changing a patient's dressing is the provision of physical care. It is not designed to assist a patient with thinking processes and behaviors that support coping.
TEST-TAKING TIP: Identify the word in the stem that is a specific determiner. The word *just* in option 2 is a specific determiner. An option with a specific determiner usually is not a correct answer.
Content Area: Psychosocial and Cultural Nursing
Integrated Processes: Caring; Communication/Documentation; Nursing Process: Intervention
Client Need: Psychosocial Integrity
Cognitive Level: Application

15. ANSWER: 3.
Rationales:
1. Although patients who sustain an amputation of a limb may believe that they are less able to provide for their own safety, it is not the human need that the nurse should anticipate to be most affected.
2. Although patients who sustain an amputation of a limb may believe that they are less able to provide for their own security, it is not the human need that the nurse should anticipate to be most affected.
3. **Body image is related to how people perceive the appearance and function of their bodies. It includes the value of the body part to a person, the importance of the body part in culture and society, and the degree to which the person's body resembles his or her ideal body. Body image is closely related to self-concept. Loss of a body part, as with an amputation of a limb, often challenges a**

person's self-concept and the way in which the *self* is viewed.

4. Although patients who sustain an amputation of a limb may believe that this event will interfere with their ability to achieve self-actualization, it is not the human need that the nurse should anticipate to be most affected.

TEST-TAKING TIP: Identify the word in the stem that sets a priority. The word *most* in the stem sets a priority. Identify the equally plausible options. Options 1 and 2 are equally plausible because Maslow's second level needs are safety and security.

Content Area: Psychosocial and Cultural Nursing
Integrated Processes: Nursing Process: Analysis
Client Need: Psychosocial Integrity
Cognitive Level: Application

16. ANSWER: 4.
Rationales:
1. Amish people, not Hispanic people, generally prefer a quiet and peaceful environment when a person is actively dying. Most often, Amish people prefer to die at home, not in a hospital.
2. Some Jewish sects, not Hispanic people, permit only a specific religious representative to touch or prepare the body for burial.
3. People of the Hindu culture, not Hispanic people, believe that expressions of happy thoughts facilitate the dying patient leaving the earth and traveling on their journey.
4. Loud moaning and expressions of grief with chanting is common in Latino and African American cultures.

TEST-TAKING TIP: Identify the options that are opposites. Options 1 and 4 are opposites. More often than not, one of the opposite options is the correct answer.

Content Area: Psychosocial and Cultural Nursing
Integrated Processes: Caring; Nursing Process: Assessment
Client Need: Psychosocial Integrity
Cognitive Level: Application

17. ANSWER: 1.
Rationales:
1. Native American tribes believe in purifying and healing chants, dances, exorcisms, and body painting performed at the bedside; they believe that it helps ward off evil spirits and promotes healing.
2. Jewish people who follow a kosher diet, not Native Americans, do not consume meat and dairy products at the same meal.
3. Native Americans are permitted to eat meat. Buddhists and Hindu people, not Native Americans, primarily are vegetarians.
4. Amish people, not Native Americans, believe that the heart is the body's soul.

Content Area: Psychosocial and Cultural Nursing
Integrated Processes: Caring; Nursing Process: Planning
Client Need: Psychosocial Integrity
Cognitive Level: Application

18. ANSWER: 2.
Rationales:
1. An observant Jewish person follows a kosher diet, not a person who is a Jehovah's Witness.

2. A person who is a Jehovah's Witness is permitted to use only artificial blood expanders because blood and blood products are prohibited. The nurse should verify with certainty that no blood products or transfusions are desired by the patient and not make the assumption that this is the patient's desire.

3. There is no rule in the Jehovah's Witness religion that prohibits a person from receiving care from a person of the opposite gender.

4. Pork and pork products are not prohibited by the Jehovah's Witness religion. Jewish people who follow a kosher diet do not eat meat and dairy products at the same meal. People who are Hindu do not eat pork or pork products.

TEST-TAKING TIP: Identify the word in the stem that sets a priority. The word *most* in the stem sets a priority.

Content Area: Psychosocial and Cultural Nursing
Integrated Processes: Caring; Communication/Documentation; Nursing Process: Implementation
Client Need: Psychosocial Integrity
Cognitive Level: Application

19. ANSWER: 3.
Rationales:
1. Although this response conveys a desire to help, it does not move toward what should be done next.
2. This response is confrontational and may escalate the patient's hostility.
3. This is the best response because it indicates that the nurse is ready to do something immediately and asks the patient to participate in making a suggestion.
4. This response is confrontational; it is a judgmental statement regarding the patient's hostility.

TEST-TAKING TIP: Identify the word in the stem that sets a priority. The word *most* in the stem sets a priority. Identify the options that are equally plausible. Options 2 and 4 are equally plausible because they are confrontational responses. Identify the patient-centered options. Options 1 and 3 are patient centered. Consider these options carefully. Identify the option that is unique. Option 3 is unique because it is the only response that actively attempts to move forward to explore a solution to the problem.

Content Area: Psychosocial and Cultural Nursing
Integrated Processes: Caring; Communication/Documentation; Nursing Process: Implementation
Client Need: Psychosocial Integrity
Cognitive Level: Application

20. ANSWER: 1, 2, 5.
Rationales:
1. Rubbing lotion on the extremities stimulates tactile sensation. Sensory stimulation helps to foster brain recovery by awakening the reticular activating system.
2. Range-of-motion exercises prevent contractures as well as stimulate kinesthetic sensation and foster brain recovery.
3. A patient with a brain injury should have interventions explained in simple, concrete terms. A thorough explanation may be too extensive to process and respond to for a person with a brain injury.
4. A radio should not provide constant background stimulation. Constant auditory stimulation may lead to sensory

overload. Stimulation interventions should be implemented in a quiet environment so that the patient can focus on the particular sense being stimulated.

5. Using a mint-flavored mouth-care agent causes gustatory stimulation, which fosters brain recovery.

TEST-TAKING TIP: Identify the option with a specific determiner. Option 4 contains the word *all*, which is a specific determiner. Generally, options with specific determiners are distractors.

Content Area: Psychosocial and Cultural Nursing
Integrated Processes: Nursing Process: Planning
Client Need: Psychosocial Integrity
Cognitive Level: Application

21. ANSWER: 4.
Rationales:
1. By giving the patient pamphlets regarding diabetes and not engaging the patient in verbal and other modalities of teaching, the nurse is assuming that the patient can learn by reading. The most effective way to educate patients is to use multimodality methods (e.g., verbal, visual, tactile).
2. This response by the nurse assumes that the patient is overwhelmed with being diagnosed with diabetes and assumes the patient will eventually learn the skills necessary to monitor and treat the diabetes. Nurses should never make assumptions.
3. This response by the nurse is nontherapeutic because it assumes the patient will find having diabetes difficult and does not allow the patient to express self-identified concerns related to having diabetes. Nurses should never make assumptions.
4. This response by the nurse offers a broad opening that allows the patient to discuss self-identified specific concerns regarding diabetes. It is important that questions and emotional needs be addressed before teaching psychomotor skills.

TEST-TAKING TIP: Identify the word in the stem that sets a priority. The word *best* in the stem sets a priority.

Content Area: Psychosocial and Cultural Nursing
Integrated Processes: Caring; Communication/ Documentation; Nursing Process: Implementation
Client Need: Psychosocial Integrity
Cognitive Level: Application

22. ANSWER: 4, 2, 5, 3, 1.
Rationales:
4. Nurses must understand their own feelings before they can provide appropriate, nonjudgmental nursing care to others.
2. Nurses must not impose their own feelings and beliefs onto patients. When nurses are nonjudgmental, they provide an accepting attitude that promotes trust and further development of the nurse-patient relationship.
5. Assessment is the first step of the nursing process. Although there are commonalities of nursing care for all the levels of anxiety, there are specific nursing interventions associated with different levels of anxiety. The patient's level of anxiety will direct the nurse toward appropriate nursing interventions.
3. If the nurse identifies that a patient is in the panic stage of anxiety, it would be unsafe to leave

the patient unattended. The patient could harm self or others.
1. This action reflects the evaluation step of the nursing process. Evaluation involves assessing a patient's status after nursing care is provided.

Content Area: Psychosocial and Cultural Nursing
Integrated Processes: Caring; Nursing Process: Planning
Client Need: Psychosocial Integrity
Cognitive Level: Analysis

23. ANSWER: 2.
Rationales:
1. This statement is premature. This service probably will not be requested by the patient or family members. Family members and other members of the Amish community usually prefer to meet their loved one's needs when dying. Also, it may increase the patient's anxiety.
2. People from the Amish community are committed to caring for its members in their homes, including when giving birth, coping with an illness, and dying.
3. People from the Amish culture are permitted to receive chemotherapy.
4. There is no indication that the patient needs skilled nursing care. Pain management can be provided in the home. Also, this may increase the patient's anxiety.

TEST-TAKING TIP: Identify the word in the stem that sets a priority. The word *most* in the stem sets a priority. Identify the options that are opposites. Option 2 and 4 are opposites. In option 2, the patient goes home, and in option 4, the patient says within a health-care facility.

Content Area: Psychosocial and Cultural Nursing
Integrated Processes: Caring; Communication/Documentation; Nursing Process: Implementation
Client Need: Psychosocial Integrity
Cognitive Level: Application

24. ANSWER: 1.
Rationales:
1. Catholics believe that a priest can transform bread and wine into the body and blood of Jesus Christ (transubstantiation); it is distributed in the form of bread wafers (Eucharist) and sips of wine.
2. This is one of the tenets of a kosher diet that is associated with the Jewish religion.
3. Catholicism does not require its male or female members to receive care from caregivers of the same gender.
4. Mormons, members of the Church of Jesus Christ of Latter-day Saints, wear a sacred undergarment that is removed only for bathing and possibly surgery. When removed, it must be treated with respect.

Content Area: Psychosocial and Cultural Nursing
Integrated Processes: Caring; Communication/ Documentation; Nursing Process: Implementation
Client Need: Psychosocial Integrity
Cognitive Level: Analysis

25. ANSWER: 3.
Rationales:
1. Caregivers of the opposite gender are permitted in the Church of Jesus Christ of Latter-day Saints. Women who

follow the Hindu or Islam religions require caregivers to be the same gender.

2. Head coverings are not worn by women in the Church of Jesus Christ of Latter-day Saints. However, they do wear a sacred undergarment that is removed only for bathing. Orthodox Jewish women wear a head scarf or a wig. Arab, Muslim, and Islamic women generally wear some form of head covering.

3. Coffee, cola, tea, and alcohol are forbidden in the Church of Jesus Christ of Latter-day Saints.

4. This statement demonstrates sensitivity for the patient's religious beliefs because people who are Mormons believe in prayer. This is an insensitive statement for a person who follows Buddhism because they do not engage in prayers for healing; they believe that illness is part of life.

Content Area: Psychosocial and Cultural Nursing
Integrated Processes: Caring; Communication/ Documentation; Nursing Process: Implementation
Client Need: Psychosocial Integrity
Cognitive Level: Application

26. **ANSWER: 2, 4, 1, 5, 3.**
Rationales:

2. First, patients have a right to know who will be providing care and what is going to be done.

4. After introducing yourself, address the patient by name and be respectful; these actions focus on the patient as an individual and promote trust.

1. After the introductory phase, interviewing techniques invite the patient to converse with the nurse. Accepting the patient's feelings promotes a nonjudgmental approach and validates the patient's feelings, both of which foster communication.

5. When a patient speaks, the nurse must listen actively to really hear what the patient is saying overtly and covertly; also, the nurse must recognize that there is a reason for all behavior because it is meeting a need of the patient.

3. After data are collected, the patient and nurse must work together to identify needs and implement interventions to progress toward recovery.

Content Area: Psychosocial and Cultural Nursing
Integrated Processes: Caring; Communication/ Documentation; Nursing Process: Planning
Client Need: Safe and Effective Care Environment; Management of Care
Cognitive Level: Analysis

27. **ANSWER: 3.**
Rationales:

1. A person with mild anxiety will be alert, relaxed, and calm and will exhibit slight muscle tension and curiosity.

2. A person in a state of panic will be erratic, combative, or withdrawn and be incoherent and scattered.

3. A person experiencing severe anxiety will have perception that is narrowed, resulting in selective attention. In addition, the person will exhibit increased motor activity and extreme muscle tension, irritability, decreased concentration, increased distractibility, and signs of the fight or flight mechanism (e.g., increased respirations, dilated pupils, and diaphoresis).

4. A person experiencing moderate anxiety will exhibit increased muscle tension, voice tremors and pitch changes, energized mood, increased respirations, and an impaired ability to focus on more than one issue.

Content Area: Psychosocial and Cultural Nursing
Integrated Processes: Nursing Process: Analysis
Client Need: Psychosocial Integrity
Cognitive Level: Analysis

28. **ANSWER: 4.**
Rationales:

1. Although this statement focuses on feelings, focusing on feelings is not the priority at this time.

2. This information is not the priority at this time.

3. Although the nurse may eventually ask this question to focus on patient-identified needs, it is not the priority at this time.

4. The patient may be experiencing command hallucinations. The nurse must identify the content of the hallucinations to ensure that they are not command hallucinations that are directing the patient to do something that will harm self or others.

TEST-TAKING TIP: Identify the word in the stem that sets a priority. The word *best* in the stem sets a priority. Identify options with clang associations. The word *voices* in the stem and in option 2 and 4 are clang associations. Examine options 2 and 4 carefully.

Content Area: Psychosocial and Cultural Nursing
Integrated Processes: Caring; Communication/ Documentation; Nursing Process: Implementation
Client Need: Psychosocial Integrity
Cognitive Level: Application

29. **ANSWER: 3.**
Rationales:

1. This is premature. This intervention is appropriate when the patient is ready to focus on positive, supportive change.

2. Identifying strengths, weaknesses, and past achievements assist a patient to develop a more positive self-image, not a positive body-image.

3. A change in body-image usually precipitates feelings of loss of "what was" and "what will never be." An exploration of these feelings will promote movement toward acceptance of a change in body-image.

4. This intervention is more appropriate for patients who are anxious.

TEST-TAKING TIP: Identify the word in the stem that sets a priority. The word *most* in the stem sets a priority.

Content Area: Psychosocial and Cultural Nursing
Integrated Processes: Caring; Nursing Process: Implementation
Client Need: Psychosocial Integrity
Cognitive Level: Application

30. **ANSWER: 2.**
Rationales:

1. Being happy or sad relates to mood. Other examples of mood include depressed, anxious, fearful, irritable, euphoric, guilty, angry, ashamed, proud, and so on.

2. When assessing thought processes, it is important to determine the length of a person's attention span. An ad-

equate attention span permits a reasonable amount of time for organized thinking.

3. Emotional expressions relate to affect, not thought processes.

4. Inhibition and disinhibition are related to impulse control, not thought processes.

Content Area: Psychosocial and Cultural Nursing
Integrated Processes: Nursing Process: Assessment
Client Need: Psychosocial Integrity
Cognitive Level: Application

31. **ANSWER: 1.**
    Rationales:

    1. **The person's inability to recall is an example of repression, which is the unconscious and involuntary forgetting of painful events, ideas, and conflicts.**

    2. There is nothing that demonstrates regression, a return to an earlier, more comfortable developmental level.

    3. There is nothing that demonstrates displacement, the shifting of feelings from an emotionally charged situation to a relatively safe substitute (usually someone or something perceived as less powerful).

    4. There is nothing that demonstrates intellectualization, the use of thinking, ideas, or intellect to avoid emotions.

    Content Area: Psychosocial and Cultural Nursing
    Integrated Processes: Nursing Process: Analysis
    Client Need: Psychosocial Integrity
    Cognitive Level: Analysis

32. **ANSWER: 2, 3, 4.**
    Rationales:

    1. Sitting quietly with the patient is most appropriate for patients who are depressed. It sends the message that the patient is worthy of the nurse's time and attention.

    2. **All people have value; therefore, each and every patient deserves to be treated with respect.**

    3. **All patients should be encouraged to express feelings and concerns. When a patient ventilates feelings and concerns the nurse collects valuable information that will assist the nurse in meeting the patient's emotional needs. It also may help to reduce the patient's anxiety.**

    4. **A nonjudgmental attitude by the nurse is an appropriate approach to be used with all patients. A nonjudgmental attitude provides an environment where patients feel accepted; this will promote a positive nurse-patient relationship.**

    5. This action is appropriate if the patient is angry or aggressive.

    Content Area: Psychosocial and Cultural Nursing
    Integrated Processes: Caring; Communication/ Documentation; Nursing Process: Implementation
    Client Need: Psychosocial Integrity
    Cognitive Level: Analysis

33. **ANSWER: 2.**
    Rationales:

    1. A variety of challenging activities will be too stimulating and will exacerbate the hyperactivity.

    2. **This patient is extremely active and easily distracted by factors in the environment. The environment should be kept calm, quiet, and nonstimulating.**

    3. Although a laudable approach, this is unrealistic. Advocating rest periods will be ineffective because a hyperactive patient has too much energy that must be expended.

    4. The patient has too much energy to engage in a quiet activity that requires focus.

    TEST-TAKING TIP: Identify the options that are opposites. Options 1 and 2 are opposites.

    Content Area: Psychosocial and Cultural Nursing
    Integrated Processes: Nursing Process: Implementation
    Client Need: Psychosocial Integrity
    Cognitive Level: Application

34. **ANSWER: 1.**
    Rationales:

    1. **These signs support the conclusion that the patient may be experiencing mild anxiety. Patients experiencing mild anxiety also may appear relaxed and alert and exhibit a slight increase in respirations and muscle tension.**

    2. These behaviors are associated with moderate anxiety.

    3. These behaviors are associated with severe anxiety.

    4. These behaviors are associated with the panic level of anxiety.

    Content Area: Psychosocial and Cultural Nursing
    Integrated Processes: Nursing Process: Analysis
    Client Need: Psychosocial Integrity
    Cognitive Level: Analysis

35. **ANSWER: 2.**
    Rationale:
    Solve the problem by using ratio and proportion.

$$\frac{\text{Desire } 100 \text{ mg}}{\text{Have } 250 \text{ mg}} = \frac{x \text{ mL}}{5 \text{ mL}}$$

$$250x = 100 \times 5$$
$$250x = 500$$
$$x = 500 \div 250$$
$$x = 2 \text{ mL}$$

Content Area: Medication Administration
Integrated Processes: Nursing Process: Planning
Client Need: Physiological Integrity; Pharmacological and Parenteral Therapies
Cognitive Level: Application

Chapter 9

Teaching and Learning

KEY TERMS

Affective domain (feeling)—Learning that deals with changes in feelings, beliefs, attitudes, and values.

Auditory learner—A person who learns by hearing.

Cognitive domain (thinking)—Learning that deals with acquiring, storing, and recalling information.

External locus of control—A desire to achieve a goal because of recognition or reward outside the self.

Goal—A desired outcome that is patient-centered, realistic, measurable, and time bound.

Internal locus of control—A desire from within the self to achieve a goal.

Kinesthetic learner—A person who learns by touch and manipulation.

Learning—An active process that involves assimilation of information that produces the acquisition of new attitudes, behaviors, or skills.

Long-term goal—Desired outcome that can be obtained within weeks to months.

Motivation—An internal drive or external stimulus that produces a thought or action.

Psychomotor domain (doing)—Learning that deals with attaining a new skill that requires both mental and physical activity.

Short-term goal—Desired outcome that can be obtained within hours or days.

Teaching—An interactive process that promotes acquisition of new information, attitudes, or skills.

Visual learner—A person who learns by processing information with the eyes.

I. Introduction

Teaching is an interactive process that promotes acquisition of new information, attitudes, or skills. It involves steps that mirror the steps of the nursing process (assessment, analysis, planning, implementation, and evaluation). Learning is an active process that involves assimilation of information that produces the acquisition of new attitudes, behaviors, or skills. These activities help to promote wellness, prevent illness, and facilitate the acquisition of coping strategies to restore health or function.

A. Purposes of Teaching and Learning
1. Wellness promotion.
   a. Presents information and skills that support and develop health practices.
   b. Examples: Information about health, nutrition, exercise, and hygiene; prenatal and parenting classes.
2. Illness prevention.
   a. Presents information and skills that promote early detection or prevention of disease and disability.

b. Examples: Information about risk factors of disease; dietary teaching to decrease the risk of cancer; information about immunizations, smoking cessation, and safe use of a car seat restraining devices for infants and children.
3. Promotion of coping strategies.
   a. Presents information and skills that enable a patient to better cope emotionally and physically with a new diagnosis, interventions, impaired function, or loss of a loved one.
   b. Examples: Information about using a walker safely, using an assistive device to eat, walking with a prosthesis, coping with role expectations, managing care for a loved one at home, coping with death and dying, administering a gastrostomy tube feeding, managing stress.
4. Restoration of health or function.
   a. Presents information and skills that enable a patient to manage a current health problem, focusing on etiology, medical condition,

treatment, and strategies to meet patient needs.

    b. Examples: Information about self-injecting insulin, employing preoperative and postoperative interventions to prevent complications of surgery, and caring for a wound drain.

B. Learning Domains

  1. People learn through three different domains.

    a. **Cognitive domain:** Thinking.

    b. **Affective domain:** Feeling.

    c. **Psychomotor domain:** Doing.

  2. Each domain requires the use of specific strategies that best promote learning. (See Table 9.1 for more information on learning domains and ways to tailor nursing strategies to those domains.)

II. Individual Factors That Influence Learning

People learn in different ways, such as by seeing, hearing, and touching. Learning is motivated by either an internal desire to achieve a goal (internal locus of control) or a desire to receive external recognition or a reward (external locus of control). In addition, people primarily use information processing functions from either the left hemisphere (logical thinking) or right hemisphere (intuitive thinking) of the brain. The way in which learning occurs is never identical for two different people and is not identical for one person in different situations. Therefore, nurses must consider these factors when engaged in the teaching/learning process.

A. Learning Styles

  1. Visual learners.

    a. Learn best by processing information with the eyes.

    b. Examples: Use of pictures, illustrations, photographs, models, and videos.

  2. Auditory learners.

    a. Learn best by processing information by listening to words.

    b. Examples: Use of verbal instructions, discussions, and videos with verbal commentary.

  3. Kinesthetic learners.

    a. Learn best when processing information by doing.

    b. Examples: Engage in physical activities and allow touching and handling of equipment.

Table 9.1 Understanding Learning Domains

Domain and Definition	Nursing Strategies

Cognitive (Thinking Domain)
• Deals with acquiring, storing, and recalling information.
• Involves intellectual thinking that demonstrates increasing complexity:
  –Knowing, such as memorizing and recalling.
  –Comprehending.
  –Analyzing.
  –Synthesizing.
  –Applying and evaluating ideas.
• Example outcome: Patient is able to verbalize the differences between regular and NPH insulin.
	• Lecture.
	• Written material.
	• Panel discussion.
	• Audiovisual materials.
	• Programmed instruction.
	• Computer-assisted instruction.
	• Case studies.
	• Care plans.
	• Evaluate learning by seeking oral or written feedback.

Affective (Feeling Domain) • Deals with changes in feelings, beliefs, attitudes, and values. • Involves increasing the depth of emotional response to tasks, receiving and responding to new ideas, demonstrating commitment to new ideas, and integrating new ideas into one's value system. • Behavioral changes commonly emerge slowly after intellectual understanding is internalized. • Example outcome: Patient maintains a diabetic diet.	• Panel discussion. • Role modeling. • One-to-one counseling. • Support groups. • Evaluate learning by observing behavioral changes that reflect beliefs, feelings and values.
Psychomotor (Skill Domain) • Deals with learning a new skill that requires both mental and physical activity. • Involves sensory awareness of cues, imitation, and performance of new skills. • Example outcome: Patient is able to self-administer insulin, maintaining principles of asepsis.	• Demonstration. • Return demonstration. • Audiovisual materials. • Printed material with illustrations. • Evaluate learning by seeking a return demonstration.

B. Locus of Control

1. Internal locus of control.
   a. Patients are motivated from within and hold themselves responsible for actions and consequences.
   b. Example: A person loses weight because of a desire to personally achieve the goals of improved health and appearance.
2. External locus of control.
   a. Patients are motivated by pressure or rewards from outside the self, not from within.
   b. Example: A person loses weight because a significant other places pressure on the patient, such as praise, guilt, or rewards.

III. Principles of Teaching and Learning and Related Nursing Care

Implementing patient education requires the nurse to assume the role of teacher. As a teacher, a nurse should use universal principles that guide patient teaching, regardless of the content being taught or the personal factors of learners. However, when a patient presents with specialized needs, these common universal principles should be augmented by individualized interventions that address the patient's specific needs.

A. Learning Takes Place Within the Learner

1. Support learning because it is a continuous process of growth throughout life.
2. Understand that learning occurs when the need to learn is relevant to the learner.
3. Assess understanding of the health problem; build a teaching plan based on developing what is already known and then moving on to the unknown. Use examples to which the patient can relate.
4. Recognize that the ability and speed at which one learns depends on the individual.
5. Match teaching strategies to the patient's learning style and learning needs.
6. Accept that a teacher only facilitates learning.

B. Motivation Facilitates Learning

1. Identify behaviors that indicate the patient's readiness to learn (motivation).
   a. Acknowledging a need and believing that the need can be met through learning.
   b. Demonstrating health-seeking behaviors, such as asking questions, attempting to participate in own care, and requesting reading material or referrals to support groups.
   c. Believing that the information to be learned has value.
   d. Believing that identified goals are attainable.
2. Identify behaviors that indicate the patient's lack of readiness to learn.
   a. Exhibiting moderate to high anxiety: Identify level of anxiety and promote expression of feelings and concerns.
   b. Exhibiting behaviors that indicate avoidance, denial, or lack of participation in own care: Accept where the patient is at and support the patient emotionally until ready to participate in the teaching/learning process.
   c. Expressing presence of pain: Medicate the patient to address pain before the teaching session or postpone the session because the patient's physiological status can impede concentration and energy.
3. Begin teaching and learning activities as soon as the need is identified by the nurse or patient and as soon as possible, such as on admission to the agency.
4. Formulate a learning contract with the patient that includes both short-term goals (desired outcomes that can be obtained within hours or days) and long-term goals (desired outcomes that can be obtained within weeks to months).
   a. Goals should be patient centered, realistic, measurable, and time bound.
   b. Short-term goals provide more opportunities for achievement that supports motivation.
   c. Learning contracts support mutual respect and responsibility.
5. Provide prompt feedback.
6. Identify progress, and employ rewards and incentives for goal achievement.
7. Understand that discussing potential complications may provoke mild anxiety that can increase motivation.
8. Avoid using fear tactics (e.g., "Unless you stop smoking you may get lung cancer.") to motivate a patient.
9. Identify and investigate the cause of nonachievement of goals. Recognize that nonadherence to a treatment regimen may be due to the presence of competing incentives rather than a lack of motivation; for example, learning new ways to achieve independence may be less important than the gains related to continuing in the sick role.
10. Modify the teaching plan accordingly based on the patient's progress and changing needs.

C. Teaching Strategies Must Be Appropriate for the Patient's Developmental and Cognitive Levels

1. According to Piaget, cognitive development progresses through three levels.
   a. Age 2 to 7 years: Find meaning through use of symbols and pictures.

MAKING THE CONNECTION

Patient Behavior and the Reason for Behavior

Many health-care professionals report that a patient is "noncompliant" or "uncooperative" when goals are not met. However, nonachievement of goals can be due to reasons other than the patient ignoring the benefits of learning. For example, economics, lack of understanding, and negative side effects of therapy can all cause a patient to not adhere to a treatment regimen. **All behavior has meaning**, and a logical connection exists between patient behavior and the reasons for the behavior. To identify the true cause of failure to meet outcome goals, nurses must first identify patient behaviors or statements that indicate nonadherence to a plan of care, and then they must explore the etiology of the nonadherence. In addition, the terms "noncompliant" and "uncooperative" should never be used when describing or documenting patient behavior; failure to meet outcome goals should be described and the reasons for the behavior should be explored and identified.

  b. Age 7 to 11 years: Have logical thinking and understand relationships.
  c. Age 11 and older: Use abstract thinking and deductive reasoning.
2. Use teaching strategies that are appropriate for the learner's gross and fine motor development when teaching psychomotor skills.
3. Use teaching strategies that are appropriate for the learner's level of intellectual ability.
4. Encourage participation in the teaching/learning process; recognize that adults prefer to be partners in this process.
5. Encourage independence; recognize that adults are more independent and self-directed than are children.
6. Reinforce that one is never too old to learn; recognize that adults may believe that they are too old to learn, fear failure, or feel threatened and therefore resist change.
7. Identify and build on positive past learning experiences; recognize that adults have previous life experiences that can hinder or enhance learning.
8. Build repetition into the teaching plan; recognize that older adults might take longer to learn than younger adults do, but they *are* able to learn.

D. Health Teaching Must Be Consistent With the Patient's Sociocultural and Religious Beliefs
1. Understand that culture and religion influence beliefs, values, and behaviors; identify factors, such as customs and taboos, that can influence content to be taught or teaching strategies to be used.
2. Identify whether the patient is the decision maker; be aware that, in some cultures, women are not allowed to make decisions and therefore the decision maker in the family should be included in teaching sessions.
3. Identify behaviors that may be culturally related, such as avoiding eye contact to demonstrate respect and smiling and nodding the head to indicate that teaching is understood, even if it is not, so as not to embarrass the nurse.
4. Respect and accept a patient's values and beliefs; incorporate them into the learning plan unless they are unsafe.
5. Use humor cautiously; the intended meaning may be lost in translation by a patient from a different culture or a patient may consider the comment condescending rather than funny.

E. Learning Occurs Best in an Environment That Is Physically and Emotionally Conducive To Learning
1. Schedule teaching so that it does not interfere with rest, meals, tests, and treatments; when appropriate, schedule sessions when a family member can be present to offer support and also learn what is being taught.
2. Determine appropriate teaching session length and frequency based on the patient's condition, such as attention span or activity tolerance.
   a. Short, more frequent sessions are better than long, infrequent sessions.
   b. Enough time should occur between sessions so that information can be absorbed and applied.
3. Provide an environment that is private, quiet, and free from distractions and interruptions.
4. Ensure that the environment is physically comfortable.
   a. Room temperature should not be too hot or too cold.
   b. Lighting should be adequate and free from glare.
5. Ensure that the environment is emotionally comfortable and provides privacy; close the door, pull the curtain, and drape the patient appropriately when teaching personal physical skills.
6. Identify the patient's level of anxiety; be aware that mild anxiety enhances motivation and learning, whereas moderate and higher levels of anxiety impede learning; teaching sessions may have to be shortened or postponed depending on the patient's level of anxiety.

⏹ 7. Emphasize what is most important to know first for a patient who is very ill because fatigue shortens teaching sessions.

8. Address the patient's fears and concerns before beginning teaching and learning activities.

F. Literacy, Language, and Communication Are Essential Components of the Teaching and Learning Process

1. Commonalities of nursing care related to literacy, language, and communication.
   a. Use a variety of teaching strategies to present information; stimulate as many of the senses as possible, such as hearing, vision, and touch.
   b. Use short, simple words and sentences; speak clearly and slowly; use words the patient understands; and avoid clichés, slang words, colloquialisms, medical jargon, abbreviations, and ambiguous words.
   c. Present information so that it progresses with increasing complexity, such as simple to complex and known to unknown.
   d. Pace teaching sessions so that learning is achieved before moving on to the next concept; identify whether teaching is too fast or too slow and modify the pace accordingly.
   e. Build repetition of information into the teaching plan; repetition reinforces learning.
   f. Provide written materials that have many drawings, photographs, and illustrations; avoid handouts with large amounts of written information.
   g. Document teaching interventions and learning progress; be aware that some facilities have teaching and learning activity forms that document progress and are signed by both teacher and learner.

2. Nursing care specific to literacy.
   a. Understand that literacy involves the ability to use print and written information to function in society to develop one's knowledge and potential and achieve one's goals.

⏹ b. Never assume that a patient is literate.

DID YOU KNOW?

Many illiterate adults in the United States hide the fact that they cannot read or write. However, illiteracy in the United States is widespread. Consider these facts: Sixty-three million adults older than age 16 do not read well enough to understand a newspaper story written at the 8th-grade level. An additional 30 million can read at only a 5th-grade level or lower. Forty-three percent of adults with the lowest literacy rates in the U.S. live in poverty.

   c. Assess a patient's ability to read.
   d. Teach at the fifth-grade level, and move up levels as appropriate.

   e. Check the reading level of presented written materials and ensure that it is at the level of the patient's ability; most educational materials are written at the high-school level, which can be challenging for some patients to read.

3. Nursing care specific to language.
   a. Determine whether the patient clearly understands English.

⏹ b. Use a professional interpreter if the patient does not understand English because patients have a right to be taught in a language that they understand. The Joint Commission mandates the use of interpreters for non-English-speaking patients.

      (1) Employ the use of a language line service, whereby a bilingual operator provides translation, if available.
      (2) Do not use family members as interpreters because information must be communicated accurately, objectively, and confidentially.
      (3) Talk to and look at the patient when using an interpreter.
   c. Provide information in written and audio formats in the patient's language.

4. Nursing care specific to communication.
   a. Understand that teaching requires effective interpersonal verbal and nonverbal interaction.
      (1) Teaching can be formal or informal.
      (2) Teaching can be planned or spontaneous.
      (3) Teaching can be performed with an individual or with a group.
   b. Ensure that nonverbal behavior is congruent with verbal language.
   c. Encourage the patient to ask questions and to write down questions that arise between teaching sessions.

G. Special Needs Populations Require Specific Teaching Strategies

1. Nursing care for patients who have visual impairments.
   a. Encourage use of prescription eyeglasses.
   b. Provide written material in large print.
   c. Provide special equipment or learning materials, such as prefilled or automatic-stop syringes, Braille learning materials, and audio learning materials.
   d. See also the section "Patients Who Are Visually Impaired" in Chapter 7, Communication, page 135.

2. Nursing care for patients who have hearing impairments.
   a. Encourage the use of hearing aids.
   b. Talk toward the patient's ear with the most acute hearing.
   c. Speak slightly louder, but do not yell.

d. Face the patient when speaking; speak slowly and enunciate each word clearly, but do not overly enunciate each word because doing so can interfere with lip reading.

e. See also the section "Patients Who Are Hearing Impaired" in Chapter 7, Communication, page 134.

3. Nursing care for patients who have sensory or motor impairments.

a. Understand that sensory and motor impairments interfere with learning psychomotor skills.

b. Plan more practice time for patients with sensory or motor impairments, such as neuropathy or hemiplegia.

c. Teach patients to use assistive devices to facilitate psychomotor skills when appropriate.

IV. Teaching Strategies

The selection of an instructional approach should be based on a patient's educational needs and personal factors, the time available for teaching, and the resources available. Each instructional approach has advantages, disadvantages, and related specific nursing actions. To maximize learning, nurses should use a variety of teaching approaches.

A. Lecture

1. Information is presented verbally and may be accompanied by written material.

2. Advantages.
   a. Is cost effective.
   b. Is easy to use with large groups.

3. Disadvantages.
   a. Does not permit individualization of the material.
   b. Is not effective in the psychomotor or affective domains.
   c. Can be a challenging format for a hearing impaired person as well as for visual learners unless written material is also provided.

4. Nursing care.
   a. Provide time for discussion at the end of the program.
   b. Provide time for additional questions and answers and to correct misconceptions.

B. One-to-One Discussion

1. Teacher and learner talk about content to be learned without interference from another learner.

2. Advantages.
   a. Allows for development of a relationship with the learner.
   b. Is learner centered.
   c. Allows time for frequent feedback.
   d. Is effective in all three learning domains.

3. Disadvantages.
   a. Can be labor intensive.
   b. Isolates the learner from others who may provide support.

4. Nursing care.
   a. Use for patients who have special learning needs, such as cognitive or sensory impairment, learning disability, mental illness, and activity intolerance.
   b. Individualize the program to meet the learner's needs.

C. Demonstration

1. Involves hands-on manipulation of equipment with time to practice a skill.

2. Advantages.
   a. Is effective for teaching psychomotor skills.
   b. Can be used with small groups.

3. Disadvantages.
   a. Is not effective with large groups.
   b. Is time consuming and labor intensive.

4. Nursing care.
   a. Demonstrate each step slowly and accurately; move on to the next step only after it is determined that the previous step is mastered via return demonstration.
   b. Allow adequate time to practice the skill within and between teaching sessions.

D. Groups (Instructional and Support)

1. Enables two or more individuals to interact, thereby enhancing learning with the exchange of information.

2. Advantages.
   a. Is effective when teaching in the affective domain.
   b. Promotes interaction among participants.

3. Disadvantages.
   a. Occurs in a less-structured environment that allows for unexpected responses by group members.
   b. Is not effective for the psychomotor domain.

4. Nursing care.
   a. Use when participant interaction is desired so that learners learn from each other; learners can share ideas, foster development of positive attitudes, solve problems, and offer solutions to each other.
   b. Function as a group facilitator to keep the group on task.

E. Role Playing

1. Stimulates interaction so that a response can be practiced in a nonthreatening environment.

2. Advantages.
   a. Offers a safe environment to rehearse and practice responses before being confronted with a real-life situation.

b. Raises issues that can be pursued through discussion.

3. Disadvantages.
   a. May be uncomfortable for people who are too embarrassed or feel awkward engaging in role playing.
   b. May increase anxiety when emotionally charged areas are explored.

4. Nursing care.
   a. Set an example by demonstrating behaviors or attitudes that should be learned.
   b. Establish the situation so that participants involved in the role playing develop an understanding of the principles to be learned.
   c. Recognize when an increase in anxiety occurs and provide emotional support.

V. Teaching Tools

The selection of a teaching tool should be based on a patient's educational needs and personal factors, the time available for teaching, and the resources available. Each teaching tool has advantages, disadvantages, and related nursing care. To maximize learning, nurses should use a variety of teaching tools.

A. Printed Materials

1. Support comprehension of complex concepts and relationships.
2. Include materials such as pamphlets, booklets, brochures, drawings, and charts.
3. Advantages.
   a. Allow for standardization of information.
   b. Can be read at learner's own pace.
   c. Are efficient.
   d. Can be provided in the patient's first language.
4. Disadvantages.
   a. Cannot be used with patients who are illiterate.
   b. Cannot be used with patients who have visual impairments.
5. Nursing care.
   a. Ensure that the learner is literate and able to see.
   b. Provide materials in the primary language of the learner.
   c. Use printed materials especially for patients who are visual learners.
   d. Ensure that printed materials are easy to read, current, and accurate.
   e. Use charts to present key points because charts provide easy retrieval of highly condensed information.

B. Programmed Instruction

1. Information is presented in a *frame* and requires a response before the learner can move onto the next frame.
2. Includes computer programs, programmed textbooks, and booklets.
3. Advantages.
   a. Allows learners to proceed at their own pace.
   b. Requires learners to be actively engaged in learning.
   c. Provides immediate feedback for right and wrong answers.
   d. Allows for efficient use of a teacher's time.
4. Disadvantages.
   a. Is not as stimulating as an audiovisual-type presentation.
   b. Requires a motivated, independent learner.
5. Nursing care.
   a. Teach the learner how to use the program.
   b. Explain that the program is a written sequential presentation of learning steps that actively engages the learner in the learning process.
   c. Teach that programmed instruction is designed so that the learner can proceed at his or her own pace as well as receive immediate feedback for right and wrong answers.

C. Audiovisual Aids

1. Present information that stimulates both the eyes and ears.
2. Include CD programs, computer apps, and movies.
3. Advantages.
   a. Stimulate the hearing and sight of the learner.
   b. Can be used with individuals or large groups.
4. Disadvantages.
   a. May require expensive equipment, such as computers, software, and projectors.
   b. Require participants to be able to hear or see material being presented.
   c. Require a large room when being presented to a large group.
5. Nursing care.
   a. Ensure that all participants have adequate hearing and vision and are positioned to see and hear the material presented.
   b. Use audiovisual aids for all patients but especially for auditory learners or individuals with literacy issues.
   c. Use audiotapes for patients who are vision impaired.

D. Equipment and Models

1. Provide hands-on items that can be observed, touched, and sometimes utilized.
   a. Models provide a two- or three-dimensional representation of subject matter that can be observed and touched.
   b. A piece of equipment may be the actual apparatus that is the focus of the teaching session.

2. Includes materials such as a skeleton, heart model, manikin for CPR, simulation manikin used to mimic clinical situations, various catheters, and syringes.
3. Advantages.
   a. Are effective in teaching kinesthetic learners.
   b. Are effective when teaching psychomotor skills.
4. Disadvantages.
   a. Are expensive.
   b. Require storage.
5. Nursing care.
   a. Use for patients who are kinesthetic learners because it allows for manipulation of objects.
   b. Use for patients who are learning psychomotor skills to promote transfer of information from the brain (cognitive learning) to the hands (psychomotor learning).
   c. Use to provide visual reinforcement of verbally presented information.
   d. Employ to teach use of new equipment and related skills presented in continuing education or in-service programs for health-care professionals.

E. Internet
   1. Provides immediate access to a vast amount of information using a computer connected to the Internet.
   2. Advantages.
      a. Is entertaining, informative, and convenient.
      b. Offers a diversity of resources, including electronic learning platforms, search engines, electronic libraries, content portals, and social networking, including chat rooms, bulletin boards, and blogs that offer sharing of information, counseling, and support.
   3. Disadvantages.
      a. Exposes the learner to information that might not be accurate, reliable, or current and content that is unregulated.
      b. May require the learner to read above a fifth-grade reading level.
      c. Can be accessed without input from a knowledgeable health-care professional.

4. Nursing care.
   a. Ensure that the learner knows how to access the Internet.
   ⓘ b. Teach the learner ways to evaluate the reliability of a site, such as by determining whether an author or organization is reputable and using readily available checklists to assess the quality of a Web site.
   c. Encourage the learner to access recommended, quality Web sites.
   d. Review the suitability of a site before making a patient referral.

F. Computer-Assisted Instruction
   1. Works like a programmed text in that a frame requires a response before the learner moves to the next frame; however, has more capabilities than a linear approach and can branch to a multiple number of responses based on the learner's response and is therefore significantly more interactive and individualized.
   2. Advantages.
      a. Allows the learner to proceed at his or her own pace.
      b. Usually includes interactive activities to engage the learner.
      c. Commonly includes pretests and posttests so that learning can be self-evaluated.
      d. Is convenient if the patient has a personal computer.
      e. Allows the teacher to design a learning prescription and/or corrective action plan that addresses a student's specific learning needs.
   3. Disadvantages.
      a. Requires access to a computer.
      b. Can be costly for an agency if it provides the computers.
   4. Nursing care.
      a. Teach the learner how to use the computer to access the learning program software.
      b. Use when a learner response pattern is desired to select future lessons.

CASE STUDY: Putting It All Together

A man who is unconscious is brought to the emergency department by his wife. The patient has type 2 diabetes and has had the flu for a week. The patient is diagnosed with ketoacidosis and is admitted to the hospital to correct fluid and electrolyte imbalances and receive insulin therapy. While being interviewed by the nurse after regaining consciousness, the patient says repeatedly, "I can't believe I have to take insulin. No one in my family who has diabetes has to take insulin." Later, the nurse has a discussion with the patient about what he knows about diabetes and gives the patient printed materials. The nurse meets with the patient every day to discuss diabetes and to explore the patient's feelings and concerns. Eventually, the nurse teaches the patient how to perform self-blood glucose monitoring (SBGM) and how to perform a subcutaneous injection using a model of an abdomen. The nutritionist performs dietary counseling, and the nurse reviews the principles of a diabetic diet with the patient at mealtimes. At discharge, the nurse schedules a follow-up visit with the diabetes counseling

CASE STUDY: Putting It All Together *cont'd*

center. The patient misses this visit, so the nurse in the counseling center telephones him and schedules a new appointment. The patient attends the appointment accompanied by his wife. He states, "My wife would kill me if I didn't come this time." When reviewing the patient's self-care diary, the nurse identifies that the patient takes the morning dose of insulin but is inconsistent with monitoring blood glucose levels and administering insulin during the day. When exploring these issues, the patient says, "My wife doesn't let me out of the house without me taking the insulin. But I am not going to give myself insulin at work where everyone can see." The patient's wife says, "He's had type 2 diabetes for several years, but he didn't take his pills consistently then and he doesn't

take his insulin consistently now, never does the finger-stick test, and eats anything he wants. I make good meals at home, but I can't control what he does at work." Most of the visit focuses on exploring the patient's feelings and concerns. Eventually, the nurse reviews and demonstrates the procedures for SBGM and self-administration of a subcutaneous injection and has the patient perform return demonstrations. At the end of the visit, the patient tells the nurse, "I learn new things better if I can actually do what I am supposed to do." The nurse gives the patient additional booklets with illustrations and a CD about these procedures. The nurse also recommends that the patient attend a support group at the counseling center and gives the patient a schedule of meetings.

Case Study Questions

A. What learning domains did the nurse address in the teaching sessions? Give examples.

1. _____
2. _____
3. _____

B. Identify and explore individual factors related to teaching and learning that the patient exhibited in this scenario.

1. _____
2. _____

C. What data demonstrated that the patient lacked readiness to learn?

1. _____
2. _____
3. _____

D. What teaching principles did the nurse use in this scenario?

1. _____
2. _____
3. _____
4. _____

E. What teaching strategies did the nurse use when teaching this patient and what were the advantages of these teaching strategies for this patient?

1. _____
2. _____
3. _____

F. What teaching tools did the nurse use and what are the advantages of each?

1. _____
2. _____
3. _____

REVIEW QUESTIONS

1. A patient is admitted to an alcohol rehabilitation unit. Which statement by the patient indicates an internal reward to achieve a goal?
   1. "I'm going to get sober for my kids."
   2. "I need to get my life back on track."
   3. "My wife is constantly on my back to give up drinking."
   4. "The judge said I can have visitation with my kids if I go to rehab."

2. A nurse is evaluating patient outcomes associated with managing a urinary retention catheter in the home. Which outcome indicates learning in the cognitive domain?
   1. Patient demonstrates effective perineal care.
   2. Patient accepts requiring a tube to empty his bladder.
   3. Patient is able to identify three actions that help reduce the risk of a urinary tract infection.
   4. Patient can empty the contents of the collection bag without contaminating the entire system.

3. A nurse is planning to educate an adult patient newly diagnosed with diabetes regarding self-blood glucose monitoring and performing an insulin injection. Which interventions are **most** helpful? **Select all that apply.**
   1. _____ Show the patient a video about self-blood glucose monitoring and then discuss the video with the patient.
   2. _____ Demonstrate self-blood glucose monitoring and then have the patient perform a return demonstration.
   3. _____ Provide a pamphlet that explains these skills and then discuss them.
   4. _____ Have another patient with this illness teach the patient these skills.
   5. _____ Use abstract statements while educating the patient.

4. Which nursing intervention **best** promotes a patient's adherence to a medication regimen?
   1. Instruct the patient to take the medication as prescribed or the primary health-care provider will discharge the patient from treatment.
   2. Provide information about the safety of the medication as indicated by the Food and Drug Administration.
   3. Warn that if the medication is not taken, the illness will get worse.
   4. Explain how the medication can reduce the patient's illness.

5. A female nurse is assessing a patient's readiness to learn a self-help skill. What patient factors alert the nurse that the teaching session should be postponed? **Select all that apply.**
   1. _____ Male gender
   2. _____ 75-year-old adult
   3. _____ High anxiety level
   4. _____ Pain of 5 on a 0-to-10 scale
   5. _____ Graduated only from grammar school

6. A nurse is caring for a patient from Spain who experienced a hypertensive crisis while on vacation in the United States. The patient knows only a few words of English. What is **most** important when planning a teaching session about nutrients that are high in sodium?
   1. Providing a professional interpreter fluent in Spanish
   2. Securing written material in Spanish from the Internet
   3. Using the technique of demonstration when teaching information
   4. Showing pictures of foods that should be avoided to lower blood pressure

7. A nurse is evaluating patient outcomes associated with learning about hypertension and self-care. Which outcome indicates success in the psychomotor domain?
   1. Patient explains how to interpret the serving size on a food label to calculate the caloric value of the nutrient.
   2. Patient is able to identify five foods high in salt that should be avoided when receiving a low sodium diet.
   3. Patient is able to accurately obtain a blood pressure reading using a sphygmomanometer.
   4. Patient adheres to a weight-reduction diet, as evidenced by a weekly 2 lb weight loss.

8. A patient is admitted to an alcohol rehabilitation program. On admission, the patient states, "I'm here because it is what I have to do to get my license back." What is motivating this patient to participate in the rehabilitation program? **Select all that apply.**
   1. _____ An internal locus of control
   2. _____ An external locus of control
   3. _____ A desire to achieve a personal goal
   4. _____ The need to fulfill a legal requirement
   5. _____ The desire to regain control over alcohol

9. A nurse is evaluating the outcome of a teaching program presented to a patient newly diagnosed with diabetes. Which outcome indicates learning in the affective domain?
   1. Maintains a diabetic diet
   2. Self-administers insulin safely
   3. Verbalizes the difference between short- and long-acting insulin
   4. Identifies clinical indicators of hyperglycemia and hypoglycemia

10. Which strategy increases the probability that learning essential information will be achieved?
    1. Postponing a teaching session if the patient appears mildly anxious
    2. Using a formal rather than an informal approach to teaching
    3. Emphasizing information that is most important first
    4. Setting room temperature on the cool side

11. A nurse is to prepare a patient who is moderately cognitively impaired for a procedure. Which approaches will be **most** effective for the nurse to plan to use with this patient? **Select all that apply.**
    1. _____ Demonstrate the procedure.
    2. _____ Describe the procedure in writing.
    3. _____ Use pictures to describe the procedure.
    4. _____ Provide a preprinted booklet that accurately describes the procedure.
    5. _____ Use group instruction with other patients who are going to have the same procedure.

12. A nurse is caring for a patient who emigrated from a foreign country. The nurse teaches the patient how to perform a wall-climbing exercise with the affected arm after a mastectomy. Later, the nurse sees the patient attempting to perform the exercise and a family member is attempting to hold her arm down. What might be the nurse's **most** accurate conclusion?
    1. Family member's place within the family system allows control over others
    2. Family member thinks that the patient is performing the exercise incorrectly
    3. Family member's cultural beliefs may not conform to the exercise regimen
    4. Family member has intimidated the patient

13. Place the following steps in the order in which they should be performed by a nurse when developing a teaching plan?
    1. Establish readiness.
    2. Select teaching tools.
    3. Determine motivation.
    4. Ascertain level of ability.
    5. Provide an appropriate environment.
    Answer: _____

14. A nurse is planning to teach a weight-loss diet to an adolescent who is obese. What concept related to adolescence is **most** important when attempting to motivate this patient to learn how to lose weight?
    1. Enjoying praise
    2. Pleasing parents
    3. Improving health
    4. Enhancing appearance

15. A nurse is teaching an obese patient how to lower the caloric content of the diet. Which statements indicate that the patient understands the teaching? **Select all that apply.**
    1. _____ "I will stop eating cake for dessert."
    2. _____ "I will use cooking spray instead of butter."
    3. _____ "I will eat three meals a day with no snacks."
    4. _____ "I will keep a diary of how many calories I eat per day."
    5. _____ "I will check the label on packaged foods for caloric content per serving."

16. A nurse is teaching a patient who was recently diagnosed with type 2 diabetes about limiting carbohydrates in the diet. Which statement indicates that the patient has learned in the cognitive domain?
    1. "I have stopped adding sugar to my coffee."
    2. "It will be difficult to stop eating chocolate."
    3. "It has not been easy to stop drinking regular sodas."
    4. "I will read the labels on food before I decide to eat them."

17. A nurse is planning to teach a patient with a newly created colostomy how to perform colostomy irrigation. What patient assessments indicate that the patient is ready to learn? **Select all that apply.**
    1. _____ Patient keeps asking questions about the procedure.
    2. _____ Patient reports pain at a level of 6 on a scale of 0 to 10.
    3. _____ Patient requested reading material about the procedure.
    4. _____ Patient refused to look at the stoma during previous care.
    5. _____ Patient states experiencing the passage of intestinal gas 2 times in the last hour.

18. A nurse is facilitating a weight-reduction program for a group of employees of a business organization. Which statement by a participant indicates an internal locus of control?
    1. "I plan to lose weight so that I improve how I look to others."
    2. "I am going to lose weight because I believe it will make me feel better."
    3. "I need to lose weight because my children are embarrassed by how heavy I am."
    4. "I hope to lose weight because my company will give me a bonus if I reach my goal."

19. A nurse is assessing a patient's motivation to follow an exercise and dietary regimen. What patient statement has the greatest influence on whether the patient will be successful?
    1. "I hope to be successful this time doing what I should be doing."
    2. "I believe that the changes I implement will make a difference."
    3. "I plan on keeping a daily diary of everything I eat."
    4. "I am going to join a gym in my neighborhood."

20. A nurse must perform a physical assessment of a 5-year-old child. What is the **best** way to prepare the child for the assessment?
    1. Answer all of the questions asked by the child.
    2. Show the child a video of another child having an examination.
    3. Have one parent explain to the child what will be done during the examination.
    4. Let the child play with the equipment that will be used during the physical assessment.

21. A patient who had type 2 diabetes for 15 years has become insulin dependent. The primary health-care provider prescribes a daily morning injection of insulin and insulin coverage a.c. and h.s. The nurse reviews the patient's demographic information and past medical history and then interviews the patient. What nursing statement is most appropriate before teaching the patient about self-injection of insulin?

Patient's Clinical Record

Demographic information

68 years old
Divorced for 4 years
Lives alone in an apartment
High school English teacher; retired 3 years ago
Has health insurance
Collecting a pension and social security

Past medical history

Right mastectomy for cancer of the breast 5 years ago
Has had type 2 diabetes for 15 years
Has stage 1 hypertension for 5 years (systolic BP between 140 and 159 mm Hg and diastolic BP between 90 and 99 mm Hg)
Taking Lasix 10 mg by mouth once a day

Patient interview

Patient states that her husband left her because she had a mastectomy and diabetes. States she was bitter, but has since made a life with her family and friends.

---

1. "What coping mechanisms did you use when confronted with past health problems?"
2. "Tell me what you were thinking when you were told you had to use insulin."
3. "How has this new diagnosis impacted on your self-image?"
4. "You must be upset now that you have to use insulin."

22. A nurse is planning to teach a 75-year-old adult how to change a surgical dressing before being discharged from the hospital. What strategy should the nurse use that takes into consideration the patient's developmental level?
    1. Incorporate repetition into the teaching plan.
    2. Obtain a return demonstration of the procedure.
    3. Include a family member in the teaching sessions.
    4. Build on the patient's past positive learning experiences.

23. A nurse is planning to educate a 13-year-old adolescent about future surgery. Which modality is **most** appropriate for the nurse to include in the teaching session?
    1. Providing a hospital brochure regarding the surgery
    2. Explaining in detail what the surgery entails
    3. Using pictures to reinforce verbal teaching
    4. Demonstrating the surgery using a doll

24. A patient is to have abdominal surgery and the primary health-care provider orders deep vein thrombosis prophylaxis to be administered 12 hours before surgery. The prescription states, enoxaparin (Lovenox) 40 mg subcutaneously 9:00 p.m. the night before surgery. The patient demonstrates a subcutaneous injection using a teaching injection pad. The nurse gives the patient a prefilled syringe of enoxaparin that states that there are 100 mg/1 mL. How much solution should the nurse teach the patient to waste before self-injecting the solution? Record your answer using 1 decimal place.
    Answer: _____ mL

25. A nurse is caring for several patients who just had surgery for a variety of pathophysiological problems. Which patient probably will benefit **most** from several teaching sessions that focus on demonstrations and return demonstrations.
    1. Adolescent who had a cast applied for a fractured femur
    2. Man who had a pacemaker inserted because of recurrent bradycardia
    3. Woman who had a vaginal hysterectomy because of multiple benign fibroids
    4. Older adult who had the creation of a colostomy because of cancer of the rectum

26. A primary health-care provider prescribes menotropins (Repronex) 100 international units to be self-administered subcutaneously once a day for 7 days as part of an infertility protocol. The vial of menotropins contains 150 international units FSH, LH. It instructs the user to add 0.8 mL of diluent to yield 1 mL. The nurse teaches the woman how to reconstitute the medication and draw up the appropriate amount prescribed. To which line should the woman fill the syringe with the correct dose of menotropins?
1. A
2. B
3. C
4. D

29. A nurse is educating an obese patient about a 1,500-calorie weight-reduction diet. Which statement by the nurse would be most effective in motivating adherence to the dietary regimen?
1. "Just think how great you will look in a bathing suit next summer."
2. "You can design your menu to include some of your food preferences."
3. "If you lose weight, you will live long enough to see your grandchildren."
4. "It is essential that you lose weight so that you reduce your blood pressure."

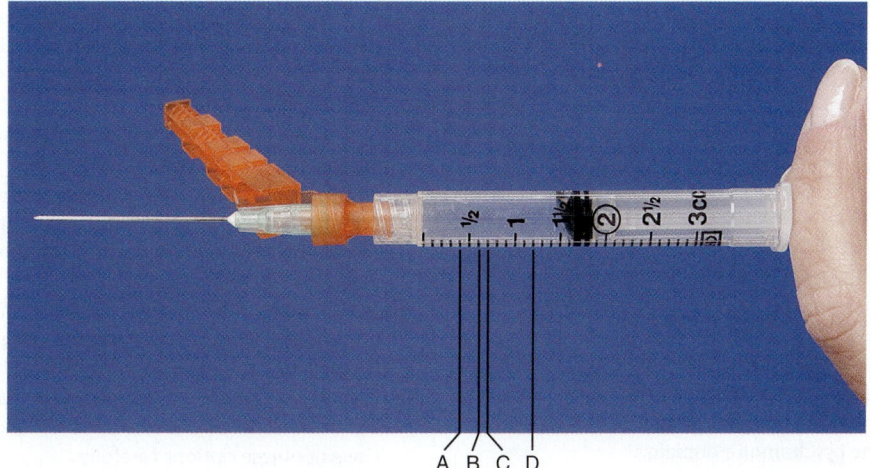

A B C D

27. A nurse plans to teach a patient how to self-administer insulin. The nurse identifies that the patient is a kinesthetic learner. Which teaching strategy should the nurse use to **best** meet this patient's learning style?
1. Encourage the patient to handle the equipment.
2. Present information using a computer-assisted program.
3. Supply written material that the patient can review at an individual pace.
4. Conduct the program in a group setting, supporting auditory exchange of information.

28. A nurse is designing a teaching plan on how to safely empty a portable wound drainage system for a patient who has impaired hearing. What nursing intervention is specific to enhance leaning for this patient?
1. Avoiding overly enunciating each word
2. Planning more time to practice psychomotor skills
3. Providing written material on a fifth-grade reading level
4. Including the patient in a group discussion about the topic

30. A nurse is preparing to educate a patient regarding self-blood glucose monitoring. Place the following interventions in the order that they should be performed.
1. Demonstrate for the patient the skill of self-blood glucose monitoring.
2. Give the patient a brief overview of the information to be covered.
3. Explain to the patient the reasons for glucose monitoring.
4. Have the patient perform self-blood glucose monitoring.
5. Determine the patient's preferred learning style.
6. Assess the patient's cognitive abilities.
Answer: _____

REVIEW ANSWERS

1. ANSWER: 2.
Rationales:
1. This statement reflects an external locus of control. The patient is going to rehabilitation for his children, not himself.
2. This statement reflects an internal locus of control. The patient is going to rehabilitation because he personally desires to regain control of his life.
3. This statement reflects an external locus of control. The patient is going to rehabilitation for his wife, not himself.
4. This statement reflects an external locus of control. The patient is going to rehabilitation to meet legal requirements.
TEST-TAKING TIP: Identify who is the central person in the question. Option 2 focuses on the patient. Options 1, 3, and 4 focus on the kids, wife, and judge, respectively.
Content Area: Teaching and Learning
Integrated Processes: Communication/Documentation; Teaching/Learning; Nursing Process: Analysis
Client Need: Health Promotion and Maintenance
Cognitive Level: Application

2. ANSWER: 3.
Rationales:
1. This outcome involves the performance of a skill that is associated with the psychomotor domain.
2. This outcome involves the affective domain because it reflects a willingness to receive and endure a particular intervention.
3. This outcome is associated with the cognitive domain. It involves knowledge and recall of information.
4. This outcome involves the performance of a skill that is associated with the psychomotor domain.
TEST-TAKING TIP: Identify the clang association. The word *urinary* in the stem and in option 3 is a clang association. Frequently options with a clang association are the correct answer. Assess option 3 carefully.
Content Area: Teaching and Learning
Integrated Processes: Teaching/Learning; Nursing Process: Evaluation
Client Need: Health Promotion and Maintenance
Cognitive Level: Application

3. ANSWER: 1, 2, 3.
Rationales:
1. Using a patient education video is an effective method of educating patients, especially when followed by a discussion.
2. Demonstration and return demonstration are effective methods of educating patients because they allow the nurse to perform a psychomotor skill and then observe the patient's performance. Actions speak louder than words.
3. Providing printed material is an effective method of educating patients, especially when combined with a discussion between the nurse and patient.
4. Having a patient educate another patient is unacceptable because the patient may teach inappropriate techniques. However, having an experienced patient talk to a newly diagnosed patient about living with diabetes is appropriate.

5. The use of abstract statements is not the method of choice because abstract words are prone to misinterpretation. When educating a patient, the nurse should use concrete terms and phrases to avoid the chance of patient misinterpretation.
TEST-TAKING TIP: Identify the word in the stem that sets a priority. The word *most* in the stem sets a priority. Identify the clang associations. The words *self-blood glucose monitoring* in the stem and in options 1 and 2 are clang associations.
Content Area: Teaching and Learning
Integrated Processes: Teaching/Learning; Nursing Process: Planning
Client Need: Health Promotion and Maintenance
Cognitive Level: Analysis

4. ANSWER: 4.
Rationales:
1. This is an authoritarian approach and a threat.
2. Although this information may be shared with the patient, it is not information personalized to the patient. The more personalized the information, the more likely it will motivate a patient.
3. This is a threat. In addition, this focuses on the negative rather than the positive.
4. Receiving information about how and why a treatment regimen is necessary and how it will improve the patient's condition is empowering, which can motivate a person to adhere to the regimen.
TEST-TAKING TIP: Identify the word in the stem that sets a priority. The word *best* in the stem sets a priority. Identify the patient-centered option. Option 4 is patient centered. It focuses on a positive outcome for the patient. Identify the options that are opposites. Options 3 and 4 are opposites. Consider these options carefully.
Content Area: Teaching and Learning
Integrated Processes: Teaching/Learning; Nursing Process: Implementation
Client Need: Health Promotion and Maintenance
Cognitive Level: Application

5. ANSWER: 3, 4.
Rationales:
1. Being male or being of the opposite sex of the nurse should not be a reason to postpone patient education.
2. Being 75 years old is not a reason to postpone patient education. The nurse's role is to assess a patient's cognitive abilities and to ensure the nurse is providing instruction where the "patient is at."
3. A high level of anxiety is a reason to postpone patient education because people with high anxiety levels have a decreased ability to focus and concentrate.
4. Pain decreases a person's ability to focus and concentrate. The teaching session should be postponed until nursing interventions reduce the patient's pain.
5. A patient's current education level is not a reason to postpone patient education; however, the nurse should tailor teaching to the patient's cognitive, emotional, and educational level.
TEST-TAKING TIP: Identify the words in the stem that indicate negative polarity. The words *teaching session should be*

postponed indicate negative polarity. The question is asking "What factors **do not** indicate a readiness to learn?" Identify the option that contains a specific determiner. The word *only* in option 5 is a specific determiner. More often than not, options with specific determiners are distractors and can be eliminated.
Content Area: Teaching and Learning
Integrated Processes: Caring; Teaching/Learning; Nursing Process: Analysis
Client Need: Health Promotion and Maintenance
Cognitive Level: Application

6. ANSWER: 1.
Rationales:
1. **The Joint Commission requires hospitals to provide professional interpreters or an interpreter service via a phone link so that patients clearly understand their condition, medical treatment, and the nursing plan of care. In addition, interpretive services must be provided when engaging a patient in teaching and learning.**
2. Although obtaining written material in Spanish from the Internet may be done, it is insufficient to meet this patient's learning needs. The patient is unable to engage in a meaningful discussion about the topic and does not have the opportunity to ask questions and receive answers.
3. Information in the cognitive or affective domain cannot be taught via demonstration.
4. Although showing pictures of food may be done, it is insufficient to meet this patient's learning needs. The patient is unable to engage in a meaningful discussion about the topic and does not have the opportunity to ask questions and receive answers.
TEST-TAKING TIP: Identify the word in the stem that sets a priority. The word *most* in the stem sets a priority. Identify the options with clang associations. The words *Spain* in the stem and *Spanish* in option 1 and 2 are clang associations. Examine options 1 and 2 carefully.
Content Area: Teaching and Learning
Integrated Processes: Communication/Documentation; Teaching/Learning; Nursing Process: Planning
Client Need: Health Promotion and Maintenance
Cognitive Level: Application

7. ANSWER: 3.
Rationales:
1. This outcome is associated with the cognitive domain on a higher level than just recalling information. It involves comprehending and applying an idea in a situation, such as interpreting and using a food label to identify the caloric value of the food.
2. This outcome involves remembering and recalling information, which are associated with the cognitive domain (thinking domain).
3. **This outcome involves the use of the hands to perform a skill, which is associated with the psychomotor domain (doing domain).**
4. Accepting limitations in life imposed by the diagnosis of hypertension and incorporating actions to support weight loss as evidenced by actual weight loss is associated with the affective domain (feeling domain).

Content Area: Teaching and Learning
Integrated Processes: Teaching/Learning; Nursing Process: Evaluation
Client Need: Health Promotion and Maintenance
Cognitive Level: Application

8. ANSWER: 2, 4.
Rationales:
1. The patient's statement does not reflect an internal locus of control. A person with an internal locus of control is motivated from within and takes responsibility for actions and consequences.
2. **The patient's statement reflects an external locus of control. A person with an external locus of control is motivated by pressure or rewards from outside the self.**
3. The patient's statement does not reflect a personal goal; it is a goal set by the legal system.
4. **The patient's statement reflects the need to participate in the rehabilitation program to meet the requirements of the legal system.**
5. The patient's statement does not reflect any interest in resolving the dependence on alcohol.
TEST-TAKING TIP: Identify the options that are opposites. Options 1 and 2 are opposites. One of these is a correct answer and one is not.
Content Area: Teaching and Learning
Integrated Processes: Communication/Documentation; Teaching/Learning; Nursing Process: Analysis
Client Need: Health Promotion and Maintenance
Cognitive Level: Analysis

9. ANSWER: 1.
Rationales:
1. **To maintain a diabetic diet, the patient has to emotionally accept the need to incorporate a diabetic diet into one's lifestyle. This requires a positive attitude and the need to value activities that promote health and wellness. Attitudes and values are associated with the affective domain.**
2. Self-administration of insulin is related to the psychomotor, not affective, domain. The psychomotor domain is related to handling equipment safely.
3. This outcome is related to learning in the cognitive, not affective, domain. The cognitive domain is associated with the acquiring of information, memorization, recall, intellectual thinking, and applying and evaluating ideas.
4. Learning the clinical indicators of hyperglycemia and hypoglycemia is associated with the cognitive, not affective, domain. Memorizing, recalling, and comprehending information are related to learning in the cognitive domain.
TEST-TAKING TIP: Identify the options that are equally plausible. Options 3 and 4 are equally plausible because they both are associated with recalling and comprehending new information. Identify the clang association. The word *diabetes* in the stem is closely related to the word *diabetic* in option 1. Consider option 1 carefully.
Content Area: Teaching and Learning
Integrated Processes: Teaching/Learning; Nursing Process: Evaluation
Client Need: Health Promotion and Maintenance
Cognitive Level: Application

10. ANSWER: 3.
Rationales:
1. A teaching session does not have to be postponed because a person is mildly anxious. Research demonstrates that a mildly anxious person is alert and focused, which enhances learning.
2. Both formal and informal approaches are effective teaching methods.
3. This is an excellent teaching strategy. This ensures that critical content is addressed first in the event that additional learning must be postponed because the patient becomes tired or experiences pain during the learning session.
4. Not all patients are comfortable in a cool environment. The temperature of the learning environment should be physically comfortable for the patient. When physically comfortable, the patient can focus on the content being learned rather than on being too cold or too hot.
TEST-TAKING TIP: Identify the word in the stem that sets a priority. The word *essential* in the stem sets a priority. Identify the obscure clang association. The word *essential* in the stem and the words *most important* in option 3 is a clang association. The words essential and most important basically have the same meaning. Examine options with a clang association carefully. More often than not, the option with a clang association is the correct answer.
Content Area: Teaching and Learning
Integrated Processes: Teaching/Learning; Nursing Process: Planning
Client Need: Health Promotion and Maintenance
Cognitive Level: Application

11. ANSWER: 1, 3.
Rationales:
1. Demonstrating the procedure is an effective method to educate a cognitively impaired patient because it allows for visual learning.
2. Describing the procedure in writing involves the use of abstract thought and symbolism, which the cognitively impaired patient may not possess.
3. Using pictures to describe a procedure is an effective method to educate a cognitively impaired patient because it allows for visual learning.
4. A preprinted book may not be an effective teaching approach because the cognitively impaired patient may not understand the written word and it does not allow for questions.
5. Group instruction for a cognitively impaired person is not a method of choice because the person may feel overwhelmed in a group setting; in addition, HIPAA laws prevent discussion of a patient's clinical condition with other patients without consent.
TEST-TAKING TIP: Identify the word in the stem that sets a priority. The word *most* in the stem sets a priority.
Content Area: Teaching and Learning
Integrated Processes: Teaching/Learning; Nursing Process: Planning
Client Need: Health Promotion and Maintenance
Cognitive Level: Application

12. ANSWER: 3.
Rationales:
1. Although this may be accurate, it is too specific an initial assumption.
2. If this were so, the nurse would expect the family member to be attempting to teach the patient, not trying to restrain her arm.
3. Although the culture is unknown, there appears to be a reason why the patient's arm is being restrained. The nurse should pursue this further because it may be related to cultural beliefs.
4. The patient would have stopped the exercise if intimidated by the family member.
TEST-TAKING TIP: Identify the words in the stem that set a priority. The word *most* in the stem set a priority.
Content Area: Teaching and Learning
Integrated Processes: Teaching/Learning; Nursing Process: Analysis
Client Need: Psychosocial Integrity
Cognitive Level: Application

13. ANSWER: 1, 3, 4, 2, 5.
Rationales:
1. The nurse must first determine if the patient realizes that there is a need to learn more.
3. After readiness to learn is established, the nurse should verify motivation by recognizing health-seeking behaviors, such as requests to participate in own care, asking for written materials or referral to a support group, and belief that interventions will precipitate desired outcomes.
4. The nurse must then establish the level at which the patient is capable of learning, such as cognitive and developmental levels, physical ability, and need for repetition.
2. The selection of teaching tools is based on the patient's level of learning and capabilities, such as visual, auditory acuity, communication skills, language, and cultural differences.
5. An environment conducive to learning enhances learning, such as appropriate time, length, and frequency of lessons, and a quiet, private, comfortable place.
Content Area: Teaching and Learning
Integrated Processes: Teaching/Learning; Nursing Process: Planning
Client Need: Safe and Effective Care Environment; Management of Care
Cognitive Level: Analysis

14. ANSWER: 4.
Rationales:
1. This is not a motivating factor for a teenager. This is associated with school-aged children.
2. This is not a motivating factor since teenagers often are in conflict with their parents because of their struggle between dependence and independence.
3. This is not a motivating factor because teenagers believe they are immortal. They live in the present and generally are uninterested in the relationship between health and maintaining a positive lifestyle.

4. Teenagers often are obsessed with their appearances and use various methods of weight loss that are unhealthy, such as bulimia, fad diets, and excessive exercise. The teenager may be motivated to lose weight by appealing to the goal of enhancing appearance.
TEST-TAKING TIP: Identify the word in the stem that sets a priority. The word *most* in the stem sets a priority.
Content Area: *Teaching and Learning*
Integrated Processes: *Teaching/Learning; Nursing Process: Analysis*
Client Need: *Health Promotion and Maintenance*
Cognitive Level: *Application*

15. **ANSWER: 4, 5.**
Rationales:
1. The chances of maintaining a diet decrease when depriving oneself of favorite foods. The calories for food preferences can be calculated into the total daily recommended caloric intake.
2. Although this may lower the caloric count of the diet, it is not as tasty or satisfying as butter. A pad of butter can be calculated into the total daily intake of calories.
3. Eating snacks between meals, provided the calories are within the recommended total intake, minimize hunger.
4. **Keeping a daily caloric intake diary is a motivating factor for staying within the recommended daily limits.**
5. **Knowing the number of calories per serving provides information for making a knowledgeable decision. This approach provides an internal locus of control and can be motivating to follow the dietary regimen.**
TEST-TAKING TIP: Identify the words in the stem and options that are clang associations. The words *caloric content* in the stem and *calories* in option 4 and *caloric content* in option 5 are clang associations. Examine these options carefully.
Content Area: *Teaching and Learning*
Integrated Processes: *Communication/Documentation; Teaching/Learning; Nursing Process: Evaluation*
Client Need: *Health Promotion and Maintenance*
Cognitive Level: *Application*

16. **ANSWER: 4.**
Rationales:
1. Sugar may be added to coffee as long as it is calculated into the dietary regimen.
2. This comment reflects the affective domain (feelings, values, attitudes, and beliefs). Chocolate may be included in the diet as long as it is calculated into the dietary regimen.
3. This comment reflects the affective domain (feelings, values, attitudes, and belief), not the cognitive domain. Regular soda may be included in the diet as long as it is calculated into the dietary regimen.
4. **The patient is indicating comprehension by verbalizing the importance of knowing how many carbohydrates are included in packaged foods.**
TEST-TAKING TIP: Identify the option that is unique. Option 4 is the only option that does not eliminate a fluid or food from the diet.
Content Area: *Teaching and Learning*

Integrated Processes: *Communication/Documentation; Teaching/Learning; Nursing Process: Evaluation*
Client Need: *Health Promotion and Maintenance*
Cognitive Level: *Application*

17. **ANSWER: 1, 3, 5.**
Rationales:
1. **Asking questions indicates interest and a readiness to learn. The patient wants answers.**
2. Pain can interfere with learning because the patient may not be able to focus beyond coping with the pain. A patient with moderate to severe pain should receive an analgesic to reduce the pain before a teaching session.
3. **Requesting information about a situation is a behavior that indicates a readiness to learn. The patient wants more knowledge.**
4. A patient who refuses to look at a colostomy may be in denial or unable emotionally or physically to learn how to care for a colostomy.
5. **Passing of intestinal gas is expected with a colostomy. It indicates that peristalsis has returned and the patient may be physically ready for colostomy irrigation.**
Content Area: *Teaching and Learning*
Integrated Processes: *Communication/Documentation; Teaching/Learning; Nursing Process: Assessment*
Client Need: *Health Promotion and Maintenance*
Cognitive Level: *Application*

18. **ANSWER: 2.**
Rationales:
1. This statement indicates that the person is influenced by what others think, which reflects an external locus of control.
2. **This statement indicates that the change in behavior is motivated by a desire from within, which reflects an internal locus of control.**
3. This statement indicates that the person wants to please or gain the respect of others, which reflects an external locus of control.
4. This statement indicates that the person is motivated by an external reward, which reflects an external locus of control.
TEST-TAKING TIP: Identify the option that is unique. Option 2 is unique because it is related to achieving a goal for personal reasons while options 1, 3, and 4 are related to influences outside the individual.
Content Area: *Teaching and Learning*
Integrated Processes: *Communication/Documentation; Teaching/Learning; Nursing Process: Analysis*
Client Need: *Health Promotion and Maintenance*
Cognitive Level: *Analysis*

19. **ANSWER: 2.**
Rationales:
1. The statement *I hope to be successful* is less emphatic than *I will be successful.* Hope is related to a desirable expectation, but it takes more than just hope to accomplish a positive outcome. Also, the words *this time* indicate that the patient may not have been successful in the past; past experiences can impact on present experiences and repeat themselves.
2. **If a patient believes that interventions will produce a beneficial outcome, the patient will more likely adhere to**

the proposed medical regimen. **This is one of the major components of the health belief model. Also, the statement reflects an internal locus of control and thinking related to the affective domain.**

3. Although it is helpful to track dietary intake, it does not ensure that the patient will follow the prescribed diet.

4. Although this is beneficial, it does not ensure that the patient will attend the gym and perform the prescribed exercises.

TEST-TAKING TIP: Identify the word in the stem that sets a priority. The word *greatest* in the stem sets a priority. Identify the options that are equally plausible. Options 3 and 4 are equally plausible because each relates to just one aspect of the regimen; one is no better than the other. These options can be deleted from consideration.

Content Area: Teaching and Learning
Integrated Processes: Communication/Documentation;
Teaching/Learning; Nursing Process: Analysis
Client Need: Health Promotion and Maintenance
Cognitive Level: Application

20. **ANSWER: 4.**
    Rationales:
    1. Although this may be done, the child may not know what questions to ask.
    2. A video is a passive activity and only stimulates the senses of vision and hearing.
    3. An explanation is a cognitive intervention that does not permit the visualization and handling of equipment.
    4. **This is an interactive way to introduce the child to the equipment that will be used. It provides visual, auditory, and kinesthetic stimulation. Anxiety usually is reduced during an assessment when familiar objects are used.**

    TEST-TAKING TIP: Identify the word in the stem that sets a priority. The word *best* in the stem sets a priority. Identify the option that contains a specific determiner. Option 1 contains the word *all*, which is a specific determiner. Identify the clang association. The words *physical assessment* in the stem and in option 4 is a clang association.

    Content Area: Teaching and Learning
    Integrated Processes: Teaching/Learning; Nursing Process: Implementation
    Client Need: Health Promotion and Maintenance
    Cognitive Level: Application

21. **ANSWER: 2.**
    Rationales:
    1. This question would be more helpful during a later session, after the patient has had an opportunity to initially process new information.
    2. **This statement focuses on the change the patient is experiencing and allows the patient to address concerns from a personal perspective. The nurse must focus on the patient's concerns before beginning teaching. The focus should be on the present situation, not the past.**
    3. This question is too direct. Initial questions should be more open ended and not focus on one factor.

4. This statement implies how the patient should have been feeling when told about the diagnosis. This assumption may not be accurate. Also, it focuses on the negative and suggests that people should be upset if they have to take insulin.

TEST-TAKING TIP: Identify the word in the stem that is a clang association. The word *insulin* in the stem and in options 2 and 4 are clang associations. More often than not, an option with a clang association is the correct answer. Examine options 2 and 4 carefully.

Content Area: Teaching and Learning
Integrated Processes: Communication/Documentation;
Teaching/Learning; Nursing Process: Implementation
Client Need: Health Promotion and Maintenance
Cognitive Level: Analysis

22. **ANSWER: 1.**
    Rationales:
    1. **Information processing speed declines with age, slowing learning and increasing the need for repetition.**
    2. A return demonstration is the primary method to evaluate a patient's ability to perform a psychomotor skill; this strategy is not age dependent.
    3. A family member may be included in a teaching session regardless of the age of the patient. The involvement of a family member requires the patient's consent.
    4. Teaching should always progress from what the patient knows to the unknown; this strategy is not age dependent.

    TEST-TAKING TIP: Identify the word in the stem that is a clang association with a word in options. The words *teach* in the stem and *teaching* in options 1 and 3 are clang associations. Consider options 1 and 3 carefully.

    Content Area: Teaching and Learning
    Integrated Processes: Communication/Documentation;
    Teaching/Learning; Nursing Process: Planning
    Client Need: Health Promotion and Maintenance
    Cognitive Level: Application

23. **ANSWER: 3.**
    Rationales:
    1. Providing a hospital brochure may facilitate education, but will not allow for questions by the adolescent.
    2. Explaining in detail what the surgery entails may create anxiety because too much information can be confusing. It is a nurse's role to assess the cognitive and emotional level of the patient before teaching.
    3. **Using pictures to reinforce the spoken word will assist the adolescent to understand what is being taught. A 13-year-old adolescent may not have the ability to think abstractly.**
    4. Using a doll with an adolescent may be beneath the adolescent's cognitive abilities; the adolescent may feel childish or become bored.

    TEST-TAKING TIP: Identify the word in the stem that sets a priority. The word *most* in the stem sets a priority. Identify the option with a clang association. The word *teaching* in the stem and in option 3 is a clang association. Examine option 3 carefully.

Content Area: Teaching and Learning
Integrated Processes: Teaching/Learning; Nursing Process: Planning
Client Need: Health Promotion and Maintenance
Cognitive Level: Application

24. **ANSWER: 0.6.**
Rationale:
Use ratio and proportion to determine the desired mL dose and then subtract this amount from the total mL of solution in the syringe to arrive at the correct answer.

$$\frac{\text{Desire 40 mg}}{\text{Have 100 mL}} = \frac{x\,\text{mL}}{1\,\text{mL}}$$
$$100x = 40 \times 1$$
$$100x = 40$$
$$x = 40 \div 100$$
$$x = 0.4\,\text{mL is the desired dose}$$

The prefilled syringe contains 1 mL. Subtract 0.4 mL from 1 mL, which yields 0.6 mL that has to be wasted. The desired dose of 0.4 mg remains in the syringe.
Content Area: Medication Administration
Integrated Processes: Teaching/Learning; Nursing Process: Planning
Client Need: Physiological Integrity; Pharmacological and Parenteral Therapies
Cognitive Level: Application

25. **ANSWER: 4.**
Rationales:
1. A patient who had a cast applied for a broken bone will be taught to keep the cast clean and dry. There is no complex care to be learned by the patient.
2. A man who had a pacemaker surgically implanted may require education regarding monitoring of the pulse and the need for routine follow-up health-care supervision; however, there is no need for learning complex self-care.
3. A woman who had a vaginal hysterectomy may require some education regarding assessment of the vaginal discharge, but will not be required to learn complex self-care.
4. **A patient with a colostomy will have to learn how to apply, remove, and empty the colostomy bag and learn how to irrigate the colostomy. Therefore, demonstration and return demonstration will be the most effective forms of teaching for this patient.**
TEST-TAKING TIP: Identify the word in the stem that sets a priority. The word *most* in the stem sets a priority.
Content Area: Teaching and Learning
Integrated Processes: Teaching/Learning; Nursing Process: Planning
Client Need: Health Promotion and Maintenance
Cognitive Level: Analysis

26. **ANSWER: 3.**
Rationales:
1. This is too small a dose. It is 0.4 mL.
2. This is too small a dose. It is 0.6 mL.

3. This is the correct dose. It is 0.7 mL.
Solve the problem by using ratio and proportion.

$$\frac{\text{Desire 100 international units}}{\text{Have 150 international units}} = \frac{x\,\text{mL}}{1\,\text{mL}}$$
$$150x = 100 \times 1$$
$$150x = 100$$
$$x = 100 \div 150$$
$$x = 0.66\,\text{mL. Round the number up to 0.7 mL.}$$

4. This is too large a dose. It is 1.2 mL.
Content Area: Medication Administration
Integrated Processes: Teaching/Learning; Nursing Process: Implementation
Client Need: Physiological Integrity; Pharmacological and Parenteral Therapies
Cognitive Level: Analysis

27. **ANSWER: 1.**
Rationales:
1. **Handling equipment best meets the learning style of kinesthetic learners. Kinesthetic learners process information by doing, engaging in physical activity, and handling equipment.**
2. Computer-assisted programs best meet the learning styles of visual and auditory learners. Visual learners learn by processing information with the eyes. Auditory learners process information by listening to words.
3. Written material best meets the learning style of visual learners. Visual learners learn by processing information with the eyes.
4. Group discussion best meets the learning style of auditory learners. Auditory learners process information by listening to words.
TEST-TAKING TIP: Identify the word in the stem that sets a priority. The word *best* in the stem sets a priority.
Content Area: Teaching and Learning
Integrated Processes: Teaching/Learning; Nursing Process: Planning
Client Need: Health Promotion and Maintenance
Cognitive Level: Application

28. **ANSWER: 1.**
Rationales:
1. **Overly enunciating each word should be avoided because it interferes with lip reading.**
2. This is unnecessary. Impaired hearing should not interfere with learning in the psychomotor domain. Demonstration and return demonstration are the most effective ways to teach and evaluate learning in the psychomotor domain.
3. This is a nursing intervention common to all patients. It is not a teaching strategy specific to a patient who is hearing impaired.
4. A hearing impaired person may not be able to follow (hear) the discussion among members of a group. Patients who are hearing impaired learn best in a one-to-one situation rather than in a group setting.

TEST-TAKING TIP: Identify the unique option. Option 1 is the only option that addresses an intervention that should be avoided. Options 2, 3, and 4 focus on interventions that should be done.
Content Area: Teaching and Learning
Integrated Processes: Communication/Documentation; Teaching/Learning; Nursing Process: Planning
Client Need: Health Promotion and Maintenance
Cognitive Level: Application

29. **ANSWER: 2.**
Rationales:
1. Looking good in a bathing suit is a potential long-term outcome. Also, the nurse is making the assumption that this factor is important to the patient.
2. This is an empowering statement because it gives the patient some control over implementing the dietary regimen. It is patient centered and focuses on the present and near future. The achievement of short-term goals is motivating.
3. Living long enough to see grandchildren is a potential long-term outcome. Also, the nurse is making the assumption that this factor is important to the patient.
4. Reducing blood pressure is a long-term outcome. Also, the nurse is making the assumption that this factor is important to the patient.
TEST-TAKING TIP: Identify the word in the stem that sets a priority. The word *most* in the stem sets a priority. Identify the unique option. Option 2 is unique. It is the only option that addresses the process of losing weight rather than a potential outcome. It is a short-term intervention rather than a long-term outcome. It focuses on the present rather than the future.
Content Area: Teaching and Learning
Integrated Processes: Communication/Documentation; Teaching/Learning; Nursing Process: Implementation

Client Need: Health Promotion and Maintenance
Cognitive Level: Application

30. **ANSWER: 6, 5, 2, 3, 1, 4.**
Rationales:
6. The patient's ability to intellectually handle the information must be assessed first. Also, this assessment will influence the level of verbal language and written materials required for this patient.
5. Information is best learned by a patient if the information is presented in the patient's preferred learning style (e.g., visual, auditory, or kinesthetic learner).
2. After the patient is assessed, then a brief overview of the teaching session puts what to come into perspective. An outline helps to provide structure for the teaching session.
3. Information in the cognitive learning domain provides the foundation for learning in the psychomotor and affective learning domains.
1. After the cognitive and affective learning domains are addressed, then the teacher can proceed to demonstrating the skill. It is important that the nurse demonstrate the skill, allow the patient to manipulate the equipment, and have the patient practice the skill.
4. After the nurse has completed the teaching of a skill and the patient has had an opportunity to practice the skill, then the patient should perform a return demonstration of the skill. This allows the nurse to evaluate whether the patient can perform the skill appropriately.
Content Area: Teaching and Learning
Integrated Processes: Teaching/Learning; Nursing Process: Planning
Client Need: Safe and Effective Care Environment; Management of Care
Cognitive Level: Analysis

Essential Components of Nursing Care

Nursing Process

Analysis—The examination of data and identification of patient problems, nursing diagnoses, and/or needs; it is the second step of the nursing process.

Assessment—The ongoing, systematic collection, validation, and documentation of data; it is the first step of the nursing process.

Critical thinking—A cognitive strategy by which one reflects on and analyzes personal thoughts, actions, and decisions.

Data—Collected information.

Delegate—Transferring the authority to act to another.

Evaluation—The comparison of planned expected outcomes with a patient's actual outcomes to determine whether patient needs have been met; it is the fifth step of the nurse process.

Goal—A broad, nonspecific statement about the status one expects a patient to achieve.

Implementation—The organization, management, and implementation of planned nursing actions that involves thinking and doing; it is the fourth step of the nursing process.

Nonverbal data—Observable behavior transmitting a message without words.

Nursing Interventions Classifications (NIC) system—A standardized classification of nursing interventions.

Nursing Outcomes Classification (NOC) system—A standardized classification of patient outcomes that respond to nursing interventions.

Nursing process—A critical thinking framework that involves assessing and analyzing human responses to plan and implement nursing care that meets patient needs as evidenced by the evaluation of patient outcomes. Consists of assessment, analysis, planning, implementation, and evaluation.

Objective data (also known as *signs*)—Overt, measurable assessments collected via the senses.

Outcome—A specific desired change in a patient's condition as a result of nursing interventions.

Planning—The identification of goals and/or outcomes and nursing interventions that address patient problems, nursing diagnoses, or needs; it is the third step of the nursing process.

Priority—Something ranked highest in terms of importance or urgency.

Subjective data (also known as *symptoms*)—Covert information, such as feelings, perceptions, thoughts, sensations, or concerns, that are shared by the patient and can be verified only by the patient.

Verbal data—Spoken or written messages.

I. Introduction to the Nursing Process

The nursing process is a critical thinking framework that involves assessing and analyzing human responses to plan and implement nursing care that meets patient needs as evidenced by evaluation of patient outcomes. Nurses use critical thinking throughout the nursing process, which involves both "thinking" and "doing," to meet complex patient needs.

A. Components of the Nursing Process
  1. Assessment.
  2. Planning.
  3. Analysis.
  4. Implementation.
  5. Evaluation.

B. Characteristics of the Nursing Process
  1. Is patient-centered.
  2. Is interpersonal.
  3. Is collaborative.
  4. Is dynamic and cyclical.
  5. Requires critical thinking.

II. Assessment

Assessment, the first step of the nursing process, is the ongoing, systematic collection, validation, and documentation of data. Nursing assessment should be comprehensive, holistic, and accurate so that it provides all the necessary information about a patient. In addition, it should reflect the patient's responses to a health problem and stressors, not disease processes. Adequate assessment depends on collecting data using various methods, collecting both subjective and objective data, verifying that data are accurate, and communicating information about assessments to other members of the health team.

A. **Methods of Data Collection**
   1. Physical examination: The use of inspection, auscultation, percussion, and palpation to collect data about a patient's physical status. (See Chapter 11, "Physical Assessment.")
   2. Interviewing.
      a. Formal approach.
         (1) Used when collecting information in a prescribed or official way, such as for a history and physical.
         (2) Usually involves direct rather than open-ended questions.

MAKING THE CONNECTION

Application of Critical Thinking to the Nursing Process: Making the Connection

Critical thinking is a cognitive strategy by which one reflects on and analyzes personal thoughts, actions, and decisions. It involves purposeful, goal-directed thinking (e.g., the nursing process); requires judgment based on facts and principles of science rather than conjecture or trial and error (e.g., evidence-based practice); and requires numerous cognitive and personal competencies. The helix of critical thinking (Fig. 10.1) demonstrates the interwoven relationship between cognitive competencies and personal competencies essential to thinking critically. Throughout the thinking process, there is constant interaction among cognitive competencies, among personal competencies, and between cognitive and personal competencies. The more cognitive competencies and personal competencies a person possesses, the greater the potential the person has to think critically (Fig. 10.2). Critical thinking has an interactive relationship with the nursing process. The nursing process is a dynamic, cyclical process in which each phase interacts with and is influenced by the other phases of the process. Critical thinking is an essential component within, between, and among the phases of the nursing process. Different combinations of cognitive and personal competencies may be used during the different phases of the nursing process (Fig. 10.3).

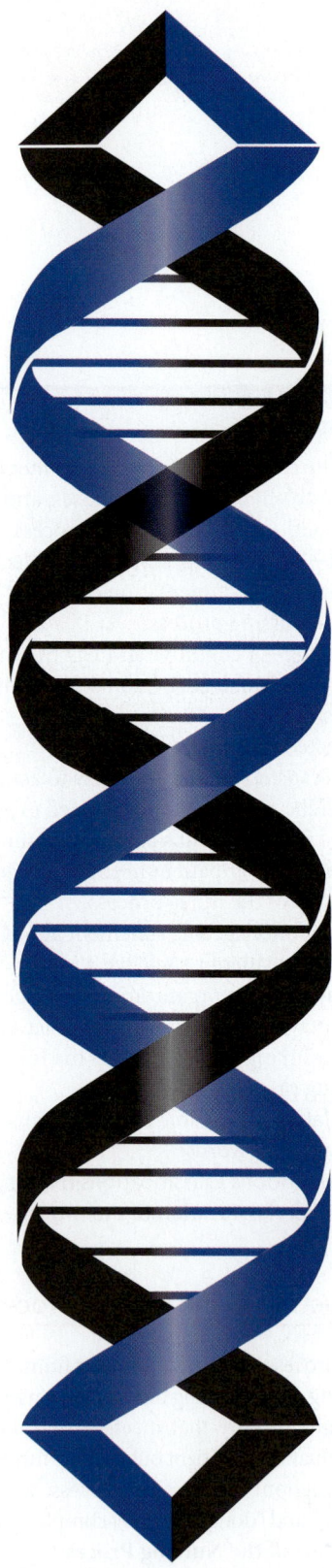

Fig 10.1 The helix of critical thinking. (From Nugent and Vitale [2012]. *Fundamentals Success,* 3rd ed. Philadelphia: F. A. Davis Company, with permission.)

Cognitive Competencies	Personal Competencies
Dissect	Tolerant of ambiguity
Modify	Think independently
Analyze	Perseverance
Interpret	Self-confident
Examine	Open-minded
Correlate	Accountable
Synthesize	Courageous
Recall facts	Imaginative
Investigate	Disciplined
Categorize	Committed
Summarize	Inquisitive
Understand	Motivated
Demonstrate	Risk taker
Self-examine	Confident
Translate data	Reflective
Query evidence	Objective
Make inferences	Authentic
Manipulate facts	Assertive
Present arguments	Intuitive
Establish priorities	Rational
Make generalizations	Creative
Compare and contrast	Humble
Determine significance	Curious
Determine implications	Honest
Determine consequences	Moral

Fig 10.2 The helix of critical thinking schematically elongated. (From Nugent and Vitale [2012]. *Fundamentals Success*, 3rd ed. Philadelphia: F.A. Davis Company, with permission.)

b. Informal approach.
  (1) Used when collecting data in a casual and more relaxed manner, such as when exploring a patient's feelings while providing other nursing care.
  (2) Usually involves open-ended questions.
c. See also Chapter 7, "Communication and Documentation."
3. Clinical record review.
  a. Involves monitoring information collected about the patient in the clinical record.
  b. Gathers information about results of laboratory examinations, diagnostic procedures, consultations by other members of the health team, and progress notes.

B. Sources of Data
1. Primary source.
  a. The patient is the only primary source of data.
  🛑 b. The patient is the most valuable source because the data collected are most recent, unique, and specific to the patient.
2. Secondary sources.
  a. These sources provide supplementary information about the patient from some place other than the patient, but within the patient's frame of reference.
  b. They include people other than the patient (e.g., family members, friends, other health team members).
  c. A patient's clinical record is also a secondary source, as it contains a vast amount of information about the patient's physical, psychosocial, and economic history as well as information about the patient's progress regarding physical and emotional responses to a health problem.

DID YOU KNOW?
Although a patient's clinical record is a secondary source, laboratory and diagnostic procedure results are direct objective measurements of the patient's status and are considered by some to be a primary source. The clinical record is an historical view of the patient and, for that reason, is less current than data collected from the patient.

3. Tertiary sources.
  a. These sources produce data from outside the patient's frame of reference.
  b. Examples include information from textbooks, surveys, medical and nursing journals, drug books, and policy and procedure manuals.

C. Types of Data
1. Objective data (also known as *signs*).
  a. Overt, measurable assessments collected via the senses, such as sight, touch, smell, or hearing, and compared to an accepted standard.

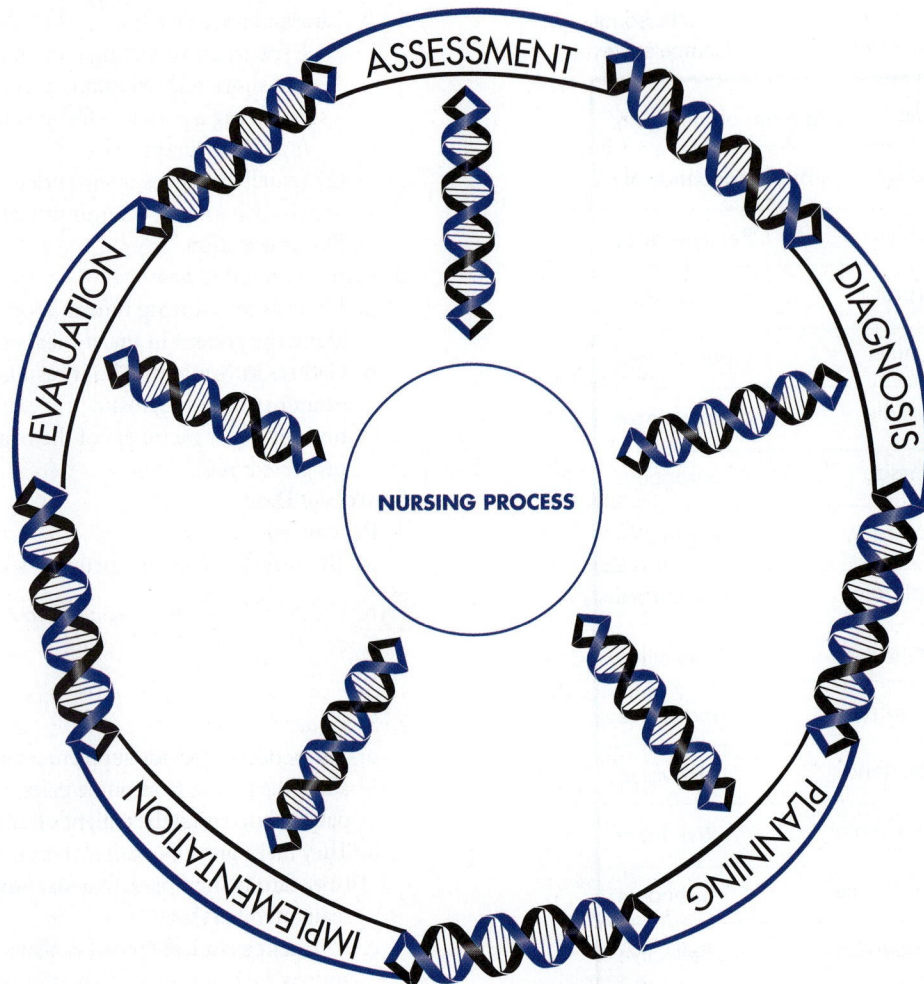

Fig 10.3 The interactive nature of the helix of critical thinking within the nursing process. (From Nugent and Vitale [2012]. *Fundamentals Success,* 3rd ed. Philadelphia: F. A. Davis Company, with permission.)

b. Examples include body temperature, pulse and respiratory rates, blood pressure, vomiting, distended abdomen, presence of edema, lung sounds, crying, skin color, and presence of diaphoresis.

2. Subjective data (also known as *symptoms*).
   a. Covert information, such as feelings, perceptions, thoughts, sensations, or concerns that are shared by the patient and can be verified only by the patient.
   b. Examples include pruritus, nausea, pain, numbness, attitudes, beliefs, values, and perceptions of the health problem and life circumstances.

3. Verbal data.
   a. Spoken or written data.
   b. Requires the nurse to listen to the pace of the communication pattern, tone of voice, vocabulary used, and presence of aggression, anxiety, or assertiveness.

c. Allows for the assessment of difficulties such as slurring, lack of clarity, flight of ideas, difficulty finding the desired word, and inability to identify an item.
   d. Examples include statements made by the patient or by a secondary source.

4. Nonverbal data.
   a. Observable behavior transmitting a message without words.
   b. Examples include patient's appearance; fearful facial expression; body language, such as posture; gestures; and eye contact or lack of eye contact.

D. Verifying Collected Data
   1. Data must be double-checked (verified) after they are collected.
   2. Ensures validity and accuracy.
   3. Ensures that the nurse does not come to a conclusion without adequate data to support the conclusion.
   4. Involves collecting additional information to support the initial data. For example, if a patient's

pulse is increased above the expected range, the nurse should take the pulse again; if it is still increased, the nurse should collect other vital signs to supplement the original information.

5. Helps to identify whether objective and subjective data are congruent or incompatible; for example:

a. When a patient has an increased blood pressure, pulse, and respiratory rate and is rubbing a shoulder, the nurse makes an inference that the patient is experiencing pain. To validate this conclusion, the nurse asks, "I noticed that you are rubbing your shoulder. Is it causing you discomfort?"

b. If a patient says, "I feel as though my bladder will burst," the nurse makes the inference that the patient might be experiencing urinary retention. To validate this, the nurse should palpate the patient's abdomen for distention. The nurse also can ask questions that clarify the patient's statement.

c. If a patient says, "I feel that I am in a big, black hole," the nurse might use the communication technique of clarification to have the patient explain in more detail what was meant, "Tell me more about this big, black hole that you feel you are in."

E. Communicating Collected Data

1. Outcomes of nursing assessments must be documented on correct forms and in appropriate places in the patient's clinical record. Many forms are used to document data and are organized by topic or body systems.

2. Communicating data ensures that pertinent and current information relative to the patient is shared with other members of the health team.

🛑 3. Data must be communicated in an objective and factual way and not be a summary of the nurse's interpretation of the data.

4. Value words, such as *good, bad, adequate, poor,* and *tolerated well,* should be avoided. For example, rather than saying that a patient's appetite is poor, the nurse should document that the patient ate half of a scrambled egg and a slice of toast. This manner of documentation communicates objective, measurable information about the patient's appetite.

5. Value words related to a patient's behavior, such as *lazy, difficult, stubborn, rude, uncooperative,* and *foolish,* should be avoided. These words reflect a value judgment made by the nurse that may be influenced by bias and personal values or beliefs. Nurses must always be nonjudgmental.

6. Subjective data should be documented in the exact words verbalized by the patient and put in quotation marks; this practice ensures that a patient's meaning is not misinterpreted or inaccurately altered by words used by the nurse to describe an event.

III. Analysis

Analysis, the second step of the nursing process, requires the nurse to use critical thinking strategies to scrutinize data. Activities associated with this step include clustering data, interpreting data, and identifying and communicating a patient's nursing diagnoses, problems, or needs.

A. Clustering Data

1. Involves grouping information into related categories, a beginning effort to organize and manage information.

2. Data can be clustered into general categories, such as physiological, sociocultural, psychological, and spiritual. Then each category may be further reduced into specific categories, such as nutrition, mobility, elimination, and oxygenation.

3. Data can be easy or difficult to cluster depending on the amount and variety of data collected.

4. Easy to cluster information commonly involves only one body system. For example, a patient reports feeling low abdominal pressure, has not voided in 8 hours, and has abdominal distension on palpation of the suprapubic area; these clinical indicators all relate to urinary elimination and lead to the interpretation that the patient may have urinary retention.

5. Difficult to cluster information may at first seem unrelated because a variety of body systems are involved. For example, a patient has a weak, thready pulse; decreased blood pressure; rapid respirations; pallor; and clammy skin; these clinical indicators cross body systems, but all are related to hypovolemic shock.

6. Inductive reasoning moves from the specific to the general. For example, if you identify that a patient has a temperature and a wound with purulent drainage, you may come to the conclusion that the wound is infected.

7. Deductive reasoning moves from the general to the specific. For example, if you know that a newly admitted patient has a wound infection, you might deduce that the patient will have a temperature, purulent drainage, and a culture and sensitivity laboratory result identifying the causative agent.

8. Data must be clustered before it can be interpreted.

9. Established frameworks are available to provide structure for organizing clustered data.

a. Abraham Maslow's hierarchy of human needs.

b. Marjory Gordon's functional health patterns.

c. NANDA International (formerly the North American Nursing Diagnosis Association), nursing diagnosis taxonomy.

10. Most health-care agencies have their own admission assessment forms, which commonly follow a systems approach to collecting and clustering data.

B. Interpreting Data

1. Interpreting data requires identifying the significance of clustered data.

2. Determining significance requires a comparison of data collected with a wide range of standards and norms (e.g., expected vital signs and laboratory values, growth and development patterns and milestones, and cause and effect relationships). The nurse must then come to a conclusion about a specific identified pattern. It also involves querying evidence, exploring alternatives, and drawing initial conclusions.

3. Conclusions are drawn after the significance of data is determined. Conclusions are the opinions, perceptions, judgments, and inferences that result from the interpretation of data.

4. More data may be necessary to support the initial conclusion. For example, a deviation from any established standard or norm is evidence that points to or supports a conclusion, but more data may be required to increase the validity and reliability of the conclusion. A nurse should ask the following questions:
   a. "Did I miss anything?"
   b. "What else do I need to know?"
   c. "Has the patient's condition or situation changed since I initially assessed the patient?"
   d. "Are there any inconsistent or conflicting data that require clarification?"
   e. "Is my data cluster complete or do I need to collect additional data to better support my conclusion?"

C. Identifying Nursing Diagnoses

1. Introduction to nursing diagnoses.
   a. Nursing diagnoses are statements of specific health problems that nurses are legally allowed to independently identify, prevent, and treat.
   b. They convert an initial conclusion into a diagnostic statement.
   c. They logically link the assessment step to the planning, implementation, and evaluation steps of the nursing process.
   d. NANDA International provides a taxonomy of diagnostic labels and etiologies.
   e. Each nursing diagnosis in the taxonomy follows the same organization for the presentation of information.
      (1) Diagnostic label (title or name): A word or phrase that is based on a pattern of interconnected data. For example, *Impaired skin integrity.*
      (2) Definition: Explains the meaning of the diagnostic label, which differentiates it from similar nursing diagnoses. For example, *Altered epidermis and/or dermis.*
      (3) Defining characteristics: Identifies clinical indicators (signs and symptoms) that support the diagnostic label. For example, *Invasion of body structures, destruction of skin layers (dermis), disruption of skin surface (epidermis).*
      (4) "Related to" factors: Situations, events, or conditions that precede, cause, affect, or are in some way associated with the diagnostic label. For example, *Related to physical immobilization.* The list of related factors in the taxonomy is not all-inclusive because it is impossible to list all possible factors.

MAKING THE CONNECTION

NANDA Taxonomy and a Nursing Diagnosis

A nurse is caring for a newly admitted patient who has paralysis of the legs as a result of a spinal cord injury several years ago. The patient sits in a wheel chair most of the day and lies in the supine position when sleeping. The nurse identifies that the patient has a shallow, round, partial-thickness loss of dermis over the sacrum. The wound bed is red with no evidence of sloughing. The nurse identifies the nursing diagnosis: *Impaired skin integrity* (diagnostic label) *related to physical immobilization* (related to factor). Because the nurse understands that there can be more than one "related to" factor, the nurse includes all the causes of the patient's impaired skin and develops this nursing diagnosis: *Impaired skin integrity related to physical immobilization, altered sensation, and pressure.* The nurse expands the nursing diagnosis to include "secondary to" information to make the etiology clearer. Often, "secondary to" information is a pathophysiological process or medical diagnosis. The new nursing diagnosis is: *Impaired skin integrity related to immobility, altered sensation, and pressure secondary to motor deficits.*

The nurse further expands the nursing diagnosis to include "evidenced by" information to make the etiology even more clear. Often, "evidenced by" information is the clinical indicators (signs and symptoms) included in the defining characteristics in the NANDA taxonomy. The final nursing diagnosis is: *Impaired skin integrity related to inactivity, altered sensation, and pressure secondary to motor deficits as evidenced by the inability to independently move the legs.*

DID YOU KNOW?

Although nursing diagnoses provide a framework for identifying a patient's nursing problems using a standardized nomenclature or language, some professionals believe that they have become too complex and abstract to be useful in everyday practice. As a result, some areas of practice are moving away from using nursing diagnoses.

D. Communicating Patient Nursing Diagnoses, Problems, or Needs
1. Nurses communicate patient nursing diagnoses, problems, or needs in a written plan of care.
2. The plan of care may be kept in a variety of places (e.g., patient's clinical record, the medication administration record, and Kardex).

IV. Planning

Planning, the third step of the nursing process, provides direction for nursing interventions. It is concerned with identifying priorities, establishing goals and expected outcomes, and selecting nursing interventions that will help the patient achieve those goals and expected outcomes. Planning begins when a patient is admitted and is ongoing to meet the changing or emerging needs of the patient. Effective planning includes collaboration with all appropriate health team members to facilitate continuity of care in a patient-centered, individualized, and coordinated manner. Planning culminates in a document about the proposed plan of care that is communicated to all members of the health team.

A. Identifying Priorities
1. A nurse must place a patient's nursing diagnoses, problems, and needs in order of importance when confronted with a variety of patient issues.
2. A nurse must have a strong foundation of scientific theory, knowledge of the commonalities and differences in response to nursing interventions, and theories to determine the priority of a patient's needs.
3. Certain theoretical bases promote the prioritization of care.
   a. Maslow's hierarchy of needs.
      (1) Needs are placed in order from the most basic needs to the highest level needs.
      (2) Physiological is the first level need, followed by safety and security, love and belonging, self-esteem, and self-actualization (see Fig. 1.3, page 7).
   b. Urgency of the health problem.
      (1) Ranks problems based on the degree of threat to the patient's life. The nurse can use the ABCs of assessment (Airway, Breathing, Circulation) when determining priorities.
      (2) A high-priority problem poses the greatest threat and should be addressed first (e.g., an impaired airway).
      (3) A medium-priority problem follows a high-priority problem. It may be related to harmful physiological responses that are not an immediate threat to life (e.g., impaired mobility).
      (4) A low-priority problem should pose the least threats and be ranked last. It may require minimal support (e.g., nausea).
   c. Patient's priorities.
      (1) Ranks patient needs based on what is most important to the patient.
      (2) Although a patient's preference should always be taken into consideration, basic life-threatening needs require urgent interventions and override less important needs.
   d. Future impact of the patient's condition.
      (1) Although a problem might not be life-threatening and is not recognized by the patient as important, the nurse may determine that it can cause future negative consequences if not addressed.
      (2) For example: A nurse identifies that a patient newly diagnosed with type 1 diabetes has dirty feet and is wearing sandals instead of shoes that enclose the feet. The nurse knows that people with diabetes are at risk for foot problems secondary to impaired circulation to the lower extremities. Therefore, the patient has a potential for skin breakdown, which can lead to infection and even amputation. The nurse ranks this issue as a priority and plans interventions to educate the patient about foot care.

B. Identifying Goals and Expected Outcomes
1. Basic concepts.
   a. A goal is a broad, nonspecific statement about the status one expects a patient to achieve.
   b. A goal generally is derived from the "diagnostic label" component of a nursing diagnosis. For example, if a patient has the nursing diagnosis *Ineffective airway clearance related to excessive respiratory secretions,* the goal might be: "The patient will maintain a patent airway."
   c. An outcome identifies a specific change in a patient's condition as a result of nursing interventions. It is commonly influenced by the "related to" component of a nursing diagnosis. Also, it provides criteria to be used in the evaluation phase of the nursing process. For example, the outcome statement using the previously state goal ("The patient will maintain a patent airway") might be: "The patient will expectorate respiratory secretions while hospitalized" (Box 10.1).

Box 10.1 Nursing Outcomes Classification (NOC) System

The Nursing Outcomes Classification (NOC) system is a standardized classification of patient outcomes that respond to nursing interventions. Each NOC outcome has a label, indicators, and measurement scale. The advantages of the NOC system are that it uses language common to all health-care professionals, it is specific, and it identifies indicators with a measurement scale to allow nurses to evaluate patient progress toward an outcome.

Example of NOC outcomes with indicators for *Impaired skin integrity:*

• Tissue integrity: Skin and mucous membranes will be intact as evidenced by the following indicators: Skin intactness/skin lesions/tissue perfusion/skin temperature.
• Rate each indicator of tissue integrity: skin and mucous membranes: 1 = severely compromised, 2 = substantially compromised, 3 = moderately compromised, 4 = mildly compromised, 5 = not compromised.

---

    d. Patients and nurses together should set goals and outcomes to ensure that these goals and outcomes are realistic, achievable, and in alignment with what the patient and nurse want to achieve.

2. Criteria for goals and outcomes.
    a. Be patient centered.
      (1) The patient is the center of the health team; therefore, the patient should be the subject of all goals and outcomes.
      (2) For example, "*The patient* will transfer from the bed to a chair safely within 1 week." Some agencies believe that the words *the patient* are understood and therefore do not include them when stating a goal.
    b. Contain an action verb.
      (1) The goal or outcome should identify the action that the patient will learn, do, or verbalize or the physical status the patient will attain.
      (2) For example: "The patient will *transfer* from the bed to chair safely within 1 week."
    c. Include performance criteria.
      (1) Actions must be specific and measurable. For example, "The patient will *transfer from the bed to chair safely* within 1 week."
      (2) Conditions may be included to describe the kind of assistance or resources needed by the patient. For example, "The patient will transfer from the bed to chair safely *with a one-person assist* within 1 week."
    d. Include a time frame.
      (1) The goal must be achievable within a set time frame.
      (2) For example, "The patient will transfer from the bed to chair safely *within 1 week.*"

Additional examples of time frames include *by discharge, within 24 hours, at all times,* and *will maintain* (the word *maintain* implies continuously).

    e. Be realistic.
      (1) The performance criteria identified must be reasonable and feasible in light of the patient's emotional and physical status.
      (2) Goals are realistic when the outcomes can be achieved in the indicated time frames.
      (3) Example of a realistic outcome for a patient who had abdominal surgery is: "The patient will exhibit bowel sounds within 3 days after surgery."
      (4) Example of an unrealistic outcome for a patient with hemiplegia due to a brain attack is: "The patient will perform active range-of-motion exercises independently within 1 week."

C. Identifying Nursing Interventions
1. Selecting appropriate interventions depends on the accuracy and thoroughness of the data collected.
2. Nursing interventions generally address the "related to" part (etiology) of the patient's problem or nursing diagnosis. For example, if a person is at risk for impaired skin integrity related to urinary incontinence and immobility, the nursing interventions selected should keep the patient clean and dry and relieve pressure.
3. Nursing interventions should include nursing assessments, nursing care to avoid complications, administration of ordered treatments and prescribed medications, and health promotion and illness prevention activities, as appropriate.
4. Selected actions should have the greatest probability of achieving the desired goal/outcome with the least risk to the patient. The nurse must consider:
    a. Cause: Planned action.
    b. Effect: Patient's response.
    c. Risk: Potential for the patient to have a negative consequence as a result of the planned action.
    d. Probability: Degree to which the patient may have a positive consequence as a result of the planned action.
    e. Value of the consequences: Significance of results of the planned action to the patient.
5. Selected interventions should be based on evidence-based practice—that is, interventions that have been proven to be effective based on rigorous scientific evidence and clinical effectiveness studies rather than tradition, intuition, or anecdotal information. Nursing practice based on evidence improves the quality of patient care and justifies nursing interventions (Box 10.2).

| Box 10.2 | **Nursing Interventions Classification (NIC) System** |

The Nursing Interventions Classifications (NIC) system is a standardized classification of nursing interventions. It includes both physiological and psychosocial interventions that can be performed across all nursing disciplines. It consists of intervention labels. Each intervention label has a definition and a list of related nursing actions. The advantages of the NIC system are it uses language common to all health-care professionals, it is specific, and it is based on evidence-based practice.

Example of NIC interventions for pressure ulcer care:
- Pressure ulcer care: Monitor color, temperature, edema, moisture, and appearance of surrounding skin; note characteristics of any drainage.

D. Communicating the Plan of Care
1. Plans of care promote communication and coordination among health team members, improving the continuity of patient care.
2. Information that should be included on a comprehensive plan of care includes:
   a. Patient nursing diagnoses, problems, or needs and related independent and dependent nursing interventions.
   b. Activities of daily living (ADLs) and basic needs.
   c. Medical orders and prescriptions and the nursing interventions required to implement them.
   d. Requirements to prepare the patient for discharge, such as teaching, equipment, and services.
3. Various types of care plans are used.
   a. Computer-generated care plans can be standardized or individualized. The nurse chooses a nursing diagnosis or health problem, and the computer presents potential goals/outcomes and nursing interventions. The nurse can then select interventions that are appropriate for the patient. The computer then generates a written printout of the plan of care.
   b. Multidisciplinary care plans (collaborative care plans, critical pathways) sequence care that is to be delivered each day during a patient's length of stay. Each day has a column and vertical boxes that address specific care that is to be delivered by each health-care discipline.

E. Modifying the Plan of Care
1. Plans of care are dynamic and require modification to keep them current and relevant.
2. The original plan of care may require changes because the original plan was inadequate or inappropriate or because additional assessments provide new information.

3. A plan of care may require modification after the evaluation step of the nursing process when it is identified that the patient did not achieve an expected outcome or because the patient's status improved.

V. Implementation

Implementation, the fourth step of the nursing process, is the actual performance of nursing actions. It is the execution of the plan of care and involves thinking and doing. Therefore, nurses must not only have a strong knowledge base of the sciences, nursing theory, nursing practice, and legal parameters of nursing interventions, but also must have the psychomotor skills to implement procedures safely. Nurses must implement only nursing actions that are described in their state's nurse practice act and conform to professional nursing standards of care.

A. Legal Parameters of Nursing Interventions
1. A nurse must know the legal parameters of nursing interventions, which include:
   a. Dependent nursing interventions.
      (1) Require an order or prescription from a health-care professional with prescriptive privileges (e.g., physicians, podiatrists, dentists, physician's assistants, nurse practitioners).
      (2) Nurses must ensure that ordered interventions and prescribed medications are appropriate to meet the needs of a patient. If a nurse implements an inappropriate order or prescription, the nurse can be held legally accountable as a contributor to the initial error made by the primary health-care provider. Nurses must question inappropriate orders or prescriptions and not follow them blindly.
      (3) Examples of dependent nursing interventions include:
         (a) Administering medications or intravenous solutions.
         (b) Implementing activity orders.
         (c) Inserting or removing a urinary retention catheter.
         (d) Providing a diet.
         (e) Implementing wound or bladder irrigations.
   b. Independent nursing interventions.
      (1) Registered nurses (RNs) can legally order and implement independent nursing interventions without supervision or direction from a person with a prescriptive license.
      (2) Each state's nurse practice act defines the scope of nursing practice within the state.

(3) Examples of independent nursing interventions include:
　(a) Assessing a patient.
　(b) Diagnosing a patient's nursing needs.
　(c) Planning, implementing, and evaluating nursing care.
　(d) Assisting with ADLs.
　(e) Teaching any subject associated with health promotion and illness prevention.
　(f) Counseling.
　(g) Advocating for a patient.
　(h) Encouraging a patient to verbalize fears and feelings.
　(i) Encouraging coughing and deep breathing.
　(j) Referring a patient to community resources.
　c. Interdependent nursing interventions.
　　(1) Nurses work in collaboration with primary health-care providers to implement dependent nursing interventions that have set parameters.
　　(2) Some settings, such as intensive care units and birthing units, have standing orders or protocols that delineate the parameters within which the nurse can implement a dependent nursing intervention.
　　(3) Examples of interdependent nursing interventions include:
　　　(a) An order says, "Out of bed as tolerated." The nurse determines whether the patient is tolerating an activity and therefore the amount of activity in which to engage the patient.
　　　(b) A prescription for a pain medication states, "Acetaminophen (Tylenol) 650 mg every 6 hours for mild lower back pain prn." The nurse assesses the level of the patient's pain and then decides whether to administer the prescribed dose.

B. Types of Nursing Interventions
　1. Assisting with ADLs.
　　a. Nurses assist patients with activities that people perform daily to promote comfort, health, and well-being.
　　b. Problems interfering with these actions can be acute or chronic, temporary or permanent, and require teaching or assistance to restore function.
　　c. Examples include helping a debilitated patient eat, ambulating a patient after surgery, providing range-of-motion exercises, turning and positioning a bed-bound patient, and administering an enema.

2. Teaching.
　a. Nurses provide teaching in relation to the cognitive, psychomotor, and affective domains.
　b. Examples include conducting a class about the signs and symptoms of hyperglycemia (cognitive domain), teaching a patient how to self-administer insulin (psychomotor domain), and facilitating a group session of adolescents discussing and role-playing how to say no when pressured to engage in alcohol or drug use (affective domain).
　c. See Chapter 9, "Teaching and Learning," for more information about the various learning domains and the nurse's role in teaching and learning.
3. Responding to life-threatening events.
　a. Nurses use clinical judgment to identify and respond to life-threatening changes in a patient's condition.
　b. The related interventions generally are associated with meeting a patient's basic physiological needs.
　c. Examples include performing abdominal thrusts for a patient who is choking, implementing cardiopulmonary resuscitation for a patient who has no palpable pulse and is not breathing, and discontinuing a blood transfusion when a patient has clinical indicators of a transfusion reaction.
4. Implementing health promotion and illness prevention activities.
　a. Nurses provide interventions that assist people to maintain health and avoid health problems.
　b. They aim to help people who are at an increased risk for illness because of their developmental level, such as neonates, young children, and older adults. They aim to help people who are at an increased risk for negative consequences of their behaviors, such as people who smoke, drink alcohol excessively, abuse drugs, have multiple sexual partners, or overeat. They also aim to help people limit exacerbations of illnesses and subsequent health problems as a result of an initial illness.
　c. Examples include administering a vaccine, teaching a class about healthy nutrition, promoting smoking cessation or weight reduction, using standard precautions, and turning and positioning an immobile patient.
5. Performing technical skills.
　a. Nurses must competently perform technical psychomotor skills associated with a procedure.
　b. The nurse should know the steps, principles, rationales, and expected outcomes relative to

nursing procedures to implement them in the appropriate situation safely.

  c. Examples include administering medications via various routes, suctioning a patient's respiratory tract, changing a wound dressing, and irrigating a colostomy.

6. Employing psychosociocultural interventions.

  a. Nurses use therapeutic interviewing techniques to encourage patients to ventilate feelings and concerns. Once the nurse identifies a patient's emotional needs, the nurse continues to support the patient emotionally while exploring potential coping strategies. In addition, the nurse uses interpersonal interventions when working as an advocate for the patient, coordinating health-care activities, and collaborating with others on the patient's behalf.

  b. Examples include using nondirective interviewing techniques, gently addressing a patient's behavior, collaborating with a patient to identify a goal, and explaining to family members that their loved one's angry behavior is associated with the anger stage of grieving in response to the diagnosis of cancer.

7. Delegating, supervising, and evaluating delegated nursing interventions.

  a. Nurses may delegate nursing care to:

  (1) Unlicensed assistive nursing personnel.

    (a) Uncomplicated, basic interventions.

    (b) Examples: Bathing a bed-bound patient, ambulating a stable postoperative patient, obtaining vital signs from patients who are stable.

  (2) Licensed practical nurse (LPN).

    (a) Routine nursing care for patients who are stable and whose care is uncomplicated.

    (b) Examples: Administering medications, changing a sterile dressing, instilling an enema.

  (3) Registered nurse (RN).

    (a) Complex nursing interventions.

    (b) Examples: Performing a physical assessment, teaching a patient how to self-administer insulin, formulating a patient's plan of care.

  b. The nurse delegating care is responsible for:

  (1) Assuming responsibility for the care that is delegated and its consequences.

  (2) Ensuring that the person implementing the care is legally permitted to provide the delegated care, is knowledgeable, and is able to deliver the care safely.

  (3) Ensuring that the care is implemented according to standards of care.

(4) Evaluating the patient's responses to the interventions implemented.

8. Reporting and documenting nursing interventions and patient responses.

  a. Nurses communicate information verbally and in writing to other members of the health team to provide continuity of patient care. Written documentation also establishes a permanent legal record of the care provided and the patient's response.

  b. Examples include documenting vital signs on a patient's graphic record, indicating the characteristics of a patient's skin integrity on a pressure ulcer flow sheet, providing a verbal report regarding the status of patients to a nurse arriving for the next shift, and documenting the administration of medications and patient responses to medications.

🛑 c. If interventions are not documented, they are considered not done.

VI. Evaluation

Evaluation, the fifth step of the nurse process, involves issues related to structure, process, and patient outcomes. The nurse first reassess the patient to identify patient responses to interventions (actual outcomes) and then compares the actual outcomes with expected outcomes to determine goal achievement. It is a continuous process that requires the plan of care to be modified as often as necessary either during or after care.

A. **Components of Evaluation of the Delivery of Nursing Care**

1. Structure.

  a. Associated with the setting and effect of organizational features on the quality or excellence of nursing care.

  b. Based on such things as policy and procedures, economic resources, available equipment, and the number, credentials, and experiential background of members of the nursing team.

  c. Example of a structure goal against which the delivery of nursing care can be assessed: *Use a controller pump for administration of intravenous medication.*

2. Process.

  a. Associated with evaluation of clinical performance of nursing team members.

  b. Example of a process goal against which the care delivered by a nurse can be assessed: *Provide for patient privacy by pulling the curtain and draping the patient when assessing a patient's wound.*

3. Patient outcome.
   a. Associated with measurable changes in a patient's status as a result of care implemented by a nurse.
   b. Example of an expected patient outcome against which an actual patient outcome can be assessed: *The patient's skin will remain clean, dry, and intact.*

B. Types of Evaluation Activities
1. Routine evaluations.
   a. Occur at preset regular time frames.
   b. For example, obtaining patients' vital signs every shift; documenting intake and output every shift and every 24 hours.
2. Ongoing evaluations.
   a. Occur during and immediately after administering nursing care or after interacting with a patient.
   b. For example, assessing a patient's response to irrigation of a colostomy; determining whether a patient understands the content in a teaching session.
3. Intermittent evaluations.
   a. Occur in specific situations.
   b. For example, obtaining daily weights to monitor a patient receiving a diuretic; assessing the degree of pain relief after a patient receives an analgesic.
4. Terminal evaluations.
   a. Occur in preparation for a patient's discharge; health-care agencies generally have a comprehensive discharge form that provides structure and consistency within an agency.
   b. For example, evaluating a patient's physical and emotional status; determining progress toward goal/outcome achievement; and formulating a plan of care to be implemented in the community setting, including topics such as medications, treatments, diet, and scheduled follow-up care.

C. Nursing Interventions to Ensure Thorough Evaluation of Patient Responses to Nursing Care
1. Reassess the patient to identify actual outcomes (patient responses).
   a. The nurse must reassess the patient to collect data, organize the data, and determine the significance of the data.
   b. Actual outcomes are then compared to the expected outcomes identified in the written plan of care to determine whether the patient successfully achieved the goals/outcomes.
2. Compare an actual outcome with an expected outcome to determine goal achievement.
   a. If they are the same, then the nurse can infer that the nursing care was effective in assisting the patient to achieve the expected outcome. In other words, a positive evaluation is indicated when an actual outcome meets the expected outcome.
   b. If they are not the same, then the nurse can infer that the nursing care was not effective in assisting the patient to achieve the expected outcome. In other words, a negative evaluation is indicated when an actual outcome does not meet the expected outcome.
   c. Once it is determined that the expected outcome was not achieved, the nurse must analyze factors that may have affected the actual outcomes of care.
3. Analyze factors that may have influenced nonachievement of expected goals/outcomes.
   a. Each step of the nursing process must be examined to determine what contributed to the failure to achieve expected goals/outcomes. For example, the nurse must ask important questions such as:
      (1) Was the data cluster thorough and accurate?
      (2) Was the nursing diagnosis, problem, or need identified correctly?
      (3) Was the goal realistic and attainable?
      (4) Were the expected outcomes specific and measurable?
      (5) Did the planned interventions address all the etiological factors of the problem?
      (6) Were the nursing interventions consistently implemented as planned?
   b. The specific reason for not achieving a goal/expected outcome should be identified. A variety of reasons may have influenced the nonachievement of a goal/expected outcome. For example, the patient might not have shared important information, the staff might not have completed all tasks as planned, the patient might not have been motivated to participate adequately in the planned care, the patient's condition may have changed.

D. Modifying the Plan of Care
1. Plans of care are dynamic and require modification to keep them current and relevant.
2. The plan of care must be modified as soon as a nurse identifies that a plan of care is ineffective.
3. The plan will have to be modified when an expected goal/outcome is met. Goals and expected outcomes advance to address evolving needs as the patient moves toward health on the health-illness continuum.
4. Once a new plan of care is implemented, the step of evaluation beings again.

CASE STUDY: Putting It All Together

A primary nurse is admitting an older adult to a surgical unit before surgery for prostate cancer. The primary health-care provider tells the nurse that the patient was admitted early to ensure that the patient is well hydrated and that electrolytes are within the expected range in preparation for surgery. The nurse assesses the patient and collects the following information:

a. Skin is pale, dry, warm, intact, and tenting when pinched.

b. Capillary refill is delayed and nail beds are pale.

c. Vital signs are: apical pulse 95 beats/minute, respirations 23 breaths/minute with a slight expiratory wheeze; temperature 97.8°F using a temporal scanner thermometer (infrared sensor), and blood pressure 160/86 mm Hg.

d. Vesicular breath sounds are present.

e. Hyperactive bowel sounds are present.

f. Slight abdominal distension is present over the suprapubic area.

g. Tympany is noted on percussion of the abdomen.

h. No lower extremity edema is present.

i. Speech is rapid and at times tremulous.

j. Patient appears clean and well groomed, with an absence of body and breath odor.

When the nurse interviews the patient, the patient's wife remains at the bedside at the patient's request. The nurse documents the following information on the nursing admission history and physical:

The patient explained, "I've been taking Hytrin 2 mg at bedtime for the past six months because I was getting up so many times at night to urinate. I started to feel bloated and uncomfortable in the abdominal area several weeks ago and did not feel that I completely emptied my bladder after urinating. I finally went to the doctor, who ran tests and said I have prostate cancer." The patient then explained that his doctor then referred him to an urologist, who planned to do a total prostatectomy in the morning. The patient stated, "Sometimes I need to go to the bathroom and I don't make it in time and I wet myself. It's embarrassing and I feel terrible. I'm afraid that I might become impotent and have incontinence after the surgery, but I trust the urologist and recognized that the surgery is necessary." The patient asked many questions about what he can expect after surgery, which were answered. He said, "Having cancer puts a big monkey wrench into my retirement plans. I hope I'll live long enough to do a little traveling." The wife stated, "I don't care if we can't travel. I don't want him to die. Also, he forgot to tell you that he is always tired because he keeps getting up at night to go to the bathroom." During the interview, the patient went to the bathroom and voided 200 mL of dark amber urine. A urine specimen was sent to the laboratory for a urinalysis. After the interview the nurse obtained a drug handbook and reviewed the side effects of Hytrin.

Case Study Questions

A. Identify the data that were collected using the following assessment techniques:

1. Inspection

a. _____

b. _____

c. _____

d. _____

e. _____

2. Auscultation

a. _____

b. _____

c. _____

d. _____

e. _____

3. Percussion

a. _____

Continued

CASE STUDY: Putting It All Together *cont'd*

———————————— **Case Study Questions** ————————————

4. Palpation

a. _____

b. _____

c. _____

d. _____

B. Identify the subjective data collected by the nurse during the patient interview.

1. _____

2. _____

3. _____

4. _____

5. _____

6. _____

7. _____

C. Identify whether the patient, wife, primary health-care provider, nurse, and volunteer are primary, secondary, or tertiary sources of data.

1. _____

2. _____

3. _____

4. _____

5. _____

D. Identify the *related to* and *secondary to* factors of the presented nursing diagnostic labels.

1. Risk for urinary retention related to _____ secondary to _____ .

2. Fear of impotence and incontinence related to _____ secondary to _____ .

3. Disturbed sleep pattern related to _____ secondary to _____ .

4. Situational low self-esteem related to _____ secondary to _____ .

5. Urge incontinence related to _____ secondary to _____ .

REVIEW QUESTIONS

1. Which activity is the nurse engaged in when identifying a nursing diagnosis?
   1. Discovering causes of diseases
   2. Documenting desired expected outcomes
   3. Planning care to meet nursing needs of a patient
   4. Identifying human responses to actual or potential health problems

2. Which is the **most** important outcome of the nursing process?
   1. Meet the nursing needs of each patient.
   2. Ensure that unit resources are allocated appropriately.
   3. Decrease the risk of an error regarding the admitting medical diagnosis.
   4. Reduce the risk of missing important data when collecting information about the patient.

3. Which nursing action is an example of the assessment step of the nursing process?
   1. Administering pain medication for a headache
   2. Taking a patient's blood pressure after ambulating
   3. Communicating information obtained from an interview
   4. Determining if a patient tolerated the change from a soft to a regular diet

4. Which action is associated with the evaluation step of the nursing process?
   1. A nurse takes the vital signs when a patient reports chest pain.
   2. A nurse determines that a patient is at risk for impaired skin integrity because of reduced mobility and malnutrition.
   3. A nurse and patient decide that within 3 days the patient will learn how to draw up and self-administer insulin safely.
   4. A nurse determines that further intervention is necessary when the patient experiences sacral edema after being turned and positioned every 2 hours.

5. A patient became short of breath and reported sudden chest pain while being transferred from the bed to a chair for the first time after surgery for a fractured hip. The nurse immediately returned the patient to bed, raised the head of the bed and started oxygen at 2 L via nasal cannula. Which step of the nursing process was **most** important in this scenario?
   1. Planning
   2. Assessing
   3. Evaluating
   4. Diagnosing

6. A 12-year-old child is transferred from the emergency department to the pediatric unit. The nurse on the pediatric unit reviews the emergency department summary note, performs an assessment, and interviews the parent.

Patient's Clinical Record

Emergency Department Summary

12-year-old child arrived in the emergency department with her mother who states her daughter has had nausea and diarrhea for 2 days. Mother reports her daughter had an oral temperature of 100°F that increased to 101.2°F today and is thirsty, but is afraid to drink fluids. Presently the temperature is 101.4°F; pulse is 72 and regular; respirations are 22 breaths per minute; blood pressure is 126/82. Child is lethargic, skin is pale and dry, and oral mucous membranes are dry. Stool specimen sent for culture and sensitivity. CBC and electrolyte panel pending. IV line inserted with normal saline infusing at 50 mL per hour. Institute oral rehydration therapy per hospital protocol.

Vital Signs on Admission to the Pediatric Unit

Temperature:	101.4°F
Pulse:	76 and regular
Respirations:	20 breaths per minute
Blood pressure:	130/78 mm Hg

Progress Notes

Mother states: "I can't believe how sick she got in such a short time. She's had nausea for several days, but the diarrhea started with a vengeance the day before yesterday. The diarrhea was so bad that she turned herself inside out. She's been afraid to drink anything because she doesn't want to throw up. I finally brought her to the hospital because I didn't know what to do for her."

What must the nurse do **next**?
   1. Institute the oral rehydration protocol.
   2. Continue to monitor the child's vital signs.
   3. Formulate a plan of care to meet the child's needs.
   4. Cluster data that have a significant interrelationship.

7. A home-care nurse identifies that a home environment is dirty and the patient's spouse appears tired and unkempt. The patient and spouse are still in pajamas, even though it is 2:00 in the afternoon. The nurse determines that these cues may indicate caregiver role strain. Which type of reasoning has the nurse used?
   1. Socratic
   2. Intuitive
   3. Inductive
   4. Deductive

8. Which statement reflects deductive reasoning?
   1. Specific information suggests a general conclusion.
   2. Research findings support the development of a theory.
   3. A suspicion moves toward identifying a clinical manifestation.
   4. Various nursing interventions are implemented until one is successful.

9. A nurse understands that inadequate activity, dietary fiber, and/or fluid intake can result in constipation. As a result, the nurse asks a patient who has hemiplegia as a result of a recent brain attack (cerebral vascular accident), "When was the last time you had a bowel movement?" Which type of reasoning has the nurse used when asking this question?
   1. Socratic
   2. Intuitive
   3. Inductive
   4. Deductive

10. A patient is admitted to the emergency department with epigastric pain. The nurse asks the patient to identify the intensity of pain using a scale of 0 to 10, with 0 being pain free and 10 reflecting excruciating pain. Which step of the nursing process does this action reflect?
    1. Analysis
    2. Planning
    3. Assessment
    4. Implementation

11. A nurse anticipates that a patient who is experiencing left hemiparesis is at risk for a plantar flexion contracture of the left foot. Which skill is the nurse using when assessing the patient for this contracture?
    1. Intuitive thinking
    2. Inductive reasoning
    3. Scientific problem-solving
    4. Trial-and-error problem-solving

12. A nurse identifies the following desired outcome: "The patient will walk 30 feet twice a day without exhibiting the signs and symptoms of activity intolerance." Which step of the nursing process does this statement reflect?
    1. Planning
    2. Assessing
    3. Evaluating
    4. Implementing

13. A nurse determines a patient's flat neck veins, inadequate skin turgor, decreased blood pressure, and dry mucous membranes are a cluster of data that is significant. Which step of the nursing process is involved when the nurse comes to this conclusion?
    1. Analysis
    2. Evaluation
    3. Assessment
    4. Implementation

14. List the following nursing interventions in the order representing the steps of the nursing process beginning with the first step and progressing to the last step.
    1. Obtaining a list of the patient's allergies
    2. Concluding that a patient has a deficient fluid volume
    3. Administering a prescribed enema to a patient who is constipated
    4. Assessing a patient's level of pain after administering an opioid analgesic
    5. Identify nursing interventions that should be implemented to meet a patient's needs
    Answer: _____

15. A nurse is evaluating a patient's response 30 minutes after administering morphine 10 mg Sub-Q. Which type of evaluation is the nurse implementing?
    1. Routine
    2. Ongoing
    3. Terminal
    4. Intermittent

16. A nurse identified the following expected outcome for a patient: "The patient will report incisional pain equal to or less than level 3 using a pain scale of 0 to 10 within 30 minutes of receiving acetaminophen (Tylenol)." Which step of the nursing process did the nurse complete?
    1. Planning
    2. Evaluation
    3. Assessment
    4. Implementation

17. A patient says, "I asked to go to the hospital because I am seeing double and everything is very blurry." Which kind of data is the patient describing?
    1. Objective data
    2. Subjective data
    3. Tertiary source of data
    4. Secondary source of data

18. The day after surgery, a patient says to the nurse, "Since surgery yesterday, I have been having bloody urine." Which type of data is this information?
    1. Objective data
    2. Subjective data
    3. Tertiary source of data
    4. Secondary source of data

19. A nurse formulates the following goal with a patient: "The patient will ambulate in the hall without experiencing activity intolerance." Which statements address the status of this goal? **Select all that apply.**
    1. _____ It is not measurable.
    2. _____ It is missing a parameter.
    3. _____ It is not patient-centered.
    4. _____ It is missing a target time.
    5. _____ It is a correctly written goal.

20. Which nurse is demonstrating the planning phase of the nursing process?
    1. A nurse who collaborates with a patient in designing a goal
    2. A nurse who observes that a patient's urine is dark amber
    3. A nurse who identifies a cluster of data as significant
    4. A nurse who provides a backrub to induce sleep

21. A patient reports to a nurse that an "accident" occurred and that the bed is wet with urine. What step in the nursing process is **most** associated with bathing the patient and changing the linen?
    1. Planning
    2. Evaluation
    3. Assessment
    4. Implementation

22. A nurse is about to administer a medication to a patient when the patient states, "I really have a hard time getting that big pill down." The nurse responds, "How about if I crush it and mix it with applesauce?" Which step of the nursing process is associated with the nurse's response?
    1. Analysis
    2. Planning
    3. Assessment
    4. Implementation

23. A nurse assists a patient to ambulate from the bed to the bathroom and back to a chair. Which step of the nursing process is associated with taking the patient's vital signs 3 minutes later?
    1. Analysis
    2. Diagnosis
    3. Evaluation
    4. Assessment

24. A nurse is collecting a health history from a patient newly admitted to the hospital. Which action associated with the data collection step of the nursing process is **most** important?
    1. Explaining to the patient's spouse that the patient's input is more significant than the spouse's input
    2. Communicating subjective data using the patient's words
    3. Using only nondirective interviewing techniques
    4. Collecting primarily objective data

25. A nurse is assessing a patient. What information collected by the nurse reflects subjective information?
    1. Clammy skin
    2. Agitated behavior
    3. Numbness of the feet
    4. Coughing after a deep breath

26. Which statement reflects inductive reasoning?
    1. Implementing various actions until one is successful
    2. Supporting the development of a theory with research
    3. Moving from specific information to a general conclusion
    4. Identifying a cue based on a suspicion or feeling without conscious analysis

27. A nurse is assessing a patient. What clinical manifestation experienced by the patient is an example of objective information?
    1. Edema
    2. Heartburn
    3. Chest pain
    4. Lightheadedness

28. Which action by a nurse is associated with the evaluation step of the nursing process?
    1. Teaching Kegel exercises to improve bladder control
    2. Securing an order for physical therapy to increase strength and endurance
    3. Having the patient use a voiding record to establish a pattern of elimination
    4. Exploring the patient's degree of satisfaction related to urinary control interventions

29. A patient has a prescription for levothyroxine 75 mcg by mouth once a day to treat hypothyroidism. The patient's previous prescription was for 25 mcg by mouth once a day. The patient wants to use up the previous tablets before filling the new prescription. The nurse teaches the patient how many tablets of the previous prescription to take. How many tablets does the patient have to take for the nurse to identify that the patient understands the teaching? Record your answer using a whole number.

Answer: _____ tablets

30. A nurse is assessing a patient for objective and subjective data. Which information should the nurse document in the patient's clinical record as subjective?
1. The patient is crying.
2. The patient is diaphoretic.
3. The patient has a bounding pulse.
4. The patient has numbness of the right hand.

REVIEW ANSWERS

1. ANSWER: 4.

Rationales:

1. Identifying the cause of disease is the responsibility of the primary health-care provider, not the nurse.

2. Identifying desired expected outcomes is part of the planning phase of the nursing process.

3. Nursing orders are associated with the planning phase of the nursing process.

4. Identifying human responses to actual or potential health problems is the definition of a nursing diagnosis. This is part of the analysis step of the nursing process.

Content Area: Nursing Process
Integrated Processes: Communication/Documentation; Nursing Process: Analysis
Client Need: Safe and Effective Care Environment; Management of Care
Cognitive Level: Comprehension

2. ANSWER: 1.

Rationales:

1. The nurse is responsible for identifying and meeting the nursing needs of each patient. Nurses identify and treat human responses to disease, illness, or injury.

2. Ensuring that unit resources are allocated appropriately is the purpose of a patient classification system that identifies the acuity of patient needs for all the patients on a unit and the amount of resources needed to provide appropriate nursing care.

3. Determining the admitting medical diagnosis is the responsibility of the primary health-care provider, not the nurse. Nurses do not make medical diagnoses.

4. A classification system, such as Gordon's functional health patterns, is a framework used by a nurse to organize the collection of important data about a patient.

TEST-TAKING TIP: Identify the word in the stem that sets a priority. The word *most* in the stem sets a priority.

Content Area: Nursing Process
Integrated Processes: Communication/Documentation; Nursing Process: Evaluation
Client Need: Safe and Effective Care Environment; Management of Care
Cognitive Level: Comprehension

3. ANSWER: 3.

Rationales:

1. Completing a nursing action, such as administering pain medication for a headache, is part of the implementation step of the nursing process.

2. Taking a patient's blood pressure after ambulating is part of the evaluation step of the nursing process.

3. Communicating information obtained from an interview is part of the assessment step of the nursing process.

4. Determining a patient's response to an intervention is part of the evaluation step of the nursing process.

Content Area: Nursing Process
Integrated Processes: Nursing Process: Assessment
Client Need: Safe and Effective Care Environment; Management of Care
Cognitive Level: Application

4. ANSWER: 4.

Rationales:

1. Taking a patient's vital signs in response to a patient's report of chest pain is an example of assessment.

2. Determining that a patient is at risk for impaired skin integrity because of reduced mobility and malnutrition is associated with the analysis/diagnosis step of the nursing process. Making a nursing diagnosis is associated with identifying human responses and contributing factors to illness, disease, or injury.

3. Identifying a desired outcome is part of the planning step of the nursing process.

4. Revising a plan of care in response to a patient not achieving a desired outcome (absence of signs and symptoms of pressure when turning and positioning a patient every 2 hours) is part of the evaluation step of the nursing process.

Content Area: Nursing Process
Integrated Processes: Nursing Process: Evaluation
Client Need: Safe and Effective Care Environment; Management of Care
Cognitive Level: Application

5. ANSWER: 3.

Rationales:

1. This scenario is not an example of the planning step of the nursing process. The planning step involves identifying goals, outcomes, and nursing interventions.

2. This scenario is not an example of the assessment step of the nursing process. Assessment is the systematic collection, validation, and documentation of data. The assessment step of the nursing process does not include the assessment that is done for the purpose of comparing actual outcomes to desired outcomes.

3. The nurse's actions were based on an evaluation of the patient's response to the nursing care being delivered. The reassessment of the patient and comparing the actual outcome to desired outcome is considered evaluation.

4. This scenario does not reflect the diagnosing step of the nursing process. However, eventually the nurse will have to progress to identifying an appropriate nursing diagnosis for this patient's changed condition.

TEST-TAKING TIP: Identify the word in the stem that sets a priority. The word *most* in the stem sets a priority.

Content Area: Nursing Process
Integrated Processes: Nursing Process: Evaluation
Client Need: Safe and Effective Care Environment; Management of Care
Cognitive Level: Analysis

6. ANSWER: 4.

Rationales:

1. Although this should be done eventually, there is something the nurse should do before this intervention.

2. Although this will be done eventually, it should be part of the patient's plan of care.

3. The plan of care cannot be formulated until the collected data are grouped significantly and a conclusion is made regarding the patient's needs.

4. The nursing process begins with the collection of data. The next step is to analyze the data and cluster significant

information to arrive at the patient's nursing diagnosis or priority needs. A nursing assessment and analysis of data corroborates the assessment and plan of action of the medical members of the health team.

TEST-TAKING TIP: Identify the word in the stem that sets a priority. The word *next* in the stem sets a priority.
Content Area: Nursing Process
Integrated Processes: Nursing Process: Assessment
Client Need: Safe and Effective Care Environment; Management of Care
Cognitive Level: Analysis

7. **ANSWER: 3.**
Rationales:
1. The nurse's conclusion does not rely on Socratic reasoning. Socratic reasoning is best used when searching for inconsistencies, examining multiple points of view, and when separating what is known from what one believes.
2. The reasoning used by the nurse does not rely on intuition. Intuition is based on recognition of a pattern or cue based on clinical experience that supports a suspicion or feeling without using conscious reasoning.
3. This scenario is an example of inductive reasoning. Inductive reasoning is used when certain information suggests an interpretation. It moves from specific information to a conclusion. If the nurse identifies a certain pattern of data and comes to a conclusion about the data, the nurse is using inductive reasoning. In this scenario the nurse identified specific information (dirty environment, spouse appears tired and unkempt) that supported a general conclusion (caregiver role strain) moving from the specific to the general.
4. Moving from a general premise to identifying data that supports the premise is an example of deductive reasoning. For example, if the nurse is concerned about caregiver role strain, the nurse should collect data to support this premise.
TEST-TAKING TIP: Identify the options that are opposites. Options 3 and 4 are opposites. Inductive reasoning moves from the specific to the general while deductive reasoning moves from the general to the specific.
Content Area: Nursing Process
Integrated Processes: Nursing Process: Analysis
Client Need: Safe and Effective Care Environment; Management of Care
Cognitive Level: Analysis

8. **ANSWER: 2.**
Rationales:
1. When a person identifies specific data and then arrives at a conclusion based on the data, the person is using inductive reasoning.
2. A research finding that support the development of a theory is an example of deductive reasoning. Deductive reasoning moves from a general premise to specific information.
3. A suspicion moving toward identifying a clinical manifestation is an example of intuitive thinking.
4. Implementing various nursing interventions until one is successful explains the process of trial-and-error reasoning.
Content Area: Nursing Process
Integrated Processes: Nursing Process: Analysis

Client Need: Safe and Effective Care Environment; Management of Care
Cognitive Level: Knowledge

9. **ANSWER: 4.**
Rationales:
1. The question in the scenario does not rely on Socratic reasoning. Socratic reasoning is best used when searching for inconsistencies, examining multiple points of view, and when separating what is known from what one believes.
2. The question in the scenario does not rely on intuition. Intuition is based on recognition of a pattern or cue based on clinical experience that supports a suspicion or feeling without using conscious reasoning.
3. The question in the scenario does not rely on inductive reasoning. Inductive reasoning moves from specific information to a generalized conclusion
4. Deductive reasoning moves from a general premise to seeking data to support the premise. The question asked in the scenario will elicit specific information as it relates to the general premise that reduced activity will increase the risk of constipation.
TEST-TAKING TIP: Identify the options that are opposites. Options 3 and 4 are opposites. Inductive reasoning moves from the specific to the general while deductive reasoning moves from the general to the specific.
Content Area: Nursing Process
Integrated Processes: Communication/Documentation; Nursing Process: Assessment
Client Need: Safe and Effective Care Environment; Management of Care
Cognitive Level: Analysis

10. **ANSWER: 3.**
Rationales:
1. Analysis is the second step of the nursing process. Analysis of information occurs after information is collected during the first step of the nursing process, assessment.
2. A plan of care is formulated after nursing assessments are conducted and conclusions made about the information collected.
3. Assessment is the first step in the nursing process, which involves the collection of information.
4. Nursing care is implemented after a plan of care is formulated in the planning step of the nursing process.
Content Area: Nursing Process
Integrated Processes: Communication/Documentation; Nursing Process: Assessment
Client Need: Safe and Effective Care Environment; Management of Care
Cognitive Level: Analysis

11. **ANSWER: 2.**
Rationales:
1. Intuitive thinking is a form of guessing based on a "feeling" about something. It does not use conscious reasoning or a scientific approach to arrive at a conclusion.
2. Inductive reasoning is used when certain information suggests an interpretation. It moves from specific data to a generalized conclusion about the data.

3. Scientific problem-solving is a systematic seven step process that starts with problem hypothesis; moves consecutively to data collection, hypothesis formation, plan of action, hypothesis testing, and interpretation of results; and ends with evaluation.

4. Trial-and-error problem-solving relates to the testing of multiple solutions until one is found to work for the identified problem.

Content Area: Nursing Process
Integrated Processes: Nursing Process: Assessment
Client Need: Safe and Effective Care Environment; Management of Care
Cognitive Level: Analysis

12. ANSWER: 1.

Rationales:

1. Identifying desired outcomes and planning actions to assist the patient in achieving the outcomes occurs in the planning step of the nursing process.

2. The assessment step includes the collection of data via physical assessment and interviewing.

3. Evaluation occurs when an actual patient outcome is compared to an expected patient outcome in an effort to determine if nursing actions have achieved the desired outcome.

4. The implementation step of the nursing process is when the nurse puts into action planned nursing interventions.

Content Area: Nursing Process
Integrated Processes: Communication/Documentation; Nursing Process: Analysis
Client Need: Safe and Effective Care Environment; Management of Care
Cognitive Level: Application

13. ANSWER: 1.

Rationales:

1. During the analysis step of the nursing process, data are critically analyzed and interpreted; cues and clusters of cues are compared to a theoretical knowledge base; inferences are made and validated; and goals and objectives are identified and prioritized.

2. The scenario in the stem does not reflect the evaluation step of the nursing process. Evaluation occurs when actual outcomes are compared to expected outcomes and establish whether the care provided reflects goal achievement or nonachievement.

3. The scenario in the stem does not reflect the assessment step of the nursing process. Assessment occurs when the nurse uses all the senses to collect data via interviewing, observation, auscultation, percussion, and palpation.

4. The scenario in the stem does not reflect the implementation step of the nursing process. The implementation step of the nursing process occurs when nursing care is delivered as planned.

Content Area: Nursing Process
Integrated Processes: Nursing Process: Analysis
Client Need: Safe and Effective Care Environment; Management of Care
Cognitive Level: Application

14. ANSWER: 1, 2, 5, 3, 4.

Rationales:

1. Collecting data from the patient is a form of assessment. Assessment is the first step of the nursing process.

2. Coming to a conclusion about collected data is part of the analysis step of the nursing process. Analysis is the second step of the nursing process.

5. Identifying nursing interventions that should be implemented is related to the planning step of the nursing process. Planning is the third step of the nursing process.

3. Administering an enema is the performance of a procedure. Procedures that require direct patient care are part of the implementation step of the nursing process. Implementation is the fourth step of the nursing process.

4. Determining a patient's response to a medication is part of the evaluation step of the nursing process. Evaluation of care is the fifth step of the nursing process.

Content Area: Nursing Process
Integrated Processes: Nursing Process: Analysis
Client Need: Safe and Effective Care Environment; Management of Care
Cognitive Level: Analysis

15. ANSWER: 2.

Rationales:

1. Routine evaluation is when patients vital signs are monitored every shift. It is not in response to a specific nursing intervention.

2. Ongoing evaluations occur during and immediately after administering nursing care or after interacting with a patient.

3. Terminal evaluations occur as the nurse implements the final evaluation just before discharge from a unit or facility. Health-care agencies generally have specific discharge forms that address an evaluation of the patient's status (progress toward goal/outcome achievement) and standing medication prescriptions and treatments.

4. Intermittent evaluation occurs at a specific time; for example, daily weights in response to a specific health problem and weekly skin assessments in a long-term care facility.

Content Area: Nursing Process
Integrated Processes: Nursing Process: Evaluation
Client Need: Safe and Effective Care Environment; Management of Care
Cognitive Level: Application

16. ANSWER: 1.

Rationales:

1. This is an expected outcome included in a patient's plan of care that involves the step of planning.

2. Evaluation is comparing a patient's planned outcome to the actual outcome identified after nursing care is implemented; evaluation activities do not include the formulation of expected outcomes.

3. Assessment is the first step in the nursing process and mainly involves collecting and clustering data; assessment activities do not include the formulation of expected outcomes.

4. Implementation is when a nurse employs various nursing interventions to assist a patient to achieve an expected

outcome; evaluation activities do not include the formulation of expected outcomes.
Content Area: Nursing Process
Integrated Processes: Communication/Documentation;
Nursing Process: Planning
Client Need: Safe and Effective Care Environment;
Management of Care
Cognitive Level: Analysis

17. **ANSWER: 2.**
Rationales:
1. The data in the statement are not objective data. Objective data are measurable, observable, or verifiable.
2. These are subjective data because only the patient can report feelings and sensations.
3. A tertiary source of data refers to sources such as a textbook, policy or procedure manual, dictionary, or medical or nursing journals.
4. A secondary source is a person who provides supplemental information about a patient.
TEST-TAKING TIP: Identify the options that are opposites. Options 1 and 2 are opposites. More often than not, options that are opposites are the correct answer. Examine options 1 and 2 carefully.
Content Area: Nursing Process
Integrated Processes: Communication/Documentation;
Nursing Process: Assessment
Client Need: Safe and Effective Care Environment;
Management of Care
Cognitive Level: Analysis

18. **ANSWER: 1.**
Rationales:
1. Hematuria is objective information because it is measurable, observable, or verifiable.
2. Subjective data are information that only the patient can report, such as feelings, sensations, or concerns.
3. A patient is a primary, not tertiary source of information. Tertiary sources of data refer to sources such as a textbook, research studies, nursing journals, or policy or procedure manuals.
4. The patient is a primary, not secondary source of data. A secondary source is someone other than the patient, such as a family member or friend.
TEST-TAKING TIP: Identify the options that are opposites. Options 1 and 2 are opposites. More often than not, options that are opposites are the correct answer. Examine options 1 and 2 carefully.
Content Area: Nursing Process
Integrated Processes: Communication/Documentation;
Nursing Process: Assessment
Client Need: Safe and Effective Care Environment;
Management of Care
Cognitive Level: Application

19. **ANSWER: 1, 2, 4.**
Rationales:
1. The words "activity intolerance" are vague. Although activity intolerance often is defined as a respiratory rate greater than 24 breaths/minute and a pulse rate greater than 95 beats/minute after 3 minutes of rest after activity,
it is not included in the goal; for example: *as evidenced by a respiratory rate below 24 breaths/minute and a pulse rate of less than 94 beats/minute.* In addition, it does not identify how many feet the patient should ambulate.
2. The goal does not identify how many feet the patient should ambulate; this is an important parameter that is missing in this goal.
3. The goal is patient-centered. It begins with: *The patient will.*
4. The goal does not identify how many times a day the patient should ambulate in the hall.
5. This goal is not correctly written. It should read: The patient will ambulate in the hall 50 feet three times a day without experiencing activity intolerance, as evidenced by a pulse rate below 94 beats/minute and a respiratory rate below 24 breaths/minute after 3 minutes of rest after ambulating.
Content Area: Nursing Process
Integrated Processes: Communication/Documentation;
Nursing Process: Analysis
Client Need: Safe and Effective Care Environment;
Management of Care
Cognitive Level: Analysis

20. **ANSWER: 1.**
Rationales:
1. Identifying goals, outcomes, and planned interventions all are part of the planning step of the nursing process.
2. Identifying urine as dark amber is part of the assessment phase; in addition, it may be part of the evaluation phase of the nursing process if the assessment is made after providing care.
3. Determining the significance of data occurs during the analysis step of the nursing process.
4. Providing nursing care occurs in the implementation phase of the nursing process.
Content Area: Nursing Process
Integrated Processes: Communication/Documentation;
Nursing Process: Planning
Client Need: Safe and Effective Care Environment;
Management of Care
Cognitive Level: Application

21. **ANSWER: 4.**
Rationales:
1. Bathing a patient and changing the linen are not part of the planning step of the nursing process. Planning involves identifying goals, outcomes, and interventions designed to meet patient needs.
2. Bathing a patient and changing the linen are not part of the evaluation step of the nursing process. Evaluation involves reassessing the patient to identify the actual outcomes and then comparing them with the expected outcomes to determine whether outcomes are achieved.
3. Bathing a patient and changing the linen are not part of the assessment step of the nursing process. Collecting data using various methods from various sources and clustering that data are what constitutes assessment activities.
4. Bathing a patient and changing the linen are associated with the implementation step of the nursing process.

The implementation step of the nursing process is when the nurse carries out planned nursing care.

TEST-TAKING TIP: Identify the word in the stem that sets a priority. The word *most* in the stem sets a priority.

Content Area: Nursing Process
Integrated Processes: Nursing Process: Implementation
Client Need: Safe and Effective Care Environment; Management of Care
Cognitive Level: Analysis

22. **ANSWER: 2.**
    Rationales:
    1. The analysis step of the nursing process includes analyzing data and identifying patient problems.
    2. The nurse's response is the planning step of the nursing process. The nurse is collaborating with the patient to design an intervention that facilitates ingestion of the prescribed medication.
    3. The assessment step of the nursing process includes the systematic collection, validation, and documentation of data.
    4. The implementation step of the nursing process includes organizing, managing, and implementing planned nursing actions.
    Content Area: Nursing Process
    Integrated Processes: Communication/Documentation; Nursing Process: Planning
    Client Need: Safe and Effective Care Environment; Management of Care
    Cognitive Level: Analysis

23. **ANSWER: 3.**
    Rationales:
    1. Taking a patient's vital signs after resting for 3 minutes after activity is not the analysis step of the nursing process.
    2. There is no step in the nursing process called diagnosis. However, during the analysis step of the nursing process the nurse may diagnose a patient's human response.
    3. Taking a patient's vital signs after resting for 3 minutes after activity is associated with evaluation of the patient's response to the activity. First, the patient is reassessed to identify the patient's actual outcome (response), which is then compared to the expected outcome to see if the expected outcome was achieved.
    4. Although the nurse is collecting data about the patient, it is being done after a nursing intervention and therefore not considered part of the assessment step of the nursing process. The assessment step of the nursing process is concerned with collecting information to identify the patient's health problems that can be treated by a nurse or provide information for the primary health-care provider.
    Content Area: Nursing Process
    Integrated Processes: Nursing Process: Evaluation
    Client Need: Safe and Effective Care Environment; Management of Care
    Cognitive Level: Analysis

24. **ANSWER: 2.**
    Rationales:
    1. This is an inappropriate comment to make to a family member. Although the patient is the primary source of

information, data provided by family members and friends may be extremely valuable.
2. Subjective data should be communicated in the words used by the patient rather than those used by the nurse to avoid any unintentional change in meaning. Communicating collected information is part of the assessment step of the nursing process.
3. When collecting information associated with a health history, the nurse generally uses a combination of direct and open-ended questions.
4. Objective and subjective data are both important when collecting data for a health history. Subjective data involves data that only patients are able to provide, such as feelings, sensations, and concerns.

TEST-TAKING TIP: Identify the word in the stem that sets a priority. The word *most* in the stem sets a priority. Identify the option with a specific determiner. Option 3 has the word *only,* which is a specific determiner. Identify the unique option. Option 2 is unique because it is the only option that reflects a nursing action after the health history is completed. The other options include actions performed during the interview with the patient.

Content Area: Nursing Process
Integrated Processes: Communication/Documentation; Nursing Process: Assessment
Client Need: Safe and Effective Care Environment; Management of Care
Cognitive Level: Application

25. **ANSWER: 3.**
    Rationales:
    1. Clammy skin is objective information. It can be verified by someone other than the patient.
    2. Agitated behavior is objective information. It can be identified and verified by someone other than the patient.
    3. Numbness of the feet is subjective information. Subjective data can be identified only by the patient.
    4. Coughing after a deep breath is observable and therefore objective information.
    Content Area: Nursing Process
    Integrated Processes: Nursing Process: Assessment
    Client Need: Physiological Integrity; Reduction of Risk Potential
    Cognitive Level: Application

26. **ANSWER: 3.**
    Rationales:
    1. Implementing various actions until one is successful explains the process of trial-and-error reasoning.
    2. When research is conducted to support a theory, thinking moves from the general to the specific; it uses deductive reasoning.
    3. Moving from specific data to a general premise is an explanation of inductive reasoning.
    4. Identifying a cue based on a suspicion or feeling, without conscious analysis, is an explanation of intuitive thinking.
    Content Area: Nursing Process
    Integrated Processes: Nursing Process: Analysis
    Client Need: Safe and Effective Care Environment; Management of Care
    Cognitive Level: Application

27. ANSWER: 1.

Rationales:

1. Edema can be measured via observation using a parameter of 1+ to 4+ and is therefore objective information.

2. Heartburn is subjective information because it can be identified only by the patient.

3. Chest pain is subjective information because it can be identified only by the patient.

4. Lightheadedness is subjective information because it can be identified only by the patient.

Content Area: Nursing Process
Integrated Processes: Nursing Process: Assessment
Client Need: Physiological Integrity; Reduction of Risk Potential;
Cognitive Level: Application

28. ANSWER: 4.

Rationales:

1. Teaching is associated with the implementation step of the nursing process.

2. Seeking an order for physical therapy is associated with the implementation step of the nursing process.

3. Having the patient complete a voiding record is associated with the implementation step of the nursing process. It involves teaching the patient how to provide self care.

4. Asking the patient about the degree of satisfaction related to urinary control interventions is one way of assessing the outcome of care. Is the patient satisfied or dissatisfied with the results of care? This is part of the evaluation step of the nursing process.

Content Area: Nursing Process
Integrated Processes: Communication/Documentation; Nursing Process: Evaluation
Client Need: Physiological Integrity; Basic Care and Comfort
Cognitive Level: Application

29. ANSWER: 3.

Rationale:

Solve the problem by using ratio and proportion.

$$\frac{\text{Desire 75 mcg}}{\text{Have 25 mcg}} = \frac{\text{x tablets}}{\text{1 tablet}}$$

$$25x = 75 \times 1$$
$$25x = 75$$
$$x = 75 \div 25$$
$$x = 3 \text{ tablets}$$

Content Area: Medication Administration
Integrated Processes: Nursing Process: Evaluation
Client Need: Physiological Integrity; Pharmacological and Parenteral Therapies
Cognitive Level: Application

30. ANSWER: 4.

Rationales:

1. Crying is an observable behavior and therefore is objective information. *Why* the patient is crying is subjective information. The *why* has to be reported by the patient.

2. Diaphoresis (sweating) is measured by observation and palpation and therefore is objective, not subjective, information.

3. A bounding pulse is objective information. A bounding pulse can be palpated by the nurse and is measurable.

4. Experiencing numbness is subjective information. Subjective data can be felt only by the patient and are not able to be measured or observed by another person.

Content Area: Nursing Process
Integrated Processes: Nursing Process: Assessment
Client Need: Physiological Integrity; Physiological Adaptation
Cognitive Level: Application

Chapter 11

Physical Assessment

Apical pulse—Number of times the ventricles of the heart contract in 1 minute when seen, felt, or auscultated over the apex of the heart.

Ataxia—Uncoordinated movements.

Auscultatory gap—A temporary loss of sound that occurs when a blood pressure cuff pressure is high, followed by the return of sounds at a lower level.

Blood pressure—Indirect measurement of the force of blood against arterial walls during cardiac contraction and cardiac relaxation.

Body temperature—The result of the amount of heat produced by the body and the amount of heat lost from the body.

Bradycardia—Heart rate less than 60 beats/minute.

Bradypnea—Respiratory rate less than 12 breaths/minute.

Cardiac output—Volume of blood that is pumped from the heart in 1 minute (about 5.6 L).

Dyspnea—Difficulty breathing.

Dysrhythmia—Irregular heart rate.

Eupnea—Normal respiratory rate of 12 to 20 breaths/minute.

Fasciculations—Localized, uncontrollable twitching of a single muscle group innervated by a single motor nerve fiber.

Febrile—Presence of a fever.

Fever (pyrexia)—Core body temperature more than a person's normal body temperature (usually 100°F orally or 101°F rectally) that is provoked by an increase in the body's temperature set point.

Gingivitis—Inflammation of the gums.

Glossitis—Inflammation of the tongue.

Hemiparesis—Weakness of an arm and a leg on same side of the body.

Hemiplegia—Paralysis of an arm and a leg on the same side of the body.

Hyperpyrexia—Core body temperature of 105.8°F (41.0°C) or more.

Hypertension—Systolic blood pressure more than 140 mm Hg or diastolic blood pressure more than 90 mm Hg on two separate occasions.

Hyperthermia—Core body temperature more than the person's normal body temperature without a change in the body's temperature set point.

Hypotension—Systolic blood pressure less than 100 mm Hg.

Hypothermia—Body temperature less than 98.6°F (36°C).

Hypoxemia (hypoxia)—Deficient oxygen in the blood.

Nonintention tremor (resting tremor)—Tremors occurring when muscles are at rest.

Orthopnea—Dyspnea relieved by assuming an upright position.

Orthostatic (postural) hypotension—A 10 to 20 mm Hg decrease between lying down and sitting blood pressures and/or a 10 to 20 mm Hg decrease between sitting and standing blood pressures caused by peripheral vasodilation without a compensatory increase in cardiac output.

Paraplegia—Paralysis of both legs.

Peripheral pulse—Rhythmic expansion of an artery that is palpated when a surge of blood occurs in response to contraction of the heart.

Peripheral vascular resistance—The amount of friction between blood flow and vessel walls.

Pulse deficit—Difference between apical and radial pulse rates.

Pulse pressure—Difference between systolic blood pressure and diastolic blood pressure.

Quadriplegia—Paralysis of both arms and both legs.

Respiration—The movement of gases into and out of the lungs, promoting an exchange of gases between the atmosphere and the capillary beds in the alveoli.

Severe hypothermia—Body temperature less than 82.4°F (28°C).

Continued

KEY TERMS—cont'd

Spasticity—Uncontrollable contractions of skeletal muscles.

Stomatitis—Inflammation of the mucous membranes of the oral cavity.

Stroke volume—Amount of blood that exits the left ventricle with each contraction of the heart (about 70 mL in a healthy adult).

Tachycardia—Heart rate more than 100 beats/minute.

Tachypnea—Respiratory rate more than 20 breaths/minute.

Tremors—Rhythmic, purposeless movements.

Vital signs—Essential clinical indicators of the physiological status of a patient; include body temperature, pulse, respirations, blood pressure, oxygen saturation, and pain.

I. Overview of Physical Assessment

Physical assessment is a major component of data collection. It is used during the initial comprehensive health assessment, routinely at periodic intervals, and when assessments are focused on a particular potential problem or emergency situation. Before performing a patient assessment, the nurse should understand developmental considerations, collect all the necessary equipment that will be used, and prepare the patient for the procedure.

A. Types of Physical Assessment
1. Initial comprehensive health assessment (database).
   a. Conducted during the initial interaction with a patient.
   b. Obtains baseline data that are global in their focus.
   c. Includes:
      (1) **Subjective data:** Data identified only by the person affected (e.g., sensations, feelings, attitudes, beliefs, and perceptions).
      (2) **Objective data:** Data that is objective and measurable against a standard (e.g., data obtained by accessing body systems, monitoring vital signs, obtaining physical measurements, and monitoring laboratory values).
2. Ongoing assessment (patient's progress).
   a. Conducted on a repetitive routine.
   b. Required because people are dynamic, not stagnant.
   c. Includes vital signs as well as focused assessments that concentrate on a particular topic, body system, or functional ability, such as daily weight, blood glucose level, and oxygen saturation level.
3. Focused assessment.
   a. Conducted when a risk factor or problem requires an in-depth assessment.
   b. Obtains information specific to a body part or system, functional ability, or topic; required for actual, potential, or suspected problems.
   c. Examples include assessing for clinical indicators that meet discharge criteria from a postanesthesia care unit, identifying rehabilitation needs as part of discharge planning, monitoring cardiac and respiratory function when a patient reports chest pain, completing an activities of daily living (ADL) scale when determining a patient's functional abilities, and using a weekly pressure ulcer assessment form to evaluate the progression of a pressure ulcer.
4. Emergency assessment.
   a. Conducted when a rapid assessment is required during a life-threatening situation.
   b. Typically focuses on the ABCs (Airway, Breathing, and Circulation).
   c. During a psychosocial crisis, focuses on identifying the patient's perception of the crisis, immediate safety needs, and coping skills.

B. Times to Perform Physical Assessment of a Patient
1. On admission to a health-care agency or service to provide a baseline of the patient's status and functional abilities against which to measure future change.
2. On an ongoing basis to assess the patient's progress.
3. When accepting responsibility for a patient at a change of shift and when a patient is transferred from an emergency department, postanesthesia care unit, or another unit within an agency.
4. When a patient's status changes.
   a. An acute onset of new signs or symptoms; for example, when a patient reports chest pain, shortness of breath, or dizziness.
   b. When signs or symptoms return or increase in intensity (**exacerbation**).
   c. When signs or symptoms subside or decrease in intensity (**remission**).
   d. When signs and symptoms persist for 6 months or more (**chronicity**).
5. To identify an issue or risk factor that may contribute to a problem.
6. When evaluating the effectiveness of medical/surgical therapy and nursing interventions; for example, level of pain relief after a patient receives an analgesic, extent of wound healing

during a dressing change, intake/output and fluid balance of a patient who is receiving a diuretic, and degree of patient comfort after administration of hygiene and a back massage.

7. When a nurse has an intuitive belief that *something is wrong*; for example, when a nurse instinctively identifies a subtle variation in a patient's condition.

C. Developmental Considerations When Performing a Physical Assessment

1. The basic techniques of physical assessment are the same regardless of the patient's age; however, the way in which the nurse approaches a patient and the additional focused assessments that should be performed vary based on the patient's age.

2. A variety of factors must be considered, such as physical changes associated with aging, cognitive level, experiential background, and age-associated health problems. (Some age-related differences specific to physical assessment are presented here, but more details about growth and development are contained in Chapter 6, "Nursing Care Across the Life Span.")

3. Infants/Toddlers.
   a. Have a parent hold an infant or toddler against the chest or have a toddler sit on the parent's lap.

   🛑 b. Place an infant or toddler on a padded examination table, but continually stay at the side of the table to prevent a fall.

   c. Convert pounds to kilograms if the childhood weight chart is expressed in kilograms. (1 kilogram is equal to 2.2 pounds. Divide the child's weight in pounds by 2.2 to determine the child's weight in kilograms.)

4. Preschoolers and school-aged children.
   a. Provide opportunities to make choices; for example, ask the child whether he or she prefers to sit in a parent's lap or to sit on the examination table.

   🛑 b. Involve the parent and child in the assessment; encourage the child to handle instruments because these actions support a sense of control that reduces anxiety.

   c. Allow the child to wear underpants when this part of the body is not being assessed.
   d. Start with the least invasive assessments, move to the more invasive assessments, and hold the most uncomfortable assessments until last; for example, examine the ear canal and oral cavity before auscultating the chest and palpating the abdomen.
   e. Provide reassurance and compliment children on how helpful they are because these actions support participation.

5. Adolescents.

   🛑 a. Ask parents to remain outside the examining room unless the adolescent prefers that the parent remain. A caregiver is more likely to receive an honest answer to a sensitive question and an adolescent is more apt to ask a sensitive question if the assessment is conducted in private.

   b. Provide privacy by pulling the curtain and draping the adolescent; recognize that adolescents are going through puberty and may be embarrassed about associated physical changes.

6. Adults.
   a. Consider the patient's developmental age, physical condition, energy level, and mobility when planning a physical assessment.
   b. Schedule extra time because the aging process may compromise energy and comprehension, requiring longer for the patient to process information and formulate an answer.

7. Older adult.
   a. Schedule physical assessments into several blocks of time so as not to exhaust a patient who is low in energy or is physically, physiologically, emotionally, or mentally compromised.
   b. Pace care and provide rest periods if needed.
   c. Modify approaches to positioning because an older adult may have arthritic joints and stiff muscles; support functional alignment with pillows.
   d. Ensure the patient wears prescribed hearing aids and eyeglasses; seek feedback to ensure that communication is understood.

   🛑 e. Use a comprehensive assessment format to identify problems common in older adults, such as the **SPICES** acronym.

       (1) Sleep disorders.
       (2) Problems with eating or feeding.
       (3) Incontinence.
       (4) Confusion.
       (5) Evidence of falls.
       (6) Skin breakdown.

   f. Assess intake of substances, such as alcohol, laxatives and cathartics, pain medications, and over-the-counter medications and supplements, because these are substances commonly used by older adults.

D. Equipment Use During a Physical Assessment and Related Nursing Responsibilities

1. Ensure that equipment is clean or sterile.
2. Verify that equipment is working properly before use.
3. Common equipment includes a drape, gloves (if exposure to blood or body fluids is anticipated),

penlight, tape measure, tongue depressor, lubricant, stethoscope, thermometer (e.g., oral, rectal, electronic, disposable, infrared sensor), sphygmomanometer or aneroid manometer, pulse oximeter, ultrasound (Doppler), scale (e.g., chair, bed, stretcher, cradle scale for infants, standing scale for weight and height), otoscope, ophthalmoscope, percussion hammer, tuning fork, pen light, cotton balls, and paper clip. (Fig. 11.1).

4. Clean or dispose of equipment or instruments after use. For example, use a separate alcohol swab to clean the diaphragm and each ear pod of a stethoscope, and place a disposable thermometer in an appropriate trash container.

🛑 5. Dedicate equipment to be left in a room when a patient is receiving transition-based precautions to reduce the risk of cross-contamination; ensure terminal cleansing of equipment when a patient is no longer in need of a device and before it is returned to general use.

E. Patient Preparation

1. Conduct assessments when the patient is amenable. If possible, avoid physical assessments when a patient is anxious, tired, hungry, or experiencing pain.
2. Respect the preference for a same-gender caregiver because of cultural or religious beliefs.

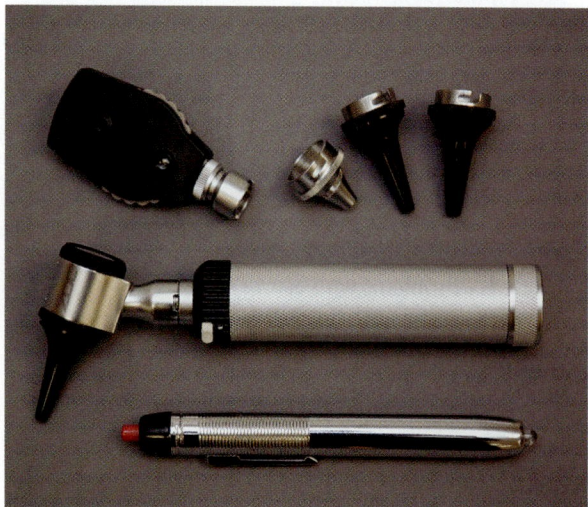

Fig 11.1 Equipment used for physical assessment. Front row: penlight. Second row: otoscope for assessing the tympanic membrane of the ear. Third row, left to right: ophthalmic head to convert otoscope to ophthalmoscope for assessing the internal eye and retina; nasal speculum for assessing the nasal passageway; two sizes of otic speculum for assessing the ear. (From Burton and Ludwig [2011]. *Fundamentals of nursing care: Concepts, connections & skills.* Philadelphia: F. A. Davis Company, with permission.)

3. Identify yourself and the patient; explain what you are going to do and why because doing so reduces anxiety, facilitates the patient's assistance, and is a patient right.
4. Encourage the patient to void, especially when planning to palpate the abdomen; an empty bladder supports comfort and facilitates accurate examination of the abdomen.
5. Allow a family member to remain present to meet developmental, cultural, or psychological needs if requested by the patient and if not detrimental to the patient.
6. Draw the bed curtain and drape the patient to avoid unnecessary exposure and to provide warmth.
7. Explain each assessment before touching the patient because doing so educates and prepares the patient, promotes rapport, and supports the development of trust.
8. Position the patient, especially infants, children, and older adults, considering their developmental age, physical condition, energy level, and mobility. Organize interventions so that several assessments are conducted during each position to reduce the number of times the patient is repositioned; use pillows to maintain functional alignment to avoid unnecessary stress and strain on muscles, joints, ligaments, and tendons.
9. Limit the amount of time a patient has to assume an uncomfortable or embarrassing position to support comfort and dignity.

II. General Survey

A general survey begins when the nurse meets the patient. The nurse makes initial observations regarding the patient's overall characteristics, gathering basic impressions of the patient's appearance, physical presence, mental status, and ability to communicate as well as generalized, nonspecific responses of the body that are the same regardless of the type of stress (general adaptation syndrome). The general survey provides information on the overall state of the patient and provides a bridge to the next stage of the physical assessment, the measurement of vital signs.

A. Appearance

1. Identify the overall personal hygiene of the patient.
   a. Is the patient clean and well groomed?
   b. Does the patient have body or breath odor?
   c. What is the patient wearing and is it appropriate for the weather?
2. Understand that appearance can deteriorate as a result of issues such as immobility, fatigue, pain, depression, and impaired cognition.

| Table 11.3 | **Routes for Obtaining a Temperature: Advantages, Disadvantages, and Specific Nursing Care—cont'd** |

Route and Normal Range	**Advantages**	**Disadvantages**	**Related Nursing Care**
Skin *Forehead skin temperature usually is 2°F to 4°F less than core temperature.* 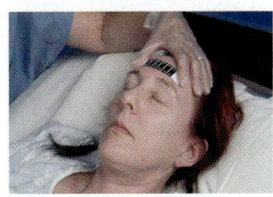	• Easily accessible: Forehead or abdomen. • Available in disposable strips.	• Less accurate and reliable than other routes; should not be used if accurate monitoring of temperature is essential. • Indicates body surface temperature only. • Perspiration interferes with measurement.	1. Draw the curtain and position the patient if the abdomen, rather than the forehead, is being used. 2. Ensure that the skin is dry. 3. Place the strip directly on skin, holding its edges firmly to the skin so that the entire strip is in contact with the skin. 4. Observe for color changes as the strip reacts to the skin temperature. 5. Read the result while the strip is still in contact with the skin. 6. Remove the strip from the skin and discard it in an appropriate trash receptacle. 7. Use another type of thermometer if the result is not within the normal range.

Photo credits: Wilkinson and Treas (2011). *Fundamentals of nursing,* Vol. 2, 2nd ed. Philadelphia: F. A. Davis Company, with permission.

G. Decreased Body Temperature (Hypothermia)
1. **Hypothermia:** A body temperature less than 98.6°F (36°C).
2. **Severe hypothermia:** A body temperature less than 82.4°F (28°C).
3. When body temperature decreases to less than 77°F (25°C), cardiac and respiratory functions cease, cells may still be viable, and death is possible.
4. Clinical indicators of hypothermia: Shivering initially; decreased, irregular pulse; decreased respirations; hypotension; reports of feeling cold and chilly; pale, cool skin; oliguria; reduced muscle coordination; disorientation; and decreased level of consciousness, progressing to coma.
5. Nursing Care.
   a. Monitor vital signs.
   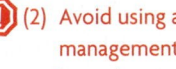 b. Monitor pulse oximetry, but do not apply a pulse oximeter probe to an appendage (e.g., finger, toe, ear lobe) that exhibits vasoconstriction because the result will be inaccurately low and may compromise skin integrity.
   c. Increase the environmental temperature.
   d. Ensure that clothing and linen are dry.
   e. Cover the patient with warm blankets, and put a hat on the patient.
   f. Position extremities close to the body.
   g. Provide warm oral fluids.
   h. Administer warm IV fluids as ordered.

i. Administer ordered procedures.
   (1) Examples: Provide a warm bath, apply an electric blanket, or position a temperature management blanket over and/or under the patient.
   (2) Avoid using an electric blanket or temperature management blanket if the patient has severe hypothermia because it may burn skin that has peripheral vasoconstriction.

H. Increased Body Temperature
1. **Hyperthermia.**
   a. Core body temperature is more than the person's normal body temperature; however, the body's temperature set point does not change. Usually, this term is used to describe increases more than 105°F (40.5°C).
   b. **Heat exhaustion:** Condition caused by excessive environmental heat and dehydration; indicated by weakness, muscle aches, headache, syncope, nausea, vomiting, paleness, dizziness, diaphoresis, and a temperature usually between 98.6°F to 103°F.
   c. **Heat stroke:** Condition generally caused by exercise in hot weather; indicated by flushed, hot, dry skin; throbbing headache; rapid, strong pulse; and a temperature of 103°F or more, progressing to impaired judgment, dizziness, delirium, unconsciousness, and seizures.

2. **Fever** (pyrexia, febrile).
   a. Core body temperature more than a person's normal body temperature (usually 100°F [37.8°C] orally or 101°F [38.3°C] rectally) that is provoked by an increase in the body's temperature set point.
   b. The higher set point is the body's attempt to establish an environment that inhibits pathogen replication. Fevers up to 102°F enhance the immune response, promote phagocytosis, hinder reproduction of many pathogens, and therefore should be permitted to achieve its objective.
   c. **Hyperpyrexia:** Core body temperature of 105.8°F (41.0°C) or more; extremely dangerous condition requiring medical intervention to avoid cell damage especially to delicate brain tissues. Clinical indicators include agitation, confusion, stupor, and coma.
   d. Stages of a fever.
      (1) Onset (cold or chill phase).
         (a) Body temperature increases, gradually or suddenly, but does not yet achieve the new set point.
         (b) Clinical indicators: Chilly feeling; increased pulse rate; increased respiratory rate and depth; pale, cold skin; absence of sweating; gooseflesh; shivering; and cyanotic nail beds.
      (2) Course (plateau phase).
         (a) Body temperature achieves the set point.
         (b) Clinical indicators: Flushing; warm, dry skin; increased pulse and respirations; thirst; mild to severe dehydration; absence of chills; glassy-eyed appearance; weakness; lethargy; and aching muscles.
      (3) Defervescence (fever abatement, flush phase).
         (a) Temperature begins to return to normal range.
         (b) Clinical indicators: Warmth and flushing due to vasodilation; diaphoresis (promotes heat loss through evaporation); possible dehydration.

MAKING THE CONNECTION

Fever and Invading Foreign Elements

A fever is caused by foreign elements (e.g., bacteria, viruses, fungi, and allergens) that enter the body and stimulate the production of phagocytes, which are specialized white blood cells (WBCs). Phagocytes consume the invaders and release pyrogens. Pyrogens stimulate the secretion of prostaglandin hormones that reset the hypothalamic thermostat to an increased temperature, called the *set point*. The body then attempts to increase the core temperature to the new set point.

e. Types of fevers.
   (1) Constant (sustained) fever.
      (a) Temperature always is higher than the normal range.
      (b) Temperature may increase or decrease by 1°F.
   (2) Intermittent fever.
      (a) Temperature is higher than the normal range.
      (b) Temperature then decreases to a normal or subnormal temperature regularly, at least once a day.
   (3) Remittent fever.
      (a) Temperature is always above the normal range.
      (b) Temperature varies by 3.6°F or higher during a 24-hour time period.
   (4) Relapsing (recurrent) fever.
      (a) Temperature in the normal range lasting for 1 to 2 days.
      (b) Followed by 1 or 2 days where the temperature is higher than the normal range.

3. Nursing care.
   a. Monitor vital signs.
   b. Assess skin temperature, color, degree of moisture, and other clinical indicators of fever.
   c. Monitor laboratory results and I&O for clinical indicators of infection and dehydration.
   d. Provide frequent oral care to maintain moist mucous membranes.
   e. Cover the patient with blankets and limit drafts when the patient reports feeling cold or when shivering (shivering increases body temperature); remove blankets when the patient feels warm.
   f. Encourage rest to reduce BMR.
   g. Encourage nutritional intake to meet energy needs because a fever increases BMR.
   h. Encourage oral fluid intake, and administer ordered IV fluids.
   i. Provide dry clothing and linens when the patient is diaphoretic during the defervescence phase.
   j. Use tepid water when providing a bath for hygiene purposes to increase heat loss through the principle of conduction; administer tepid sponge baths as ordered by the primary health-care provider. Avoid causing shivering because shivering increases body temperature.
   k. Avoid rapid lowering of body temperature because doing so causes vasoconstriction and a delay in decreasing the core temperature.
   l. Administer ordered antipyretics, generally for a fever higher than 102°F. Antipyretics are

prescribed to prevent a fever from becoming dangerously high and/or to minimize discomfort.

🛑 m. Teach the patient and family members interventions to prevent negative consequences from hot environmental temperatures.

    (1) Teach people, especially older adults, to drink adequate fluids, avoid alcohol and caffeine, take cool showers or baths, and use a fan or stay in an air-conditioned space.

    (2) Encourage family members to check on older adult family members and neighbors at least twice a day to ensure that they are safe.

V. Measurement of Pulse

A **pulse** (heart rate) reflects the waves of pressure throughout the arterial vessels generated by contractions of the ventricles of the heart that occur within 1 minute. In addition to rate, the characteristics of a pulse also are identified. These assessments provide information about the status of the heart and circulatory system. Nurses measure a patient's pulse to obtain baseline information, to assess the progression of an illness, and/or to monitor a response to therapy. Measuring a patient's pulse requires the use of the fingers, a stethoscope, or an instrument that magnifies sounds (Doppler). Nurses must understand the commonalities of nursing care for all sites of assessment and the differences for specific sites when obtaining a pulse. The site selected for measurement requires nursing judgment because the pulse rate is influenced by such factors as characteristics of the site, method used to obtain the pulse, as well as the patient's developmental level and pathophysiological condition.

A. Physiology Related to Pulse

1. **Apical pulse:** Central pulse auscultated over the apex of heart; reflects heart rate.
2. **Peripheral pulse:** Rhythmic expansion of an artery that is palpated when a surge of blood occurs in response to contraction of the heart; reflects heart rate and adequacy of circulation to a part of the body beyond the heart, such as an extremity.
3. **Pulse deficit:** Difference between apical and radial rates (apical rate minus radial rate).
4. **Stroke volume:** Amount of blood that exits the left ventricle with each contraction of the heart; about 70 mL in a healthy adult.
5. **Cardiac output:** Volume of blood that is pumped from the heart in 1 minute; about 5.6 L/minute; it is the product of the stroke volume multiplied by the heart rate per minute.

B. Factors That Affect the Pulse (Heart Rate)

1. Age.
   a. As age increases, heart rate gradually decreases.
   b. Variations by age.
      (1) Newborns: 120 to 160 beats/minute.
      (2) 1 to 2 years of age: 90 to 120 beats/minute.
      (3) 3 to 18 years of age: 80 to 100 beats/minute.
      (4) Adults: 60 to 100 beats/minute.
2. Gender: After puberty, the heart rate of males generally is slightly slower than the heart rate of females.
3. Circadian rhythm (diurnal variations).
   a. Rate is slowest from predawn to dawn hours.
   b. Rate progressively increases toward evening.
4. Blood volume.
   a. Increased blood volume (hypervolemia).
      (1) Pulse is full and bounding; rate may increase.
      (2) Commonly caused by fluid volume excess or excess IV fluids.
   b. Decreased blood volume (hypovolemia).
      (1) Pulse is weak or thready; rate increases to transport more oxygen to body cells.
      (2) Commonly caused by decreased fluid volume related to dehydration or hemorrhage.
5. Body temperature.
   a. Increased body temperature: With a fever, each degree of Fahrenheit increases the heart rate by 10 beats/minute to compensate for the decreased blood pressure associated with vasodilation and increased BMR.
   b. Decreased body temperature: When the body cools, each degree of Fahrenheit decreases the heart rate by 10 beats/minute because BMR slows.
6. Exercise.
   a. Rate increases because of the increase in the metabolic rate and the increased demand for oxygen and nutrients at the cellular level; stroke volume and cardiac output increase.
   b. Rate of increase in athletes may be less than the average adult because of larger cardiac size, strength, efficiency, and endurance.
7. Rest, sleep, and biofeedback activities: These activities decrease the body's metabolic rate and subsequently the heart rate.
8. Stress, emotions, and hormones.
   a. Sympathetic nervous system releases epinephrine and norepinephrine, resulting in constriction of peripheral blood vessels and an increase in the metabolic rate, force of cardiac contractions, and heart rate.
   b. Increased thyroid hormones (hyperthyroidism) increase the heart rate and decreased thyroid hormones (hypothyroidism) decrease the heart rate.

9. Medications.
   a. Some medications increase the heart rate (e.g., epinephrine, theophylline, and atropine).
   b. Some medications decrease the heart rate (e.g., digoxin, antihypertensives, and opioids).
10. Ingested or inhaled substances.
    a. Ingestion of food increases the heart rate slightly for several hours.
    b. Caffeine, nicotine, and illegal drugs, such as cocaine, increase the heart rate.
11. Pathological processes.
    a. Any condition that influences cardiac, respiratory, or neurological functioning may alter the heart rate.
    b. For example, obstructive pulmonary diseases and hypoxia increase the heart rate; increased intracranial pressure (ICP) decreases the heart rate and may make it irregular; cardiovascular disease may increase or decrease the heart rate or make it irregular.

C. Commonalities of Nursing Care When Obtaining a Pulse Regardless of the Site
1. Perform hand hygiene.
2. Introduce yourself, and explain what is to be done and why.
3. Identify the patient using two identifiers (e.g., hospital identification number, name, birth date).
4. Provide privacy by closing the door, pulling the curtain, and draping the patient to expose only the site being assessed.
5. Use anatomical landmarks to locate the site to be assessed.
6. Count the number of beats of a pulse within a time frame.
   a. Apical rate for 1 minute.
   b. Peripheral pulse for 30 seconds and then multiply result by 2.
7. Identify characteristics of the pulse (e.g. rate, rhythm, volume, and symmetry).
8. Perform focused assessments if results are outside the norm.
🛑 9. Notify the rapid response team and primary healthcare provider if results are significantly outside the norm or indicate a concern.
10. Document the results in the patient's clinical record.

D. Sites for Obtaining a Pulse and Related Nursing Care
1. Apical pulse.
   a. Auscultate over the apex of the heart, known as the *point of maximum impulse* (Fig. 11.3).
      (1) Find the angle of Louis (bump below the sternal notch where the manubrium and sternum meet) and slide your finger into the

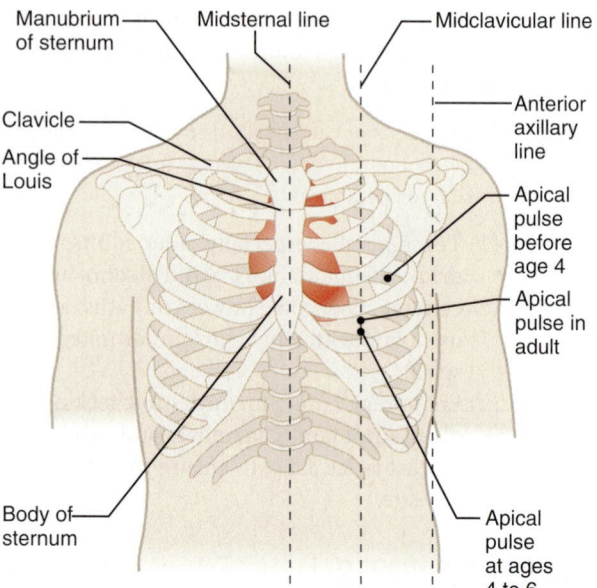

Fig 11.3 Location of apical pulse for adults and children. (From Wilkinson and Treas [2011]. *Fundamentals of Nursing*, Vol. 1, 2nd ed. Philadelphia: F. A. Davis Company, with permission.)

second intercostal space on the left side of the sternum.
      (2) Place one finger in each intercostal space, moving down to the fifth intercostal space.
      (3) Slide your finger to the midclavicular line over the apex of the heart (Fig. 11.4).
   b. Place the diaphragm of a stethoscope over the site and count the rate of heart contractions for 1 minute.
   c. Adjust the patient's position or stethoscope placement if apical beats are difficult to hear

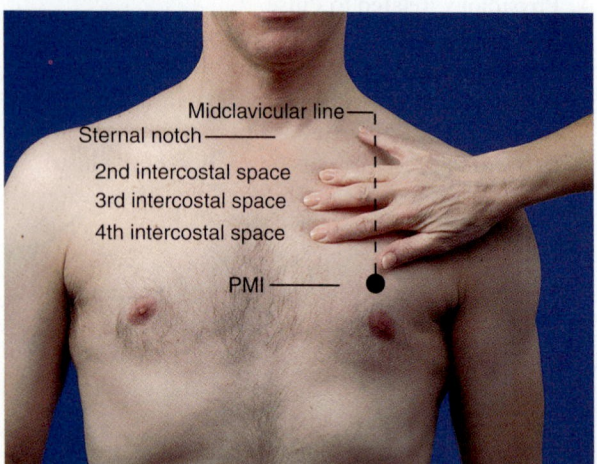

Fig 11.4 Technique to identify point of maximum impulse. (From Wilkinson and Treas [2011]. *Fundamentals of nursing*, Vol. 2, 2nd ed. Philadelphia: F. A. Davis Company, with permission.)

because of large pectoral muscles or large or dense mammary tissue. Have the patient tilt forward while in a sitting position; turn the patient to the left lateral position and move the stethoscope to the fifth or sixth intercostal space in the left midaxillary line.

    d. Use the apical pulse to assess heart rate, particularly in children younger than age 3 years and patients with a cardiac problem.

2. Peripheral pulse sites.

    a. Identify the site to be palpated by using anatomical landmarks (Fig. 11.5 and Table 11.4).

    b. Apply gentle pressure to compress the artery between the fingers and an underlying bone.

    c. Count each pulsating, tapping, or throbbing sensation as one beat; assess the presence and characteristics of the pulsations.

    d. Perform assessment with a Doppler ultrasound machine if difficult to assess pulse via palpation.

    e. Use to assess heart rate (e.g., radial), assess circulation to a body part (e.g., dorsalis pedis, posterior

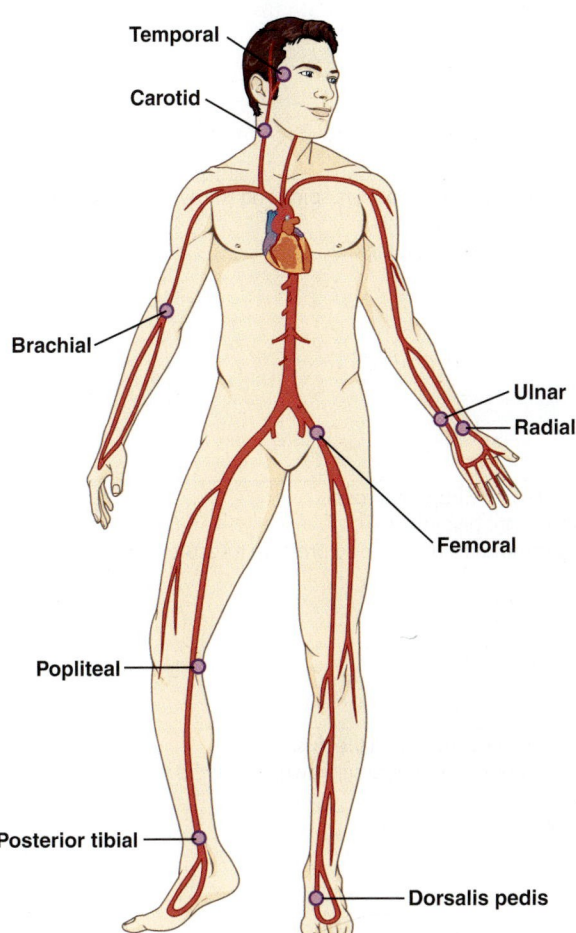

Fig 11.5 Peripheral pulse sites. (From Wilkinson and Treas [2011]. *Fundamentals of nursing,* Vol. 1, 2nd ed. Philadelphia: F. A. Davis Company, with permission.)

tibial), and identify a site for blood pressure measurement (e.g., brachial, popliteal).

E. Characteristics of a Pulse and Related Nursing Care

1. Rate.

    a. Identify the number of beats of a pulse within a specific time frame.

       (1) Apical rate: Count the number of heart beats while auscultating over the point of maximum intensity; two sounds, *lub* and *dub* together, are counted as one beat. Count the number of beats for a full minute.

       (2) Peripheral rate: Count each pulsating, tapping, or throbbing sensation as one beat when palpating over an artery. Count the pulsations for at least 30 seconds and multiple the result by 2; some advocate counting the beats for 15 seconds and multiplying by 4, but this results in less accurate counts. An irregular rate should be counted for a full minute.

    b. Assess distal peripheral pulses, such as the dorsalis pedis and posterior tibial, for their presence and quality rather than their rate because this assessment is done to assess the presence of circulation to the feet rather than assess the heart.

    c. Determine the significance of the rate obtained in an adult.

       (1) Expected rate: 60 to 100 beats/minute; for additional heart rates by age, see "Factors That Affect the Pulse (Heart Rate), Age" on page 251.

       (2) **Bradycardia:** Pulse rate less than 60 beats/minute.

       (3) **Tachycardia:** Pulse rate more than 100 beats/minute.

2. Rhythm.

    a. Identify rhythm by comparing the intervals between beats.

    b. Determine the significance of the intervals obtained.

       (1) Regular rhythm: Intervals are equal in length.

       (2) Irregular rhythm (**dysrhythmia**): Intervals vary in length.

    c. Identify the pattern of an irregular rhythm.

       (1) Regularly irregular: Lengths of intervals between beats are repetitive and predictable (e.g., short delay after every third beat).

       (2) Irregularly irregular: Lengths of intervals between beats are unpredictable (e.g., delays after beats with no identifiable pattern).

🛑 d. Count the number of beats for a full minute when an irregular rhythm is identified.

Table 11.4 Peripheral Pulse Sites and Related Nursing Care

Site	Related Nursing Care
Brachial Pulse 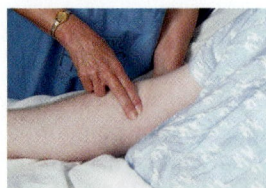	1. Palpate the inner aspect of the antecubital fossa. 2. Have the patient turn the palm downward if the pulse is difficult to obtain because doing so moves the brachial artery over a bony prominence. 3. Use to assess heart rate in children or obtain a blood pressure measurement.
Carotid Pulse 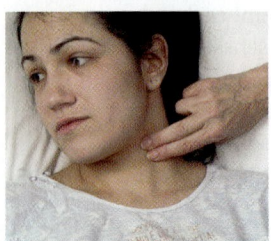	1. Palpate in the groove between the trachea and sternocleidomastoid muscle. 2. Palpate gently to avoid obliteration of the pulse, which decreases blood flow to the brain or stimulates the carotid bodies, precipitating a decrease in heart rate and blood pressure. 3. Never palpate both arteries at the same time. 4. Use only during cardiopulmonary resuscitation (CPR) or when assessing the presence of circulation to the brain.
Dorsalis Pedis Pulse 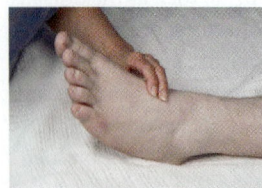	1. Palpate in the groove between the big toe and first toe and move toward the top of the foot. 2. Use to assess circulation to the foot.
Femoral Pulse 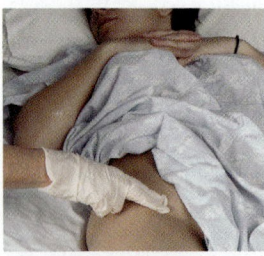	1. Palpate the groin halfway between the anterosuperior iliac spine and the symphysis pubis. 2. Requires deep palpation to feel pulse in an adult. 3. Use to assess circulation to the leg; may be used during CPR.
Popliteal Pulse 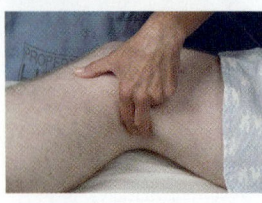	1. Palpate behind the knee in the center of the popliteal fossa. 2. Flex the patient's knee slightly to facilitate palpation. 3. Use to assess circulation to the leg or obtain a thigh blood pressure measurement.
Posterior Tibial Pulse 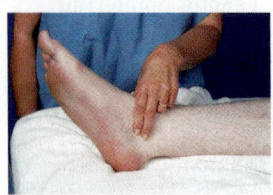	1. Palpate the inner side of the ankle below the medial malleolus. 2. Avoid deep palpation to prevent obliteration of the pulse; however, may be necessary to use deeper palpation in some people. 3. Use to assess circulation to the foot.

Table 11.4 Peripheral Pulse Sites and Related Nursing Care—cont'd

Site	Related Nursing Care
Radial Pulse 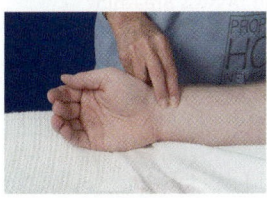	1. Ensure the arm is in a resting position, such as flexed across the chest or lying on the bed or table to eliminate muscles contraction that can interfere with accurate assessment. 2. Palpate in the groove on the thumb side of the wrist over the radial artery. 3. Begin with light pressure and increase pressure until pulse is felt.
Temporal Pulse 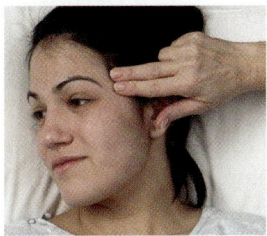	1. Palpate over a temporal bone on the side of the face, lateral and superior to the eye. 2. Use for infants.

Photo credits: Wilkinson and Treas (2011). *Fundamentals of nursing,* Vol. 2, 2nd ed. Philadelphia: F. A. Davis Company, with permission.

3. Quality of volume.
   a. Assess the force produced by blood surging through the artery (pulse volume).
   b. Recognize that the rating scale is somewhat subjective (Table 11.5).
   c. Assess adequacy of contractions and arterial circulation.
      (1) Adequate strength of contractions of the heart produces a palpable pulse with a rating scale of bounding (3+) or strong (2+).
      (2) Inadequate strength of contractions of the heart or impaired arterial circulation to the site produces a palpable pulse with a rating scale of weak (1+) or thready, or an absent pulse (0). These indicate inadequate perfusion, resulting in decreased oxygen and nutrients to body cells adjacent to and distal to the pulse site.
   d. Assess next proximal pulse in the extremity when a distal peripheral pulse volume is 1+ or absent.
   e. Perform additional peripheral vascular assessments when pulses are 1+, thready, or absent to assess circulation to the site. (See Table 11.11, "Peripheral Neurovascular Assessments.")
4. Symmetry of characteristics.
   a. Determine whether all pulse characteristics are equal bilaterally by comparing results of unilateral assessments; assessments may be done concurrently or one after the other.
   b. Perform focused assessments, such as neurovascular assessments (see Table 11.11, "Peripheral Neurovascular Assessments"), ECG, and cardiac enzymes if unequal results are identified.

VI. Measurement of Respirations

Respiration involves the movement of gases into and out of the lungs, promoting an exchange of gases between the atmosphere and the capillary beds in the alveoli. The

Table 11.5 Quality of Pulse Volume Rating Scale

Rating Scale	Description of Pulse
3+ Bounding	• Feels strong and full. • Not obliterated with moderate pressure. • Easily detected and counted.
2+ Strong	• Feels strong. • Obliterated with moderate pressure. • Easily detected and counted.
1+ Weak	• Feels weak. • Obliterated with slight pressure.
Thready Feeble	• Feels very weak. • Obliterated with slight pressure. • Difficult to detect; may require use of a Doppler ultrasound machine.
0 Absent	• Not detectable via palpation or use of a Doppler ultrasound machine.

measurement of respirations involves observing and counting the number of inhalations (breathing in) and exhalations (breathing out) within a specific time frame. Although breathing is usually an involuntary act, people can actively control respirations. Therefore, nurses must know how to perform accurate assessments. Assessment of respirations also includes the characteristics of respirations, including depth, rhythm, and effort. (See Chapter19, "Oxygenation," for details about the structures and functions of the respiratory system, factors that influence respiratory functioning, breathing patterns, and auscultation of breath sounds.)

A. Assess Respirations Discreetly
  1. Respirations are under both involuntary and voluntary control.
  2. Assess respirations without the patient's awareness to ensure that the respirations counted are under involuntary control.
     a. Position the patient's arm across the diaphragm and palpate over the patient's radial pulse site at the same time respirations are being assessed. The patient will assume you are obtaining a pulse and not feel self-conscious and voluntarily alter the respiratory rate.
     b. Observe the rate and characteristics of respirations while the patient is resting or sleeping.

B. Count the Respiratory Rate
  1. One respiration consists of one inhalation and one exhalation.
  2. Observe them by the rise and fall of the chest or abdomen or palpate them with the palm of the hand on the chest, diaphragm, or abdomen.
  3. Count respirations for a minimum of 30 seconds and multiply the result by 2.
  4. Assess the respiratory rate.
     a. **Eupnea:** Normal respiratory rate of 12 to 20 breaths/minute.
     b. **Bradypnea:** Less than 12 breaths/minute.
     c. **Tachypnea:** More than 20 breaths/minute.

C. Identify the Depth of Respirations
  1. "Depth" refers to the observed amount of chest expansion; it is directly related to the volume of air inhaled.
  2. Depth can be described as shallow, normal, or deep; this is a somewhat subjective observation by the nurse.
  3. Amount of air inhaled in one breath is between 300 and 500 mL (tidal volume).

D. Identify the Rhythm and Pattern of Respirations
  1. Rhythm is determined by identifying the length of intervals between respirations.
     a. Regular rhythm: Evenly spaced intervals between respirations.
     b. Irregular rhythm: Unevenly spaced intervals between respirations.

2. Assess irregular rhythms for a full minute.

3. Assess irregular rhythms further to identify patterns associated with Cheyne-Stokes, Biot, and Kussmaul respirations. (See the section "Assess Breathing Patterns" in Chapter 19, "Oxygenation," page 574.)

E. Identify the Degree of Respiratory Effort
  1. Respiratory effort is the amount of work required to breathe.
  2. The act of breathing should be effortless.
  3. Difficulty breathing (**dyspnea**) can be observed by another; the feeling of not being able to catch your breath (**shortness of breath**) is a subjective symptom that only the patient can describe.
  4. Clinical indicators of respiratory distress (see the section "Assess Breathing Patterns" in Chapter 19, "Oxygenation," page 574, for more information about respiratory distress).
     a. Use of accessory muscles of respiration, such as intercostal, trapezius, and abdominal muscles, to help expand the thoracic cavity.
     b. Sinking of intercostal, supraclavicular, and subcostal tissues during inspiration (**retractions**).
     c. Widening of the nares during inhalation (**nasal flaring**) to reduce resistance to airflow; occurs more often in infants and children.
     d. Closed glottis immediately before exhalation, causing grunting; a closed glottis promotes exchange of gases in alveoli.
     e. Exhaling through the mouth with lips shaped like a small O to lengthen exhalation (**pursed-lip breathing**); helps keep airways open and prevents trapping of air in the alveoli.
     f. Wide-eyed, startled look or other signs of fear related to an inability to breathe.
     g. Dyspnea relieved by assuming an upright position (**orthopnea**).
     h. Leaning forward while in a sitting position (**orthopneic position**).

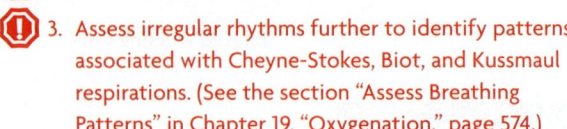

VII. Measurement of Blood Pressure

Blood pressure is an indirect measurement of the force of blood against arterial walls during cardiac contraction and cardiac relaxation. Numerous factors (determinants) influence blood pressure, including physiological factors, such as cardiac output, blood volume, peripheral vascular resistance, and viscosity of the blood and personal factors, such as age, activity, body weight, medications, and lifestyle behaviors. To obtain accurate blood pressure measurements and analyze measurement results, a nurse must not only know how to perform the skill of obtaining a blood pressure measurement but also understand the physiological and personal determinants that influence blood pressure.

A. Physiological Determinants of Blood Pressure
1. Cardiac output.
   a. The volume of blood that is pumped from the heart in 1 minute (about 5.6 L).
   b. It increases as a result of an increase in heart rate, an increase in heart contractility, and an increase in circulating blood volume.
2. Blood volume.
   a. The amount of blood within the intravascular compartment.
   b. When the amount of circulating blood increases within the intravascular compartment, the pressure in that space also increases because the blood exerts more pressure against the vessel walls.
   c. As the amount of circulating blood decreases, blood pressure decreases.
3. Peripheral vascular resistance.
   a. The amount of friction between blood flow and vessel walls.
   b. It is influenced by the thickness of the blood (viscosity), elasticity of arterial walls, and width of arterial lumens.
   c. Decreased elasticity of arterial walls, decreased width of arterial lumens, and increased blood viscosity all increase blood pressure.
   d. Increased elasticity of arterial walls, increased width of arterial lumens, and decreased blood viscosity all decrease the blood pressure.

B. Personal Determinants of Blood Pressure
1. Age.
   a. Infants have a mean systolic blood pressure (SBP) of approximately 75 mm Hg.
   b. Blood pressure increases with age and arrives at the expected adult values at puberty; continues to rise slightly during adulthood.
   c. Both systolic and diastolic blood pressures increase in older adults because of decreased arterial wall elasticity.
2. Gender.
   a. After puberty, women tend to have lower blood pressures than men of the same age.
   b. After menopause, blood pressure may increase due to a decrease in estrogen.
3. Diurnal rhythms.
   a. Blood pressure usually is lowest in the morning, increases during the day, and is highest in the late afternoon or evening.
   b. These changes are related to the body's metabolic rate.
4. Race (men in the United States).
   a. Evidence supports the fact that people of specific ethnicities may have a higher or lower risk of developing certain illnesses; whether this difference is caused by some genetic component or due to cultural circumstances is unclear.
   b. For example, some believe that the higher rate of hypertension among men of African American heritage (43 percent) versus men of white European heritage (27.8 percent) may be due to a genetically based salt sensitivity. In addition, men of African American heritage have a higher rate of kidney disease, which can increase blood pressure. American men of Asian or Pacific Islander heritage have a 9.7 percent rate of hypertension. These statistics hold constant across independent research, suggesting a genetic component.
5. Exercise: Activity increases metabolic rate and cardiac output, thereby increasing blood pressure.
6. Stress.
   a. The sympathetic nervous system response to stress increases cardiac output and constricts blood vessels; therefore, blood pressure increases.
   b. Acute pain increases blood pressure; however, chronic pain might not.
7. Obesity: An additional vascular supply is necessary to perfuse excessive body mass, resulting in increased peripheral resistance; thus, blood pressure increases.
8. Lifestyle behaviors: Excessive dietary sodium, smoking tobacco, and three or more alcoholic beverages a day may increase the blood pressure.
9. Medications.
   a. Blood pressure may decrease with use of opioids, antihypertensives, antidysrhythmics, and diuretics.
   b. Blood pressure may increase with use of some over-the-counter medications, herbal preparations, and illicit drugs.
10. Diseases: Any condition that affects the circulatory system or any major organ of the body (e.g., kidneys, thyroid gland, and brain) may affect the blood pressure.
11. Body position: Blood pressure is higher when a person is standing rather than sitting or lying; when the arm being used for measurement is held higher than the heart; when sitting, when the feet are dangling rather than on the floor; and when the legs are crossed at the knees when sitting.

C. **Nursing Care to Obtain a Blood Pressure Measurement**

1. Perform hand hygiene.
2. Collect appropriate equipment for measuring blood pressure (BP).
   a. Sphygmomanometer: May have a dial that registers the BP by a pointer attached to a spring (Fig. 11.6a) or an electronic machine that can detect either sounds or pressure waves as blood flows through an artery (Fig. 11.6b).

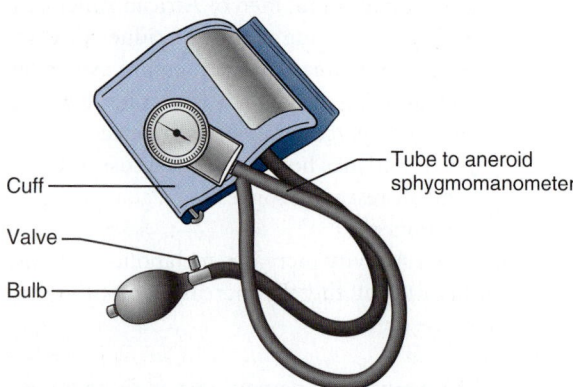

Cuff
Valve
Bulb
Tube to aneroid sphygmomanometer

Fig 11.6a Aneroid sphygmomanometer. (Adapted from Wilkinson and Treas [2011]. *Fundamentals of nursing,* Vol. 1, 2nd ed. Philadelphia: F. A. Davis Company, with permission.)

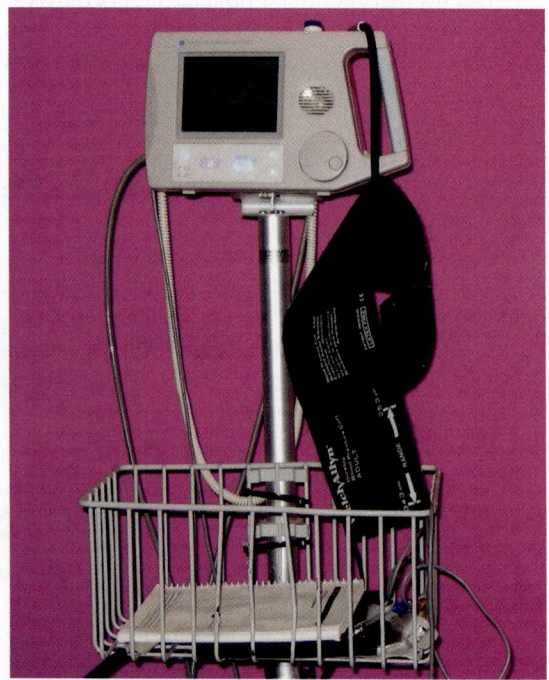

Fig 11.6b Electronic sphygmomanometer. (From Wilkinson and Treas [2011]. *Fundamentals of nursing,* Vol. 1, 2nd ed. Philadelphia: F. A. Davis Company, with permission.)

DID YOU KNOW?

In 1998, the U.S. Environmental Protection Agency and the American Hospital Association signed a memorandum of understanding regarding the virtual elimination of mercury from hospitals by 2005. In addition, mercury waste is regulated under the Resource Conservation Recovery Act. Handlers of hazardous waste must be specially trained and use special equipment to manage a spill and agencies must meet standards for storage, handling, disposal, tracking, and reporting regulations. Significant fines can be collected if regulations are not met. It is interesting to note that, based on a study by the California Department of Health Services in September 2000, the sources of mercury in hospitals were 46.5 percent sphygmomanometers, 42.3 percent gastroenterology equipment, 0.66 percent thermometers, 2.69 percent other clinical sources, and 8.17 percent nonclinical sources.

   b. Blood pressure cuff: The width and length of the bladder of the cuff being used must be appropriate for the limb used and the patient's size (Fig. 11.7).
      (1) Width of bladder: Should cover about two-thirds of the length of the person's upper arm (Fig. 11.8).
      (2) Length of bladder: Should encircle 80 percent of the upper arm (Fig. 11.9).
      🛑 (3) If the cuff is too small, the BP result will be inaccurately high. If the cuff is too large, the BP result will be inaccurately low.
   c. Stethoscope: The diaphragm or bell of a stethoscope may be used to auscultate the sounds associated with a blood pressure (Fig. 11.10). Clean each area of the stethoscope (e.g., bell, diaphragm, and ear pieces) with a separate alcohol wipe before and after use.

DID YOU KNOW?

Most nurses use the diaphragm of a stethoscope to auscultate blood pressure. However, evidence-based practice supports the use of the bell rather than the diaphragm because diastolic pressure (low-pitched sounds) can be heard more accurately using the bell.

Blood pressure cuff

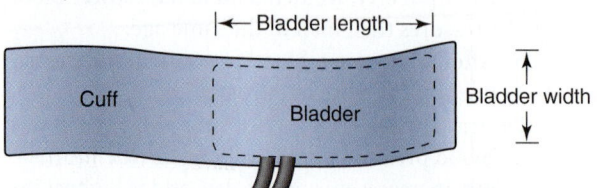

Bladder length
Cuff
Bladder
Bladder width

Fig 11.7 Blood pressure cuff. (Adapted from Wilkinson and Treas [2011]. *Fundamentals of nursing,* Vol. 1, 2nd ed. Philadelphia: F. A. Davis Company, with permission.)

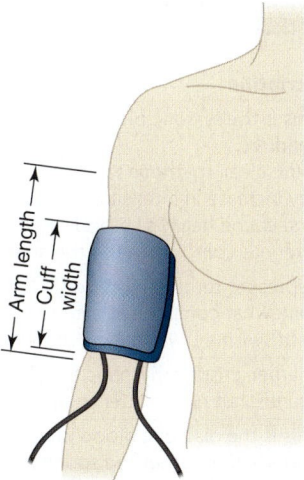

Fig 11.8 Width of bladder of blood pressure cuff. (Adapted from Wilkinson and Treas [2011]. *Fundamentals of nursing,* Vol. 1, 2nd ed. Philadelphia: F. A. Davis Company, with permission.)

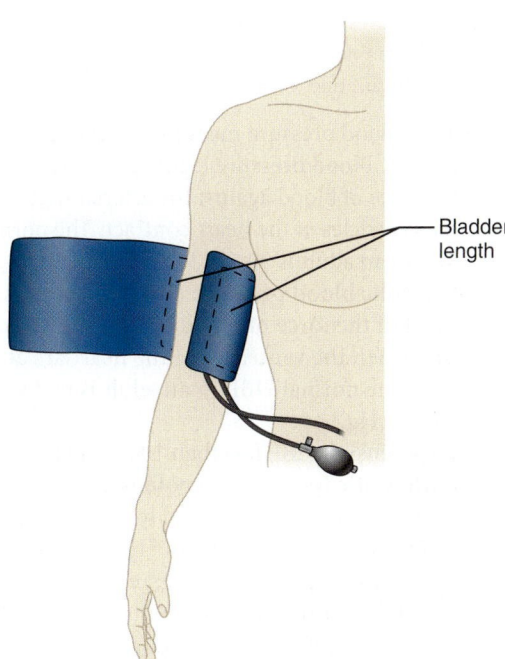

Fig 11.9 Length of bladder in blood pressure cuff. (Adapted from Wilkinson and Treas [2011]. *Fundamentals of nursing,* Vol. 1, 2nd ed. Philadelphia: F. A. Davis Company, with permission.)

3. Ensure that equipment is working properly before using it with a patient and charged if it is an electronic device.
4. Introduce yourself, identify the patient, explain what you are going to do, and provide privacy by closing the door or pulling the curtain.

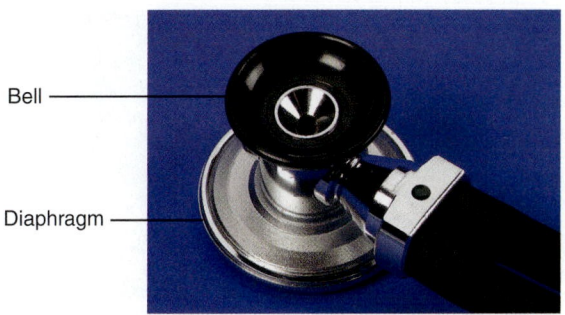

Fig 11.10 Stethoscope. (Adapted from Burton and Ludwig [2011]. *Fundamentals of nursing care: Concepts, connections & skills.* Philadelphia: F. A. Davis Company, with permission.)

5. Identify the site to be used and position the patient accordingly.
    a. Arm.
        (1) Contraindications for obtaining a BP in an arm include: presence of an intravenous infusion or renal dialysis shunt; presence of a cast, brace, or dressing; amputation, trauma, or surgery of the arm being considered; and mastectomy or therapy to the breast on the side of the arm being considered.
        (2) Place the patient in the low-, semi-, or high-Fowler position or sitting position; support the arm at the level of the heart.
        (3) Place the cuff above (proximal) the antecubital fossa (area opposite to the elbow) when auscultating over the brachial artery (Fig. 11.11) or around the forearm when auscultating over the radial artery.
    b. Thigh.
        (1) Contraindications for obtaining a BP in a thigh include: upper or lower amputation of the extremity, presence of edema, capillary refill more than 3 seconds, and any inflammation, infection, lesions, or trauma in the leg.
        (2) Place the patient prone or supine with the leg in a slightly flexed position.

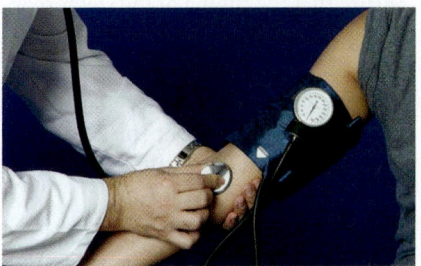

Fig 11.11 Placement of a blood pressure cuff on the arm. (From Wilkinson and Treas [2011]. *Fundamentals of nursing,* Vol. 2, 2nd ed. Philadelphia: F. A. Davis Company, with permission.)

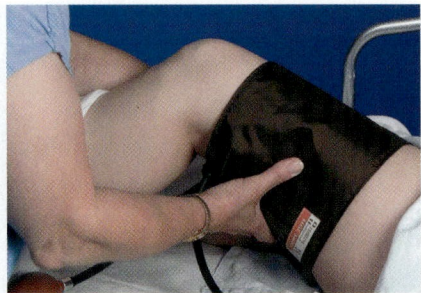

Fig 11.12 Placement of a blood pressure cuff on the thigh. (From Wilkinson and Treas [2011]. *Fundamentals of nursing*, Vol. 2, 2nd ed. Philadelphia: F. A. Davis Company, with permission.)

    (3) Place the cuff just above the knee around the thigh while auscultating over the popliteal artery in the popliteal fossa (area behind the knee). (Fig. 11.12.)

6. Determine systolic blood pressure (SBP) by palpation.
   a. A palpable pulse provides an indication of the approximate level of the systolic BP.
   b. This technique prevents erroneously underestimating the systolic BP by beginning the BP measurement during an auscultatory gap.
      (1) An **auscultatory gap** is the temporary loss of sound when the cuff pressure is high followed by the return of sounds at a lower level.
      (2) It occurs more often in patients with excessively high blood pressures.
   c. Palpating BP can be done when BP is difficult to hear; however, it reveals only the systolic BP.
   d. Palpate the artery, inflate the cuff rapidly to 80 mm Hg, and continue to inflate the cuff in 10 mm Hg increments until the pulse can no longer be felt. Note the level of the systolic BP.
   e. Deflate the cuff and wait 2 minutes before obtaining the auscultated BP.
7. Determine the systolic and diastolic BP by auscultation.
   a. Place the bell or diaphragm of the stethoscope over the artery without touching the cuff and ensure that the tubing of the stethoscope and sphygmomanometer are not touching anything; these actions eliminate interfering sounds.
   b. Inflate the cuff 30 mm Hg above the level of the palpated systolic BP. This ensures that the first sound associated with a BP will be heard accurately.
   c. Release the pressure within the cuff slowly (2 to 3 mm Hg per second) to allow the return of blood flow to the arm. As blood begins and continues to flow through the artery, listen for a variety of sounds (Korotkoff sounds). (Table 11.6)

Table 11.6	Korotkoff Sounds
Sound	**Description**
First	• This is the systolic blood pressure in adults and children. • Faint, clear, rhythmic tapping sounds that gradually increase in intensity. • First sound heard as blood begins to flow through artery as compression of the artery is released.
Second	• Represent turbulent blood flow through the somewhat compressed artery. • Soft, swishing, whooshing sounds.
Third	• Sharper, crisper, rhythmic and more intense sounds, but not as intense as first sounds.
Fourth	• This is the diastolic blood pressure in children. • Soft, rhythmic, muffled sounds. • Compression of the artery is lessening.
Fifth	• This is the diastolic blood pressure in adults. • Last sound is heard. • Followed by silence.

🛑 8. Wait 2 minutes before reinflating a cuff if a second assessment is necessary to prevent a falsely elevated diastolic result due to venous congestion.

9. Analyze blood pressure measurement results.
   a. **Systolic blood pressure** (SBP): Measurement of the force of blood against the arterial wall when the ventricles of the heart contract. The normal SBP in an adult is 90 to 120 mm Hg.
   b. **Diastolic blood pressure** (DBP): Measurement of the force of blood against the arterial wall when the ventricles of the heart are at rest. The normal DBP in an adult is 60 to 80 mm Hg.
   c. **Hypotension:** SBP less than 100 mm Hg.
   d. **Orthostatic (postural) hypotension:** A 10 to 20 mm Hg decrease between lying down and sitting and/or a 10 to 20 mm Hg decrease between sitting and standing; results from peripheral vasodilation without a compensatory increase in cardiac output.
   e. **Prehypertension:** SBP 120 to 139 mm Hg or DBP 80 to 89 mm Hg.
   f. **Hypertension:** SBP 140 mm Hg or higher or DBP 90 mm Hg or higher on two separate occasions.
      (1) High blood pressure—Stage I: SBP 140 to 159 or DBP 90 to 99 mm Hg.
      (2) High blood pressure—Stage II: SBP ≥160 mm Hg or DPB ≥100 mm Hg.
   g. **Pulse pressure:** Difference between SBP and DBP; reflects the volume of blood exiting the left ventricle; should be no more than one-third the SBP.

10. Record the BP measurement in the patient's clinical record.
    a. Adult: The SBP is the first sound heard; the DBP is the last sound heard.
    b. Child: The SBP is the first sound heard; the DBP is when the sound becomes muffled (fourth sound heard).
    c. Some advocate recording the level of three sounds: the first sound heard, the muffling of the sound, and the last sound heard.

VIII. Measurement of Arterial Blood Oxygen Saturation

An arterial blood oxygen saturation level provides vital information about a person's cardiopulmonary status and, therefore, is now considered one of the vital signs. Oxygen entering the body binds with hemoglobin in red blood cells (RBCs) and is transported via the circulation to body cells. **Pulse oximetry** is a noninvasive technique that estimates the percentage of hemoglobin molecules carrying oxygen in circulating RBCs. It detects the presence of deficient oxygen in the blood (**hypoxemia**) before visible signs develop. Expected normal values are between 95 and 100 percent. Nurses must understand factors that affect oxygen saturation results, factors indicting the need for monitoring oxygen saturation, clinical manifestations of alterations in oxygen saturation, and ways to perform pulse oximetry to assess blood oxygen saturation.

A. Factors That Affect Oxygen Saturation and Related Nursing Care
  1. Amount of RBCs/hemoglobin: Oxygen saturation measurement will be within the normal range when the circulating hemoglobin is fully saturated. However, if the patient has a low RBC count (**anemia**), all the hemoglobin may be saturated, but the patient may have inadequate oxygen reaching body tissues. Consider the patient's laboratory value for RBCs when analyzing results.

🛑 2. If the circulation under the sensor is impaired, the reading will be inaccurately low; distal appendages that have thickened nails, edema, or a capillary refill more than 3 seconds should not be used for placement of the sensor.

  3. Patient activity: Excessive movement or shivering interferes with accurate readings; place the probe on an ear lobe, nose, or forehead instead of a finger or toe.
  4. Acrylic nails and dark nail polish interfere with an accurate assessment; remove nail polish or use an alternate placement site for the sensor.
  5. Moisture and oils on the skin: Excessive perspiration can interfere with accurate readings; clean the site with alcohol and dry it before sensor placement.

B. Patient Factors Indicating the Need for Monitoring Oxygen Saturation
  1. Acute or chronic impaired respiratory or cardiac functioning.
  2. Recovery from any type of anesthesia or conscious sedation.
  3. Any trauma, including surgery.
  4. Ventilatory dependency.
  5. Receipt of supplemental oxygen.

C. Clinical Manifestations of Altered Oxygen Saturation
  1. Altered respiratory rate, depth, or rhythm.
  2. Dyspnea and use of accessory muscles of respiration (see the section "Assess Breathing Patterns" in Chapter 19, "Oxygenation," page 574).
  3. Adventitious breath sounds (see the section "Abnormal Breath Sounds" in Chapter 19, "Oxygenation," page 580).
  4. Pallor or cyanosis of the lips, mucous membranes, nail beds, and skin.
  5. Restlessness, irritability, confusion, and decreased level of consciousness.

D. Measurement of Arterial Blood Oxygen Saturation via Pulse Oximetry (See the section "Pulse Oximetry" in Chapter 19, "Oxygenation," page 578.)

IX. Measurement of Pain

Pain is an unpleasant, emotional or sensory experience related to potential or actual tissue damage. It is a physiological compensatory mechanism that signals that something is not right with the body and, therefore, is now considered one of the vital signs. Although pain is a universal phenomenon, the experience of pain is unique to each individual. It is a subjective symptom that only the patient can describe—*pain is what and where the patient says it is.* Therefore, a thorough comprehensive assessment of pain must be conducted when a patient reports feeling pain. (See Chapter 23, "Pain, Comfort, Rest, and Sleep," for a thorough discussion of pain, including measurement of pain and related nursing care.)

X. Techniques of Physical Assessment Used By Nurses

After performing a general survey of the patient and obtaining vital signs the nurse should perform a comprehensive physical assessment. Before performing this assessment, the nurse must understand information specific to the techniques of physical assessment and must also understand that the techniques used should progress from least invasive to most invasive so as not to influence subsequent assessments. These techniques should begin with inspection and progress to auscultation, percussion, and finally palpation.

A. Inspection

1. Performed first because it is the least invasive physical assessment technique.
2. Use of the naked eye to visually observe and examine the patient.
3. Also involves using the sense of smell.
4. Principles of inspection.
   a. Begin inspection immediately on visual contact with the patient and continue while conducting the general survey; move to a focused inspection when you identify a specific problem.
   b. Provide adequate lighting to ensure that the colors of the curtains and walls do not influence visual assessments.
   c. Use equipment to enhance vision, such as a penlight to examine pupil reaction to light or to examine the oral cavity and an otoscope to examine inside the nose, ear canals, and tympanic membranes.
   d. Position and drape the patient appropriately to ensure that the part of the body being inspected can be seen in its entirety.
   e. Examine the body for size, shape, symmetry, position, movement, and color.
   f. Compare one side of the body with the other side to determine whether they are the same (**symmetry**) or different. For example, one leg may be pink and the other pale, indicating impaired circulation to the pale leg or the patient may be able to move one side of the body but not the other side, indicating a neurological problem.

B. Auscultation

1. Performed after inspection because it is more invasive than inspection and before percussion and palpation because these steps can alter the results of auscultation.
2. Use of the ears to listen for sounds produced by the body.
3. Principles of auscultation.
   a. Listen to sounds.
      (1) Directly: Use unaided ears for audible sounds, such as burping, passing flatus, snoring, loud wheezing, and a grating sound when moving a joint.
      (2) Indirectly: Use a device (e.g., stethoscope, electronic Doppler) to magnify the sound when sounds are not audible outside the body.
      (3) To detect sounds in different parts of the body: Lungs (e.g., normal and adventitious breath sounds), heart (e.g., rate, rhythm, murmurs, rubs, or gallops), intestines (e.g., bowel sounds [borborygmi]), uterus (e.g., fetal heart rate and blood flowing through uterine arteries of a pregnant woman [soufflé]).
   b. Assess the characteristics of the sounds heard.
      (1) Pitch: Quality of a sound based on its frequency.
      (a) High-pitched sounds have more vibrations per minute.
      (b) Low-pitched sounds have fewer vibrations per minute.
      (2) Intensity: Amplitude of the sound (e.g., loud or soft).
      (3) Quality: Characteristics of the sound (e.g., musical, gurgling, or grating).
      (4) Duration: Length of time the sound is heard (e.g., short, medium, or long).
      (5) Precipitating factors: Sound caused by or associated with some condition (e.g., pleural friction rub heard at the height of inspiration, wheezes heard on exhalation).
      (6) Relieving factors: Factors that minimize or eliminate the sound (e.g., bowel sounds decrease after flatus is expelled).

C. Percussion

1. Performed after auscultation because it is more invasive than auscultation and before palpation because palpation can alter the results of percussion.
2. Use of fingers to strike a patient's body part directly to elicit a sound or vibration.
3. Can involve the use of a small rubber-tipped hammer (e.g., for assessment of deep tendon reflexes).
4. Principles of percussion.
   a. Use the middle finger of one hand to firmly and rapidly strike the middle finger of the other hand that is placed in direct contact with the patient's skin to elicit a sound or vibration (Fig. 11.13).

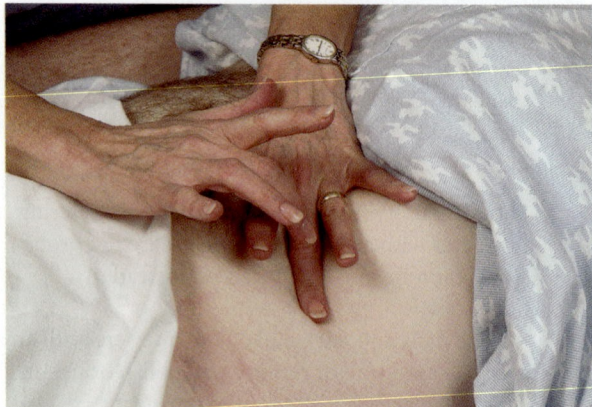

Fig 11.13 Percussion. (From Burton and Ludwig [2011]. *Fundamentals of nursing care: Concepts, connections & skills.* Philadelphia: F. A. Davis Company, with permission.)

b. Assess the sounds produced to determine the location, dimension, or density (e.g., solid, hollow, filled with air) of underlying body structures.

(1) Flatness: Dull sound generated by very dense tissue, such as bone and muscle.

(2) Dullness: Thud-like sound generated by dense tissue, such as the liver, heart, or spleen; fluid-filled abdominal cavity (**ascites**); or distended bladder.

(3) Resonance: Hollow sound generated by a normal lung.

(4) Hyperresonance: Abnormal booming sound heard when percussing a lung of a patient with emphysema.

(5) Tympany: Musical sound associated with air in the stomach or intestines.

D. Palpation

1. Performed last after percussion.

2. Use of the fingers or hands to apply pressure to the external surface of the body to feel for deviations in the skin or determine underlying structures below the skin.

a. Light palpation depresses the skin 1 to 2 cm; for example, assessing extent of edema (see Fig. 21.8), bladder distention, and a peripheral pulse.

b. Deep palpation depresses the skin 3 to 5 cm; performed only by a skilled practitioner because excessive pressure can injure an organ; not usually done during a routine nursing assessment.

(1) One-handed technique: One hand compresses the skin (Fig. 11.14).

(2) Two-handed technique: One hand supports the body while the other hand palpates the organ (Fig. 11.15).

3. Principles of palpation.

a. Keep fingernails short.

b. Perform hand hygiene and warm the hands before touching the patient.

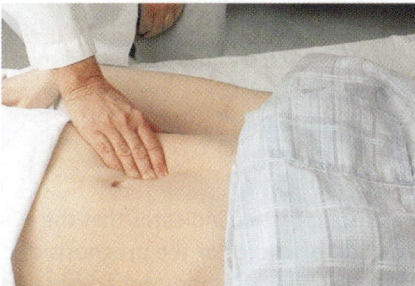

Fig 11.14 Deep palpation: one-handed technique. (From Wilkinson and Treas [2011]. *Fundamentals of nursing,* Vol. 2, 2nd ed. Philadelphia: F. A. Davis Company, with permission.)

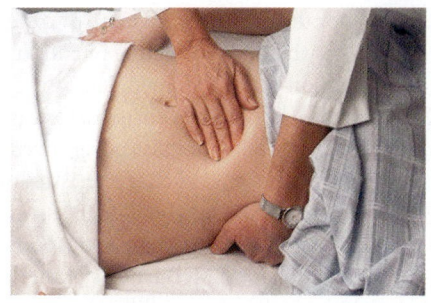

Fig 11.15 Deep palpation: two-handed technique. (From Wilkinson and Treas [2011]. *Fundamentals of nursing,* Vol. 2, 2nd ed. Philadelphia: F. A. Davis Company, with permission.)

c. Implement light palpation first, followed by deep palpation if qualified to perform this technique.

d. Palpate tender or painful areas last; observe for grimacing, response to initiation or release of pressure, and reports of discomfort or pain.

e. Assess all four quadrants of the abdomen.

4. Assessment sites.

a. Assess the status of the skin for texture, turgor, moisture, and temperature; use the back of the fingers where skin is thinner to assess for surface temperature (Fig. 11.16). Assess both legs at the same time for symmetry.

b. Assess the rate and quality of arterial pulses.

c. Assess the status of muscle relaxation or rigidity (e.g., tense muscles indicate muscle contraction, board-like abdomen, or compartment syndrome).

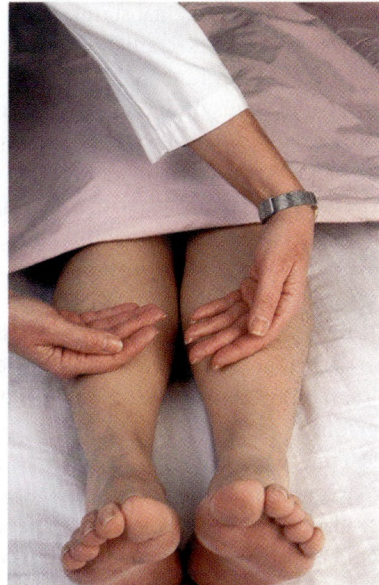

Fig 11.16 Assessing skin temperature. (From Burton and Ludwig [2011]. *Fundamentals of nursing care: Concepts, connections & skills.* Philadelphia: F. A. Davis Company, with permission.)

d. Assess for the presence of fluid (e.g., distention of the urinary bladder, indicating retention of urine, or distention of the abdomen, indicating ascites.

e. Determine the location, consistency, size, and movability of organs or masses (e.g., liver, spleen).

f. Assess the location and characteristics of pain in response to pressure (e.g., pain associated with appendicitis that occurs in response to pressure applied to McBurney's point, located in right lower quadrant of the abdomen halfway between the anterior iliac crest and the umbilicus) or tensing of abdominal muscles or pain that occurs when moderate pressure is applied to the abdomen, held, and then quickly released (**rebound tenderness**).

XI. Perform a Physical Assessment

After performing a general survey of the patient and obtaining vital signs, the nurse should assess the patient's physical status in more detail. Physical assessment should follow a systematic, thorough, and consistent approach. For this discussion, assessment is performed in relation to the systems of the body (e.g., neurological, integumentary, respiratory, cardiovascular, GI, genitourinary, and so on).

A. Neurological System

1. The anatomy of the nervous system includes the brain (cerebrum, cerebellum, brainstem, and cranial nerves), spinal cord and spinal tracks, and spinal nerves. There are 31 pairs of spinal nerves that arise from the spinal cord and exit at each intervertebral foramen (vertebrae include 8 cervical, 12 thoracic, 5 lumbar, and 5 sacral).

2. Assessment involves mental status, level of consciousness, reflexes, cranial nerves, sensory function, and motor function.

3. Assess mental status: Indicates functioning of the cerebrum.
   a. Language: Ability to send and receive messages in verbal, written, or behavioral forms.
      (1) **Expressive aphasia:** Inability to express oneself by verbal or written words or behavioral signs.
      (2) **Receptive aphasia:** Inability to comprehend spoken or written words or behavioral signs.
   b. Orientation: Ability to identify time, place, and person.
      (1) Time: Knows the year, month, day of the week, or time of day. Ask, "What day is it?"
      (2) Place: Knows location. Ask, "Where are you?"
      (3) Person: Knows own name and recognizes or knows names of significant others. Self-identity remains the longest when there is dysfunction with time, place, and person. Ask, "What is your name?"

c. Memory: Ability to recall information.
   (1) Immediate recall: Remembers information given seconds before tested. State three numbers and immediately have patient recall the numbers.
   (2) Recent memory: Remembers information within hours and days. Ask, "What did you have for breakfast?"
   (3) Long-term memory: Remembers information within months to years. Ask, "Where were you born?"
d. Cognitive skills: Ability to focus on a mental task. Ask, "How much is three plus three?" or "Start with the number 100 and count backward in intervals of five."

4. Assess level of consciousness.
   a. Determines the patient's level of arousal.
      (1) Alert: Follows commands.
      (2) Lethargic: Is drowsy, drifts off to sleep.
      (3) Stuporous: Requires vigorous stimulation for a response.
      (4) Comatose: Does not respond to verbal or painful stimuli.
   b. Use a stimulus to precipitate a response from the patient. Progressively move to the next type of stimulus if the previous stimulus does not evoke a response.
      (1) Verbal: Responds to spoken stimulus. State, "Open your eyes."
      (2) Tactile: Responds to touch. Gently shake the patient's shoulder or stroke the arm.
      (3) Painful stimulus: Responds to uncomfortable stimulus (e.g., pressure, pain). Press on the sternum or over a fingernail bed or squeeze the trapezius muscle.
   c. Use a standard reference for assessing level of consciousness when assessing a patient with a head injury; decreasing level of consciousness is one of the first indications of increased intracranial pressure (ICP).
      (1) Glasgow Coma Scale: Assesses patient's eye response, motor response, and verbal response to stimuli.
      (2) Full Outline of UnResponsiveness (FOUR) score: Assesses the patient's respirations, brainstem reflexes, eye response, and motor response to stimuli.

DID YOU KNOW?

Evidence-based practice indicates that the FOUR score is a good predictor of the prognosis of critically ill patients and has important advantages over the Glasgow Coma Scale. In addition to assessing eye response and motor response, the FOUR score also assesses respirations and brainstem reflexes.

5. Assess reflexes: A **reflex** is an automatic response to a stimulus that does not require conscious thought.
   a. Indicate the integrity of sensory and motor pathways of the reflex arc and spinal cord segments.
   b. Are either.
      (1) Superficial reflexes: Abdominal, anus, cremasteric, and plantar (Table 11.7); result graded as positive or negative.
      (2) Deep tendon reflexes: Biceps, triceps, brachioradialis, patellar, Achilles (Table 11.8); results graded as 0 = no response, +1 = diminished, +2 = normal response, +3 = increased but not pathologic, +4 = hyperactive or involuntary contraction and relaxation of skeletal muscle (clonic).
6. Assess the cranial nerves.
   a. The 12 cranial nerves are peripheral nerves that arise from the brain rather than from the spinal cord.
   b. They control numerous sensory and motor functions (Table 11.9).
7. Assess sensory functions.
   a. Assess the patient's ability to perceive sensations of light touch, pain, and temperature while the eyes are closed.
      (1) Use a wisp of cotton; use the sharp end of a toothpick or paper clip (do not use an object, such as a needle, that will break the skin); use test tubes filled with hot and cold water.
      (2) Assess distal areas first and then proximal areas; if the distal area is intact, you need not test the proximal area. If pain sensation is intact, you need not test for temperature because these stimuli are transmitted along the same spinal tracks.
      (3) Monitor for expected patient responses: patient should feel light touch, pain, and temperature variations in all extremities; assess for symmetry.
      (4) Monitor for deviations from expected responses; dysfunction will relate to areas

Table 11.7 **Evaluating Superficial Reflexes**		
Reflex	**Expected Response**	**Deviation**
Abdominal: Stroke each abdominal quadrant toward the umbilicus. 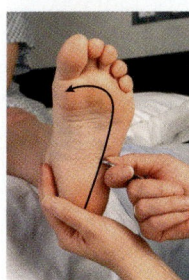	• Positive: Umbilicus moves toward stimulus.	• Negative: No response indicates problem involving T8, T9, or T10.
Anus: Touch the side of the anus with a gloved finger.	• Positive: Anus puckers.	• Negative: No response indicates problem involving S3, S4, or S5.
Cremasteric: Stroke the inner aspect of a male's thigh.	• Positive: Elevation of testes.	• Negative: No response indicates problem with L1 or L2.
Plantar (Babinski): With a thumb or dull instrument, stroke the sole of the foot from the heel up the lateral side toward and then across the ball of the foot to the great toe.	• Negative: All toes curl downward or no response; positive response is normal until age 2 years or until child is walking.	• Positive: Dorsiflexion of great toe with or without fanning of other toes indicates problem with upper motor neurons.

Photo credits: Dillon (2007). *Nursing health assessment: Clinical pocket guide,* 2nd ed. F. A. Davis Company, with permission.

Table 11.8 **Evaluating Deep Tendon Reflexes**

Reflex	Expected Response	Deviation
Biceps: Support the patient's elbow with your thumb over the biceps tendon and strike the percussion hammer on your thumb.	• +2; feel biceps contract under your thumb; observe slight flexion of the elbow.	• Increased or decreased response indicates problem with C5 or C6.
Triceps: Abduct the patient's shoulder; flex the elbow, letting the arm hang down; and strike the triceps tendon 1 to 2 inches above the olecranon process.	• +2; observe and feel extension of the elbow.	• Increased or decreased response indicates a problem with C7 or C8.
Brachioradialis: Rest the arm on the patient's leg, strike 1 to 2 inches above the bony prominence of the wrist on the side by the thumb.	• +2; observe flexion of the elbow and supination of the forearm.	• Increased or decreased response indicates a problem with C5 or C6.
Patellar: Place the patient in a sitting position with the legs dangling, strike the patellar tendon just below the patella.	• +2; observe extension of the knee.	• Increased or decreased response indicates a problem with L2, L3, or L4.
Achilles: Strike the Achilles tendon 2 inches above the heel.	• +2; observe plantar flexion of the foot.	• Increased or decreased response indicates a problem with S1 or S2.

Photo credits: From Dillon (2007). *Nursing health assessment: Clinical pocket guide*, 2nd ed. F. A. Davis Company, with permission.

Table 11.9 Assessment of Cranial Nerves

Cranial Nerve (CN) and Assessment Technique	Expected Response	Significant Deviations
I: Olfactory—Sense of smell.		
• Have the patient discriminate between odors (e.g., orange, peanut butter, coffee).	• Ability to discriminate odors.	• Impaired or absent ability to discriminate odors.
II: Optic—Sense of sight.		
• Test far vision with a Snellen chart.	• Visual acuity of 20/20.	• Inability to read Snellen chart accurately.
• Test near vision with a Rosenbaum chart.	• Ability to read Rosenbaum chart.	• Inability to read Rosenbaum chart accurately.
• Ask the patient to describe boundaries of visual field while eyes are in a fixed forward position.	• Peripheral vision of 50° in superior field, 70° in inferior field, 60° in nasal field, and 90° to 110° in temporal field.	• Limited peripheral vision **(tunnel vision)**.
III: Oculomotor—Movement of eyeballs, position of lids, and constriction of pupils.		
IV: Trochlear—Moves eyeball downward and laterally.		
VI: Abducens—Moves eyeball laterally.		
• Have the patient follow your finger moving through all fields of gaze (up-down, left-right, at an angle up right to lower left, and at an angle up left to lower right).	• Movement of eyes through all fields of gaze equally.	• Lack of eye symmetry when moving through fields of gaze; rapid involuntary rhythmic eye movements **(nystagmus)**.
• Place your finger 12 inches in front of the patient's eyes and move toward the eyes.	• Pupils constriction and both eyes turn inward toward the nose as the person focuses on the finger.	• Failure of one or both pupils to accommodate or slow accommodation.
• Inspect location of lids.	• No lid lag.	• Drooping of eyelid (ptosis).
• Shine light on pupil.	• Pupils equal, round, reactive to light and accommodation (PERRLA).	• Slow pupil constriction or lack of constriction.
V: Trigeminal—Muscle strength, facial sensation, corneal reflex.		
• Have the patient clench the jaw while your hands are on the sides of the face.	• Firm and symmetrical muscle tone.	• Deviation of jaw to one side; uncoordinated twitching of muscles **(fasciculations)**.
• Touch the side of the face at the scalp, cheek, and chin with the point of a paperclip, alternating with a wisp of cotton; do not follow a predictable pattern.	• Ability to distinguish between the sharp versus light sensation.	• Inability to distinguish between the sharp versus light sensation.
• Touch a wisp of cotton to the cornea (usually not performed on a conscious patient).	• Symmetrical blink reflex.	• Absent blink reflex or asymmetrical blink reflex.
VII: Facial—Facial expression, muscle strength, and taste.		
• Have the patient smile, wrinkle the forehead, puff out the cheeks, purse the lips, squeeze the eyes shut, and bear the teeth.	• Symmetrical facial movements.	• Asymmetrical facial movements (e.g., mouth droops, nasolabial fold flattens, or lower eyelid sags).
• Test taste by placing various foods on the anterior two-thirds of the tongue (e.g., sugar—sweet; lemon juice—sour; table salt—salty).	• Ability to distinguish among sweet, sour, and salt stimuli.	• Difficulty with or inability to distinguish among sweet, sour, and salt stimuli.

Continued

Table 11.9 Assessment of Cranial Nerves—cont'd

Cranial Nerve (CN) and Assessment Technique	Expected Response	Significant Deviations
VIII: Auditory—Hearing acuity, sound conduction, and equilibrium.		
• Stand behind the patient and whisper or place a ticking clock by the patient's ear. • Place a vibrating tuning fork on the top of the patient's head (Weber test). 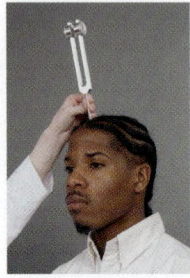	• Ability to hear the voice or ticking clock. • Sound heard equally in both ears.	• Diminished or absent ability to hear voice or ticking clock. • Sound louder in an impaired ear with conductive hearing loss and louder in an unaffected ear if sensorineural hearing loss is present.
• Place a vibrating tuning fork on the mastoid bone (Rinne test) and record the length of time it takes the patient to no longer hear the sound (A); then place the fork next to the ear and again have the patient indicate when the sound is no longer heard (B). 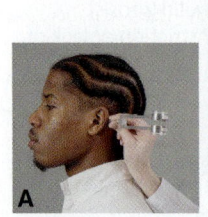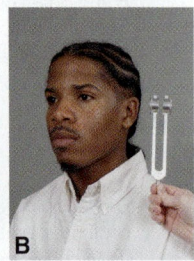	• The length of time that sound is heard via air conduction is twice as long as sound heard by bone conduction.	• Sound heard longer by air conduction with sensorineural hearing loss and sound heard longer by bone conduction with conductive hearing loss.
• Assess equilibrium by having the patient stand with feet together and arms at the sides; done with eyes open and then closed (Romberg test).	• Maintenance of balance with minimal swaying.	• Swaying or loss of balance.
IX: Glossopharyngeal—Taste, swallowing, gag reflex, tongue movement, and secretion of saliva. *X: Vagus—Swallowing, movement of vocal cords, peristalsis, digestive secretions, sensory in cardiac, respiratory, and blood pressure reflexes.*		
• Listen to the patient speak. • Assess ability to swallow. • Assess ability to cough. • Depress the tongue with a tongue blade and observe the soft palate while the patient says "ah." • Touch the back of the pharynx with a tongue blade. • Test taste by placing sweet, sour, and salty foods on posterior one-third of tongue.	• Strong, clear voice. • Swallowing with ease. • Coughing with ease. • Symmetrical rising of uvula and soft palate. • Elicits gag reflex. • Ability to distinguish among sweet, sour, and salt stimuli.	• Hoarseness. • Impaired ability to swallow. • Impaired ability to cough. • Asymmetrical movement of uvula and soft palate. • Absence of gag reflex. • Difficulty with or inability to distinguish among sweet, sour, and salt stimuli. May be diminished in older adults.

Table 11.9 Assessment of Cranial Nerves—cont'd

Cranial Nerve (CN) and Assessment Technique	Expected Response	Significant Deviations
XI: Accessory—Head movement and elevation of shoulders.		
• Have the patient turn the head from side to side against resistance. • Place your hands on the patient's shoulders and ask the patient to raise the shoulders against resistance.	• Full range of symmetrical movement without pain. • Ability to raise shoulders symmetrically.	• Asymmetrical movement, limited or absent movement, or pain. • Asymmetrical movement, limited or absent movement, or pain.
XII: Hypoglossal—Tongue movement.		
• Have the patient protrude the tongue and move it from side to side. • Ask the patient to say *"l, t, d, n."*	• Ability to move the tongue easily. • Ability to articulate letters easily.	• Limited ability to move the tongue. • Difficulty articulating letters.

Photo credits: Wilkinson and Treas (2011). *Fundamentals of nursing,* Vol. 2, 2nd ed. Philadelphia: F. A. Davis Company, with permission.

innervated by specific spinal nerves (dermatomes).

  (a) **Hyperalgia:** Increased pain sensation.
  (b) **Analgesia:** No pain sensation.
  (c) **Paresthesia:** Numbness and tingling.

  b. Assess ability to identify an object via touch (**stereognosis**): Have the patient close the eyes, place a familiar object in the patient's hand, and then have the patient identify the object (e.g., key, coin, paperclip). Abnormal finding indicates problem with sensory cortex or posterior column of spinal cord.

  c. Assess ability to identify the position or movement of the body (**kinesthesia**): Move a patient's finger from one position to another and ask the patient to describe the direction of movement. An abnormal finding indicates damage to peripheral nerves or the posterior column of the spinal cord.

  d. Assess for human responses to both sensory deprivation and sensory overload (e.g., irritability, confusion, reduced attention span, drowsiness, decreased problem solving ability).

    (1) Assess for adaptations specific to sensory overload (e.g., fatigue, inability to concentrate, disorientation, anxiety, increased muscle tension).
    (2) Assess for adaptations specific to sensory deprivation (e.g., depression, preoccupation with somatic ailments, delusions, hallucinations).

 8. Assess motor functions.
  a. The cerebellum helps coordinate muscle movement, posture, equilibrium, and body positioning.

  b. Assess coordination; all movements should be smooth and rhythmical.

    (1) Have the patient extend the arms out to the side and then alternately touch each index finger to the nose with the eyes closed.
    (2) Have the patient touch the thumb to each fingertip in rapid sequence.
    (3) Place the patient in the supine position and, with the ball of the patient's foot in your hand, ask the patient to repeatedly tap your hand with the foot.

  c. Assess balance.

    (1) Have the patient perform the Romberg test (see Table 11.9, cranial nerve VIII).
    (2) Have the patient stand on one foot with the eyes closed and the arms at the side; should maintain balance for ≥5 seconds with just slight swaying.
    (3) Have the patient walk a straight line, alternating the feet while placing the heel of one foot directly in front of the toes of the other foot.

B. Integumentary System

For a thorough assessment of the skin (including temperature, moisture, texture, and primary and secondary lesions), hair, and nails, see the section "Assessment of Skin" in Chapter 16, "Hygiene."

 1. The anatomy of the integumentary system includes the skin, mucous membranes, hair, and nails.
 2. Mucous membranes consist of an epithelial membrane that lines body surfaces opening directly to the exterior of the body (e.g., oral cavity, rectum, nose, urethra) and the entire GI tract from the mouth to the anus; these membranes secrete mucus, a thick, slippery material that keeps the membranes moist and protected.

3. Assessment of these tissues reveals changes in oxygenation, circulation, nutrition, and hydration.
4. Assess the mouth and oropharynx by inspection.
   a. Lips: Should be pink or color of the person's skin, smooth, moist, intact, and free from lesions. Abnormalities include dryness, fissures, pallor, cyanosis, involuntary movement, and drooping.
   b. Inner surface of mouth, buccal mucosa, roof of mouth, and floor of mouth: Same assessments results as lips. Note if the mucosa of the oral cavity is inflamed (**stomatitis**).
   c. Tongue: Should be shiny, pink, and moist, with an even distribution of papillae organized in an inverted "V." Note dryness, fissures, or inflammation of the tongue (**glossitis**).
   d. Uvula and tonsils: Uvula should be in midline and rise when patient says "ah." Tonsils should be pink, smooth, with no discharge, and be behind the tonsillar pillars. Note if the tonsils are inflamed (**tonsillitis**).
   e. Teeth and gums: Teeth should be free from tarter, hardened deposits of plaque (debris from bacteria, saliva, epithelial cells, and leukocytes). Note if the gums are inflamed (**gingivitis**).

C. Cardiovascular System
1. The anatomy of the cardiovascular system consists of the heart, great vessels (e.g., aorta, superior and inferior vena cava, pulmonary arteries, and pulmonary veins), and peripheral circulation (e.g., arteries, capillaries, and veins).
2. Assessment involves determining the blood pressure; rate and rhythm of heart contractions; rate, volume, and symmetry of peripheral arteries; and inspection of veins and condition of peripheral tissues.
3. Assess blood pressure (see the section "Measurement of Blood Pressure" earlier in this chapter).
4. Auscultate heart sounds using a systematic progression; begin at the aortic area and end at the mitral area.
   a. Apical pulse: See "Measurement of Pulse" and Figures 11.3 and 11.4 for detailed information about assessing the heart rate.
   b. Auscultate over cardiac auscultation sites (Fig. 11.17).
      (1) Aortic valve: Second intercostal space (ICS) at right sternal border.
      (2) Pulmonic valve: Second ICS at left sternal border.
      (3) Tricuspid valve: Fourth ICS at left sternal border.
      (4) Mitral valve: Fifth ICS at midclavicular line.
   c. Heart sounds (Table 11.10).

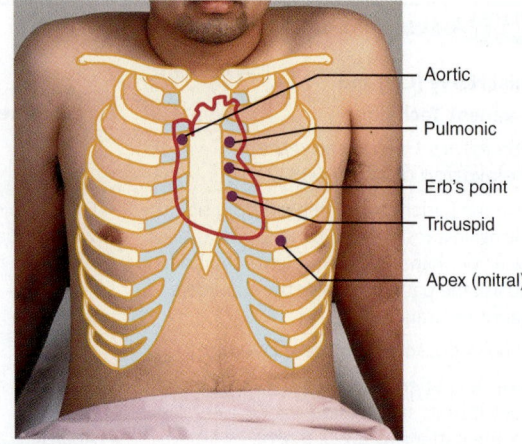

Fig 11.17 Auscultation of heart sounds. (Adapted from Wilkinson and Treas [2011]. *Fundamentals of nursing*, Vol. 1, 2nd ed. Philadelphia: F. A. Davis Company, with permission.)

   d. Identify the presence of a heart murmur.
      (1) A soft, muffled, swooshing prolonged heart sound rather than a clear S_1 or S_2.
      (2) Caused by turbulence of blood flow through a heart valve that does not close completely.
      (3) Aortic murmurs are best heart over Erb's point.
   e. Identify the presence of pericardial friction rub.
      (1) A short, scratchy, grating sound.
      (2) Caused by roughened pericardial membranes rubbing against each other; specific for pericarditis.
      (3) Heard at the apex, left of the sternum.
5. Assess the carotid arteries.
   (1) Auscultate over the artery to identify the presence of a whooshing sound due to narrowing of the lumen (**bruit**).
   (2) Palpate the artery lightly if a bruit is auscultated to identify vibrations from turbulent blood flow (**thrill**).

   🛑 (3) **Do not palpate both carotid arteries at the same time because doing so can impair cerebral blood flow.**

6. Assess the external jugular veins.
   (1) Return blood flow from the brain to the superior vena cava and then the heart.
   (2) Reflect functioning of the right side of the heart and circulating fluid volume.
   (3) Place the patient in the semi-Fowler (45° angle) position and then inspect for distention of the veins.
      (a) No neck vein distention expected.
      (b) Distended veins suggest a condition such as hypervolemia, right-sided heart failure, and tricuspid stenosis.
7. Assess peripheral circulation (Table 11.11).

Table 11.10 Cardiac Auscultation Sites

Heart Sound	Location	Physiology	Description
First: S_1	Mitral and tricuspid areas while sitting.	• Beginning of systole.	• *lub:* Dull, low-pitched sound.
Second: S_2	Aortic and pulmonic areas while sitting.	• Closure of valves between the ventricles and the arteries exiting the heart (semilunar valves).	• *dub:* Higher in pitch and shorter in length than S_1.
Third: S_3	Apical site with patient in left-lateral position.	• Early in diastole. • Immediately after S_2. • Produced by rapid ventricular filling.	• *ee:* Gallop tempo when combined S_1 and S_2: *lub-dub-ee.* • Disappears when patient is sitting. • Failure to disappear when sitting indicates hypervolemia or heart failure.
Fourth: S_4	Apical site with patient in left-lateral position.	• Late in diastole. • Immediately before S_1. • Produced by rapid ventricular filling.	• Presystolic gallop that has a rhythm like the word *FLOrida.* • Heard in some athletes and older adults. • Associated with hypertension, coronary artery disease, and pulmonic stenosis.

Table 11.11 Peripheral Neurovascular Assessments

Assessment	Expected Response	Deviations in Circulation
Volume of arterial pulses	• Strong. • Obliterated with moderate pressure.	• Weak, thready, or absent. • Bounding (see Table 11.5).
Capillary refill	• Blanching on compression of nail bed or tip of toe. • Return of usual skin color in ≤3 seconds (up to 5 seconds in an older adult) when compression is released, as capillaries refill with blood.	• Return to original color in >3 seconds (5 seconds in older adults).
Color and texture of nails	• Variation of pink. • Translucid.	• Yellow, thick, and brittle.
Color, texture, and temperature of skin	• Similar in color to skin on rest of body. • Smooth and supple texture. • Warmth to touch.	• Arterial: Color pale, mottled, or dependent rubor; texture rough and dry; temperature cool to touch; ulcers of toes or heels. • Venous: Brownish discoloration due to breakdown of hemoglobin and deposition of ferrous sulfate; distended, tortuous, and palpable veins; edema; venous stasis ulcers around ankles and calves.
Sensation	• Ability to distinguish dull and sharp stimuli (e.g., cotton ball versus pointed object).	• Diminished or absent ability to distinguish dull and sharp stimuli.
Mobility	• Ability to move joints through full range of motion.	• Limited ability to move joints through full range of motion.

D. **Respiratory System:** See Chapter 19, "Oxygenation," for a thorough review of the structures and functions of the respiratory system, factors that influence respirations, and assessment of the respiratory system. Assessment topics encompass inspection (including breathing patterns), auscultation (including normal and abnormal breath sounds), percussion, and palpation.

E. **Gastrointestinal (GI) System:** See Chapter 22, "Gastrointestinal," for a thorough review of the structures and functions of the GI system, factors affecting bowel elimination, nursing assessments (including characteristics of normal and abnormal stool), and common human responses related to the GI system (including diarrhea, constipation, fecal incontinence, hemorrhoids, and flatulence).

1. The GI system includes the mouth, esophagus, stomach, small intestine, and large intestine.
2. Accessory organs (e.g., pancreas, liver, gall bladder, and appendix) are often considered in a GI assessment.
3. Inspect the abdomen.
   a. Follow a systematic pattern and include the four abdominal quadrants (Fig. 11.18).

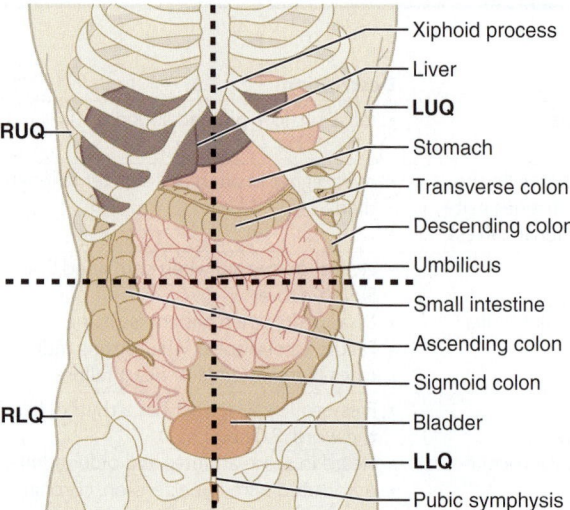

Fig 11.18 Four abdominal quadrants. (From Wilkinson and Treas [2011]. *Fundamentals of nursing,* Vol. 1, 2nd ed. Philadelphia: F. A. Davis Company, with permission.)

b. Assess color and integrity.
   (1) Normal findings: Uniform color; unblemished; silverish white stretch marks (**striae**); possible surgical scars.
   (2) Deviations: Tense, glistening skin, possibly indicating edema, ascites, or flatulence; purple striae, possibly indicating rapid weight loss or gain or Cushing's syndrome; rashes; other lesions.
c. Assess contour.
   (1) Normal findings: Flat; round (convex); scaphoid (concave).
   (2) Deviations: Abdominal distension, which requires a further focused assessment (e.g., measure the abdominal girth with a tape measure around the body at the level of the umbilicus, auscultate for bowel sounds, and assess for ascites by placing the hands on each side of the abdomen while pushing against the abdomen with one hand and feeling for the presence of fluid exerting pressure against the other side of the abdomen [**fluid wave test**]).
d. Assess symmetry: Have the patient take and hold a deep breath.
   (1) Normal findings: Symmetrical appearance.
   (2) Deviations: Enlarged liver and spleen become more prominent; localized protrusions may indicate an umbilical or inguinal hernia or a tumor.
e. Assess vascular pattern, including the presence of prominent veins.
   (1) Normal findings: No visible vascular pattern.
   (2) Deviations: Dilated veins visible; associated with ascites, liver disease, and venocaval obstruction.

4. Auscultate the abdomen for bowel sounds.
   a. Follow a logical sequence, listening in several areas in all four quadrants.
   b. Disconnect nasogastric tube suctioning during the assessment if present.
   c. Record the results of assessment of bowel sounds.
      (1) Normal findings: High-pitched, irregular musical sounds or gurgles (**borborygmi**) that occur every 5 to 15 seconds and last 1 to several seconds.
      (2) Deviations.
         (a) Absent sounds: No sounds heard after listening for 5 minutes.
         (b) Hypoactive sounds: Soft, infrequent sounds occurring approximately one per minute; caused by decreased intestinal peristalsis associated with anesthesia, abdominal surgery, or conditions such as bowel infections, obstruction, or impaired innervation.
         (c) Hyperactive sounds: Loud, frequent sounds occurring approximately every 2 to 3 seconds; caused by increased intestinal peristalsis associated with diarrhea, gastroenteritis, and early bowel obstruction.
5. Auscultate the abdomen for vascular sounds.
   a. Listen over major blood vessels in the abdomen (Fig. 11.19).
   b. Listen for the presence of a whooshing sound due to turbulent blood flow; associated with narrowing of the lumen (**stenosis**) or dilation of a lumen (**aneurysm**). Immediately notify the primary health-care provider if you identify this whooshing sound because it indicates a life-threatening situation.
6. Percuss the abdomen.
   a. Use indirect percussion (see Fig. 11.13) in several areas in each quadrant using a systematic sequence (Fig. 11.20).

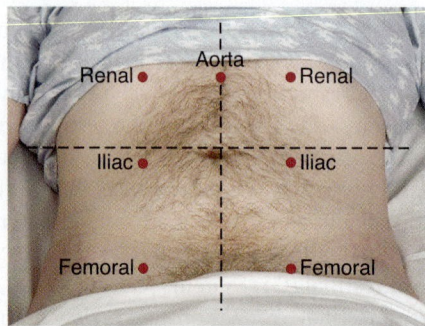

Fig 11.19 Auscultation of abdomen for vascular sounds. (From Wilkinson and Treas [2011]. *Fundamentals of nursing,* Vol. 2, 2nd ed. Philadelphia: F. A. Davis Company, with permission.)

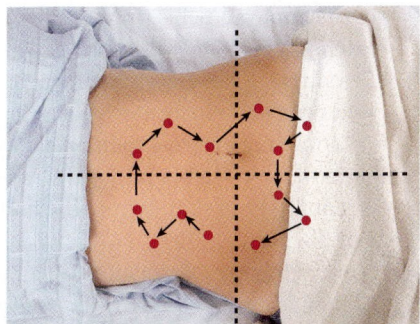

Fig 11.20 Percussion of abdomen. (From Wilkinson and Treas [2011]. *Fundamentals of nursing,* Vol. 2, 2nd ed. Philadelphia: F. A. Davis Company, with permission.)

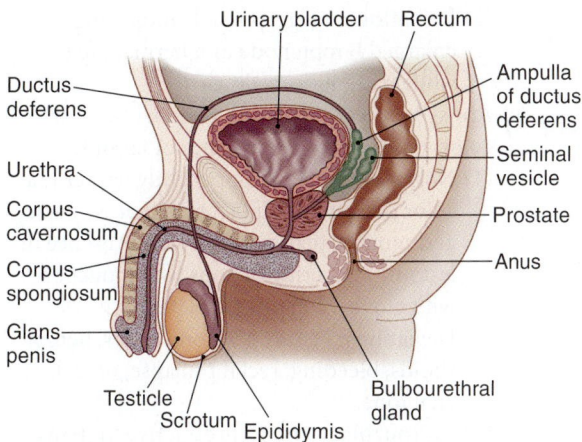

Fig 11.21 Male genitourinary and reproductive systems. (From Wilkinson and Treas [2011]. *Fundamentals of nursing,* Vol. 1, 2nd ed. Philadelphia: F. A. Davis Company, with permission.)

b. Normal findings: Tympany over the stomach and gas-filled intestine; dullness over the liver, spleen, and full bladder; no tenderness.

c. Deviations: High-pitched tympany heard with distention; large dull areas associated with organ enlargement, tumors, and presence of fluid.

7. Palpate the abdomen.

🛇 a. Do not palpate when large pulsations are present, in a patient who had an organ transplant, or when a Wilms' tumor is suspected.

b. Perform light palpation.
   (1) Palpate in several areas in each quadrant using a systematic sequence.
   (2) Press down 1 to 2 cm with a slight circular motion.
   (3) Normal findings: Abdomen is soft, not tender, and without palpable masses.
   (4) Deviations: Tenderness, guarding, and rigidity may indicate peritonitis; presence of masses.

F. Male Genitourinary and Reproductive Systems

See Chapter 20, "Urinary Elimination," for a thorough review of the anatomy and physiology of the urinary system, factors affecting urinary function, characteristics of normal and abnormal urine, and nursing assessments related to urinary status.

1. The male genitourinary system includes the structures of the urinary system and the reproductive system. The reproductive system has both internal and external structures (Fig. 11.21).

2. Inspect and palpate external genital structures while wearing gloves and with the patient standing, followed by the supine position.

   a. Pubic hair: Assess distribution, amount, and characteristics.
      (1) Normal findings: Triangular distribution of thick hair above the penis, spreading up toward the abdomen and possibly extending onto the thighs.
      (2) Deviations: Thin texture; sparse or absent hair; presence of parasites.

   b. Penis: Assess the shaft, glans, and urethral meatus.
      (1) Normal findings: Color similar to patient's skin; skin intact, slightly wrinkled. Absence of foreskin if circumcised and presence of foreskin if uncircumcised; ability to retract foreskin, revealing small amount of thick white material (**smegma**). Smooth and semifirm shaft. Absence of discharge from urethral meatus at tip of glans if gently compressed.
      (2) Deviations: Presence of lesions, nodules, pimples, warts, rash, ulceration, or thickening; tenderness; inability to retract foreskin (**phimosis**); urethral meatus on underside of shaft (**hypospadias**) or upper side of shaft (**epispadias**); white, green, or yellow discharge from urethral meatus, possibly indicating a sexually transmitted infection (if present, obtain specimen for examination).

   c. Scrotum: Assess condition, size, position, and symmetry.
      (1) Normal findings: Intact skin, numerous wrinkles (**rugae**), and darker in color than patient's skin. Size and shape varies but in proportion to penis; smooth, rubbery, and free of nodules; symmetrical but left scrotal sac usually lower than the right.
      (2) Deviations: Discolorations; tightening of skin with few rugae, possibly indicating edema, fluid, infection, torsion, or a mass; small, hard lump; rash caused by fungal infection (*tinea cruris*).

   d. Inguinal area: Assess the inguinal canal while the patient bears down or coughs.
      (1) Normal findings: Area free from bulges and swelling.

(2) Deviations: Bulge, possibly indicating an enlarged lymph node or a hernia if felt while patient bears down.

e. Anus: Assess the anus and perianal skin for color, intactness, and presence of lesions.

  (1) Normal findings: Color slightly darker than color of buttocks. Intact skin that is coarser and moister than perianal skin. Absence of lesions. Puckering of anus when touched with gloved finger (**anal reflex**).

  (2) Deviations: Fissures, lesions, warts, hemorrhoids, bleeding, rectal prolapse, or lack of anal tone.

G. **Female Genitourinary and Reproductive Systems**

See Chapter 20, "Urinary Elimination," for a thorough review of the anatomy and physiology of the female urinary system, factors affecting urinary function, characteristics of normal and abnormal urine, and nursing assessments related to urinary status.

1. The female genitourinary system includes the structures of the urinary system and the reproductive system. The reproductive system has both internal and external structures (Fig. 11.22).

2. Inspect and palpate the external genital structures while wearing gloves and with the patient in the lithotomy position (Fig. 11.23).

a. Pubic hair: Assess distribution, amount, and characteristics.

  (1) Normal findings: Triangular shaped, course, full, symmetrical over pad of fatty tissue over symphysis pubis (**mons pubis**); may extend toward inner thighs.

  (2) Deviations: Sparse, asymmetrical, or excessive; presence of parasites.

b. Labia (consist of external folds [**labia majora**] and internal folds [**labia minora**]). Assess color, condition of skin, symmetry, and presence of discharge.

  (1) Normal findings: Color similar to patient's skin; intact skin; symmetrical; no discharge.

  (2) Deviations: Presence of erythema, ecchymosis, swelling, rash, lesions, firm mass, and warts; asymmetrical; and presence of discharge.

c. Clitoris: Inspect for size and position.

  (1) Normal findings: 2 cm long and 0.5 cm wide; no redness, swelling, or lesions.

  (2) Deviations: Enlargement may be due to excess androgen; swelling may be due to trauma or inflammation; absence may be due to female circumcision (ritual associated with some African countries and some Muslim groups).

d. Urethral meatus: Assess color, shape, size, and position.

  (1) Normal findings: Slit-like opening midline below clitoris and above vagina; pink; moist.

  (2) Deviations: Displacement of urethral meatus; erythema; swelling; lesions; presence of discharge.

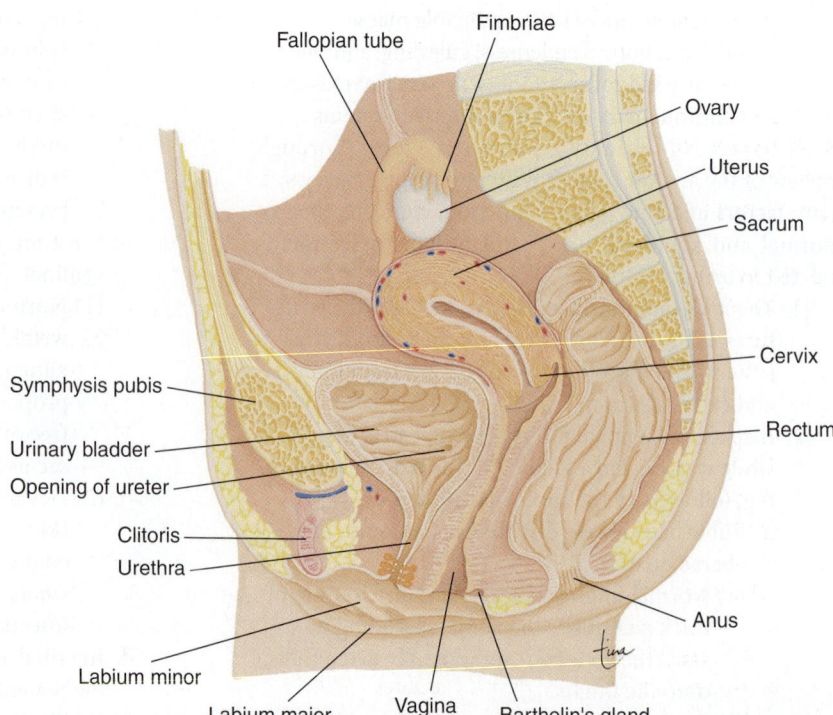

Fig 11.22 Female genitourinary and reproductive systems. (From Wilkinson and Treas [2011]. *Fundamentals of nursing*, Vol. 1, 2nd ed. Philadelphia: F. A. Davis Company, with permission.)

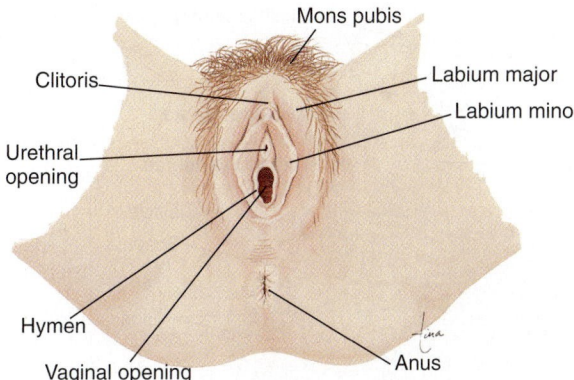

Fig 11.23 Female external genitalia. (From Scanlon [2007]. *Essentials of anatomy and physiology,* 5th ed. Philadelphia: F. A. Davis Company, with permission.)

Labels: Mons pubis, Clitoris, Urethral opening, Hymen, Vaginal opening, Labium major, Labium minor, Anus

   e. Vaginal introitus: Assess color, shape, and size.
   (1) Normal findings: Pink; moist with clear to white odorless discharge; patent with no bulging or tenderness when the patient bears down.
   (2) Deviations: Pale and dry, possibly caused by aging or topical steroids; any color discharge with a foul odor, possibly indicating a sexually transmitted infection; fissures, swelling, and ecchymosis, possibly indicating trauma or abuse; bulging of anterior vaginal wall (**cystocele**); bulging of posterior vaginal wall (**rectocele**).
   f. Anus: Same as for male genitourinary system.
   3. Inspection and palpation of internal structures such as cervix, vaginal wall, uterus and ovaries (pelvic examination) should be performed only by an experienced practitioner.

H. Musculoskeletal System
See Chapter 17, "Mobility," for a review of the physiology of movement (e.g., skeletal system, nervous system, and muscles). Included in the discussion is information related to balance, body alignment, coordination, joint mobility, gait, abnormal gaits, and range of motion of all joints of the body.
   1. The musculoskeletal system consists of bones, joints, connecting structures (e.g., tendons, ligaments, bursae, and cartilage), and muscles.
   2. The skeletal system, consisting of 206 bones, provides shape and support for the body, protects internal organs, produces constituents of the blood (e.g., RBCs, WBCs, platelets), and stores calcium and phosphorus (Fig. 11.24).
   a. Axial bones: Skull, vertebral column, and rib cage.
   b. Appendicular bones: Arms, shoulder girdle, legs, and pelvic girdle.

   3. An interrelationship among the nervous system, skeletal system, connecting structures, and muscles provide for movement.
   4. Posture: Assess body and head position.
   a. Normal findings: Posture erect; head midline.
   b. Deviations: Posture slumped or tilted.
   5. Spinal curves: Assess the symmetry of shoulders, scapula, and iliac crests. Assess cervical, thoracic, lumbar, and sacral curves.
   a. Normal findings: Symmetrical shoulders, scapula, and iliac crests. Cervical–concave; thoracic–convex; lumbar–concave; sacral–convex (Fig. 11.25).
   b. Deviations: Accentuated thoracic curve (**kyphosis**); accentuated lumbar curve (**lordosis**); lateral "S" spinal deviation (**scoliosis**) (Fig. 11.26).
   6. Gait: Assess arm swing, cadence, width of feet apart, stride length, and toe position.
   a. Normal findings: Smooth, rhythmic movements with arms swinging in opposition; width of feet apart is 2 to 4 inches; length of stride is 12 to 14 inches; toes point forward.
   b. Deviations: Uncoordinated movements; lack of arm swing (associated with Parkinson disease); wide base of support and shortened stride associated with muscle weakness, joint stiffness, central nervous system dysfunction (usually cerebellum), and problems with balance. Extending arms to the side with a wide base of support and shortened stride, indicating problems with balance. See the section "Abnormal gaits" (e.g., waddling, propulsive, spastic, steppage) in Chapter 17, "Mobility," page 479.
   7. Balance: See "c. Assess balance" under the section "Assess Motor Functions," earlier in this chapter (page 269); see also Table 11.9, "Assessment of Cranial Nerves," cranial nerve VIII (Romberg test).
   a. Normal findings: Coordinated; ability to maintain balance with minimal swaying.
   b. Deviations: Difficulty maintaining balance related to cerebellar disorder or dorsal column problem.
   8. Muscles: Assess tone while muscles are at rest and when contracted; hand strength via grip; leg strength via foot push/leg rise against resistance; and movements.
   a. Normal findings: Muscles soft and pliable at rest; muscles firm when contracted; hand grip and foot push/leg rise strong and equal; no involuntary movements.
   b. Deviations.
   (1) Strength in arm and legs weak, unequal, or absent.

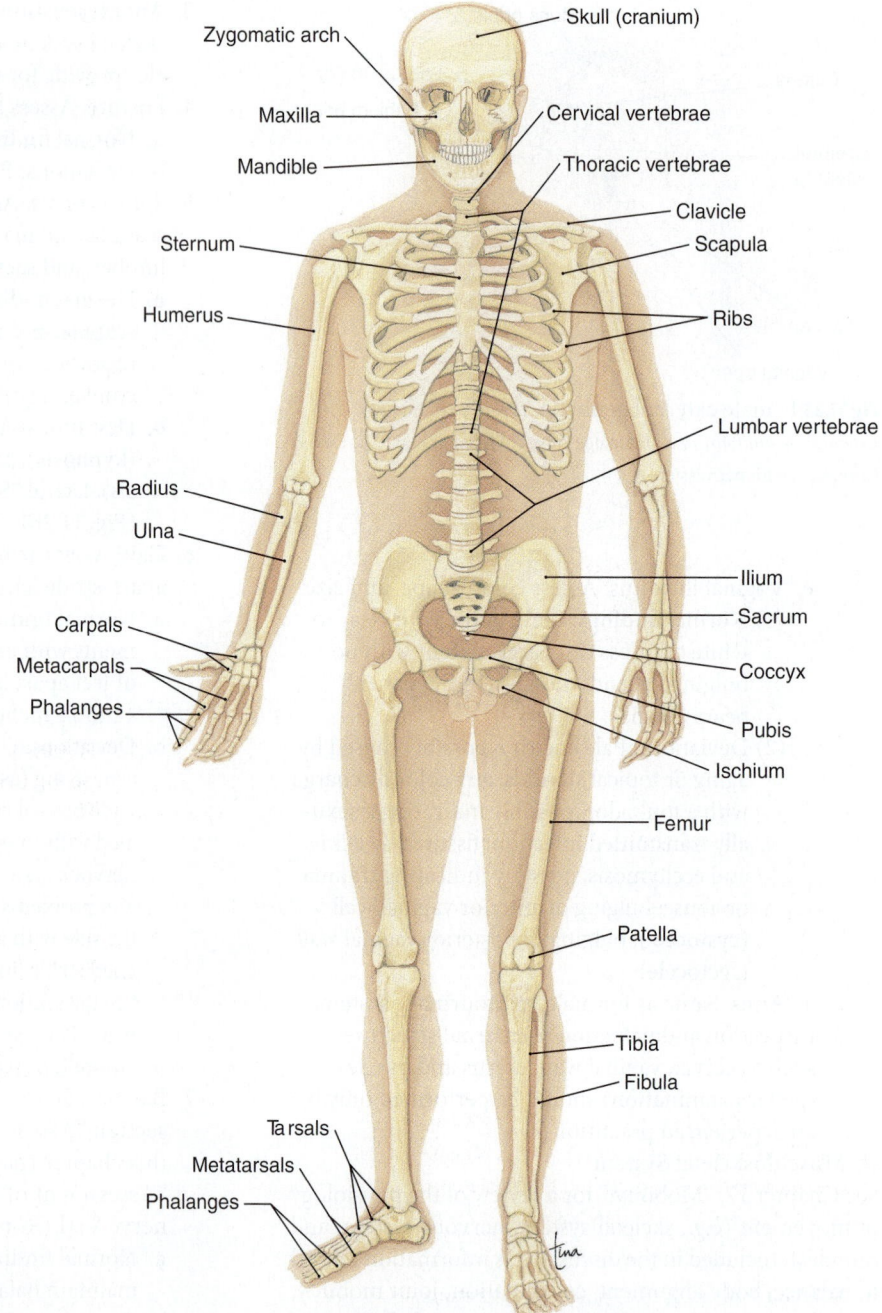

Fig 11.24 Skeletal system. (From Scanlon [2007]. *Essentials of anatomy and physiology,* 5th ed. Philadelphia: F. A. Davis Company, with permission.)

(2) Deviations in muscle tone.
   (a) **Atony:** Lack of muscle tone.
   (b) **Hypotony:** Decreased muscle tone.
   (c) **Hypertony:** Excessive tone.

(3) Deviations in movement.
   (a) **Ataxia:** Uncoordinated movements.
   (b) **Spasticity:** Uncontrolled contractions of skeletal muscles.
   (c) **Hemiparesis:** Weakness in arm and leg on same side of body.
   (d) **Hemiplegia:** Paralysis in arm and leg on same side of body.
   (e) **Paraplegia:** Paralysis of both legs.

   (f) **Quadriplegia:** Paralysis of both arms and both legs.
   (g) **Tremors:** Rhythmic, purposeless movements.
   (h) **Intention tremor:** Tremors occurring when attempting voluntary movement.
   (i) **Nonintention tremor** (resting tremor): Tremors occurring when muscles are at rest.
   (j) **Fasciculations:** Localized, uncontrollable twitching of a single muscle group innervated by a single motor nerve fiber.

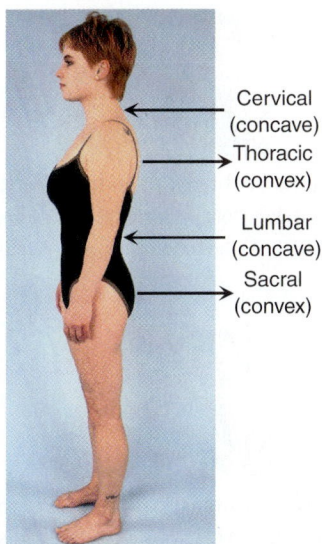

Fig 11.25 Normal spine curves. (From Wilkinson and Treas [2011]. *Fundamentals of nursing,* Vol. 2, 2nd ed. Philadelphia: F. A. Davis Company, with permission.)

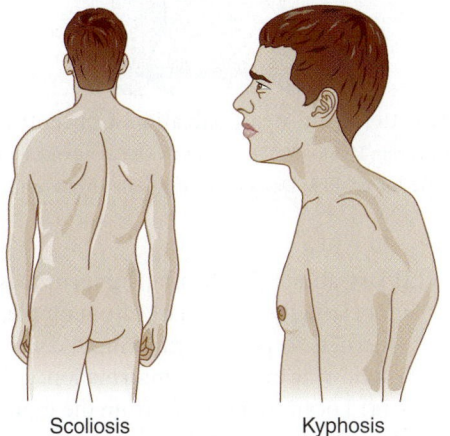

Scoliosis   Kyphosis

Fig 11.26 Scoliosis and kyphosis. (From Wilkinson and Treas [2011]. *Fundamentals of nursing,* Vol. 2, 2nd ed. Philadelphia: F. A. Davis Company, with permission.)

9. Bones: Assess length, shape, and symmetry.
   a. Normal findings: Length between arms and length between legs less than 1 cm; expected skeletal configuration reflected in shape of all bones; absence of sound on movement.
   b. Deviations: Asymmetrical lengths; grating sound (**crepitus**) on movement; deformities of shape:
      (1) Rheumatoid arthritis: Boutonnière deformity—proximal interphalangeal joint flexion and distal interphalangeal joint hyperextension of the fingers; swan-neck deformity—proximal interphalangeal joint hyperextension and distal interphalangeal joint flexion of the fingers; ulnar drift— long axis of fingers deviates towards the ulnar side of the hand.

(2) Osteoarthritis: Heberden nodes—enlarged distal interphalangeal joints of fingers; Bouchard nodes—enlarged proximal interphalangeal joints of fingers.
(3) Gouty arthritis: Sodium urate deposits in tissues (**tophi**) of outer ear, hands, feet, elbows, or knees.

I. Assessment of the Breasts
1. The breasts of both males and females consist of glandular, fibrous, and adipose tissue. Glandular and lymphatic tissue in women is concentrated in the upper outer quadrant and extends into the ax- illa (tail of Spence) (Fig. 11.27a and Fig. 11.27b).
2. Assess the breasts via inspection for size, shape, symmetry, color, and condition of skin.
   a. View breasts with the patient standing or sitting with arms at the sides, followed by pressing

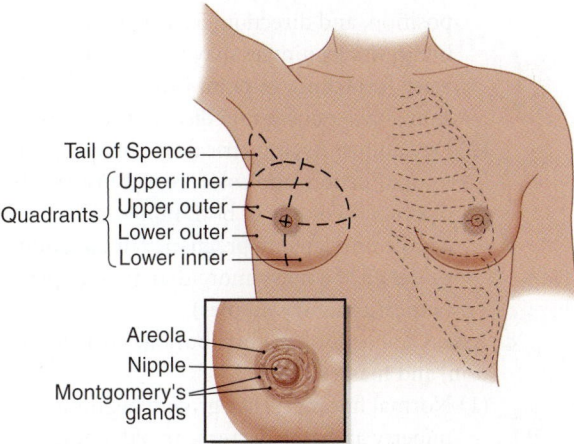

Fig 11.27a Female breast. External breast structures and quadrants. (From Dillon [2007]. *Nursing health assessment: Clinical pocket guide,* 2nd ed. F. A. Davis Company, with permission.)

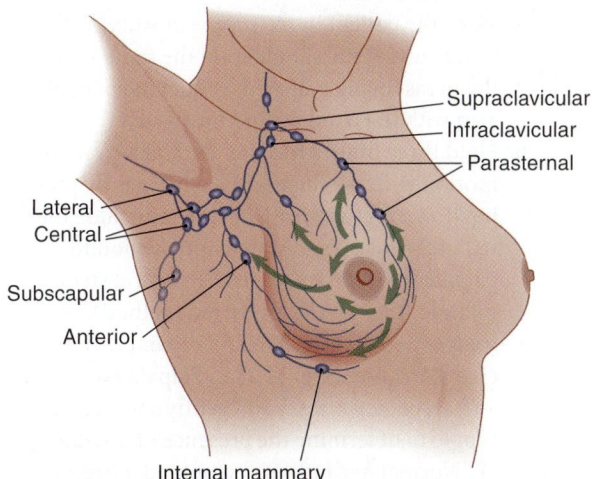

Fig 11.27b Female breast. Lymph nodes. (From Dillon [2007]. *Nursing health assessment: Clinical pocket guide,* 2nd ed. F. A. Davis Company, with permission.)

hands down on hips, pressing palms of hands together with elbows flexed, holding arms over head, and leaning forward.

    (1) Normal findings: Size and shape vary depending on individual; symmetrical, but one breast may be slightly larger than the other; skin color lighter than exposed skin surfaces; smooth skin texture; male breast even with chest wall.

    (2) Deviations: Swelling, edema, and erythema, possibly indicating infection; asymmetry, puckering, lesions, and dimpled skin texture (*peau d'orange*), possibly indicating cancer; enlargement of breasts in males (**gynecomastia**), possibly due to obesity, hormone imbalances, cancer, or estrogen therapy.

  b. Assess nipples and areolae for size, shape, position, direction, symmetry, discharge, and masses.

    (1) Normal findings: Symmetrical size, shape, position, and direction; darker color than breast tissue; nipples may be flat, point outward (eversion), or point inward (inversion) since puberty; no discharge or masses.

    (2) Deviations: Asymmetrical size, shape, position, direction, and color; recent inversion or eversion of one or both nipples; discharge unrelated to pregnancy or lactation; presence of a mass; more than two nipples (**supernumerary nipples**).

  c. Assess axillae for hair distribution, skin condition, and masses.

    (1) Normal findings: Hair growth begins at puberty and may decrease in older adults; intact skin with no masses.

    (2) Deviations: Rashes, redness, or unusual pigmentation, possibly related to infection or allergy to deodorants.

3. Palpate the breasts.

  a. Place the patient in the supine position with a wedge under the shoulder on the same side as the breast being palpated; abduct the patient's arm with the hand behind the head.

  b. Hold three fingers together and make a rotary motion with the finger pads while gently pressing down on the breast; ensure to include the tail of Spence. Use a systematic method to palpate the breast, such as the vertical strip method (Fig. 11.28a, preferred method), pie wedge method (Fig. 11.28b), or concentric circles method (Fig. 11.28c). Palpate the nipple and areola for masses and gently squeeze the nipple to determine the presence of discharge.

    (1) Normal findings: Soft, nontender breast; elastic, nontender nipples; no masses or discharge from nipples.

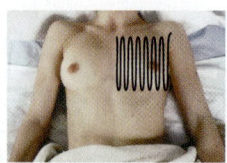

Fig. 11.28a Patterns for breast palpation. Vertical strip method. (From Dillon [2007]. *Nursing health assessment: Clinical pocket guide,* 2nd ed. F. A. Davis Company, with permission.)

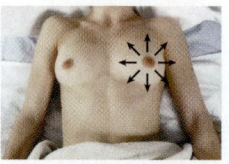

Fig 11.28b Patterns for breast palpation. Pie wedge method. (From Dillon [2007]. *Nursing health assessment: Clinical pocket guide,* 2nd ed. F. A. Davis Company, with permission.)

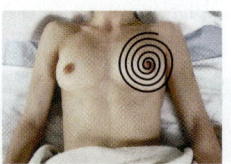

Fig 11.28c Patterns for breast palpation. Concentric circles method. (From Dillon [2007]. *Nursing health assessment: Clinical pocket guide,* 2nd ed. F. A. Davis Company, with permission.)

    (2) Deviations: Thickening, lump, or mass; loss of elasticity or discharge from nipple; tenderness. If you identify a mass, collect the following additional information.

      (a) Location: Distance from the nipple and distance from the tail of Spence; use a clock position to identify the location of the deviation around the nipple.

      (b) Size: Approximate width, length, and thickness in centimeters.

      (c) Shape: Regular, irregular, round, or oval.

      (d) Consistency: Hard or soft.

      (e) Mobility: Mobile or fixed.

      (f) Nipple: Normal or displaced, retracted; color of discharge (e.g., bloody, serous, purulent, and gray).

      (g) Tenderness: Level of discomfort when palpated.

4. Palpate the axillae.

  a. Place the patient in the sitting position while abducting the arm on the side the breast is being assessed; support the patient's arm on your forearm.

  b. Use flattened fingertips of four fingers to palpate all lymph nodes around the breast, above the clavicle, tail of Spence, and upper part of the arm (see Fig. 11.27b).

(1) Normal findings: Nonpalpable nodes; nontender.

(2) Deviations: Enlarged, tender nodes, usually indicating infection; enlarged nontender nodes, usually malignancy.

DID YOU KNOW?

The National Cancer Institute predicted that 226,870 women and 2,190 men will be diagnosed with breast cancer in 2012. Men account for approximately 1 percent of breast cancer diagnoses. This percentage is low because men obviously have less breast tissue than women. The incidence of female breast cancer in the United States is highest in the upper outer quadrant of the breast because this is the location of the most amount of breast tissue and it is closest to lymph nodes. Eight out of 10 breast cancers in women are diagnosed as infiltrating ductal carcinoma.

J. **Assessment of the Eyes**

1. Assess acuity of near vision and far vision, and boundaries of peripheral vision (see Table 11.9, "Assessment of Cranial Nerves," cranial nerve II).

2. Assess fields of gaze, accommodation, and pupillary reaction to light (see Table 11.9, "Assessment of Cranial Nerves," cranial nerves III, IV, and VI).

3. Assess color perception: Have the patient identify the color bars on the Snellen Eye Chart or distinguish colors using Ishihara cards.

a. Normal findings: Color perception is intact.

b. Deviations: Inability to distinguish colors; be aware that some older adults have difficulty distinguishing pastels and purples.

4. Assess external structures via inspection (Fig. 11.29).

a. Eyes for size, alignment, and protrusion.

(1) Normal findings: Symmetrical size; clear and bright; parallel alignment; no protrusion beyond frontal bone.

(2) Deviations: Unequal size and alignment; glazed eyes, possibly indicating excessive tearing or fever; sunken appearance related to dehydration or a decrease in periorbital fat associated with older adults; eyes protruding out of the orbit (**exophthalmos**) is associated with hyperthyroidism; visible sclera between iris and upper lids (**sun-set eyes**) is associated with hydrocephalus.

b. Eyelids for shape, position, and movement and distribution of eyelashes.

(1) Normal findings: Symmetrical opening between margins of upper and lower lids; no lid lag; ability to open and close lids; even distribution of eyelashes.

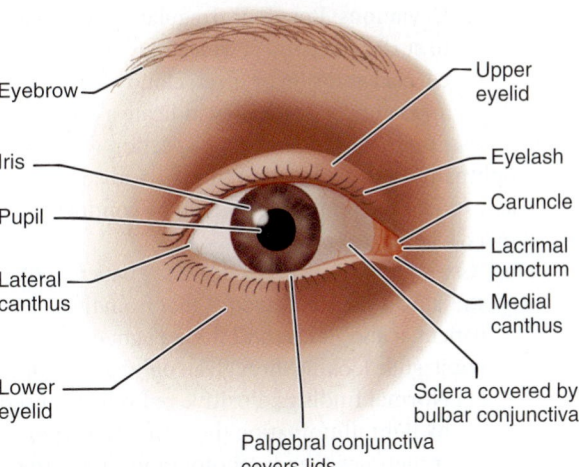

Fig 11.29 External structures of the eye. (From Wilkinson and Treas [2011]. *Fundamentals of nursing*, Vol. 1, 2nd ed. Philadelphia: F. A. Davis Company, with permission.)

(2) Deviations: Asymmetry of lids; drooping lid (**ptosis**) due to malfunction of cranial nerve III; ptosis of one lid may indicate brain attack and ptosis of both lids may indicate myasthenia gravis; absence of eyelashes, possibly reflecting alopecia.

c. Conjunctivae for color, moisture, and lesions.

(1) Normal findings: Clear; pink; moist; smooth; no lesions.

(2) Deviations: Redness, swelling, drainage, and tenderness, possibly indicating infection (**conjunctivitis**); pale pink color, possibly indicating anemia.

d. Sclerae for color, moisture, and lesions.

(1) Normal findings: White; glistening; smooth with no lesions. Dark-skinned patients may have sclera with a yellowish cast in the periphery.

(2) Deviations: Redness ("bloodshot" appearance), indicating inflammation of the sclera; yellow, indicating jaundice (**icterus**).

e. Iris for color, shape, and symmetry.

(1) Normal findings: Uniform color (e.g., blue, brown, green, or a combination of these colors); round and symmetrical.

(2) Deviations: Pigment degeneration in older adults; partial or total absence of iris, a congenital anomaly.

f. Cornea (colorless portion of eye covering the pupil and iris) and lens for clarity, texture, and moisture. Shine a light at an angle to the eye while the patient looks straight ahead.

(1) Normal findings: Clear, smooth, and glistening cornea and lens.

(2) Deviations: Rough or irregular appearance to surface of cornea, which may indicate corneal abrasion or ulcer; cloudy lens appearance, which may indicate a cataract.

5. Assess internal structures via inspection with an ophthalmoscope. Note that this is an advanced assessment technique that should be conducted in a darkened room.

   a. Assess for red light reflex: Have the patient look straight ahead, stand about 1 foot from the patient at a 15° angle, and shine a light on one pupil while looking through an ophthalmoscope.

   (1) Normal findings: Positive red reflex caused by light illuminating the retina (red eyes sometimes seen in photographs when the flash of a camera illuminates the retina).

   (2) Deviations: Opacity of the lens; hemorrhage into vitreous humor.

   b. Assessment of other internal structures (e.g., retina, choroid, optic nerve disc, macula, fovea centralis, and retinal vessels) is not conducted by most nurses. These structures can be assessed by advanced practice nurses.

K. Assessment of the Ears

1. Assess hearing acuity, sound conduction (Weber test, Rinne test), and balance (Romberg test). See Table 11.9, "Assessment of Cranial Nerves," cranial nerve VIII.

2. Assess the external ear.

   a. Auricle: Assess size, shape, position, angle of attachment, and symmetry.

   (1) Normal findings: 4 to 10 cm in length; all structures present (e.g., helix, antihelix, antitragus, tragus, and lobule) (Fig. 11.31); top of ears level with eyes; ears vertical with 10° posterior tilt and symmetrical.

MAKING THE CONNECTION

Auditory Stimuli and Interpretation of Sound

An auditory stimulus (sound) occurs. The external ear, consisting of the auricle and external auditory canal, collects and transmits the sound to the middle ear. The middle ear consists of the tympanic membrane, eustachian tube (connection between middle ear and nasopharynx), and three auditory bones (malleus, incus, and stapes). The tympanic membrane transmits the sound to the three auditory bones, and they in turn transmit the sound to the inner ear (labyrinth). The labyrinth consists of the vestibule and semicircular canals (both of which are concerned with balance) and the cochlea (which is concerned with hearing). The organ of Corti within the cochlea has specialized microvilli that contain endings of the cochlear branch of cranial nerve VIII that transmits the sound impulses to the temporal lobes of the cerebral cortex of the brain, where the sound is interpreted (Fig. 11.30).

   (2) Deviations: Size <3 cm or >10 cm, absent external structures, low-set ears, exaggerated posterior tilt, asymmetrical ears.

   b. External auditory canal: Use an otoscope to visualize the walls of the canal and tympanic membrane. Pull the auricle (**pinna**) up and back to straighten the canal of an adult, and pull the lobule down and back to straighten the canal of a child younger than age 3 years.

   (1) Normal findings: Walls of canal light in color, patent, with a small amount of earwax (**cerumen**); no drainage. Tympanic

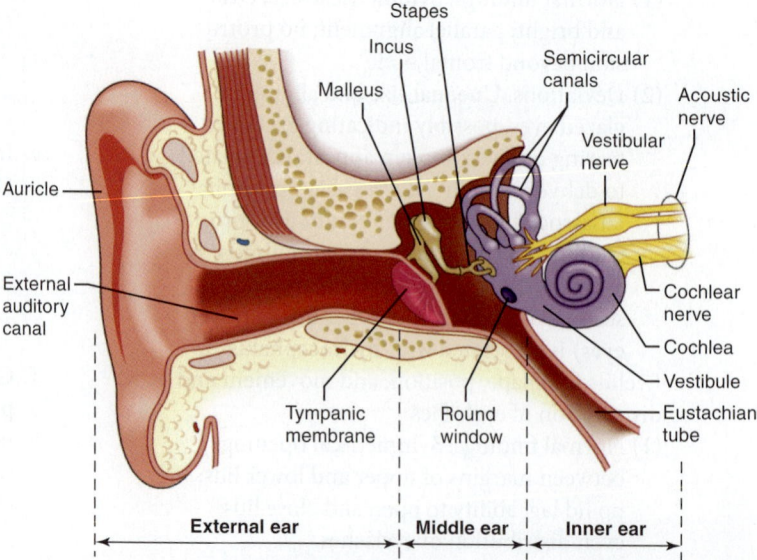

Fig 11.30 Cross section of the ear. (From Wilkinson and Treas [2011]. *Fundamentals of nursing,* Vol. 1, 2nd ed. Philadelphia: F. A. Davis Company, with permission.)

Stapes
Incus
Malleus
Semicircular canals
Acoustic nerve
Vestibular nerve
Auricle
Cochlear nerve
Cochlea
Vestibule
External auditory canal
Tympanic membrane
Round window
Eustachian tube
External ear | **Middle ear** | **Inner ear**

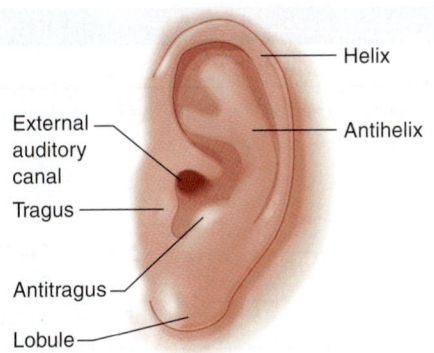

Fig 11.31 External structures of the ear. (From Wilkinson and Treas [2011]. *Fundamentals of nursing,* Vol. 2, 2nd ed. Philadelphia: F. A. Davis Company, with permission.)

membrane pearly gray, shiny, semitransparent, and mobile.

(2) Deviations: Excessive and/or dry cerumen, possibly obscuring the tympanic membrane; redness of walls, possibly indicating infection; bloody drainage, indicating trauma; purulent drainage, indicating infection; clear drainage, possibly indicating spinal fluid from a head injury; tympanic membrane that is pink, red, yellow, amber, white, or blue; is dull or somewhat opaque; has limited mobility; and appears bulging or retracted.

CASE STUDY: Putting It All Together

An older adult with a history of peripheral arterial disease and osteoarthritis is admitted to a hospital with a diagnosis of pneumonia. The nurse obtains the patient's vital signs and performs a physical assessment, including the patient's lungs, eyes, and ears. Some of the results of these assessments are: temperature—102.4°F; apical pulse—96 beats/minute and regular; respirations—26 breaths/minute, shallow, and use of accessory muscles of respiration; blood pressure—146/88 mm Hg; oxygen saturation— 88 percent; breath sounds—crackles in both lungs; eyes—glazed, limited red eye reflex; ears—difficulty hearing, excessive cerumen in both ears; abdomen— distended, hypoactive bowel sounds, tympany. The patient reports feeling short of breath and having tingling in the feet.

Case Study Questions

A. What instruments did the nurse use to perform these assessments and what was the nurse assessing by using the instruments?

1. _____

2. _____

3. _____

4. _____

5. _____

6. _____

B. What techniques of physical assessment did the nurse use and what was the nurse assessing by using the techniques?

1. _____

2. _____

3. _____

4. _____

Continued

CASE STUDY: Putting It All Together cont'd

___ **Case Study Questions** ___

C. The patient has a history of peripheral arterial disease and reports feeling tingling in the feet. Describe the focused assessment the nurse should perform to collect additional information.

1. _____

2. _____

3. _____

4. _____

5. _____

6. _____

D. What is the priority commonality of assessment when auscultating a patient's heart sound, lung sounds, and bowel sounds and why?

1. _____

REVIEW QUESTIONS

1. A nurse is obtaining a patient's radial pulse and identifies that its rhythm is irregular. What should the nurse do **next**?
1. Notify the patient's primary health-care provider.
2. Obtain the patient's blood pressure.
3. Take the pulse in the other arm.
4. Assess the apical pulse.

2. Which patient should the nurse perform a focused assessment on **first**?
1. A patient with obstructive pulmonary disease who is using pursed lip breathing
2. A patient returning from a walk down the hall who is exhibiting nasal flaring
3. A patient with dyspnea who abruptly assumes the orthopneic position
4. A patient with asthma who is wheezing

3. A nurse is taking a patient's temperature using the thermometer in the photograph. Which action is important when using this thermometer?

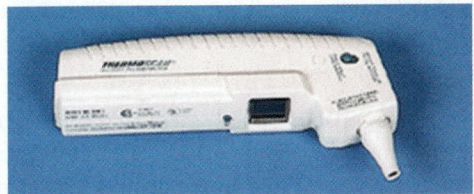

1. Clean the probe before and after use.
2. Use a new probe cover for each patient.
3. Slide the probe medially to laterally across the forehead to the temple.
4. Pull the pinna of the ear upward when inserting the probe into the ear of an infant.

4. A nurse identifies that a patient's abdomen is distended. What assessment should the nurse perform **next**?
1. Weigh the patient.
2. Obtain the vital signs.
3. Measure the girth of the abdomen.
4. Inspect the characteristics of the next stool.

5. A nurse is performing a breast examination as part of a patient's physical assessment. What technique should the nurse employ during this examination?
1. Use the finger pads to palpate breast tissue.
2. Assess the nipples before palpating the breasts.
3. Inspect the breasts while the patient is in the supine position.
4. Follow only a circular sequence of palpation of a breast from the nipples outward.

6. A nurse analyzes data collected about a patient, including temperature, 101°F; apical pulse, 104 beats/minute; radial pulse, 72 beats/minute; respirations, 22 breaths/minute; pulse oximetry, 95 percent; and blood pressure, 138/72 mm Hg. What is the patient's pulse deficit?
Answer: _____

7. Which patient assessment documented by the nurse in the patient's clinical record indicates a period of remission?
1. "Patient continues to experience dull pain in the joints from osteoarthritis."
2. "Patient's response indicates a variation from the response that one would expect."
3. "Patient's readmission to the hospital was due to a return of signs and symptoms of leukemia."
4. "Patient continues to experience freedom from pain in the left foot after receiving a cortisone injection for plantar fasciitis."

8. A nurse is taking a tympanic temperature of an adult patient who is in a right lateral position. Place the following steps in the order in which they should be implemented.
1. Return the tympanic unit to its storage unit for recharging.
2. Attach a disposable probe cover to the tympanic temperature unit.
3. Use the left hand and gently pull the pinna of the right ear upward and backward.
4. Remove the unit from the patient's ear and discard the probe cover without contaminating the environment.
5. Press the probe gently into the patient's ear canal and hold the temperature button until a green light flashes and a temperature is displayed.
Answer: _____

9. A nurse is caring for a patient in the postanesthesia care unit who had surgery for a coronary artery bypass graft. The patient has an intravenous catheter in the right forearm, a urinary retention catheter, and a nasogastric tube in place to low intermittent suction. Where should the nurse place the oxygen saturation sensor?
1. Right nostril
2. Left ear lobe
3. Right great toe
4. Left index finger

10. A nurse performs the following techniques when assessing a patient. Which assessment uses the technique of percussion?
    1. Pressing down on the symphysis pubis to determine the presence of urinary retention
    2. Placing a stethoscope on the abdomen to assess the extent of bowel sounds
    3. Using a rubber-tipped hammer to elicit a deep tendon reflex
    4. Touching the skin over an artery to obtain a pulse rate

11. A nurse is caring for an older adult who was just transferred to the unit after being in the intensive care unit for the last 72 hours. The nurse is concerned about the patient experiencing sensory overload. For which clinical manifestations of sensory overload should the nurse assess the patient? **Select all that apply.**
    1. _____ Pain
    2. _____ Fatigue
    3. _____ Confusion
    4. _____ Restlessness
    5. _____ Scattered attention
    6. _____ Hearing impairment

12. When assessing a patient's radial pulse, a nurse is unable to feel pulsations. What should the nurse do **first**?
    1. Release the pressure of the fingers slightly while compressing the artery.
    2. Apply more pressure when palpating the artery.
    3. Assess an artery in the other arm.
    4. Use a Doppler to assess the artery.

13. A nurse is completing an assessment of several newly admitted patients to a nursing home. For which patients should the nurse assess clinical indicators of sensory deprivation? **Select all that apply.**
    1. _____ The patient who was recently cared for in an intensive care unit
    2. _____ The patient who recently sustained an injury causing blindness
    3. _____ The patient who is experiencing quadriplegia
    4. _____ The patient who has a history of depression
    5. _____ The patient who is experiencing acute pain

14. A nurse is assessing a patient's ability to focus on a mental task. What question is appropriate for the nurse to ask the patient in relation to this assessment?
    1. "What day of the week is it?"
    2. "What did you have for lunch today?"
    3. "What is the result when you multiply 2 times 2?"
    4. "What city did you live in when you were 20 years old?"

15. A nurse is assessing a patient's oculomotor nerve, cranial nerve III. How should the nurse assess the functioning of this nerve?
    1. Instruct the patient to smile.
    2. Shine a light onto the patient's pupil.
    3. Ask the patient to raise the shoulders against resistance.
    4. Place a padded tongue blade gently against the patient's posterior oropharynx.

16. A nurse analyzes data collected about a patient, including temperature, 98.6°F; apical pulse, 90 beats/minute; radial pulse, 60 beats/minute; respirations, 24 breaths/minute; pulse oximetry, 98 percent; and blood pressure, 110/60 mm Hg. What is the patient's pulse pressure?
    Answer: _____

17. A patient with diabetes is admitted to the hospital with the concurrent diagnosis of peripheral vascular disease. Which patient assessment indicates that the vascular impairment is arterial rather than venous?
    1. Skin of the lower extremities is pale with mottling.
    2. Distal capillary refill is less than three seconds.
    3. Toenails on both feet are translucid.
    4. Skin of the feet is warm to touch.

18. A nurse is collecting a past medical history of a newly admitted patient with chest pain. Which information should the nurse include in this assessment? **Select all that apply.**
    1. _____ Allergies
    2. _____ Vital signs
    3. _____ Prior surgeries
    4. _____ Immunizations
    5. _____ Childhood illnesses
    6. _____ Present signs and symptoms

19. A nurse is assessing a female patient's external genitalia. Which finding should be reported to the primary health-care provider?
    1. The vaginal introitus has a discharge that is clear and odorless.
    2. The pubic hair extents to the upper inner thighs.
    3. The urethra is midline below the clitoris.
    4. The clitoris is 4 cm long and 2 cm wide.

20. A nurse is assessing a patient who was admitted to the hospital with a history of hemiparesis. Which physical assessment supports this diagnosis?
    1. Paralysis of both arms and both legs
    2. Uncontrolled contractions of skeletal muscles
    3. Rhythmic purposeless movements of the extremities
    4. Weakness in an arm and leg on the same side of the body

21. At which site should the nurse position a stethoscope when assessing the apical pulse rate for an adult?

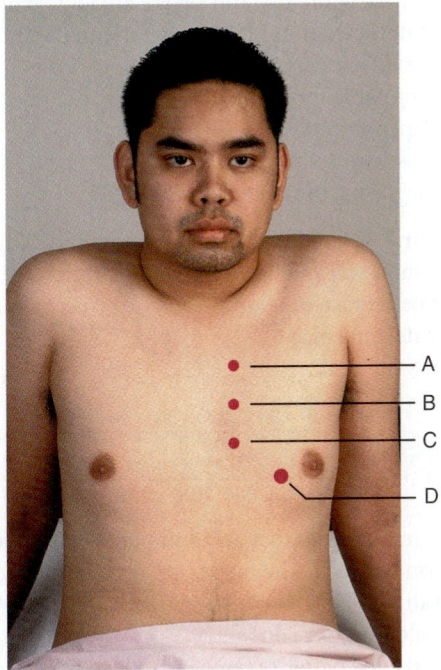

1. A
2. B
3. C
4. D

22. A nurse is obtaining a patient's blood pressure. What is reflected by the diastolic blood pressure?
1. Contraction of the left ventricle
2. Volume of cardiac output
3. Resting arterial pressure
4. Pulse pressure

23. A primary health-care provider asks the nurse for a report on the quality of a patient's pulse. Which information collected by the nurse will answer this question posed by the primary health-care provider?
1. The pulse rate is 65 beats/minute.
2. The pulse volume is full and bounding.
3. The pulse rate is slower than the heart rate.
4. The pulse has 2 beats that repeatedly occur close together.

24. A parent brings a 4-year-old child to the urgent care center stating, "I think she has a bad cold." The nurse takes the child's vital signs, performs an inspection, and interviews the parent.

Patient's Clinical Record

Vital Signs

Temperature: 100.4°F, temporal scanner
Pulse: 94 beats/minute, regular rhythm, radial
Respirations: 30 breaths/minute

Inspection

Facial flushing, slight supraclavicular and intercostal retractions, nonproductive cough, restless, sitting in the tripod position on bed. Abdomen appears soft, no signs of guarding noted.

Parental Interview

Mother states, "She started coughing about 2 days ago, but the cough is getting worse. She is not bringing up phlegm, but she keeps coughing. I kept her home from school thinking that it was just a cold and she would get better, but she has gotten worse. She doesn't want to drink and her urine is very dark. When her face got so red, I got scared and brought her here."

What assessment should the nurse perform **next**?
1. Auscultate the lungs.
2. Palpate the abdomen.
3. Obtain the apical heart rate.
4. Ask the child where it hurts.

25. Which site should the nurse use when monitoring the heart rate prior to administering a cardiac medication?
1. Brachial
2. Carotid
3. Apical
4. Radial

26. A patient is experiencing the onset of a fever. Which nursing action is appropriate during this phase?
1. Applying cloth covered ice packs to the groin
2. Covering the patient with a blanket
3. Lowering the heat in the room
4. Ensuring that bed linen is dry

27. A primary health-care provider orders a dose of a medication for a child at 2 mg/kg of body weight. The child weighs 64 pounds. Before determining the prescribed dose, the nurse must convert the child's weight from pounds to kilograms. How many kilograms does this child weigh? Record your answer using a whole number.
Answer: _____ kilograms

28. A nurse is assessing a male patient's external genitalia. Which assessment should be reported to the primary health-care provider?
1. The urethral meatus has a white discharge.
2. The foreskin can be retracted back from the glans.
3. The anus constricts when touched with a gloved finger.
4. The scrotum is darker than the rest of the patient's skin.

29. A nurse is caring for a variety of patients. Place the patients in the order in which they should be attended to by the nurse. Begin first with the patient who has the highest priority and progress to the patient who has the lowest priority.
1. A patient who just returned from the operating room with a temperature of 100°F
2. A patient who returned from rigorous physical therapy who has a temperature of 99°F
3. A patient who had surgery three days ago and has developed a temperature of 100.2°F
4. A patient who received 2 intravenous antibiotic doses in the last 24 hours for a urinary tract infection and has a temperature of 100.6°F
5. A patient who was admitted to the hospital after receiving multiple bruises as a result of an automobile collision and has a temperature of 100.4°F
Answer: _____

30. A nurse is performing a complete physical assessment of an adolescent. What is an important approach to use with the patient?
1. Pull the curtain so that the parents are beyond the curtain during the examination.
2. Limit questions from the adolescent to after the examination is completed.
3. Allow the adolescent to keep underpants on during the examination.
4. Have the parents remain outside the room during the examination.

31. A nurse is caring for an infant who has a core body temperature of 104.8°F. The infant has a prescription for acetaminophen 10 mg/kg PO every 6 hours prn for a temperature more than 102°F. Place the following nursing interventions in priority order from highest priority to lowest priority.
Answer: _____
1. Obtain all vital signs.
2. Institute seizure precautions.
3. Remove the blanket that is covering the infant.
4. Administer acetaminophen as per the prescription.
5. Inform the primary health-care provider of the infant's status.

32. A nurse is caring for a patient who is presenting with diarrhea, abdominal cramps, diaphoresis, shortness of breath, and severe anxiety. Which thermometer should the nurse use to obtain this patient's temperature?
1. Tympanic thermometer
2. Paper strip thermometer
3. Plastic rectal thermometer
4. Electronic oral thermometer

33. A nurse obtains a patient's temperature using an oral thermometer indicated in the illustration. What is the patient's temperature? Record your answer using one decimal place.
Answer: _____ °F

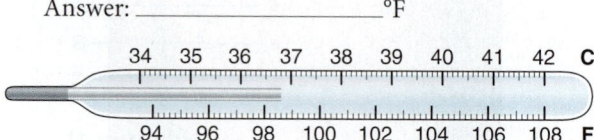

34. A nurse assesses that an adult patient's skin feels warm to touch. The nurse obtains a tympanic temperature of 97.2°F via the patient's right ear. What should the nurse do?
1. Take the patient's temperature in the other ear while pulling the pinna upward and back.
2. Retake the patient's temperature in the same ear while pulling the pinna upward and back.
3. Take the patient's temperature in the other ear while pulling the pinna downward and back.
4. Retake the patient's temperature in the same ear while pulling the pinna downward and back.

35. A nurse in the emergency department is obtaining the temperatures of several patients using a temporal scanner thermometer. Which patients should the nurse identify as requiring an alternate route for the assessment of body temperature? **Select all that apply.**
1. _____ Patient who is diaphoretic
2. _____ Patient who is a mouth breather
3. _____ Patient who is wearing a ski hat
4. _____ Patient who is exhibiting male pattern baldness
5. _____ Patient who is sleeping in the side-lying position with the head on a pillow

1. **ANSWER: 4.**
   Rationales:
   1. This is premature. The nurse should obtain additional data about the patient's status.
   2. Although obtaining the blood pressure may eventually be done, it is premature at this time.
   3. Although assessing the radial pulse in the other arm may eventually be done, it is premature at this time.
   4. **The nurse should first assess the apical pulse and rhythm and then determine the pulse deficit. These assessments provide valuable information about the rate and rhythm of the patient's apical and radial pulse rates.**
   TEST-TAKING TIP: Identify the word in the stem that sets a priority. The word *next* in the stem sets a priority. Identify options that contain a clang association. The word *pulse* in the stem and in options 3 and 4 are clang associations. Consider options 3 and 4 carefully.
   Content Area: Physical Assessment
   Integrated Processes: Nursing Process: Assessment
   Client Need: Physiological Integrity; Reduction of Risk Potential
   Cognitive Level: Application

2. **ANSWER: 3.**
   Rationales:
   1. Although this patient should be assessed frequently, pursed lip breathing is a technique that may be used constantly by patients with obstructive pulmonary disease. Pursed lip breathing prolongs exhalation, preventing collapse of alveoli and small bronchial passages, which promotes gas exchange.
   2. Although additional assessments may be performed to assess this patient's response to physical exertion, this patient is not the priority from among the patient situations presented. Nasal flaring commonly is associated with physical effort because it reduces the friction of air entering and exiting the body.
   3. **A patient who has difficulty breathing and assumes an upright leaning forward position is attempting to expand the thoracic cavity to promote respirations. This patient should be assessed first because medical intervention may be necessary to relieve this patient's respiratory distress.**
   4. Although this patient should be monitored closely for an escalation of the wheezing, wheezing is associated with asthma because of constricted airways.
   TEST-TAKING TIP: Identify the word in the stem that sets a priority. The word *first* in the stem sets a priority. Use the ABCs (**A**irway, **B**reathing, and **C**irculation) of physical assessment when considering the options in this question.
   Content Area: Physical Assessment
   Integrated Processes: Nursing Process: Assessment
   Client Need: Safe and Effective Care Environment; Management of Care
   Cognitive Level: Analysis

3. **ANSWER: 2.**
   Rationales:
   1. The probe does not have to be cleaned before and after use unless it is touched by the patient or is contaminated by touching something in the environment that is contaminated.
   2. **The use of a new probe sheath for each patient is an infection control practice that prevents the transmission of microorganisms from one patient to another. Each used probe sheath is ejected into a trash container or onto a paper towel, which is then discarded into a trash container.**
   3. This technique is used when using a temporal artery thermometer.
   4. The pinna should be pulled upward and backward when using a tympanic thermometer to obtain the temperature of an adult. The pinna should be pulled backward or downward and backward when using a tympanic thermometer to obtain the temperature of a child less than 3 years of age. These actions straighten the ear canal, which allows the probe to access the tympanic membrane.
   Content Area: Physical Assessment
   Integrated Processes: Nursing Process: Implementation
   Client Need: Health Promotion and Maintenance
   Cognitive Level: Analysis

4. **ANSWER: 3.**
   Rationales:
   1. Although this should be done, it is premature to weigh the patient at this time.
   2. Although this should be done, it is premature to obtain the vital signs at this time.
   3. **Measuring the abdominal girth with a tape measure around the body at the level of the umbilicus is an objective measurement of the circumference of the abdomen. Repeat assessments can be compared with the first assessment to determine progression of the distention.**
   4. This is unrealistic. It could take hours or days before the patient has a bowel movement. Abdominal distension usually is related to gas in the intestine (flatus) or fluid in the abdominal cavity (ascites). Assessing bowel sounds may provide information related to flatus and a fluid wave test may provide information related to ascites.
   TEST-TAKING TIP: Identify the word in the stem that sets a priority. The word *next* in the stem sets a priority. Identify the clang association. The word *abdomen* in the stem and in option 3 is a clang association.
   Content Area: Physical Assessment
   Integrated Processes: Nursing Process: Assessment
   Client Need: Physiological Integrity; Reduction of Risk Potential
   Cognitive Level: Application

5. **ANSWER: 1.**
   Rationales:
   1. **Placing the pads of three fingers flat against the patient's breast is the correct technique for palpation of the breast. There are numerous nerve endings in the pads of the fingers that promote the sense of touch.**
   2. This sequence of assessment is not required.
   3. The patient should be sitting or standing during breast inspection. The patient should be instructed to assume several positions; hold the hands at the side and then over the head;

press the hands down on the hips and then together with the elbows flexed; and leaning forward. These positions accentuate retraction of tissue that may occur with pathological changes.

4. Any systematic method can be used: concentric circles, vertical strip, or pie wedge. The vertical strip method is the preferred method.

TEST-TAKING TIP: Identify the options with specific determiners. Option 4 contains the word *only*, which is a specific determiner; this option can be eliminated from consideration.

Content Area: Physical Assessment
Integrated Processes: Nursing Process: Assessment
Client Need: Health Promotion and Maintenance
Cognitive Level: Application

6. **ANSWER: 32.**

The pulse deficit is calculated by subtracting the radial pulse rate from the apical pulse rate. Therefore, $104 - 72 = 32$.

Content Area: Physical Assessment
Integrated Processes: Nursing Process: Analysis
Client Need: Physiological Integrity; Reduction of Risk Potential
Cognitive Level: Application

7. **ANSWER: 4.**

Rationales:

1. The statement in option 1 indicates the concept of chronicity, not remission; Chronicity (chronic disease) refers to a disease of long duration or demonstrating progressive deterioration over a long period of time.

2. The statement in option 2 indicates the concept of deviation or deviance, not remission. Deviation or deviance refers to a departure from the norm.

3. The statement in option 3 indicates the concept of exacerbation, not remission. Exacerbation refers to a return of symptoms or increase in the severity of symptoms.

4. **The statement in option 4 indicates the concept of remission, a period whereby symptoms abate or there is an absence of the underlying disease.**

Content Area: Physical Assessment
Integrated Processes: Communication/Documentation; Nursing Process: Assessment
Client Need: Physiological Integrity; Physiological Adaptation
Cognitive Level: Application

8. **ANSWER: 2, 3, 5, 4, 1.**

Rationales:

2. A disposable probe cover reduces the spread of microorganisms between patients.

3. Using the right hand to hold the unit when using the left ear and using the left hand to hold the unit when using the right ear helps to attain the best angle for a good seal when the probe is placed in the ear. Pulling the pinna upward and backward for an adult helps to straighten the ear canal and provide better access to the tympanic membrane. This helps to attain an accurate reading.

5. Pressing the probe gently into the patient's ear canal facilitates a seal and helps to attain an accurate reading. A flashing green light and the display of a temperature reading indicate that the reading is complete.

4. Once the reading is established the unit is then removed from the patient's ear and the probe cover discarded in an appropriate trash receptacle to prevent cross-contamination.

1. The unit should be returned to its base unit for recharging for future use.

Content Area: Physical Assessment
Integrated Processes: Nursing Process: Planning
Client Need: Health Promotion and Maintenance
Cognitive Level: Analysis

9. **ANSWER: 2.**

Rationales:

1. This placement would be uncomfortable because the patient already has a nasogastric tube in place.

2. **The ear lobes have many capillary beds that are appropriate for placement of an oxygen saturation sensor. The ear lobes are not distal appendages that may be affected by a decreased cardiac output.**

3. The patient had cardiac surgery because of inadequate cardiac output. The capillary refill time in the toes may be prolonged, which will interfere with accurate oxygen saturation results.

4. The patient had cardiac surgery because of inadequate cardiac output. The capillary refill time in the fingers may be prolonged, which will interfere with accurate oxygen saturation results.

TEST-TAKING TIP: Identify the equally plausible options. Options 3 and 4 are equally plausible because both are distal points on the extremities. One is no better than the other. Eliminate both from further consideration.

Content Area: Physical Assessment
Integrated Processes: Nursing Process: Assessment
Client Need: Health Promotion and Maintenance
Cognitive Level: Application

10. **ANSWER: 3.**

Rationales:

1. Using the fingers to assess for distention of the urinary bladder employs the technique of palpation.

2. Listening to sounds produced within the body by use of a stethoscope employs the assessment technique of auscultation.

3. **Striking a patient's body part with the fingers or a rubber-tipped hammer to elicit a sound, vibration, or response involves the assessment technique of percussion.**

4. Measuring a pulse rate by using the fingers employs the assessment technique of palpation.

Content Area: Physical Assessment
Integrated Processes: Nursing Process: Assessment
Client Need: Health Promotion and Maintenance
Cognitive Level: Application

11. **ANSWER: 2, 3, 4, 5.**

Rationales:

1. Pain is a contributing factor, not a clinical manifestation, of sensory overload.

2. **Fatigue is a common clinical manifestation of sensory overload. Sensory overload prevents the brain from ignoring environmental stimuli, interfering with the ability to sleep.**

3. Confusion occurs because many stimuli cause difficulty recognizing the environment in a way that makes sense.

4. Constant stimuli attack the both the physical and emotional domains of the patient, contributing to restlessness.

5. As a result of constant stimuli, a patient's mind can race in many directions, contributing to scattered attention.

6. Hearing impairment is a contributing factor, not a clinical manifestation, of sensory deficit, not sensory overload.

Content Area: *Physical Assessment*
Integrated Processes: *Nursing Process: Assessment*
Client Need: *Safe and Effective Care Environment; Safety and Infection Control*
Cognitive Level: *Analysis*

12. **ANSWER: 1.**

Rationales:

1. **Excessive compression of an artery sometimes will obliterate a pulse. Releasing pressure of the fingers slightly will allow the blood to flow through the artery.**

2. This will further compound the problem of obstructing blood flow through the artery, obliterating the pulse.

3. Assessing an artery in the other arm may eventually be done; however, the nurse's assessment technique should be adjusted first.

4. Using a Doppler may eventually be done; however, the nurse's assessment technique should be adjusted first.

TEST-TAKING TIP: Identify the word in the stem that sets a priority. The word *first* in the stem sets a priority. Identify options that are opposites. Options 1 and 2 are opposites. Examine options 1 and 2 carefully.

Content Area: *Physical Assessment*
Integrated Processes: *Nursing Process: Assessment*
Client Need: *Health Promotion and Maintenance*
Cognitive Level: *Application*

13. **ANSWER: 2, 3, 4.**

Rationales:

1. A person in an intensive care unit (ICU) may experience sensory overload, not deprivation. A patient in an ICU is exposed to an increase in the quantity and/or intensity of internal and/or external stimuli and can become overwhelmed, resulting in ICU psychosis. The clinical manifestations of ICU psychosis include confusion, disorientation, fatigue, irritability, anxiety, restlessness, reduced ability to problem-solve, increased muscle tension, and scattered attention span.

2. A person experiencing sudden blindness may require several months or more to develop compensatory coping behaviors to deal with the loss of vision. This person can no longer watch television, read a book, or recognize others by sight, resulting in sensory deprivation. Fear of new environments and depression may occur, maximizing the initial isolation caused by blindness.

3. The person who is experiencing quadriplegia and other patients with impaired mobility may have less exposure to stimulating environments and activities because of the effort it takes to become involved or to leave the home.

4. A patient with a history of depression is at risk for sensory deprivation because of the emotional and physical withdrawal from others.

5. The patient with acute pain is more likely to experience sensory overload, not sensory deprivation. The patient with chronic, not acute, pain is more likely to experience sensory deprivation because the patient may not have the stamina or interest to engage in stimulating and socializing activities.

Content Area: *Physical Assessment*
Integrated Processes: *Nursing Process: Assessment*
Client Need: *Safe and Effective Care Environment; Safety and Infection Control*
Cognitive Level: *Analysis*

14. **ANSWER: 3.**

Rationales:

1. This question assesses the person's orientation to time. It is part of the assessment of time, place, and person.

2. This question assesses short-term memory.

3. **This question requires the patient to perform a mathematical calculation, which is a cognitive skill.**

4. This question assesses long-term memory.

Content Area: *Physical Assessment*
Integrated Processes: *Communication/Documentation; Nursing Process: Assessment*
Client Need: *Physiological Integrity; Reduction of Risk Potential*
Cognitive Level: *Analysis*

15. **ANSWER: 2**

Rationales:

1. The facial nerve, cranial nerve VII, promotes facial expressions, facial muscle strength, and taste. The patient should be instructed to smile, wrinkle the forehead, puff out the cheeks, purse the lips, squeeze the eyes shut, and bear the teeth. Deviations from expected responses indicate impairment of the facial nerve.

2. **Shining a light onto the patient's pupil should cause the pupil to constrict. If it is slow to constrict or does not constrict then the oculomotor nerve, cranial nerve III, is impaired.**

3. The accessory nerve, cranial nerve XI, is associated with raising the shoulders and turning the head from side to side. Asymmetrical movements, limited or absent movements, or pain indicate an impaired accessory nerve.

4. The glossopharyngeal nerve, cranial nerve IX, is involved with the gag reflex, swallowing, tongue movements, taste, and secretion of saliva. Absence of the gag reflex, dysphagia, impaired tongue movements, alterations in taste, and dry mouth all indicate malfunctioning of the glossopharyngeal nerve.

Content Area: *Physical Assessment*
Integrated Processes: *Nursing Process: Assessment*
Client Need: *Physiological Integrity; Reduction of Risk Potential*
Cognitive Level: *Analysis*

16. **ANSWER: 50.**

Rationales:

Pulse pressure is calculated by subtracting the diastolic blood pressure from the systolic blood pressure. Therefore, 110 – 60 = 50.

Content Area: *Physical Assessment*
Integrated Processes: *Nursing Process: Analysis*
Client Need: *Physiological Integrity; Reduction of Risk Potential*
Cognitive Level: *Application*

17. ANSWER: 1.

Rationales:

1. Inadequate circulation to the legs and feet causes the tissues to appear pale with patches of variations in color. When the legs are dependent they may develop a dusky red color known as *dependent rubor.*
2. When blanching returns to pink after release of compression of peripheral tissues it indicates that cardiac output and circulation to the feet are adequate. Capillary refill that takes longer than 3 seconds or longer than 5 seconds in an older adult indicates impaired cardiac or peripheral vascular functioning.
3. Healthy toenails are translucid (not transparent but allows for slight penetration by light rays) or have variations of pink. Arterial insufficiency will cause the toenails to be yellow, thick, and brittle.
4. The skin of the feet should feel warm to touch because adequate peripheral circulation brings warm blood to the capillary beds of the feet. The feet will feel cool to touch when there is impaired peripheral arterial circulation to the feet.

Content Area: Physical Assessment
Integrated Processes: Nursing Process: Assessment
Client Need: Physiological Integrity; Reduction of Risk Potential
Cognitive Level: Analysis

18. ANSWER: 1, 3, 4, 5.

Rationales:

1. Allergies are information that is associated with a past medical history.
2. Vital signs are associated with the current health problem; current vital signs are not part of a past medical history.
3. Prior surgeries are information that is associated with a past medical history.
4. Immunizations are information that is associated with a past medical history.
5. Childhood illnesses are information that is associated with a past medical history.
6. Present signs and symptoms are associated with the current health problem, not data related to a past medical history.

Content Area: Physical Assessment
Integrated Processes: Communication/Documentation; Nursing Process: Assessment
Client Need: Physiological Integrity; Physiological Adaptation
Cognitive Level: Analysis

19. ANSWER: 4.

Rationales:

1. A clear discharge can occur because the vaginal canal is lined with mucous membranes.
2. Pubic hair is coarse, full, and symmetrical over the mons pubis and can extend to the inner upper thighs.
3. The normal location of the urethra is midline below the clitoris and above the vagina.
4. The expected size of the clitoris is 2 cm long and 0.5 cm wide. An enlarged clitoris may indicate excess androgens and therefore should be reported to the primary healthcare provider.

TEST-TAKING TIP: Identify the words in the stem that indicate negative polarity. The words *should be reported* in the stem indicate negative polarity. The question is asking "What physical assessment is not within the normal range?" Identify the option that is unique. Option 4 is unique because it is the only option that contains numbers. Consider option 4 carefully.

Content Area: Physical Assessment
Integrated Processes: Communication/Documentation; Nursing Process: Assessment
Client Need: Physiological Integrity; Reduction of Risk Potential
Cognitive Level: Application

20. ANSWER: 4.

Rationales:

1. Paralysis of both arms and legs is known as quadriplegia.
2. Uncontrolled contractions of skeletal muscles are known as spasticity.
3. Rhythmic purposeless movements of the extremities are known as tremors.
4. Weakness or partial paralysis in an arm and leg on the same side of the body is known as hemiparesis.

Content Area: Physical Assessment
Integrated Processes: Nursing Process: Assessment
Client Need: Physiological Integrity; Reduction of Risk Potential
Cognitive Level: Application

21. ANSWER: 4.

Rationales:

1. This is not the site for assessing an apical pulse rate in an adult. This is the site to assess heart sounds generated at the pulmonic valve. It is two or three fingerbreadths below the clavicular notch at the second intercostal space.
2. This is not the site for assessing an apical pulse rate in an adult. This is Erb's point. This is the left third intercostal space and is used to assess heart sounds generated at the mitral valve.
3. This is not the site for assessing an apical pulse rate in an adult. This is the left lateral sternal border. It is used to assess heart sounds generated at the tricuspid valve.
4. This is the point of maximum impulse. It is the apex of the heart, where the heart contraction is the strongest, and is the site for assessing an apical pulse rate in an adult. It is located at the end of the left ventricle, which is near the fifth intercostal space and 3 to 4 inches to the left of the sternum at the midclavicular line.

Content Area: Physical Assessment
Integrated Processes: Nursing Process: Assessment
Client Need: Health Promotion and Maintenance
Cognitive Level: Analysis

22. ANSWER: 3.

Rationales:

1. Contraction of the left ventricle is reflected by the systolic pressure.
2. The volume of cardiac output is computed by multiplying the stroke volume by the number of heart beats per minute.
3. Diastole is the period when the ventricles are relaxed and reflects the pressure in the arteries when the heart is at rest.

4. Pulse pressure is the difference between the systolic and diastolic pressures.

TEST-TAKING TIP: Identify options with a clang association. The word *pressure* in the stem and in options 3 and 4 are clang associations. Examine options 3 and 4 carefully.
Content Area: Physical Assessment
Integrated Processes: Nursing Process: Assessment
Client Need: Physiological Integrity; Reduction of Risk Potential
Cognitive Level: Comprehension

23. ANSWER: 2.
Rationales:
1. The rate is not related to the quality of a pulse. It is related to the number of beats per minute.
2. The amount of circulating blood volume will influence the quality of the pulse. An increased circulating blood volume will result in a bounding pulse. A decreased circulating blood volume will result in a weak, thready pulse.
3. This is known as a pulse deficit. It is related to the rate of a pulse and reflects either a dysrhythmia or a decrease in the strength of ventricular contractions.
4. Two beats repeatedly occurring close together (bigeminy) is related to a dysrhythmia, not quality of the pulse.
Content Area: Physical Assessment
Integrated Processes: Communication/Documentation; Nursing Process: Assessment
Client Need: Health Promotion and Maintenance
Cognitive Level: Application

24. ANSWER: 1.
Rationales:
1. The nurse should perform a focused assessment. The child is in respiratory distress and the lungs should be auscultated to determine the presence of wheezes and/or crackles. The expected respiratory rate of a 6-year-old child is 21 breaths/minute. The child is exhibiting retractions when breathing and is assuming the tripod position, indicating dyspnea. Facial flushing is one of the clinical manifestations of asthma, along with the respiratory signs of dyspnea.
2. Although abdominal palpation should be done eventually, the data collected via inspection and the parental interview do not indicate that the child is in pain or is experiencing urinary retention. Another assessment is the priority.
3. Although the apical heart rate should be obtained eventually, the radial rate is sufficient initially. Another assessment is the priority.
4. Although asking the child where it hurts may be done eventually, the data collected via inspection and the parental interview do not indicate that the child is in pain. Another assessment is the priority.

TEST-TAKING TIP: Identify the word in the stem that sets a priority. The word *next* in the stem sets a priority.
Content Area: Physical Assessment
Integrated Processes: Nursing Process: Assessment
Client Need: Physiological Integrity; Reduction of Risk Potential
Cognitive Level: Analysis

25. ANSWER: 3.
Rationales:
1. The brachial site generally is assessed when assessing the heart rate of an infant during cardiopulmonary resuscitation. It is also used when obtaining a blood pressure in an arm.
2. The carotid site generally is used when preforming cardiopulmonary resuscitation and assessing circulation to the brain.
3. The apical pulse is assessed at the apex of the heart. It is the most accurate because the pulse rate is generated by the contraction of the left ventricle of the heart as blood is pumped away from the heart.
4. The radial pulse generally is used for routine assessment of the heart rate. However, due to various factors, there may be a difference between the heart rate and radial pulse rate (pulse deficit) and therefore is not as accurate as another site.
Content Area: Physical Assessment
Integrated Processes: Nursing Process: Assessment
Client Need: Health Promotion and Maintenance
Cognitive Level: Application

26. ANSWER: 2.
Rationales:
1. Ice packs to the groin during the onset phase can cause excessive chilling and shivering, which will cause the temperature to increase, not decrease.
2. When the temperature increases and the body has not yet reached the new set point, the patient usually feels chilly and may shiver. A blanket helps prevent a patient from shivering. Shivering should be avoided because it can increase body temperature.
3. Decreasing the temperature in the room is associated with the second phase (course) of a fever when the temperature reaches the new set point and the patient generally feels flushed and warm.
4. Keeping bed linen dry is important when the patient is experiencing diaphoresis that accompanies the third phase (defervescence or crisis phase) of a fever.
Content Area: Physical Assessment
Integrated Processes: Nursing Process: Implementation
Client Need: Safe and Effective Care Environment; Reduction of Risk Potential
Cognitive Level: Application

27. ANSWER: 29.
Rationale:
Recall that 1 kilogram equals 2.2 pounds. Divide the child's weight in pounds by 2.2 to determine the child's weight in kilograms. 64 ÷ 2.2 = 29 kilograms. The formula for ratio and proportion also can be used to solve this problem.

$$\frac{\text{Desire 64 pounds}}{\text{Have 2.2 pounds}} = \frac{\text{x kilograms}}{\text{1 kilogram}}$$

$$2.2x = 64 \times 1$$

$$2.2x = 64$$

$$x = 64 \div 2.2$$

$$x = 29 \text{ kilograms}$$

Content Area: Physical Assessment
Integrated Processes: Nursing Process: Planning
Client Need: Physiological Integrity; Pharmacological and Parenteral Therapies
Cognitive Level: Application

28. ANSWER: 1.
Rationales:
1. There should be no discharge from the urethral meatus. A white, yellow, or green discharge may indicate the presence of a sexually transmitted infection.
2. This is done when performing perineal care for an uncircumcised patient. The primary health-care provider should be notified if the foreskin cannot be retracted.
3. This is an expected response and is called the anal reflex.
4. This is expected. The scrotum in most men is darker than the rest of their skin.
TEST-TAKING TIP: Identify the words in the stem that indicate negative polarity. The words *should be reported* in the stem indicate negative polarity. The question is asking "What physical assessment is not within the range of normal?"
Content Area: Physical Assessment
Integrated Processes: Nursing Process: Assessment
Client Need: Physiological Integrity; Reduction of Risk Potential
Cognitive Level: Application

29. ANSWER: 3, 5, 1, 2, 4.
Rationales:
3. An increased temperature three days after surgery indicates a potential postoperative infection. The nurse should assess this patient immediately (e.g., vital signs, characteristics of the incision) and notify the primary health-care provider of the patient's status.
5. Having a temperature of 100.4°F is expected after receiving multiple bruises in an automobile collision. However, this patent should be monitored for other possible sequela of the event.
1. Having a low-grade fever immediately after surgery is not unusual; it occurs as a result of an increased metabolic rate in response to the trauma of surgery.
2. Having a low-grade fever after rigorous physical therapy is not uncommon because of the increased metabolic rate. The patient should be assessed to ensure that the other vital signs have returned to the expected range.
4. The patient's urinary tract infection is being treated. The patient's increased temperature may persist for several days until the antibiotics take full effect.
Content Area: Physical Assessment
Integrated Processes: Nursing Process: Planning
Client Need: Safe and Effective Care Environment; Management of Care
Cognitive Level: Analysis

30. ANSWER: 4.
Rationales:
1. Although pulling the curtain provides some privacy, the parents will still be able to hear the conversation between the nurse and adolescent.

2. This is an authoritative and restrictive approach. The adolescent should be encouraged to ask a question whenever desired.
3. This is unrealistic. Physical assessment includes inspection of the genitalia because of the development of secondary sexual characteristics during adolescence.
4. An adolescent is more likely to give an honest answer to a sensitive question and is more apt to ask the nurse a sensitive question if the examination is conducted in private. Privacy also promotes a trusting relationship between the nurse and adolescent.
TEST-TAKING TIP: Identify the options that are opposites. Options 1 and 4 are opposites because in option 1 the parents are within hearing distance of the interaction between the adolescent and the primary health-care provider and in option 4 the parents are not in hearing distance. Consider options 1 and 4 carefully because more often than not one of the opposites is the correct answer.
Content Area: Physical Assessment
Integrated Processes: Caring; Nursing Process: Assessment
Client Need: Psychosocial Integrity
Cognitive Level: Application

31. ANSWER: 2, 1, 3, 4, 5.
Rationales:
2. An infant with a temperature of 104.8°F is at high risk for seizures and therefore should be placed on seizure precautions to prevent injury if a seizure does occur. Seizure precautions include padding raised bed rails, ensuring the bed is in the lowest position, and communicating the infant's status to other members of the health-care team providing direct patient care.
1. Obtaining a full set of vital signs is important to gain more data. The vital signs must be taken before administration of the acetaminophen because acetaminophen will lower the temperature, thus providing artificially low temperature readings. Before contacting the patient's primary health-care provider, the nurse should always take the patient's vital signs.
3. Removing the infant's blanket will help slightly to reduce the child's temperature through radiation.
4. Administering acetaminophen (Tylenol) will help reduce the temperature, although not immediately.
5. Informing the infant's primary health-care provider should be done after the previous interventions. The patient is the center of the health team and the patient's needs must be met first.
Content Area: Physical Assessment
Integrated Processes: Nursing Process: Planning
Client Need: Safe and Effective Care Environment; Management of Care
Cognitive Level: Analysis

32. ANSWER: 1.
Rationales:
1. A tympanic thermometer is the preferred thermometer to use in this scenario. It will not impose on the patient's respiratory or gastrointestinal system and it should not increase the patient's anxiety because it is not invasive.

2. A paper strip thermometer is contraindicated for a patient with diaphoresis because it will not adhere to the skin, resulting in an inaccurate result.

3. A rectal thermometer is contraindicated for a patient with a potential intestinal problem. A rectal thermometer may irritate the mucous membranes of the anus and rectum.

4. Any type of oral thermometer is contraindicated for a patient who is short of breath. People who are short of breath frequently become mouth breathers and will be unable to seal the lips around the thermometer to ensure an accurate result.

Content Area: Physical Assessment
Integrated Processes: Nursing Process: Implementation
Client Need: Health Promotion and Maintenance
Cognitive Level: Analysis

33. **ANSWER: 98.6.**
    Each short line above 98 is equal to 2 tenths. The line of the temperature indicator is almost at the third short line after the line indicating 98. The result should be moved up to the next nearest line. Therefore, the patient's temperature is 98.6°F.
    Content Area: Physical Assessment
    Integrated Processes: Nursing Process: Assessment
    Client Need: Health Promotion and Maintenance
    Cognitive Level: Analysis

34. **ANSWER: 1.**
    Rationales:
    1. **The other ear should be used because the patient may have excessive ear wax (cerumen) in the right ear that is causing an inaccurate low reading. Pulling the pinna upward and back in an adult straightens the ear canal so that the sensor can assess the tympanic membrane.**
    2. Pulling the pinna upward and back is the appropriate technique for straightening the external ear canal in an adult. However, the same ear should not be used because the temperature was below the expected range, indicating that excessive cerumen may be interfering with an accurate assessment.
    3. Although it is appropriate to access the other ear, pulling the pinna downward and back will not straighten the external ear canal in an adult. This technique is appropriate for children less than 3 years of age.

4. The other ear should be used because the patient may have excessive cerumen in the right ear that is interfering with an accurate reading. Pulling the pinna downward and back is the appropriate technique to straighten the external ear canal of children less than 3 years of age, not an adult.

TEST-TAKING TIP: Identify the options with duplicate facts. Four concepts are presented: taking the temperature in the same ear, taking the temperature in the other ear, pulling the pinna upward and back, and pulling the pinna downward and back. If you know just one of these concepts in relation to the question you can eliminate 2 options from consideration.

Content Area: Physical Assessment
Integrated Processes: Nursing Process: Assessment
Client Need: Physiological Integrity; Reduction of Risk Potential
Cognitive Level: Application

35. **ANSWER: 1, 3, 5.**
    Rationales:
    1. **Excessive perspiration may interfere with contact between the skin and the temporal scanner probe, resulting in an inaccurate result.**
    2. Being a mouth breather will not interfere with obtaining an accurate temperature with a temporal scanner probe.
    3. **A hat helps retain surface body heat and may result in an inaccurate high result when using a temporal scanner probe.**
    4. Obtaining an accurate temperature is not influenced by a patient who has male pattern baldness. Excessive hair that flows over the forehead may help retain surface body heat, producing an inaccurate high result when using a temporal scanner probe.
    5. **Sleeping in the side-lying position with the head on a pillow may result in the retention of surface body heat that may result in an inaccurate high result when using a temporal scanner probe.**

TEST-TAKING TIP: Identify the words that indicate negative polarity. The words *requiring an alternate route* indicate negative polarity. The questions is asking, "Which patients are not candidates for the use of a temporal scanner?"

Content Area: Physical Assessment
Integrated Processes: Nursing Process: Assessment
Client Need: Health Promotion and Maintenance
Cognitive Level: Analysis

Chapter 12

Infection Control and Wound Care

KEY TERMS

Active immunity—Antibodies are formed within the body.

Bacterium—Single-celled microorganism that replicates independently outside of cells with the appropriate environment.

Carrier—Person who harbors a microorganism capable of causing disease while not exhibiting clinical manifestations of the disease.

Fomite—Any substance (e.g., food, water, object) that conveys a microorganism to a portal of entry.

Fungus—Microorganism that requires nutrients from decaying organic matter; includes yeasts and molds.

Immune response—Extent of resistance to a pathogen.

Immunizations (vaccines)—Administration of an antigen that precipitates the immune system to produce antibodies that protect the individual from a specific disease.

Infection—Invasion and multiplication of a pathogenic organism within the body.

Mode of transmission—Method by which a microorganism is transferred from an infectious agent to a host.

Parasite—Organism living in or on another living being and feeding off its cells and tissues.

Passive immunity—Antibodies acquired from a source other than the individual's body.

Pathogenicity—Ability to produce pathophysiological changes and disease.

Sterile—Absence of microorganisms.

Sterilization—Process by which microorganisms are destroyed.

Toxigenicity—Ability to produce harmful substances.

Vector—Animal or insect that transports microorganisms to a portal of entry.

Virulence—Degree of pathogenicity possessed by a microorganism.

Virus—Tiny microorganism that lives inside a host cell and takes over metabolism of the cell to replicate.

I. Body's Defenses Against Infection

The human body fights infection on three levels. Primary defenses involve body systems or parts of body systems that resist or confine invading pathogens. Secondary defenses are physiological responses to toxins produced by invading pathogens. Tertiary defenses are immune responses that react to the presence of an antigen and precipitate protective mechanisms or act directly against antigenic cells. Nurses must not only understand the way in which this three-level defense system helps to protect the body from infection but also the types of immunity, the role of immunizations (vaccines) that produce immunity to communicable diseases, and nursing care specific to these issues.

A. Primary Defenses
1. Skin and mucous membranes.
   a. Sebum on skin protects the skin.
   b. Ongoing desquamation of skin cells removes microorganisms.
   c. Low pH limits microbial growth.
   d. Mucous membranes produce mucus that traps microorganisms.
   e. Macrophages and lysozymes destroy bacteria on mucous membranes.

2. Respiratory system.
  a. Cilia capture and move microorganisms out of the respiratory tract.
  b. Mucous membranes secrete lysozymes that destroy microorganisms.
3. Gastrointestinal (GI) system.
  a. Saliva contains microbial inhibitors, such as lysozymes, lactoferrin, and immunoglobulin A (IgA).
  b. Low pH (acetic) of stomach and high pH of small intestine create inhospitable environments for microorganisms.
  c. Goblet cells lining the GI system produce secretions that prevent penetration by microorganisms and destroy (lyse) the cell walls of microorganisms.
  d. Peristalsis moves microorganisms out of the anus.
4. Circulatory system.
  a. Blood carries components of the inflammatory response (e.g., fibrinogen; thromboplastin; platelets; and white blood cells [WBCs], including neutrophils and monocytes).
  b. Blood carries components of the immune response (e.g., immunoglobulins, T cells, and antibodies).
5. Eyes.
  a. Tears and blinking flush microorganisms out of the eyes.
  b. Tears contain lysozymes that destroy microorganisms.
6. Genitourinary system.
  a. The vagina has a low pH that creates an inhospitable environment for microorganisms.
  b. The low pH of urine and flushing action of urination limits microbial growth.

B. Secondary Defenses
1. Fever.
  a. Products of pathogenic microorganisms (**pyrogens**) stimulate production of prostaglandins that reset the body's temperature thermostat in the hypothalamus to a higher level.
  b. An elevated temperature facilitates some immune reactions and inhibits the action of pathogens (exact mechanisms are still being debated).
2. Complement cascade.
  a. Proteins in the blood trigger chemicals that destroy pathogens by rupturing their cell membranes.
  b. Proteins in the blood stimulate basophils, a type of WBC, to release histamine, which is involved in the inflammatory response.
3. Inflammatory response: Local adaptation syndrome (LAS)—Hans Selye.
  a. A cellular response to irritation, injury, or infection attempts to neutralize pathogens and repair body tissues.

  b. A similar response occurs regardless of the stressor.
    (1) Physical, such as heat, cold, radiation, and pressure, resulting in ischemia.
    (2) Pathogens, such as bacteria and viruses.
    (3) Chemicals, such as acid or alkaline burns.
    (4) Internal body factors, such as enzymes leaking into the abdomen, antigen-antibody reactions, and autoimmune diseases.

DID YOU KNOW?
Infection is always accompanied by the inflammatory response, but the inflammatory response can occur without the presence of infection.

  c. Nursing care can help to detect or disrupt the inflammatory response. (Table 12.1)
C. Tertiary Defenses
1. **Immune response:** Body's reaction to and interaction with substances identified by the body as being foreign.
  a. Humoral immunity.
    (1) The humoral immune response reacts to the presence of an antigen (e.g., toxins, foreign substances, or particulates, such as bacteria, viruses, and proteins originating from within the body).
    (2) Macrophages and helper T cells stimulate B lymphocytes to produce antibodies, also called *immunoglobulins* (e.g., IgM, IgG, IgA, IgD, IgE).
    (3) Antibodies target antigens and destroy them through a variety of processes, such as phagocytosis, neutralization, agglutination, and activation of the complement cascade.
  b. Cellular immunity.
    (1) T cells act directly against antigenic cells.
    (2) Cytotoxic (killer) T cells attack and destroy cells infected with pathogens.
    (3) Helper T cells stimulate B cells in humoral immune responses.
    (4) Memory T cells form in response to an antigen and increase the speed and extent of T cell responses to subsequent invasion by the same antigen.
    (5) Suppressor T cells interrupt the immune response when infection is contained, acting like a feedback loop.
2. Types of immunity.
  a. Active immunity: Antibodies are formed within the body.
    (1) Natural-active immunity.
      (a) Antibodies are formed during the course of the disease.
      (b) Usually produces life-long immunity, such as to measles, chickenpox, and smallpox.

Table 12.1 Stages of the Inflammatory Response and Related Nursing Care

Commonalities of Nursing Care for Patients Experiencing the Inflammatory Response

1. Collect information to identify the causative factor.
2. Use standard precautions.
3. Perform physical assessment to identify the stage of the inflammatory response.
4. Inspect the site and surrounding area to determine the presence of lymphatic streaking.
5. Obtain vital signs to identify potential progression to sepsis, such as hyperthermia, tachycardia, and tachypnea.
6. Obtain specimens for culture and sensitivity, if necessary, before initiating antibiotics.
7. Institute transmission-based precautions if the patient has a known or suspected communicable infection or infestation.
8. Implement ordered interventions, such as application of warm soaks and administration of antibiotics or other medications.

Stage	Physiological Response	Specific Nursing Care
Vascular Response	• Initially, blood vessels briefly constrict (vasoconstriction) at the site of injury. • Histamine is released at the site of injury, causing blood vessel dilation (vasodilation) and increasing blood flow to the site. • Kinins released by destroyed cells make capillaries permeable and fluid moves into the interstitial compartment at the site of injury.	• Assess the site for paleness when blood vessels are constricted. • Assess the site for redness (hyperemia) and heat when blood vessels are dilated. • Assess the site for swelling (edema), pain, and loss of function.
Cellular Response	• Blood flow slows in dilated vessels. • White blood cells (WBCs), specifically neutrophils and monocytes, migrate to the site of injury and pass into tissues. • WBCs engulf foreign material, damaged cells, and microorganisms and destroy them (phagocytosis). • Bone marrow responds by increasing the number of WBCs in circulation (leukocytosis).	• Monitor continuation of signs of redness, heat, edema, pain, and loss of function. • Assess WBC count (expected level is 5,000 to 10,000/mm³; rate may increase to 15,000 to 20,000/mm³).
Exudate Formation	• A fluid forms that contains protein and cellular debris as a result of the inflammatory response (exudate). • Fibrinogen, thromboplastin, platelets, and WBCs may make a barrier around the site to limit the injury (abscess). • Abscesses contain thick liquid made up of cellular debris, destroyed tissue, phagocytic cells, and microorganisms (pus); they are generally associated with infection. • The nature and amount of exudate depends on the type and extent of injury. *Serous:* Clear, watery liquid that is like plasma. *Sanguineous:* Fluid that is red like blood. *Serosanguineous:* Pink, watery fluid; a mixture of serous and sanguineous fluid. *Purulent:* Thick fluid that appears yellow, green, tan, or brown; may be free flowing or contained in an abscess.	• Assess the amount and characteristics of exudate. • Perform irrigations and dressing changes as ordered.
Reparative Phase	*Healing by primary intention* • Wounds with approximated edges and minimal tissue destruction heal with minimal scar formation. • Tissue is replaced by identical or similar cells to original tissue (regeneration). *Healing by secondary intention* • Wounds with extensive tissue damage that do not have approximated edges heal from the inner layer to the outer surface. • Initially fragile, gelatinous tissue made up of newly formed capillaries forms (granulation). • Eventually, capillaries constrict, the tissue shrinks, collagen fibers contract, and firmer fibrous tissue remains (scar). *Healing by tertiary intention* • Two surfaces of granulated tissue are brought together and sutured in the absence of edema, foreign matter, or infection.	• Assess for fragile, gelatinous tissue that appears pink or red at the base of the injury. • Assess for shrinkage of tissue because, as it occurs, bleeding may recur. • Perform irrigations and dressing changes as ordered.

(2) Acquired-active immunity.
    (a) Antigen (e.g., vaccine or toxoid) is administered to stimulate the formation of antibodies.
    (b) Usually produces life-long immunity or requires revaccination to maintain titers.
b. Passive immunity: Antibodies are acquired from a source other than the individual's body.
    (1) Natural-passive immunity.
        (a) Passage of antibodies occurs from a mother to a fetus via the placenta or to a neonate via colostrum.

        (b) Provides immunity for 6 months to 1 year.
    (2) Acquired-passive immunity.
        (a) Antibodies produced from another source (immune serum) are injected into a person.
        (b) Provides immunity for 2 to 3 weeks.
3. Immunizations (vaccines).
    a. Administration of a specific substance that precipitates the immune system to produce antibodies (antigen) that protect an individual from a specific disease.
    b. Administered at specific developmental timetables (Figs. 12.1 and 12.2).

Recommended Immunization Schedule for Persons Aged 0 Through 18 Years – United States – 2013

See the original source for footnotes and recommendations associated with these immunizations and the schedule for those whose immunizations fall behind or start late (www.cdc.gov/vaccines/schedules/hcp/imz/child-adolescent.html).

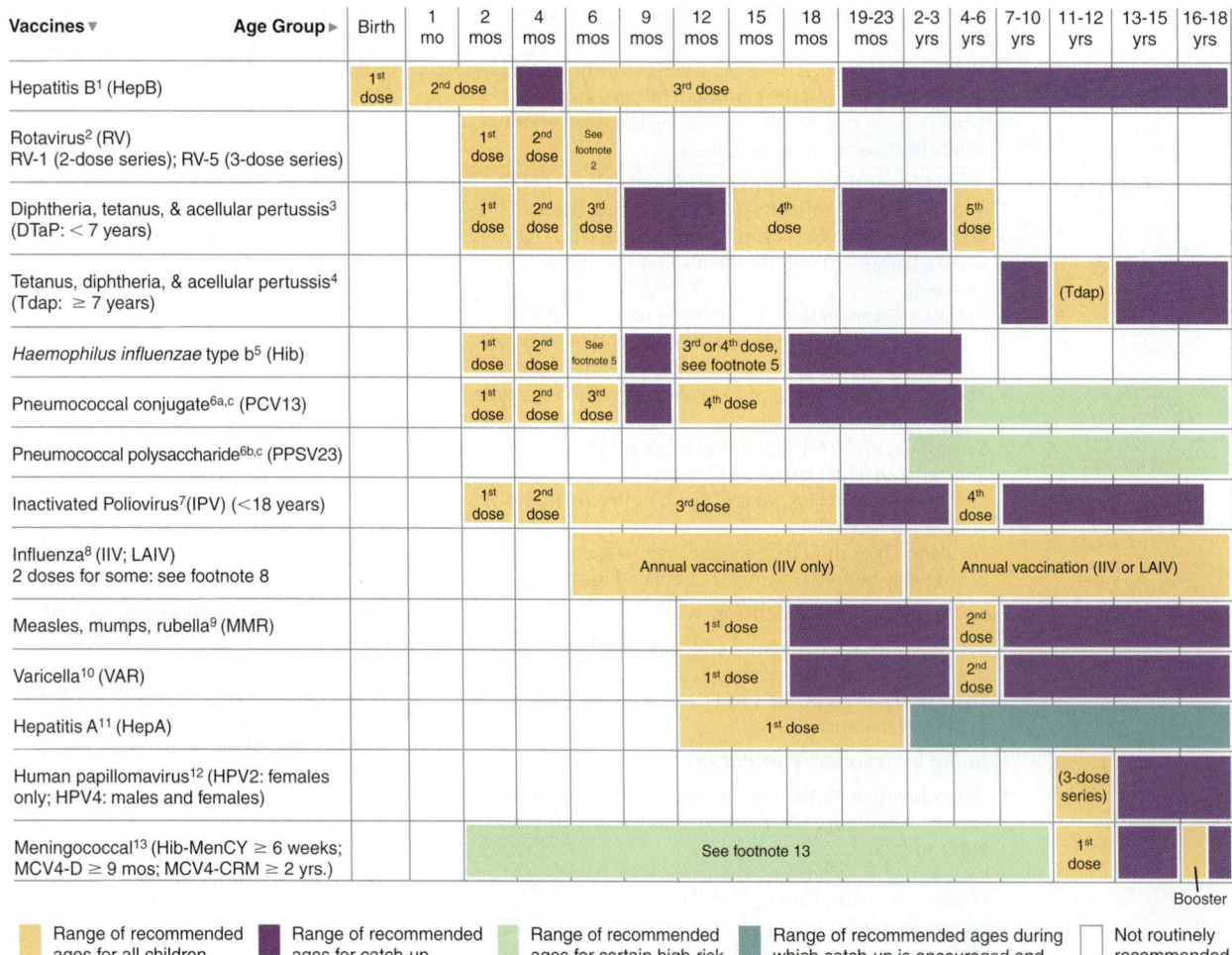

Fig 12.1 Recommended immunization schedule for persons aged 0 through 18 years—United States, 2013. (From Centers for Disease Control and Prevention [2013]. *Recommended Immunization Schedule for Persons Aged 0 Through 18 Years—United States, 2013.* Retrieved June 22, 2013, from www.cdc.gov/vaccines/schedules/download/child/0-18years-schedule.pdf.)

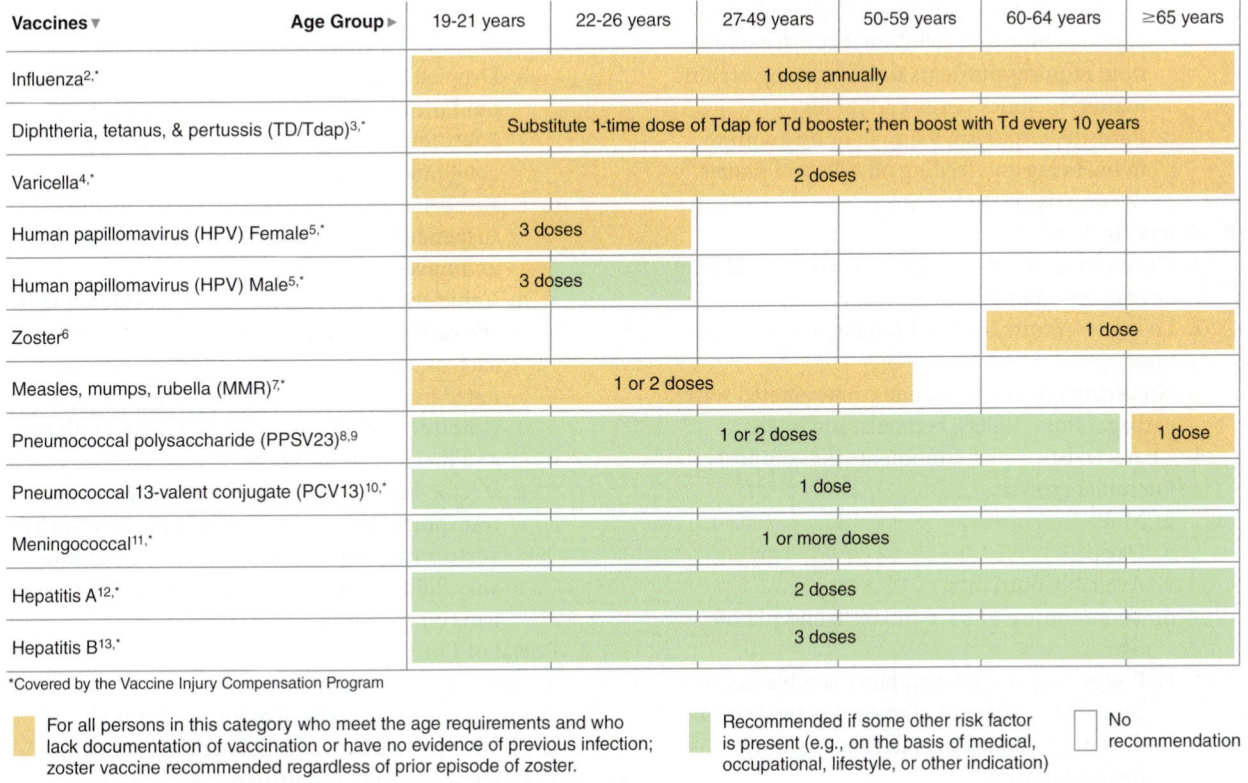

Recommended Adult Immunization Schedule – United States – 2013

See the original source for footnotes and recommendations associated with these immunizations and the schedule
for those who have high risk physiological conditions (www.cdc.gov/vaccines/schedules/hcp/imz/adult.html).

Vaccines ▼	Age Group ▶	19-21 years	22-26 years	27-49 years	50-59 years	60-64 years	≥65 years
Influenza[2,*]		1 dose annually					
Diphtheria, tetanus, & pertussis (TD/Tdap)[3,*]		Substitute 1-time dose of Tdap for Td booster; then boost with Td every 10 years					
Varicella[4,*]		2 doses					
Human papillomavirus (HPV) Female[5,*]		3 doses					
Human papillomavirus (HPV) Male[5,*]		3 doses					
Zoster[6]							1 dose
Measles, mumps, rubella (MMR)[7,*]		1 or 2 doses					
Pneumococcal polysaccharide (PPSV23)[8,9]		1 or 2 doses					1 dose
Pneumococcal 13-valent conjugate (PCV13)[10,*]		1 dose					
Meningococcal[11,*]		1 or more doses					
Hepatitis A[12,*]		2 doses					
Hepatitis B[13,*]		3 doses					

*Covered by the Vaccine Injury Compensation Program

For all persons in this category who meet the age requirements and who lack documentation of vaccination or have no evidence of previous infection; zoster vaccine recommended regardless of prior episode of zoster.

Recommended if some other risk factor is present (e.g., on the basis of medical, occupational, lifestyle, or other indication)

No recommendation

Fig 12.2 Recommended adult immunization schedule—United States, 2013. (From Centers for Disease Control and Prevention [2013]. *Recommended Adult Immunization Schedule—United States, 2013*. Retrieved June 22, 2013, from www.cdc.gov/vaccines/schedules/hcp/imz/adult/html.)

II. Chain of Infection

An **infection** is the invasion and multiplication of a pathogenic organism within the body. The transmission of an infection requires an uninterrupted cycle that consists of an infectious agent, a reservoir, a portal of exit, a mode of transmission, a portal of entry, and a susceptible host (Fig. 12.3).

A. **Infectious Agent** (Microorganism)
   1. Extent to which a microorganism can cause an infection.
      a. **Pathogenicity:** Ability to produce pathophysiological changes and disease.
      b. **Virulence:** Degree of pathogenicity possessed by a microorganism, including invasiveness, such as ability to survive in the environment, method of transfer to another host, ability to grow once attached to the new site, and ability to produce harmful substances (**toxigenicity**).
      c. Amount of microorganisms present.
   2. Type of microorganism.
      a. **Virus:** Tiny microorganism that lives inside a host cell and takes over metabolism of the cell to replicate.

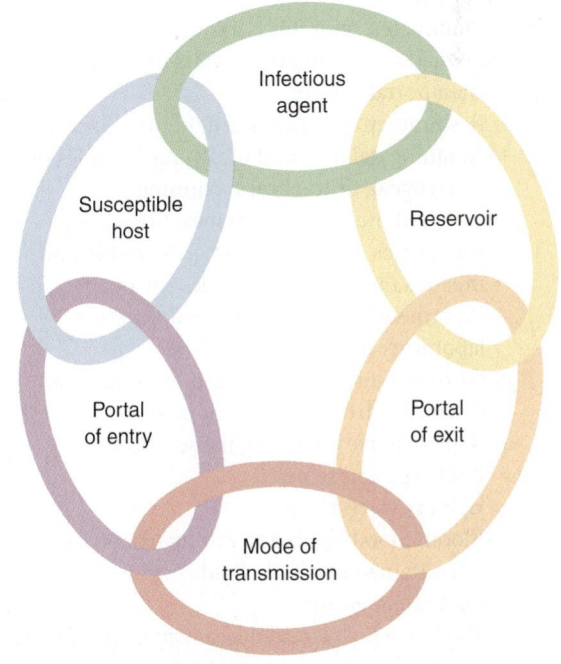

Fig 12.3 Chain of infection. (From Wilkinson and Treas [2011]. *Fundamentals of nursing*, Vol. 1, 2nd ed. Philadelphia: F. A. Davis Company, with permission.)

b. **Bacterium:** Single-celled microorganism that replicates independently outside of cells with the appropriate environment.

c. **Fungus:** Microorganism with cell walls that contain chitin and cellulose that resist destruction; requires nutrients from decaying organic matter; includes yeasts and molds.

d. **Parasite:** Organism living in or on another living being and feeding off cells and tissues, causing tissue destruction.

B. **Reservoir** (Source)

1. Place where microorganism can survive and may or may not multiply.
2. Living reservoirs include humans, animals, and insects.
3. Nonliving reservoirs include contaminated water, garbage, sinks, toilets, bed rails, and linens.
4. Characteristics of environments that support microbial growth.
   a. Moist.
   b. Dark.
   c. Available nutrients.
   d. Temperature of 68°F to 109°F and pH of 5 to 8.
   e. Presence of oxygen (supports aerobic microorganisms) or absence of oxygen (supports anaerobic microorganisms), depending on type of microorganism.
5. **Carrier:** Person who harbors a microorganism capable of being transmitted and causing disease in another while not exhibiting clinical manifestations of the disease.

C. **Portal of Exit**

1. Contaminated reservoir is a source of infection only when a microorganism exits the reservoir.
2. Human portals of exit.
   a. Respiratory tract (nose and mouth): Sneezing, coughing, talking, and breathing; includes oral, pharyngeal, or tracheal suctioning.
   b. Skin and mucous membranes: Breaks (e.g., tears, sores, fissures) in integrity of skin and mucous membranes; includes site of an IV catheter, injection, or blood draw for laboratory tests.
   c. GI tract: Saliva, vomitus, and feces; includes discharges from GI tubes or ostomies.
   d. Reproductive tract: Vaginal secretions or discharge and semen.
   e. Urinary tract: Urine.
   f. Blood: Blood or plasma exiting from a wound or contained in a body fluid.

D. **Mode of Transmission**

1. Method by which a microorganism is transferred from an infectious agent to a host.

2. Depends on characteristic of the microorganism and the disease it produces.
   a. Direct: Transfer of microorganism via contact between the infectious agent and host via touching, sexual intercourse, or kissing.
   b. Droplet: Transfer of large microorganisms in fluid droplets that can travel a maximum of 3 feet through activities such as sneezing, coughing, and talking.
   c. Airborne: Transfer of small microorganisms suspended in air for extended periods of time and travel via air currents.
   d. Vehicle-borne: Transfer via any substance that conveys a microorganism to a portal of entry, such as contaminated food or water; contaminated inanimate object that acts as a vehicle (**fomite**), such as tissues, toys, linens, clothing, and medical equipment.
   e. Vector-borne: Animal or insect (**vector**) that transports microorganisms to a portal of entry; vectors may deposit feces on skin, inject salivary fluid during biting, or carry microorganisms on their legs.

E. **Portal of Entry**

1. Microorganisms can enter the body through the same routes as portals of exit from the body.
2. Human portals of entry include the respiratory, GI, reproductive, and urinary tracts and the skin and mucous membranes.
3. Protecting patients from infection involves maintaining protective tissues (e.g., mucous membranes of the mouth, nose, vagina, urethra, anus and rectum) in the host.

F. **Susceptible Host**

1. Person who is at risk for infection because of inadequate defenses against microorganisms, such as the very young, very old, or immunocompromised; those with multiple chronic illnesses, inadequate nutrition, tissue destruction related to trauma or medical or surgical interventions; and people who smoke cigarettes.
2. Susceptibility depends on the extent of resistance to a pathogen (immune response).
3. Defenses protect the body from infection. (See Section IV, "Defenses Against Infection.")

III. Nursing Care to Interrupt the Chain of Infection

Microorganisms are transmitted when the chain of infection progresses without interruption. However, the transmission of microorganisms can be prevented if the chain is broken by practices performed by nurses, other healthcare providers, and patients. Each link of the chain of infection necessitates specific interventions to prevent transmission of an infectious agent.

A. Infectious Agent (Microorganism)

1. Use soap and water or disinfectant to decrease microorganisms on the skin.
2. Teach patients to:
   a. Avoid taking antibiotics unless absolutely necessary to prevent antibiotic resistant mutations and superinfections.

🛑 b. Complete the full course of prescribed antibiotics to avoid resistance.

   c. Not share antibiotics with others.

B. Reservoir (Source)

1. Ensure potentially contaminated surfaces, such as sinks, toilets, and overbed tables, are regularly cleaned.
2. Change bed linens regularly or whenever contaminated.
3. Use medical asepsis, such as fluid impervious garbage bags and linen hampers, and avoid touching sinks and toilets in public restrooms.
4. Clean and change water in covered water jugs every 8 hours.

5. Empty suction and drainage bottles at regular intervals (e.g., every 8 hours, end of each shift).
6. Teach patients to:
   a. Store food in a cool environment.
   b. Regularly clean surfaces where food is prepared.
   c. Regularly perform hand hygiene, particularly before and after handling food.

C. Portal of Exit

1. Maintain the integrity of closed systems, such as urinary catheters, portable wound drainage systems, and wound dressings.
2. Limit talking when performing sterile procedures, such as dressing changes.
3. Teach patients to:
   a. Cough and sneeze into an elbow or upper arm.
   b. Formula feed infants if mother is HIV positive because breast milk may contain the HIV.

D. Mode of Transmission

1. Maintain isolation precautions, including standard- and transmission-based precautions. (Table 12.2)

Table 12.2 Isolation Precautions and Related Nursing Care

Commonalities of Nursing Care for Patients Receiving Isolation Precautions

1. Institute specific precautions as indicated (e.g., with a health-care provider's order or when a patient's condition meets the criteria identified in agency protocol).
2. Explain to the patient the nature of the condition, the need for precautions, and the specifics of required interventions.
3. Involve the patient in the plan of care and provide the patient with choices to support independence.
4. Ensure that the patient understands how to use the call bell to summon health team members, if necessary.
5. Demonstrate a supportive, nonjudgmental attitude about the need for precautions; ensure that verbal and nonverbal communication does not convey negative feelings, such as disgust or revulsion.
6. Schedule time to converse with and provide nursing care to the patient on a regular basis; use touch appropriately after donning personal protective equipment (PPE).
7. Assess the need for stimulation and encourage the patient to engage in activities within abilities, such as watching television, reading a book, sitting in a chair, or walking around the room.
8. Assess for clinical manifestations of sensory deprivation, such as boredom, apathy, anxiety, increased sleeping, and disorganized thoughts.
9. Screen visitors to prevent entry of a person who may place patients or visitors at risk, such as a visitor with a respiratory tract infection or an unimmunized person.
10. Instruct visitors about specific precautions they must use.
11. Dedicate patient-care equipment to prevent transmission of microorganisms to others.
12. Limit patient movement outside of the room for essential reasons.

Tier 1 Precautions

Type	Description	Nursing Care
Standard Precautions	• Used for all patients regardless of absence of, suspicion of, or confirmed presence of infection. • Based on the concept that blood, body fluids, body secretions and excretions (except sweat), mucous membranes, and nonintact skin contain microorganisms. • Limit risk of transmission of microorganisms from a patient with an unrecognized or confirmed infection.	• Clean hands with an alcohol-based (minimum of 60%) antimicrobial gel; after application briskly rub hands together until dry. • Wash with soap and warm water if hands are visibly soiled or after caring for patients with suspected or known infectious diarrhea; wash vigorously with friction for a minimum of 15 seconds and then rinse and dry hands. • Use PPE (e.g., gloves, gown, and eye, nose, and mouth protection with a mask and goggles or a face shield) when a potential for exposure to body fluids exists.

Continued

Table 12.2 Isolation Precautions and Related Nursing Care—cont'd

Tier 1 Precautions

Type	Description	Nursing Care
		• Use respiratory hygiene and cough etiquette, such as covering the mouth and nose when coughing or sneezing, disposing of tissues in no-touch receptacles, and performing hand hygiene after hands come in contact with respiratory secretions. • Limit visitors with suspected respiratory infections or require them to wear masks. • Use safe injection practices, such as surgical asepsis, cleaning access diaphragms of vials with 70 % alcohol, and using single-use syringes, vials, and infusion sets.

Tier 2: Transmission-Based Precautions

Type	Description	Nursing Care
Airborne Precautions	• Used for patients suspected or known to be colonized or infected with an infectious agent that is transmitted via the air. • Based on the concept that droplet nuclei smaller than 5 mcg can remain suspended in the air and travel air currents. • Examples: Pulmonary tuberculosis, measles, chickenpox (varicella), and disseminated varicella zoster.	• Place in a private airborne infection isolation room (AIIR) with the door closed with negative-pressure air flow of 6 to 12 air exchanges per hour via HEPA filtration or discharged to outside air. • Wear a particulate filter mask (N95 respirator) when in the room. • Place a surgical mask on the patient during transport for essential reasons. • Ensure nonimmune people do not enter rooms of patients with vaccine-preventable airborne diseases, such as measles, chickenpox, and smallpox.
Droplet Precautions	• Based on the concept that microorganisms larger than 5 mcg within 3 feet of the patient can be transmitted to others through direct contact with the patient or via contaminated objects. • Examples: Rubella, influenza virus, adenovirus, rhinovirus, and group A streptococcus.	• Place the patient in a private room or cohort with another patient who has the same microorganism after consultation with infection control personnel. • Wear a mask for close contact with the patient. • Place a surgical mask on the patient during transport for essential reasons.
Contact Precautions	• Based on the concept that microorganisms can be transmitted by direct contact with the patient or indirect contact with contaminated objects in the patient's environment. • Examples: *Clostridium difficile*, respiratory syncytial virus, methicillin-resistant *Staphylococcus aureus* (MRSA), vancomycin-resistant enterocci (VRE), scabies, and conditions in which excretions or secretions are difficult to contain, such as draining wounds and fecal incontinence.	• Place in a private room or cohort with another patient who has the same microorganism after consultation with infection control personnel. • Wash hands before entering and when leaving the patient's room. • Don gloves and a gown before entering the patient's room. • When leaving the room, while still inside the room, remove gloves first and then the gown; untie ties of mask and ties in back of gown at neck and waist because they are considered clean; remove the gown by touching only the inside of the gown. • Wear additional PPE if splashing of body fluids is anticipated (e.g., goggles, face shield).

Protective Environmental Precautions

Type	Description	Nursing Care
Reverse isolation, protective isolation, neutropenic precautions	• Based on the concept that immunocompromised individuals are at risk for contracting invasive environmental infections, such as *aspergillosis*. • Examples: Patients who have a neutrophil count ≤500 cells/mL; are receiving immunosuppressive therapy, such as chemotherapy, radiation, antirejection agents, or allogeneic hematopoietic stem cell transplant; and those with chronic illnesses.	• Use transmission-based precautions as ordered. • Ensure air quality of the environment (e.g., HEPA filtration of incoming air, positive room air pressure relative to corridor, 12 air exchanges per hour, well-sealed room). • Ensure strategies to limit dust, such as wet dusting solid surfaces daily. • Ban dried and fresh flowers and potted plants from the patient's room. • Place a N95 respirator on the patient during transport for essential reasons.

2. Wash hands in sinks with foot pedals, keep hands above the level of the sink; if faucet has handles, shut off faucets with a clean, dry paper towel.
3. Perform hand hygiene after touching contaminated articles.
4. Keep fingernails short and avoid wearing artificial nails, fingernail polish, and jewelry with stones.

DID YOU KNOW?

The Centers for Disease Control and Prevention (CDC) recommend that nurses "not wear artificial fingernails or extenders when having direct contact with patients at high risk" and that they "keep natural nail tips less than 1/4-inch long." The CDC documents that studies indicate that persons wearing artificial nails or long nails have been epidemiologically implicated in outbreaks of infection related to gram-negative bacilli and yeasts. In addition, studies indicate that chipped nail polish may support the growth of larger numbers of organisms on fingernails even after careful hand washing.

5. Wear clean gloves when potential exposure to blood or body fluids exists.
6. Use additional PPE, such as a mask, a face shield, a fluid impervious gown, and gloves, when there is potential for splashing of body fluids or if a patient is receiving transmission-based precautions.
7. When removing soiled linen, fold the linen into itself.
8. Put contaminated linen in a fluid impervious hamper.
9. Provide fluid impervious bags at the bedside for disposal of used tissues.
10. Keep all items off the floor and off closet floors.
11. Routinely disinfect items that act as fomites, such as stethoscopes, clamps, eyeglasses, pens, and telephones.
12. Place needles and needleless systems into puncture-proof containers (sharps containers).
13. Dispose of urine and feces in appropriate receptacles, such as a patient's toilet.
14. Ensure the patient's immediate area is kept clean, including overbed tables.
15. Arrange for the area to be disinfected between patients.
16. Clean spills immediately.
17. Teach patients to:
    a. Use insect repellent and wear long-sleeve shirts and long pants when in areas where insect-causing diseases are endemic.
    b. Dispose of used tissues into a fluid impervious bag.
    c. Use a sharps container for used puncture devices associated with self-blood glucose

monitoring or needles and syringes for injection of medication.

E. Portal of Entry

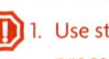 1. Use sterile technique when performing invasive procedures, such as injections, urinary catheterizations, dressing changes, and catheter irrigations.

2. Ensure all drainage tubes and drainage containers are kept below the insertion site.
3. Change dressings as soon as they become moist.
4. Provide or encourage perineal care with soap and water daily and when necessary, such as after toileting.
5. Teach patients to:
    a. Perform perineal care after toileting and to wash the genital area with soap and water daily.
    b. Maintain medical or surgical asepsis concerning tubes that enter the body (e.g., urinary catheter, portable wound drainage systems) and procedures that must be performed (e.g., dressing changes, injections).

F. Susceptible Host

1. Implement protective environmental precautions when the patient is immunocompromised (see Table 12.2).
2. Ensure the patient has received all age-appropriate immunizations (see "Immunizations" under "Body's Defenses Against Infection," page 295).
    a. Provide a vaccine information statement, including the safety, benefits, and risks concerning immunizations.
    b. Correct misconceptions regarding immunizations.
    c. Teach the parents potential adverse effects and appropriate interventions (e.g., prescribed dose of acetaminophen to minimize discomfort).
    d. Do not administer live virus vaccines (e.g., measles, mumps, and rubella [MMR] and varicella [chickenpox]) to a person with a depressed immune system or a temperature within the last 24 hours or a person who lives in a home with very young children, received another vaccination within the last month, or had an allergic reaction to the vaccination in the past.

3. Teach patients to follow a healthy lifestyle.
    a. Avoid tobacco-related habits.
    b. Eat a healthy diet.
    c. Drink adequate fluids daily (e.g., 2 to 3 L/day).
    d. Cough and deep breathe hourly when at an increased risk for stasis of respiratory secretions (e.g., when sedentary or on bed rest, after receiving anesthesia).
    e. Maintain the integrity of the skin and mucous membranes, such as by bathing, using moisturizing lotions, performing oral care, and alternating positions.

Chain of Infection and Nursing Care to Interrupt the Chain of Infection

To help prevent the spread of infection, nurses must make the connection between an organism's chain of infection and nursing actions that interrupt the chain at each point. For example, pulmonary tuberculosis is caused by the bacterium *Mycobacterium tuberculosis* (infectious agent). It lives and multiplies in the body of an infected person (reservoir). The infectious agent exits the respiratory tract via respiratory secretions from an infected person (portal of exit). It is transmitted via respiratory secretions that are released into the air when an infected person exhales, coughs, sneezes, or talks. The secretions are aerosolized and carried by air currents (mode of transmission). Generally, the infectious agent is inhaled in through the nose as aerosolized nuclei from an infected person (portal of entry). People with reduced immunity because of receiving chemotherapy for cancer, acquired immunodeficiency syndrome, chronic alcohol abuse, or advanced age are at an increased risk for contracting the disease if exposed to the agent (susceptible host). To help prevent the spread of tuberculosis, nurses should be involved in activities that interrupt the chain of infection at each point along the chain. For example:

- **Infectious agent:** Obtain a sputum specimen to send to the laboratory to identify the presence of *M. tuberculosis*.
- **Reservoir:** Screen using purified protein derivative (PPD) to identify people who have been exposed to tuberculosis and may be harboring the *M. tuberculosis* bacterium. Verify the presence of *M. tuberculosis* via a sputum culture.
- **Portal of exit:** Place a mask on a patient when transported outside a negative pressure room for essential purposes.
- **Mode of transmission:** Institute airborne transmission-based precautions. Maintain the patient in a negative pressure room with multiple air exchanges per hour.
- **Portal of entry:** Wear a high-efficiency particulate air (HEPA) respirator when in the patient's room.
- **Susceptible host:** Do not allow people with immature or inadequate immune systems to visit a patient with active tuberculosis.

IV. Sterile Technique (Surgical Asepsis)

Sterile technique (surgical asepsis) involves interventions that prevent the introduction of microorganisms into an area (e.g., sterile field) or body part (e.g., skin). The situations in which a nurse must use sterile technique are numerous. Regardless of the sterile procedure being performed, certain principles should be employed to maintain sterility. This section discusses these issues and relates nursing care associated with each principle.

A. Introduction
1. **Sterile** means absence of microorganisms.
2. **Sterilization** is a process that destroys microorganisms (e.g., moist heat, gas, boiling water, and radiation).
3. Human skin harbors many microorganisms, is not sterile, and cannot be sterilized; however, techniques can be used to limit the number of microorganisms, such as the use of hand washing, alcohol-based antimicrobial gels, and surgical scrubs.
4. Sterile technique involves using practices to prevent the introduction of microorganisms into an area.
5. Sterile technique is used in a variety of instances, including:
   a. When intentionally piercing a patient's skin, such as inserting an intravenous catheter into a vein or creating a surgical incision.
   b. When a patient's skin or membranes are breached or not intact, such as with burns, wounds, postoperative incisions, and childbirth.
   c. When inserting catheters into body cavities, such as a urinary catheter or tracheobronchial suctioning.
   d. When providing care in specialty environments, such as a birthing room, an operating room, and certain diagnostic procedure rooms, such as cardiac catheterization laboratories.

B. Principles of Surgical Asepsis (Table 12.3)

V. Wounds and Wound Care

A wound is a disruption in the integrity of the skin. Wounds can be classified by duration of healing, amount of microorganisms present, depth of injury, and integrity of the skin. They heal by primary, secondary, or tertiary intention; however, many factors can delay wound healing. Nurses must know how to collect a specimen of exudate, assess wounds, and provide care for all types of wounds. These topics are reviewed in this section.

A. Classification of Wounds
1. By duration of healing.
   a. Acute.
      (1) Healing occurs over a short duration, such as a surgical incision.
      (2) Most commonly heals by primary intention.
   b. Chronic.
      (1) Healing occurs over a long duration.
      (2) Healing is delayed due to the presence of infection, ischemia, edema, impaired circulation, or another underlying disease process, such as diabetes.
      (3) Generally heal by secondary intention.

Table 12.3 Principles of Surgical Asepsis and Related Nursing Care

Principle	Nursing Care
• All objects placed on a sterile field must be sterile and be kept sterile.	• Keep sterile objects in a clean, dry storage area. • Check sterile packages for intactness, dryness, and expiration dates and discard torn, wet, or outdated packages. • Check sterile packages for indication of sterilization (e.g., the word "STERILE" is on a closure tape that changes color when sterilized). • Place sterile objects inside a 1-inch margin of all edges of a drape because this area is considered sterile; the 1-inch border around the entire edge of the drape is considered unsterile. • The flat surface of a sterile field is considered sterile; draping material falling over the side of the surface is considered unsterile.
• Sterile objects remain sterile when touched by something sterile.	• Manipulate objects on a sterile filed with sterile forceps or hands wearing sterile gloves. • Touch only sterile equipment with sterile gloved hands. • Change sterile gloves if they become contaminated.
• Sterile objects become unsterile when touched by unsterile, clean, or contaminated objects or fluid.	• Discard sterile objects that come in contact with unsterile, clean, or contaminated objects; discard object when sterility is questionable. • Refrain from reaching over a sterile field with ungloved hands or moving unsterile objects over a sterile field. • Keep the lip of a bottle of liquid several inches above a sterile receptacle when pouring sterile liquid because the edge of the bottle is considered unsterile. • Use a moisture-proof barrier between the table and sterile objects. • Discard a sterile field that is pervious to liquid if it becomes wet by fluid from under or on the sterile field because capillary action will draw microorganisms onto the field. • Hold wet swabs with forceps held downward to keep fluid from flowing up toward the hands and becoming contaminated. • Hold hands above the elbows during a surgical hand scrub to prevent contaminated fluid from flowing onto the hands. • Wear surgical caps in operating rooms and birthing and burn units.
• Sterile objects become contaminated by exposure to air.	• Limit air currents in the room by closing the door, closing the bed curtain, and limiting unnecessary movement of people in the room. • Prepare the sterile field immediately before use. • Limit talking over the sterile field, and avoid laughing, sneezing, or coughing in the room. • Avoid walking between a sterile field and the patient.
• Sterile objects are considered unsterile when out of the nurse's sight or below the nurse's waist.	• Prepare and hold sterile objects above the waist. • Keep sterile objects and sterile gloved hands in the line of vision. • Never leave a sterile field unattended.

2. By presence and extent of microorganisms in the wound.
   a. *Clean wound:* Uninfected wound.
   b. *Clean-contaminated wound:* Surgical incision that penetrates the GI, respiratory, or genitourinary tract, and areas that commonly harbor pathogenic microorganisms.
   c. *Contaminated wound:* Colonized with microorganisms but has not progressed to an infection; generally associated with traumatic breaks in the skin; usually less than 100,000 organisms per gram of tissue.
   d. *Infected wound:* Colonized with bacteria causing erythema, swelling, and warmth around the wound; foul odor; drainage; and discomfort or pain; presence of greater than 100,000 organisms per gram of tissue; however, any number of beta-hemolytic streptococci present is considered an infection.

3. By depth of the wound.
   a. *Superficial wound:* Involves loss of only the epidermal layer (e.g., a superficial excoriation caused by friction); may take several days to a week to heal.
   b. *Partial-thickness wound:* Involves loss of the epidermis and possibly partial loss of the dermis (e.g., a partial-thickness burn); may take 2 to 3 weeks to heal.
   c. *Full-thickness wound:* Involves loss of the epidermis and dermis; may extend into deeper structures, such as subcutaneous tissue, muscle, joint, and bone, which are nonregenerative (e.g., a stage III or IV pressure ulcer); may take months or years to heal; some chronic full-thickness wounds may never heal because of underlying pathology, such as inadequate circulation secondary to a peripheral occlusive disorder or diabetes.

4. By integrity of the skin.
   a. *Open wound.*
      (1) Caused by a surgical incision or break in the skin for a therapeutic intervention, such as an intravenous infusion, spinal anesthesia, removal of fluid from the abdomen (paracentesis), or removal of fluid from the thoracic cavity (thoracentesis).
      (2) Provides a portal of entry.
   b. *Closed wound.*
      (1) Caused by an external blow or crushing force usually associated with a fall, automobile collision, or physical assault, causing damage to soft tissue and underlying structures while the skin remains intact.
      (2) May involve internal hemorrhage.

B. Types of Healing (Fig. 12.4) (see Reparative Phase in Table 12.1 Stages of the Inflammatory Response and Related Nursing Care)
1. Primary intention.
2. Secondary intention.
3. Tertiary intention.

C. Factors That Delay Wound Healing or Increase the Risk of a Wound Infection
1. Increased age.
   a. Aging skin loses elasticity.
   b. Collagen replacement is diminished.
   c. Circulation, phagocytic, and immune responses are reduced.
   d. Wound contraction occurs slowly.
   e. Scars are less strong.
2. Chronic illness and impaired health.
   a. The essential factors needed to facilitate wound healing are absent.

Primary intention

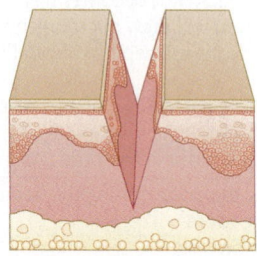 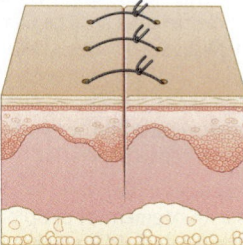 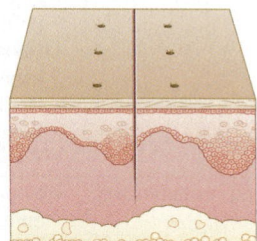

Clean wound · Sutured early · Results in hairline scar

Secondary intention

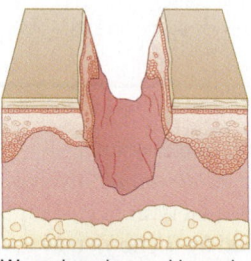 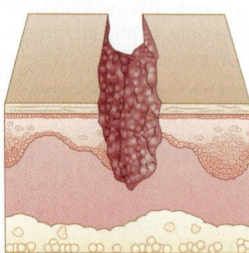 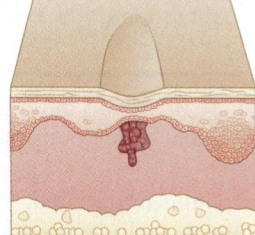

Wound gaping and irregular · Granulation occurring · Epithelium fills in scar

Tertiary intention

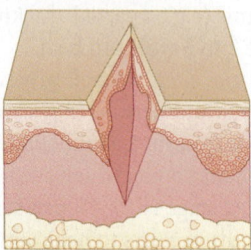 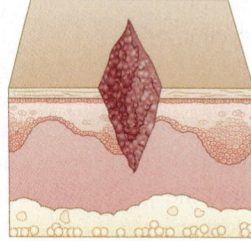 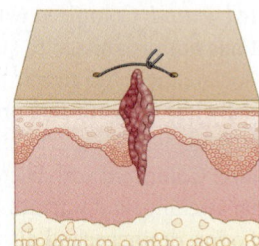

Wound not sutured · Granulation partially fills in wound · Granulating tissue sutured together

Fig 12.4 Types of healing. (From Burton and Ludwig [2011]. *Fundamentals of nursing care: Concepts, connections & skills.* Philadelphia: F. A. Davis Company, with permission.)

b. The immune system is depressed because of the illness or therapy (e.g., radiation, chemotherapy).

3. Edema.
   a. Fluid in the interstitial space increases the distance from the circulation to body cells.
   b. Edematous tissue reduces transport of nutrients to a wound and removal of debris from a wound.

4. Fever.
   a. Fever increases the metabolic rate and the demand for oxygen on a cellular level.
   b. Fever may precipitate dehydration, which limits the amount of circulating blood volume to the injured area.

5. Infection.
   a. Infection interferes with the inflammatory response and causes edema.
   b. Pathogenic organisms increase the extent of exudate in the wound.

6. Lifestyle.
   a. Personal behaviors, such as inadequate nutrition, do not provide the vitamins and proteins needed for adequate wound healing.
   b. Smoking (nicotine) constricts blood vessels, reducing the oxygen needed for healing.

7. Medications.
   a. Anti-inflammatory drugs, such as steroids and aspirin, impair the inflammatory process.
   b. Antineoplastics are cellular toxic and depress the bone marrow, resulting in decreased leukocyte production, which increases the risk of infection.

8. Multiple wounds.
   a. Multiple wounds compete for nutrients, such as enzymes and protein, needed for tissue repair.
   b. Multiplicity of stressors increases the demand on the sympathetic nervous system, precipitating hormonal and metabolic changes that interfere with the synthesis of inflammatory mediators.

9. Nutrition.
   a. Inadequate calories, protein, zinc, fluid, and vitamins C, A, and E impair healing.
   b. Vitamin C is needed for collagen synthesis, capillary growth, and fibroblast and immunologic function.
   c. Protein is needed for tissue growth, angiogenesis, collagen formation, immune function, and wound remodeling.
   d. Overeating results in obesity; excessive adipose tissue has fewer blood vessels, predisposing a person to wound complications.

10. Tissue perfusion.
    a. Impaired perfusion to a wound decreases the delivery of nutrients and oxygen to the area (e.g., lung and heart disease, anemia, peripheral edema, or peripheral artery disease).
    b. Impaired perfusion away from a wound decreases the removal of waste, carbon dioxide, and cellular debris (e.g., peripheral venous disease or peripheral edema).

11. Radiation.
    a. The initial stages of the inflammatory response are severely inhibited.
    b. Radiation breaks down underlying connective tissue and bone marrow.
    c. Radiation slows the growth of granulation tissue and the reepithelialization process.

12. Wound tension.
    a. Vomiting, coughing, sneezing, and obesity strain wound edges, which may cause them to pull apart.
    b. Tension can lead to wound dehiscence or evisceration (see the sections on dehiscence and evisceration in "Postoperative Wound Complications" in Chapter 24, "Perioperative Nursing," page 770).

D. Culture and Sensitivity Testing
1. Culture and sensitivity.
   a. Identifies microorganisms present in a specimen.
   b. Identifies antibiotics that are most effective in destroying an identified microorganism.

🛑 c. Requires the nurse to obtain a specimen before initiating antibiotic therapy.

2. Nursing care for obtaining a wound specimen.
   a. Wash hands.
   b. Collect the appropriate equipment (e.g., clean gloves, sterile culturette tube that contains a cotton-tipped swab).
   c. Confirm the patient's identity.
   d. Explain the procedure.
   e. Provide for the patient's privacy.
   f. Don PPE as indicated, such as a gown, a face shield, and clean gloves.
   g. Place the patient in a position that provides easy access to the wound.
   h. Assess the characteristics of the wound and drainage.
   i. Irrigate the wound surface with sterile normal saline solution to remove surface bacteria.
   j. Rotate the tip of the sterile swab from a culturette tube in the wound bed, avoiding areas that have drainage or necrotic tissue and the wound edges (Fig. 12.5).
   k. Place the sterile swab back into the culturette tube and then seal the tube.
   l. Place identifying information on the culturette tube and outside of the fluid-impervious bag before sending the specimen to the laboratory.
   m. Document all assessments, interventions, and patient responses.

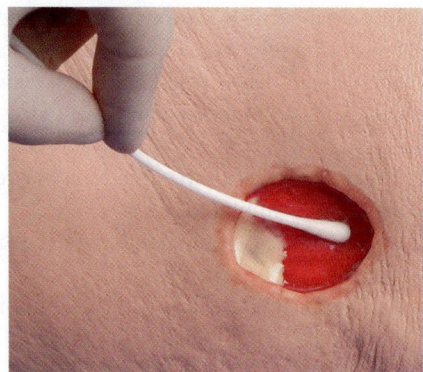

Fig 12.5 Obtaining a specimen from a wound for culture and sensitivity. (From Burton and Ludwig [2011]. *Fundamentals of nursing care: Concepts, connections & skills.* Philadelphia: F. A. Davis Company, with permission.)

E. Nursing Care Common to Patients With All Types of Wounds
  1. Support the patient emotionally.
     a. Encourage the patient to verbalize feelings about the wound and its implications.
     b. Identify whether the patient is anxious or fearful about the size, location, appearance, or odor of the wound; accept the patient's feelings about the wound.
     c. Avoid excessive exposure of the patient to the wound until the patient is ready to look at the wound or participate in wound care.
     d. Avoid body language that may communicate a negative reaction to the wound.
     🛑 e. Help the patient to maintain a positive body-image when the body is altered due to such events as mastectomy, colostomy, burns, or facial scarring.
  2. Monitor the patient's vital signs, including temperature, pulse, respirations, blood pressure, and pain.
  3. Assess the characteristics of the wound.
     a. Identify the location of the wound.
     b. Measure the dimensions of the wound, including length, width, and depth and amount of undermining and tunneling, using an objective measuring device.
     c. Describe the wound edges, such as approximation; signs of infection (e.g., reddened edges, slightly swollen, and warm to touch).
     d. Assess the condition of the surrounding skin for clinical indicators of a problem, such as infection, maceration, and edema.
     e. Identify type of exudate. (See also the interventions under "Exudate Formation" in Table 12.1.)
     f. Document the number of saturated gauze or abdominal pads; document output from wound drains in milliliters (mLs); and, if two or more drains are present, ensure that they are numbered.

  g. Describe the status of the wound using the Red, Yellow, and Black classification system.
     (1) Red.
         (a) Reflects newly granulating tissue.
         (b) Care involves gentle cleaning and a moist dressing (transparent or hydrocolloid).
     (2) Yellow.
         (a) Reflects oozing exudate, which may be purulent.
         (b) Care includes cleansing or irrigating the wound; using a wet-to-moist dressing, foam absorptive dressing, hydrogel, or alginate to debride the wound; and possibly seeking an order for a topical antimicrobial.
     (3) Black.
         (a) Indicates necrotic tissue (**eschar**); color variations of eschar include grey, tan, or brown.
         (b) Care involves removal of eschar (**debridement**) (see the section below on debridement in "Nursing Care for Patients With a Wound That May Be Infected, Is Infected, or Requires Debridement").
  h. Identify the stage of the wound by indicating the tissue layers involved when assessing wounds healing by secondary or tertiary intention (see Table 17.4, "Pressure Ulcer Stages," in Chapter 17, "Mobility," page 492).
  i. Identify pain or discomfort associated with the wound using an objective rating scale, and administer an analgesic as prescribed 30 minutes before a dressing change if pain is anticipated.

F. Nursing Care for Patients With a Wound That May Be Infected, Is Infected, or Requires Debridement
  1. Assess and implement nursing care related to caring for a patient with a wound infection (see the section "postoperative wound complications" under "Manage the Patient's Operative Site", in Chapter 24, "Perioperative Nursing", page 766).
  2. Clean the wound as ordered (see the section "clean a wound" under "Manage the Patient's Operative Site", in Chapter 24, "Perioperative Nursing", page 766).
  3. Irrigate the wound as ordered (see the section "irrigate a wound as ordered" under "Manage the Patient's Operative Site", in Chapter 24, "Perioperative Nursing", page 766).
  4. Promote debridement of the wound, if ordered.
     a. Assist the primary health-care provider with surgically cutting away devitalized tissue with a scalpel or scissor (surgical debridement) at the bedside. Wear a gown, mask, face shield, and sterile gloves. If the wound is large, expect this procedure to be completed in an operating room.

b. Employ other debridement methods, such as scrubbing the wound with gauze (mechanical debridement), using collagenase enzyme products (chemical debridement), or using a dressing that promotes the body to generate enzymes to break down eschar (autolytic debridement).

c. Apply ointment or paste to the skin surrounding the wound to protect the skin from contact with exudate, which can macerate tissue.

5. Apply the dressing ordered by the primary health-care provider and according to the manufacturer's instructions (Table 12.4).

6. Apply and secure a secondary dressing (e.g., generally 4″ X 4″ gauze or an abdominal pad) over the primary dressing using either the three tape method or window method (see Fig. 24.12 and Fig. 24.13 in Chapter 24, "Perioperative Nursing," page 768).

VI. Medications Related to Infection and Infestation

When a person is diagnosed with an infection caused by a bacteria, virus, or fungus or is diagnosed with an infestation of a parasite or helmintic, the primary health-care provider prescribes appropriate medication to cause death of the invading agent. Nurses need to know the mechanisms of action, therapeutic and nontherapeutic effects, and nursing care related to common antibiotics, anti-infectives, antivirals, antiretrovirals, antifungals, antiparasitics, and anthelmintics. (Table 12.5)

Table 12.4 Types of Wound Dressings and Related Nursing Care

A dressing facilitates healing.
- Keeps the wound dry (dry sterile dressing) for an approximated incision or laceration.
- Keeps the wound bed continuously moist (wet to moist dressing) for wounds with unapproximated edges to promote granulation in the wound bed.
- Controls exudate without dehydrating or drying the wound bed.
- Fills the wound cavity and undermining areas to avoid dead space.
- Keeps surrounding intact skin dry because it prevents maceration and skin impairment.

The nursing care provided for a patient with a wound dressing varies by the type of dressing used.

Type of Dressing	Nursing Care
Transparent Dressing • See-through, film-like, thin sheet that is semipermeable, allowing for an interchange of oxygen between the wound and the environment. • Self-adhesive. • Elastic and pliable, making it comfortable. • Used over intact skin to reduce shearing or to protect a small, superficial wound, such as a blister, stage I or II pressure ulcer, abrasion, skin tear, IV site, or minor burn. • Used for a wound that has minimal drainage. • Maintains a moist wound bed. • Protects the wound from contamination. • Examples: Op-Site, Tegaderm, Acu-derm, Bioclusive, and Polyskin.	• Clean the wound as ordered and then thoroughly dry the skin around the wound. • Apply the dressing to a dry skin surface. • Do not stretch or wrinkle the dressing when applying it to the area which will prevent pulling on the skin and promote adherence. • Remove and replace the dressing if its edges roll, its seal breaks, or after 24 to 72 hours, depending on manufacturer's instructions. • Assess the area daily for clinical indicators of a problem.
Hydrocolloid Dressing • Occlusive adhesive dressing that adheres to wet and dry sites. • Available in many sizes and shapes that contour to fit different body parts. • Also available as a paste, granules, or powder that can be applied to the wound cavity. • Becomes an absorbent gel on contact with drainage. • Protects the wound from contamination, serving as an excellent microbial barrier. • Is moisture retentive. • Cushions the wound. • Serves as a thermal insulator. • Used for wounds with light to moderate drainage; contraindicated with heavy drainage because this type of dressing absorbs drainage slowly. • Used for shallow to medium depth skin ulcers and donor sites and with packing for small cavity wounds.	• Ensure a 1-inch margin of healthy skin around the wound when sizing the dressing. • Round off the edges to reduce the likelihood of the edges catching on gowns or linens. • Warm the dressing by rubbing it between the hands before application to improve adhesion if it is an adhesive product. • Apply to dry skin with a secondary dressing if indicated (a secondary dressing is unnecessary if it is an adhesive dressing). • Avoid applying the dressing by stretching the product or using too much tension to prevent a tourniquet effect; do not reinforce it with tape. • Remove and replace the dressing if the edges roll, the seal breaks, after 3 to 7 days according to the manufacturer's directions or whenever necessary. • Assess for maceration of the skin around wound margins.

Continued

Table 12.4 Types of Wound Dressings and Related Nursing Care—cont'd

Type of Dressing	Nursing Care
• Some can be used on intact skin and others in the presence of dry eschar, necrosis, or slough. • Facilitates autolytic debridement. • Does not permit visualization of the wound. • Contraindicated for infected wounds, wounds with exposed tendon or bone, and foot ulcers associated with diabetes mellitus. • Examples: DuoDERM, Intact, IntraSite, Ultec, Comfeel, Restore, and Tegasorb.	

Hydrogel Dressing

• Available in flexible sheets or as a powder, beads, or paste. • Is 80% to 90% glycerin or water, adding moisture to a wound. • Devitalizes tissue to assist with autolytic debridement. • Forms a gelatinous mass when in contact with exudate to maintain a moist wound environment. • Does not adhere to the wound. • Pads the wound, increasing comfort and reducing shearing. • Softens eschar (autolytic debridement). • Used for partial-thickness and full-thickness wounds, necrotic wounds, and superficial burns. • Contraindicated with wounds that are infected, have excessive exudate, or are bleeding. • Examples: Aquasorb, Vigilon, IntraSite Gel, Nu-Gel, and Hypergel.	• Gently insert the flexible sheet to fill the contour of the wound; apply powder, beads, paste, or spray as indicated by the manufacturer's instructions to fill the wound cavity; avoid skin surrounding the wound. • Apply a secondary dressing over the hydrogel product. • Change the dressing every 8 to 48 hours as indicated by the manufacturer's instructions. • Irrigate the hydrogel residue from the wound; then reapply a new dressing. • Assess the skin around the wound for clinical indicators of maceration or infection; however, do not be confused with expected gel residue that looks like pus and is malodorous.

Alginate Dressing

• Made of soft, nonwoven fibers developed from seaweed in the form of pads, ropes, or ribbons for application to various shaped wounds. • Becomes a gel on contact with exudate and absorbs 20 times its weight. • Used for wounds with moderate to high amounts of drainage. • Used for partial-thickness and full-thickness wounds, venous status ulcers, pressure ulcers, diabetic ulcers, graft sites, traumatic and surgical wounds, and infected wounds. • Contraindicated in dry wounds and full-thickness wounds with exposed tendons or bone. • Examples: Sorbsan, AlgiDerm, Curasorb, Kaltostat, and Dermacea, SeaSorb, and Melgisorb.	• Cut or fold the dressing so that it fits the wound; do not overlap the wound margins. • Secure the dressing with a nonocclusive secondary dressing. • To change the dressing, gently remove the secondary dressing; if the area looks dry, saturate it with sterile normal saline solution, gently remove the alginate, and then discard it appropriately. • Irrigate the wound with a wound cleanser as ordered before applying a new dressing. • Change the dressing as needed (possibly every 24 hours depending on the volume of exudate).

Foam Dressing

• A highly absorbent dressing that wicks exudate off the wound, decreasing maceration of surrounding tissue. • Available in many shapes to fit the contours of the body. • Protects the wound. • Maintains wound moisture. • May have hemostatic, debriding, antimicrobial, and odor-controlling activities and inactivate proteolytic enzymes in chronic wounds. • May be adhesive. • Used for heavily exudating wounds, such as deep cavity wounds, weeping ulcers, and chronic wounds. • Used in wound vacuum-assisted closure systems. • Contraindicated for wounds with little drainage because of its drying effect. • Examples: FOAM, POLYDERM, CURAFOAM, Mepilex, and Allevyn.	• Clean the wound as ordered. • Place the foam over the wound, extending over the wound margins or cut it to fit the wound cavity. • Secure the dressing in place with tape, elastic gauze, or tube gauze if the dressing is not adhesive; avoid excessive tightness because, as foam absorbs moisture, it will place increased pressure on the wound bed. • Leave the dressing in place for 2 to 7 days, per the manufacturer's directions or when evidence indicates that the foam is full of exudate (e.g., dressing becomes heavy). • For nursing care related to vacuum-assisted closure, see the section "Negative Pressure Wound Therapy" in Chapter 24, "Perioperative Nursing," page 770.

Growth Factor–Impregnated Dressing

• Growth factors are small protein hormones that enhance wound healing at various places along the healing cascade. • Attract immune cells to fight infection, promote production of connective tissue, facilitate new blood vessel growth to nourish the area, and promote remodeling.	• Apply a growth factor–impregnated dressing as prescribed. • Apply growth factor directly to a wound bed and cover with a dressing as prescribed.

Table 12.4 **Types of Wound Dressings and Related Nursing Care—cont'd**

Type of Dressing

Growth Factor–Impregnated Dressing (cont'd)

- May be impregnated into a dressing or applied topically and covered with a dressing.
- Most common growth factors.
  - Platelet-derived growth factor (PDGF).
  - Epidermal growth factor (TGF).
  - Transforming growth factor-beta (TGF-Beta).
  - Vascular endothelial growth factor (VEGF).
  - Insulin growth factor-1 (IGF-1).
- Each works differently; for example, PDGF recruits stem cells to the wound site, promotes angiogenesis, and initiates tissue regeneration and remodeling.

Table 12.5 **Medications That Control Infection or Infestation**

Antibiotics and Anti-infectives

Decrease growth of or destroy susceptible microorganisms.

Mechanism of Action	Examples	Nontherapeutic Effects
Anti-infectives • Decrease protein and DNA synthesis, bacteriocidal, trichomonacidal, and amebicidal.	metronidazole (Flagyl)	• Nausea and vomiting. • Diarrhea. • Hypersensitivity reactions, such as skin rash and anaphylaxis. • Possibly, hepatotoxicity, nephrotoxicity, and bone marrow depression.
Aminoglycosides • Decrease protein synthesis.	azithromycin (Zithromax) clarithromycin (Biaxin) gentamicin (Garamycin)	
Cephalosporins • Bind to cell wall, causing cell death.	cefazolin (Ancef) cephalexin (Keflex)	
Penicillins • Bind to cell wall, causing cell death.	amoxicillin (Amoxil) penicillin V (Veetids, Pen-Vee)	
Quinolones • Decrease DNA synthesis.	ciprofloxacin (Cipro) levofloxacin (Levaquin)	
Sulfonamides • Decrease protein synthesis.	doxycycline (Vibramycin)	

NURSING CARE

- Obtain a specimen for culture and sensitivity testing before administering the first dose of medication.
- Assess for and teach about clinical manifestations of infection.
- Administer evenly spaced doses to maintain therapeutic blood levels of the medication.
- Teach the patient to complete the entire antibiotic regimen to prevent resistance.
- Teach the patient not to chew or crush extended-release tablets.
- Assess for clinical manifestations of superinfection, such as furry overgrowth on the tongue, vaginal discharge, and foul-smelling stool.
- Obtain a blood specimen 1 to 3 hours after a dose to measure the peak level (depends on medication's half-life). A **peak level** is the highest blood concentration of a medication.
- Obtain a blood specimen 30 to 60 minutes before the next dose to measure the trough level. A **trough level** is the lowest blood concentration of a medication.

Antifungals

Decrease fungal growth.

Mechanism of Action	Examples	Nontherapeutic Effects
Systemic • Impair fungal plasma membrane.	clotrimazole (Mycelex) fluconazole (Diflucan) nystatin (Mycostatin)	• Nausea and vomiting. • Diarrhea. • Hypersensitivity reactions, such as rash and anaphylaxis.

Continued

Table 12.5 Medications That Control Infection or Infestation—cont'd

Mechanism of Action	Examples	Nontherapeutic Effects
Antifungals (cont'd)		• Possible harm to fetus if woman being treated is pregnant (teratogenic). • Ototoxicity. • Hepatotoxicity. • Nephrotoxicity.
Topical • Disrupt fungal cell wall and cell metabolism.	clotrimazole (Lotrimin) ketoconazole (Nizoral) nystatin (Mycostatin) amphotericin B	• Burning and irritation at the site of application.

NURSING CARE

Systemic

- Teach the patient to refrain from intercourse to prevent pregnancy during therapy.
- Teach the patient to complete the entire regimen.
- Monitor for ototoxicity, nephrotoxicity, and hepatotoxicity.

Topical

- Clean the skin with tepid water before application.
- Monitor for skin or mucous membrane irritation.
- Teach the patient how to insert a vaginal suppository or cream.
- Teach the patient how to insert a rectal suppository.
- Teach the patient difference between "swish and spit" and "swish and swallow."

Antiparasitics and Anthelmintics

Cause death of a parasite or helmintic

Mechanism of Action	Examples	Nontherapeutic Effects
Parasiticidal • Absorbed into parasites and eggs. • Used for scabies and lice.	lindane (Kwell)	• Central nervous system toxicity. • Seizures.
	permethrin (Nix)	• Tingling. • Pruritus.
Antihelmintic • Prevents worm growth and reproduction. • Used for pinworms.	mebendazole (Vermox)	• Hypersensitivity, such as skin rash and anaphylaxis. • Abdominal pain.

NURSING CARE

- Teach the patient to wash linens and clothing in hot water and dry in a dryer.
- Teach the patient to seal nonwashables in plastic bags for a minimum of 2 weeks.
- Teach the patient to vacuum carpets and furniture daily.
- Ensure that all persons living within the household are treated.

For Pinworms

- Obtain a specimen via cellophane tape test in the morning before a bowel movement.
- Monitor for GI distress and for irritation of the perianal area.

For Head Lice

- Teach the patient to wash hair for 5 minutes with an antiparasitic shampoo.
- Teach the patient to comb hair with fine-tooth comb to remove eggs (nits).
- Teach the patient to assess for the continued presence of nits at the base of hair shafts, particularly hair at the nape of the neck and behind the ears.
- Maintain contact precautions (e.g., gown and gloves; hair covering is recommended) when providing patient care before treatment and for 24 hours after initiation of topical treatment.

For Scabies

- Maintain contact precautions (e.g., gown and gloves; hair covering is recommended) when providing patient care before treatment and for 24 hours after initiation of topical treatment.
- Teach the patient to scrub the body with soap and water, dry, and apply antiparasitic medication, avoiding the face, eyes, mucous membranes, and open wounds.

Table 12.5 **Medications That Control Infection or Infestation—cont'd**

Antivirals

Decrease severity of infections (not curative).

Mechanism of Action	Examples	Nontherapeutic Effects
Anti-Herpes Agents • Decrease viral DNA synthesis.	acyclovir (Zovirax) famciclovir (Famvir) valacyclovir (Valtrex)	• Anorexia. • Nausea and vomiting. • Diarrhea. • Headache. • Dizziness.
Anti-Cytomegalovirus (CMV) Agents • Decrease viral DNA synthesis.	cidofovir (Vistide) ganciclovir (Cytovene) valganciclovir (Valcyte)	• Insomnia. • Moniliasis or vaginitis. • Nephrotoxicity. **Anti-CMV agents**
Anti-Hepatitis Agents • Depending on the drug, cause viral DNA death by inhibiting viral replication and phagocytizing cells.	adefovir (Hepsera) interferon (Intron A) lamivudine (Epivir HBV)	• Hepatotoxicity. • CNS and bone marrow depression. • Teratogenicity. **Interferon**
Anti-Influenza Agents • Prevent penetration of virus into host cells or inhibit the neuramidase enzyme needed for viral replication.	amantadine (Symmetrel) oseltamivir (Tamiflu) rimantadine (Flumadine) zanamivir (Relenza)	• Clinical depression. **Anti-Influenza agents** • Headache. • Dizziness. • Fatigue.

NURSING CARE

• Obtain a specimen for culture and sensitivity testing before the first dose is administered.
• Teach the patient to take the medication exactly as prescribed to maintain therapeutic blood levels.
• Teach the patient to drink adequate fluids to prevent nephrotoxicity.
• Assess for and teach the patient about clinical manifestations of nephrotoxicity, hepatotoxicity, and bone marrow and CNS depression.
• Employ safety interventions if the patient is experiencing headache, dizziness, or fatigue.
• Teach the patient to avoid pregnancy if the medication can harm a fetus (teratogenic).

Anti-Herpes Agents

• Teach the patient to take the medication when pain or pruritus occurs because these precede eruptions.
• Teach the patient to avoid sexual activity during exacerbations to prevent transmission of the virus.
• Teach the patient the need for continued health-care supervision because of the increased risk of cervical cancer.

Antiretrovirals

Prevent or decrease severity of viral infections (e.g., HIV and AIDS).

Mechanism of Action	Examples	Nontherapeutic Effects
Nucleoside Reverse Transcriptase I (NRTIs) • Inhibit activity of reverse transcriptase, terminating the cellular DNA chain.	ABC: abacavir (Ziagen) FTC: emtricitabine (Emtriva) 3TC: lamivudine (Epivir) ZDV: zidovudine (AZT, Retrovir)	• Nausea and vomiting. • Diarrhea. • Headache. • Dizziness. • Insomnia. • Moniliasis or vaginitis. **Effects depending on drug**
Non-Nucleoside Reverse Transcriptase Inhibitors (NNRTIs) • Inactivate reverse transcriptase, preventing conversion of HIV RNA to HIV DNA.	EFV: efavirenz (Sustiva) TDF: tenofovir (Viread)	• Confusion. • Skin lesions. • Allergic reactions. • Neuropathies. • Nephrotoxicity.
Protease Inhibitors • Inhibit HIV protease, preventing virus maturation.	LPV/r: lopinavir/ritonavir (Kaletra) RTV: ritonavir (Norvir)	• Hepatotoxicity. • Bone marrow and CNS depression.
Multiple Drug Regimens for Naïve Patients • First time on highly active antiretroviral therapy **(HAART)**: EFV + (3TC or FTC) + (ZDV or TDF) LPV/r + (3TC or FTC) + ZDV.	Atripla: EFV + TDF + FTC Combivir: AZT + 3TC Epzicom: ABC + 3TC Kaletra: (LPV/r + RTV) Trizivir (AZT + 3TC + ABC) Truvada (FTC + TDF)	

Table 12.5	Medications That Control Infection or Infestation—cont'd

Antiretrovirals (cont'd)

NURSING CARE

- Teach the patient to take the medication exactly as prescribed (95% adherence is required to prevent resistance) and to avoid over-the-counter medications unless first approved by the primary health-care provider.
- Refer the patient to the manufacturer's insert regarding the need to take the drug with or without food and what to do if a dose is missed.
- Explain to the patient that GI nontherapeutic effects and insomnia will resolve in 3 to 4 weeks after the initiation of therapy.
- Encourage routine primary health-care provider supervision and blood studies.
- Assess for and teach the patient about the clinical manifestations of nephrotoxicity, hepatotoxicity, and bone marrow and CNS depression.
- Assess for and teach the patient about the clinical manifestations of opportunistic infections.
- Encourage the use of safer sexual practices to prevent virus transmission.

CASE STUDY: Putting It All Together

An older adult female is admitted to a hospital with extensive weeping lesions over her scalp, neck, axillae, and groin and under her breasts. The patient says that she has experienced many rashes over the years and generally uses home remedies that her mother had used when she was a child; however, this time nothing worked to eliminate the rash and itching. She went on to say that, when the lesions spread to her chest and looked like they were infected, she became frightened and short of breath and immediately went to the emergency department. The primary health-care provider admits the patient with a diagnosis of atopic dermatitis R/O methicillin-resistant *Staphylococcus aureus* (MRSA) infection. The patient's 45-year-old daughter is notified of her mother's admission to the hospital and plans to visit after work.

Primary health-care provider orders:

- Regular diet.
- OOB ad lib.
- Contact precautions.
- IV 0.9% sodium chloride, 100 mL/hour.
- C&S of lesion exudate.
- Wash scalp with fluocinolone acetonide 0.01% (Capex shampoo) daily. Massage into the scalp, allow to stay on for 5 minutes, and then rinse thoroughly.
- Apply a thin layer of desonide 0.05% (Desonate) topical gel to lesions on the neck, chest, axillae, and groin BID.
- Solu-Cortef 60 mg IVPB times 1 dose, then Solu-Cortef 30 mg IVPB every 8 hours.
- Benadryl 50 mg IVPB times 1, then Benadryl 50 mg PO every 6 hours.
- Vancomycin 1g IVPB times 1 dose; then check vancomycin level to determine frequency.

Case Study Questions

A. Which nursing action should the nurse implement first and why?

_____

B. When caring for this patient, what standard precautions should the nurse implement, what personal protective equipment should the nurse wear, and what other special precautions should the nurse employ that are associated with contact precautions?

1. _____

2. _____

3. _____

4. _____

5. _____

6. _____

7. _____

CASE STUDY: Putting It All Together   *cont'd*

___ **Case Study Questions** ___

C. What teaching points should the nurse cover with people who are visiting this patient?

1. _____

2. _____

3. _____

4. _____

5. _____

D. Can alcohol-based and nonalcohol-based hand sanitizers be used to reduce the risk of transmission of MRSA when soap and water are not available?

_____

REVIEW QUESTIONS

1. A nurse is caring for an older adult who sustained a skin tear on the forearm. What type of dressing should the nurse anticipate the primary health-care provider might order for this injury?
   1. Hydrogel dressing
   2. Dry sterile dressing
   3. Wet-to-moist dressing
   4. Transparent film dressing

2. A nurse is assessing a patient who has a wound on the leg as the result of a bicycle accident. Which clinical manifestation indicates a localized inflammatory response?
   1. Body temperature is 101.4°F.
   2. Heart rate is 102 beats/minute.
   3. Area around the wound is swollen.
   4. Exudate from the wound is greenish yellow in color.

3. A nurse is caring for a patient with gastroenteritis who is receiving contact precautions. Which actions are required when caring for this patient? **Select that apply.**
   1. _____ Keeping visitors 3 feet away from the patient
   2. _____ Wearing gloves when entering the patient's room
   3. _____ Wearing a gown when entering the patient's room
   4. _____ Wearing an eye protective surgical mask if working within 3 feet of the patient
   5. _____ Placing the patient in a private room or cohort with another patient with the same organism

4. A nurse is assessing a patient. Which assessment indicates that the patient may be at risk for infection because a primary defense is impaired?
   1. Oral mucous membranes are pink.
   2. Hair can be seen in the nostrils.
   3. Eyes appear moist.
   4. Skin is dry.

5. Which action is unique to maintaining airborne precautions for a patient with a diagnosis of suspected primary tuberculosis?
   1. Maintaining negative air pressure in the room
   2. Wearing a surgical mask when in the room
   3. Donning a gown when entering the room
   4. Wearing gloves when entering the room

6. A group of women who are positive for HIV are attending a program about how to prevent the transmission of the virus. Which activity should the nurse teach them to avoid?
   1. Hugging
   2. Breastfeeding
   3. Shaking hands
   4. Using public toilet seats

7. A nurse is administering a vaccination to a female patient. Which questions should the nurse ask the patient before administering the vaccination? **Select all that apply.**
   1. _____ "Are you menstruating?"
   2. _____ "Do you live in a home with very young children?"
   3. _____ "Have you had a temperature within the last 24 hours?"
   4. _____ "Have you received another vaccination within the last month?"
   5. _____ "Did you ever have an allergic reaction to this vaccination in the past?"

8. A nurse is assessing several patients with a variety of wounds. Which type of wound should the nurse anticipate will heal by secondary intention?
   1. Paper cut
   2. Pressure ulcer
   3. Abdominal incision from surgery
   4. Superficial slash caused by a knife

9. A nurse is assessing a patient who had numerous stitches several days ago for a traumatic injury to the base of the right index finger. Which assessment of the site indicates that the inflammatory response has progressed to an infectious process?
   1. Yellow discharge
   2. Swelling around the site
   3. Inability to flex the finger
   4. Feeling of heat when touched

10. A nurse is counseling a sexually active male patient newly diagnosed with HIV about the ways it is transmitted. Which situations that increase the risk of transmitting HIV should the nurse discuss with this patient? **Select all that apply.**
    1. _____ Unprotected anal sex with another person
    2. _____ Unprotected sex with a menstruating woman
    3. _____ Receiving unprotected oral sex from another person
    4. _____ Unprotected sex when the receiver has a genital lesion
    5. _____ Sharing intravenous drug equipment with another person

11. A nursing staff development educator is monitoring the sterile technique of a newly hired nurse in a simulation laboratory. What behavior by the newly hired nurse alerts the nurse educator that further teaching is necessary?
    1. Wears a mask because of a seasonal cold
    2. Opens sterile gauze packages with ungloved hands
    3. Uses a bottle of normal saline that was opened fourteen hours ago
    4. Discards sterile gauze that may have touched the edge of the sterile field

12. A nurse is working in a long-term care facility. Which resident should the nurse assess **first**?
    1. The resident who reports nausea after eating lunch
    2. A newly admitted resident who says that under her breasts are itchy
    3. A resident who just sustained an uncomfortable scratch on the forearm
    4. The older adult resident who reported feeling dizzy when moving from lying to sitting while in bed

13. A nurse is removing personal protective equipment when exiting an isolation room. Place the following steps in the order in which they should be implemented.
    1. Untie the gown at the waist.
    2. Release the ties of the mask and dispose of the mask in an appropriate trash container.
    3. Place fingers of the dominant hand inside cuff of the other sleeve and pull gown sleeve over the nondominant hand.
    4. Remove one glove by touching the outside of the glove with the other gloved hand and without contaminating oneself; dispose of it in an appropriate trash container.
    5. With the ungloved hand, slip a finger inside the cuff of the other glove and remove it without contaminating oneself and dispose of it in an appropriate trash container.
    6. With gown covered hand, pull gown down over the dominant hand, folding the gown inward and gathering it together as it is pulled down; dispose of it in an appropriate container.
    Answer: _____

14. A nurse is working on a medical unit in an acute care agency. For which patient should the nurse institute transmission-based droplet precautions?
    1. HIV infection
    2. MRSA infected wound
    3. Pulmonary tuberculosis
    4. *Streptococcal* pneumonia

15. A nurse's assessment of a patient's wound that is healing by secondary intention indicates the presence of some raw-looking red tissue with extensive necrosis. How should the nurse classify the wound using the color classification system?
    1. Red
    2. Black
    3. Green
    4. Yellow

16. A nurse in a home health-care agency is teaching a class about infection control to a group of nursing assistants. Which interventions did the nurse include that interrupts the chain of infection at the mode of transmission stage? **Select all that apply.**
    1. _____ Maintain a urinary collection bag below the level of the patient's bladder.
    2. _____ Shut off the handles of water faucets with a clean, dry paper towel.
    3. _____ Clean bedside tables routinely with a disinfectant.
    4. _____ Reposition patients every 2 hours.
    5. _____ Keep your fingernails short.

17. A nurse is caring for a patient with *Staphylococcus aureus* who is to receive an antibiotic. Which statement should the nurse include in a teaching session that **best** explains the reason for the medication?
    1. "This medication should eradicate the organism that is causing your symptoms."
    2. "This medication will help to avoid a recurrence of your infection in the future."
    3. "The intention of this medication is to support normal body function."
    4. "The principle purpose of this medication is palliative."

18. A primary health-care provider orders DuoDERM, a hydrocolloid dressing, for a patient with a break in the skin that has a small amount of drainage. What should the nurse do when applying this dressing?
    1. Stretch the dressing while placing it over the wound.
    2. Apply tape around all 4 sides of the dressing after its application.
    3. Warm the dressing between the hands before applying the dressing.
    4. Ensure a 1/4-inch margin of healthy skin around the wound when sizing the dressing.

19. A patient is admitted to a medical unit from the emergency department with the diagnosis of pneumonia. The patient is in the high-Fowler position and is receiving oxygen 2 L via nasal cannula. The nurse obtains the patient's vital signs, performs a focused assessment, and verifies the primary health-care provider's orders.

Patient's Clinical Record

Vital Signs

Temperature: 101.4°F, orally.
Pulse: 98 beats/minute, regular rhythm, radial.
Respirations: 28 breaths/minute, shallow, regular rhythm.
Blood pressure: 138/84 mm Hg.

Primary Health-Care Provider's Orders

Bed rest.
Regular diet.
Droplet precautions.
Culture and sensitivity of sputum.
Clarithromycin (Biaxin) 500 mg twice a day by mouth.
Guaifenesin (Mucinex) 200 mg every 6 hours by mouth.
Acetaminophen (Tylenol) 650 mg every 6 hours for a temperature more than 101°F.
IVF: 0.9% sodium chloride at 100 mL/hour.
Oxygen 2L via nasal cannula.
Incentive spirometer.
Monitor vital signs and pulse oximetry every 4 hours.

Physical Assessment

Reports shortness of breath, a feeling of tightness in the chest when breathing in, and excessive coughing after a deep breath. Coughing is frequent and produces thick yellow sputum. Breaths are rapid and shallow. Crackles in lower lobes bilaterally and bronchial wheezes heard on auscultation. Dull percussion over lower lobes bilaterally.

What should be the nurse's **next** intervention?
1. Suction the patient's airway.
2. Administer the clarithromycin as ordered.
3. Obtain a sputum specimen for culture and sensitivity.
4. Insert a circulatory access device and administer the ordered intravenous fluids.

20. A nurse teaches a patient about a health-related regimen associated with acquired-active immunity. For which patient is the nurse providing teaching?
1. A parent of a child who has chickenpox
2. A woman who is learning how to breastfeed
3. An older adult who is to receive a medication to prevent pneumonia
4. An adolescent with an inadequate history of immunization who stepped on a rusty nail

21. A nurse is assessing several patients with a variety of wounds. Which wound should the nurse anticipate will heal by primary intention?
1. Infected abrasion as a result of a bicycle accident
2. Ulcer on the greater trochanter as a result of pressure
3. Sore on a toe as a result of impaired arterial perfusion
4. Abdominal incision as a result of gastrointestinal surgery

22. Which actions are associated with droplet precautions? **Select all that apply.**
1. _____ Keeping the door of the patient's room closed.
2. _____ Keeping visitors three feet away from the patient.
3. _____ Wearing gloves when entering the patient's room.
4. _____ Wearing a surgical mask when working within three feet of the patient.
5. _____ Placing a surgical mask on the patient when transporting for procedures.

23. A primary health-care provider orders mechanical debridement of a patient's wound. Which action should the nurse perform to implement this order?
1. Scrubbing the wound with gauze
2. Placing a collagenase enzyme product into the wound
3. Assisting with cutting away devitalized tissue from the wound with a scalpel
4. Applying a dressing to the wound that promotes the body to generate enzymes

24. A nurse is providing teaching to a patient who is taking antibiotics for a bacterial infection. What is important for the nurse to teach the patient to do to help prevent resistance to the medication in the future?
1. "Eat some food when taking the medication."
2. "Complete the entire regimen of pills ordered."
3. "Assess yourself for signs of a superinfection."
4. "Take the pills evenly spaced around the clock."

25. A primary health-care provider orders a nasal specimen for culture and sensitivity. Place the following steps in the order in which they should be implemented.
1. Check the nasal passage with a flashlight.
2. Offer the patient a tissue to clean or blow the nose.
3. Gently rotate culture swab at site of purulent/inflamed tissue.
4. Position the patient in a semi-Fowler position with head hyperextended.
5. Insert culture swab into nasal passage without touching nasal structures.
6. Remove swab without touching nasal structures and insert into culture tube.
Answer: _____

26. During the initial assessment of a newly admitted patient, the nurse observes several small red excoriated lines on the patient's wrists. What is the nurse's **best** intervention at this time?
    1. Place the patient on contact precautions.
    2. Place the patient in a negative pressure room.
    3. The patient should be oriented to the assigned bedroom.
    4. The patient's condition should be communicated to the primary health-care provider.

27. A nurse is changing a patient's sterile dressing and performing wound irrigation. Which action by the nurse maintained sterile technique?
    1. Used the piston syringe from the previous time the wound was irrigated
    2. Dried the skin on either side of the wound by using one gauze pad for each swipe
    3. Held sterile gloved hands below the waist as much as possible during the procedure
    4. Poured fluid from an opened bottle of normal saline sitting on the patient's bedside table

28. An adult is diagnosed with an infection and the primary health-care provider prescribes penicillin G 1,000,000 units every 6 hours via an intermittent infusion. The vial instructions state to add 1.8 mL of sterile water to yield 250 mg/mL. How many mL should the nurse prepare to add to the intravenous infusion? Record your answer using a whole number.
    Answer: _____ mL

29. A nurse is collecting equipment for several procedures that need to be performed. For which procedure should the nurse wear sterile gloves?
    1. Collecting a urine specimen from a closed drainage system for a culture and sensitivity test.
    2. Instilling solution into a nasogastric tube to reestablish patency of the catheter.
    3. Suctioning the oropharynx to maintain airway patency.
    4. Obtaining a specimen for blood glucose monitoring.

30. A primary health-care provider orders protective isolation (neutropenic precautions) for a patient who is immunocompromised. What should the nurse do?
    1. Wear gloves when entering the patient's room.
    2. Remove fresh flowers from the patient's room.
    3. Have people with a respiratory infection wear a mask when in the patient's room.
    4. Ensure that housekeeping staff use a dry mop when cleaning the floor of the patient's room.

31. A patient is to begin a regimen of cephalexin (Keflex) by mouth for a pneumococcal infection. What actions should the nurse take to help the patient avoid complications from this medication? **Select all that apply.**
    1. _____ Suggest that the patient eat an active culture yogurt while taking the medication.
    2. _____ Tell the patient to inform the clinic if the tongue develops a white coating.
    3. _____ Inform the patient to call the clinic if there is blood in the stool.
    4. _____ Advise the patient to take the medication with food.
    5. _____ Encourage the patient to drink more fluids.

32. A school nurse is planning a health class for seniors in high school about interrupting the chain of infection at the reservoir stage. What should the nurse include in the teaching plan?
    1. Store food in a cool environment.
    2. Obtain age-appropriate immunizations.
    3. Cover a cough by coughing into an elbow.
    4. Wear long pants in an area where ticks are endemic.

33. Which action is essential when maintaining standard precautions?
    1. Putting on a gown when changing soiled linen
    2. Wearing goggles when changing a dry sterile dressing
    3. Wearing gloves during contact with a patient's body fluids
    4. Donning a mask with an eye shield when entering a patient's room

34. Place the photographs in the order in which the steps should be implemented when donning sterile gloves.

1.

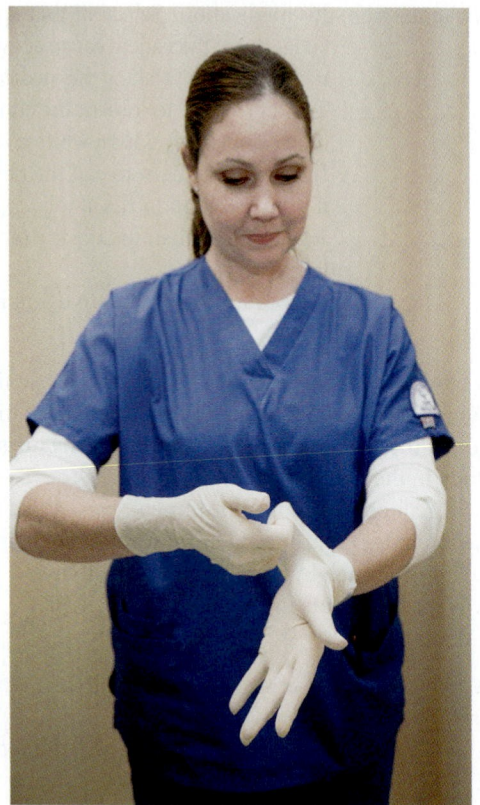

3.

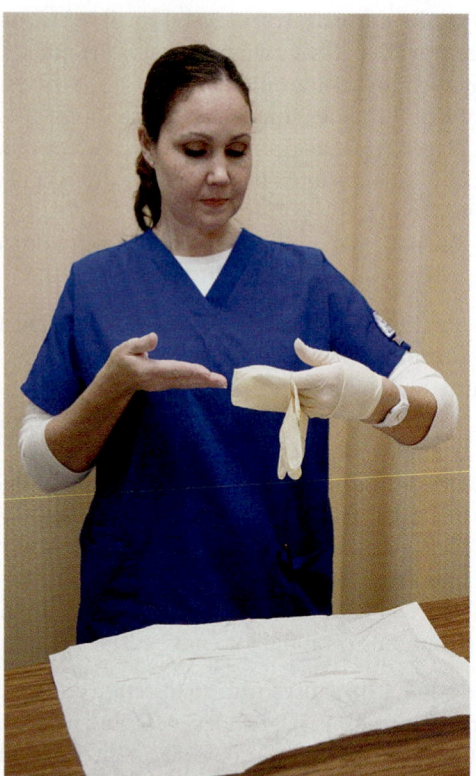

2.

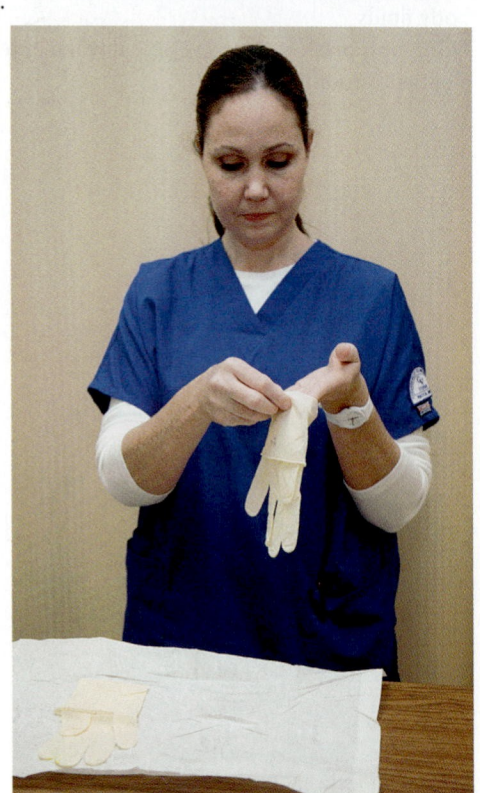

4.

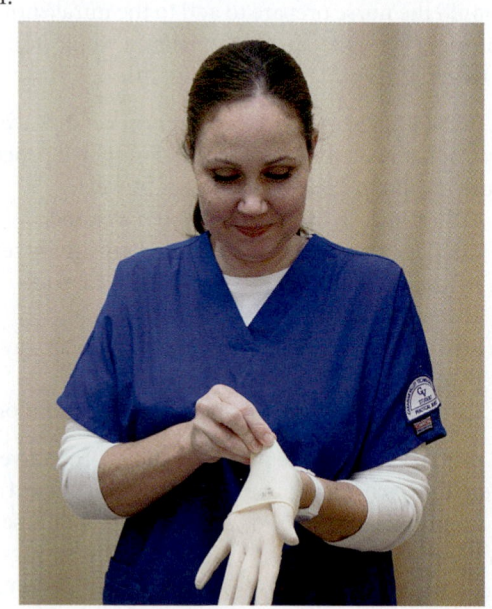

5.

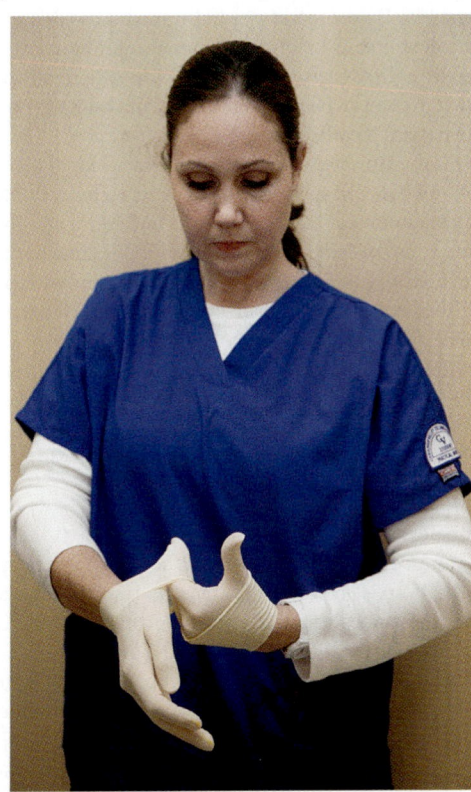

Answer: _____

35. A patient has a wound that is healing by secondary intention. The nurse is using sterile technique to irrigate the wound before applying a wet to damp dressing. What step of this procedure is required to maintain sterile technique?
1. Wipe the outside of edges of the wound first.
2. Wash the hands again after setting up the sterile field.
3. Place the irrigating solution on the side of the field farthest from the patient.
4. Direct the flow of sterile irrigating solution to the inside top of the patient's wound.

36. A nurse is caring for a patient who is to have a midstream urine specimen collected. Which action interrupts the chain of infection at the mode of transmission?
1. Giving the patient a sterile container for the collection of urine
2. Cleansing the urethral orifice with an antiseptic solution soaked cotton ball
3. Instructing the patient to collect the specimen after initiating the urine stream
4. Placing the urine specimen container into a transport bag using aseptic technique

37. A patient is diagnosed as having herpes simplex type 2 and the primary health-care provider prescribes acyclovir (Zovirax) during outbreaks of lesions. Which statement indicates that the patient understands the nurse's instructions about this medication?
1. "I should discontinue the medication if I develop dizziness."
2. "I have to increase fiber in my diet because the medication may cause constipation."
3. "I must take my pulse before I take this medication because it can increase my heart rate."
4. "I need to take this medication as soon as I feel tingling in the area where I get the lesions."

38. A child is diagnosed with a head lice infestation and the primary health-care provider prescribes permethrin (Nix). What should the nurse recommend that the parents do to help control this infestation?
1. Soak bed linens in cold water daily.
2. Brush the hair vigorously twice a day.
3. Clean nonwashable items with alcohol.
4. Ensure that everyone in the family is treated.

39. Which actions should nurses take to reduce the risk of transmitting microbes in a hospital setting? **Select all that apply.**
1. _____ Wash the hands when entering a patient's room.
2. _____ Bring the linen hamper into a patient's room.
3. _____ Use alcohol-based hand cleaners.
4. _____ Avoid wearing dangling apparel.
5. _____ Keep fingernails short.

40. A nurse is assessing the vaccines received by an infant. Which vaccine should have been received at least twice by 4 months of age?
1. Varicella vaccine
2. Influenza vaccine
3. Inactivated poliovirus vaccine
4. Measles, mumps, and rubella vaccine

REVIEW ANSWERS

1. ANSWER: 4.

Rationales:

1. A hydrogel dressing helps to maintain a moist wound environment and should be covered with other dressing materials, which makes it too bulky for a superficial injury such as a skin tear. Hydrogel dressings are most often used on pressure ulcers with moderate drainage.

2. A dry sterile dressing is inappropriate for a skin tear because it will dry out the wound, interfering with wound healing.

3. A wet-to-moist dressing is inappropriate for a skin tear. It is more often used for a larger wound. Also, excess moisture will cause maceration of tissue around the wound, inhibiting wound healing.

4. **Transparent film dressings have an adhesive side that adheres to dry tissue but not moist tissue. It provides a protective barrier and moist inner surface that facilitates epithelialization of a wound. They are not used for stage III and IV pressure ulcers; draining wounds; infected, puncture, or arterial wounds; or full-thickness burns.**

Content Area: Infection Control and Wound Care
Integrated Processes: Nursing Process: Planning
Client Need: Physiological Integrity; Physiological Adaptation
Cognitive Level: Analysis

2. ANSWER: 3.

Rationales:

1. An increased body temperature is a systemic, not local, response that is associated with infection, not inflammation.

2. An elevated heart rate is a systemic, not localized, response that is associated with infection, not inflammation.

3. **A localized swelling around a wound indicates the presence of edema. Vasodilation and increased permeability of the capillaries promote the shift of fluid from the intravascular compartment to the interstitial compartment.**

4. Greenish-yellow exudate from a wound indicates infection, not inflammation. A clear, watery (serous) discharge is associated with the inflammatory response.

TEST-TAKING TIP: Identify the clang associations. The word *wound* in the stem and in options 3 and 4 are clang associations. Examine options 3 and 4 carefully.

Content Area: Infection Control and Wound Care
Integrated Processes: Nursing Process: Assessment
Client Need: Physiological Integrity; Reduction of Risk Potential
Cognitive Level: Analysis

3. ANSWER: 2, 3, 5.

Rationales:

1. The need to keep a visitor, without a surgical mask, further than 3 feet from the patient refers to droplet precautions, not contact precautions. As long as the visitor wears gloves and a gown and wears a mask if splashing with blood or body fluids is likely, the visitor may enter the patient's room as well as move within three feet of the patient.

2. **Gloves always must be worn when entering a room when a patient is on contact precautions. Gloves protect the hands from exposure to the patient's pathogens.**

3. **A gown must be worn when entering the room of a patient who is on contact precautions who has diarrhea, has a colostomy, is incontinent, has a wound not contained by a dressing, or when giving direct patient care. A gown protects a person's clothing from being exposed to the patient's pathogens.**

4. A mask with eye protection is necessary only if there is a likelihood of being splashed with a patient's body fluids.

5. **A patient on contact precautions must either be in a private room or have a roommate with the same pathogenic microorganism; this contains pathogens within a controlled environment protecting noninfected patients.**

Content Area: Infection Control and Wound Care
Integrated Processes: Nursing Process: Implementation
Client Need: Safe and Effective Care Environment; Safety and Infection Control
Cognitive Level: Application

4. ANSWER: 4.

Rationales:

1. The mucous membranes have an abundant capillary network that carries blood to the area; as a result, the mucous membranes appear pink. Also, the mucous membranes produce mucus that traps microorganisms.

2. Hair in the nostrils and cilia and mucus in the respiratory tract capture and move microorganisms out of the respiratory tract.

3. Tears contain lysosomes that destroy microorganisms. Tears and blinking flush microorganism out of the eyes.

4. **Sebum, a secretion of the sebaceous glands of the skin, is an oily substance that softens and lubricates the skin; it also has a bactericidal effect that protects the skin from microorganisms.**

TEST-TAKING TIP: Identify the words in the stem that indicate negative polarity. The words *primary defense is impaired* indicate that the stem has negative polarity.

Content Area: Infection Control and Wound Care
Integrated Processes: Nursing Process: Assessment
Client Need: Physiological Integrity; Safety and Infection Control
Cognitive Level: Application

5. ANSWER: 1.

Rationales:

1. **A private room that has negative air pressure (6 to 12 exchanges of air per hour, or discharge of air to the outside, or a filtration system for the air in the room) is required for airborne precautions.**

2. A respiratory device (N95 respirator), not a surgical mask, is necessary to protect a caregiver from the *M. tuberculosis* or *M. bovis* emanating from the patient's respiratory tract.

3. Donning a gown is necessary only when the caregiver is at risk for coming into contact with the patient's body fluids, contaminated items, or nonintact skin.

4. Gloves are only necessary when it is likely that the nurse will come into contact with the patient's body fluids, contaminated items, nonintact skin, or mucous membranes.

Content Area: Infection Control and Wound Care
Integrated Processes: Nursing Process: Implementation
Client Need: Safe and Effective Care Environment; Safety and Infection Control
Cognitive Level: Analysis

6. ANSWER: 2.
Rationales:
1. HIV is not spread casually through hugging.
2. Breast milk can transmit HIV to a newborn.
3. HIV is not spread casually through hand shaking.
4. HIV is not spread through the use of public toilet seats.
TEST-TAKING TIP: Identify the word in the stem that indicates negative polarity. The word *avoid* indicates a stem with negative polarity. The test-taker is being asked, "What behavior *should not* be performed to help prevent the transmission of HIV?"
Content Area: *Infection Control and Wound Care*
Integrated Processes: *Nursing Process: Implementation*
Client Need: *Safe and Effective Care Environment; Safety and Infection Control*
Cognitive Level: *Application*

7. ANSWERS: 2, 3, 4, 5.
Rationales:
1. Menstruation has no effect on the administration of vaccinations.
2. If the person has very young children, the primary health-care provider should be consulted because the vaccine may contain a live virus or bacterium that has the potential for causing an infection in young children.
3. A temperature is a contraindication for receiving a vaccination because the body is fighting an infection. Vaccines are stressors that challenge the immune system.
4. If a patient had another vaccination within the last month, the patient should be referred to the primary health-care provider to ensure that the two vaccines will not interact.
5. If a patient had an allergic reaction to a vaccine or any of its ingredients (e.g., eggs), the patient should not receive the vaccine again without consultation with the primary health-care provider.
Content Area: *Infection Control and Wound Care*
Integrated Processes: *Communication/Documentation; Nursing Process: Assessment*
Client Need: *Physiological Integrity; Pharmacological and Parenteral Therapies*
Cognitive Level: *Analysis*

8. ANSWER: 2.
Rationales:
1. A paper cut will heal by primary intention because the injury is superficial and the wound edges are approximated. Primary intention healing involves minimal formation of granulated tissue and scarring.
2. A pressure ulcer does not have approximated wound edges. Pressure ulcers usually involve the epidermis and dermis that require healing by secondary intention. Secondary intention healing occurs from inner skin layers to outer skin layers. Fragile granulated tissue fills in the wound and eventually the capillaries constrict, tissue shrinks, collagen fibers contract, and firmer fibrous tissue remains (scar).
3. Although internally there may have been extensive surgery, surgery is conducted using sterile technique and the abdominal incision has approximated wound edges. An abdominal incision usually heals by primary intention.

4. A superficial slash will heal by primary intention because it has minimal tissue destruction and approximated wound edges.
Content Area: *Infection Control and Wound Care*
Integrated Processes: *Nursing Process: Analysis*
Client Need: *Physiological Integrity; Safety and Infection Control*
Cognitive Level: *Analysis*

9. ANSWER: 1.
Rationales:
1. Purulent drainage, which may be yellow, green, tan, or brown, indicates the presence of an infectious process. The discharge contains cellular debris, destroyed tissue, phagocytic cells, and microorganisms (pus). The discharge associated with the inflammatory response usually is clear (serous) and contains cellular debris proteins, and plasma fluid; it also may contain blood (e.g., serosanguineous, sanguineous).
2. This is part of the local inflammatory response. Histamine released at the site of the trauma causes vasodilation, and kinins released by destroyed cells increase capillary permeability; both allow fluid to move from the intravascular compartment into the interstitial compartment, resulting in an accumulation of fluid (edema).
3. This is part of the local inflammatory response. Edema and pain interfere with the ability to flex the finger.
4. This is part of the local inflammatory response. Dilation of blood vessels brings more warm blood to the site and there is an increase in metabolic processes at the site; both increase heat at the site of the injury.
Content Area: *Infection Control and Wound Care*
Integrated Processes: *Nursing Process: Evaluation*
Client Need: *Physiological Integrity; Safety and Infection Control*
Cognitive Level: *Application*

10. ANSWER: 1, 2, 3, 4, 5.
Rationales:
1. Semen containing the HIV and trauma to mucous membranes that may result in bleeding increase the risk of transmission of the HIV during anal sex.
2. Unprotected sex with a menstruating woman who is HIV positive exposes the partner to the HIV because the virus resides in blood.
3. Providing unprotected oral sex to another person places the provider at risk because of mucous membrane contact with potentially infected body fluids.
4. The risk of contracting the HIV from unprotected sex with an infected person is greater when the person has a genital lesion because the skin or mucous membrane is not intact.
5. Sharing intravenous equipment exposes the second person using the equipment to the blood of a potentially HIV infected individual.
Content Area: *Infection Control and Wound Care*
Integrated Processes: *Nursing Process: Implementation*
Client Need: *Safe and Effective Care Environment; Safety and Infection Control*
Cognitive Level: *Application*

11. ANSWER: 1.

Rationales:

1. This was not an appropriate decision on the part of the nurse. A nurse who has an upper respiratory infection should not be caring for any patient, especially a patient with a wound. Although this was just a simulation, the nurse should have said to the educator, "I cannot put patients at risk by caring for them when I have a cold. I will proceed as if I did not have a cold for the purpose of this simulation."

2. The outside of sterile gauze packages are not sterile; they can be touched with the hands.

3. An opened and recapped bottle of sterile normal saline can be used again for the same patient but must be discarded after 24 hours. When a bottle of sterile normal saline is opened for the first time the nurse should write on the label the date and time that the bottle was opened along with the nurse's initials.

4. If a sterile item is believed to have touched a nonsterile surface or item, the sterile item must be discarded as contaminated. The outer one inch of a sterile field is always considered contaminated.

TEST-TAKING TIP: Identify the words in the stem that indicate negative polarity. The words *further teaching is necessary* in the stem indicate negative polarity. The question is asking, "What is unacceptable technique when changing a sterile dressing?"

Content Area: Infection Control and Wound Care
Integrated Processes: Teaching/Learning; Nursing Process: Evaluation
Client Need: Safe and Effective Care Environment; Management of Care
Cognitive Level: Application

12. ANSWER: 2.

Rationales:

1. Although it is important to assess a resident experiencing nausea, this situation is not the priority.

2. The newly admitted resident may have scabies. This is a condition where a mite burrows under the skin; it generally involves the wrists, auxiliary area, and/or under the breasts. Scabies are contagious and contact precautions should be instituted until the resident is assessed. If scabies is diagnosed, contact precautions should be maintained for 24 hours after the resident receives treatment.

3. Although it is important to address this resident's needs because the scratch may become a portal of entry for microorganisms, this situation is not the priority.

4. It is not uncommon to experience orthostatic hypotension when moving from a lying to a sitting position. Although it is important to assess this resident, this situation is not the priority.

TEST-TAKING TIP: Identify the word in the stem that sets a priority. The word *first* in the stem sets a priority.

Content Area: Infection Control and Wound Care
Integrated Processes: Nursing Process: Planning
Client Need: Safe and Effective Care Environment; Safety and Infection Control
Cognitive Level: Analysis

13. ANSWER: 1, 4, 5, 2, 3, 6.

Rationales:

1. The tie at the waist is released first while still wearing gloves. The tie at the waist is considered contaminated because it is at or below the level of the waist which is always considered contaminated.

4. The gloves are removed next so as not to contaminate the hands or the environment. The first glove is removed by only touching the outside of the gloves.

5. After the first glove is removed, the second glove is removed by only touching the inside of the contaminated glove.

2. The ties of the mask can be untied with the hands because the ties are considered clean.

3. The gown is removed by only touching the inside of the gown. A hand can be used by placing the fingers of one hand up the inside of the other sleeve and pulling the sleeve down over the hand.

6. With the other hand inside the gown the gown should be folded downward and gathered inward to itself. The gown acts as a barrier and protects the nurse from contact with the contaminated outer surface of the gown. Gathering the soiled gown together as it is pulled down contains the contaminated surface of the gown. A paper gown is then placed in an appropriate trash container while a material gown is placed in a designated linen hamper. Before leaving the patient's room, the hands are washed.

Content Area: Infection Control and Wound Care
Integrated Processes: Nursing Process: Planning
Client Need: Safe and Effective Care Environment; Safety and Infection Control
Cognitive Level: Analysis

14. ANSWER: 4.

Rationales:

1. HIV is transmitted via blood, semen, vaginal secretions, and breast milk. Standard precautions, which are instituted for all patients, should be followed.

2. Methicillin-resistant *Staphylococcus aureus* (MRSA) in a wound is transmitted by contact with the infected individual or a MRSA contaminated surface or object. Contact precautions should be instituted.

3. *Mycobacterium tuberculosis* microorganisms are transmitted via airborne nuclei. Airborne precautions should be instituted.

4. *Streptococcal* pneumonia is transmitted by large particle respiratory droplets. Droplet precautions should be instituted.

TEST-TAKING TIP: Identify the unique option. Option 4 is unique. It is the only option that contains an italicized word.

Content Area: Infection Control and Wound Care
Integrated Processes: Nursing Process: Implementation
Client Need: Safe and Effective Care Environment; Safety and Infection Control
Cognitive Level: Analysis

15. ANSWER: 2.

Rationales:

1. A wound with newly granulating tissue is classified as red. This is a sign of the reparative stage of wound healing.

2. Necrotic tissue indicates cell death caused by the progressive degradative action of enzymes. Wounds exhibiting necrotic tissue are classified as black.

3. The color green is not part of the color classification system of wounds.

4. A wound with purulent exudate is classified as yellow. It usually indicates the presence of infection.

Content Area: Infection Control and Wound Care
Integrated Processes: Nursing Process: Assessment
Client Need: Physiological Integrity; Safety and Infection Control
Cognitive Level: Analysis

16. **ANSWER: 2, 3, 5.**
Rationales:
1. Keeping a urinary collection bag below the level of the patient's bladder will prevent the backflow of urine into the urinary bladder. This will prevent microorganisms from entering the bladder. Portals of entry in humans include the respiratory, gastrointestinal, reproductive, and urinary tracts and the skin and mucous membranes.
2. **This action interrupts the chain of infection at the mode of transmission stage. Microorganisms thrive on the handles of water faucets and are transmitted to others when touched.**
3. **The mode of transmission stage of the chain of infection is related to how a microorganism is transferred from an infectious agent to the portal of entry of a host. Microorganisms can thrive on surfaces that the patient uses and be transmitted to a portal of entry in the patient.**
4. Repositioning a patient every two hours maintains skin integrity. This interrupts the chain of infection at the susceptible host stage.
5. **Microorganisms thrive under fingernails because the area is warm, dark, and moist. Therefore, they should be kept short to prevent the harboring of microorganisms. Also, artificial nails and nail polish should be avoided.**

Content Area: Infection Control and Wound Care
Integrated Processes: Teaching/Learning; Nursing Process: Implementation
Client Need: Safe and Effective Care Environment; Safety and Infection Control
Cognitive Level: Analysis

17. **ANSWER: 1.**
Rationales:
1. **Antibiotics are used to destroy disease-producing pathogens. Antibiotics are curative in nature.**
2. Antibiotics will not prevent a recurrence of the infection.
3. Antibiotics are not classified as health maintenance drugs. Drugs that support normal body function are called "substitutive" medications or provide for "health maintenance" (e.g., levothyroxine [Synthroid] for an underactive thyroid gland).
4. Antibiotics are not drugs that are palliative in nature. A palliative drug is used to relieve signs or symptoms of disease, not cure the disease (e.g., acetaminophen to relieve a fever).

TEST-TAKING TIP: Identify the word in the stem that sets a priority. The word *best* in the stem sets a priority.
Content Area: Infection Control and Wound Care
Integrated Processes: Teaching/Learning; Nursing Process: Implementation

Client Need: Physiological Integrity; Pharmacological and Parenteral Therapies
Cognitive Level: Application

18. **ANSWER: 3.**
Rationales:
1. Avoid applying the dressing by stretching the product or using too much tension to prevent a tourniquet effect.
2. This is unnecessary; it is a self-adhesive dressing.
3. **Warming the dressing between the hands before application improves adhesion of the dressing to the patient's skin.**
4. The nurse should ensure that there is a 1-inch margin of healthy skin around the wound when sizing the dressing.

Content Area: Infection Control and Wound Care
Integrated Processes: Nursing Process: Implementation
Client Need: Physiological Integrity; Safety and Infection Control
Cognitive Level: Application

19. **ANSWER: 3.**
Rationales:
1. Although the patient has excessive respiratory secretions, the patient is capable of clearing the airway as evidenced by the productive cough. Suctioning can be traumatic to the mucous membranes when it is unnecessary.
2. Although this should be done eventually, administering the clarithromycin first is inappropriate.
3. **A sputum specimen must be obtained before antibiotic therapy is instituted. The results of the culture and sensitivity may be inaccurate if an antibiotic is administered before the sputum specimen is obtained.**
4. Although this should be done, it is not the priority. This intervention will take time that will delay another intervention that is more important.

TEST-TAKING TIP: Identify the word in the stem that sets a priority. The word *next* in the stem sets a priority.
Content Area: Infection Control and Wound Care
Integrated Processes: Nursing Process: Implementation
Client Need: Physiological Integrity; Reduction of Risk Potential
Cognitive Level: Analysis

20. **ANSWER: 3.**
Rationales:
1. A person with a disease develops immunity to the disease in the future because the body produced antibodies in response to the original antigen. This is known as natural-active immunity.
2. A breastfeeding mother transmits antibodies to her infant through colostrum in breast milk. This is known as natural-passive immunity.
3. **A medication that stimulates the production of antibodies that prevent future infection is called an immunization or vaccine. This is known as acquired-active immunity.**
4. An adolescent who stepped on a rusty nail and has an inadequate immunization history will be treated with an antitoxin that contains antibodies (human tetanus immune globulin—TIG). This is known as acquired-passive immunity.

Content Area: Infection Control and Wound Care
Integrated Processes: Teaching/Learning; Nursing Process: Implementation

Client Need: Health Promotion and Maintenance
Cognitive Level: Analysis

21. ANSWER: 4.
Rationales:
1. An abrasion is an area of skin that is denuded by a mechanical process, such as friction. An abrasion does not have wound edges that are approximated and therefore heals by secondary intention. An infection interferes with the inflammatory response and causes edema. In addition, pathogenic organisms in a wound increase the extent of exudate. Edema and increased exudate interfere with wound healing.
2. A pressure ulcer usually involves the epidermis and dermis resulting in a crater that does not have approximated wound edges. It heals by secondary intention. In addition, a pressure ulcer results from impaired capillary perfusion due to pressure, which also delays wound healing.
3. An ulcer on a toe as a result of impaired arterial circulation can injure the epidermis, dermis, and underlying structures, such as muscle and bone. Wounds with impaired circulation can become chronic, are difficult to heal, and usually heal by secondary intention.
4. An abdominal incision is created under sterile conditions and the wound edges are approximated and sutured in place. Incisions usually heal by primary intention.
Content Area: Infection Control and Wound Care
Integrated Processes: Nursing Process: Analysis
Client Need: Physiological Integrity; Reduction of Risk Potential
Cognitive Level: Application

22. ANSWER: 2, 4, 5.
Rationales:
1. The door to a patient's room must be kept closed with airborne, not droplet, precautions.
2. Keeping visitors three feet away from the patient is required with droplet precautions to protect visitors from large-particle droplets emanating from the patient's respiratory tract.
3. Gloves are necessary only when coming into contact with body fluids, such as excretions and secretions, mucous membranes, or nonintact skin.
4. Wearing a mask within three feet when working with the patient is required with droplet precautions to protect the caregiver from large-droplet particles emanating from the patient's respiratory tract.
5. Placing a surgical mask on the patient when transporting the patient is required with droplet precautions to protect others and the environment from contamination with large-droplet particles emanating from the patient's respiratory tract.
Content Area: Infection Control and Wound Care
Integrated Processes: Nursing Process: Implementation
Client Need: Safe and Effective Care Environment; Safety and Infection Control
Cognitive Level: Application

23. ANSWER: 1.
Rationales:
1. Scrubbing a wound with gauze uses friction to remove devitalized, necrotic tissue. This type of debridement is known as mechanical debridement. A nurse can

implement this procedure at the direction of a primary health-care provider.
2. The use of a collagenase enzyme product to remove devitalized, necrotic tissue is known as chemical debridement. A nurse can implement this procedure after receiving a prescription from a primary health-care provider.
3. Removal of devitalized, necrotic tissue with a scalpel or scissor is known as surgical debridement. A nurse does not perform this intervention independently but assists a primary health-care provider.
4. The application of a dressing that promotes the body to generate enzymes to break down necrotic tissue is known as autolytic debridement. A nurse can apply this dressing after receiving an order from a primary health-care provider.
TEST-TAKING TIP: Identify the options that are equally plausible. Options 2 and 4 both involve enzymes to debride the wound. More often than not, equally plausible options are distractors and can be eliminated from consideration.
Content Area: Infection Control and Wound Care
Integrated Processes: Nursing Process: Implementation
Client Need: Physiological Integrity; Physiological Adaptation
Cognitive Level: Application

24. ANSWER: 2.
Rationales:
1. Taking an antibiotic with food prevents gastric irritation, not resistant bacteria. Not all antibiotics should be administered with food because some are absorbed more efficiently on an empty stomach.
2. Taking the entire regimen of antibiotic eradicates the pathogens that have invaded the body. Stopping the medication early promotes the development of resistant bacteria.
3. A superinfection is an infection occurring in a person who already is experiencing an infection. These signs generally include furry overgrowth on the tongue, vaginal discharge, and foul-smelling stool. A pathogen causing a superinfection usually is resistant to the medication being administered.
4. Evenly spacing doses of antibiotic medication maintains a therapeutic blood level of the drug, it does not prevent bacterial resistance.
Content Area: Infection Control and Wound Care
Integrated Processes: Teaching/Learning; Nursing Process: Implementation
Client Need: Physiological Integrity; Pharmacological and Parenteral Therapies
Cognitive Level: Analysis

25. ANSWER: 4, 1, 5, 3, 6, 2.
Rationales:
4. Positioning the patient in a semi-Fowler position with the head hyperextended ensures access to the nose to obtain a specimen.
1. Before inserting the culture swab, the nurse should visualize the nasal passage for patency. This is done to ensure that there is no obstruction. Inserting a culture swab in the presence of a nasal obstruction may cause trauma to the nasal passage.

5. Not touching nasal structures while inserting the culture swab prevents contamination of the swab with resident bacteria before reaching the material to be swabbed.

3. Gently rotating the culture swab while coming into contact with purulent/inflamed structures exposes the swab to pathogenic microorganisms.

6. Removing the swab without touching nasal structures prevents contamination of the specimen with resident bacteria. The swab is then inserted into the culture tube and the ampule within the culture medium is crushed. The nurse must ensure that the culture medium saturates the end of the swab. The culture medium is designed to support growth of microorganisms collected on the swab.

2. The patient should be offered a tissue to clean or blow the nose after the procedure. This provides for physical comfort.

Content Area: Infection Control and Wound Care
Integrated Processes: Nursing Process: Planning
Client Need: Physiological Integrity; Reduction of Risk Potential
Cognitive Level: Analysis

26. ANSWER: 1.
Rationales:

1. These lines can be an indication of scabies, which are highly contagious; therefore, the patient should be placed on contact precautions.

2. Excoriated lines on a patient do not indicate tuberculosis or any other disease requiring a negative pressure room.

3. The nurse should orient the patient to the room after another intervention is performed.

4. The nurse should inform the patient's primary healthcare provider of the assessment findings after another intervention is performed.

TEST-TAKING TIP: Identify the word in the stem that sets a priority. The word *best* in the stem sets a priority.

Content Area: Infection Control and Wound Care
Integrated Processes: Nursing Process: Implementation
Client Need: Safe and Effective Care Environment; Safety and Infection Control
Cognitive Level: Application

27. ANSWER: 2.
Rationales:

1. This is unsafe. This piston syringe is considered contaminated.

2. This maintains sterile technique. One gauze pad should be used for each swipe because it prevents cross contamination.

3. This violates sterile technique. Sterile gloved hands should be held above the waist and within the line of site at all times.

4. This violates sterile technique. The nurse has no knowledge about the sterility of the bottle of normal saline.

TEST-TAKING TIP: Identify the clang associations. The word *wound* in the stem and in options 1 and 2 are clang associations. Examine these options carefully.

Content Area: Infection Control and Wound Care
Integrated Processes: Nursing Process: Evaluation

Client Need: Safe and Effective Care Environment; Safety and Infection Control
Cognitive Level: Application

28. ANSWER: 4.
Rationale:

Solve the problem by using ratio and proportion.

$$\frac{\text{Desire } 1{,}000{,}000 \text{ units}}{\text{Have } 250{,}000 \text{ units}} = \frac{x \text{ mL}}{1 \text{ mL}}$$
$$250{,}000x = 1{,}000{,}000 \times 1$$
$$250{,}000x = 1{,}000{,}000$$
$$x = 1{,}000{,}000 \div 250{,}000$$
$$x = 4 \text{ mL}$$

Content Area: Medication Administration
Integrated Processes: Nursing Process: Planning
Client Need: Physiological Integrity; Pharmacological and Parenteral Therapies
Cognitive Level: Application

29. ANSWER: 3.
Rationales:

1. Sterile equipment (e.g., sterile syringe and sterile specimen container) and clean gloves should be used by the nurse to perform this procedure.

2. This is not a sterile procedure. Clean gloves should be worn by the nurse while performing this procedure.

3. This is a sterile procedure. A foreign object is being placed into the oropharynx, which makes the patient vulnerable to being exposed to microorganisms.

4. This is not a sterile procedure. Clean gloves should be worn by the provider of care during this procedure.

Content Area: Infection Control and Wound Care
Integrated Processes: Nursing Process: Planning
Client Need: Safe and Effective Care Environment; Safety and Infection Control
Cognitive Level: Analysis

30. ANSWER: 2.
Rationales:

1. Wearing gloves is unnecessary. The nurse does not have to be protected from the patient.

2. Fresh flowers and potted plants harbor molds. They should be removed from the patient's room to limit exposure to microorganisms that could harm the patient.

3. People with respiratory infections should not be permitted in the patient's room with or without a mask.

4. Although the floor should be cleaned, it should be wet mopped, not dry mopped. Wet mopping will limit dust and help prevent microorganisms from becoming aerosolized.

Content Area: Infection Control and Wound Care
Integrated Processes: Nursing Process: Implementation
Client Need: Safe and Effective Care Environment; Safety and Infection Control
Cognitive Level: Application

31. ANSWERS: 1, 2, 3, 4.
Rationales:

1. Oral antibiotics can interfere with the normal gastrointestinal (GI) flora. An active culture yogurt will help maintain proper GI flora.

2. A white tongue may indicate a super infection and appropriate medical intervention is warranted.

3. Blood in the stool may indicate pseudomembranous colitis requiring medical intervention.

4. Taking Keflex with food will limit GI irritation.

5. An increased fluid intake will not alter the potential side effects of Keflex.

Content Area: Infection Control and Wound Care
Integrated Processes: Nursing Process: Implementation
Client Need: Physiological Integrity; Pharmacological and Parenteral Therapies
Cognitive Level: Application

32. ANSWER: 1.

Rationales:

1. The reservoir stage of the chain of infection is where microorganisms survive (e.g., people, animals, insects, food, and surfaces). Cool environmental temperatures help to minimize microbial growth. Microorganisms survive best in environments with a temperature between 68°F and 109°F.

2. Immunizations protect an individual by stimulating the production of antibodies. This interrupts the chain of infection at the susceptible host stage.

3. Covering a cough will interrupt the chain of infection at the portal of exit stage.

4. Wearing long pants in areas where ticks are endemic interrupts the chain of infection at the mode of transmission stage.

Content Area: Infection Control and Wound Care
Integrated Processes: Teaching/Learning; Nursing Process: Planning
Client Need: Safe and Effective Care Environment; Safety and Infection Control
Cognitive Level: Application

33. ANSWER: 3.

Rationales:

1. A gown is not necessary to maintain standard precautions when changing soiled linen. However, the nurse should wear gloves and hold the linen away from one's uniform to prevent contamination.

2. Eye protection is not necessary when changing a dry sterile dressing because splashing with the patient's blood or body fluids is not likely.

3. **A caregiver must always wear clean gloves when there is a likelihood of coming into contact with a patient's body fluids, such as secretions, excretions, nonintact skin, mucous membranes, or contaminated items.**

4. A mask with eye protection is only necessary if the caregiver is at risk for being splashed with the patient's body fluids. A surgical mask is required within three feet of a patient receiving droplet precautions and an N95 respirator mask is required when entering a room with airborne precautions.

TEST-TAKING TIP: Identify the word in the stem that sets a priority. The word *essential* in the stem is asking the test-taker to identify a priority.

Content Area: Infection Control and Wound Care
Integrated Processes: Nursing Process: Implementation
Client Need: Safe and Effective Care Environment; Safety and Infection Control
Cognitive Level: Application

34. ANSWER: 2, 4, 3, 5, 1.

Rationales:

2. Picking up the first sterile glove, touching only the inside of the folded cuff edge, and inserting the dominant hand into the sterile glove is the first step in donning sterile gloves.

4. After the dominant hand is inside the sterile glove, the nurse uses the ungloved hand to pull the glove on until it fits snuggly, touching only the inside cuff of the sterile glove.

3. The sterile gloved hand is then slipped underneath the cuff of the second sterile glove. The second sterile glove touches only the sterile surface of the first glove. The nondominant hand is inserted into the second glove.

5. The nurse then pulls the second glove on until it fits snuggly, touching only sterile surface to sterile surface.

1. Last, the nurse uses the nondominant hand to pull up the cuff of the first glove, touching only sterile surface to sterile surface.

Content Area: Infection Control and Wound Care
Integrated Processes: Nursing Process: Planning
Client Need: Safe and Effective Care Environment; Safety and Infection Control
Cognitive Level: Analysis

35. ANSWER: 4.

Rationales:

1. This will bring microorganisms on the skin toward the wound opening; the opposite should be done. In addition, the center of a wound healing by secondary intention should not be wiped to prevent dislodging granulated tissue.

2. This is not necessary. The nurse should perform hand hygiene before collecting the equipment for the procedure and positioning the patient and then again just before beginning the procedure.

3. This violates a principle of sterile technique. If the solution is farthest from the patient, the irrigating solution may drip on and contaminate the sterile field when it is time to irrigate the wound.

4. **This is appropriate sterile technique because it prevents microorganisms on the skin from being carried into the wound.**

TEST-TAKING TIP: Identify the word in the stem that sets a priority. The word *required* in the stem sets a priority. Identify the options with clang associations. The word *sterile* in the stem and in options 2 and 4 are clang associations. The word *wound* in the stem and in options 1 and 4 are clang associations. The word *irrigate* in the stem and *irrigating* in options 3 and 4 are clang associations. Examine option 4 carefully because it contains all 3 clang associations.

Content Area: Infection Control and Wound Care
Integrated Processes: Nursing Process: Implementation
Client Need: Safe and Effective Care Environment; Safety and Infection Control
Cognitive Level: Application

36. ANSWER: 4.

Rationales:

1. A sterile container will help prevent the contamination of the urine specimen, but it will not interrupt the chain of

infection at the mode of transmission, thereby protecting others from infection.

2. This action will interrupt the portal of entry step in the chain of infection. In addition, it will help prevent the contamination of the specimen from microorganisms that are on the skin and mucous membranes. It will not prevent transmission of microorganisms to others.

3. Instructing the patient to collect the specimen midstream prevents contamination of the specimen by flushing microorganisms from the urethra first, but it does not prevent the transmission of microorganisms to others.

4. **Placing the urine specimen container into a transport bag using aseptic technique will interrupt the chain of infection at the mode of transmission step. Containing the specimen container in a bag prevents transmission of microorganisms that may be on the outside of the specimen container. This action protects others from the transmission of microorganisms.**

TEST-TAKING TIP: Identify the clang associations. The word *urine* in the stem and in options 1 and 4 are clang associations. The word *specimen* in the stem and in options 3 and 4 are clang associations. Option 4 has 2 clang associations, *urine* and *specimen*. Examine this option carefully.
Content Area: Infection Control and Wound Care
Integrated Processes: Nursing Process: Implementation
Client Need: Safe and Effective Care Environment; Safety and Infection Control
Cognitive Level: Analysis

37. **ANSWER: 4.**
Rationales:
1. A medication should not be discontinued without collaboration with the primary health-care provider. Safety precautions should be taken if the patient develops dizziness or fatigue.
2. Acyclovir (Zovirax) will not precipitate constipation; it may cause anorexia, nausea, vomiting, and diarrhea.
3. Taking the pulse before the administration of acyclovir (Zovirax) is unnecessary; it does not influence the heart rate.
4. **Acyclovir (Zovirax) should be taken at the first indication of an outbreak, such as tingling, itching (pruritus), or pain at the site where lesions develop (usually the perineal area).**
Content Area: Infection Control and Wound Care
Integrated Processes: Communication/Documentation; Teaching/Learning; Nursing Process: Evaluation
Client Need: Physiological Integrity; Pharmacological and Parenteral Therapy
Cognitive Level: Application

38. **ANSWER: 4.**
Rationales:
1. Bed linens should be washed in hot, not cold, water and dried in a dryer to kill lice and their eggs (nits).
2. The hair should be treated with the prescribed medication and then combed with a fine-tooth comb to remove dead lice and nits.
3. Alcohol will not eradicate this infestation. Nonwashable items should be placed in plastic bags for a minimum of 2 weeks to kill lice and their eggs.

4. **Head lice are an easily transmitted infestation. All members of the household must be treated to prevent repeated cross contamination.**
TEST-TAKING TIP: Identify the unique option. Option 4 is unique. Option 4 relates to the prescribed medication, while options 1, 2, and 3 include recommendations to promote lice and nit removal or their death.
Content Area: Infection Control and Wound Care
Integrated Processes: Teaching/Learning; Nursing Process: Implementation
Client Need: Physiological Integrity; Pharmacological and Parenteral Therapies
Cognitive Level: Application

39. **ANSWER: 1, 3, 4, 5.**
Rationales:
1. **Hand washing is the single most important way to prevent the transmission of microbes. Soap, water, friction, and rinsing the hands limit the amount of microorganisms on the hands.**
2. The linen hamper should not be brought into a patient's room because it is a vector that can transmit microorganisms. The linen hamper should be left in the hall just outside a patient's room.
3. **Although not as effective as washing with soap and water, alcohol-based hand cleaners are effective in limiting the amount of most microorganism on the hands.**
4. **Dangling apparel has the potential of touching a patient's clothing or bed linens. Contaminated apparel can act as a vector when the health-care provider visits another patient.**
5. **Keeping fingernails short can help prevent the spread of microbes by eliminating areas where they can collect and multiply.**
Content Area: Infection Control and Wound Care
Integrated Processes: Nursing Process: Implementation
Client Need: Physiological Integrity; Safety and Infection Control
Cognitive Level: Application

40. **ANSWER: 3.**
Rationales:
1. The varicella vaccine should be administered at the minimum age of 12 months and is known as the VAR vaccine. The second dose may be administered before 4 years of age, provided that at least 3 months have elapsed since the first dose.
2. The influenza vaccine is not administered until an infant is at least 6 months of age and then yearly.
3. **The inactivated poliovirus should have been administered at least twice by 4 months of age. Four or more doses should be administered before age 4 years and an additional dose should be administered at age 4 through 6 years of age.**
4. The MMR vaccine consists of the measles, mumps, and rubella vaccines and should be administered at the minimum age of 12 months.
Content Area: Infection Control and Wound Care
Integrated Processes: Nursing Process: Evaluation
Client Need: Health Promotion and Maintenance
Cognitive Level: Application

Chapter 13

Safety

KEY TERMS

Allergy—Hypersensitivity precipitated by exposure to an allergen that causes a harmful immunologic reaction with subsequent exposures.

Anaphylaxis—Severe, sudden immune response that involves a decrease in blood pressure and can cause shock, unconsciousness, and death if untreated.

Aspiration—Inhalation of a substance into the respiratory tract.

Drowning—Filling of the lungs with fluid, which prevents gas exchange and results in suffocation.

Orthostatic hypotension—Lack of adequate autonomic vasoconstriction of peripheral blood vessels when moving from a lying to a sitting or standing position, resulting in a temporary decrease in blood pressure and inadequate circulation to the brain.

Restraint—Devices used to limit movement of a body limb or body activity.

  Level 1 restraint—Restraint used to protect the patient from injuring self or others while receiving acute medical or surgical care.

  Level 2 restraint—Restraint used to manage violent behavior to protect a patient from injuring self or others.

Safety—Freedom from physical or emotional trauma or injury.

Suffocation (asphyxiation)—Failure of air to reach the lungs, causing lack of oxygen, excess carbon dioxide, loss of consciousness, cessation of breathing, and death.

Syncope—Temporary loss of consciousness due to an inadequate level of oxygen in the brain.

I. Patient Safety and Nursing Care

To remain safe is a basic expectation and right of all patients. A health-care environment, whether it is in a health-care agency or created in the home, can be frightening, unfamiliar, and stressful for a patient. Nurses must focus on the basic needs of safety and security so that patients do not experience accidents or sustain injuries.

A. Introduction
  1. **Safety** is freedom from physical or emotional trauma or injury.
  2. Safety and security are second level needs, after physiological needs, according to Maslow's hierarchy of needs.
  3. According to the Centers for Disease Control and Prevention, unintentional injuries are the fifth leading cause of death in the United States.
  4. Nursing interventions for promoting safety for all patients involve:
     a. Assessing for factors that can jeopardize safety.
     b. Maintaining a safe environment in a health-care facility.
     c. Providing patient teaching about maintaining safety in the home.
  5. The Joint Commission has identified goals and requirements to provide for patient safety; they include:
     a. Identify patients correctly.
     b. Improve communication among health-care workers.
     c. Administer pharmaceuticals safely.
     d. Identify patients at risk for injury.
     e. Prevent infection.
     f. Prevent falls.
     g. Prevent pressure ulcers.
     h. Reduce the risk of influenza and pneumococcal disease in older adults.
     i. Implement preprocedure verification processes.
     j. Improve responses to changes in a patient's status.
     k. Encourage patient involvement in own safety care.
  6. Unfortunately, accidents do occur in health-care facilities and they are documented in an incident

report. An **incident report** documents details of a situation that caused or has the potential to cause harm to a patient, health-care provider or visitor. These reports record the facts, provide data for overseeing agencies, and help identify trends and influence the development of measures to limit similar events in the future.

B. **Nursing Interventions to Maintain Patient Safety in Health-Care Environments**

1. Ensure personal knowledge of agency policies and procedures that relate to safety.
2. Be knowledgeable about the use of equipment and information concerning medications.
3. Continuously assess for physical, biological, and chemical hazards in the environment.
4. Perform a risk for injury assessment on all patients, including developmental and individual factors.
5. Ensure that each patient has an identity band on his or her wrist.
6. Ensure that, as applicable, the patient has individual risk factor bands on his or her wrist, such as for an allergy, a risk of falls, or an alert to avoid trauma to an arm (e.g., arm on the side of a mastectomy, presence of fistula for dialysis).
7. Orient the patient to the environment.
8. Maintain a clutter-free environment.
9. Keep the call bell and personal items within the patient's reach.
10. Keep the bed in the lowest position with one to four side rails raised, as required by the patient.
11. Keep wheels on moveable objects locked.
12. Maintain adequate lighting in the environment for day, evening, and night.
13. Explain to the patient what is to be done before and/or during an activity.
14. Immediately answer call bells and check equipment that set off alarms.
15. Inspect all equipment before use.
16. Ensure that tubing (e.g., IV catheters, chest tubes, urinary catheters, electrocardiogram lines, and portable would drainage systems) is coiled on the bed with no dependent loops and is safeguarded during activities, particularly during transfers and when the patient is ambulating.
17. Instruct the patient to seek assistance when ambulating as needed.
18. Employ the use of assistive devices to transfer patients safely as needed.
19. Protect oneself from harm, such as by using sharps containers; following infection control guidelines, particularly hand hygiene; and using transfer devices, such as a mechanical lift.

II. Factors That Influence Patient Safety

A. **Age**
1. Significance.
   a. Each age-group has unique developmental factors (e.g., physical, emotional, and cognitive) that influence the ability to remain safe.
   b. Nurses must understand these age-related factors to anticipate safety precautions necessary for patients in each age-group.
      (1) Infants.
         (a) Depend on others for care.
         (b) Initially cannot turn over.
         (c) Put things in mouths to explore the world.
         (d) Able to manipulate small objects.
         (e) Have immature body systems (e.g., neurological and musculoskeletal systems).
         (f) Lack judgment due to limited experiences and immature cognition.
         (g) Gain mobility, such as turning over, crawling, and walking.
      (2) Toddlers.
         (a) Increase in mobility, such as walking and climbing.
         (b) Lack judgment due to limited experiences and immature cognition.
         (c) Have increasing curiosity (e.g., intrigued by stairs).
      (3) Preschoolers.
         (a) Desire independence.
         (b) Have continuing curiosity.
         (c) Play in areas beyond the house, such as in pools, playgrounds, and front yards.
         (d) Engage in magical thinking that overestimates their abilities.
         (e) Still lack judgment but are a little more aware of physical dangers.
         (f) Trust authority figures, which may increase the risk of being abducted.
      (4) School-aged children.
         (a) Are less fearful than toddlers and preschoolers, such as attempting new skills without instruction.
         (b) Use tools and household items that can cause harm, such as knives and lawn mowers.
         (c) Have increased involvement with the environment, such as traveling to school, staying at school for activities, and playing team sports on weekends.
         (d) Are involved in more active and competitive play; often overestimate personal abilities.
         (e) Begin learning to be wary of strangers but trusting authority figures still persists.

(5) Adolescents.

    (a) Are at peak of physical, sensory, and psychomotor abilities.

    (b) Believe they are invincible.

    (c) Engage in risk-taking behaviors, such as smoking, drug and alcohol abuse, driving fast, and unprotected sex.

    (d) Desire to be independent and in control.

    (e) Are exposed to increased peer relationships and pressure and decreased parental influence.

    (f) Begin driving; tend not to wear seat belts.

(6) Adults.

    (a) Have progressively declining physical, sensory, and psychomotor abilities.

    (b) Engage in lifestyle habits that increase risk, such as smoking, alcohol and drug abuse, and unprotected sex.

    (c) Have increased stress due to career, family responsibilities, and financial demands.

    (d) May be at risk for injury at work (e.g., using heavy machinery, working at heights, or engaging in repetitive motions).

(7) Older adults.

    (a) Have decreased musculoskeletal strength and mobility.

    (b) Have declining voluntary and autonomic reflexes.

    (c) Have declining sensory functions, such as impaired hearing, vision, and sensation.

    (d) May have declining cognitive awareness or ability to manage multiple incoming stimuli simultaneously.

    (e) May engage in polypharmacy, which can precipitate overdoses or drug interactions.

2. Nursing care: See safety-related nursing interventions under each age-group in Chapter 6, "Nursing Care Across the Life Span."

B. Impaired Vision

1. Significance.

    a. Impaired vision limits or eliminates visual cues regarding the environment that can result in patient injury.

    b. An inability to detect relevant visual stimuli and perceive spacial relationships can cause postural instability, increased sway, and impaired balance, resulting in a fall.

    c. Impaired depth perception, judgment of distance, and contrast sensitivity contribute to an inability to identify hazards and, therefore, avoid obstacles in the environment.

2. Nursing care.

    a. Assess the patient's visual acuity to determine the extent of the patient's risk of injury and the level of assistance required by the patient (see the section "Assessment of the Eyes" in Chapter 11, "Physical Assessment," page 279).

    b. Encourage the use of prescription eyeglasses, contact lenses, tinted eyeglasses, a magnifying glass, and other visual devices.

    c. Provide adequate room lighting and a small light at night.

    d. Use shades or blinds on windows during the day to reduce glare.

    e. Describe and maintain the placement of furniture in the room.

    f. Use a clock arrangement for placement of food on a plate or tray.

    g. Ensure that food and liquids are warm, not hot.

    h. Provide care standing on the side of the patient's most effective vision.

    i. When walking with the patient, be next to and slightly in front of the patient with the patient holding your arm.

    j. Provide or encourage the use of objects with large print, such as clocks, phones, and computers.

C. Impaired Hearing

1. Significance.

    a. Impaired hearing limits the reception of auditory stimuli, which can result in patient injury.

    b. Nurses must understand that impaired hearing also impacts a patient's ability to communicate and, therefore, nursing interventions must facilitate communication.

2. Nursing care.

    a. Assess the patient's hearing ability to determine the extent of the patient's risk of injury and the level of assistance required by the patient (see the section "Assessment of the Ears" in Chapter 11, "Physical Assessment," page 280).

    b. Encourage the use of a prescribed hearing aid.

    c. Decrease background noise when communicating with the patient, such as by turning off the TV and closing the door.

    d. Face the patient and speak clearly.

    e. Encourage the use of devices that amplify sound or use motion or lights to communicate a message, such as a smoke detector, phone, and doorbell.

🛑 f. Ensure that the patient hears and understands communication, especially instructions concerning activities.

D. Impaired Mobility
1. Significance.
   a. Mobility relates to body alignment, joint flexibility, gait, and balance, which includes center of gravity and base of support. Impairment in any one of these areas can result in a fall.
   b. Falls are a major concern because they can cause injury, loss of function, and mortality.
   c. Falls are the leading cause of injury resulting in death in older adults.
2. Nursing care.
   a. Assess the patient for factors that increase the risk of falls; preferably use a measurement tool (e.g., The Morse Fall Scale).
      (1) History of falls.
      (2) Secondary medical diagnosis (e.g., cardiopulmonary, musculoskeletal, endocrine diseases).
      (3) Use of ambulatory aids.
      (4) Presence of one or more objects that hamper mobility (e.g., urinary catheter, IV, oxygen tubing, and venous compression device).
      (5) Impaired gait, balance, or weight-bearing ability of lower extremities.
      (6) Impaired cognition or judgment.
      (7) Impaired vision.
      (8) Hypotension, orthostatic hypotension, or dizziness.
      (9) Medications that depress the central nervous system, such as sedatives and opioids, or promote hypotension, such as antihypertensives and diuretics.
      (10) Age more than 65 years.
   b. Perform the "Get Up and Go Test."
      (1) Have the patient move from a sitting to a standing position without using the arms for support.
      (2) Instruct the patient to walk several steps, turn, and return to the chair.
      (3) Have the patient sit down in the chair without using the arms for support.
      (4) Perform a follow-up assessment if the test reveals that the patient is unsteady.
         (a) Have the patient move from a sitting to a standing position without using the arms for support.
         (b) Have the patient stand in place with eyes closed for several seconds.
         (c) Push gently on the sternum while the patient has his or her eyes closed.
         (d) Instruct the patient to walk several steps, turn, return to the chair, and sit down without using the arms for support.

   c. Use monitoring devices that alert others when the patient attempts to get out of a bed or chair; use two, three, or four side rails, as indicated.
   d. Have the patient use an assistive device to maintain a wide base of support, such as a walker or cane.
   e. Implement hourly rounding on patients to reduce patient anxiety and attend to personal needs.
   f. Ensure the patient has well-fitted footwear with nonskid soles.
   g. Instruct the patient to rise slowly to a standing position and allow time for blood pressure to adjust to change in position; encourage the patient to sit down if dizzy.
   h. Use assistive devices when transferring patients, such as a transfer belt (Fig. 13.1), mechanical lift (Fig. 13.2), or sit-to-stand lift (Fig. 13.3).
   i. Arrange physical therapy sessions in the morning before the patient becomes fatigued.
   j. Assist the patient if the patient begins to fall.
      (1) Place the feet apart and project the hip and leg closest to the patient, allowing the patient to slide down the care-giver's leg to the floor (Fig. 13.4).
      (2) Protect the patient's head.
      (3) Call for assistance.

MAKING THE CONNECTION

Making Hourly Rounds and Reducing the Rate of Falls

Falls are the leading cause of injury and death among people who are 65 years of age and older. In fact, in 2009, 2.2 million fall injuries requiring treatment in emergency departments occurred among people age 65 and older. Twenty-five percent of these individuals required hospitalization. Traumatic brain injuries accounted for almost half of the fatal falls. In addition, 90 percent of hip fractures are caused by falls. However, performing hourly rounds (intentional checking of patients at hourly intervals) can help reduce the risk of falls. When the results of nine studies were examined that implemented hourly rounds, seven of the nine studies indicated that fall rates were reduced. In eight of the nine studies, improvements in overall patient satisfaction with attention to personal needs and timeliness of nurses' response were identified. Hourly rounds helped to reduce patients' anxiety about getting needs met and patients learned to trust the process. One study documented a 52 percent reduction in falls, 37 percent reduction in the use of call lights, and 14 percent reduction in the development of pressure ulcers.

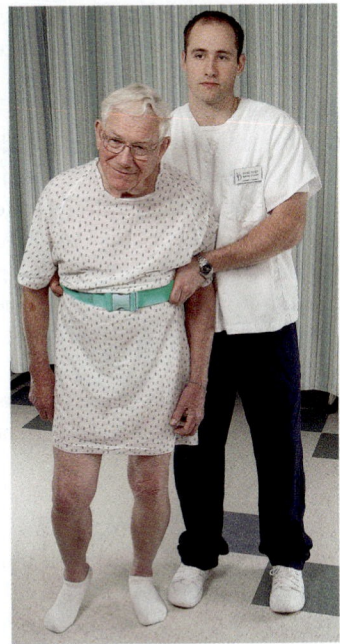

Fig 13.1 Transfer belt. (From Wilkinson and Treas [2011]. *Fundamentals of nursing*, Vol. 1, 2nd ed. Philadelphia: F. A. Davis Company, with permission.)

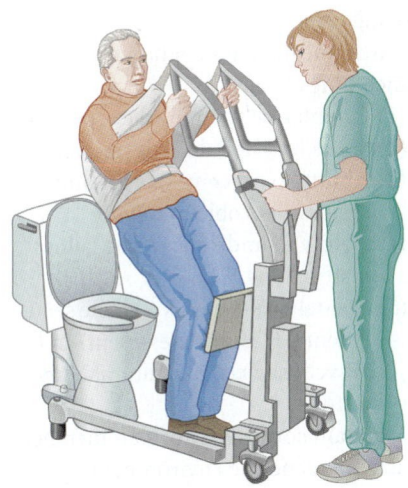

Fig 13.3 Sit-to-stand lift. (From Burton and Ludwig [2011]. *Fundamentals of nursing care: Concepts, connections & skills.* Philadelphia: F. A. Davis Company, with permission.)

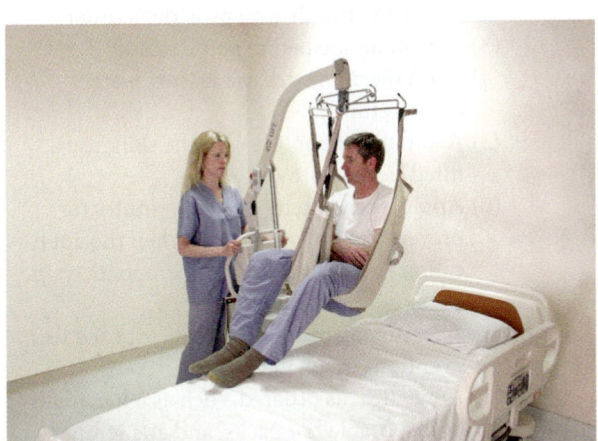

Fig 13.2 Mechanical lift. (From Wilkinson and Treas [2011]. *Fundamentals of nursing*, Vol. 1, 2nd ed. Philadelphia: F. A. Davis Company, with permission.)

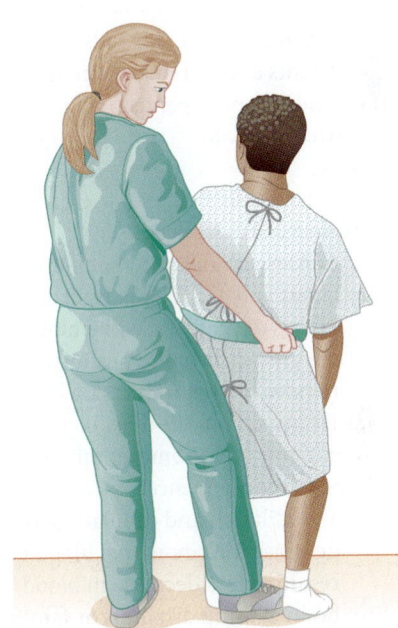

Fig 13.4 Guiding a falling patient. (From Wilkinson and Treas [2011]. *Fundamentals of nursing*, Vol. 1, 2nd ed. Philadelphia: F. A. Davis Company, with permission.)

(4) Have the patient examined by a health-care provider for injury.

(5) Document the event and complete an incident report.

E. Impaired Cognition (Confusion, Disorientation, Impaired Memory, Lack of Judgment)

1. Significance.

   a. The ability to perceive external stimuli and react appropriately requires intact cognition, which includes the thought processes of thinking, problem-solving, judgment, and insight; level of consciousness; memory; and orientation to time, place, and person.

   b. Issues such as lack of sleep, impaired memory, an altered level of consciousness, disorientation, confusion, or taking medications that influence the central nervous system, such as narcotics, hypnotics or sedatives, can impair thought processes.

   c. When thought processes are impaired, a patient is unable to perceive risk factors or use judgment to maintain safety, thereby increasing the risk of injury.

2. Nursing care.
   a. Assess the patient's cognitive functioning, including.
      (1) Orientation to time, place, and person.
      (2) Short-term and long-term memory.
      (3) Ability to perceive danger and use judgment and problem-solving.
      (4) Ability to understand and follow instructions.
      (5) Mental health status (see the section "Mental Health Assessment" in Chapter 8, "Psychosocial and Cultural Nursing," p. 160).
   b. Maintain consistency of staff members, activities, and the environment.
   c. Use color as environmental clues.
   🛑 d. Use position monitoring devices that alert others when the patient attempts to get out of a bed or chair.
   e. Use two, three, or four side rails as indicated.
   f. Use restraints as ordered and needed.
   g. Assign one-to-one supervision if necessary.

F. Exposure to Heat or Cold
1. Significance.
   a. Heat.
      (1) Positive consequences.
         (a) Causes vasodilation that increases circulation and capillary permeability.
         (b) Brings oxygen and white blood cells to the area to promote healing and help remove waste products.
         (c) Decreases muscle tension and joint stiffness and promotes relaxation.
      (2) Negative consequences.
         (a) Vasodilation and capillary permeability decrease the circulating blood volume, resulting in a decrease in blood to the brain causing dizziness or fainting (**syncope**).
         (b) Decreased muscle tension and relaxation may result in muscle weakness or lack of attention to personal abilities or factors in the environment, which may result in injury.
         (c) The addition of moisture increases the intensity of heat.
         (d) Excessive heat can cause tissue injury and cell death (thermal burn).
   b. Cold.
      (1) Positive consequences.
         (a) Causes vasoconstriction that decreases circulation and capillary permeability.
         (b) Reduces muscle tension and cell metabolism.

            (c) Limits inflammation, pain, edema, oxygen requirements at the cellular level, and bleeding.
      (2) Negative consequences.
         (a) Vasoconstriction may limit the transport of adequate oxygen and nutrients necessary for muscle contraction resulting in weakness.
         (b) Cold anesthetizes nerve endings, which diminishes the ability to perceive sensations, such as placement of feet on the floor.
         (c) Excessive cold can cause tissue injury and cell death because of ischemia (cold burn).
2. Nursing care.
   a. Commonalities of care for patients exposed to interventions involving either heat or cold.
      (1) Identify patients at increased risk for nontherapeutic results, such as the very young and very old, those with sensory impairments, and those with injuries on highly vascular areas (e.g., hand, face, perineum), traumatized skin, or involvement of large surface areas.
      (2) Verify the health-care provider's order.
      (3) Assess the site before application.
      (4) Use a thermometer to measure water temperature.
      (5) Avoid direct contact with the skin; use a fitted sleeve or towel.
      (6) Apply intermittently for 15 minutes to prevent the opposite effect when the application reaches maximum therapeutic value (rebound phenomenon).
   b. Specific nursing care for patients exposed to interventions involving heat.
      (1) Apply heat as ordered, such as a heating pad or disposable hot packs, and at a temperature of 105°F to 115°F; sitz bath should not exceed 110°F.
      (2) Assess for nontherapeutic responses, such as extreme redness, cyanosis, blanching, blistering, and decreased blood pressure.
   c. Specific nursing care for patients exposed to interventions involving cold.
      (1) Apply cold as ordered, such as a cool sponge bath, cold compresses, ice collar, or disposable ice packs, and at the recommended temperature; cool sponge bath should be 65°F to 90°F.
      (2) Reduce the temperature extreme or discontinue treatment if the patient begins to shiver because shivering increases body temperature.

(3) Assess for nontherapeutic responses, such as blanching, mottled skin, numbness, pain, blisters, shivering, and increased blood pressure.

G. Allergies

1. Significance.
   a. An **allergy** is a hypersensitivity precipitated by exposure to a stimulus (**allergen**) that can cause harmful immunologic reactions within the body.
   b. Mild and moderate reactions involve uncomfortable responses, such as sneezing, coughing, itching eyes, and conjunctivitis.
   c. A rapid severe reaction (unrelated to an initial mild or moderate reaction) may include hives, swelling of respiratory passages that causes difficulty breathing, and wheezing and can progress to anaphylaxis.
   d. Anaphylaxis involves a decrease in blood pressure and can cause shock, unconsciousness, and death if untreated.

2. Nursing care.
   a. Assess for a history of allergies, such as to drugs (prescription and over the counter), foods (especially seafood), tape, skin care products, animals, and insects; obtain a description of the patient's response to each.
   b. Identify the risk of a latex allergy. An increased risk is associated with asthma; allergies to bananas, kiwi, chestnuts, or avocados; and repeated exposure to latex in medical care settings. Use latex-free gloves and equipment.
   c. Assess for clinical indicators of mild to moderate allergic responses, such as a skin rash, urticaria, pruritus, nausea, vomiting, diarrhea, rhinitis, and lacrimal tearing.
   d. Assess for clinical indicators of anaphylaxis, such as wheezing, dyspnea, angioedema, tachycardia, hypotension, and circulatory collapse.
   🛑 **e. Apply an allergy alert wristband (usually red in color) that itemizes the offending agents.**

   f. Communicate the allergy to other health team members, such as by documenting it in the medication administration record, history and physical, front of the clinical record, and the patient's plan of care.
   g. Ensure that the patient is not exposed to any known offending agents.
   h. Encourage the patient to wear a medical alert band at all times.
   i. Encourage the patient to carry or have readily available an epinephrine auto-injector (EpiPen), if prescribed.

H. Increased Risk of Aspiration, Drowning, or Suffocation

1. Significance.
   a. **Aspiration** is the inhalation of a substance (e.g., foreign material, vomitus, blood, saliva) into the respiratory tract.
   b. **Drowning** occurs when the lungs fill with fluid, preventing gas exchange and resulting in suffocation.
   c. **Suffocation (asphyxiation)** occurs when no air reaches the lungs, causing lack of oxygen, excess carbon dioxide, loss of consciousness, stoppage of breathing, and death. It can be caused by gas or smoke inhalation, strangulation, a foreign body in the trachea, drowning, and electric shock and also occurs when an infant's face is pressed against a sleeping caregiver, mattress, stuffed toy, or blanket.
   d. Nursing interventions for promoting safety in relation to these issues involve direct nursing interventions and health teaching for patients and parents.

2. Nursing care.
   a. Teach parents to:
      (1) Ensure that cribs meet regulations, such as slats less than 2⅜ inch apart and stationary side rails.
      (2) Keep cords out of reach, such as from mobiles, venetian blinds, neck ties, and sweatpants.
      (3) Ensure that toys are larger than a fist and have no small removable parts.
      (4) Store plastic bags out of reach.
      (5) Cut food (e.g., grapes, hot dogs, and cheese) into small pieces.
      (6) Do not give children chewing gum, hard candy, nuts, popcorn, marshmallows, or peanut butter.
      (7) Supervise play with balloons and discard broken balloons immediately.
      (8) Ensure pools have appropriate safety precautions, such as a high fence, pool cover, and splash sensor.
      (9) Supervise children around water, such as tubs, pools, buckets, and toilets; provide Coast Guard–approved flotation devices.
   b. Provide specific nursing care for patients at risk for aspiration.
      (1) Assess for risk factors, such as dysphagia, dentures, and impaired cognition.
      (2) Position the patient in a sitting position for meals, and ensure the patient swallows food before giving the next spoonful.
      (3) Teach the patient to cut food into small pieces.

(4) Teach the patient to chew food thoroughly.

(5) Use a thickening product to thicken liquids.

(6) Identify whether a patient with a neurological impairment has retained food in the buccal cavity (**cheeking**) to prevent aspiration.

c. Teach the patient to check the depth of water before jumping or diving.

d. Teach older children and adults the universal choking sign. (see Fig. 19.23, page 588.)

III. Safety of Health-Care Providers

Nursing is a profession that exposes its members to numerous work-related stressors that can impact their health. New devices have been developed, such as needleless syringes, passive guards on syringes, and sit-to-stand lifts, to address some workplace stressors. However, nurses are increasingly caring for more patients who are obese, acutely ill, and physically dependent and those receiving a variety of radiation and/or intravenous therapies that raise new concerns in relation to the safety of nurses. In addition, nurses must cope with patients who become verbally and physically aggressive due to delirium, cognitive impairment, mental illness, grief, jealousy, caregiver role strain, and drug or alcohol abuse. The potential for musculoskeletal injuries, radiation exposure, puncture injuries, and violence toward nurses and other health-care providers still exists.

A. Introduction

1. The American Nurses Association (ANA), Occupational and Safety and Health Administration (OSHA), Joint Commission (JC), American Hospital Association (AHA), and Environmental Protection Agency (EPA) all issue guidelines and regulations that address safety in health-care settings to protect health-care providers, patients, and visitors.

2. Agency policies and procedures must address such safety issues as infection control, handling of chemical and biological agents, disposal of sharps, equipment for moving patients, badges for measuring level of radiation exposure, and ways to manage violence in the workplace.

B. Hazards to Health-Care Providers

1. Back injury.

   a. Most commonly result from activities that require bending and twisting the torso, such as lifting patients up in bed, transferring patients from a bed to a chair, and changing linens.

   b. Preventive measures.

      (1) Use appropriate body mechanics (see the section "Body Mechanics" in Chapter 17, "Mobility," page 478.)

(2) Use patient handling devices when necessary, such as mechanical lifts (see Fig. 13.2), transfer boards, and sit-to-stand lifts (see Fig. 13.3).

2. Exposure to a patient receiving radiation therapy.

   a. Types of radiation therapy.

      (1) Internal radiation therapy (brachytherapy).

         (a) Interstitial implants (e.g., needle, seeds, wire).

         (b) Intracavitary implants (e.g., radioactive source contained within an applicator that is inserted into a body cavity).

      (2) External radiation therapy (teletherapy): Radiation dose administered by a machine.

      (3) Radiopharmaceutical therapy: Radioactive medication administered orally or intravenously.

   b. Preventive measures to protect nurses caring for patients receiving internal radiation therapy.

      (1) Perform all care based on the concept of "As Low As Reasonably Achievable" (ALARA).

         (a) Understand that ALARA means making all reasonable efforts regarding controlling time, distance, and shielding to minimize exposure to ionizing radiation.

         (b) Monitor radiation dosimeter (badge) to ensure that it does not exceed the U.S. annual occupational dose limit of 5,000 millirem (5 rem); many agencies advocate exposure to less than 500 millirem yearly.

         (c) Ensure that pregnant women and women attempting to become pregnant do not routinely care for patient's receiving internal radiation.

      (2) Control time.

         (a) Wear a radiation dosimeter (badge) when providing care if regularly exposed to radiation to measure the extent of radiation exposure.

         (b) Organize care to minimize the amount of time at the patient's bedside, meeting only essential needs; keep time to less than 30 minutes in an 8-hour period per care giver.

         (c) Rotate care among nurses.

      (3) Control distance.

         (a) Place the patient in a private room.

         (b) Stand as far away from the patient as possible (at least 6 feet) unless giving direct care.

(c) Provide care by standing at the head or foot of the bed as indicated, such as head and side of the patient's bed for vaginal or prostate implants or seeds and foot of the bed if seeds are in the neck or tongue.

(4) Control shielding.

(a) Wear a lead apron and protective shoe covers and gloves when in the room with the patient.

(b) Ensure that an internal radiation device is in place.

(c) Inspect linens for displacement of radioactive seeds.

(d) Maintain the patient in the position ordered to prevent displacement and promote comfort, such as supine for a vaginal implant and semi-Fowler's position for seed implants in the neck or tongue.

(e) Notify the appropriate radiation team immediately if a radioactive device or seed is displaced; use a long-handled forceps to place a dislodged radioactive device in a lead container only if trained in this technique.

🛑 (f) **Never touch radioactive implant devices or seeds with the hands.**

c. Preventive measures to protect nurses when caring for a patient receiving external radiation therapy.

(1) Wear a radiation dosimeter (badge) when providing care if regularly exposed to radiation to measure the extent of radiation exposure.

(2) Stand behind the designated shield/door or wear full body lead clothing during diagnostic tests that emit radiation.

d. Preventive measures to protect nurses and others when caring for a patient receiving radiopharmaceutical therapy.

(1) Follow recommendations for time, distance, and shielding depending on the radioactive material used for diagnostic or therapeutic procedures. Recommendations depend on the half-life of the radioactive material.

(2) Teach patients and family members about precautions that should be followed when a patient is discharged home after receiving radiopharmaceutical therapy (e.g., ^{131}I: oral and close contact with others should be avoided, urine and vomitus should be disposed of in a toilet and the toilet flushed twice, meticulous hand washing should be performed after urinating, and eating utensils should be washed thoroughly with soap and water).

3. Puncture injuries.

a. Can occur when handling anything sharp enough to pierce the skin; most occur as a result of the penetration of a needle of a syringe, hence the sometimes interrelated term *needle-stick injury.*

b. Preventive measures.

(1) Encourage the adoption of needleless systems.

(2) Use devices that passively activate a safety guard over a needle rather than requiring the nurse to activate the guard.

(3) Use caution when working with sharp objects, such as scissors, clamps, scalpels, and syringes with needles.

(4) See also Box 14.2, "Preventing Needlestick Injuries" in Chapter 14, "Medication Administration," p. 382.

4. Violence.

a. Can be precipitated by physical stressors (e.g., delirium, cognitive impairments, alcohol or drug use) and emotional stressors (e.g., manic episodes of bipolar disorder, grief, jealousy, and caregiver role strain).

b. Preventive measures.

(1) Stay with the patient.

(2) Listen attentively and validate the patient's feelings.

(3) Provide an atmosphere of caring and empathy.

(4) Remain calm and communicate in short, clear sentences.

(5) Give the patient choices if possible and if the patient is capable of decision making.

(6) Limit environmental stimuli, such as by reducing noise and people in the room.

(7) Identify whether the patient's level of anxiety is escalating; be aware that behavior usually progresses to verbal and then physical aggression, such as agitation, pacing, pressured speech, gesturing wildly, sarcasm, swearing, verbal threats, pushing, and hitting.

🛑 (8) **Protect self and others when a patient or visitor is angry.**

(a) Know how to access the help of agency safety control officers.

(b) Do not go into the room alone.

(c) Keep the door open and stand between the patient and the door.

(d) Remain at least 3 feet away from and do not turn your back on an angry patient.

(e) Do not wear anything that can be used to inflict harm, such as a stethoscope, dangling jewelry, and pointed objects.

(f) Avoid threatening, aggressive verbal or nonverbal communication; do not respond to anger with anger.

(g) Do not touch the patient without permission.

(h) Offer first and then administer prescribed sedatives if necessary, using a calm, reassuring approach.

(i) Use mechanical restraints as ordered and necessary to prevent injury to self and others.

(9) Ensure safety in home-care settings.

(a) Carry a cell phone and a minimal amount of money.

(b) Exit the car after determining the safety of the surroundings, such as adequate lighting and nonthreatening behavior of residents; drive away if you do not deem the area safe.

(c) Remain close to an exit after entering a home.

(d) Request that animals and visible weapons be kept in another room.

(e) Leave immediately if you suspect substance use, drug dealing, or drunken behavior.

(f) Leave immediately if a domestic argument occurs; do not attempt to intervene.

(g) Request a security escort if the area is considered potentially unsafe.

(h) Report to the appropriate authorities (depends on state law and local agencies) suspected child, domestic partner, or elder abuse.

IV. Restraints

Restraints are devices used to limit movement of a body limb or body activity. They should be used only as a last resort to prevent injury to the patient or others after other less-restrictive measures have failed.

A. **Introduction**

1. Two levels of restraints are used.

   a. Level 1 restraints are used to protect a patient from injuring self and others while receiving acute medical or surgical care.

   b. Level 2 restraints are used to manage violent behavior to protect a patient from injuring self and others.

2. Less-restrictive means to provide for patient safety that should be attempted before restraint use include:

   a. Orienting the patient to the environment.

   b. Planning nursing care with the patient and explaining all procedures.

   c. Monitoring the patient frequently.

   d. Keeping the bed in the lowest position.

   e. Keeping two side rails up and using additional rails cautiously because the patient may attempt to climb over the rails if feeling confined.

DID YOU KNOW?

Raising all side rails is considered a restraint that requires an order from a primary health-care provider. If all side rails are raised at the request of a patient it is not considered a restraint and does not require an order.

   f. Using verbal interventions.

   g. Using a weight or position-sensitive device to alert caregivers of a patient's attempt to ambulate.

   h. Using seclusion (e.g., locked, padded room) in a mental health setting.

   i. Providing one-to-one supervision.

3. Patient rights include freedom from physical restraints or psychoactive medications for the purpose of discipline or convenience.

4. Restraints should be used only as a last resort because they can cause injury, actually do not reduce falls, and make patient care more time consuming.

5. Orders for as-needed restraints or seclusion are not acceptable.

B. **Types of Restraints**

1. Physical restraints immobilize a limb or movement of a body part; examples include wrist restraint, ankle restraint, cloth vest, and material mitt (Table 13.1).

2. Environmental restraints confine a person to an area; examples include side rails, a wheel chair with an immovable tray, and a seclusion room.

3. Chemical restraints alter disruptive and aggressive behavior so that the patient cannot cause harm to self or others; examples include sedatives and psychotropic medications.

C. **Nursing Care for Patients Who Are Restrained**

1. Follow agency policies, state laws, and professional guidelines.

2. Use less-restrictive interventions first; document their use and the patient's response.

3. Use restraints as last resort to protect the patient and others from harm.

4. Before application, obtain a health-care provider's order for the least restrictive restraint, except in an emergency.

Table 13.1	**Types of Physical Restraints**

Type of Restraint	Nursing Care
Mitt Restraint • Limits use of fingers. • Prevents removal of tubes and scratching. 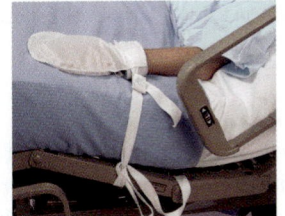	• Apply to one or both hands, as ordered. • Tie to an immobile object. • Ensure that the patient can flex and extend the fingers. • Ensure that two fingers can be slid under the wrist strap to ensure that it is not too tight. • Remove the restraint every 2 hours to perform a neurovascular assessment and put the entire extremity through full range-of-motion (ROM) exercises.
Vest and Jacket Restraints • Prevent getting out of bed or chair. • Permit turning from side to side. 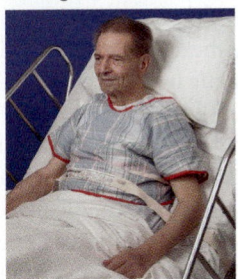	• Place the device on with the *V* in the front and the closure at the back. • Ensure that the device does not impair breathing. • Ensure that the patient can turn from side to side. • Encourage the patient to cough and deep breathe every hour. • Remove the restraint every 2 hours and assess skin integrity.
Wrist and Ankle Restraints • Prevent removal of tubes. • Prevent hitting or kicking others. 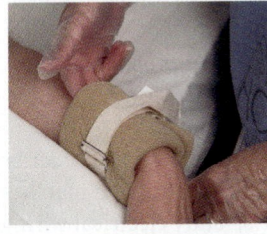	• Apply the restraints as ordered, such as two-point (both arms) or four-point (all extremities) restraints. • Place padding around the wrists or ankles before applying the straps. • Make the straps tight enough to prevent removal without impairing circulation (but ensure that two fingers can be slid under the strap). • Remove the restraint every 2 hours to assess neurovascular status and tissue integrity and put the extremity through full ROM exercises. • Follow guidelines for use of four-point restraints: limit use to 4 hours; continuously assess response, monitor for safety, and reevaluate need; ensure the patient is assessed by a primary health-care provider within 1 hour of institution of the restraint.

Photo credits: Wilkinson and Treas (2011). *Fundamentals of nursing,* Vol. 2, 2nd ed. Philadelphia: F. A. Davis Company, with permission.

🛑 5. **Secure the restraint using a quick-release knot (Fig.13.5), which should not constrict or slip with patient movements but will untie rapidly in an emergency; tie the knot to the bed frame, not a movable object such as a bed rail, because doing so could injure a patient when the rail moves.**

6. Maintain supervision of a patient in restraints or seclusion based on agency policy and procedures (e.g., observe every 15 minutes if in a seclusion room, check the site of a restraint every 30 minutes).

7. Release restraints every 2 hours or more frequently, especially if used for behavioral problems, to assess the site of application for impaired circulation, tissue injury, or nerve compression; perform range-of-motion (ROM) exercises to the limbs; and provide skin care.

8. Document all interventions and the patient's response. Document continued need for restraints every several hours for a patient in a mental health agency, according to state mental health laws, and at least every 24 hours in other health-care agencies; discontinue use as soon as possible.

9. Delegate application and reapplication of restraints only to assistive personnel who are educated to performed this skill; however, retain the responsibility to evaluate the patient's response, which should be performed only by a registered professional nurse.

10. Meet hydration, nutrition, elimination, and emotional needs while the patient is restrained or secluded.

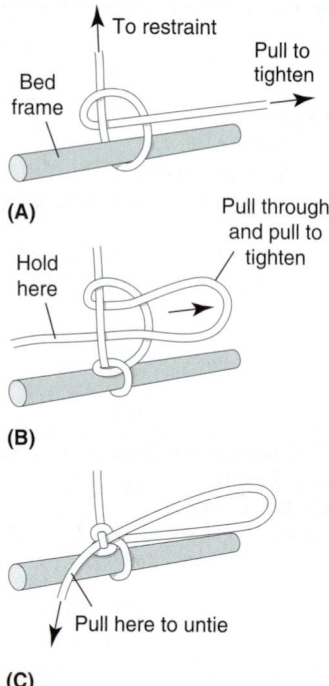

(A)

(B)

(C)

Fig 13.5 Quick release knot. (From Burton and Ludwig [2011]. *Fundamentals of nursing care: Concepts, connections & skills.* Philadelphia: F. A. Davis Company, with permission.)

V. Fire Safety

Fire is a risk in all health-care environments and in the home. Fires in health-care environments sometimes occur due to the presence of flammable gases and materials as well as electrical equipment. Oxygen supports combustion of flammable materials and intensifies the severity of a fire. Incapacitated or immobile individuals are particularly at risk for injury from a fire because they may be unable to evacuate themselves.

A. Fire Prevention Measures
1. Ensure all electrical equipment have three-pronged grounded plugs.
2. Test electrical equipment before use.
3. Avoid overloading outlets.
4. Remove an electric plug by gripping the plug, not pulling on the cord.
5. Inspect electrical plugs and wires for signs of loss of integrity, such as visible damage and frayed wires.
6. Decommission damaged electrical equipment; discard, send home with family, or forward to appropriate maintenance department.
7. Keep rooms and halls free from clutter.
8. Participate in educational programs regarding fire prevention and safety measures.
9. Participate in routine fire drills, and know the protocol for evacuating a home or unit.

10. Know the location of fire alarms, chart of bell codes, exists, and fire extinguishers.
11. Know how to locate a fire using a bell code chart.
🛑 12. Know how to report a fire per agency protocol.
🛑 13. Ensure caregivers are aware of where and when oxygen is in use and the location of oxygen shut-off valves in a facility.

B. Agency Fires
🛑 1. Follow the RACE mnemonic.
   a. Rescue: Remove patients in the vicinity of a fire; evacuate patients beyond a fire safety door if necessary; evacuate laterally and then horizontally. Do not use elevators.
   b. Alarm: Activate the first alert, usually by pulling an alarm or via telephone; indicate the type and location of the fire and identify yourself; then, activate the agency-wide call-bell system and automatic notification of the fire department.
   c. Confine: Close all doors and windows on the unit; ensure that fire safety doors that close automatically have closed; shut off all oxygen valves after ensuring patients' oxygen needs.
   d. Extinguish: Extinguish the fire using the appropriate fire extinguisher.
2. Respond to a fire if you are on the fire brigade; usually one person from each unit of the agency in addition to maintenance personnel are members of the fire brigade.
   a. Bring your assigned equipment.
   b. Use the stairs, not an elevator.

C. Home Fires
1. Be aware that home fires sometimes occur because of careless disposal of cigarettes and matches as well as kitchen grease, faulty electrical wiring, and defective heating equipment.
2. Teach individuals to.
🛑 a. Install smoke alarms, and change the batteries once a year.
   b. Have and practice a home fire escape plan.
🛑 c. Keep the fire department's number on home phones.
   d. Keep a fire extinguisher readily available, especially in a kitchen or workshop.
   e. Avoid smoking inside or near the entrances and exits to the home.
   f. Attend to fireplace fires, hot barbeque fires, and burning candles at all times.
   g. Store flammable liquids in appropriate containers.
   h. Never pour water on a grease fire.
   i. Unplug electrical appliances that give a shock or are on fire.

D. Fire Extinguishers
1. Types.
   a. A: Used for materials that burn, such as wood, cloth, and paper.
   b. B: Used for flammable materials, such as liquids, gases, grease, tar, solvents, and paint.
   c. C: Used for fires involving electrical equipment, such as toasters and electric stoves.
   d. ABC: Used for all types of fires.
2. Nursing interventions.
   a. Determine the type of fire and select the appropriate extinguisher; most agencies now use ABC fire extinguishers.
   b. Position yourself between the fire and an exit.
   c. Follow the **PASS** mnemonic when using a fire extinguisher.
      (1) **P**ull the pin on the fire extinguisher.
      (2) **A**im the nozzle at the base of the flames.
      (3) **S**queeze the handles of the fire extinguisher.
      (4) **S**weep the nozzle from side to side at the base of the flames.

CASE STUDY: Putting It All Together

A 72-year-old widow is admitted to the hospital to receive treatment for a fracture of the neck of the left femur. This is the second admission for the patient, who was admitted 4 months ago for a right brain attack (cerebrovascular accident, stroke). She has residual left-sided hemiparesis, a sling on her left arm to prevent subluxation of the shoulder, and a below-the-knee foot brace on the lower left leg for foot drop and to facilitate ambulation. She has been receiving furosemide (Lasix) daily for hypertension. When interviewed, the patient says that she heard the doorbell ring, got up quickly, stood at the side of the bed, slipped on the scatter rug next to the bed, and fell to the floor. She was able to activate her safety alert necklace to summon help. An x-ray confirms a fracture in the intertrochanteric area, below the neck of the left femur. The patient is admitted to the surgical unit so that orthopedic surgery can be performed to stabilize the femur. When assessing the patient after transfer from the postanesthesia care unit to her room after the surgery, the primary nurse on the surgical unit identifies that the patient's dressing is dry and intact, vital signs are within expected limits, and urine output is more than 50 mL/hour (according to the hourly urine output

via a urinary retention catheter). The patient states that she has pain and rates it as a level 3 on a 0-to-10 pain scale. She is able to state her name but does not recognize that she is in the hospital or that she had surgery and that it is the afternoon. The patient states, "Why is everyone trying to kill me?" In addition, the patient is attempting to get out of bed.

Postoperative orders
- Position on back and left side.
- Vital signs every 4 hours.
- Neuro checks every 4 hours for 24 hours.
- Bed rest and range-of-motion exercises to all unaffected extremities BID.
- Full liquid diet; advance to regular diet as tolerated.
- Elevate left leg on two pillows.
- IV fluids: 0.9% normal saline solution 60 mL/hr.
- Heparin 5000 units Sub-Q every 12 hours.
- Dilaudid 2 mg Sub-Q every 4 hours prn for severe pain.
- Percocet 5/325 mg, tab for mild pain and 2 tabs for moderate pain, PO every 6 hrs prn
- Colace 100 mg po BID.
- Senokot 86 mg per tab, 2 tabs PO at bedtime prn for constipation.

Case Study Questions

A. What factors increased the risk of the patient falling at home?

1. _____

2. _____

3. _____

4. _____

B. Which of the following concerns is the priority and what data support the nurse's conclusion: potential for hemorrhage, fluid balance, patient safety, or pain management?

_____

CASE STUDY: Putting It All Together

cont'd

Case Study Questions

C. Identify common nursing actions that should be implemented to ensure the safety of this patient?

1. _____
2. _____
3. _____
4. _____
5. _____
6. _____
7. _____
8. _____
9. _____

D. Identify additional nursing interventions specific to this patient that the nurse should implement before seeking an order for a restraint.

1. _____
2. _____
3. _____
4. _____
5. _____

E. Because nonrestrictive measures are ineffective in providing for the patient's safety, the primary health-care provider writes an order for a vest restraint. What actions should the nurse implement when caring for this patient while she is in the vest restraint?

1. _____
2. _____
3. _____
4. _____
5. _____
6. _____
7. _____
8. _____
9. _____
10. _____

REVIEW QUESTIONS

1. A nurse is teaching new parents about care of their newborn. What should the nurse teach them to do to prevent the leading cause of accidental death in infants?
   1. Give your infant toys that are bigger than an adult's clenched fist.
   2. Place your infant in a four-point infant seat when in an automobile.
   3. Support your infant when placed on an elevated surface.
   4. Position your infant on the back when sleeping.

2. A nurse has an order from a primary health-care provider to apply wrist restraints to maintain a patient's safety. What should the nurse do **first** when applying this type of restraint?
   1. Remove the wrist restraints to provide skin care every 3 hours.
   2. Ensure that the wrists are well padded when applying wrist restraints.
   3. Permit 3 finger-widths to slide between the patient's wrists and the restraints.
   4. Tie the tales of the wrist restraints to the frame of the bed using a square knot.

3. Which is an important step when transferring a patient using a mechanical lift?
   1. Position the chair as close as possible to the bed.
   2. Remove the sling after the patient is moved to the chair.
   3. Position the sling at the middle of the patient's back to the ankles.
   4. Attach the longer belts to the lower grommets on each side of the sling.

4. A patient who is legally blind says to the nurse, "I once was able to see a little bit, but now I can't see anything." What should the nurse encourage the patient to do while hospitalized?
   1. Wear dark-tinted eyeglasses.
   2. Keep a light on in the room at all times.
   3. Close the window blinds during the day.
   4. Call for assistance when getting out of bed.

5. A nurse is caring for an older adult who is cognitively impaired and has a history of pulling out tubes and falling. List the following safety devices in the order of least restrictive to most restrictive that may be employed to ensure the safety of this patient.
   1. Cloth vest
   2. Two wrist straps
   3. Four side rails up
   4. Bed exiting alarm device
   5. Four-point restraint tied to the bed frame
   Answer: _____

6. A patient who is cognitively impaired is admitted to the hospital for pneumonia. The patient has a history of wandering at night. What should the nurse do to ensure the safety of this patient?
   1. Encourage a family member to remain with the patient every night.
   2. Obtain a sedative to be administered to the patient at bedtime.
   3. Apply a vest restraint when the patient plans to go to sleep.
   4. Activate the bed alarm on the patient's bed.

7. An 87-year-old adult is admitted to the hospital after a fall in the home. The patient was admitted for diagnostic tests and intravenous rehydration therapy. The next day the patient's order for "out of bed to chair" twice daily was changed to "out of bed ad lib."

Patient's Clinical Record

Medical History

Diagnosed with hypothyroidism for 10 years and hypertension for 5 years. Taking levothyroxine (Synthroid) 100 mcg once a day PO and hydrochlorothiazide 25 mg PO once a day. Came to the emergency department twice in the past year because of falls in the home. Both times blood work and x-rays were normal. Both times treated for cuts and bruises and discharged.

Serum Electrolyte Levels

Potassium: 3.4 mEq/L.
Sodium: 134 mEq/L.
Calcium: 9.6 mEq/L.

Progress Note

Out of bed to chair for 1 hour twice between 8:00 a.m. and 8:00 p.m. Required minimal assistance and did not experience lightheadedness or syncope. States, "I'm afraid to walk because I was admitted to the hospital when I fell walking from the living room to the bedroom." IVF 5% dextrose in water at 75 mL/hour.

What should the nurse do before getting the patient out of bed?
   1. Test the strength of the patient's legs.
   2. Take the blood pressure while the patient is supine.
   3. Give the patient oxygen via a nasal cannula for several minutes.
   4. Disconnect the patient's intravenous tubing from the venous access device.

8. A health team member is using a type C fire extinguisher to put out a fire in a health-care facility. What kind of fire is the health team member attempting to extinguish because a type C fire extinguisher is the only extinguisher that should be used in this situation?
   1. Burning material in a garbage can
   2. Smoke from a rag in a maintenance closet
   3. Smoldering sparks from a patient's mattress
   4. Flames emanating from a toaster in a pantry

9. What nursing intervention can give a patient a sense of control regarding personal safety? **Select all that apply.**
   1. _____ Inform the patient why an identification band should be worn.
   2. _____ Instruct the patient how to lock the wheels on a wheel chair.
   3. _____ Keep the patient's bed in the lowest position.
   4. _____ Teach the patient how to use the call bell.
   5. _____ Orient the patient to the environment.

10. A nurse is caring for a patient who has a vaginal radiation implant. What essential action should the nurse implement when caring for the patient?
   1. Maintain the patient in the semi-Fowler position.
   2. Talk while standing at the foot of the patient's bed.
   3. Have the patient wear a detection badge while receiving care.
   4. Wear a lead apron when providing direct nursing care to the patient.

11. A school nurse is planning a class about safety precautions for a group of parents who have children between the ages of 7 and 10 years. What information should the nurse include in the teaching plan? **Select all that apply.**
   1. _____ "Supervise stretching exercises before your child engages in physical activities."
   2. _____ "Check your child's toys to ensure that they are larger than a clenched fist."
   3. _____ "Select activities that are appropriate for your child's developmental level."
   4. _____ "Provide a four-point safety seat for your child when in the car."
   5. _____ "Ensure that your child wears a seat belt when in the car."

12. A nurse in the emergency department hears a patient and a family member arguing with each other in a room at the end of the unit. What should the nurse do **first**?
   1. Get another staff member and go to the room together.
   2. Have a security guard handle the situation.
   3. Ask what is going on and then set limits.
   4. Go to the room and attempt to intervene.

13. A primary health-care provider orders warm compresses to be applied to the site of an intravenous catheter that had become red and inflamed. What should the nurse explain to the patient is the desired outcome of this therapy?
   1. "The area will feel less tense, which will decrease the risk of bleeding."
   2. "Circulation to the area will increase, which will promote healing."
   3. "Circulation to the area will decrease, which will limit edema."
   4. "The area will feel numb, which will decrease discomfort."

14. A nurse is caring for a patient who has an order for a vest restraint. Which action should the nurse implement?
   1. Provide skin care every 3 hours.
   2. Tie the restraint to the bed frame.
   3. Check the restraint every 2 hours.
   4. Release the restraint every 4 hours.

15. A nurse is teaching a class on home safety to a group of parents of children younger than 4 years of age. Which intervention is essential that the nurse should include in the class?
   1. Cut up firm foods into half inch pieces.
   2. Ensure that crib slats are greater than three inches apart.
   3. Supervise balloon play and discard burst balloons immediately.
   4. Monitor toddlers when they eat marshmallows, popcorn, or grapes.

16. A nurse is teaching a group of high school students on the golf team how to provide for safety during an electrical storm. Which suggestion should be included in the program?
   1. Do not hold golf clubs.
   2. Take off shoes with cleats.
   3. Move toward water hazards.
   4. Seek shelter under the nearest tree.

17. A nurse is planning a class about safety precautions for a group of parents who have toddlers. What information should the nurse include in the teaching plan? **Select all that apply.**
   1. _____ Position them on the back when sleeping.
   2. _____ Attend toddlers when on elevated surfaces.
   3. _____ Use a rear-facing car seat until 4 years of age.
   4. _____ Keep plastic inserts in unused electrical outlets.
   5. _____ Turn pot handles toward the back of stove when cooking.

18. Which intervention is **most** effective in reducing the major cause of injury in the hospital setting for patients who are older adults?
    1. Assist all older adults with toileting activities.
    2. Elevate all bedside rails of older adults at night.
    3. Place a fall precautions sign on the door to a room with an older adult.
    4. Identify medications taken by an older adult that may increase the risk of falls.

19. A nurse just finished a complete bath for a patient with limited mobility. Which action is **most** important for the nurse to perform before leaving the bedside of the patient?
    1. Raise all of the bedside rails.
    2. Ensure that the water pitcher has fresh water.
    3. Lower the height of the bed to the lowest position.
    4. Position the bedpan in easy reach under the covers.

20. A nurse is caring for a patient who is in the intensive care unit. Which action should the nurse implement to prevent sensory overload? **Select all that apply.**
    1. _____ Organize care into blocks of time.
    2. _____ Provide objects that are pleasant to touch.
    3. _____ Maintain frequent meaningful interaction.
    4. _____ Medicate for pain immediately when it occurs.
    5. _____ Explain the meaning of sounds in the environment.

21. Which nursing intervention is **most** essential to provide for patient safety, regardless of the patient's individual health issue?
    1. Keep the patient's bed in the lowest position.
    2. Ensure the call bell is within reach.
    3. Raise the 4 side rails when in bed.
    4. Check the patient every 2 hours.

22. A nurse is caring for a patient who is hearing impaired and legally blind. What should the nurse do to prevent a sensory deficit? **Select all that apply.**
    1. _____ Encourage the patient to wear prescribed hearing aids.
    2. _____ Provide a telephone, radio, and talking books.
    3. _____ Encourage purchase of a talking watch.
    4. _____ Provide a foot bath and back massage.
    5. _____ Speak in a high tone of voice.

23. A nurse educator is preparing a health curriculum for high school students. Which content should be included in the program that addresses the leading cause of physical injury during adolescence?
    1. Driver education
    2. Anger management
    3. Alcohol and drug use
    4. Irresponsible water safety

24. A nurse is preparing a health promotion and illness prevention class for a group of parents of young school-aged children. Which information should the nurse include in the program to help prevent sensory disturbances in children in this age-group? **Select all that apply.**
    1. _____ Obtain rubella, mumps, and measles vaccinations at recommended ages.
    2. _____ Discourage sports that use sticks, such as hockey and lacrosse.
    3. _____ Seek regular eye examinations to screen for eye problems.
    4. _____ Allow use of pointed scissors only when sitting at a table.
    5. _____ Encourage the use of sunglasses with UV protection.

25. A nurse is caring for a 60-year-old adult who is a resident in a rehabilitation center recovering from a right-sided brain attack (cerebrovascular accident, stroke). The patient has orders for out of bed ambulating with assistance as tolerated. Which intervention is **most** important?
    1. Assessing balance
    2. Using a bed alarm
    3. Encouraging the use of a walker
    4. Teaching to rise slowly from a lying to sitting position

26. A nurse is caring for a patient who is blind. What should the nurse do to facilitate patient safety?
    1. Encourage the patient to have a bed bath rather than a shower.
    2. Walk about a foot ahead and have the patient grasp your arm.
    3. Provide a small light in the room and bathroom at night.
    4. Provide cold rather than hot drinks.

27. A nurse is caring for a patient who fell by the side of the bed when attempting to use the commode. What should the nurse do **first** when completing responsibilities associated with this situation?
    1. Initiate an incident report.
    2. Notify the nursing supervisor of the event.
    3. Document the incident in the patient's clinical record.
    4. Have a primary health-care provider examine the patient immediately.

28. Which nursing action is **most** important when ambulating a patient with a gait belt?
    1. Position yourself slightly in front of and next to the patient when ambulating a patient with a gait belt.
    2. Adjust the gait belt so that no fingers can be inserted between the belt and the patient's waist.
    3. Assess for activity intolerance while ambulating a patient with a gait belt.
    4. Hold the gait belt in the middle of the patient's back.

29. A school nurse is teaching a group of high school students about safety precautions. What should the nurse include in the teaching session that addresses the leading cause of accidental deaths in adolescents?
    1. Use a seat belt when riding in a car.
    2. Engage in sports that are within your physical abilities.
    3. Wear a life preserver when engaging in water-related activities.
    4. Resist peer pressure to participate in experimenting with illegal drugs.

30. A nurse is caring for a patient with wrist restraints. Which action is **most** important when caring for this patient?
    1. Release the restraints every 3 hours and provide skin care.
    2. Offer fluids and assist the patient to toilet each time the restraints are released.
    3. Check on the patient every hour and ensure that circulation is not impaired by the restraints.
    4. Ensure that every 48 hours the primary health-care provider assesses the need for the restraints.

31. A nurse working on the night shift in a long-term care facility identifies a small fire in a magazine rack in the corner of a community lounge. Because all of the residents are in their rooms, the nurse activates the fire alarm and then instructs staff members to close all doors on the unit. The nurse then obtains a type A extinguisher to fight the fire. Place the following steps in the order in which they should be implemented.
    1. Pull the pin on the extinguisher.
    2. Drag the extinguisher on the floor to the area of the fire.
    3. Aim the nozzle of the extinguisher at the base of the flames.
    4. Squeeze the handles together to discharge water from the extinguisher.
    5. Sweep the nozzle of the extinguisher back and forth at the base of the flames.
    Answer _____

32. A nurse is preparing a safety program for parents about accidental poisoning. What information should the nurse include concerning what to do in the event a toddler ingests a poison?
    1. Have the child drink salt water.
    2. Administer Ipecac immediately.
    3. Take the child to an emergency department.
    4. Seek guidance from a poison control center.

33. A nurse is completing a patient assessment for the purpose of determining factors that place the patient at risk for falls. Which factor should cause the **most** concern when completing this assessment?
    1. Uses a walker
    2. Has a history of falls
    3. Takes a diuretic twice a day
    4. Has a urinary retention catheter

34. A school nurse is teaching a third-grade class about safety precautions. What should the nurse include in the teaching session? **Select all that apply.**
    1. _____ Run in the opposite direction if approached by a stranger to go someplace.
    2. _____ Take a bicycle safety course when you get a two-wheeled bicycle.
    3. _____ Get instructions before using equipment for the first time.
    4. _____ Use a regular car seat belt when you reach 50 pounds.
    5. _____ Stop, drop, and roll if your clothes are on fire.

35. A nurse is preparing a program regarding health promotion for individuals who are middle-aged adults. Which information is **most** important to include regarding the prevention of injury?
    1. Avoiding alcohol when planning to drive
    2. Learning to use meditation to reduce stress
    3. Doing warm-up exercises before engaging in sports
    4. Maintaining an exercise program to increase endurance

36. A nurse is teaching a health promotion class for a group of recently retired older adults. Which information should be included to help reduce the risk of the major cause of physical injury in older adults?
    1. Remove throw rugs from the home.
    2. Look both ways before crossing a street.
    3. Do warm-up exercises before engaging in sports.
    4. Read the label of an over-the-counter drug before taking it.

37. A nurse is teaching a group of children about the importance of firearm safety because of the severity of unintentional firearm injuries involving children. Place the steps in order that children should take when they see a gun.
1. Tell an adult.
2. Don't touch it.
3. Leave the area.
4. Stop the activity.
5. Identify the presence of a gun.
Answer _____

38. A nurse is teaching a class for a community group about how to prevent the most common cause of fatal accidents in the home. Which information is **most** important to include that addresses this concern?
1. Remove scatter rugs from the home.
2. Check for the presence of lead paint.
3. Use gates at the bottom and top of stairs.
4. Store cleaning products in a locked cabinet.

39. An older adult who has left-sided weakness as the result of a brain attack (stroke, cerebrovascular accident) has the need to urinate several times during the night. What should the nurse do to ensure patient safety?
1. Encourage the use a bedpan at night.
2. Keep the light on in the room at night.
3. Assist the patient to a commode at night.
4. Encourage the patient to use a walker at night.

40. An older adult is admitted to the hospital in heart failure. The primary health-care provider orders an IV of dextrose 5% water to infuse at 50 mL/hour. The nurse uses a microdrip infusion set that has a drop factor of 60. At what rate should the nurse administer the intravenous solution? Record your answer using a whole number.
Answer _____ drops per minute

41. A nurse is teaching a class to parents of toddlers about how to reduce the risk of suffocation, asphyxiation, or drowning. What information is essential to include in this program?
1. Ensure that slats of cribs are more than 2⅜ inches wide.
2. Provide toys that are at least 2 inches in diameter.
3. Keep venetian blind cords out of reach.
4. Use only light blankets when sleeping.

42. A public health nurse is visiting a patient recently discharged from the hospital to the home. The patient has a history of violence. What is **most** important for the nurse to do when caring for this patient?
1. Apply restraints if the patient engages in threatening behavior.
2. Administer a prescribed sedative before providing patient care.
3. Identify when the level of anxiety is elevating.
4. Use gentle touch communicating acceptance.

43. A nurse is transferring a weak, older adult from a bed to a toilet using the apparatus in the illustration. What is the **most** important reason why a nurse uses this device rather than a gait belt to transfer a patient to a toilet?
1. Encourage independence
2. Protect the nurse from injury
3. Promote muscle development
4. Support psychological well-being

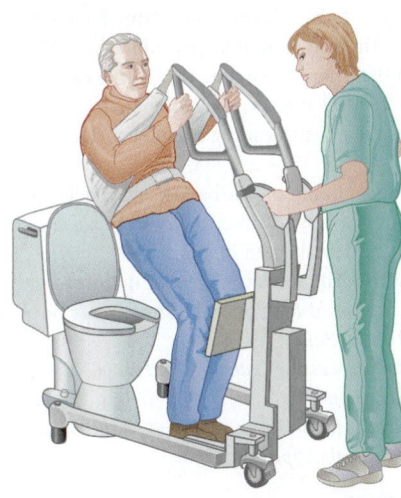

44. A patient is confused and trying to pull out an indwelling urinary catheter. The nurse tried various interventions to protect the patient from pulling out the catheter to no avail. The nurse notifies the primary health-care provider and asks for an order for a restraint. What type of restraint should the nurse anticipate will be ordered?
1. Belt
2. Mitt
3. Vest
4. Wrist

45. A nurse is teaching a group of older adults about safety precautions. What instruction should the nurse give them to prevent the leading cause of injuries in older adults?
1. Have your vision evaluated yearly.
2. Limit drinking alcohol to one glass a day.
3. Rise slowly when moving from a sitting to a standing position.
4. Wash your hands with an antimicrobial soap several times a day.

REVIEW ANSWERS

1. ANSWER: 2.

Rationales:

1. Avoiding small objects and providing toys that are bigger than a clenched fist help prevent airway obstruction accidents. Although the risk for choking is the greatest between 6 months and 3 years of age, it is not the leading cause of accidental deaths in infants.

2. The leading cause of death in infants is motor vehicle accidents. A four-point infant car seat provides the necessary support to help limit injuries during a motor vehicle accident. The seat should be placed in the back seat of the car with the infant facing the rear of the car.

3. Although this intervention will help limit injuries from falls, falls are not the leading cause of accidental deaths in infants.

4. Placing an infant on the back to sleep helps prevent sudden infant death syndrome; however, this is not the leading cause of accidental death in infants.

TEST-TAKING TIP: Identify the word in the stem that sets a priority. The word *leading* in the stem sets a priority.

Content Area: Safety

Integrated Processes: Teaching/Learning; Nursing Process: Implementation

Client Need: Health Promotion and Maintenance

Cognitive Level: Application

2. ANSWER: 2.

Rationales:

1. These actions should take place at least every 2, not 3, hours and more frequently if is determined to be necessary. In addition, when restraints are released, they should be removed and skin care provided.

2. This helps to prevent injury to the wrists and is the first thing that the nurse should do of the options presented.

3. Three finger-widths would make the restraint too loose. Two finger-widths are sufficient to ensure that the patient's circulation is not impaired and yet tight enough for the restraints to remain secured around the patient's wrists.

4. A slip, not square, knot should be used to permit a quick release of the ties in the event of an emergency.

TEST-TAKING TIP: Identify the word in the stem that sets a priority. The word *first* in the stem sets a priority. Identify the clang association. The words *apply wrist restraints* in the stem and *applying wrist restraints* in option 2 is a clang association. Examine option 2 carefully.

Content Area: Safety

Integrated Processes: Nursing Process: Implementation

Client Need: Safe and Effective Care Environment; Safety and Infection Control

Cognitive Level: Application

3. ANSWER: 4.

Rationales:

1. It is not necessary to position the chair as close as possible to the patient's bed. Mechanical lifts are designed to move a patient completely across a room safely.

2. The sling remains under the patient after the transfer. It would be difficult or even impossible to remove and then reposition the sling if the patient were obese or immobile.

3. The sling should start at the shoulders and end at the knees. This completely supports the patient for the transfer. If it is too high, the patient could slide out from the bottom of the sling. If it is too low, the patient could slide out from the top of the sling.

4. This is correct. When the longer belts/chains are attached to the bottom of the sling and the shorter belts/chains are attached to the top of the sling, the patient will be raised to a sitting position when the lift raises the sling and the patient up and off the bed.

Content Area: Safety

Integrated Processes: Nursing Process: Implementation

Client Need: Safe and Effective Care Environment; Safety and Infection Control

Cognitive Level: Analysis

4. ANSWER: 4.

Rationales:

1. Dark-tinted eyeglasses will not benefit a patient who "can't see anything."

2. Keeping a light on in the room may help a patient with partial vision, but it will be insignificant for a patient who "can't see anything."

3. Closing window blinds will be beneficial for a patient with partial vision who is affected by glare; this intervention will not benefit a patient who "can't see anything."

4. A patient who is in a strange environment and who has a visual impairment is at an increased risk for falls. The patient should seek assistance with transfers and ambulating until the patient feels comfortable engaging in these activities and the nurse determines that the patient is safe to perform this activity unassisted.

TEST-TAKING TIP: Identify the option with a specific determiner. Option 2 contains the specific determiner *all.* Identify the unique option. Option 4 is unique because it is the only option that involves another person and it is the only option that does not engage in adjusting the light in the room. Identify options that are equally plausible. Option 1 and 3 are equally plausible. Both reduce light that meets the eye. Option 1 is no better than option 3. Eliminate both from further consideration.

Content Area: Safety

Integrated Processes: Communication/Documentation; Nursing Process: Implementation

Client Need: Safe and Effective Care Environment; Safety and Infection Control

Cognitive Level: Application

5. ANSWER: 4, 3, 1, 2, 5.

Rationales:

4. A bed exiting alarm device will signal caregivers when the patient attempts to exit the bed. These devices do not curtail the patient's movement but will alert staff members that the patient needs supervision. This is a safety device that does not require an order from a primary health-care provider.

3. Although four side rails will curtail the patient to the bed, the patient is still able to turn and sit up with ease.

1. A cloth vest permits turning from side to side and sitting up but physically restricts the patient to the bed by the use of straps tied to the bed frame.

2. Two wrist restraints curtail the movement of the upper extremities and prevent turning from side to side; also, they curtail the patient to the bed because the straps are tied to the bed frame.

5. This is the most restrictive physical restraint because the extremities are for all practical purposes immobilized; all four extremities are tied to the bed frame.

Content Area: Safety
Integrated Processes: Nursing Process: Analysis
Client Need: Safe and Effective Care Environment; Safety and Infection Control
Cognitive Level: Analysis

6. **ANSWER: 4.**
   Rationales:
   1. Expecting a family member to remain with the patient every night is an unrealistic suggestion. The nurse, not the patient's family members, is responsible for maintaining patient safety.
   2. A chemical restraint should be used as a last resort. Patients have a right to have the least restrictive restraint used to promote safety.
   3. A vest restraint is too restrictive a device to use before a less restrictive method is proven unsuccessful.
   4. **A bed-exiting device (e.g., position sensor on the leg, weight sensor under the mattress of a bed) should be used to alert caregivers when the patient is attempting to exit the bed. A health team member should immediately assist the patient and maintain safety when the alarm sounds.**
   TEST-TAKING TIP: Identify the option that contains a specific determiner. Option 1 contains the word *every*, which is a specific determiner. Identify equally plausible options. Option 2 (chemical) and 3 (physical) are both restraints. Option 1 is no better than option 2. Eliminate both from consideration.

   Content Area: Safety
   Integrated Processes: Nursing Process: Implementation
   Client Need: Safe and Effective Care Environment; Safety and Infection Control
   Cognitive Level: Application

7. **ANSWER: 1.**
   Rationales:
   1. **The patient's serum sodium (expected range 135 to 145 mEq/L) and potassium (expected range 3.5 to 5.0 mEq/L) are both low, which precipitate muscle weakness. The strength of the patient's legs should be assessed to determine if the patient can bear the body's weight. While the patient is lying in bed, the patient can be asked to exert pressure against the nurse's hands that are pressed against the soles of the patient's feet. The nurse should assess the strength of the pressure exerted by the patient. While the patient is sitting on the side of the bed, the patient can be instructed to extend the knee of one leg and hold it in extension for 15 seconds. Then the other leg should be assessed in the same manner. If the patient can hold the legs in extension, then the patient probably has the strength to bear the body's weight.**
   2. This assessment is incomplete. When assessing the blood pressure to determine a patient's risk of falls, the nurse should obtain orthostatic blood pressures. The patient's blood pressure should be obtained while lying in bed, sitting

up, and when standing. The patient is experiencing orthostatic hypotension when the blood pressure drops to the level where it causes transient hypotension resulting in lightheadedness and dizziness (syncope).
   3. The administration of oxygen is a dependent function of a nurse. Nurses may administer oxygen in an emergency situation, but this is not an emergency situation.
   4. It is not necessary to interrupt the intravenous infusion. A patient can be ambulated safely while receiving intravenous fluid therapy.

   Content Area: Safety
   Integrated Processes: Nursing Process: Implementation
   Client Need: Safe and Effective Care Environment; Safety and Infection Control
   Cognitive Level: Analysis

8. **ANSWER: 4.**
   Rationales:
   1. Material in a garbage can usually is paper or textiles; these items are extinguished with a type A or type ABC fire extinguisher.
   2. A maintenance closet commonly contains flammable liquids; flammable materials are extinguished with a type B or type ABC fire extinguisher.
   3. A mattress consists of cloth covered in plastic; these materials are extinguished with a type A or type ABC fire extinguisher.
   4. **A toaster is an electrical appliance; fire involving live electrical wires or equipment is extinguished with a type C or type ABC fire extinguisher.**

   Content Area: Safety
   Integrated Processes: Nursing Process: Implementation
   Client Need: Safe and Effective Care Environment; Safety and Infection Control
   Cognitive Level: Analysis

9. **ANSWER: 2, 4, 5.**
   Rationales:
   1. Although wearing an identification band will provide for patient safety, it does not give the patient a sense of control.
   2. **This information allows the patient to ensure that the wheels of a wheel chair are locked.**
   3. Keeping the patient's bed in the lowest position will not give the patient a sense of control.
   4. **The ability to call for help when needed gives the patient a sense of control.**
   5. **Having an understanding of the environment (e.g., how to use a call bell, how to raise and lower the bed, and how to use the side rails when turning or transferring) gives the patient a sense of control.**

   Content Area: Safety
   Integrated Processes: Teaching/Learning; Nursing Process: Implementation
   Client Need: Safe and Effective Care Environment; Safety and Infection Control
   Cognitive Level: Analysis

10. **ANSWER: 4.**
    Rationales:
    1. The semi-Fowler position may result in dislodgement of the implant, inappropriately exposing the nurse and

patient to the source of radiation. The supine position will help maintain the implant in the vaginal vault.

2. When in the room the nurse should stand across the room or at the head of the bed when giving care. When possible, the nurse should talk with the patient through an intercom outside the room or from the doorway. These actions adhere to the principles of distance and shielding.

3. The nurse, not the patient, should wear a radiation film badge.

4. **A lead apron provides a barrier between the nurse and the source of the radiation; it adheres to the principle of shielding.**

TEST-TAKING TIP: Identify the word in the stem that sets a priority. The word *essential* in the stem sets a priority.

Content Area: Safety
Integrated Processes: Nursing Process: Implementation
Client Need: Safe and Effective Care Environment; Safety and Infection Control
Cognitive Level: Application

11. ANSWER: 1, 3, 5.

Rationales:

1. **School-aged children become more involved in physical activities and team sports as they progress through school. Stretching exercises before physical activities help to limit musculoskeletal injuries.**

2. Checking that toys are smaller than a clenched fist is appropriate for infants, toddlers, and preschoolers. The risk for choking is greatest between 6 months and 3 years of age.

3. **Children's physical skills vary depending on the developmental age and individual abilities; these factors must be considered before engaging in activities such as skiing, bicycle riding, and skate boarding.**

4. A four-point safety car seat is appropriate for infants, toddlers, and preschoolers. School-aged children usually transition to using a booster seat or a regular car seat belt.

5. **Motor vehicle collisions are the highest cause of accidental deaths in school-aged children. Wearing a seat belt in a car helps to reduce morbidity and mortality.**

TEST-TAKING TIP: Identify options that are opposites. Options 4 and 5 are opposites. More often than not, a correct answer is one of the opposites.

Content Area: Safety
Integrated Processes: Teaching/Learning; Nursing Process: Planning
Client Need: Safe and Effective Care Environment; Safety and Infection Control
Cognitive Level: Application

12. ANSWER: 1.

Rationales:

1. **The situation needs to be assessed, but a health team member should never enter a volatile situation alone. When entering the room the health team members should stand between the patient/visitor and the door.**

2. This is premature and may cause the situation to escalate

3. The nurse is in a vulnerable, unsafe position when going to a volatile situation alone. Setting limits may be unnecessary or may escalate an already volatile situation. Setting limits should not be attempted without adequate staff members readily available.

4. The nurse is in a vulnerable, unsafe position when going to a volatile situation alone. Attempting to intervene may result in harm to the nurse.

TEST-TAKING TIP: Identify the word in the stem that sets a priority. The word *first* in the stem sets a priority. Identify options that are opposites. Option 1 and 4 are opposites. In option 1 the nurse gets another staff member to go to the room together. In option 4 the nurse goes to the room alone.

Content Area: Safety
Integrated Processes: Nursing Process: Implementation
Client Need: Safe and Effective Care Environment; Safety and Infection Control
Cognitive Level: Application

13. ANSWER: 2.

Rationales:

1. The application of heat causes vasodilation, which may increase the potential for bleeding. Cold applications cause vasoconstriction, which decreases the risk for bleeding.

2. **Heat causes vasodilation, which increases circulation and capillary permeability in the area; this brings oxygen, nutrients, and WBCs to the area and removes toxic wastes.**

3. Circulation to the area decreases with an application of cold, not heat.

4. The application of cold, not heat, influences nerve endings and precipitates an anesthetic effect, which decreases pain.

TEST-TAKING TIP: Identify options that are opposites. Options 2 and 3 are opposites.

Content Area: Safety
Integrated Processes: Communication/Documentation; Nursing Process: Evaluation
Client Need: Safe and Effective Care Environment; Safety and Infection Control
Cognitive Level: Application

14. ANSWER: 2.

Rationales:

1. Skin care should be provided every 2, not 3, hours when a restraint is removed and range-of-motion exercises provided.

2. **A restraint should be tied to the bed frame. If tied to the bed rail the patient may be injured or the restraint may become too tight and impair respirations when the rail is lowered. If the rail is raised, the restraint will become too loose.**

3. A patient with a restraint should be checked every 30 minutes, not every 2 hours, to ensure patient safety. The restraint should not be too tight or too loose. The nurse should check the patient's circulation and ensure that there is room to insert 2 finger-widths between the restraint and the patient.

4. Restraints should be released every 2, not 4, hours so that the patient can receive exercise and skin care.

TEST-TAKING TIP: Identify the unique option. Option 2 is the only option without a time frame. In addition, it is the only option that does not end with the word *hours*. Identify options with specific determiners. Options 1, 3, and 4 contain the word *every*, which is a specific determiner. Rarely are options with specific determiners the correct answer.

Content Area: Safety
Integrated Processes: Nursing Process: Implementation
Client Need: Safe and Effective Care Environment; Safety and Infection Control
Cognitive Level: Application

15. ANSWER: 3.
Rationales:
1. Food should be cut up into tiny, not half inch, pieces. Food items are the main cause of nonfatal choking events in children younger than 4 years of age.
2. Crib slats should be less than 2⅜ inches (6 cm) apart and the mattress should fit the bed frame snuggly. This prevents an infant or child from getting the head caught between slats, which could cut off the airway, or from suffocation between the mattress and bed frame.
3. Balloon play should be supervised. Latex balloons and plastic bags are the main cause of suffocation deaths in young children.
4. Young children should not eat marshmallows, popcorn, grapes, nuts, hard candy, or chewing gum because of the increased risk of a choking event in this age-group. These types of food can obstruct the small airway of a child.
TEST-TAKING TIP: Identify the word in the stem that sets a priority. The word *essential* in the stem sets a priority. Identify equally plausible options. Option 1 and 4 both have to do with food. Option 1 is no better than option 4. Eliminate options 1 and 4 from further consideration. Identify the obscure clang association. The word *essential* in the stem and the word *immediately* in option 3 are both words that indicate a priority, a necessity or a fundamental element, and is a clang association.
Content Area: Safety
Integrated Processes: Teaching/Learning; Nursing Process: Implementation
Client Need: Safe and Effective Care Environment; Safety and Infection Control
Cognitive Level: Application

16. ANSWER: 1.
Rationales:
1. Objects with metal parts, such as golf clubs and fishing gear, should be dropped immediately because they attract lightening. Then the person should immediately seek shelter in a building.
2. It is not necessary to take off shoes with cleats because most cleats are hard plastic, not metal.
3. Water hazards generally are in open places, which should be avoided. A standing person in an open place may attract lightening.
4. Tall objects attract lightening. Trees should be avoided, especially if they are not around other trees.
TEST-TAKING TIP: Identify the clang association. The word *golf* in the stem and in option 1 is a clang association. Identify the unique option. Option 1 is unique because it is an instruction that tells the students *what not to do*. Options 2, 3, and 4 instruct students regarding what they *should do*.
Content Area: Safety
Integrated Processes: Teaching/Learning; Nursing Process: Implementation

Client Need: Safe and Effective Care Environment; Safety and Infection Control
Cognitive Level: Application

17. ANSWER: 2, 4, 5.
Rationales:
1. Positioning on the back when sleeping is recommended for infants, not toddlers, because it decreases the risk of sudden infant death syndrome. Toddlers have the ability to change position and turn from front to back and back to front when in bed.
2. Toddlers can be rambunctious and lack judgment because of limited experiences; their position should be guarded/supported when on elevated surfaces (e.g., changing tables, playground equipment) to prevent falls.
3. Toddlers can transition to forward-facing car seats when they are 2 years of age or they reach the maximum weight specified by the car seat manufacturer.
4. Electrical outlets stimulate the curiosity of toddlers; plastic inserts keep toddlers from inserting fingers or objects into outlets.
5. Toddlers like to role play the activities of adults; reachable pot handles may result in accidental burns.
TEST-TAKING TIP: Identify the clang association. The word *toddler* in the stem and in option 2 is a clang association.
Content Area: Safety
Integrated Processes: Teaching/Learning; Nursing Process: Planning
Client Need: Safe and Effective Care Environment; Safety and Infection Control
Cognitive Level: Application

18. ANSWER: 4.
Rationales:
1. This action is not patient centered. Not all older adults need to be assisted with toileting activities. This promotes dependence and violates the patient's right to privacy if assistance is unnecessary.
2. This action is not patient centered. Not all older adults need all side rails raised at night. Side rails are considered a restraint when all of them are raised. Unless it is requested by the patient, the use of all side rails requires an order from a primary health-care provider for a specific reason that is documented.
3. This action is not patient centered. Not all older adults require fall precautions beyond the average interventions implemented to maintain physical safety for all adult patients.
4. Assessment is the first step in the nursing process. Assessments should be completed before making a nursing diagnosis and planning and implementing care. Older adults often experience one or more chronic illness and receive a variety of medications. Polypharmacy is a risk factor for adverse reactions and drug interactions that may cause an older adult to fall.
TEST-TAKING TIP: Identify the word in the stem that sets a priority. The word *most* in the stem sets a priority. Identify options with specific determiners. Options 1 and 2 contain the word *all*, which is a specific determiner. More often than not, options with specific determiners are distractors. Identify options that deny patient's feelings, concerns, and

needs. Options 1 and 2 deny patient's the right to be independent. Identify the option that is patient centered. Option 4 is patient centered because it involves an assessment specific to the patient. Identify the unique option. Option 4 is unique. Options 1, 2, and 3 are interventions designed to reduce a fall. Option 4 is the only option that is an assessment. Assessment is the first step of the nursing process.

Content Area: *Safety*
Integrated Processes: *Nursing Process: Assessment*
Client Need: *Safe and Effective Care Environment; Safety and Infection Control*
Cognitive Level: *Application*

19. **ANSWER: 3.**

Rationales:

1. Raising all the side rails on a bed is considered a restraint. It can be requested by the patient or ordered by the primary health-care provider if necessary. This order must be rewritten every 24 hours. A progress note must address the reasons for the restraint and what other measures were tried that were ineffective.
2. Although it is important for a patient to have fresh water and ice if preferred and permitted, it is not as important as another option.
3. **All patients should have their beds maintained in the lowest position unless a member of the health-care team is providing direct care. This supports patient safety. It enables mobile patients to more easily enter and exit the bed. Also, if a patient should fall out of bed accidentally, the bed is closer to the floor, which may minimize patient injury.**
4. A patient with limited mobility generally will not be able to use a bedpan unassisted.

TEST-TAKING TIP: Identify the word in the stem that sets a priority. The word *most* in the stem sets a priority. Identify the option with a specific determiner. Option 1 contains the word *all,* which is a specific determiner.

Content Area: *Safety*
Integrated Processes: *Nursing Process: Implementation*
Client Need: *Safe and Effective Care Environment; Safety and Infection Control*
Cognitive Level: *Application*

20. **ANSWER: 1, 4, 5.**

Rationales:

1. **Organizing care into blocks of time minimizes the need to interrupt rest or sleep to complete a task.**
2. Touching pleasant objects is an intervention to prevent sensory deficit, not overload.
3. The patient should not be awakened or rest interrupted to engage the patient in conversation. This is an intervention that is used to prevent sensory deficit, not overload.
4. **Pain is a contributing factor to interrupted rest and sleep. The patient in pain should receive care that addresses the patient's pain appropriately.**
5. **Sounds that are not understood can be frightening. When a person is frightened, the patient often is afraid to sleep, which contributes to sensory overload. When sounds are understood, the patient can organize them mentally, and the sounds are less confusing and more easily overlooked and disregarded.**

TEST-TAKING TIP: Identify opposite options. Options 1 and 3 are opposites. Option 1 attempts to minimize the frequency of interactions and option 3 attempts to increase the frequency of interactions. Eliminate one of these options.

Content Area: *Safety*
Integrated Processes: *Nursing Process: Implementation*
Client Need: *Safe and Effective Care Environment; Safety and Infection Control*
Cognitive Level: *Application*

21. **ANSWER: 1.**

Rationales:

1. **There is always a potential to fall even when in bed; keeping the bed in the lowest position allows the feet to touch the floor before standing and if a fall occurs, the potential for injury probably will be less than from a higher height.**
2. Although important, not all patients have the physical or cognitive abilities to use a call bell.
3. The use of 4 side rails is not indicated for all patients; in addition, it may lead to falls if the patient attempts to climb over the rails. Four elevated side rails constitute a restraint unless the use of four rails is requested by the patient or ordered by a primary health-care provider.
4. The frequency of checking a patient should be individualized; some patients may need more frequent or continuous monitoring.

TEST-TAKING TIP: Identify the key word in the stem that sets a priority. The word *most* is the word in the stem that sets a priority. Identify the option that denies a patient's rights. Option 3 denies the patient's right not to be restrained. When all four side rails are raised, it is considered a restraint and requires an order by the primary health-care provider or the patient's consent.

Content Area: *Safety*
Integrated Processes: *Nursing Process: Implementation*
Client Need: *Safe and Effective Care Environment; Safety and Infection Control*
Cognitive Level: *Application*

22. **ANSWER: 1, 2, 3, 4.**

Rationales:

1. **Hearing aids will enhance hearing, which should help prevent the sense of isolation.**
2. **A telephone, radio, and talking books will help to stimulate the patient (e.g., hearing, thinking, socialization).**
3. **When a button is pushed, a talking watch reports the time. This will help to keep the patient oriented to time, which is stimulating.**
4. **A foot bath and back massage will provide for tactile interaction with the caregiver, increasing stimulation.**
5. Hearing impaired people tend to have a reduced ability to hear high pitched tones. The nurse should use a lower tone when speaking with a patient who is hearing impaired.

TEST-TAKING TIP: Identify the clang association. The word *hearing* in the stem and in option 1 is a clang association. Examine option 1 carefully.

Content Area: *Safety*
Integrated Processes: *Communication/Documentation; Nursing Process: Implementation*

Client Need: Psychosocial Integrity
Cognitive Level: Application

23. ANSWER: 3.
    Rationales:
    1. Motor vehicle accidents are the leading cause of death, not injury, during adolescence.
    2. Although a class in anger management is important, anger is not the leading cause of physical injury in adolescence.
    3. Alcohol and drug use is the root cause of most physical injuries that occur in adolescence. Alcohol and drugs impair judgment, leading to reckless driving (leading cause of death in adolescence); fuels anger, which can lead to homicide (second leading cause of death in adolescence); and irresponsible behavior regarding water sports (drowning and paralysis).
    4. Although a class about responsible water safety is important, drowning and diving incidents are not the leading cause of injury in adolescence.
    TEST-TAKING TIP: Identify the word in the stem that sets a priority. The word *leading* in the stem sets a priority. Identify the unique option. Option 3 is unique. It is the only option with two parts separated by the word *and.*
    Content Area: Safety
    Integrated Processes: Teaching/Learning; Nursing Process: Planning
    Client Need: Health Promotion and Maintenance
    Cognitive Level: Application

24. ANSWER: 1, 3, 5.
    Rationales:
    1. Rubella, mumps, and measles can cause hearing loss. Children should be immunized against these diseases.
    2. Children can engage in sports that involve sticks if they are taught the proper use of sports equipment and wear protective gear (e.g., helmets, eye shields).
    3. Regular eye examinations help identify problems early so that they can be treated.
    4. Young school-aged children always should use round, not sharp, tipped scissors.
    5. Sunglasses with UV protection help avoid damage from ultraviolet rays. In addition, the nurse should encourage parents to teach their children to never look directly into the sun.
    TEST-TAKING TIP: Identify the specific determiner in an option. The word *only* in option 4 is a specific determiner. Rarely are options with specific determiners correct answers. Eliminate option 4 from further consideration.
    Content Area: Safety
    Integrated Processes: Teaching/Learning; Nursing Process: Planning
    Client Need: Health Promotion and Maintenance
    Cognitive Level: Application

25. ANSWER: 1.
    Rationales:
    1. Assessment is the first step of the nursing process. The nurse must first assess the patient for the presence of problems with strength and balance before moving a patient out of bed. People with problems with balance may not be able to maintain the sitting position while sitting on the side of the bed.

    2. A bed alarm is unnecessary. There is no information in the stem that indicates that the patient is confused or unwilling to call for assistance when getting out of bed.
    3. This is implementing an intervention before the patient's needs are assessed.
    4. Although this should be done, it is not as critical as another option. Even though a patient may become dizzy when moving from a lying to sitting position, the patient is in bed and has little risk of falling out of bed. The upper rails should be raised to provide for the patient's safety.
    TEST-TAKING TIP: Identify the word in the stem that sets a priority. The word *most* in the stem sets a priority. Identify the option that is unique. Option 1 is the only option that is an assessment. Options 2, 3, and 4 identify actions to prevent a fall.
    Content Area: Safety
    Integrated Processes: Nursing Process: Implementation
    Client Need: Safe and Effective Care Environment; Safety and Infection Control
    Cognitive Level: Application

26. ANSWER: 2.
    Rationales:
    1. With guidance or supervision, a blind patient can shower safely.
    2. This is the proper way to assist a blind patient with ambulation. By walking slightly ahead and with the patient holding the nurse's arm, the nurse is able to guide the patient around obstacles.
    3. The patient is blind. A nightlight will not help a blind patient see.
    4. Blind patients have a right to have hot drinks, such as coffee, tea, or soup. With guidance, a blind patient can be instructed regarding the location of hot drinks. In addition, suggesting the use of a commuter cup is a reasonable accommodation to help prevent spilling a hot drink, which may cause a burn.
    Content Area: Safety
    Integrated Processes: Nursing Process: Implementation
    Client Need: Safe and Effective Care Environment; Safety and Infection Control
    Cognitive Level: Application

27. ANSWER: 4.
    Rationales:
    1. This is not the priority intervention when a patient falls. However, this should be done eventually.
    2. Although a nursing supervisor should be notified, it is not the first nursing responsibility associated with a patient falling.
    3. This is not the priority intervention when a patient falls. However, eventually the incident should be documented on the patient's clinical record.
    4. This is the first action that the nurse should implement. The patient needs to be examined by a primary health-care provider to ensure that the patient has not sustained an injury.
    TEST-TAKING TIP: Identify the words in the stem and an option that is a clang association. The word *first* in the stem and *immediately* in option 4 is an obscure clang. These words are closely related because they both are associated with the concept of a priority.

Content Area: Safety
Integrated Processes: Nursing Process: Implementation
Client Need: Safe and Effective Care Environment; Management of care
Cognitive Level: Application

28. ANSWER: 3.
Rationales:
1. The care giver should walk next to and slightly behind, not in front of, the patient being ambulated with a gait belt. This enables the caregiver to hold the belt handles, one arm around the patient's back with the hand grasping the handle on the far side of the patient and the other hand grasping the handle of the belt closest to the caregiver.
2. A belt this tight may cause discomfort and impair breathing. Three fingers should be able to be positioned between the belt and the patient.
3. Patients who need a gait belt when being ambulated generally have impaired balance or are weak and, therefore, must be assessed for clinical indicators of activity intolerance. It is not acceptable to just make this assessment after the completion of ambulation.
4. Holding a gait belt just at the location of the patient's back does not provide leverage and control of the patient's stability.
TEST-TAKING TIP: Identify the word in the stem that sets a priority. The word *most* in the stem sets a priority. Identify clang associations. The words *ambulating a patient with a gait belt* in the stem and in options 1 and 3 are clang associations. Identify the option that is unique. Option 3 is the only option that is an evaluation of the patient's response to the activity. Options 1, 2, and 4 are actions that violate principles associated with ambulation of a patient with a gait belt. Examine option 3 carefully.
Content Area: Safety
Integrated Processes: Nursing Process: Evaluation
Client Need: Safe and Effective Care Environment; Safety and Infection Control
Cognitive Level: Application

29. ANSWER: 1.
Rationales:
1. Motor vehicle accidents are the leading cause of death in the adolescent age group. Many adolescents believe that they are invincible and do not wear seat belts when riding in a car. Seat belts do limit morbidity and mortality associated with motor vehicle accidents.
2. Although this is appropriate advice, sports related injuries are not the leading cause of accidental deaths in adolescents.
3. Although this may be advisable, water-related accidents are not the leading cause of accidental deaths in adolescents.
4. Although this is excellent advice, the use of illegal drugs is not the leading cause of accidental deaths in adolescents. Role-playing appropriate behaviors is more beneficial than giving advice.
TEST-TAKING TIP: Identify the word in the stem that sets a priority. The word *leading* in the stem sets a priority.
Content Area: Safety
Integrated Processes: Teaching/Learning; Nursing Process: Implementation

Client Need: Health Promotion and Maintenance
Cognitive Level: Application

30. ANSWER: 2.
Rationales:
1. Restraints must be released every 2, not 3, hours.
2. When a restraint is removed every 2 hours, the nurse should assess for the presence of edema, capillary refill, sensation, function, skin integrity, and erythema. In addition, the patient should be offered fluids and the opportunity to go to the bathroom. Finally, skin care and range-of-motion exercises should be provided and the patient's position changed before restrains are reapplied.
3. Circulation should be checked every 30 minutes, not every hour. The restraint is removed every 2 hours.
4. A primary health-care provider must renew the order for restraints every 24 hours. In addition, a progress note should indicate why the restraint is still needed.
TEST-TAKING TIP: Identify the word in the stem that sets a priority. The word *most* in the stem sets a priority. Identify the option that is unique. Option 2 is the only option that does not indicate a time frame. Identify the options with specific determiners. Options 1 and 4 contain the word *every*, which is a specific determiner. Rarely is an option with a specific determiner a correct answer.
Content Area: Safety
Integrated Processes: Nursing Process: Implementation
Client Need: Safe and Effective Care Environment; Safety and Infection Control
Cognitive Level: Application

31. ANSWER: 2, 1, 3, 4, 5.
Rationales:
2. An extinguisher can be heavy and it is an acceptable practice to drag a fire extinguisher on the floor to the site of a fire.
1. Follow the acronym PASS. Pulling the pin between the handles is the first step when using an extinguisher and prepares the extinguisher for use.
3. Follow the acronym PASS. Aiming the nozzle of the extinguisher at the base of the flames is the second step when using an extinguisher. The base of a fire is the source of the flames.
4. Follow the acronym PASS. Squeezing the handles together to discharge water from the extinguisher is the third step when using an extinguisher.
5. Follow the acronym PASS. Sweeping the nozzle of the extinguisher back and forth across the base of the flames is the fourth step in using an extinguisher. This ensures that water from the extinguisher makes contact with the entire source of the fire.
Content Area: Safety
Integrated Processes: Nursing Process: Planning
Client Need: Safe and Effective Care Environment; Safety and Infection Control
Cognitive Level: Analysis

32. ANSWER: 4.
Rationales:
1. Salt water induces vomiting. The ingested poison may cause additional damage to the esophagus and mouth if vomiting is induced.

2. Ipecac is an emetic that induces vomiting. The ingested poison may cause additional damage to the esophagus and mouth if vomiting is induced.

3. This action could delay an immediate response that may help minimize a negative consequence.

4. Poison control centers provide immediate instructions regarding what to do for the specific poison ingested. **Never employ a home remedy without directions from a poison control center.**

TEST-TAKING TIP: Identify the clang association. The words *poisoning* and *poison* in the stem and the word *poison* in option 4 are clang associations. Examine an option with a clang association carefully.

Content Area: Safety
Integrated Processes: Teaching/Learning; Nursing Process: Planning
Client Need: Safe and Effective Care Environment; Safety and Infection Control
Cognitive Level: Application

33. **ANSWER: 2.**
Rationales:

1. Although a patient using a walker is a concern in relation to safety, it is a less significant predictor of the potential for a fall than another option.

2. Most assessment tools indicate that a history of a recent fall is a significant factor regarding the risk for a future fall. A tool such as the Morse Fall Scale identifies 6 factors to examine: history of falls, secondary diagnosis, use of an ambulatory aid, intravenous infusion, gait and transfer ability, and mental status. Two factors on this scale (*history of a fall within the last 3 months* and *uses furniture as an ambulatory aid*) independently identify a patient as a level 2 risk potential out of 3 levels of concern (1–preventing, 2–modified risk, 3–strict fall risk).

3. Although a patient receiving a diuretic is at risk for hypotension, which is a concern, it is a less significant predictor of the potential for a fall than another option.

4. Although a urinary retention catheter is a concern in relation to safety, it is a less significant predictor of the potential for a fall than another option.

TEST-TAKING TIP: Identify the word in the stem that sets a priority. The word *most* in the stem sets a priority. Identify the clang association. The word *fall* in the stem and in option 2 is a clang association. Examine option 2 carefully.

Content Area: Safety
Integrated Processes: Nursing Process: Assessment
Client Need: Safe and Effective Care Environment; Safety and Infection Control
Cognitive Level: Application

34. **ANSWER: 1, 2, 3, 5.**
Rationales:

1. Children tend to be naive and trustful of others, including strangers. They should be taught about self-protection and what to do if approached by a stranger.

2. School-aged children develop gross motor skills and balance and progress from a three-wheeled bicycle to a two-wheeled bicycle. Learning to ride a two-wheeled bicycle should include instruction about safety precautions, physical support, and practice.

3. School-aged children are less fearful than infants and preschoolers, which results in an increase in risk-taking behaviors with inadequate information to perform the skills safely. Students should be reminded to get directions before using new equipment.

4. School-aged children should transition to using regular car seatbelts when they reach 60 pounds, can sit against the back of the seat with the legs hanging off the seat while bent at the knees, or are at least 8 years of age. School-aged children should sit in the back seat until 13 years of age.

5. These interventions help limit the amount of oxygen feeding the base of the flames, which helps to put out the fire.

Content Area: Safety
Integrated Processes: Teaching/Learning; Nursing Process: Implementation
Client Need: Health Promotion and Maintenance
Cognitive Level: Application

35. **ANSWER: 1.**
Rationales:

1. Motor vehicle accidents, often linked to alcohol use, are the leading cause of death and injury to middle-aged adults. This is the reason why this topic is most important to include in a discussion of injury prevention.

2. Although meditation may help to manage the stress of family and work place responsibilities, it is not as important as a topic in another option.

3. While it is important to teach middle-aged adults to do warm-up exercises before engaging in sports because middle-aged weekend athletes have an increased risk of sports injuries, it is not as important as a topic in another option

4. Although discussing a daily exercise program to increase endurance will help minimize the barely perceptible physical decline of aging during middle adulthood, it is not as important as a topic in another option.

TEST-TAKING TIP: Identify the word in the stem that sets a priority. The word *most* in the stem sets a priority.

Content Area: Safety
Integrated Processes: Teaching/Learning; Nursing Process: Planning
Client Need: Health Promotion and Maintenance
Cognitive Level: Application

36. **ANSWER: 1.**
Rationales:

1. Falls are the major cause of injury in this age-group. Removing throw/scatter rugs minimizes the risk of a fall.

2. Although most older adults experience a decline in hearing and vision and may be victims of pedestrian accidents, this type of accident is not the major cause of injury in this age-group.

3. Although older adults engage in sports, such as golf and bowling, and may experience a sports injury because of inadequate *warming up*, it is not the major cause of injury in this age-group.

4. Polypharmacy is a concern because older adults may take several prescription drugs plus over-the-counter drugs, placing them at risk for toxicity and drug interactions; however, injury from these chemical stressors are not the major cause of injury in this age-group.

Content Area: Safety
Integrated Processes: Teaching/Learning; Nursing Process: Implementation
Client Need: Health Promotion and Maintenance
Cognitive Level: Application

37. ANSWER: 5, 4, 2, 3, 1.
Rationales:
5. Recognizing that a gun is present is the first step in preventing accidental firearm injuries.
4. Stopping what one is doing immediately interrupts the activity; it gives the child time to remember the next 3 steps that should be implemented to provide for one's own safety and the safety of others.
2. If the gun is not touched, it cannot be fired accidentally.
3. Leaving the vicinity places distance between the child and the gun in the event another person touches the gun.
1. Reporting the presence of the gun to an adult enables the adult to intervene and secure the gun in a locked area so that it cannot be accessed.
Content Area: Safety
Integrated Processes: Teaching/Learning; Nursing Process: Planning
Client Need: Safe and Effective Care Environment; Safety and Infection Control
Cognitive Level: Analysis

38. ANSWER: 4.
Rationales:
1. Although it is important to remove scatter rugs from the home to prevent falls, falls are not the leading cause of accidental deaths in the home.
2. Although it is important to check for the presence of lead paint in the home, it is not one of the top five leading causes of accidental death.
3. According to the National Safety Council, falls are the third leading cause of accidental death. It is important to teach the use of gates at the bottom and top of stairs until children can negotiate stairs safely.
4. Accidental poisoning and unintentional overdose are the *leading* causes of death in the *home* and are the *second* leading cause of death after motor vehicle accidents *overall*. Household cleaners are followed by medicine, houseplants, cosmetics, pesticides, kerosene, gasoline, furniture polish, lighter fluid, and other chemicals. The five leading causes of accidental death are motor vehicle accidents, poisoning (accidental or unintentional), falls, choking/suffocation, drowning, and fire/flames/smoke.
TEST-TAKING TIP: Identify the word in the stem that sets a priority. The word *most* in the stem sets a priority.
Content Area: Safety
Integrated Processes: Teaching/Learning; Nursing Process: Implementation
Client Need: Health Promotion and Maintenance
Cognitive Level: Application

39. ANSWER: 3.
Rationales:
1. Using a bed pan limits mobility, does not let the patient assume the best position for voiding, and unnecessarily places the patient in a dependent situation.

2. This does not provide for the patient's safety needs; the patient has a problem with mobility, not vision.
3. The nurse should assist patients who are unstable or have impaired mobility. A commode at the bedside limits the energy the patient needs to expend at night when the risk for falls escalates.
4. Although a walker may help with patient stability, the patient should not be performing this activity independently, especially at night when the risk for falls escalates.
Content Area: Safety
Integrated Processes: Nursing Process: Implementation
Client Need: Safe and Effective Care Environment; Safety and Infection Control
Cognitive Level: Application

40. ANSWER: 50.
Rationale:
A microdrip infusion set is more accurate and safer to use than a macrodrip infusion set when administering small volumes of intravenous solutions. A microdrip infusion set delivers 60 drops per milliliter, whereas a macrodrip infusion set delivers 10 or 15 drops per milliliter, depending on the manufacturer.
Solve the problem using the following formula.

$$\frac{\text{Volume to be infused} \times \text{drop factor}}{\text{Total time in minutes}}$$

$$\frac{50\ (\text{mL}) \times 60\ (\text{drop factor})}{60\ (\text{minutes in 1 hour})} = \frac{3{,}000}{60} = 50 \text{ drops per minute}$$

Content Area: Medication Administration
Integrated Processes: Nursing Process: Planning
Client Need: Physiological Integrity; Pharmacological and Parenteral Therapies
Cognitive Level: Application

41. ANSWER: 3.
Rationales:
1. Slats of cribs should be less, not more, than 2⅜ inches in width to prevent a toddler's head from becoming wedged between the slats of a crib.
2. Toys should be much larger than 2 inches in diameter. Toys should be larger than the closed fist of an adult to minimize the risk of aspirating a toy.
3. This is essential to protect a toddler from accidentally causing self-strangulation.
4. Toddlers should be placed in a blanket sleeper and not under even a light blanket when sleeping to prevent the risk of suffocation.
TEST-TAKING TIP: Identify the word in the stem that sets a priority. The word *essential* in the stem sets a priority. Identify the option with the specific determiner. The word *only* in option 4 is a specific determiner. Rarely are options with a specific determiner the correct answer.
Content Area: Safety
Integrated Processes: Teaching/Learning; Nursing Process: Implementation
Client Need: Safe and Effective Care Environment; Safety and Infection Control
Cognitive Level: Application

42. ANSWER: 3.

Rationales:

1. The nurse should not attempt to apply restraints in a patient's home. The nurse should immediately leave the patient's home and/or call 911 if the nurse feels in imminent danger.

2. This is not the first action of the nurse. Although the patient has a history of violence, it does not mean that the patient will be violent during this home visit.

3. This is the most important nursing action. Assessment is the first step of the nursing process. A patient with a history of violence may resort to violence when coping with anxiety. As soon as a nurse identifies that the patient's level of anxiety is elevating, the nurse should leave and return when the patient is less anxious.

4. The nurse should never touch a person with a history of violence without permission. Touch may be perceived as a threat and may precipitate a violent patient reaction.

Content Area: Safety
Integrated Processes: Nursing Process: Assessment
Client Need: Safe and Effective Care Environment; Safety and Infection Control
Cognitive Level: Application

43. ANSWER: 2.

Rationales:

1. Although the patient participates to some degree in a transfer with a sit-to-stand lift by partially bearing weight and holding on to the handles of the device, encouraging independence is not its primary purpose.

2. Both the nurse and patient are protected from injury when the nurse uses this device to transfer the patient from a chair/bed to a chair/commode/toilet. It is designed for individuals who can bear some weight in an upright position, but who are weak or recovering from surgery.

3. Although weight bearing in the upright position and holding onto the handles of the sit-to-stand device may require muscle contraction promoting muscle strengthening, it is not its primary purpose.

4. Although the patient participates to some degree in a transfer with a sit-to-stand lift by partially bearing weight and holding onto the handles of the device, encouraging independence and psychological well-being, it is not its primary purpose.

TEST-TAKING TIP: Identify the word in the stem that sets a priority. The word *most* in the stem sets a priority. Identify options that are equally plausible. Options 1 and 4 are equally plausible because they both address the psychosocial domain. Option 1 is no better than option 4. Eliminate both from further consideration. Identify the unique option. Option 2 is unique. It is the only

option that addresses the nurse's need. Options 1, 3, and 4 address the patient's needs.

Content Area: Safety
Integrated Processes: Nursing Process: Planning
Client Need: Safe and Effective Care Environment; Safety and Infection Control
Cognitive Level: Application

44. ANSWER: 2.

Rationales:

1. A belt restraint is applied around a patient's abdomen and tied to the base of a bed or behind a chair to prevent a patient from getting out of a bed or chair without assistance. The upper and lower extremities have free range of motion. It does not protect a patient from pulling out a catheter.

2. Mitt restraints are the least restrictive of the restraints presented in the options and are most appropriate for this patient. A mitt restraint permits the patient to move the upper extremities but will not permit the patient to grasp a tube.

3. A vest restraint does not protect a patient from pulling out a catheter. It protects the patient from leaving a bed or chair without assistance. The upper arms and hands have free range of motion.

4. A wrist restraint is more restrictive than a restraint presented in another option. Although a wrist restraint may prevent pulling out a catheter, it unnecessarily prevents free range of motion of the upper extremities.

Content Area: Safety
Integrated Processes: Communication/Documentation; Nursing Process: Planning
Client Need: Safe and Effective Care Environment; Management of Care
Cognitive Level: Analysis

45. ANSWER: 3.

Rationales:

1. Although this may be advisable, diminished vision is not the leading cause of falls in older adults.

2. The influence of alcohol is not the leading cause of falls in older adults.

3. The leading cause of injuries in older adults is falls that usually occur when moving from sitting to standing or when transferring from a bed to a chair.

4. Washing the hands with an antimicrobial soap helps prevent infections, not injuries.

TEST-TAKING TIP: Identify the word in the stem that sets a priority. The word *leading* in the stem sets a priority.

Content Area: Safety
Integrated Processes: Teaching/Learning; Nursing Process: Implementation
Client Need: Health Promotion and Maintenance
Cognitive Level: Application

Chapter 14

Medication Administration

KEY TERMS

Aerosol—Aqueous product that is delivered as a fine mist into the nose or mouth and absorbed in the upper airway.

Ampule—Characteristically shaped glass container that has a pre-scored, generally colored, ring around a constricted neck that contains a sterile parenteral solution.

Caplet—Gelatin-coated tablet that is easy to swallow and dissolves in the stomach.

Capsule—Product encased in a hard or soft container or gelatin shell that dissolves in the stomach.

Drop factor—The number of drops it takes for specific tubing to deliver 1 mL of fluid.

Elixir—Product that is dispersed in a solution of alcohol containing glycerin or sweeteners.

Emulsion—Liquid product that is distributed as small droplets in another liquid.

Enteric-coated—Product that is encased in a substance that dissolves in the intestine.

Parenteral—Other than the alimentary canal (gastrointestinal tract).

Polypharmacy—Administration of many medications together.

Prn—Whenever necessary.

STAT—Immediately.

Suspension—Product that dissolves in a liquid when shaken vigorously.

Sustained-release—Product that gradually is released, ensuring a constant blood level of the product.

Syrup—Product that is dispersed in a sugar liquid.

Tablet—Product molded into a disk or cylinder that is swallowed, chewed, or melted under the tongue.

Time-release—Product that is further enclosed in smaller casings that release a dose over time.

Vial—Glass rubber-sealed container covered with a metal cap that contains a sterile parenteral solution.

I. The Rights of Medication Administration and Related Nursing Care

A nurse should focus on five elements when administering medications. These elements are called the "Five Rights of Medication Administration" and include the right patient, right medication, right dose, right route, and right time. A nurse should consider these five elements when administering each medication because they have proven to be valuable in reducing medication errors.

A. Right Patient

1. Check the patient's name against two verifiers, following agency policy. For example, ask the patient to state his or her name and birth date and verify the name against the medication administration record (MAR) and patient's wristband; if applicable, use a computer scanner to verify the patient's wristband bar code.
2. Follow alert procedures when two patients have a similar last name (e.g., place them in different rooms, flag their MARs and the fronts of their charts, and place wristbands issuing the alert).

B. Right Medication

1. Know the normal dose for commonly administered medications.
2. Check a resource about a medication for which you are unsure.
3. Verify the medication against the primary healthcare provider's order.
4. Use a computer scanner to verify the medication package bar code.

C. Right Dose
1. Ensure that the prescribed dose is appropriate for the patient. Use a pediatric calculation formula for infants and children.
2. Calculate the dose carefully and double-check all math calculations.
3. Use a computer scanner to verify the medication package bar code.
4. Question the primary health-care provider about a dose outside the expected range.

D. Right Route
1. Give the medication via the prescribed route.
2. Ensure that the route is safe for the patient (e.g., rectal route is contraindicated in patients with rectal bleeding; oral route is contraindicated when a patient is vomiting).

E. Right Time
1. Give the medication at the prescribed time, ensuring that it is less than 60 minutes before or after the scheduled time (e.g., numerous patients receiving care from one nurse cannot all receive 10:00 medications at the same time).
2. Ensure that the medication is administered at the prescribed frequency (e.g., once a day, twice a day, three times a day).

DID YOU KNOW?

The five rights of medication administration are so effective in reminding a nurse of the significant elements to consider when preparing and administering medications that an additional five rights were identified. They include right education, right assessment, right to refuse, right documentation, and right evaluation. These additional five rights reflect the fact that medication administration is not just the physical process of preparing and administering a prescribed medication. Nursing responsibilities also include educating the patient, ensuring that the medication is still appropriate for the patient, evaluating patient responses, maintaining legal records through documentation, and respecting that a patient has a right to refuse a prescribed medication.

F. Right Education
1. Provide the patient with information about the medication, including its name, action, expected therapeutic response, and associated precautions.
2. Ask whether the patient has any questions and correct misconceptions.

G. Right Assessment
1. Implement all assessments required before medication administration (e.g., pulse rate and/or blood pressure [BP] for cardiac medications).
2. Administer medications based on parameters identified by the primary health-care provider that require a specific assessment (e.g., give a specific

number of units of insulin to "cover" a particular blood glucose level).
3. Ensure that the medication is still appropriate for the patient.

H. Right to Refuse
1. Explore the patient's reason for refusing to take a medication.
2. Implement teaching regarding the necessity of the medication and correct patient misconceptions.
3. Accept the patient's right to refuse to take a medication.
4. Document the patient's stated reason for refusing a medication.
5. Notify the primary health-care provider of the patient's refusal to take a prescribed medication.

I. Right Evaluation
1. Reassess the patient and compare the actual outcome with the expected outcome to determine medication effectiveness.
2. Be alert for nontherapeutic effects.
3. Notify the primary health-care provider of nontherapeutic effects and seek new orders as needed.
4. Document the patient's response to all medications in the clinical record.

J. Right Documentation
1. Document all medications given in the MAR *after* they are given, never before.
2. Maintain appropriate legal documents concerning controlled medications.
3. Follow agency policy when a medication is not administered; for example, circle, initial, or highlight the dose on an electronic chart and document why the medication was not given (e.g., patient refused medication, BP beyond parameters).
4. Complete an incident report if a prescribed medication was not administered properly, such as not on time, missed dose, or inaccurate dose.

II. Medication Dispensing Systems

Until the 1960s, medications were prepared in a medication room using little cards with the information for each medication for each patient. Medications were dispensed from large bottles of medications into a small paper cup accompanied by its appropriate cards. All the medications were delivered to patients on one tray. This outdated system presented many opportunities for errors to occur. The introduction of individual packaging of medications (unit-dose) and the use of a medication cart with a drawer for each patient provided a better system to secure, store, prepare, and deliver medications to patients, reducing medication errors. Automated dispensing systems have added an additional level of safety by requiring a user password and providing a computer database that records all pertinent information when a medication is administered.

The most recent safety measure is the use of a computer sensor to scan a bar code to verify the patient's name and the medication to be administered; it also documents the medications administered. Multiple checks and balances help to maintain patient safety concerning medication administration.

A. Medication Cart
  1. Lockable, rolling cabinet that contains medications for patients on a specific unit.
      a. Must be locked whenever the nurse steps away.
      b. Can be opened only by a key or access code.
  2. Should be wheeled to outside each patient's room when administering medications and left locked outside an open doorway to a patient's room when giving medications to a patient.
  3. Generally are stored in or near the nurse's station when not in use, although some facilities require them to be locked to the wall of the nurse's station or stored in a locked medication room.
  4. Generally contains the following contents.
      a. Top of the cart provides a work surface and holds important equipment and supplies, such as the MAR, pitcher of water, medicine cups, pill crusher, and possibly a computer.
      b. A sharps container, trash container, and light may be built into the top or attached to the side of the cart.
      c. Handles are provided for steering and for holding equipment, such as a stethoscope.
      d. The top drawer may contain straws, tongue blades, gauze, alcohol wipes, and other supplies.
      e. Small drawers correlate to the room number and beds on the unit; they are labeled with patients' names and contain the medications that each patient is to receive for 24 hours.
      f. A large drawer may contain bulkier items, such as bottles of liquids.
      g. Another large drawer may contain stock medications, such as aspirin, ibuprofen, acetaminophen, and docusate sodium (Colace).
      h. Another drawer with divided compartments may contain different sized syringes and gauge needles.
  5. Medications in drawers are restocked by a pharmacist.
  6. Generally contain medications in unit-dose packages, with each package stating the medication name, dose, and expiration date.

B. Medication Room
  1. Generally, contains controlled medications in a locked cabinet or an automated medication dispensing cabinet. (Box 14.1.)
  2. Used to prepare intravenous solutions before transport to a patient's room or preparation of subcutaneous (Sub-Q) or intramuscular (IM)

Box 14.1 Managing Controlled Drugs

Management and administration of controlled drugs are highly regulated by federal law. Be aware of these nursing considerations when working with controlled drugs.
- Store controlled drugs in a double-locked cabinet, medication room, cart, or computer-automated drug dispensing system.
- Use a secure identification code to access computer-automated drug dispensing systems.
- Count opioids and controlled drugs at specific times, such as at change of shift (a nurse completing a shift counts the controlled drugs together with a nurse coming on duty). If a computer-automated dispensing system runs a continuous count, manual counting at the end of a shift is unnecessary.
- Account for each dose of an opioid or controlled drug on a controlled substance record, which includes the name of the patient, amount of drug used, time the drug was administered, name of the prescribing primary health-care provider, and name of the nurse administering the drug.
- Ensure that stock doses remaining equal the number of doses available on the controlled-drug record before preparing a controlled drug.
- Immediately report a discrepancy in a controlled drug count to an administrative nurse and the pharmacy, depending on facility policy.
- Employ efforts to help identify the source of the discrepancy immediately.
- Have a second nurse act as a witness if all or part of a controlled drug needs to be discarded; both nurses must sign the controlled drug sheet.

---

injections, which are then capped and transported individually to each patient.
  3. May have a refrigerator dedicated only for the storage of medications that must be kept cool, such as some vaccines and skin test agents.

C. Automated Medication Dispensing Cabinet
  1. Computer access system that controls the distribution, management, and control of medications.
  2. Usually contains controlled medications, but some agencies are moving toward using an automated medication dispensing cabinet for all patient medications.
  3. Requires the password of the caregiver, requires the nurse to access a patient's name and select a medication, dispenses the medication, and records the entire transaction.

III. Medication Orders

Administration of a medication requires an order by a primary health-care provider and is a dependent function of the nurse. The nurse must ensure that all components of an order are contained in the order before administering the medication. Primary health-care providers can write various types of orders, such as *standing, as needed (PRN), single-dose, immediately (STAT),* and *now orders.* Nurses must know the policies and procedures associated with the communication of medication orders, such as transcription of medication orders and reception of verbal and telephone orders. These legal requirements and policies and procedures are designed to ensure safety and reduce errors associated with the delivery of medications.

A. Parts of a Medication Order
1. Patient's full name.
2. Date and time the order is written.
3. Name of the medication.
4. Dosage of the medication.
5. Route of administration.
6. Frequency of administration.
7. Situation (e.g., when an as-needed medication should be administered, parameters for when a medication should be held).
8. Primary health-care provider's signature.

DID YOU KNOW?

A nurse must call the primary health-care provider to discuss concerns if a medication order is incomplete, ambiguous, contraindicated, inappropriate, or unusual. A nurse should document in the clinical record that the primary health-care provider was called about the medication order, including details about the discussion and response.

B. Types of Medication Orders
1. Standing (routine).
   a. Medication order that is carried out until it is discontinued or the required number of days has lapsed.
   b. Nursing care.
      (1) Know facility policies regarding automatic discontinuation of medications.
      (2) Be aware that standing orders must be reordered after surgery or transfer to a different service.
      (3) Administer a medication as prescribed until it is discontinued, the number of prescribed days lapse, or according to facility policy, such as 5 to 14 days for specific antibiotics.
      (4) Evaluate the patient's response to the medication.
2. As-needed (PRN).
   a. Order for a medication to be given only when it is needed; must include circumstances in which the medication is to be given (e.g., morphine sulfate 2 mg IV PRN *every 3 hours for incisional pain*).
   b. Nursing care.
      (1) Document assessments that indicated the need for the medication in the clinical record.
      (2) Check the MAR to identify when a medication was last given to ensure that adequate time has lapsed since the previous dose.

(3) Document administration in the PRN section of the MAR.
(4) Evaluate the patient's response to the medication.
3. Single-dose (one-time only).
   a. Order for a medication to be given only once, such as a medication given before a diagnostic test or before surgery.
   b. Nursing care.
      (1) Administer the medication one time only.
      (2) Document administration of the medication in the single-dose section of the MAR.
      (3) Evaluate the patient's response to the medication.
4. Immediately (STAT).
   a. Order for a single dose of a medication to be given immediately.
   b. Often ordered in emergency situations.
   c. Nursing care.
      (1) Administer a STAT medication immediately.
      (2) Document administration in the single-dose section of the MAR.
      (3) Evaluate the patient's response to the medication.
5. Now order.
   a. Order for a single dose of a medication that is to be given quickly but not as quickly as a STAT order.
   b. Nursing care.
      (1) Administer a "now" order within 90 minutes.
      (2) Document administration in the single-dose section of the MAR.
      (3) Evaluate the patient's response to the medication.

C. Communication of Medication Orders
1. Written order: A primary health-care provider writes an order following the protocol established by the agency. It may be written in an order book or in the patient's clinical record, using a computer order form or standard order form with specific orders indicated with checkmarks.
   a. Ensure that medication orders contain all required elements.
   b. Notify the pharmacy of the new medication order; this may be done manually, by fax, or automatically when the order was initiated on a computer; computer orders help to minimize errors by automatically notifying the pharmacy and generating an MAR.
   c. Transcribe to or verify medication order on the MAR; this may be done manually or by a computer; recheck it several times to ensure accuracy.

2. Verbal order: Medication order given by a primary health-care provider verbally in person.
   a. Accept only in emergency situations, when there is no time to put an order in writing.
   b. Repeat the order back to the primary health-care provider for confirmation.
   c. Ensure that the primary health-care provider countersigns the order as soon as possible and no later than 24 hours after the event.
3. Telephone order: Medication order given by a primary health-care provider via the telephone; generally used in emergency situations when a primary health-care provider is not present.
   a. Use only in situations in which a written or verbal order is not possible.
   b. Follow policy as to who can receive telephone orders, such as a primary nurse or supervisor.
   c. Repeat the order back to the primary health-care provider for confirmation.
   d. Make sure that two nurses listen to the order and have both nurses countersign the order.
   e. Ensure that the primary health-care provider countersigns the order within 24 hours.

IV. Nursing Care Related to Medication Administration

Preparing and administering medications involves more than just removing medication from a package and giving it to a patient. It involves critical thinking throughout the process to ensure that the rights of medication administration are addressed as well as the general considerations associated with medication administration. When administering any medication, irrespective of the route, the nurse should follow specific guidelines to ensure that medications are prepared and administered safely. This process is complex and requires that the nurse remain focused without interruptions because it is too easy to become distracted and confused. Accuracy and patient safety are the expected outcomes of medication administration.

A. **General Considerations When Administering Medications**
   1. Complete or review the medication reconciliation form, including prescribed medications, over-the-counter medications, supplemental herbs, and vitamins, to ensure the patient is receiving prescribed medications and help prevent nontherapeutic medication-medication interactions or an excess of medication intake.
   2. Identify food and medication allergies and communicate them according to facility policies and procedures, such as on the MAR, on the front of the clinical record, on a wristband, in the plan of care, and by notification of the pharmacy.

Doing so prevents allergic responses and ensures continuity of care.
   3. Identify factors that impact medication therapy (e.g., age, disease, gender, body mass, diet) and perform a health history and physical examination as needed to ensure patient factors are taken into consideration when determining the appropriateness of a medication.
   4. Administer oral medications with food or between meals as indicated by the pharmacy and the medication manufacturer to facilitate absorption (e.g., taking ferrous sulfate [Feosol] with ascorbic acid [citrus juice] or taking certain medications, such as levothyroxine [Synthroid], on an empty stomach) and to help minimize gastric irritation for certain medications (e.g., ibuprofen [Advil, Motrin]).
   5. Assess patient understanding of prescribed medications and provide information to ensure accurate knowledge, including medication name; therapeutic action; rationale; nontherapeutic effects; parameters associated with the medication, such as pulse rate or BP; and actions to take in case of an adverse reaction or missed dose. Doing so ensures the patient is knowledgeable about prescribed medications and supports participation in the medication regimen.
   6. Assess pregnancy status if a prescribed medication is teratogenic to reduce the risk of injury to a developing fetus. Determine whether a mother is breastfeeding to reduce the risk of transfer of medication ingredients to a breastfeeding infant.
   7. Perform (e.g., blood glucose monitoring) or review results (e.g., peak and trough levels) of diagnostic tests that impact on medication administration to ensure administration of a safe dose of a medication.
   8. Hold a medication that indicates a peak level higher than the therapeutic level to ensure prevention of excessive medication levels.
   9. Notify the primary health-care provider of medication levels outside the established parameters to ensure that the primary health-care provider can order a corrective action if necessary.

B. **Common Nursing Interventions When Administering Medications**
   1. Perform hand hygiene per policy and procedure, such as using soap and water or a hand sanitizer, to remove debris and minimize the number of microorganisms on the hands, thereby reducing the risk of infection.
   2. Position the medication cart outside the patient's room. Lock the cart when it is unattended and when away from the cart giving medications to a patient to minimize contamination of the cart and prevent unauthorized access to medications.

3. Verify that the medication being prepared is prescribed for the patient (right patient and right medication), is the prescribed dose (right dose), is being administered via the ordered route (right route), and is being given at the prescribed time (right time). This verification should be performed three times (triple check) to reduce the risk of medication errors.
   a. *First check:* When removing the medication from a drawer.
   b. *Second check:* When preparing the medication, such as placing an unopened oral medication in a medicine cup, pouring a liquid, or filling a syringe.
   c. *Third check:* Just before opening the package of an oral medication at the bedside or just after preparation of a liquid or parenteral medication.
4. Verify the expiration date on a medication package and return the medication to the pharmacy if it is expired because expired medications can lose their potency.
5. Introduce yourself and state that you are there to administer medications. This supports a patient's right to know who is providing care and what is to be done.
6. Ask the patient to state his or her name and birth date and verify the response against the MAR and wristband; follow the verification policy and procedure of the facility (e.g., a medication package bar code must be verified against the bar code on the patient's wristband).
7. Teach about the medications being administered and ask whether the patient has any questions to ensure understanding about the medications being administered and support motivation to take the medication.
8. Establish whether a patient's status is within prescribed or expected parameters before administering a medication (e.g., pulse rate greater than 60 beats/minute for digoxin or BP within parameters set by a policy or the primary health-care provider).
9. Hold a medication and inform the primary health-care provider when a patient's status does not meet set parameters to prevent an excessive level of the medication and promote an appropriate response by the primary health-care provider.
10. Assess for therapeutic and nontherapeutic responses to a medication before administering another dose (e.g., stools are not loose when receiving a stool softener or laxative.)
11. Hold a medication if it is no longer appropriate or if an adverse response occurred to prevent patient injury.

12. Notify the primary health-care provider if a nontherapeutic response occurs that is more serious than a minor side effect. Doing so ensures immediate attention to nontherapeutic responses that require medical intervention or a change in a medication order.
13. Assist the patient into a comfortable position for the prescribed route, such as sitting or Fowler's for oral medications or side lying for IM injections. The upright position uses gravity to facilitate ingestion of oral medications; the side-lying position provides access to the dorsogluteal and ventrogluteal muscles for an IM injection.
14. Allow the patient to self-administer medications when appropriate. Assist those who need assistance, such as with positioning, holding a cup, or inserting an oral medication into the mouth. Doing so supports independence, allows the patient to set the pace, and facilitates medication ingestion.
15. Document administration of medications, only after medications are administered, in the clinical record or MAR or according to facility policy and procedure. Doing so ensures accurate and complete documentation of medication administration in a permanent record.
16. Document nonadministration of a medication in the MAR or the clinical record progress notes or according to facility policy and procedure. Doing so ensures documentation of the event.

C. Nursing Interventions When Administering Medications to Patients at Risk for Complications
1. Introduction.
   a. A nurse must assess all patients to determine whether they are at risk for complications associated with medication administration. For example, a nurse should assess the patient's developmental level (particularly age) and health status (particularly the ability to swallow, presence of the gag reflex, and efficiency of kidney function).
   b. Once the potential for complications are identified, the nurse should implement additional interventions that specifically address the patient's needs.
2. Older adults and related nursing care.
   a. May have difficulty swallowing tablets due to dry mouth.
      (1) Crush tablets that are crushable.
      (2) Give water before, during, and after medication administration.
      (3) Stroke under the chin to promote swallowing.
      (4) Seek an order for a liquid form of the medication.

b. May process information more slowly, have slower physical movements, and/or experience decreased strength and reflexes.

(1) Allow more time to provide information about medications.

(2) Keep explanations simple.

🛑 (3) Allow more time to administer medications; do not hurry the patient.

🛑 (4) Teach the patient to avoid childproof safety tops on medication containers to facilitate easier handling of containers and to support independence if unable to open safety top containers. If children are in the home keep medications in a locked cabinet.

(5) Assess the patient's ability to self-administer medications, such as eye drops and injections.

(6) Explore strategies for assistance, such as having a visiting nurse or family member assist with medication administration in the home.

c. May be more forgetful, omitting doses or taking excessive doses of medications.

(1) Construct a calendar of days and times medications are taken.

(2) Instruct the patient to place medications or signs in a prominent place in the home.

(3) Teach the patient how to use a divided pill container (e.g., if the a.m. section is empty in the evening, it confirms the morning medications were taken) to support the medication regimen and minimize errors.

d. May have decreased visual acuity.

(1) Write out the medication calendar in large letters or containers with raised letters.

(2) Suggest using a large-labeled or braille divided pill container.

(3) Suggest using a syringe that has a preset volume control feature to ensure an accurate dose when self-administering a parenteral medication.

e. May not be able to afford prescribed medications.

(1) Suggest that the primary health-care provider prescribe the generic form of the medication if available or a less costly medication.

(2) Seek funding resources.

DID YOU KNOW?

Older adults are requesting primary health-care providers to write prescriptions for medications at twice the required dose. The patient then divides the tablets into two doses in an effort to reduce the cost of prescribed medications. This practice is unsafe because the consistency of the dose may vary and dividing doses increases the risk of contaminating the tablets. Nurses should teach patients why this practice is discouraged and assist patients to seek funding resources instead.

f. Have decreased rate of medication metabolism and excretion, which increases the risk of toxicity.

(1) Ensure that the prescribed dose takes into consideration the aging process to minimize the risk of an excessive dose.

(2) Explore whether the patient can manage with a lower dose than that for younger adults to avoid medication toxicity.

(3) Assess for clinical indicators of medication toxicity.

(4) Monitor blood levels of medications to ensure early identification of medication accumulation and promote early intervention to prevent toxicity.

(5) Teach the patient not to exceed the recommended doses of medications.

g. Are at increased risk for medication interactions due to the intake of multiple medications (**polypharmacy**) necessary for treatment of chronic illnesses.

(1) Assess for clinical indicators of medication interactions.

(2) Encourage the primary health-care provider to periodically review the medication reconciliation form to promote discontinuation of unnecessary medications or to reduce a dose.

MAKING THE CONNECTION

Polypharmacy and Aging

A nurse must understand the connection between the risks associated with the intake of multiple drugs and the factors related to aging. Because of the aging process, older adults are less able to metabolize and excrete medications, placing them at greater risk for drug toxicity. In addition, polypharmacy associated with the treatment of multiple chronic illnesses increases the risk of unfavorable drug interactions. According to the Centers for Disease Control and Prevention, by 2030, the number of U.S. adults age 65 years and older will double to about 71 million. That means, one out of every five people will be over the age of 65. Currently, 80 percent of older adults have one chronic illness and 50 percent of older adults have at least two chronic illnesses. Heart disease, cancer, brain attack (cerebrovascular accident, stroke), chronic obstructive pulmonary disease, and diabetes are the five most common causes of chronic illness in older adults. The essential challenge is to help older adults to remain healthy by preventing and/or minimizing these chronic diseases and their complications, thereby requiring fewer medications.

3. Infants and children and related nursing care.
   a. Infants and children vary in size, weight, and surface area and pass through various stages of growth and development.
      (1) Carefully calculate and recheck medication dosages using a pediatric calculation formula.
      (2) Assess developmental level and adjust interventions based on the child's physical, emotional, and cognitive levels.
   b. Infants and children are at risk for aspirating or choking on liquid medications.
      (1) Position the child in sitting or semi-sitting position.
      (2) Use a needless syringe or dropper.
      (3) Place the liquid between the lower gum and cheek.
      (4) Instill the medication slowly to avoid giving too much liquid at once.
   c. Young children may not be able to ingest tablets.
      (1) Crush tablets that are crushable and mix them with applesauce or secure a liquid form of the medication.
      (2) Offer the child a choice of a spoon, syringe, or dropper to support a sense of control.
      (3) Use a medication nipple for infants so that they can suck the medication.
   d. Young children are not moved by logic; saying, "This medication will make you feel better" will not work if the child does not like the taste.
      (1) Admit that the medication might not taste good, but that it will be followed with a nice-tasting juice to facilitate trust.
      (2) Give an ice pop just before giving an unpleasant tasting medication to numb the taste buds.
      (3) Avoid using an important food or liquid to mask the taste of a medication to prevent an unpleasant association and subsequent refusal of the important food or liquid.
   e. Children may be afraid of injections because they are associated with pain or the unfamiliar.
      (1) Awaken a sleeping child for an injection because doing so is less frightening and supports trust.
      (2) Admit that the injection might be uncomfortable, but that it will be over quickly to support trust.
      (3) Apply a topical anesthetic cream before an injection to minimize the discomfort of needle insertion.
      (4) Offer a toy to play with during and after the injection to distract the child.
      (5) Use the vastus lateralis muscle for children who are not walking yet because gluteal muscles are not fully developed.

      (6) Obtain the assistance of another health team member, rather than a parent, to restrain the child if necessary to avoid associating the parent with an unpleasant event.
      🛑 (7) Cuddle or have the parent cuddle the child after an injection to provide comfort.

4. Patients at risk for aspiration and related nursing care.
   a. The patient may have difficulty chewing and swallowing or have an impaired gag reflex.
      (1) Assess the patient's ability to swallow and cough and the presence of the gag reflex.
      (2) Place the patient in an upright position if possible.
      (3) Thicken liquids or offer fruit nectars with oral medications to make fluid easier to control.
      (4) Avoid the use of a straw because fluid is harder to control when using a straw than when using a cup.
      (5) Crush tablets that are crushable and mix them with a teaspoon of applesauce or secure an order for an alternate route.
      (6) Allow the patient to hold PO medications and a cup of water and to set the pace; do not hurry the patient.
      (7) Administer medications on the strong side of the mouth for a patient with weakness or hemiparesis of the oral cavity.
      (8) Administer PO medications one at a time and ensure that each is swallowed before giving the next.
   b. The patient may have an altered level of consciousness.
      (1) Seek an order for an alternate route for oral medications.
      (2) Explain what is being done and why, with the assumption that the patient hears and understands.

V. Routes of Medication Administration

The route of administration refers to where the medication enters the body. It is included as one of the parts of a medication order. The route of administration selected depends on such factors as the characteristics of the pharmacological product (e.g., insulin is destroyed in the gastrointestinal [GI] system and therefore is administered subcutaneously); the purpose of the medication (e.g., local or systemic effect); and patient characteristics (e.g., patient is unconscious, is vomiting, or has an impaired GI system). Routes of administration include oral, enteral tubes, oral mucous membranes (e.g., sublingual, buccal, swish and spit, swish and swallow), skin, eye, ear, rectum, vagina, upper or lower respiratory tract, and parenteral (e.g., intramuscular, subcutaneous, intradermal, and intravenous). Each route has its indications for use, advantages and disadvantages, and specific techniques that must be employed to deliver the medication appropriately to the patient. Nurses must be knowledgeable about these issues and possess the necessary skills to administer medications safely via a variety of routes.

A. Oral
1. Introduction.
   a. Product is administered through the mouth or a tube into the stomach.
   b. Product is absorbed in the stomach or intestines.
2. Types of oral medication preparations.
   a. **Capsule:** Product encased in a hard or soft container or gelatin shell that dissolves in the stomach.
   b. **Caplet:** Gelatin-coated tablet that is easy to swallow and dissolves in the stomach.
   c. **Tablet:** Product molded into a disk or cylinder that is swallowed, chewed, or melted under the tongue (sublingual) and comes in different types.
      (1) **Enteric-coated:** Product encased in a substance that dissolves in the intestine.
      (2) **Sustained-release:** Product that is gradually released, ensuring a constant blood level of the drug.
      (3) **Time-release:** Product further enclosed in smaller casing that releases a dose over time.
   d. **Liquid:** Substance that flows readily.
      (1) **Aerosol:** Aqueous product that is delivered as a fine mist into the nose or mouth and absorbed in the upper airway.
      (2) **Elixir:** Product in a solution of alcohol containing glycerin or sweeteners.
      (3) **Emulsion:** Liquid product that is distributed as small droplets in another liquid.
      (4) **Suspension:** Powder or particle that is dissolved in a liquid when shaken vigorously.
      (5) **Syrup:** Product that is dispersed in a sugar liquid.
3. Advantages.
   a. Convenient.
   b. Comfortable for the patient.
   c. Chewable forms that appeal to children.
   d. Seldom causes patient anxiety.
   e. Easy to administer.
   f. Economical and cost effective; does not require expensive equipment.
   g. Can cause a local effect.
   h. Can cause a systemic effect.
4. Disadvantages.
   a. Slower action than other routes.
   b. Can irritate the oral and gastric mucosa, stain teeth, or have an objectionable taste.

   c. Contraindicated for some patients.
      (1) Patients who have impaired GI function.
      (2) Patients who are unconscious or cognitively impaired and cannot swallow.
      (3) Patients who are nauseated, vomiting, on nothing-by-mouth (NPO) status, or receiving gastric decompression.
      (4) Patients at high risk for aspiration.
5. Commonalities of nursing interventions specific to administering oral medications.
   a. Verify whether the patient is receiving a restricted diet, is having intake and output (I&O) measured, or is on NPO status to ensure that fluid intake is permitted and should be documented.
   b. Assess the presence of contraindications for administering a medication via the oral route, such as decreased level of consciousness, depressed gag reflex, presence of nausea or vomiting, and NPO status. Seek an order for an alternate route if any contraindications are present. Doing so ensures that the patient can receive the medication via an alternate route without interruption of therapy.
   c. Encourage the patient to drink 5 oz of water with ingestion of the medication to facilitate dissolution and absorption of the medication.
   d. Cut scored tablets with a cutting device or held within a tissue when splitting by hand. Ensure both halves of a tablet are equal in size to produce two equal doses (a cutting device is more effective than splitting tablets by hand) and ensures an accurate dose.
   e. Follow agency policy regarding using or discarding unadministered split tablets.
   f. Crush crushable tablets and mix with applesauce when necessary to facilitate swallowing. Use only as much applesauce as necessary to mix with the medication to ensure ingestion of the entire dose.
   g. Observe the patient while he or she is ingesting the medication.
   h. Inspect the mouth for "pocketed" medications (e.g., under the tongue or in the buccal cavity) after administration when ingestion is questionable, such as with difficulty swallowing, confusion, hoarding, or unilateral weakness, to ensure that the medication was ingested and reduce the risk of aspiration of an unswallowed medication.

 i. Do not leave medications at the bedside to be taken later to prevent the medication from becoming lost, not being taken, being taken without supervision, or being hoarded for a nontherapeutic purpose.

6. Nursing interventions specific to administering enteric-coated, time-release, and sustained-release capsules.
   a. Do not crush enteric-coated drugs to avoid deactivation by gastric juices and ensure delivery to the intestine, where it dissolves and is absorbed.
   b. Do not open time-release or sustained-release capsules to prevent the entire dose from being activated at one time, resulting in an overdose.
   c. Assess for the therapeutic effect of the medication over the length of time expected.
   d. Notify the primary health-care provider if a patient is unable to ingest a medication whole.
7. Nursing interventions specific to administering liquid medications (aerosols, elixirs, emulsions, suspensions, and syrups).
   a. Follow the manufacturer's directions regarding whether a container should be vigorously shaken to ensure even distribution of constituents.
   b. Place an opened top of a container on a surface with the inside lid facing up to prevent contamination of the inside of the lid and subsequent contamination of the bottle when the lid is returned and closed.
   c. Measure oral liquids accurately.
      (1) Measure oral liquids in a calibrated medication cup at eye level.
      (2) Use a syringe without a needle to measure oral liquid volumes less than 5 mL and transfer them to a medication cup.

   🛑 (3) Avoid keeping oral liquid medications in a syringe to prevent accidental administration of an oral liquid via the parenteral route.

   d. Pour liquids with the label against the palm of the hand to allow a view of the label to facilitate the three checks of medication administration and prevent the liquid from dripping on and obscuring the label.
   e. Wipe the outside rim of the bottle with a clean paper towel before replacing the top.
   f. Use measures to make unpleasant tasting medications more palatable.
      (1) Refrigerate unpleasant tasting liquids unless contraindicated to lessen objectionable taste and odor.
      (2) Offer ice chips before giving unpleasant tasting medications to numb the taste buds.
      (3) Use a needleless syringe to place unpleasant tasting medications on the back of the tongue to minimize unpleasant taste.
      (4) Provide oral hygiene after administration of unpleasant tasting medications.

B. GI Tubes
1. Introduction.
   a. Tube inserted into the stomach or intestine.
   b. Can be used to remove stomach secretions (gastric decompression) or intestinal secretions (intestinal decompression).
   c. Can be used to deliver formula feedings to the stomach or small intestine to meet nutritional needs.
   d. Can be used to deliver liquid, powder, or crushed medications even when the tube is being used for decompression or for formula feedings.
2. Types of GI tubes.
   a. Nasogastric (NG).
      (1) Tube passed through a nostril, the nasopharynx, and the esophagus with the distal end placed in the stomach.
      (2) Used for patients who are unable to ingest substances through the mouth or esophagus due to impaired swallowing, an absent gag reflex, or recent head and neck surgery or for decompression after abdominal surgery.
   b. Jejunostomy.
      (1) Tube passed through the nose, the esophagus, and the stomach with the distal end placed in the jejunum.
      (2) Used for patients with impaired gastric functioning so that formula feedings can directly enter the small intestine or to promote intestinal decompression in patients with a small bowel obstruction.
   c. Percutaneous endoscopic gastrostomy (PEG) or percutaneous endoscopic jejunostomy (PEJ).
      (1) Tube surgically or laparoscopically inserted through the skin and abdominal wall into the stomach or jejunum and sutured in place to maintain placement. Also held in place by an internal retention balloon and flat external bumper.
      (2) Traditionally used for long-term (6 to 8 weeks or longer) nutritional support but now used more frequently for short-term support because of ease of insertion.
3. Advantages.
   a. Provide a route for administering medication that otherwise would need to be delivered parenterally.
   b. PEG tube considered the most comfortable feeding tube.
4. Disadvantages.
   a. Increased risk of aspiration that can lead to pneumonia, infection, abscess formation, and respiratory distress syndrome (RDS); risk is greater with an NG tube than with gastrostomy

or jejunostomy tubes because an NG tube can curl up within the esophagus and enter the trachea and bronchi.

b. Requires use of an enteral tube and a piston syringe for insertion of medication, which is more costly than most other routes.

c. Requires shutting off a tube used for decompression for 30 minutes after medication administration to allow time for absorption.

d. Does not permit administration of enteric-coated, time-release, or sustained-release medications because they would require crushing a tablet or emptying a capsule, which would expose the patient to the entire dose at once.

e. Requires more time for administration than do other routes.

5. Nursing interventions specific to administering medications via GI tubes.

a. Administer liquid forms of medication when available to prevent clogging the tube.

b. Crush crushable tablets into a fine powder and mix with 30 mL of warm water; avoid administering whole or undissolved medications to prevent clogging the tube.

🛑 c. Identify placement of the tube in the stomach or intestine before medication administration. Doing so ensures that medication is administered into the appropriate place rather than into the respiratory system. (See the section "Ensure accurate placement of the tube using several methods" in Chapter 18, "Nutrition," page 544.)

d. Flush the tube with 15 to 30 mL of water before medication administration to ensure tube patency.

e. Give each medication separately and flush with 15 to 30 mL of water between each and after the last medication. If necessary, modify the procedure if the patient has a fluid restriction. (Fig. 14.1.)

🛑 f. Shut off a nasogastric tube used for decompression for 30 minutes after medication administration to enhance medication absorption and then reestablish decompression.

C. Oral Mucous Membranes (Sublingual, Buccal, Swish and Spit, Swish and Swallow)

1. Introduction.

a. The mucous membranes of the oral cavity line the entire cavity, including inside the lips, under the tongue (sublingual), between the gum and cheeks (buccal cavity), and the posterior oropharyngeal area, including the uvula and tonsils.

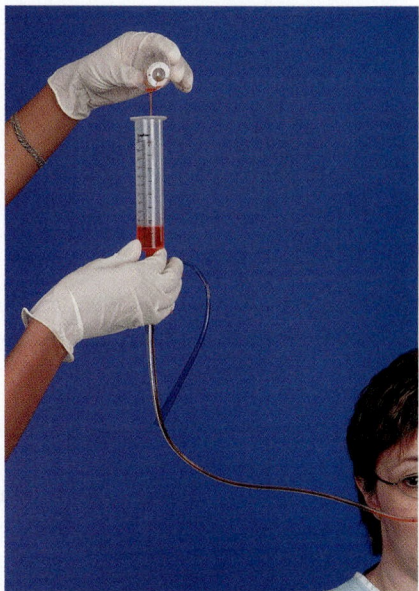

Fig 14.1 Medication via an enteral tube. (From Burton and Ludwig [2011]. *Fundamentals of nursing care: Concepts, connections & skills.* Philadelphia: F. A. Davis Company, with permission.)

b. Products for these routes are designed to dissolve or circulate in the mouth and produce either a local or a systemic effect.

c. Sublingual (Fig. 14.2): Tablet is dissolved under the tongue (e.g., nitroglycerine).

d. Buccal cavity (Fig. 14.3): Troche or lozenge is dissolved between a cheek and the gum.

e. Swish and spit/swish and swallow: Solution dispersed throughout the oral cavity and esophagus (when swallowed).

2. Advantages.

a. Same as oral route, plus information below.

b. Sublingual.

(1) Enters the blood, bypassing the liver and allowing for a quick effect.

(2) Administered for a systemic effect.

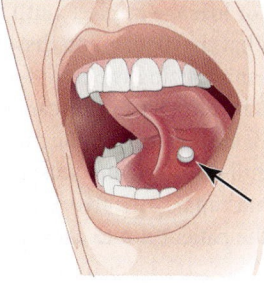

Fig 14.2 Sublingual route. (From Burton and Ludwig [2011]. *Fundamentals of nursing care: Concepts, connections & skills.* Philadelphia: F. A. Davis Company, with permission.)

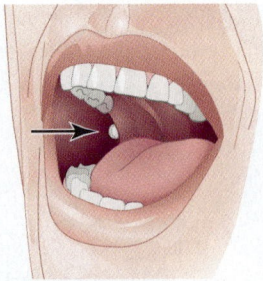

Fig 14.3 Buccal route. (From Burton and Ludwig [2011]. *Fundamentals of nursing care: Concepts, connections & skills.* Philadelphia: F. A. Davis Company, with permission.)

    c. Buccal.
      (1) Dissolves slowly between the cheek and gum to affect the mucous membranes of the oral cavity.
      (2) Administered for a local effect.
    d. Swish and spit/swish and swallow.
      (1) Solution circulated in the mouth and expelled or swallowed.
      (2) Administered for a local effect (e.g., mucous membranes of the mouth and esophagus if swallowed).

3. Disadvantages.
    a. Contraindicated for individuals who are unable to maintain a tablet in place until dissolved or unable to follow directions regarding dispersing a solution throughout the oral cavity.
    b. Sublingual: Must remain under the tongue until completely dissolved for best effect.
    c. Buccal: Must remain in the buccal cavity until completely dissolved for best effect and may cause irritation of the mucous membranes.
    d. Swish and spit/swish and swallow: Patient may accidentally aspirate the solution or swallow the solution meant to be expelled.

4. Commonalities of nursing interventions specific to administering medications via oral mucous membranes.
    a. Ensure that the patient is physically able and mentally aware of the need to keep the tablet, troche, or lozenge in place until dissolved to ensure that the medication dissolves in the mouth, minimizing the risk of aspiration.
    b. Inform the primary health-care provider if the patient is unable to keep the medication in place until dissolved and seek an order for a route that can be tolerated.
    c. Teach the patient not to chew or swallow the tablet.
    d. Assess the mucous membranes for irritation; inform the primary health-care provider if any occurs, and suggest a change in route.

5. Nursing interventions specific to administering medications via the sublingual route.
    a. Instruct the patient to hold the tablet under the tongue until the medication dissolves.
    b. Assess for a therapeutic effect immediately to promote evaluation and documentation of the patient's response (sublingual route has a quick absorption rate).

6. Nursing interventions specific to administering medications via the buccal route.
    a. Instruct the patient to place the troche or lozenge against the mucous membrane of the cheek and gum until it dissolves.

    🛑 b. Ensure that the patient stays awake until the troche or lozenge dissolves to reduce the risk of aspiration.

    c. Advise the patient to alternate cheeks when taking additional doses to minimize the risk of mucosal irritation.

7. Nursing interventions specific to administering medications via swish and spit/swish and swallow.
    a. Instruct the patient to keep the lips closed and puff the cheeks in and out to ensure that the solution is dispersed to all mucous membranes in the oral cavity.
    b. Instruct the patient to expel the solution from the mouth for swish and spit to ensure that the solution is in contact with only the oral mucous membranes.
    c. Instruct the patient to swallow the solution for swish and swallow to ensure that the solution is in contact with the mucous membranes of the oral cavity and the esophagus.

D. Skin
1. Introduction.
    a. Skin is the largest organ of the body (integumentary system); it protects underlying tissue, helps to regulate body temperature, secretes sebum, transmits sensations through nerve endings, and produces and absorbs vitamin D.
    b. The product is designed to be absorbed through the skin and produce either a local or systemic effect.
      (1) **Topical:** Applied to the skin to provide a local or systemic effect, depending on the site, but usually used for a local effect.
      (2) **Transdermal:** Applied to the skin for a systemic effect.

2. Types of preparations.
    a. **Liniment:** Alcohol, oil, or soapy emollient containing a medicated substance.
    b. **Lotion:** Medication in a liquid suspension often used to clean, cool, or protect the skin.
    c. **Ointment (salve or cream):** Semisolid substance containing a medication.

d. **Paste:** Thick ointment that is absorbed slowly through the skin and is generally used for skin protection.
   e. **Transdermal patch:** Impregnated sheath that releases a controlled amount of medication to produce a systemic response.
3. Advantages.
   a. Topical.
      (1) Easy to apply.
      (2) Generally painless.
   b. Transdermal.
      (1) Provides a prolonged systemic effect (1 to 7 days, depending on the medication).
      (2) Convenient when used for 72 hours or longer.
      (3) Replaces daily administration of a medication.
4. Disadvantages.
   a. Topical.
      (1) Risk for fast absorption and a systemic effect in the presence of impaired skin integrity, such as excoriation or a break in the skin.
      (2) May irritate the skin.
      (3) May cause adverse systemic effects.
      (4) May leave oily matter on the skin that can soil clothing.
   b. Transdermal.
      (1) May require shaving of hair to facilitate adherence of the patch.
      (2) May cause skin irritation.
5. Commonalities of nursing interventions specific to administering medications via the skin.
   a. Follow standard precautions (e.g., don gloves) when applying topical medications to prevent exposure to the medication and contact with blood and body fluids.
   b. Maintain sterile technique if the patient's skin lacks integrity to reduce the risk of infection.
   c. Assess for irritation at the site and report to the primary health-care provider if any occurs.
6. Nursing interventions specific to administering liniments, lotions, ointments, and pastes.
   a. Clean the skin with soap and water before application to improve medication absorption.
   b. Place the lid of a container on a surface with the inside facing upward to prevent contamination of the inside of the lid.
   c. Use a separate sterile tongue blade each time when obtaining paste from a container to maintain the sterility of the inside of the jar.
   d. Apply in a thin or thick layer, according to the manufacturer's directions.
   e. Apply onto the skin with the degree of rubbing recommended by the manufacturer.

7. Nursing interventions specific to administering medications via a transdermal patch.
   a. Follow standard precautions when administering a patch.
   🛑 b. Remove the previous patch before applying a new one to minimize the risk of overdose.
   c. Contain and dispose of a used patch to protect others from exposure to the active substance still on the patch.
   d. Wash and dry the skin after removing a used patch. Doing so removes any lingering medication from the skin and minimizes the risk of overdose.
   e. Shave hair on the skin with the patient's consent if the hair interferes with patch adherence.
   f. Apply the patch and gently compress the patch with a gloved hand for 10 seconds to facillitate adherence.
   g. Write the date, the time, and your initials on a patch.
E. Eye
1. Introduction.
   a. **Ophthalmic medications:** Medicinal substances administered into an eye.
   b. Ophthalmic medications produce a local effect.
2. Advantages.
   a. Provides medication directly to the desired site.
   b. Allows medication of one or both eyes.
3. Disadvantages.
   a. Difficult to self-administer, particularly if the patient has impaired vision.
   b. Damage may occur to the eye if the tip of the dropper or tube touches the eye or drops fall directly on the cornea.
   c. Infection may occur if the tip of the dropper or tube touches the eye because this contaminates the medication container.
4. Nursing interventions specific to administering eye medications.
   a. Clean the eyelid and lashes with sterile normal saline solution–soaked cotton balls. Use a new one for each stroke, moving from the inner canthus to outer canthus. Doing so cleans the eye and reduces the risk of debris entering the lacrimal duct.
   b. Tilt the patient's head slightly back and toward the eye being medicated to prevent the solution from flowing toward the other eye.
   c. Have the patient look up to reduce the risk of blinking.
   d. Place a finger just below the lower eyelashes and exert gentle downward pressure over the bony prominence of the cheek to expose the conjunctival sac (Fig. 14.4).

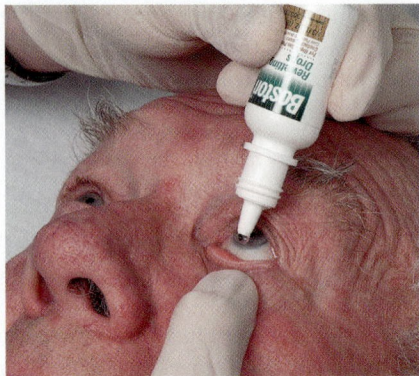

Fig 14.4 Administering eye drops. (From Burton and Ludwig [2011]. *Fundamentals of nursing care: Concepts, connections & skills.* Philadelphia: F. A. Davis Company, with permission.)

e. Hold the dropper close to the eye without touching it and administer the prescribed number of drops so they fall into the conjunctival sac and not on the eyeball.

f. Apply ointment along the edge of the lower conjunctival sac without touching the eye with the tube to maintain the sterility of the ointment tube.

g. Release the lower lid and instruct the patient to close the eyes gently to prevent the medication from being squeezed out of the eye.

h. Apply gentle pressure over the inner canthus to prevent medication from flowing into the lacrimal duct.

i. Teach the patient not to rub the medicated eye to avoid irritation and contamination of the hands, which may contaminate the other eye, surfaces in the environment, and other people.

F. Ear
1. Introduction.
   a. **Otic medications:** Medicinal substances administered into an ear.
   b. Otic medications produce a local effect.
2. Advantages.
   a. Provides medication directly to the desired site.
   b. Allows medication of one or both ears.
3. Disadvantages.
   a. May require removal of earwax (cerumen) for the medication to reach the involved tissue.
   b. May cause damage if drops fall directly onto the tympanic membrane.
4. Nursing interventions specific to administering ear medications.
   a. Warm the solution to room temperature by holding the container of medication in the palm of a hand for several minutes to minimize discomfort.
   b. Clean the external ear of drainage with normal saline solution–moistened cotton balls.

c. Place the patient in the side-lying position with the affected ear facing toward the ceiling to help retain the drops in the ear.

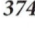 d. Gently pull up and back on the cartilaginous part of the pinna for an adult and a child older than 3 years of age. Pull the cartilaginous part of the pinna down and back for an infant or child younger than age 3 years (Fig. 14.5).

e. Place the drops on the side of the ear canal so that the drops flow down the wall of the ear canal, but avoid touching the canal with the dropper to protect the dropper from contamination and avoid injury to the tympanic membrane.

f. Release the pinna and gently press on the tragus several times to move the medication along the canal to the tympanic membrane.

g. Maintain the patient in the side-lying position with the affected ear facing the ceiling for 5 minutes after medication administration. Doing so uses gravity to ensure drug contact with the structures within the ear canal.

h. Loosely insert a cotton ball into the external canal, if prescribed, to prevent the drug from leaking out of the ear canal.

G. Rectum
1. Introduction.
   a. The rectum is the last 7 to 8 inches of the large intestine. The last inch of the rectum is called the *anal canal* and the opening itself is called the *anus.*
   b. Products must be inserted through the anus and anal canal to reach the rectum.

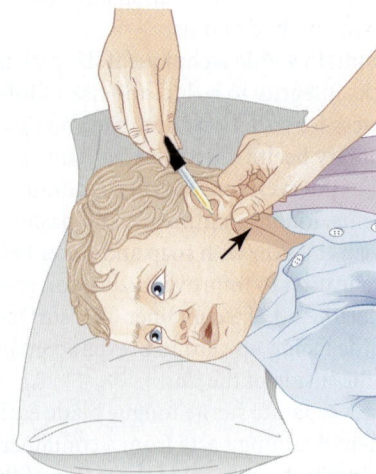

Fig 14.5 Administering ear drops to a child younger than 3 years of age. (From Burton and Ludwig [2011]. *Fundamentals of nursing care: Concepts, connections & skills.* Philadelphia: F. A. Davis Company, with permission.)

c. Products include creams that are inserted with an applicator or a cone-shaped, firm substance (suppository) that can be inserted with a gloved finger.

d. Products are designed to dissolve and be absorbed through the mucous membranes of the rectum.

2. Advantages.

a. Provides for a local or systemic effect, depending on the medication (e.g., laxative or anti-inflammatory for a local effect; sedative or analgesic for a systemic effect).

b. Allows medication to be released at a slow, steady rate.

c. Provides an alternate administration site when the patient is vomiting or oral medication has an objectionable taste.

3. Disadvantages.

a. Rates of absorption are unpredictable.

b. Is contraindicated if the patient had rectal surgery or has rectal bleeding.

c. May be perceived by the patient as unpleasant or cause patient embarrassment.

d. May soil or stain clothing.

4. Nursing interventions specific to administering medications via the rectum.

a. Store foil-wrapped suppositories in a refrigerator to help the suppository retain its form for ease of insertion.

b. Follow standard precautions, including donning gloves, to prevent exposure to body fluids.

c. Close the door and pull the curtain around the bed to provide privacy.

d. Position the patient in the lateral position.

e. Drape the patient with a sheet exposing only the perianal area to provide privacy.

f. Identify whether the patient has a fecal mass in the rectum. If a mass is present, the product must be inserted between the fecal mass and the rectal wall to promote its effect.

🛑 g. Lubricate the suppository and the index finger of your gloved hand to facilitate insertion and prevent tissue trauma.

h. Direct insertion toward the umbilicus, using the full length of an index finger. Doing so ensures placement past the anal canal, anal sphincter, and anal-rectal ridge, which promotes retention of the suppository (Fig. 14.6).

i. Instruct the patient to remain in the lateral or supine position for 10 to 20 minutes after insertion to keep the suppository in place, which facilitates absorption.

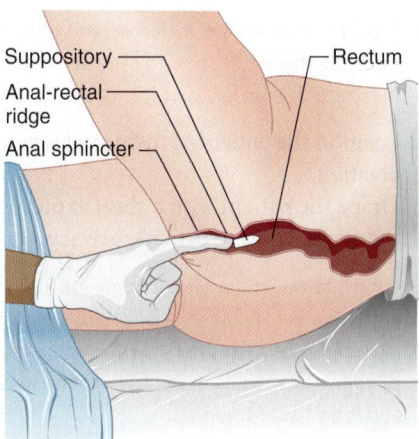

Fig 14.6 Inserting a rectal suppository. (From Burton and Ludwig [2011]. *Fundamentals of nursing care: Concepts, connections & skills.* Philadelphia: F. A. Davis Company, with permission.)

H. Vagina

1. Introduction.

a. The vagina is a 3-inch long area (vaginal canal) extending from the cervix of the uterus to the vaginal opening (vaginal introitus).

b. Products must be inserted through the vaginal introitus and be placed deep within the vaginal canal.

c. Products include creams, foams, jellies, or tablets that are inserted with an applicator or a cone-shaped, firm substance (suppository) that can be inserted with a gloved finger.

d. Products are designed to dissolve and be absorbed through the mucous membranes of the vagina.

2. Advantages.

a. Provides a local effect.

b. Provides an alternate route for a contraceptive other than oral or intradermal.

3. Disadvantages.

a. May be perceived by the patient as unpleasant or cause patient embarrassment.

b. May soil or stain clothing.

4. Nursing interventions specific to administering medications via the vagina.

a. Store foil-wrapped suppositories in a refrigerator to help the suppository retain its form for ease of insertion.

b. Follow standard precautions, including donning gloves to prevent exposure to body fluids.

c. Have the patient void before insertion of the medication to eliminate the pressure of a full bladder, which may cause discomfort during insertion.

d. Close the door and pull the curtain around the bed to provide privacy.

> **(!)** e. Provide perineal care with soap and water before inserting the medication to remove debris and minimize the presence of microorganisms.

f. Position the patient in the dorsal recumbent position.
g. Drape the patient with a sheet exposing only the vaginal area to provide privacy.

> **(!)** h. Lubricate the tablet and your gloved index finger with a water-soluble jelly or expel a small amount of vaginal cream at the tip of the applicator supplied by the manufacturer to facilitate insertion and limit tissue trauma.

i. Direct insertion downward and backward using the full length of the applicator or index finger. Doing so follows the contour of the vaginal anatomy and ensures that the medication is inserted deep in the vaginal canal (Fig. 14.7).
j. Use a rolling motion when inserting a cream with an applicator. Doing so spreads lubricant along the vaginal lining, easing insertion.
k. Fully compress the plunger of the applicator to ensure disbursement of the cream or placement of the tablet deep in the vaginal canal.
l. Remove the applicator slowly to prevent tissue trauma.
m. Instruct the patient to remain in a supine position for 10 to 20 minutes after insertion to keep the medication in place, which facilitates absorption.

I. Upper and Lower Respiratory Tract
1. Introduction.
   a. The upper respiratory tract consists of the nose, nasopharynx, sinuses, oropharynx, laryngopharynx, and larynx.
   b. The lower respiratory tract consists of the trachea, all segments of the bronchial tree, and the alveoli.

c. Medications are introduced into the upper respiratory tract through the nose via drops or sprays.
d. Medications are introduced into the lower respiratory tract usually through the mouth via a fine spray, fog, powder, or mist.
e. Most medications are delivered to achieve a local effect, improving ventilation and oxygenation (e.g., bronchodilators, anti-inflammatory agents, antihistamines, and nasal decongestants).
f. Intranasal mists may be given for a systemic effect (e.g., flu vaccine).

2. Types of respiratory tract medication delivery systems (Fig. 14.8).
   a. Upper respiratory tract.
      (1) **Drops:** Drops of medicated solution are introduced into a nostril by a dropper.
      (2) **Nasal sprays:** Sprays suspend droplets of medication that are propelled into the nose by depressing a cartridge adaptor or squeezing the container.
   b. Lower respiratory tract.
      (1) **Metered-dose inhaler (MDI):** A pressurized container propels medication as a fine spray through a mouthpiece that is then inhaled into the lower respiratory tract.
      (2) **Nonpressurized aerosol (handheld nebulizer):** Medication is changed to a fine mist or fog so that it can be inhaled deep into the lower respiratory tract; generally administered via a mouthpiece but can be delivered with a mask to infants or children or an adult who has difficulty using the mouthpiece.

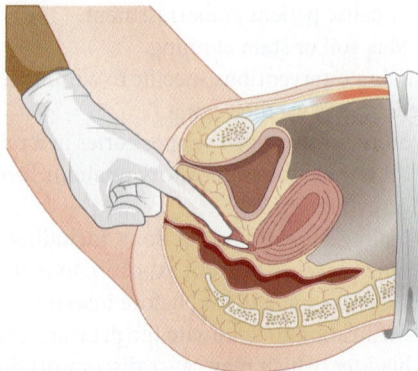

Fig 14.7 Inserting a vaginal suppository. (From Wilkinson and Treas [2011]. *Fundamentals of nursing,* Vol. 2, 2nd ed. Philadelphia: F. A. Davis Company, with permission.)

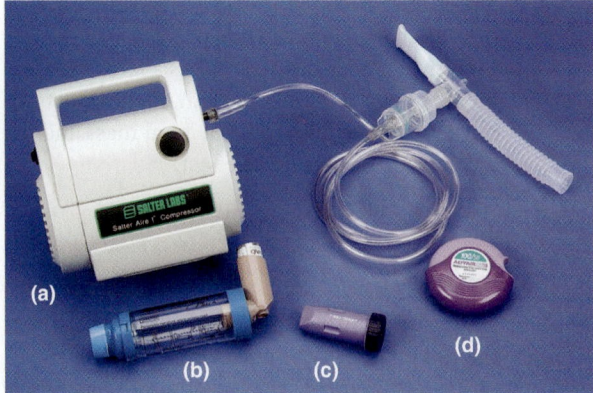

Fig 14.8 Types of inhalers: a. An ultrasonic nebulizer delivers medication and humidity as a fine mist. b. A metered-dose inhaler delivers measured doses. This one has a spacer. c. A dry-powder inhaler (Turbuhaler). d. A Diskhaler. (From Burton and Ludwig [2011]. *Fundamentals of nursing care: Concepts, connections & skills.* Philadelphia: F. A. Davis Company, with permission.)

(3) **Dry powder disk inhaler:** Multiple-dose disks deliver dry powder to the lower respiratory tract when inhaled through the mouth.

3. Advantages.
   a. Lower respiratory tract delivery systems: Promote inhalation of medication deep into respiratory passages.
   b. Have a rapid, efficient local effect due to the highly vascular nature of airways and alveoli.
   c. Some can be administered to an unconscious patient.

4. Disadvantages.
   a. Requires sufficient inhalation flow rates to deliver inhaled medication to the lower respiratory tract.
   b. Metered-dose and dry powder disk inhalers require coordination with device activation and inhalation.
   c. May cause unwanted systemic effects (e.g., tachycardia and palpitations with some bronchodilators) or irritate the mucous membranes of the respiratory tract, depending on the medication.
   d. Some delivery systems cannot be used for children and cognitively impaired persons who cannot follow directions.
   e. Requires the use of special equipment that needs to be cleaned.

5. Commonalities of nursing interventions specific to administering mediations via the upper and lower respiratory tract.
   a. Assess respiratory function.
      (1) Rate, rhythm, and effort.
      (2) Sounds: crackles, rhonchi, stridor, wheezing, diminished.
      (3) Use of accessory muscles.
      (4) Nasal flaring.
      (5) Orthopnea.
      (6) Pulse oximetry: 95 percent and higher for normal.
      (7) Cough: Productive or nonproductive; characteristics.
      (8) Secretions: Amount; color; odor; and consistency.
      (9) Nasal congestion.
      (10) Gross abnormalities of the visible mucosa, such as lesions, irritation, or inflammation.
   b. Wear gloves if contamination is likely to prevent exposure to blood and body fluids.
    c. Encourage the patient to blow the nose and cough up respiratory tract secretions. Doing so clears excess secretions from the respiratory tract and permits the medication to reach the mucous membrane.
   d. Position the patient's head as indicated for the specific delivery system to facilitate distribution of the medication to the appropriate site.

e. Avoid sharing sprays, droppers, and inhalers to minimize the risk of cross-contamination.
f. Clean equipment after each use or weekly, based on the manufacturer's recommendations, to minimize the risk of bacterial contamination of equipment and prepare the equipment for the next dose.
g. Discard expired inhalers, sprays, and drops.
 h. Instruct the patient to rinse the mouth after administration to remove any unpleasant taste, if present, and minimize the risk of candidiasis (with steroidal agents).

6. Nursing interventions specific to administering medications via a metered-dose inhaler (MDI). Teach the patient to:
   a. Shake the canister before each depression to mix the propellant with the medication.
   b. Attach the mouthpiece to the medication canister.
   c. Exhale slowly and completely through pursed lips to ensure air is exhaled fully from the lower lobes of the lungs and prepare the lungs for full inhalation.
   d. Hold the inhaler 2 cm from the mouth (Fig. 14.9a: Open-mouth method) or insert the mouthpiece beyond the teeth and instruct the patient to form a tight seal with the lips (Fig. 14.9b: Closed-mouth method).
   e. Depress the device while inhaling slowly and deeply and hold the breath for 5 to 10 seconds at the height of inhalation. Doing so disperses the medication deep in the respiratory tract and prolongs contact of the medication with the respiratory mucosa.
   f. Exhale slowly and completely through pursed lips to keep the smaller airways open during exhalation.

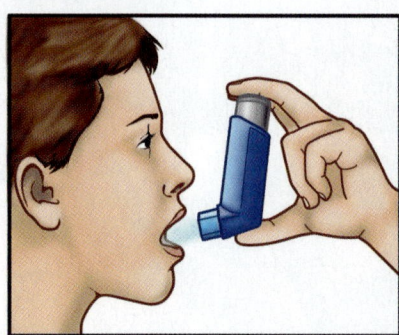

Fig 14.9a Metered-dose inhaler: Open-mouth method.
(From Wilkinson and Treas [2011]. *Fundamentals of nursing,* Vol. 2, 2nd ed. Philadelphia: F. A. Davis Company, adapted with permission.)

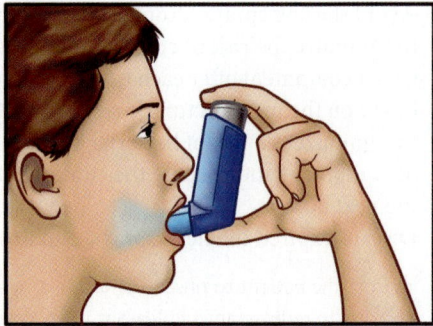

Fig. 14.9b Metered-dose inhaler: Closed-mouth method. (From Wilkinson and Treas [2011]. *Fundamentals of nursing,* Vol. 2, 2nd ed. Philadelphia: F. A. Davis Company, adapted with permission.)

g. Use a spacer device for better results because the medication is released into the spacer and is then inhaled via a mouthpiece (Fig. 14.10). Doing so eliminates the need to coordinate inhalation with canister compression and promotes larger droplets to fall to the bottom of the spacer and increases the volume of smaller droplets reaching the lungs.

7. Nursing interventions specific to administering medications via a nasal spray. Teach the patient to:
   a. Insert the tip of the nasal device into one nostril while occluding the other by gently pressing on the nostril toward the midline. Doing so minimizes the aerosol from entering the other nostril.
   b. Press the adapter cartridge or squeeze the container while inhaling through the accessed nostril to discharge a measured dose into the accessed nostril.

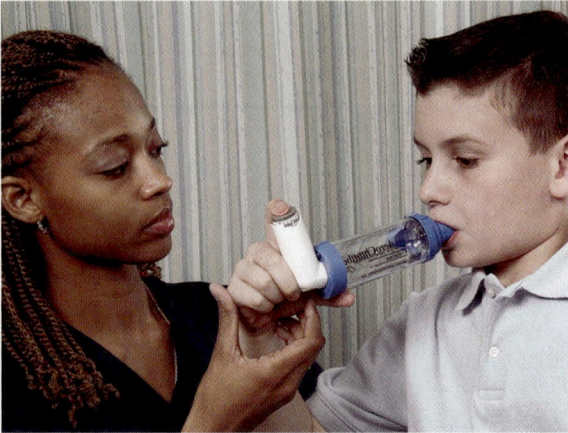

Fig 14.10 Metered-dose inhaler with spacer. (From Wilkinson and Treas [2011]. *Fundamentals of nursing,* Vol. 2, 2nd ed. Philadelphia: F. A. Davis Company, with permission.)

c. Exhale slowly through the mouth to help retain the medication in the nasal passage.
d. Insert the tip into the other nostril and, while breathing in slowly through the nose, squirt the spray into the nostril; do not occlude the first nostril. Dong so discharges one measured dose in the accessed nostril; occluding the first nostril may expel previously administered medication.
e. Exhale slowly through the mouth to help retain medication in the nasal passage.
f. Tilt the head backward to allow the spray to reach the back of the nose.
g. Wait 1 minute before administering a prescribed second dose to allow time for the first dose to take effect.
h. Clean the outside of the container weekly according to the manufacturer's recommendations to minimize the risk of bacterial contamination of equipment.

🛑 i. Avoid excessive use of OTC nasal decongestants; limit use to 7 days. Increased congestion can occur after the therapeutic effect subsides with excessive use **(rebound congestion).**

8. Nursing interventions specific to administering medications via an aerosol handheld nebulizer. Teach the patient to:
   a. Place the medication and a small volume of saline (if required) in a cup connected to a handheld nebulizer that has a mouthpiece. Doing so mixes the medication and saline, preparing it for aerosolization.
   b. Attach the nebulizer to wall oxygen or a nebulizer compressor to propel oxygen or air through the medication cup, changing the medication solution to a mist (see Fig. 14.8a).
   c. Sit in an upright position to promote thoracic excursion by allowing the abdominal organs to drop by gravity.
   d. Insert the mouthpiece beyond the teeth and form a tight seal with the lips (Fig. 14.11) to ensure that the mist does not escape from the mouth.
   e. Inhale and exhale slowly and deeply through the mouth without removing the mouthpiece to deliver the medication deep into the small respiratory airways.
   f. Tap the side of the nebulizer occasionally to dislodge the solution from the sides of the cup down to where it can be misted.

🛑 g. Continue for several minutes until the misting stops to ensure the entire dose is delivered.

h. Disassemble the nebulizer, mouthpiece, and cup; clean them with soap and water; and reassemble when dry to minimize the risk of infection.

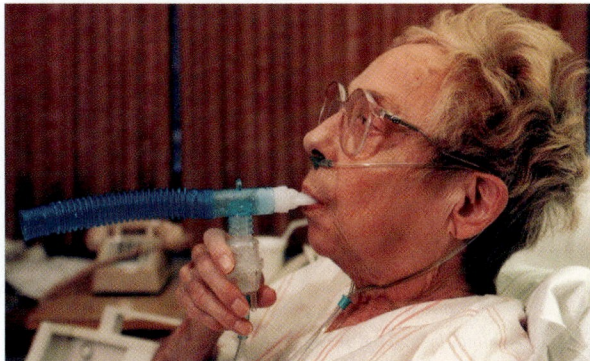

Fig 14.11 Hand-held nebulizer. (From Williams and Hopper [2011]. *Understanding medical surgical nursing,* 4th ed. Philadelphia: F. A. Davis Company, with permission.)

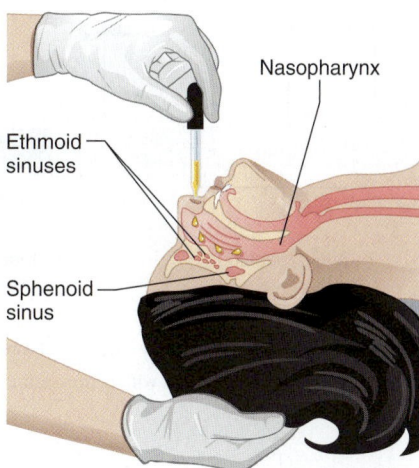

Fig 14.12 Instilling nose drops. (From Wilkinson and Treas [2011]. *Fundamentals of nursing,* Vol. 2, 2nd ed. Philadelphia: F. A. Davis Company, with permission.)

9. Nursing interventions specific to administering medications via a dry powdered disk inhaler. Teach the patient to:
    a. Hold the disk horizontal in one hand throughout administration; put the thumb in the notch and push it away from the body until the mouthpiece appears. Doing so accesses the mouthpiece of the inhaler.
    b. Use a thumb to slide the lever away from the body until it clicks to ensure the medication is ready for delivery.
    c. Seal the lips around the mouthpiece and breathe in quickly and deeply through the mouth to move medication into the respiratory tract.
    d. Remove the disk from the mouth and hold the breath for 5 to 10 seconds to lengthen the time the medication is in contact with the respiratory mucosa.
    e. Use the thumb to slide the notch back to shut the disk, preparing it for the next dose.
10. Nursing interventions specific to administering nose drops. Teach the patient to:
    a. Hyperextend the head slightly (place a rolled towel behind the shoulders or place the head over the edge of the bed) (Fig. 14.12) to promote distribution of the solution over the surfaces of the nasal mucosa.
    b. Hold the dropper over the nostril without touching the nose to avoid contamination of the dropper.
    c. Apply the prescribed number of drops.
    d. Avoid swallowing the medication to ensure that the medication stays in contact with the nasal mucosa.
    e. Maintain the head tilt for a few minutes after insertion of drops to prevent the solution from exiting the nose via gravity.

    f. Return the dropper to the bottle and then close the bottle tightly to maintain the integrity of the medication and dropper.
J. **Parenteral Routes**
  1. Introduction.
    a. **Parenteral**: Means other than the alimentary canal (GI tract).
    b. Parenteral medications are administered intramuscularly, subcutaneously, intradermally, or intravenously.
  2. Advantages.
    a. Avoids the GI tract when the GI tract is impaired, the medication is too irritating to the mucosa, or the GI tract inactivates the medication.
    b. Has more rapid onset than the oral route.
    c. Is more predictable results than other routes.
    d. Can be administered to unconscious patients.
  3. Disadvantages.
    a. Punctures the skin, increasing the risk of infection.
    b. May cause tissue injury if the solubility or pH of the medication is inappropriate for the tissue being accessed.
    c. Requires sterile equipment and is a more complex procedure than oral or topical medication administration (e.g., use of sterile technique, multiplicity of sites than can be used, safe disposal of equipment).
  4. Characteristics of syringes and needles.
    a. Type of syringe.
      (1) Consists of a barrel, plunger, hub, needle (cannula, shaft), and safety device to prevent a needlestick injury; measurement calibrations are on the barrel (Fig. 14.13).

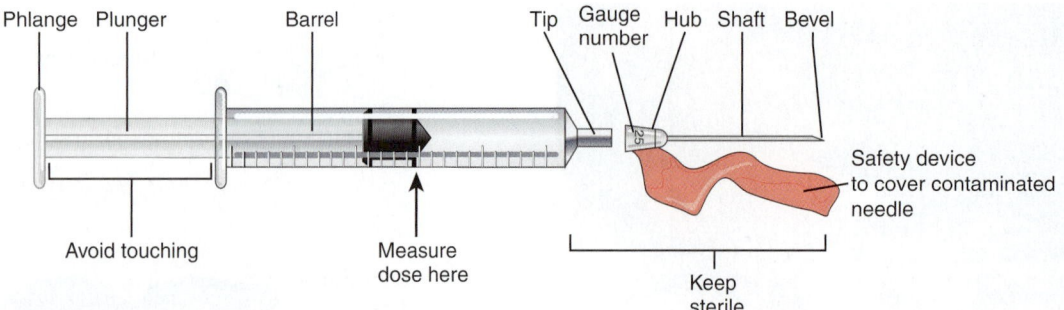

Fig 14.13 Parts of a syringe and safety needle. (From Burton and Ludwig [2011]. *Fundamentals of nursing care: Concepts, connections & skills.* Philadelphia: F. A. Davis Company, with permission.)

(2) Generally packaged with an attached needle; however, the needle should be changed after drawing up a caustic drug or when a more appropriate needle gauge or length is desired.

(3) **Luer-Lok syringe:** Marked in 0.1 (tenths); requires a special needle that twists on the tip of the syringe and locks into place (Fig. 14.14).

(4) **Tuberculin syringe:** Marked in 0.01 (hundredths) for doses less than 1 mL and has a very narrow barrel (Fig. 14.15).

(5) **Insulin syringe:** Marked in either 50 or 100 units and has a short barrel (Fig. 14.16).

(6) **Prefilled single-dose syringe:** May require a drug calculation before administering the correct dose; larger volumes of the drug than that which is prescribed may have to be wasted (Fig. 14.17).

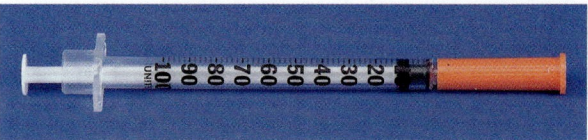

Fig 14.16 Insulin syringe. (From Burton and Ludwig [2011]. *Fundamentals of nursing care: Concepts, connections & skills.* Philadelphia: F. A. Davis Company, with permission.)

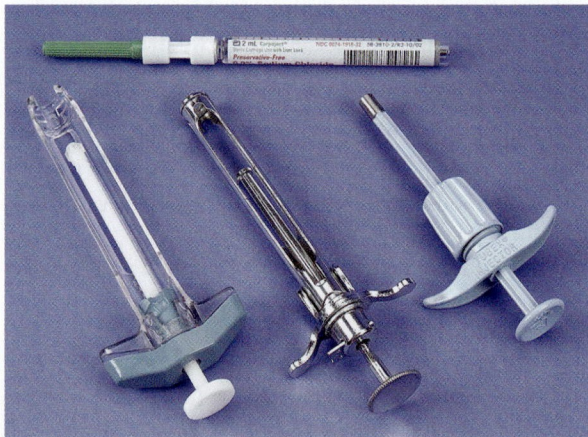

Fig 14.17 Prefilled single-dose syringe and three types of holders. (From Burton and Ludwig [2011]. *Fundamentals of nursing care: Concepts, connections & skills.* Philadelphia: F. A. Davis Company, with permission.)

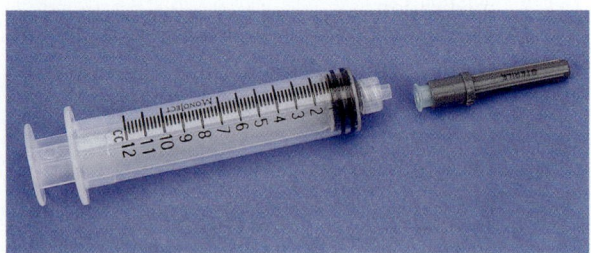

Fig 14.14 Luer-Lok syringe. (From Burton and Ludwig [2011]. *Fundamentals of nursing care: Concepts, connections & skills.* Philadelphia: F. A. Davis Company, with permission.)

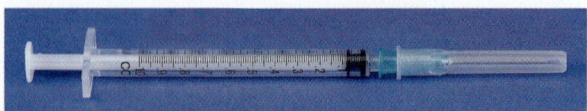

Fig 14.15 Tuberculin syringe. (From Burton and Ludwig [2011]. *Fundamentals of nursing care: Concepts, connections & skills.* Philadelphia: F. A. Davis Company, with permission.)

b. Volume of syringe (Fig. 14.18).

(1) Sizes vary with volumes, from 0.5 mL to 60 mL.

(2) Syringes with volumes of 1 mL or less usually are used for subcutaneous (Sub-Q) injections.

(3) Syringes with volumes of 3 mL usually are used for IM injections.

(4) Syringes with volumes larger than 3 mL are used to administer intravenous (IV) medications, add solutions to IV bags, or irrigate tubes or wounds.

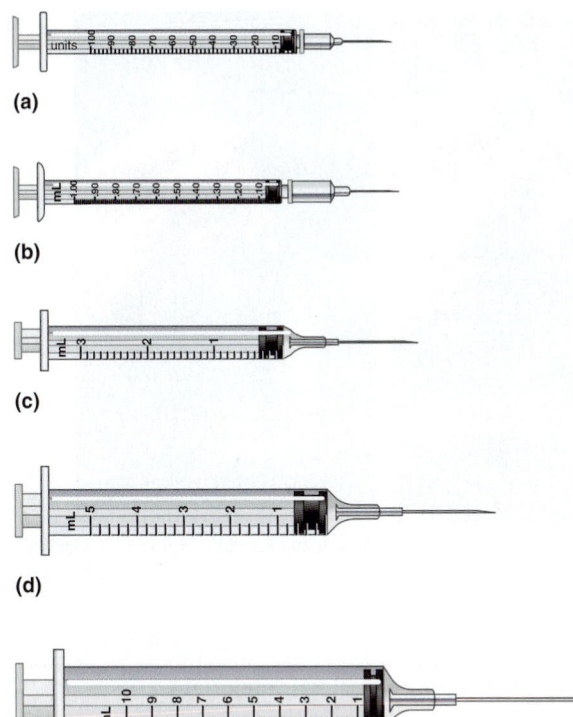

Fig 14.18 Syringe sizes: (a) U-100 syringe marked in units, of which there are 100/mL. (b) 1-mL tuberculin syringe marked in 0.01 mL (1/100th of a milliliter) and minims (16 minims equals 1 mL). (c) 3-mL standard syringe marked in whole milliliters and 0.1 mL (1/10th of a milliliter). (d) 5-mL standard syringe marked in whole milliliters and 0.2 mL (2/10ths of a milliliter). (e) 10-mL standard syringe marked in whole milliliters and 0.2 mL (2/10ths of a milliliter). (From Burton and Ludwig [2011].
Fundamentals of nursing care: Concepts, connections & skills.
Philadelphia: F. A. Davis Company, with permission.)

c. Needle (shaft) length.
  (1) Vary in length from ¼ to 3 inches.
  (2) Shorter needles (⅝, ½, and 1 inch) are used for infants, children, and thin adults and for subcutaneous injections.
  (3) Longer needles (1½ inch) are used for IM injections.
  (4) Needles longer than 1½ inches in length are used for obese patients and invasive procedures that require insertion of a needle, such as biopsies, paracentesis, and thoracentesis.
  (5) Needles in different size gauges and lengths are packaged in individual sterile sheaths or come attached to a packaged syringe.
  (6) Syringe needles can be replaced with a different gauge or length needle as necessary.

d. Needle gauge (diameter of shaft).
  (1) **Gauge:** Diameter of a needle; varies in size from #18 to #28 gauge.
  (2) The smaller the needle gauge, the larger the diameter of the needle; the larger the needle gauge, the smaller the diameter of the needle.
  (3) Larger gauge needles cause less tissue damage when inserted.
  (4) Viscous solutions require a smaller gauge needle.
e. Needle bevel.
  (1) Tips of needles are slanted (beveled) to create a narrow slit in the skin when inserted; when the needle is removed, the slit in the skin closes to prevent leakage of fluid.
  (2) Long-beveled needles are more pointy and sharp; generally used for IM and Sub-Q injections.
  (3) Short-beveled needles are used for intradermal and IV injections because the risk of the bevel becoming occluded is less likely.
5. Commonalities of nursing interventions specific to administering medications via all parenteral routes.
  a. Perform hand hygiene to prevent infection.
  b. Select an appropriate-size syringe, needle gauge, and needle length to ensure that the medication is deposited at the correct tissue depth.
  c. Maintain sterile technique (the outside of the barrel and tip of the plunger can be touched but not the inside of the barrel, the hub, or the shaft of the plunger).
  d. Aspirate the prescribed volume of solution (see "Withdrawing fluid from an ampule," page 383; "Withdrawing fluid from a vial," page 383; and "Mixing two medications in one syringe," page 384).
  e. Recap the sterile needle using a hands-free method (Fig. 14.19) to prevent a needlestick injury and maintain the sterility of the needle.
  f. Close the door and curtain to provide privacy.
  g. Put on clean gloves to prevent contact with blood and body fluids.
  h. Select the injection site.
    (1) Check the MAR for the site of the last injection and select a new site; systematically rotate sites to minimize underlying tissue damage, which may decrease absorption.
    (2) Inspect the potential injection site for bruises, inflammation, edema, and signs of prior injections; avoid the area if any of these signs are present because they can interfere with absorption.

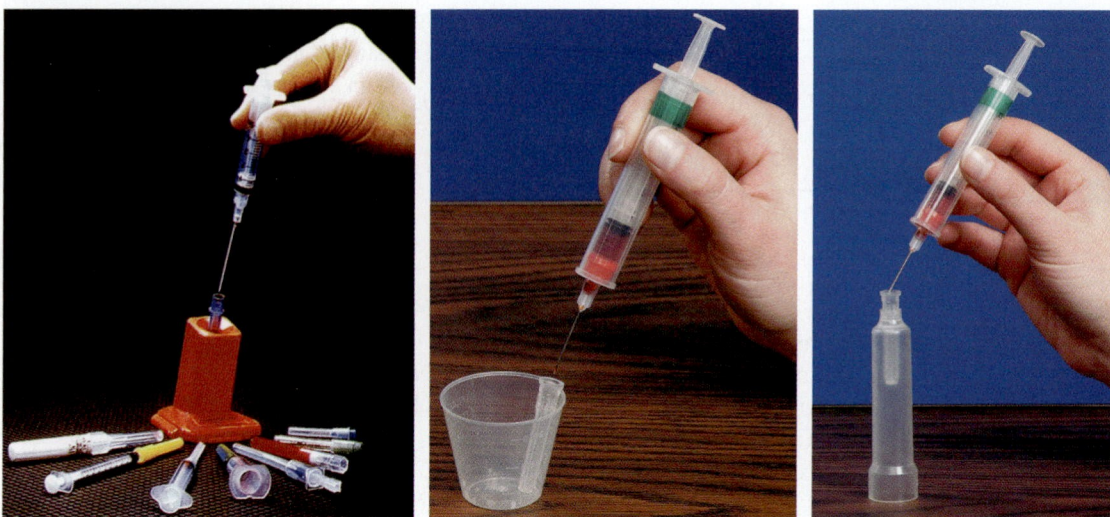

Fig. 14.19 Recapping a sterile needle. (From Wilkinson and Treas [2011]. *Fundamentals of nursing*, Vol. 2, 2nd ed. Philadelphia: F. A. Davis Company, with permission.)

(3) Use landmarks to select a site to minimize trauma to underlying structures, such as nerves and bones.

i. Assist the patient into a comfortable position that permits access to the selected injection site.

j. Drape the patient to expose only the injection site to provide for privacy.

k. Clean the injection site with an alcohol wipe in a circular motion from the center outward to minimize the risk of infection.

l. Pinch or spread the skin, based on the injection type, to position the skin and underlying tissue for insertion of the needle into the correct tissue layer.

m. Insert the needle at a 10- to 90-degree angle to the skin, depending on the type of injection.

n. Stabilize the syringe with your nondominant hand; use your other hand to depress the plunger smoothly and slowly to reduce discomfort and inject the medication into the tissue.

o. Aspirate or avoid aspiration, depending on the type of injection; see IM, Sub-Q, and intradermal injections for specifics regarding aspiration.

p. Move the nondominant hand away from the site slightly; apply pressure with an antiseptic swab but not too close to the needle; quickly but carefully withdraw the needle in one smooth motion along the line of insertion to minimize discomfort and reduce the risk of a needlestick injury.

q. Massage the area if directed by the medication's instructions to increase drug distribution and absorption and stimulate circulation. Avoid massaging when administering insulin or anticoagulants to limit bleeding and bruising.

r. Institute precautions to prevent a needlestick injury (Box 14.2).

Box 14.2 Preventing Needlestick Injuries

- Use safety syringes that are designed to actively (A) or passively (B) cover used needles to protect the caregiver. Be aware that many facilities use needleless equipment (C).

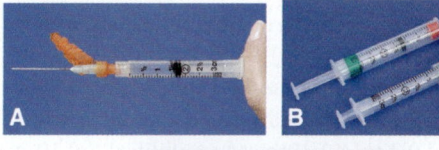

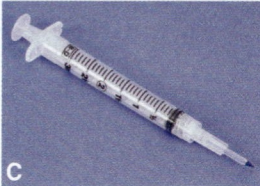

- Dispose of ampules, needles, and sharps (e.g., broken glass, lancets, razors, and any other disposable sharp instruments) in a sharps container, which is usually positioned in strategic locations, such as on medication carts, in medication rooms, in patient rooms, and in dirty utility rooms. Place a used syringe in an emesis basin to transport it to a sharps container if a sharps container is not easily accessible.
- Never recap a used needle or put it in a pocket, in a wastebasket, or on a surface at the bedside; never break or bend needles before disposal.
- For a needle containing a substance that is to be transported to a laboratory, use a safety device that grips the needle cap and holds it so that the needle can be recapped, minimizing the risk of a needlestick injury. The method for recapping a sterile needle can be employed to safely recap a used needle/syringe in preparation for transport to a laboratory (see Fig. 14.19).

Photo credits: Burton and Ludwig (2011). *Fundamentals of nursing care: Concepts, connections & skills*. Philadelphia: F. A. Davis Company, with permission.

6. Withdrawing fluid from an ampule.
   a. Introduction.
      (1) **Ampule:** Characteristically shaped glass container that has a prescored, generally colored ring around a constricted neck.
      (2) Ampules generally hold a single dose of a drug but may hold up to 10 mL or more.
   b. Nursing interventions.
      (1) Flick the top of the ampule repeatedly if fluid is trapped to move the fluid below the constricted neck to ensure the entire dose is in the ampule for withdrawal.
      (2) Position a plastic ampule opener over the top of the constricted neck and snap off the top to protect the hands from injury.

   🛑 (3) Use a filter needle to aspirate the fluid into the syringe to prevent aspiration of glass particles.

      (4) Aspirate fluid into the syringe.
         (a) Invert the ampule, place the needle into the liquid, and aspirate the required volume (Fig. 14.20a). Doing so allows surface tension to hold the solution inside the ampule until the syringe's negative pressure pulls the solution into the syringe.
         (b) Place the ampule on a counter, insert the needle, and aspirate the solution (Fig. 14.20b).
      (5) Change the filter needle to a needle suitable for the injection.
      (6) Dispose of the used ampule, glass top, and filter needle in a sharps container to prevent a puncture injury.

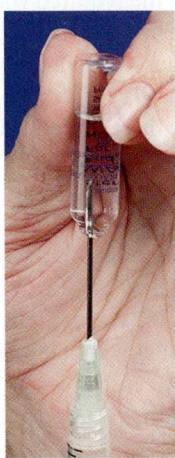

Fig 14.20a Removing fluid from an ampule. Invert the ampule and insert a sterile needle into the ampule, keeping the needle tip below the fluid level. (From Burton and Ludwig [2011]. *Fundamentals of nursing care: Concepts, connections & skills.* Philadelphia: F. A. Davis Company, with permission.)

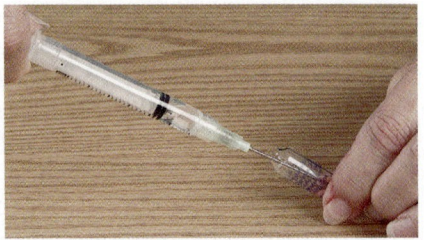

Fig 14.20b Removing fluid from an ampule. Tilt the ampule for medication removal. (From Burton and Ludwig [2011]. *Fundamentals of nursing care: Concepts, connections & skills.* Philadelphia: F. A. Davis Company, with permission.)

7. Withdrawing fluid from a vial.
   a. Introduction.
      (1) **Vial:** Glass rubber-sealed container covered with a metal cap that maintains sterility of the seal until the metal cap is removed.
      (2) Vials hold single or multiple doses.
      (3) Medication is supplied as a liquid or a powder that requires reconstitution because it is stable only for a short period of time when in solution.
   b. Nursing interventions.
      (1) Remove the metal cap that keeps the rubber seal sterile to provide access to the top seal of the vial.
      (2) Clean the rubber seal by wiping its surface with a 70 percent alcohol swab in a firm circular motion from the center, working outward when accessing a multiple-dose vial that has no metal cap, to ensure sterility of the seal.
      (3) Dissolve a medication supplied as a dry powder (**reconstitution**).
         (a) Instill fluid into the vial (**diluent**) with a syringe, following the manufacturer's instructions on the label of the vial for the type and amount of fluid in milliliters.
         (b) Remove the syringe and then gently roll the vial between the palms of the hands to prevent the formation of bubbles, which may result in withdrawal of an inaccurate dose.
         (c) Indicate on the label of a multidose vial the amount of solution that provides a specific dose, along with the date, time, and your initials if you plan to use the vial again in the near future.
         (d) Be aware that some reconstituted drugs must be given within 15 minutes of preparation to prevent degradation of the medication.

   🛑 (e) Do not use a vial that has been reconstituted by another nurse. Only use vials that you have reconstituted to ensure that you know the accuracy of the dose per milliliter.

(4) Select an appropriate syringe and needle and draw air into the barrel to the calibration mark indicating the volume of desired medication. Doing so ensures that an equal volume of air is injected into the vial to ease removal of the same volume of medication.

(5) Insert the needle into the vial above the level of the solution and slowly inject the air to prevent turbulence that can cause bubbles.

(6) Invert the vial and gently pull on the plunger until the calibration mark indicates that the desired volume of medication is withdrawn; keep the tip of the needle below the surface of the solution (Fig. 14.21) to prevent air from being aspirated into the syringe.

(7) Remove the needle from the vial and replace it with an appropriate needle for the situation. Doing so provides a sharp, capped needle and eliminates medication on the outside of the needle that could irritate tissue along the needle tract during insertion.

(8) Administer the medication immediately to prevent errors and degradation of the medication if it was reconstituted.

8. Mixing two medications in one syringe.
   a. Introduction.
      (1) Two medications can be mixed in one syringe, if compatible, to limit the number of injections.

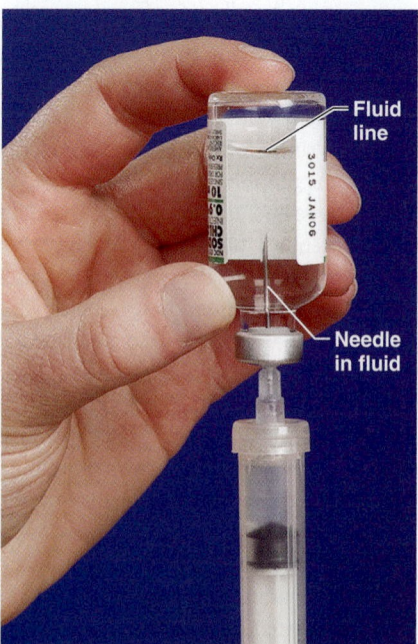

Fig 14.21 Removing fluid from a vial. (From Burton and Ludwig [2011]. *Fundamentals of nursing care: Concepts, connections & skills.* Philadelphia: F. A. Davis Company, with permission.)

(2) Do not mix more than two drugs in one syringe to minimize the risk of medication incompatibility.

(3) Ensure medications are compatible by reading package inserts or consulting with a pharmacist, medication formulary, or textbook; administer drugs separately if compatibility is undetermined to prevent an incompatibility reaction.

b. Commonalities of nursing interventions when mixing two medications in one syringe.
   (1) Determine the volume of each medication as well as the total volume to ensure that the right volume of each medication when added together equals the expected total volume of medication.
   (2) Maintain sterile technique throughout the procedure to reduce the risk of contaminating the medication and reduce the risk of infection.
   (3) Observe the combined solution in the syringe for cloudiness or precipitate formation, which indicates an incompatibility; discard the solution if this occurs and prepare the doses in separate syringes.
   (4) Recap the sterile needle using a safety capping device or a hands-free method to prevent a needlestick injury and maintain the sterility of the needle.
   (5) Administer the medication immediately to prevent drug degradation.

9. Preparing a dose from one multidose vial and one single-dose vial.
   a. Insert air into both vials to facilitate aspiration of the medication from the vials.
   b. Withdraw the required volume from the multidose vial first to prevent contamination of the multidose vial with medication from the single-dose vial.
   c. Withdraw the required volume from the single-dose vial last.

10. Preparing a dose from one multidose vial and an ampule.
    a. Withdraw the required volume from the multidose vial first. By drawing the solution from the multidose vial first, medication from the ampule will not contaminate the multidose vial.
    b. Withdraw the required volume from the ampule last.

11. Preparing a dose from two multidose vials (e.g., insulin).
    a. Identify which medication should be in vial 1 and which should be in vial 2: Vial 1 is the

medication that should not be diluted accidentally with medication from vial 2 (e.g., regular insulin is vial 1 and NPH insulin is vial 2).

b. Instill air into the NPH insulin first and then the regular insulin.

c. Withdraw the prescribed dose from the regular insulin first and then the NPH insulin (Fig. 14.22).

K. Intramuscular (IM) Injections

1. Introduction.

a. **IM injection:** Insertion of medication into a muscle below the subcutaneous layer.

b. The volume of solution injected depends on the site being used and patient characteristics (e.g., age, weight).

(1) Up to 3 mL can be inserted in a large muscle, such as the ventrogluteal site, in a well-developed adult.

(2) Divide the dose when more than 3 mL are prescribed.

(3) Insert only 1 to 2 mL in less-developed muscles associated with children, older adults, and thin patients.

(4) Insert only 0.5 to 1.0 mL in the deltoid muscle in an adult.

c. The length of the needle depends on the site being used and the patient's age and weight.

(1) Adults: Use a 1-inch length needle for the deltoid muscle and $1\frac{1}{2}$-inch for all other intramuscular sites.

(2) Obese adults: May have to use a 2-inch needle to pass through the layer of fatty tissue above the subcutaneous tissue to reach the muscle.

(3) Infants and children: Generally use a $\frac{5}{8}$- to 1-inch length needle, depending on size and depth of the muscle at the selected site.

d. The gauge of the needle depends on the viscosity of the solution (e.g., #20 for thick [viscid] solutions and #22 for thin solutions).

2. Advantages.

a. Can use two medications in one syringe.

b. Allows rapid absorption because of more ample blood supply in the muscles than in the subcutaneous tissue.

3. Disadvantages.

a. Carries a risk of tissue injury if landmarks are not used to select the site.

b. Is more painful than a Sub-Q injection because it uses a smaller gauge and longer needle.

c. May cause fibrosis, abscess, nerve damage, pain, tissue necrosis, and muscle contraction when administered at all sites except the ventrogluteal muscle.

d. Has variable absorption depending on the adequacy of circulation at the injection site.

4. Selection of an IM injection site depends on multiple variables (e.g., advantages, disadvantages, and patient characteristics) (Table 14.1).

5. Nursing interventions specific to administering an IM injection.

a. Select the appropriate gauge needle to ensure the needle gauge is strong enough to pass through the tissue and reach the muscle.

b. Select the appropriate needle length to permit passage through the tissue to penetrate a deep muscle.

c. Alternate sites among the deltoid, vastus lateralis, and ventrogluteal muscles, when appropriate, to minimize tissue injury and facilitate absorption.

d. Position the patient in a comfortable, appropriate position and identify landmarks to ensure

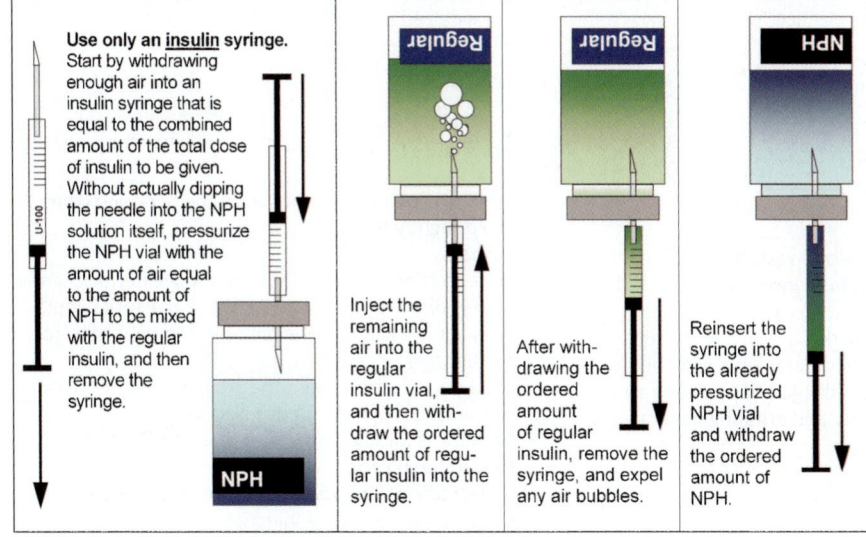

Use only an <u>insulin</u> syringe. Start by withdrawing enough air into an insulin syringe that is equal to the combined amount of the total dose of insulin to be given. Without actually dipping the needle into the NPH solution itself, pressurize the NPH vial with the amount of air equal to the amount of NPH to be mixed with the regular insulin, and then remove the syringe.

Inject the remaining air into the regular insulin vial, and then withdraw the ordered amount of regular insulin into the syringe.

After withdrawing the ordered amount of regular insulin, remove the syringe, and expel any air bubbles.

Reinsert the syringe into the already pressurized NPH vial and withdraw the ordered amount of NPH.

Fig 14.22 Mixing insulin. (From Myers [2006]. *RNotes,* 2nd ed. Philadelphia: F. A. Davis Company, with permission.)

Table 14.1 **Intramuscular Injection Sites: Advantages, Disadvantages, and Nursing Care**

Advantages and Disadvantages	Nursing Care

Deltoid

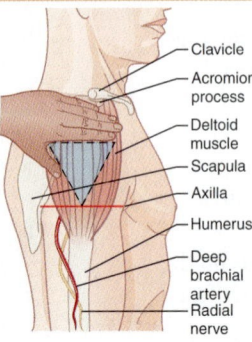

Advantage
- Easily accessible.

Disadvantages
- Generally not used for infants and children because the deltoid is not well developed.
- Carries risk of injury to radial and ulnar nerves and brachial artery.

1. Position the patient standing with the arm at the side; sitting with the lower arm on lap; or supine with the lower arm across the abdomen.
2. **Landmark:** Make an inverted triangle between two to three finger widths below the acromion process and a line from the anterior to posterior axillary crease.

Vastus Lateralis

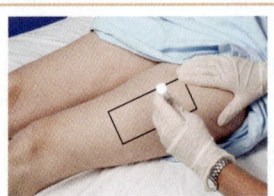

Advantages
- Lacks major nerves and blood vessels.
- Easily accessible.
- Used often for infants, toddlers, and children for immunizations until ventrogluteal muscles develop.

Disadvantage
- None.

1. Position the patient supine with knee slightly flexed.
2. Determine the angle of insertion, which depends on the volume of subcutaneous tissue and needle length.
3. **Landmark:** The muscle extends from a handbreadth above the knee to a handbreadth below the greater trochanter of the femur on the anterior lateral aspect of the thigh.

Ventrogluteal (VG) Gluteus Medius Muscle

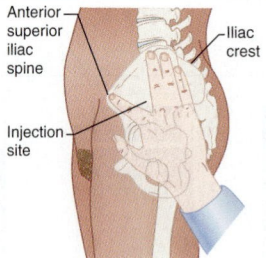

Advantages
- Provides greatest muscle thickness.
- Is located away from major nerves and blood vessels.
- Carries a reduced risk of contamination from incontinent patients or infants.
- Is easily located by obvious bony landmarks.
- Is a deep, well developed muscle even in older infants and children; is the preferred site for children 7 months of age and older and adults.
- Desirable for larger volume, more viscous, and irritating medications.

Disadvantage
- None.

1. Position the patient laterally or on the back with knee and hip slightly flexed.
2. **Landmark:**
   - Place the heel of your hand over the greater trochanter with your wrist perpendicular to the patient's femur; use your left hand for the right hip and right hand for the left hip.
   - Point your thumb toward the groin and index finger toward the anterior superior iliac spine.
   - Extend the middle finger back along the iliac crest toward the buttock.
   - The middle of the triangle between the middle and index fingers marks the injection site.

Figure credits: Burton and Ludwig (2011). *Fundamentals of nursing care: Concepts, connections & skills.* Philadelphia: F. A. Davis Company, with permission.

the needle is inserted into the muscle, avoiding undesirable body structures.

e. Spread the skin taut between the index finger and thumb to facilitate needle insertion and minimize discomfort.

f. Insert the needle at a 90-degree angle (Fig. 14.23) to ensure that the needle tip reaches muscle tissue.

g. Aspirate by pulling the plunger back gently; check the manufacturer's instructions to determine whether aspiration is contraindicated.

(1) If no blood appears, continue with the procedure because the needle is outside a blood vessel.

🛑 (2) If blood appears, withdraw the needle because it is in a blood vessel; prepare a new syringe.

h. Inject the medication.

(1) Inject the medication quickly for a child or an infant to minimize discomfort.

(2) Inject the medication over 5 to 10 seconds for an adult to minimize discomfort and allow time for drug dispersal.

6. Nursing interventions specific to administering an IM injection via the Z-track method.

a. Change the needle after drawing the medication into the syringe to prevent tissue irritation caused by the drug adhering to the outside of the needle.

b. Use the ulnar side of the hand or thumb of the nondominant hand to pull the skin laterally 1 to 1.5 inches (2.5 to 3.5 cm) (Fig. 14.24); hold until the dominant hand injects the medication if there was no blood return on aspiration; remove the needle after 10 seconds and then release the skin. Doing so ensures that a zigzag path is established before needle insertion, which seals the needle track as the tissue planes slide across each other upon release, confining the drug in the muscle, minimizing irritation, and preventing tissue discoloration caused by some medications.

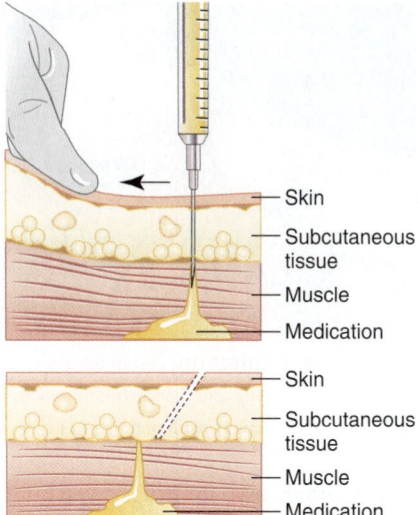

Fig 14.24 Z track method. (From Burton and Ludwig [2011]. *Fundamentals of nursing care: Concepts, connections & skills.* Philadelphia: F. A. Davis Company, with permission.)

L. Subcutaneous (Sub-Q) Injections

1. Introduction.

a. **Sub-Q injection:** Insertion of medication between the dermis and muscle.

b. The volume of solution injected should be less than 1 mL.

c. The length of the needle depends on the angle of needle insertion; for example, usually a ⅜- or ½-inch needle for a 90-degree angle and ⅝- or 1-inch needle for a 90-degree angle (Fig. 14.25).

d. The gauge of the needle usually is #25 to #30.

e. The type of syringe used depends on the type of medication (e.g., an insulin syringe should be used for insulin).

2. Advantages.

a. Is more comfortable than an IM injection because it uses a larger gauge and shorter length needle.

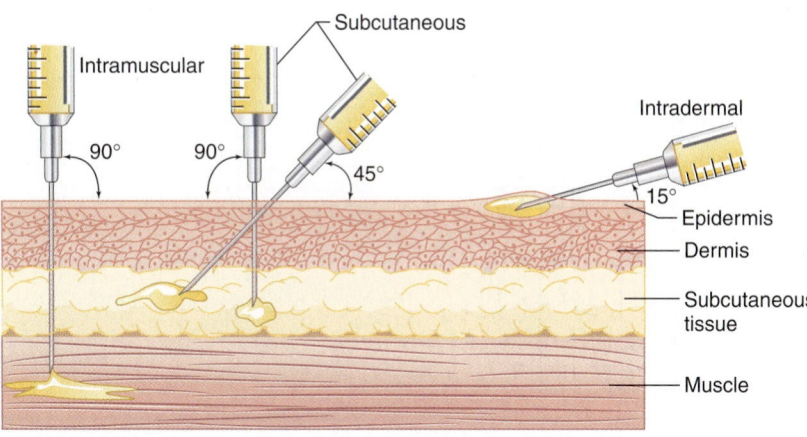

Fig 14.23 Needle insertion angles. (From Burton and Ludwig [2011]. *Fundamentals of nursing care: Concepts, connections & skills.* Philadelphia: F. A. Davis Company, with permission.)

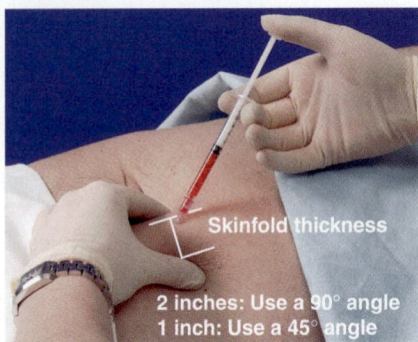

Fig 14.25 Subcutaneous injection. (From Burton and Ludwig [2011]. *Fundamentals of nursing care: Concepts, connections & skills.* Philadelphia: F. A. Davis Company, with permission.)

b. Is commonly used for drugs given multiple times daily, such as heparin and insulin.
c. Allows slower absorption of drugs than IM route because of less-rich blood supply in subcutaneous tissue versus muscle.

3. Disadvantages.
   a. Allows administration of a maximum of only 1 mL of solution.
   b. Cannot be used for many drugs because they are irritating to subcutaneous tissue.
4. Selection of a Sub-Q injection site depends on multiple variables (e.g., advantages, disadvantages, and type of medication) (Table 14.2).
5. Nursing interventions specific to administering a Sub-Q injection.
   a. Select the appropriate gauge needle.
   b. Select the appropriate length needle (should be half the width of the pinched skinfold) to ensure the drug is inserted into the subcutaneous layer.
   c. Select the appropriate site.
   d. Alternate the site from recent injections; use a body flow chart to identify various sites by number. Doing so minimizes tissue injury, facilitates absorption, and minimizes lipodystrophy and lipohypertrophy.

Table 14.2 Subcutaneous Injection Sites: Advantages, Disadvantages, and Nursing Care

Advantages and Disadvantages	Nursing Care
Abdomen	
Advantages	1. Position the patient in any position but prone.
• Has a large subcutaneous layer that allows for rotation of injections within one site.	2. **Landmark**
• Allows medication to be absorbed more evenly than thighs and buttocks, which are affected by activity.	• **Abdomen:** Left and right of the umbilicus and below the umbilicus on the left, right, and middle; avoid 2 inches around the umbilicus to reduce the risk of bleeding. (see figure below, green dots.)
• Is the best site for insulin and anticoagulant administration because of a quicker absorption rate than other sites.	• **"Love handles":** Tissue around the midsection on the sides of the lower waist and lower back. (see figure below, red dots.)
Anterolateral and posterolateral abdominal wall ("love handles")	• **Areas of subcutaneous tissue:** (see figure below, blue dots.)
• Best site for low-molecular-weight anticoagulants, such as enoxaparin (Lovenox), because of its deep subcutaneous layer.	
Disadvantages	
• None.	
Outer, Posterior Aspect of Upper Arms; Anterior Thighs; and Upper Buttocks	
Advantage	1. Position the patient so that each site is accessible. (see figure below, blue dots.)
• Have large subcutaneous tissue layers that allow for rotation of injections within one site.	
Disadvantages	
• Absorption may be uneven because areas are affected by activity.	
• Should not be used for low-molecular-weight heparin because of increased risk of bruising.	

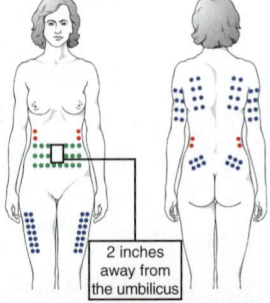

2 inches away from the umbilicus

Figure credit: Adapted from Vitale (2013). *NCLEX-RN notes: Core review and exam prep,* 2nd ed. Philadelphia: F. A. Davis Company, with permission.

e. Position the patient so the site is accessible and the patient is comfortable to provide accessibility to the injection site and relax the patient for needle insertion.

f. Pinch a fold of skin between your fingers and thumb to elevate subcutaneous tissue and insert the needle at a determined angle using a smooth movement (see Figs. 14.23 and 14.25). The angle depends on the volume of subcutaneous tissue and needle length.

   (1) If you can pinch 2 inches of tissue, use a 90-degree angle.

   (2) If you can pinch only 1 inch of tissue, use a 45-degree angle.

   (3) For obese adults, inject deep into the tissue fold to avoid injecting the medication into adipose tissue.

g. Release the pinch and hold the syringe steady with the nondominant hand to minimize discomfort. Push the plunger slowly with the dominant hand to limit tissue discomfort and damage (see the information below on anticoagulants regarding holding a pinch); aspiration is not necessary because piercing a blood vessel is rare.

🛑 h. Follow the drug manufacturer's instructions regarding massage of the site to limit local tissue trauma; do not massage for insulin and anticoagulants.

6. Nursing interventions specific to administering insulin.

🛑 a. Check the patient's blood glucose level before administration to evaluate response to insulin therapy and guide the next dose.

b. Generally, use a large gauge, short needle to minimize trauma and discomfort (a larger gauge needle is less painful than a smaller gauge needle).

c. Check documentation of the previous site and rotate sites to support absorption and minimize the risk of lipodystrophy and lipohypertrophy.

d. Leave the needle in place for 5 seconds after the injection of solution to ensure complete delivery of the insulin dose.

7. Nursing interventions specific to administering an anticoagulant (e.g., heparin, low-molecular-weight heparin).

a. Observe injection sites daily for signs of complications, such as bleeding, bruising, pain, swelling, and heat; hold the medication and notify the primary health-care provider if any are present.

🛑 b. Check coagulation laboratory results, such as International Normalized Ratio (INR); notify the primary health-care provider if findings are outside the expected parameters.

c. Have protamine sulfate (antidote for heparin) readily available if the patient is receiving heparin.

d. Add 0.2 mL of air when preparing the correct dose. Do not expel the air bubble in a prefilled syringe; allow the air bubble to follow the medication into the needle tract, which limits bleeding and bruising.

e. Select the appropriate site.

   (1) Heparin: Inject in the abdomen, level with the iliac crest at least 2 inches from the umbilicus.

   (2) Low-molecular-weight heparin: Inject in the anterolateral and posterolateral abdominal wall ("love handles").

f. Hold the pinch throughout the procedure and insert the full length of the needle to ensure the solution enters the subcutaneous tissue; do not aspirate.

g. Inject solution slowly over 30 seconds, including the air bubble, to allow for drug dispersal and minimize pain and bleeding.

h. Leave the needle in place for 10 seconds after the injection of solution to ensure delivery and dispersement of the anticoagulant dose.

i. Keep the plunger depressed while removing the needle to ensure that the bubble stays in the needle track.

j. Do not massage the site to minimize trauma and bleeding.

k. Document the site used to promote rotation of sites.

l. Institute sharps precautions, such as avoiding the use of blade razors, to protect the patient from injury.

m. Avoid giving and tell the patient to avoid taking aspirin and other over-the-counter drugs that can decrease platelet aggregation, causing bruising and bleeding.

M. **Intradermal (ID) Injections**

1. Introduction.

a. **ID injection:** Insertion of medication into the dermis, which is just below the epidermis and above the subcutaneous tissue.

b. The volume of solution generally is 0.01 to 0.1 mL of solution.

c. The length of the needle generally is ¼- to ⅝-inch.

d. The gauge of the needle generally is #25 to #28.

e. The type of syringe used generally is a 1 mL or tuberculin syringe.

2. Advantages.
   a. Avoids the need to use more invasive and risky anesthetic agents when used as a local anesthetic.
   b. Is less expensive than other methods for testing for TB or allergens.
3. Disadvantages.
   a. Local inflammatory response may be uncomfortable or painful.
   b. Can cause an anaphylactic reaction to allergens being injected.
4. Nursing interventions specific to administering an ID injection.
   a. Select a tuberculin syringe with a gauge of #25 to #28 and a needle length of ¼- to ⅝-inch to ensure the needle is inserted into the intradermis.
   b. Select the appropriate site: Choose the inner aspect of the forearm, upper chest, or upper back; avoid pigmented areas or areas with excessive hair.
   c. Use your nondominant hand to stretch the skin over the site with your forefinger and thumb to facilitate needle insertion.
   d. Insert the needle slowly at a 5- to 15-degree angle no more than ⅛ inch below the surface of the skin with the bevel facing upward (see Fig. 14.23) to ensure the solution is injected upward within the dermis rather than down toward the subcutaneous tissue.
   e. Slowly inject the solution until a small bleb forms under the surface of the skin (Fig. 14.26), indicating the solution was deposited into the dermis.

   🛑 **f. Do not massage the area; massage will disperse solution into local tissue, which may alter test results.**

   g. Draw a circle around the site to identify the site for future analysis.
   h. Instruct the patient to return to the primary health-care provider at the time indicated (usually 24 to 48 hours); measure the area of redness and induration in millimeters and document the results.

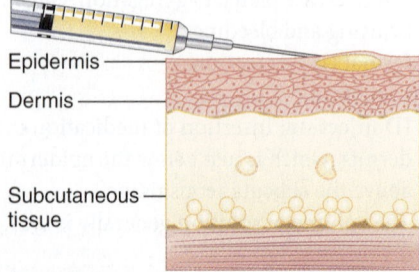

Fig 14.26 Intradermal injection. (From Wilkinson and Treas [2011]. *Fundamentals of nursing,* Vol. 2, 2nd ed. Philadelphia: F. A. Davis Company, with permission.)

N. Intravenous (IV) Medication Administration
(see also the section "Administration of IV Solutions" in Chapter 21, "Fluids and Electrolytes," page 659.)
1. Introduction.
   a. IV medications are administered directly into a vein.
   b. Methods of administration.
      (1) Addition of a medication, such as potassium chloride or vitamins, to a large volume bag of IV fluid that is running continuously.
      (2) **Bolus ("push"):** Single dose of a medication in a syringe or in a small amount of IV fluid administered through a primary IV line or a venous access device, such as a heparin or saline lock. Heparin or saline locks are used for intermittent IV medications to allow the patient more freedom of movement.
      (3) **"Piggyback" infusion:** Single dose of medication mixed with a small volume of fluid in its own IV bag administered via secondary tubing attached to a current IV line (primary line).
         (a) May be administered concurrently through the primary line.
         (b) May interrupt the primary line solution while the medication solution is administered.
   c. Method of IV medication preparation.
      (1) Most large-volume bags of IV fluid that contain medication are prepared and labeled by the manufacturer or pharmacy.
      (2) Most piggyback infusions are prepared and labeled by the pharmacy.
      (3) Some piggyback infusions and most bolus infusions are prepared by the nurse administering the medication.
2. Advantages.
   a. Is rapid acting, making it useful in an emergency.
   b. Used for patients who cannot take drugs via the oral route.
   c. Avoids barriers to drug absorption associated with other routes.
   d. Allows larger volumes to be administered than by IM or Sub-Q routes.
   e. Provides for slow administration of a drug when required.
   f. Is more comfortable than administering an irritating drug into a muscle or subcutaneous tissue.
   g. Provides for a continuous blood level of a drug.
3. Disadvantages.
   a. Carries a greater risk of adverse reactions because of rapid action and is difficult to reverse if the patient has an adverse reaction or received

an excessive dose; bolus method is most dangerous because the medication is not diluted in a larger volume of solution.

b. May irritate the blood vessel, particularly with a bolus dose.

c. Carries a greater risk of complications, such as bleeding, infection, fluid overload, and extravasation as well as phlebitis and thrombosis, which cause discomfort and pain. (see Table 21.4 in Chapter 21, "Fluids and Electrolytes," page 666.)

4. Nursing interventions common to administering all intravenous medications.

🛑 a. Double-check all calculations to ensure accuracy and prevent dosage errors.

b. Assess the IV site for signs of infiltration, such as swelling and edema, and check whether the flow rate is accurate.

c. Assess the IV site for clinical indicators of phlebitis, such as redness, swelling, and heat.

5. Nursing interventions specific to administering medication via a large-volume infusion.

a. Spike the IV bag with appropriate tubing, flush the air out of the tubing (prime the tubing), and connect it to the venous access device. Doing so prepares the tubing and ensures that air is flushed from the tubing.

b. Ensure that the IV fluid is compatible with the medication to be added to prevent drug and fluid incompatibilities.

c. Prepare the syringe with the prescribed drug.

d. Wipe the IV additive port with an alcohol wipe to reduce the risk of infection.

e. Insert the needle or needleless syringe into the center of the IV additive port and inject the medication; then withdraw the syringe (Fig. 14.27). Doing so allows the IV additive port to self-seal; using the sides of a port may produce leaks and cause fluid contamination.

f. Gently turn the IV bag end to end to mix the solutions without causing bubbles.

g. Attach the label with the patient's name, medication, dose, date, time, and nurse's initials.

h. Hang the IV bag and open the roller clamp on the tubing to the ordered rate of infusion if administered by gravity OR use an infusion pump and set the rate accordingly.

6. Nursing interventions specific to administering medication via a bolus infusion ("IV push").

a. Ensure that medication is administered by a registered nurse; do not delegate this procedure to a licensed practical nurse.

b. Determine the rate of solution administration by considering the volume of solution to be

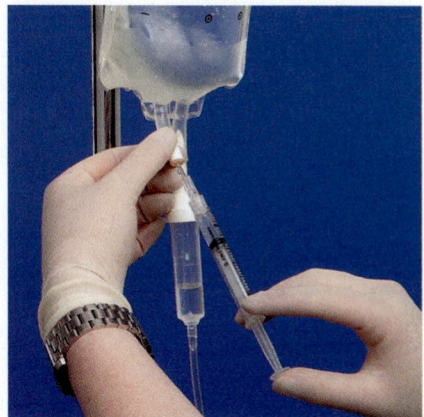

Fig 14.27 Instilling a medication into an IV bag. (From Burton and Ludwig [2011]. *Fundamentals of nursing care: Concepts, connections & skills.* Philadelphia: F. A. Davis Company, with permission.)

administered in relation to the amount of time the medication is to be given, such as 4 mL over 2 minutes (therefore, instill 0.5 minims every 30 seconds). Doing so ensures the medication is diluted slowly in the patient's blood, preventing excessive intake in a short amount of time that may irritate the vein or cause an unwanted reaction.

c. Cleanse the insertion port with an alcohol wipe to limit the risk of infection.

d. Access the insertion port.

(1) Heparin or saline lock.

(a) Follow agency policy and procedure for identifying patency and flushing the venous access device before a bolus dose.

(b) Insert the syringe into the venous access device and instill the medication.

(c) Withdraw the syringe, activate the needle safety feature to prevent a needlestick injury, and follow agency policy and procedure for flushing the venous access device after the bolus dose to ensure that the entire dose is received and that the venous access device is free from medication.

(2) Currently running IV infusion (Fig. 14.28).

(a) Pinch the IV tubing just above the injection port closest to the venipuncture site to stop the flow of IV fluid from the IV bag temporarily, which allows the drug to be instilled toward the patient rather than up the tubing.

(b) Insert the syringe into the port and aspirate until a slight amount of blood appears in the syringe or tubing to

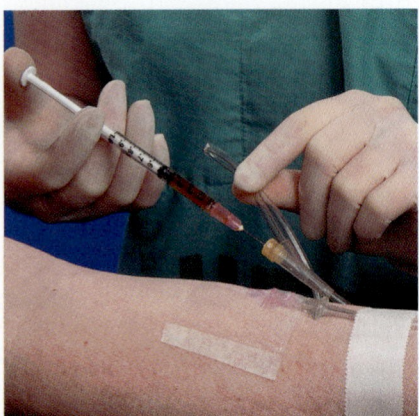

Fig 14.28 IV push. (From Burton and Ludwig [2011]. *Fundamentals of nursing care: Concepts, connections & skills.* Philadelphia: F. A. Davis Company, with permission.)

ensure that the device is in a vein and that the bolus will be injected into the vein.

    (c) Inject the medication at the ordered rate.

    (d) Remove the syringe, activate the needle safety feature to prevent a needlestick injury, and release the pinch in the tubing to allow the primary solution to begin to flow.

  e. Dispose of syringe(s) in the nearest sharps container; do not recap the needle if there is no passive or active needle safety feature to prevent a needlestick injury.

  f. Monitor the patient closely for adverse drug reactions.

7. Nursing interventions specific to administering a medication via an intermittent (piggyback) infusion.

  a. Ensure the medication bag has a label with the patient's name, medication, dose, time/frequency, date, and nurse's initials.

  b. Attach the tubing to the medication bag; prime the tubing without losing more than 1 drop of the solution. Doing so prepares the equipment for use, removes air from the tubing, and ensures that the patient receives the entire dose.

  c. Wipe the insertion port with alcohol to prevent infection.

  d. Access the insertion port.

    (1) Heparin or saline lock: Attach the medication tubing directly to the venous access device or use a needless piercing device.

    (2) Currently running IV (primary) line.

      (a) When a primary line is not interrupted to deliver a piggyback (Fig. 14.29a): Use the tubing port closest to the insertion site; keep both bags at the same height; open the clamp on the medication bag; control the flow of solution from both bags using the clamp on the primary tubing.

      (b) When a primary line is interrupted to deliver a piggyback (Fig. 14.29b): Use the tubing port furthest from the insertion site; drop the primary infusion bag lower than the medication bag; open the clamp on the medication tubing and control the flow using the clamp on the primary tubing. Doing so ensures that the primary infusion will flow (via gravity) after the medication bag is empty.

  e. Depending on the critical nature of the medication, use an infusion pump to ensure an accurate flow rate.

  f. Reestablish the prescribed flow rate of the primary infusion, if one is present, to maintain continuity of IV fluid administration.

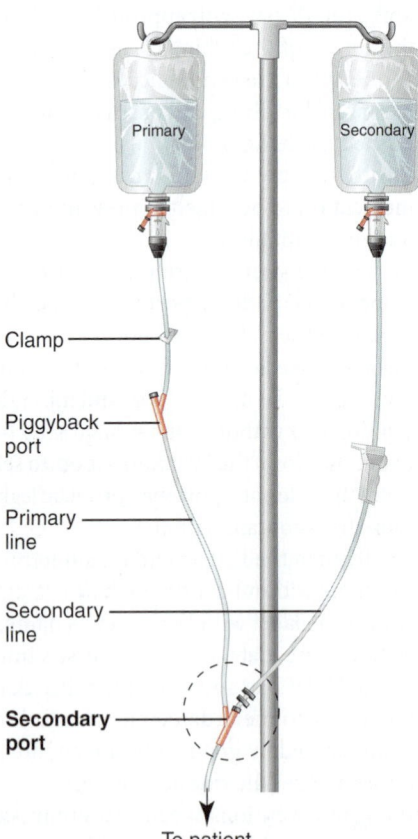

Fig 14.29a Intermittent (piggyback) infusion. Tandem (secondary) setup. (From Wilkinson and Treas [2011]. Fundamentals of nursing, Vol. 1, 2nd ed. Philadelphia: F. A. Davis Company, with permission.)

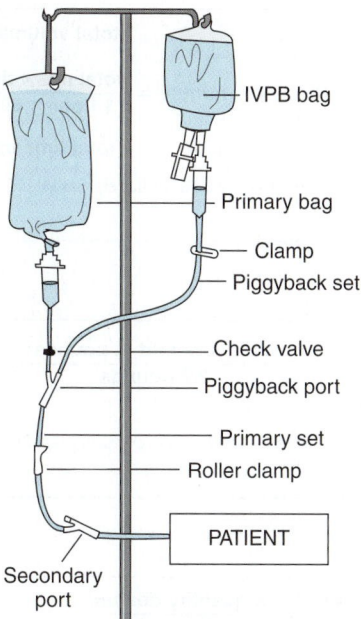

Fig 14.29b Intermittent (piggyback) infusion. Piggyback setup. (From Vitale [2013]. *NCLEX-RN notes: Content review & exam prep,* 2nd ed. Philadelphia: F. A. Davis Company, with permission.)

8. Nursing interventions specific to administering IV medication via a volume-controlled infusion set (Fig. 14.30).
   a. Prepare a syringe with the prescribed medication.
   b. Fill the set by opening the clamp between the set and main IV tubing until the desired volume of IV fluid enters the set and then clamp the main IV tubing.
   c. Cleanse the injection port on the set with an alcohol wipe to reduce the risk of infection.
   d. Inject the medication into the medication port of the set and gently mix the solutions to ensure even distribution of medication in the IV fluid and prevent formation of bubbles.
   e. Open the clamp below the set, and adjust it to the prescribed flow rate (usually delivered over 30 to 60 minutes).

VI. Medication Calculation Formulas

A. **IV Drop Rate Formula** (Fig. 14.31)
   1. IV tubing drop factor: The number of drops it takes for specific tubing to deliver 1 mL of fluid.

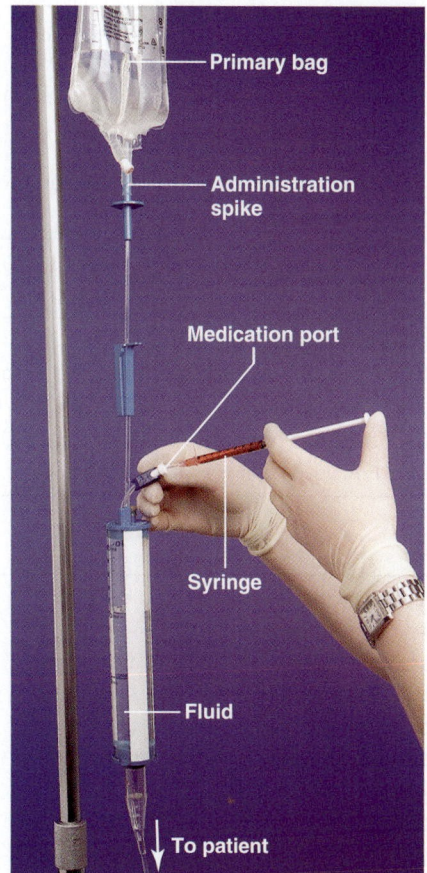

Fig 14.30 Volume-controlled administration set. (From Wilkinson and Treas [2011]. *Fundamentals of nursing,* Vol. 2, 2nd ed. Philadelphia: F. A. Davis Company, with permission.)

   2. The drop factor is a component of the formula when calculating the IV flow rate when using a specific IV set.
   3. Drop factors are indicated on the tubing box. For example:
      a. Macro-drops: Drop factor of 10 delivers 10 drops/1 mL; drop factor of 15 = 15 drops/1 mL; drop factor of 20 = 20 drops/1 mL.
      b. Micro-drops: Drop factor of 60 = 60 drops/1 mL.
B. **Conversion of Pounds to Kilograms (Kg)** (Fig. 14.32)
C. **Ratio and Proportion Formulas** (Fig. 14.33)
D. **Weight Based Method to Calculate a Pediatric Dose** (Fig. 14.34)
E. **Body Surface Area (BSA) Method to Calculate a Pediatric Dose for Infants and Children ≤12 Years of Age** (Fig. 14.35)

- Multiply the numerators (total mL × drop factor).
- Multiply the denominators (1 hour × 60 minutes).
- Divide the numerator by the denominator to obtain the drops per minute.

$$\text{Drops per minute} = \frac{\text{total mL} \times \text{drop factor (total volume in drops)}}{\text{1 hour} \times \text{60 minutes (total time in minutes)}}$$

Fig 14.31 IV drop rate formula. (From Vitale [2013]. *NCLEX-RN notes: Content review & exam prep,* 2nd ed. Philadelphia: F. A. Davis Company, with permission.)

- Solve for X by cross multiplying.
- Divide both sides of resulting equation by the number in front of the X.
- Reduce to lowest terms to achieve child's weight in kg.

$$\frac{\text{child's weight in pounds}}{\text{2.2 pounds}} = \frac{\text{X kg}}{\text{1 kg}}$$

Fig 14.32 Conversion of pounds to kilograms (Kg). (From Vitale [2013]. *NCLEX-RN notes: Content review & exam prep,* 2nd ed. Philadelphia: F. A. Davis Company, with permission.)

- Ordered dose and dose on hand must be in the same unit of measure.
- Formulas 1 and 2: Solve for X by cross multiplying.
- Formula 3: Solve for X by multiplying the means and the extremes.
- Divide both sides of all resulting equations by the number in front of the X.
- Reduce to lowest terms to achieve the quantity of dose.

#1 $\dfrac{\text{desired}}{\text{have}} = \dfrac{\text{ordered dose}}{\text{dose on hand}} = \dfrac{\text{X quantity desired}}{\text{quantity on hand}}$

#2 $\dfrac{\text{quantity on hand}}{\text{dose on hand}} = \dfrac{\text{X quantity desired}}{\text{ordered dose}}$

#3 dose on hand : quantity on hand : : ordered dose : X quantity desired
(extremes)   (means)   (means)   (extremes)

Fig 14.33 Ratio and proportion formulas. (From Vitale [2013]. *NCLEX-RN notes: Content review & exam prep,* 2nd ed. Philadelphia: F. A. Davis Company, with permission.)

- Divide the numerator (child's weight in kg) by the denominator (50 kg).
- Multiply the result by the adult dose in mg.

$$\text{Pediatric dose in mg} = \frac{\text{Child's weight in kg}}{\text{50 kg}} \times \text{Adult dose in mg}$$

Fig 14.34 Weight-based method to calculate a pediatric dose. (From Vitale [2007]. *NCLEX-RN notes: Core review & exam prep,* 1st ed. Philadelphia: F. A. Davis Company, with permission.)

$$\text{Pediatric dose in mg} = \frac{\text{*Child's BSA in square meters (m}^2\text{)}}{\text{1.73 m}^2} \times \text{Adult dose in mg}$$

- *Estimate the child's BSA in square meters (m^2) by using a BSA chart (nomogram).
- The BSA chart consists of three columns. The left column is height, the middle column is body surface area, and the right column is weight. These numbers increase from the bottom to the top of each column.
- Draw a straight line from the child's height in the left column to the child's weight in the right column. The number found where the line crosses the middle column is the child's estimated BSA.
- The BSA should be used in the formula for the body surface area method to calculate a pediatric dose.

Fig. 14.35 Body surface area (BSA) method to calculate a pediatric dose for infants and children ≤12 years of age. (From Vitale [2013]. *NCLEX-RN notes: Content review & exam prep,* 2nd ed. Philadelphia: F. A. Davis Company, with permission.)

CASE STUDY: Putting It All Together

An 80-year-old man is admitted to the emergency department. He states that he has lived alone since his wife passed away a few years ago but that his son visits about once a month. He says, "I'm on a tight budget because my only income is Social Security. I hoped that I would get better and not have to pay for an emergency room visit. I finally came because I couldn't breathe and my legs were very swollen." The patient shares that, at times, he gets a little forgetful and does not remember to take his medication every day. The patient brought all the containers of the medications that he takes daily. The nurse identified the following medications that the patient is taking at home and why and documented the medications on the medication reconciliation form.
- Lasix 20 mg PO, daily (diuretic)
- Colace 100 mg PO, bid (stool softener)
- Pepcid 20 mg PO, bid (antiulcer agent for gastroesophageal reflux disease)
- 1 Tab Centrum Silver for Men daily (multivitamin for men)
- Toprol XL 50mg PO, daily (beta-blocker for hypertension)

The patient states that he has a history of hypertension. His blood pressure on admission is 180/90 mm Hg. He says that he does not always take the Lasix when he has to go out in the morning to do errands because he has to stop so often to urinate. He also has some urinary frequency, urinary urgency, and nocturia because of an enlarged prostate. When talking, the patient stops frequently to catch his breath. Respirations are 30 breaths/minute, the patient is using accessory muscles to breathe, and capillary refill is longer than 3 seconds. Oxygen saturation is 90 percent.

The primary health-care provider writes and signs the following orders:
- I&O
- 2-g sodium diet
- OOB to chair every shift with assistance
- VS (vital signs) every 8 hours
- IV lock—flush with 10cc NS every 8 hours
- 2 L oxygen via nasal cannula
- Lasix 40 mg IVPB
- Pepcid 20 mg bid
- Colace 1 tab PO, bid
- Toprol XL 50 mg PO, daily

After 6 hours, the patient still has not voided, his abdomen is distended, and he says, "I feel a lot of pressure in my lower belly and I have to urinate, but I can't." The nurse calls the primary health-care provider, who orders the following interventions via a telephone order.
- Insert urinary retention catheter to bedside drainage
- Flomax 0.4 mg PO daily after a meal

Case Study Questions

A. Discuss the factors identified by the nurse that place the patient at risk for complications related to a medication regimen?

1. _____

2. _____

3. _____

B. What nursing interventions should the nurse implement to help the patient manage his forgetfulness associated with his medication regimen?

1. _____

2. _____

3. _____

Continued

CASE STUDY: Putting It All Together   *cont'd*

_____ **Case Study Questions** _____

C. Which medication prescriptions are incomplete? Also indicate what information the primary health-care provider must include to make the prescriptions complete.

1. _____

2. _____

3. _____

D. When taking the telephone order for the urinary retention catheter and Flomax, what procedural steps should the nurse implement to ensure accuracy?

1. _____

2. _____

3. _____

REVIEW QUESTIONS

1. A nurse plans to administer an intramuscular injection to an obese patient. What muscle should the nurse consider the least desirable site for an intramuscular injection in an obese adult?
1. Vastus lateralis
2. Rectus femoris
3. Dorsogluteal
4. Deltoid

2. A primary health-care provider prescribes 0.75 g of an antibiotic intramuscularly for a patient with an infection. The vial of the medication contains 1 gram of the medication and it must be reconstituted. The vial has instructions to instill 1.8 mL of diluent to yield 2 mL of solution. How much solution should the nurse administer?
1. A
2. B
3. C
4. D

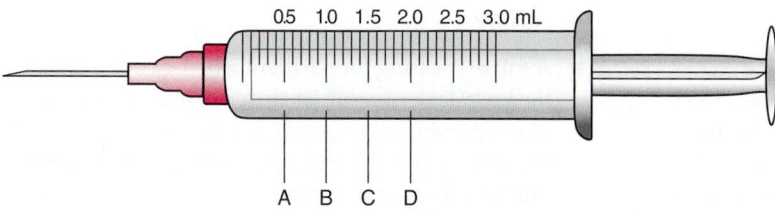

A B C D

3. A nurse must administer a rectal suppository. Which should the nurse do when administering the suppository?
1. Use the full length of a gloved lubricated index finger when inserting the suppository to ensure it is beyond the rectal sphincters.
2. Explain the need to remain seated for several minutes after insertion of the suppository to promote its retention in the rectum.
3. Take the suppository out of the refrigerator a half hour before insertion to allow it to warm to room temperature.
4. Place the patient in the supine position to allow easy access to the anus when inserting the suppository.

4. A nurse is interviewing a newly admitted patient as part of a nursing history and physical. What information should be included in the medication reconciliation form? **Select all that apply.**
1. _____ Vitamins
2. _____ Drug allergies
3. _____ Food supplements
4. _____ Over-the-counter herbs
5. _____ Prescribed medications

5. A nurse must administer 3 mL of a distasteful liquid medication to a 3-year-old child. Which should the nurse do to promote ingestion of the medication?
1. Dilute it in several ounces of the child's favorite fruit juice and then give it to the child.
2. Use a needleless syringe and instill it all at the same time into the child's buccal cavity.
3. Mix it in a glass of water and have the child sip the medication through a straw.
4. Have the child eat an ice pop and then administer the medication to the child.

6. A nurse observed another nurse administering an injection via the Z-track technique. Which action by the nurse indicated that the technique was performed correctly?
1. Obtained a syringe with a 25 gauge needle for the procedure
2. Used the same needle for drawing up and administering the medication
3. Attached a needle with a 1-inch length after the medication was drawn into the syringe
4. Pulled the skin laterally before insertion of the needle and removed the needle at the same angle of its insertion

7. A nurse is to administer eyedrops to a patient. The nurse verifies the primary health-care provider's prescription, washes the hands, and collects the medication following the five rights and three checks associated with medication administration. The nurse places the patient in a supine position with the head extended and then dons clean gloves. Place the following steps in the order in which they should be implemented.
   1. Instruct the patient to look up toward the ceiling without moving the head.
   2. Direct the patient to gently close eyelids but avoid squeezing the eyes shut.
   3. Instruct the patient to press firmly on the naso-lacrimal duct for 30 to 60 seconds.
   4. Wash each eye from inner to outer canthus using a different moistened cotton ball for each eye.
   5. Place a finger of the nondominant hand below the lower lid and gently pull the skin down to reveal the conjunctival sac.
   6. Place the dominant hand on the forehead, approach the eye from the side with the eye dropper 1 to 2 cm above the conjunctival sac, and instill the ordered number of drops.

   Answer: _____

8. A nurse is to administer 1 mL of a liquid medication to a 3-month-old infant. Which is the **best** way to administer this medication?
   1. Use a needless syringe to instill the medication on the back of the infant's tongue.
   2. Use a dropper to insert the medication into the infant's buccal cavity.
   3. Use a medicine cup to allow the infant to sip the medication slowly.
   4. Use a medication nipple so that the infant can suck the medication.

9. A nurse is to administer one nose drop to each nostril of a school-aged child. Which action should the nurse perform as part of this procedure?
   1. Position the child in the supine position with the head tilted backward when inserting the drops
   2. Position the tip of the medication dropper within a nostril when expelling the drop
   3. Instruct the child to breathe deeply through the nose after the drop is inserted
   4. Return the unused nose drops in the dropper to the medication bottle

10. A nurse is to administer an intradermal injection for a tuberculin test to an adult. The nurse verifies the primary health-care provider's order, washes the hands, and collects the medication following the five rights and three checks associated with medication administration. The nurse then dons clean gloves. Place the following steps in the order in which they should be implemented.
    1. Draw a 1-inch circle around the wheal.
    2. Position the patient with the forearm supinated.
    3. Stabilize tissue on both sides of the puncture site as the needle is quickly removed at the same angle of insertion.
    4. Clean the site with an alcohol wipe using a circular motion moving from the center outward and allow the site to dry.
    5. Inject the solution with slow, even pressure so that a small wheal (raised welt, bleb) of fluid becomes apparent under the skin.
    6. Insert a ¼- to ⅝-inch, 25- to 27-gauge needle with the bevel up just below the skin surface at a 10- to 15-degree angle until the bevel is no longer visible.

    Answer: _____

11. A nurse is caring for a patient who was admitted to the hospital as a result of an accidental double dose of a prescribed medication. Which strategy should the nurse suggest that the patient use to **best** prevent this from happening again?
    1. Teach the patient how to use a medication organizer system.
    2. Set an alarm clock to ring at the time a drug is to be taken as a reminder.
    3. Suggest that a family member call to remind the patient when to take medications.
    4. Hang a calendar in a significant place that indicates the drug name, dose, and time it is to be taken.

12. A primary health-care provider prescribes a medication based on a child's weight. The pediatric nurse identifies that the prescribed dose is for a child weighing 10 lb more than the weight of the child for whom the drug dose was prescribed. What should the nurse do?
    1. Call the primary health-care provider and discuss the excessive dose.
    2. Recalculate the dose using the actual weight and give the recalculated dose.
    3. Ask the pharmacist about the weight difference and whether it is necessary to change the dose.
    4. Notify the nurse manager and seek support to confront the primary health-care provider about the dose.

13. Which site is appropriate for the nurse to use for the administration of heparin?

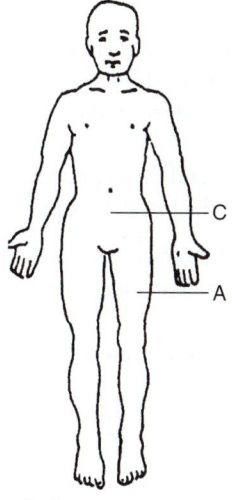 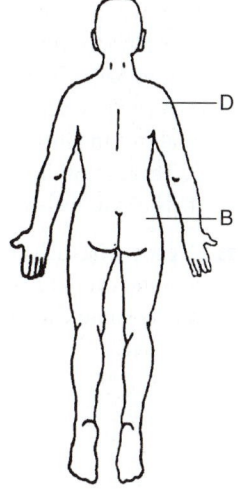

1. A
2. B
3. C
4. D

14. Which nursing action is indicated when administering a heparin injection?
1. Rubbing the site after the injection
2. Placing the needle just under the epidermis
3. Spreading the skin during insertion of the needle
4. Cleaning the site with a disinfectant before the injection

15. A patient has an order for IVF: 0.9% sodium chloride to infuse at 80 mL/hour. The nurse has an infusion set that has a drop factor of 10 drops/mL. At how many drops per minute should the nurse set the infusion rate?
Answer: _____ drops per minute

16. A patient with moderate dementia, who lives at home with a relative, insists on being as independent as possible. The patient frequently forgets to take the prescribed morning medications. Which action should the nurse discuss with the patient and relative?
1. The relative should verbally explain to the patient which medications to take each morning.
2. A divided medication dispensing system should be used for all of the patient's medications.
3. A written list of the medications that must be taken should be left on the patient's bedside table.
4. The relative should place the medications in a medication cup by the patient's toothbrush in the bathroom each morning.

17. A nurse must administer 2 mL of a medication via the intramuscular route. Which syringe should the nurse use for this injection?
1. A
2. B
3. C
4. D

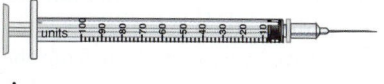

A

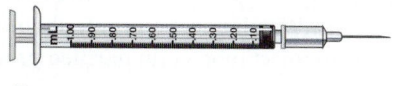

B

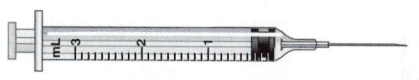

C

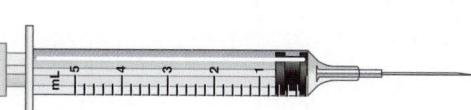

D

18. A nurse in a hospital receives a telephone order from a patient's primary health-care provider. What action must the nurse take before hanging up the telephone?
1. Insert the order into the patient's clinical record.
2. Recite the order back to the primary health-care provider.
3. Confirm that the ordered medication is available in the hospital pharmacy.
4. State that the primary health-care provider must sign the order within forty-eight hours.

19. A primary health-care provider orders a medication to be administered every 6 hours prn. What should the nurse teach the patient about this medication?
1. "I will give this medication over 6 hours."
2. "I can give you this medication every 6 hours if you need it."
3. "I must wait 6 hours before administering this medication to you."
4. "I have to give you this medication every 6 hours around the clock."

20. A patient has a prescription for 2 drops of a medication to be placed into an eye. What is an important nursing action associated with this procedure?
   1. Having the patient look down while the medication is inserted
   2. Applying slight pressure over the inner canthus of the eye after drop administration
   3. Placing a finger on the top lid while simultaneously pulling the lid toward the forehead
   4. Cleansing the eye by wiping gently from the outer canthus to the inner canthus with a cotton ball

21. A nurse is caring for a patient who is to be screened for tuberculosis. Which injection route should the nurse use to inject tuberculin purified protein derivative?

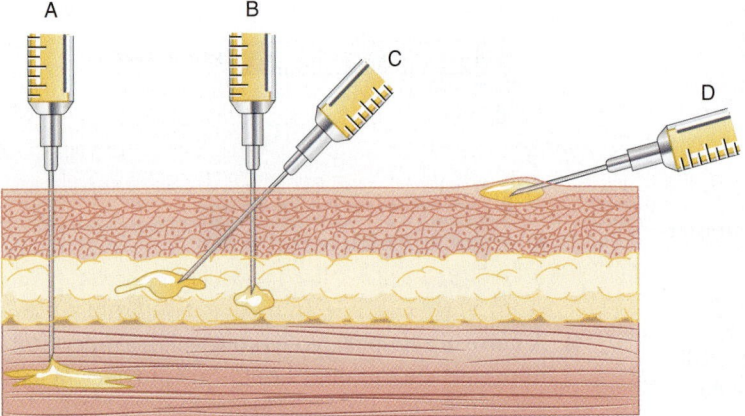

   1. A
   2. B
   3. C
   4. D

22. A nurse reconstituted and drew up a medication from a vial. Which nursing action compromised the ability to withdraw an accurate dose?
   1. Injected air into the vial with the bevel of the needle below the level of the solution
   2. Placed slightly more air into the vial than the volume of solution to be removed
   3. Rolled the vial in the palms of the hands after the diluent was added to the vial
   4. Instilled the diluent into the vial slowly

23. A nurse is to administer an intramuscular injection into the deltoid muscle. What bony landmark should the nurse use to help locate the appropriate site?
   1. Knee
   2. Greater trochanter
   3. Acromion process
   4. Anterior superior iliac spine

24. A nurse is monitoring a patient's IV site that is on the forearm just below the antecubital fossa. Which clinical manifestation alerts the nurse that an infiltration may have occurred?
   1. A blood return occurs when the intravenous solution bag is lowered below the insertion site.
   2. A red line under the skin extends several inches above the insertion site.
   3. There is swelling of tissue around the insertion site.
   4. The skin feels warm around the insertion site.

25. A patient has an order for IVF: 1,000 mL of 5% dextrose in water every 12 hours. At what rate should the nurse set the volume infusion device?
   Answer: _____ mL/hour

26. A nurse is monitoring a patient's intravenous insertion site that is in the right forearm just below the antecubital fossa. The nurse identifies that an infiltration has occurred and removes the intravenous catheter. What should the nurse do **next**?
   1. Keep the right arm dependent.
   2. Restart the infusion in the patient's left forearm.
   3. Apply the standing ordered warm soak to the right forearm.
   4. Reinsert the infusion distal to the previous site in the patient's right arm.

27. What should the nurse do to **best** prevent needlestick injuries when administering injections?
   1. Bend the needle of the syringe before disposal.
   2. Recap the needle while transporting it to a sharps container.
   3. Use a syringe with a device that automatically covers the needle after its use.
   4. Dispose of a syringe with its attached needle into the closest sharps container.

28. A patient has a prescription for 22 units of NPH insulin and 8 units of regular insulin once daily at 8 a.m. The nurse teaches a patient how to draw up and self-administer these insulins. Which amount of solution depicted in the illustration indicates that the patient prepared the correct dose?
1. A
2. B
3. C
4. D

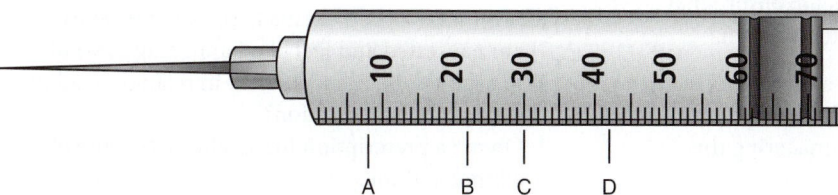

29. A patient has an intravenous infusion running at 30 drops/minute by gravity. The nurse must administer hydromorphone (Dilaudid) IV push via an infusion port in this line. What should the nurse do to ensure that the patient receives the full effect of the dose?
1. Use the port furthest from the insertion site.
2. Pinch the tubing above the port as the medication is instilled.
3. Double the flow rate of the solution for a half hour after the drug is given.
4. Shut the roller clamp off on the tubing before administering the medication.

30. A nurse is planning to piggyback an intermittent infusion of a medication (IVPB) to an existing primary infusion set that is delivering normal saline at 100 mL per hour. What steps should the nurse perform to administer this medication appropriately? **Select all that apply.**
1. _____ Warm the bag of solution with the medication before administration.
2. _____ Hang the secondary infusion bag lower than the primary infusion bag.
3. _____ Wipe the port with alcohol before connecting the secondary infusion tubing.
4. _____ Prime the secondary infusion line before attaching it to the primary infusion line.
5. _____ Open the clamp on the secondary infusion tubing and use the clamp on the primary infusion tubing to control the flow.

31. A nurse is teaching a parent how to administer eardrops to a 2-year-old child with an ear infection. What instruction should the nurse give the parent?
1. "Dispense the drops while holding the dropper several inches above your child's ear canal."
2. "Keep the medication refrigerated until just before you are going to give your child the drops."
3. "Pull your child's pinna up and backward to straighten the ear canal before inserting the drops."
4. "Have your child lie with the ear facing the ceiling while inserting the drops and for five minutes after the drops are inserted."

32. A nurse is applying a transdermal patch to a patient's upper arm. Which nursing actions are essential for every patient to complete this procedure? **Select all that apply.**
1. _____ Wear clean gloves when removing and applying a medicated patch.
2. _____ Shave body hair in the area that the medicated patch is to be applied.
3. _____ Wash and dry the area where the previous medicated patch was removed.
4. _____ Compress the medicated patch against the skin for 10 seconds after it is applied.
5. _____ Remove the previous medicated patch one hour after applying the new medicated patch to the patients.

33. A nurse is to administer an antibiotic capsule orally but first asks the patient, "What is your name and date of birth." What should the nurse do **next** after receiving this information?
    1. Give the patient a glass of apple juice to take with the oral medication.
    2. Compare the response to the patient's identification bracelet to verify the information.
    3. Raise the head of the patient's bed to allow gravity to facilitate swallowing the oral dose.
    4. Check the patient's allergy bracelet to ensure that the patient is not allergic to the medication.

34. A nurse is preparing to administer a medication that is known to be teratogenic. What should the nurse say to the patient before administering this medication?
    1. "Are you pregnant?"
    2. "Do you have an allergy to gluten?"
    3. "You must eat some food just before taking this drug."
    4. "I have to obtain blood for a culture and sensitivity test before you take this drug."

35. A patient had multiple surgical procedures as a result of extensive injuries sustained in a motor vehicle collision. The patient has type 1 diabetes and an order for blood glucose monitoring before meals and at the hour of sleep with related insulin coverage. The nurse obtains the patient's blood glucose level, verifies the prescription for insulin coverage, and assesses the patient.

■ Patient's Clinical Record

Blood Glucose Level

190 mg/dL

Primary Health-Care Provider's Orders

Blood glucose monitoring before meals and hour of sleep with regular insulin coverage via subcutaneous route.
150 to 200 mg/dL—2 units regular insulin.
201 to 225 mg/dL—4 units regular insulin.
226 to 275 mg/dL—8 units regular insulin.
276 to 300 mg/dL—12 units regular insulin.
>300—notify primary health-care provider.

Progress Notes

Bilateral above the knee amputations with compression dressings; an abdominal incision that extends from the sternum to the symphysis pubis and a new colostomy stoma in the left lower quadrant of the abdomen. Patient lying in the low-Fowler position. Dependent edema 2+ noted. The patient states, "There is no way anyone is going to give me another injection in my arms. I've had it!"

Which should the nurse do in this situation?
1. Administer 2 units of regular insulin in the deltoid site.
2. Administer 8 units of regular insulin into the vastus lateralis site.
3. Administer 2 units of regular insulin into the love handles on the right side.
4. Administer 8 units of regular insulin several inches away from the colostomy.

36. A nurse enters a patient's room to administer a drug that is in the form of a tablet. The patient states, "I am nauseated and feel like I am going to vomit." What should the nurse do **next** in relation to administration of the medication?
    1. Obtain a prescription for an alternate route of administration.
    2. Give the medication and hope that the patient does not vomit.
    3. Obtain a liquid form of the prescribed medication and give it to the patient.
    4. Hold the medication for an hour and a half and then attempt to give it again.

37. A nurse is administering a medication via the buccal route. What should the nurse instruct the patient to do?
    1. "Swish this solution around in your mouth and then swallow it."
    2. "Hold the tablet between your cheek and gum until it dissolves."
    3. "Extend your forearm and I will inject a small amount of fluid under your skin."
    4. "Roll on your side with your knees bent and I will insert a suppository into your rectum."

38. A patient has a prescription for the insertion of a vaginal cream. Which steps should the nurse perform when administering this medication? **Select all that apply.**
    1. _____ Have the patient void before the procedure.
    2. _____ Clean the perineal area before inserting the cream.
    3. _____ Withdraw the applicator rapidly after the cream is inserted.
    4. _____ Place the patient in the supine position with the legs extended.
    5. _____ Direct the insertion of the applicator upward toward the umbilicus.
    6. _____ Press the plunger to expel a small amount of cream at the tip of the applicator before insertion.

39. A nurse is evaluating a patient's ability to self-administer a medication to both nasal passages via a nasal spray. What action by the patient indicates that the nurse must provide additional teaching?
    1. Compressing the other nostril while initiating the spray into the first nostril
    2. Exhaling slowly through the nose after initiating the spray
    3. Tilting the head backward after inhaling the spray
    4. Inhaling the spray while squeezing the container

40. A patient with diabetes who is on insulin coverage has been receiving 3 to 4 injections of insulin a day. What is important for the nurse to do when administering these injections?
    1. Alternate injection sites to minimize tissue injury.
    2. Spread the skin to facilitate entry of the needle through the skin.
    3. Instill the medication over 5 seconds to promote absorption of the medication.
    4. Use a syringe with a needle that is 1½-inches long to ensure access of subcutaneous tissue.

41. A primary health-care provider orders 1,000 mL of 0.9% sodium chloride with 20 mEq of KCl to be administered at 75 mL/hour. The nurse finds only 250 mL bags of 0.9% sodium chloride on the unit. What should the nurse do in this situation?
    1. Use a 1,000 mL bag of dextrose 5% in water with 20 mEq of KCl until the appropriate bag of solution is obtained.
    2. Withhold starting the intravenous infusion until a 1,000 mL bag of the appropriate solution is obtained.
    3. Insert 20 mEq of KCl into a 250 mL bag of 0.9% sodium chloride and set it at 25 mL/hour.
    4. Insert 5 mEq of KCl into a 250 mL bag of 0.9% sodium chloride and set it at 75 mL/hour.

42. A primary health-care provider prescribes clindamycin palmitate hydrochloride (Cleocin) oral suspension 60 mg three times a day for 10 days for a young child. The bottle of medication indicates that there are 75 mg per 5 mL of solution. How many milliliters of solution should the nurse plan to administer for each dose? Record your answer using a whole number.
    Answer: _____ mL

43. A nurse withdrew fluid from an ampule. What did the nurse do to ensure that the entire dose was withdrawn?
    1. Placed a plastic cover over the top of the ampule before snapping the constricted neck
    2. Changed the needle on the syringe after aspirating the solution from the ampule
    3. Flicked the ampule above the constricted neck several times
    4. Used a filter needle to aspirate solution from the ampule

44. In what section of the medication administration record should a nurse document a STAT drug given in an emergency?
    1. PRN section
    2. Single-dose section
    3. Progress note section
    4. Standing drugs section

45. During report, a nurse is informed that an assigned patient has diabetes mellitus with insulin coverage before meals and before going to sleep at night. The nurse tests the patient's blood glucose level before lunch and identifies that it is elevated. Place the interventions in the order in which the nurse should perform them.
    1. Wash the hands with soap and water.
    2. Don gloves and administer the prepared insulin.
    3. Draw up the prescribed amount of insulin to be administered.
    4. Compare the patient's blood glucose level to the insulin prescription.
    5. Verify the primary health-care provider's prescription for insulin coverage.
    Answer: _____

REVIEW ANSWERS

1. ANSWER: 3.

Rationales:

1. The vastus lateralis site is appropriate for an intramuscular injection in an obese individual as long as the amount of fluid injected is 3 mL or less.

2. The rectus femoris is an appropriate site for an intramuscular injection in an obese individual as long as the amount of fluid injected is 3 mL or less.

3. The dorsogluteal muscle has a thick fat layer, and an intramuscular injection will deposit the medication into subcutaneous tissue rather than a muscle.

4. The deltoid is an appropriate muscle for an intramuscular injection in an obese individual as long as the amount of fluid injected is 2 mL or less.

TEST-TAKING TIP: Identify the word in the stem that indicates negative polarity. The word *least* in the stem indicates negative polarity.

Content Area: Medication Administration
Integrated Processes: Nursing Process: Planning
Client Need: Physiological Integrity; Pharmacological and Parenteral Therapies
Cognitive Level: Application

2. ANSWER: 3.

Rationales:

1. This is an inaccurate dose; it is only 0.5 mL, which is less than the prescribed dose.

2. This is an inaccurate dose; it is only 1 mL, which is less than the prescribed dose.

3. This is the accurate dose. The markings on the syringe indicate that it contains 1.5 mL of solution. Solve the problem by using ratio and proportion and then identify the place on the syringe that indicates 1.5 (1½) mL.

$$\frac{\text{Desire 0.75 grams}}{\text{Have 1 gram}} = \frac{x \text{ mL}}{2 \text{ mL}}$$
$$1x = 0.75 \times 2$$
$$1x = 1.5$$
$$x = 1.5 \div 1$$
$$x = 1.5 \text{ mL}$$

4. This is an inaccurate dose; it is 2 mL, which exceeds the prescribed dose.

Content Area: Medication Administration
Integrated Processes: Nursing Process: Planning
Client Need: Physiological Integrity; Pharmacological and Parenteral Therapies
Cognitive Level: Application

3. ANSWER: 1.

Rationales:

1. A gloved lubricated index finger and suppository moves the suppository 3- to 4-inches into the rectum past the external and internal rectal sphincters. Lubrication with a water-soluble jelly prevents trauma to the mucous membranes of the intestines.

2. Assuming the sitting position after a suppository is inserted will allow it to move out of the rectum and anus via gravity. The patient should remain in the supine or a side-lying position for 15 to 20 minutes after insertion to allow the suppository to melt in the rectum, where the medication will be absorbed through the mucous membranes.

3. A warm suppository will soften or melt and be impossible to insert into the anus. A suppository should be administered immediately after removal from the refrigerator while it is still firm.

4. The supine position will not allow access to the anus. The patient should be placed in the left lateral position to permit access to the anus and allow the suppository to follow the contour of the rectum and sigmoid colon once inserted.

TEST-TAKING TIP: Identify clang associations. The word *rectal* in the stem and in option 1 and *rectum* in option 2 are clang associations. Examine options 1 and 2 carefully.

Content Area: Medication Administration
Integrated Processes: Nursing Process: Implementation
Client Need: Physiological Integrity; Pharmacological and Parenteral Therapies
Cognitive Level: Application

4. ANSWER: 1, 2, 3, 4, 5.

Rationales:

1. Vitamins are a medication and should be included on a medication reconciliation form. An accurate list of all the drugs that a patient is taking (including drug name, dose, route, and frequency) should be reconciled on admission and during transitions (e.g., transfer between units, when new medication administration records are implemented, and at discharge). This list should be compared to new medications prescribed and education provided to the patient about each medication.

2. Most drug reconciliation forms contain a section that records drug allergies.

3. Food supplements are considered medications because they contain ingredients that may interact with medicinal products.

4. Over-the-counter herbs are considered medication because they contain ingredients that may interact with medicinal products.

5. Prescribed medications should be included on a medication reconciliation form.

Content Area: Medication Administration
Integrated Processes: Communication/Documentation; Nursing Process: Implementation
Client Need: Safe and Effective Care Environment; Management of Care
Cognitive Level: Application

5. ANSWER: 4.

Rationales:

1. Administering a distasteful medication in a child's favorite fruit juice should not be done because it may result in the child refusing to ingest the juice in the future.

2. This is unsafe. Instilling 3 mL of medication at one time may overwhelm the child's ability to safely swallow the dose, resulting in aspiration.

3. This is unsafe. Sipping liquid through a straw makes it difficult to control the flow of fluid being delivered to the back of the oral cavity. It is safer to drink out of a cup.

4. An ice pop numbs the nerve endings in the taste buds of the tongue, limiting the experience of distasteful medication.

TEST-TAKING TIP: Identify the option with a specific determiner. Option 2 contains the word *all,* which is a specific determiner. Rarely is an option with a specific determiner the correct answer. Identify clang associations. The word *medication* in the stem and in options 1 and 4 are clang associations. Examine options 1 and 4 carefully.
Content Area: Medication Administration
Integrated Processes: Nursing Process: Implementation
Client Need: Physiological Integrity; Pharmacological and Parenteral Therapies
Cognitive Level: Application

6. **ANSWER: 4.**
Rationales:
1. The Z-track technique is used for an intramuscular injection. A 25-gauge needle is too thin and fragile as well as too short (usually is ½- to 1-inch in length) for an intramuscular injection. In addition, medications administered via the Z-track technique are thick (viscous) and require a needle gauge of 18 to 22.
2. This is unsafe because medication clinging to the outside of the needle can irritate tissue along the needle tract. The Z-track technique is used for medications that are known to irritate or discolor subcutaneous tissue. Therefore, the needle should be changed so that there is no medication residue on the needle during insertion.
3. A 1-inch needle is used for subcutaneous injections. The Z-track technique is used for an intramuscular injection. Therefore, a needle length of 1½ inches should be used to ensure access to a muscle.
4. **Pulling the skin and subcutaneous tissue to the side establishes a zigzag path before needle insertion; when the skin is released after insertion of the medication the tissue planes slide across each other confining the medication in the muscle and preventing it from flowing back up the needle track.**
TEST-TAKING TIP: Identify the unique option. Option 4 is unique. Options 1, 2, and 3 all address information concerning the type of needle to be used for the procedure. Option 4 addresses the actual technique of administering the injection to the patient.
Content Area: Medication Administration
Integrated Processes: Nursing Process: Evaluation
Client Need: Physiological Integrity; Pharmacological and Parenteral Therapies
Cognitive Level: Application

7. **ANSWER: 4, 1, 5, 6, 2, 3.**
Rationales:
4. **Washing the eyes before administering eyedrops removes crusts and microorganisms and facilitates medication absorption. Using separate cotton balls for each eye reduces the risk of cross-contamination and wiping from the inner to outer canthus limits entrance of microorganisms into the lacrimal duct.**
1. **Looking upward helps reduce the likelihood of blinking or squinting during the procedure.**
5. **Exposing the conjunctival sac reduces the risk of touching the cornea with the dropper when instilling eyedrops.**

6. **Placing the dominant hand on the forehead stabilizes hand movement. Approaching the eye from the side minimizes blinking. Instilling the drop 1 to 2 cm above the conjunctival sac eliminates the danger of corneal injury by either a drop falling directly on the cornea or the dropper touching the cornea.**
2. **Gently closing the eyes spreads the medication over the eyeball. Squeezing the eyes shut should be avoided because this can cause injury to the eye and force the medication out.**
3. **Pressing firmly on the nasolacrimal duct for 30 to 60 seconds prevents medication from draining out of the eye and to the nasopharynx. Also, it may help to prevent an unpleasant taste.**
Content Area: Medication Administration
Integrated Processes: Nursing Process: Planning
Client Need: Physiological Integrity; Pharmacological and Parenteral Therapies
Cognitive Level: Analysis

8. **ANSWER: 4.**
Rationales:
1. This is unsafe. The infant may be unable to manage liquid instilled in this location and it can result in aspiration of the medication.
2. Although this can be done, it is not the best method to administer a liquid medication to an infant.
3. This is unsafe. A 3-month-old infant is unable to manage sipping fluid from a cup.
4. **This technique uses a method that is familiar to an infant. Infants obtain milk by sucking on a human nipple or a nipple of a bottle containing formula. They become proficient at sucking the milk at a rate that they can manage without causing aspiration of the liquid.**
TEST-TAKING TIP: Identify the word in the stem that sets a priority. The word *best* in the stem sets a priority.
Content Area: Medication Administration
Integrated Processes: Nursing Process: Implementation
Client Need: Physiological Integrity; Pharmacological and Parenteral Therapies
Cognitive Level: Application

9. **ANSWER: 1.**
Rationales:
1. **This facilitates dispersing the medication to all of the nasal surfaces via gravity. This position should be maintained for 1 minute after insertion of the medication so that it does not flow out of the nostril.**
2. This violates an infection control practice. The tip of the dropper may touch the mucous membranes of the nose, contaminating the dropper. The tip of the dropper should be held just outside the opening to the nostril.
3. This will move the medication to the posterior oropharynx and trachea, which are undesirable outcomes. The child should be instructed to breathe through the mouth after insertion to help keep the medication in contact with the nasal mucosa.
4. This violates an infection control practice. The unused medication should be wasted and the empty dropper should be returned to the medication bottle.

TEST-TAKING TIP: Identify clang associations. The word *child* in the stem and in options 1 and 3 are clang associations. The word *nose* in the stem and in options 3 and 4 are clang associations. The words *drop* and *drops* in the stem and *drop* in options 2 and 3 and *drops* in options 1 and 4 are clang associations. The word *nostril* in the stem and in option 2 is a clang association. All options contain clang associations. This test-taking tip will not help you focus on the correct answer.
Content Area: Medication Administration
Integrated Processes: Nursing Process: Implementation
Client Need: Physiological Integrity; Pharmacological and Parenteral Therapies
Cognitive Level: Application

10. **ANSWER: 2, 4, 6, 5, 3, 1.**
Rationales:
2. The forearm allows for easier insertion of the solution into the dermis which is just below the epidermis and above the subcutaneous tissue. It is easily accessible and permits visualization of the pateint's response to the injection.
4. Cleaning the site with an alcohol wipe decreases microorganisms.
6. Using a small gauge, short needle with the bevel up facilitates needle placement just below the epidermis.
5. Slow, steady insertion of the medication allows time to stop the procedure if a systemic reaction occurs. The formation of a wheal (raised welt, bleb) confirms correct drug administration.
3. Stabilizing the tissue on both sides of the puncture site as the needle is quickly removed minimizes the skin from dragging on the needle as it is removed. Removing the needle along the insertion angle prevents tissue trauma.
1. Drawing a 1-inch circle around the wheal identifies the site for assessment purposes. The site should be not be massaged and the patient should be instructed not to rub the area.
Content Area: Medication Administration
Integrated Processes: Nursing Process: Planning
Client Need: Physiological Integrity; Pharmacological and Parenteral Therapies
Cognitive Level: Analysis

11. **ANSWER: 1.**
Rationales:
1. Many accidental drug overdoses result from a person forgetting that a medication was ingested and therefore taking another dose. A drug organizer has 7 horizontal rows of boxes and up to four vertical rows of boxes for 4 different times during the day (a.m., noon, afternoon, p.m.). Each box holds the tablets/pills that are to be taken on a particular day and at a particular time. This is a safe way to know if drugs prescribed for a particular day or time were taken. If the box is empty, they were taken. If the box is still full, they were not taken. Some patients may need assistance in filling the boxes on a weekly basis to ensure accuracy.
2. Setting an alarm clock may help to take the medication initially, but it will not help if the patient later has difficulty remembering if the drug was taken.

3. Relying on a family member can be a burden for the family member. Also, it takes the responsibility away from the patient, contributing to dependence.
4. Making a calendar may help to take the medication initially, but it will not help if the patient later has difficulty remembering if the drug was taken.
TEST-TAKING TIP: Identify the word in the stem that sets a priority. The word *best* in the stem sets a priority. Identify the clang association. The word *medication* in the stem and in options 1 and 3 are clang associations.
Content Area: Medication Administration
Integrated Processes: Teaching/Learning; Nursing Process: Implementation
Client Need: Health Promotion and Maintenance
Cognitive Level: Application

12. **ANSWER: 1.**
Rationales:
1. The nurse is required to question orders or prescriptions when they are outside normal, expected parameters. If the nurse blindly follows orders and administers an excessive dose of a medication, the nurse compounds the initial error and is also liable for damages.
2. Administering a medication is a dependent function of the nurse. It is not within the nurse's scope of practice to change a prescribed dose without a prescription from a primary health-care provider.
3. It is unnecessary to call the pharmacist because it is within the nurse's role to manage this situation.
4. A nurse does not need to seek the support of a nurse manager to initially discuss an excessive dose of a medication with a primary health-care provider. It is wise to inform the nurse manager of the problem if the primary health-care provider refuses to adjust the prescription and the nurse in turn refuses to administer the excessive dose of the medication.
TEST-TAKING TIP: Identify the clang associations. The words *primary health-care provider* in the stem and in options 1 and 4 are clang associations. The word *weight* in the stem and in options 2 and 3 are clang associations. Using the test-taking tip, identify clang associations, does not help you to focus on a potential correct answer because all 4 options contain a clang association.
Content Area: Medication Administration
Integrated Processes: Communication/Documentation; Nursing Process: Implementation
Client Need: Safe and Effective Care Environment; Management of Care
Cognitive Level: Application

13. **ANSWER: 3.**
Rationales:
1. This site is the vastus lateralis. This site is not recommended for the injection of heparin. It is used mainly for intramuscular injections. This is the second site after the ventrogluteal site for the injection of 1 mL or larger. Also, it is used for newborns and infants who have not yet developed the gluteal or deltoid muscles.
2. This is the ventrogluteal site. This site is not recommended for the administration of heparin.
3. This site is the abdomen. It is the best site to inject heparin because the abdomen has a large subcutaneous

layer under the skin and above the muscle. A subcutaneous injection into the abdominal area must avoid a 2-inch area around the umbilicus.

4. This site is the deltoid and is not recommended for the administration of heparin. It has a small subcutaneous layer and arm activity hastens absorption, which is not desired.

Content Area: Medication Administration
Integrated Processes: Nursing Process: Implementation
Client Need: Physiological Integrity; Pharmacological and Parenteral Therapies
Cognitive Level: Analysis

14. ANSWER: 4.
Rationales:
1. This is contraindicated. Rubbing the site can cause bleeding and bruising because heparin is an anticoagulant.
2. Placing the needle just under the epidermis is the technique used for an intradermal injection. Heparin is administered via the subcutaneous route.
3. This is contraindicated. Spreading the skin may permit the needle to enter a muscle rather than subcutaneous tissue.
4. **The needle pierces the skin and enters subcutaneous tissue during an injection of heparin. A disinfectant, such as alcohol, will minimize microorganisms on the skin before the needle pierces the skin. This will limit the development of an infection at the site of the injection.**
TEST-TAKING TIP: Identify the option with a specific determiner. Option 2 contains the word *just,* which is a specific determiner. Identify clang associations. The word *injection* in the stem and in options 1 and 4 are clang associations. Examine options 1 and 4 carefully.
Content Area: Medication Administration
Integrated Processes: Nursing Process: Implementation
Client Need: Physiological Integrity; Pharmacological and Parenteral Therapies
Cognitive Level: Application

15. ANSWER: 13.
Rationale:
Arrive at the answer to this question using the following formula.

$$\frac{\text{Total mL to be infused} \times \text{drop factor}}{\text{Total time in minutes}}$$

$$\frac{80 \text{ (mL)} \times 10 \text{ (drop factor)}}{60 \text{ (minutes)}} = \frac{800}{60} = 13.33$$

Round down to 13 drops per minute because 0.3 is less than 0.5.

Content Area: Medication Administration
Integrated Processes: Nursing Process: Planning
Client Need: Physiological Integrity; Pharmacological and Parenteral Therapies
Cognitive Level: Application

16. ANSWER: 4.
Rationales:
1. Verbal interactions, particularly if they involve complex information or instructions concerning the future, may

not be understood or remembered by a patient who is cognitively impaired.
2. How to use a plastic box with multiple sections may not be understood by a patient who is cognitively impaired.
3. Writing involves the use of symbols that may not be able to be read or understood by a patient who is cognitively impaired.
4. **Placing medications next to the patient's toothbrush provides a reminder for the patient to take them. It allows the person a sense of independence. Repetitive, routine activities that have been performed throughout life, such as brushing the teeth, usually can be performed by a person with moderate dementia.**
TEST-TAKING TIP: Identify the option with a specific determiner. Option 2 contains the word *all,* which is a specific determiner. Identify clang associations. The word *relative* in the stem and in options 1 and 4 are clang associations. Examine options 1 and 4 carefully.
Content Area: Medication Administration
Integrated Processes: Teaching/Learning; Nursing Process: Implementation
Client Need: Physiological Integrity; Pharmacological and Parenteral Therapies
Cognitive Level: Application

17. ANSWER: 4.
Rationales:
1. This is a U 100 syringe marked in units, of which there are 100 per 1 mL. It has a needle that is a $\frac{1}{2}$-inch in length, which is not long enough to reach a muscle. This syringe is used for insulin injections.
2. This is a 1 mL tuberculin syringe marked in 0.01 mL (1/100th of a milliliter) and minims (16 minims = 1 mL). It has a needle that is a $\frac{1}{2}$-inch in length, which is not long enough to reach a muscle. This syringe is used for intradermal injections, such as instillation of allergens for allergy testing and purified protein derivative (PPD) to identify exposure to the pathogen causing tuberculosis.
3. This is a 3 mL standard syringe marked in whole milliliters and 0.1 mL (1/10th of a milliliter). It has a needle that is $\frac{5}{8}$-inch in length, which is not long enough to reach a muscle. This syringe is used for subcutaneous injections.
4. **This is a 5 mL standard syringe marked in whole milliliters and 0.2 mL (2/10th of a milliliter). It has a needle that is $1\frac{1}{2}$-inches long, which is capable of reaching a muscle. This syringe is used for intramuscular injections.**
Content Area: Medication Administration
Integrated Processes: Nursing Process: Planning
Client Need: Physiological Integrity; Pharmacological and Parenteral Therapies
Cognitive Level: Analysis

18. ANSWER: 2.
Rationales:
1. Inserting the order into the patient's clinical record can be done after the telephone call.
2. **This action is essential. It repeats the message for the primary health-care provider and ensures that the order was understood correctly.**

3. It is unnecessary to confirm that the medication is available in the hospital pharmacy before the telephone call is completed. The nurse can contact the primary health-care provider if the medication is unavailable.

4. A telephone order usually is required to be signed by the primary-health care provider within 24 hours.

TEST-TAKING TIP: Identify clang associations. The words *primary health-care provider* in the stem and in options 2 and 4 are clang associations. Examine options 2 and 4 carefully.

Content Area: *Medication Administration*
Integrated Processes: *Nursing Process: Implementation*
Client Need: *Physiological Integrity; Pharmacological and Parenteral Therapies*
Cognitive Level: *Application*

19. ANSWER: 2.
Rationales:

1. This direction usually is not indicated in a prescription. This information usually is included in directions from the pharmacist, in literature distributed by the manufacturer of the medication, or in a reputable drug book that includes the medication.

2. **The letters prn mean *as needed* or *when necessary*. The prescription basically states that the medication may be taken by the patient every 6 hours if needed. Frequently, additional parameters are stipulated by the primary health-care provider, such as every 6 hours prn for severe pain or every 6 hours prn for diarrhea.**

3. This instruction is not related to the patient's prescription.

4. This information is related to a standing (routine) order. A routine prescription might state, "Give aspirin 325 mg by mouth every 6 hours." This order is carried out by a nurse until it is discontinued by the primary health-care provider, a hospital policy stipulates that it should be discontinued, or a nurse determines that it is placing the patient in jeopardy. The primary health-care provider should be notified when a medication is discontinued or when a patient is in jeopardy.

Content Area: *Medication Administration*
Integrated Processes: *Teaching/Learning; Nursing Process: Implementation*
Client Need: *Physiological Integrity; Pharmacological and Parenteral Therapies*
Cognitive Level: *Application*

20. ANSWER: 2.
Rationales:

1. The patient should look up during medication insertion to limit the risk of blinking.

2. **Pressure over the inner canthus prevents medication from entering the lacrimal duct.**

3. A finger should be placed just below the lower eyelashes while simultaneously exerting downward pressure toward the cheek.

4. Debris around the eye should be removed before medication insertion and excess medication removed after medication insertion by wiping from the inner to the outer canthus with a cotton ball.

TEST-TAKING TIP: Identify the options with a clang association. The word *eye* in the stem and in options 2 and 4 are clang associations. Examine these options carefully. More often than not, an option with a clang association is the correct answer.

Content Area: *Medication Administration*
Integrated Processes: *Nursing Process: Implementation*
Client Need: *Physiological Integrity; Pharmacological and Parenteral Therapies*
Cognitive Level: *Application*

21. ANSWER: 4.
Rationales:

1. This is the intramuscular route. The intramuscular route is not used to test for tuberculosis or allergies.

2. This is the subcutaneous route. The subcutaneous route is not used to test for tuberculosis or allergies. When a $\frac{1}{2}$-inch or $\frac{5}{8}$-inch needle is used to administer a medication via the subcutaneous route, the needle is inserted at a 90-degree angle to ensure that the medication is injected into subcutaneous tissue and not muscle.

3. This is the subcutaneous route. The subcutaneous route is not used to test for tuberculosis or allergies. When a 1-inch needle is used to administer a medication via the subcutaneous route, the needle is inserted at a 45-degree angle to ensure that the medication is injected into subcutaneous tissue and not muscle.

4. **This is the intradermal route. It is used mainly for testing for tuberculosis and allergies.**

Content Area: *Medication Administration*
Integrated Processes: *Nursing Process: Implementation*
Client Need: *Physiological Integrity; Pharmacological and Parenteral Therapies*
Cognitive Level: *Analysis*

22. ANSWER: 1.
Rationales:

1. **Injecting air with the bevel of the needle below the level of the solution will cause turbulence resulting in bubbles. Bubbles in the solution will result in the withdrawal of a dose less than the prescribed dose.**

2. Instilling slightly more air into the vial than the amount of solution to be withdrawn will increase pressure within the vial, but it will not result in an inaccurate dose.

3. Rolling the vial between the palms of the hands to disperse the diluent is an action that will not cause bubbles. Shaking the vial will cause bubbles that will result in withdrawal of an inaccurate dose.

4. Instilling the solution slowly limits turbulence that causes bubbles.

TEST-TAKING TIP: Identify the word in the stem that indicates negative polarity. The word *compromised* in the stem indicates negative polarity. The question is asking, "What is an inappropriate action when withdrawing medication from a vial?"

Content Area: *Medication Administration*
Integrated Processes: *Nursing Process: Evaluation*
Client Need: *Physiological Integrity; Pharmacological and Parenteral Therapies*
Cognitive Level: *Application*

23. ANSWER: 3.
Rationales:
1. The vastus lateralis site extends from one handbreadth above the knee to one handbreadth below the greater trochanter of the femur on the anterior lateral aspect of the thigh.
2. The greater trochanter is one of several bony landmarks used to locate the ventrogluteal site.
3. **The deltoid is located by making an inverted triangle approximately 2 to 3 finger widths below the acromion process and a line from the anterior to the posterior axillary crease.**
4. The anterior superior iliac spine is one of several bony landmarks used to locate the ventrogluteal site.
Content Area: Medication Administration
Integrated Processes: Nursing Process: Implementation
Client Need: Physiological Integrity; Pharmacological and Parenteral Therapies
Cognitive Level: Application

24. ANSWER: 3.
Rationales:
1. This is an expected response when an intravenous catheter is in a vein.
2. This is a sign of inflammation of a vein (phlebitis), not infiltration.
3. **Swelling of tissue occurs with an infiltration because the intravenous solution is entering the interstitial compartment.**
4. The site will be cool to the touch with an infiltration because the solution infusing into the subcutaneous tissue is at room temperature, which is lower than body temperature. Warmth may indicate the presence of inflammation or infection.
Content Area: Medication Administration
Integrated Processes: Nursing Process: Evaluation
Client Need: Physiological Integrity; Pharmacological and Parenteral Therapies
Cognitive Level: Application

25. ANSWER: 83.
Rationale:
A volume control device is programmed at mL per hour. Therefore, to answer the question, divide 12 hours into 1,000 mL to determine the hourly rate. 1000 ÷ 12 = 83.33 mL per hour. Round the answer down to 83 because 0.3 is less than 0.5.
Content Area: Medication Administration
Integrated Processes: Nursing Process: Planning
Client Need: Physiological Integrity; Pharmacological and Parenteral Therapies
Cognitive Level: Application

26. ANSWER: 2.
Rationales:
1. The arm should be elevated on a pillow above the level of the heart. This will promote venous return and facilitate resorption of the intravenous solution in the interstitial compartment.
2. **Restarting the infusion in the patient's left arm allows the right arm to recover from the trauma of the infiltration.**

Also, the infusion should be restarted as soon as possible to limit the interruption of the IV fluid order. Once the infusion is restarted, the flow rate should be set at the ordered rate. It should not be increased to make up the amount of solution that was not administered. An increased flow rate could cause an excessive amount of fluid in the intravascular compartment (hypervolemia).
3. The preparation of a warm soak will take time, causing a delay in meeting the patient's primary need. This is a dependent function of the nurse and requires an order from a person with a prescriptive license or a standing order of the facility.
4. When an infusion is restarted in an extremity that had an infiltration, the site should be proximal to the site of the infiltration; this prevents trauma at the site of the infiltration. The use of the same arm is discouraged but may be used when an alternate site is unavailable.
TEST-TAKING TIP: Identify the word in the stem that sets a priority. The word *next* in the stem sets a priority. Identify the options that are opposites. Options 2 and 4 are opposites. In option 2, the infusion is restarted in the left arm and in option 4, the infusion is restarted in the right arm. Consider these options carefully. Often, when there are opposites, one of them is the correct answer. Identify the options that have a clang association. The stem contains the word *forearm* and options 2 and 3 both contain the word *forearm*. Identify the option that is unique. Option 2 is the only option that addresses the left arm. Options 1, 3, and 4 address the right arm.
Content Area: Medication Administration
Integrated Processes: Nursing Process: Implementation
Client Need: Physiological Integrity; Pharmacological and Parenteral Therapies
Cognitive Level: Application

27. ANSWER: 3.
Rationales:
1. Bending the needle of a syringe is unsafe and could result in a needle stick injury.
2. A used needle should never be recapped, particularly when walking, because it may precipitate a needle stick injury.
3. **Many syringes are designed to actively or passively cover used needles to protect the caregiver from needle stick injuries.**
4. Although this should be done, it does not protect the nurse if the needle is not covered when walking from the patient to the location of a sharps container.
TEST-TAKING TIP: Identify the word in the stem that sets a priority. The word *best* in the stem sets a priority.
Content Area: Medication Administration
Integrated Processes: Nursing Process: Implementation
Client Need: Physiological Integrity; Pharmacological and Parenteral Therapies
Cognitive Level: Application

28. ANSWER: 3.
Rationales:
1. This is an inaccurate dose. This is 8 units, which reflects the amount of solution required if just the regular insulin were to be administered.

2. This is an inaccurate dose. This is 22 units, which reflects the amount of solution required if just the NPH insulin were to be administered.

3. This is the correct volume of solution (30 units) when the NPH insulin dose (22 units) is added to the regular insulin dose (8 units). These medications can safely be administered in the same syringe.

4. This volume of solution is 42 units, which exceeds the combined volume of the prescribed insulins.
Content Area: Medication Administration
Integrated Processes: Nursing Process: Evaluation
Client Need: Physiological Integrity; Pharmacological and Parenteral Therapies
Cognitive Level: Analysis

29. **ANSWER: 2.**
Rationales:
1. If this port is used, some of the medication will mix with the larger volume of fluid in the tubing and will not reach the patient for a longer period of time. The port closest to the insertion site should be used.

2. Pinching the tubing above the insertion port ensures that the medication being instilled flows toward the patient rather than backward up the intravenous tubing; the port closest to the patient should be used.

3. Increasing the flow rate is unsafe and not within the legal role of the nurse. The nurse should set the flow rate as prescribed. The administration of intravenous fluids is a dependent function of the nurse.
4. This is not necessary.
TEST-TAKING TIP: Identify clang associations. The word *port* in the stem and in options 1 and 2 are clang associations. Examine options 1 and 2 carefully.
Content Area: Medication Administration
Integrated Processes: Nursing Process: Implementation
Client Need: Physiological Integrity; Pharmacological and Parenteral Therapies
Cognitive Level: Application

30. **ANSWER: 3, 4, 5.**
Rationales:
1. Warming the solution is unnecessary; it can be administered at room temperature.
2. When hanging an IVPB, the primary infusion bag must be hung lower than the secondary infusion bag. Hanging the secondary infusion bag lower than the primary infusion bag will cause fluid from the primary infusion bag to enter the secondary infusion tubing and bag. This occurs because the pressure in the primary infusion set is higher than the pressure within the secondary infusion set, and the secondary infusion set does not have a check valve that prevents fluid from flowing up the secondary tubing into the bag.
3. Wiping the port with alcohol is a necessary infection control intervention. This is a sterile procedure because the port has direct access to the patient's circulatory system.
4. Priming the secondary line removes air from the tubing, which will prevent the introduction of air into the patient's circulatory system.
5. Opening the clamp on the secondary infusion tubing and using the clamp on the primary infusion tubing to

control the flow ensures that the primary infusion will flow after the secondary infusion bag is empty.
Content Area: Medication Administration
Integrated Processes: Nursing Process: Implementation
Client Need: Physiological Integrity; Pharmacological and Parenteral Therapies
Cognitive Level: Application

31. **ANSWER: 4.**
Rationales:
1. The pressure of the falling drops may injure the tympanic membrane. The dropper should be held close to but not touching the ear canal and the drops should be directed to the side of the canal so that the drops do not fall directly on the tympanic membrane.
2. The medication should be administered close to body temperature. The nurse should hold the medication bottle in a hand for several minutes until it is warm. Medication for the ear usually is stored at room temperature.
3. The pinna should be pulled up and backward to straighten the ear canal of an adult or child older than 3 years of age. The pinna should be pulled down and backward to straighten the ear canal of a child younger than 3 years of age.
4. Gravity will facilitate the flow of medication into the ear and retain it in contact with structures within the ear canal when the child is in a position with the ear facing the ceiling. A cotton ball can be placed gently into the external canal, if prescribed, to prevent the drug from leaking out of the ear canal when sitting up.
TEST-TAKING TIP: Identify the option with a specific determiner. Option 2 contains the word *just,* which is a specific determiner. An option with a specific determiner usually is an incorrect answer.
Content Area: Medication Administration
Integrated Processes: Teaching/Learning; Nursing Process: Implementation
Client Need: Physiological Integrity; Pharmacological and Parenteral Therapies
Cognitive Level: Application

32. **ANSWER: 1, 3, 4.**
Rationales:
1. Gloves should be worn when removing and applying medicated patches to protect the nurse from being exposed to the medication.
2. Shaving hair on the skin is necessary only if the hair is interfering with adherence of the patch. This action is not necessary for every patient. The nurse must receive consent from the patient when hair must be shaved.
3. Washing and drying the skin after removing a used patch removes lingering drug on the skin and minimizes the risk of an overdose.
4. Compressing the medicated patch against the skin for 10 seconds after it is applied ensures that it is attached to the patient's skin.
5. An excessive amount of medication may be administered if both patches are on at the same time. The previous patch should be removed and the area cleansed at the time that a new patch is applied. The new patch should be applied to a different area.

Content Area: Medication Administration
Integrated Processes: Nursing Process: Implementation
Client Need: Physiological Integrity; Pharmacological and Parenteral Therapies
Cognitive Level: Application

33. **ANSWER: 2.**
Rationales:
1. Although this should be done eventually, offering the patient apple juice next to take with the medication is premature.
2. **Administering a medication to the *right patient* is one of the ten rights of medication administration. Before administering a medication, the nurse should check the patient's stated name and date of birth against an objective source of this information.**
3. Although the head of the bed should be raised before administering oral medications to a patient, this action is premature at this time.
4. Although this should be done eventually, checking for the patient's allergies next is premature.
TEST-TAKING TIP: Identify the word in the stem that sets a priority. The word *next* in the stem sets a priority.
Content Area: Medication Administration
Integrated Processes: Communication/Documentation; Nursing Process: Implementation
Client Need: Physiological Integrity; Pharmacological and Parenteral Therapies
Cognitive Level: Application

34. **ANSWER: 1.**
Rationales:
1. **A drug that is teratogenic may negatively affect a fetus, producing a congenital anomaly. Drugs that are known to be teratogenic should not be administered to pregnant women.**
2. Gluten, the protein of wheat and other grains, is unrelated to drugs that are teratogenic.
3. Eating food before receiving a medication that is teratogenic is unnecessary. Food should be taken with medications that are known to be gastrointestinal irritants.
4. Obtaining a blood specimen for a culture and sensitivity test is required before administering an antibiotic so that the antibiotic does not influence the test results.
TEST-TAKING TIP: Identify the option with a specific determiner. Option 4 contains the word *just* which is a specific determiner.
Content Area: Medication Administration
Integrated Processes: Communication/Documentation; Nursing Process: Implementation
Client Need: Physiological Integrity; Pharmacological and Parenteral Therapies
Cognitive Level: Analysis

35. **ANSWER: 3.**
Rationales:
1. The nurse can be sued for battery when performing an injection into a site against the patient's wishes.
2. The vastus lateralis sites are beneath the compression dressings at the site of the amputations. They cannot be

accessed for an injection. Also, the dose being administered is inaccurate.
3. **Two units of regular insulin is the accurate dose to be administered as per the primary health-care provider's prescription (150 to 200 mg/dL—2 units regular insulin). The lateral sides of the waist just above the iliac crests (love handles) are alternate injection sites for a subcutaneous injection. The side opposite to the colostomy ensures that the injection will not traumatize the area around the colostomy. The ventral gluteal and scapular areas should not be used because of 2+ dependent edema. Dependent edema, when a patient is in the low-Fowler position, will occur in the back and sacrum. The vastus lateralis sites are inaccessible because of compression bandages.**
4. Performing injections close to a new colostomy may be traumatic and should be avoided. Also, the dose being administered is inaccurate.
TEST-TAKING TIP: Identify duplicate facts in options. Options 1 and 3 have a duplicate fact (2 units) and options 2 and 4 have a duplicate fact (8 units). If you know the correct dose to be administered, you can reduce the options to be considered to just 2 options. By doing this, you increase your chances of selecting the correct answer from 25 to 50 percent.
Content Area: Medication Administration
Integrated Processes: Nursing Process: Implementation
Client Need: Physiological Integrity; Pharmacological and Parenteral Therapies
Cognitive Level: Analysis

36. **ANSWER: 1.**
Rationales:
1. **Administering medication is a dependent function of the nurse. The nurse should notify the primary health-care provider of the patient's status and obtain a prescription for an alternate route of administration.**
2. This is unsafe because it may precipitate vomiting.
3. Although substituting the liquid form of the drug for the tablet form of the drug is acceptable practice, in this instance, any form of the drug administered orally may precipitate vomiting and should be avoided.
4. This is outside the legal practice of nursing. Administering medications is a dependent function and a nurse cannot make this decision independently. A drug may be held for one hour because administering drugs one hour before or one hour after the prescribed time of administration is acceptable nursing practice. This practice is acceptable because all the medications due at a certain time cannot feasibly be administered to all the patients on a unit at the same exact time.
TEST-TAKING TIP: Identify the word in the stem that sets a priority. The word *next* in the stem sets a priority. Identify the option with a clang association. The word *administration* in the stem and in option 1 is a clang association. Identify the option that is unique. Option 1 is unique; it is the only option that does not contain the word *medication*.
Content Area: Medication Administration
Integrated Processes: Communication/Documentation; Nursing Process: Implementation
Client Need: Safe and Effective Care Environment; Management of Care
Cognitive Level: Application

37. ANSWER: 2.
Rationales:
1. Swirling a solution around the oral cavity and swallowing it is called *swish and swallow.*
2. **The buccal cavities are the spaces between the cheek and gum on either side of the mouth. The mucous membranes in a buccal cavity are warm and moist and a tablet will melt slowly.**
3. Inserting a small amount of medicated fluid under the skin is known as an intradermal injection.
4. Inserting a suppository through the anus into the rectum utilizes the rectal route.
Content Area: Medication Administration
Integrated Processes: Communication/Documentation; Nursing Process: Implementation
Client Need: Physiological Integrity; Pharmacological and Parenteral Therapies
Cognitive Level: Application

38. ANSWER: 1, 2, 6.
Rationales:
1. **An empty bladder limits the discomfort that may be experienced when the medication is inserted into the vagina.**
2. **Cleaning removes debris and reduces the amount of microorganisms in the perineal area; this limits the risk of infection.**
3. The applicator should be removed slowly to prevent tissue trauma.
4. This position will not allow access to the vagina. The patient should be placed in the dorsal recumbent (supine with hips and knees flexed) or Sims (side lying with the top hip and knee flexed) position to allow visualization of and access to the vagina.
5. This is unsafe; it will traumatize the delicate mucous membranes of the vagina. The applicator should be inserted downward and backward toward the cervix. Insertion of a catheter toward the umbilicus is the technique used when inserting a catheter to perform an enema.
6. **Expelling a small amount of cream at the tip of the applicator will act as a lubricant to facilitate insertion of the applicator and limit tissue trauma.**
Content Area: Medication Administration
Integrated Processes: Nursing Process: Implementation
Client Need: Physiological Integrity; Pharmacological and Parenteral Therapies
Cognitive Level: Application

39. ANSWER: 2.
Rationales:
1. This is a correct technique. When administering a nasal spray to both nostrils the patient should compress the opposite nostril while administering the nasal spray into the first nostril; this prevents the medication from entering the other nostril. When instilling the nasal spray into the second nostril the patient should not compress the first nostril; compressing the first nostril may expel the previously administered medication from the first nostril.
2. **This is an undesirable practice. Exhaling through the nose will facilitate leakage of medication out of the nasal**

passage, minimizing its contact with the mucous membranes of the nose.
3. This is a correct technique. Tilting the head backward will help retain the medication in the nasal passage.
4. This is a correct technique. Compressing the container discharges a dose and inhaling the spray ensures that it enters the nostril.
TEST-TAKING TIP: Identify the words in the stem that indicate negative polarity. The words *provide additional teaching* indicate negative polarity. The question is asking, "What is *not acceptable* when self-administering a nasal spray?"
Content Area: Medication Administration
Integrated Processes: Teaching/Learning; Nursing Process: Evaluation
Client Need: Physiological Integrity; Pharmacological and Parenteral Therapies
Cognitive Level: Application

40. ANSWER: 1.
Rationales:
1. **The administration of numerous injections in one site may cause tissue injury, such as degradation of adipose tissue (lipodystrophy). Lipodystrophy is less of a problem since the advent of human insulin. The nurse should rotate sites and document them on the medication administration record so that there can be continuity of care among the nurses administering insulin to the patient.**
2. Insulin is administered via a subcutaneous injection, which often involves pinching the skin while inserting the needle. Spreading the skin is done with an intramuscular injection.
3. Insulin does not have to be administered over 5 seconds. Usually, a dose of insulin is a small volume that can be instilled over 1 to 2 seconds. However, the needle should remain in place for 5 seconds after instillation to ensure complete delivery of the solution.
4. Insulin is administered via a subcutaneous injection. The needle should be $\frac{1}{2}$-inch, $\frac{5}{8}$-inch, or 1-inch in length. A $1\frac{1}{2}$-inch needle is used for an intramuscular injection.
TEST-TAKING TIP: Identify the clang association. The word *injections* in the stem and the word *injection* in option 1 is a clang association. More often than not, an option with a clang association is the correct answer. Examine option 1 carefully.
Content Area: Medication Administration
Integrated Processes: Nursing Process: Implementation
Client Need: Physiological Integrity; Pharmacological and Parenteral Therapies
Cognitive Level: Application

41. ANSWER: 4.
Rationales:
1. This is unsafe and outside the legal role of the nurse. The administration of intravenous fluids is a dependent function of the nurse and the nurse should administer only the fluid ordered by the primary health-care provider.
2. This is unsafe. The time it takes to obtain the correct bag of solution will deprive the patient of the ordered therapy. The primary health-care provider ordered intravenous fluids that the nurse should institute as soon as possible.

3. This is an excessive dose of KCl and could harm the patient. Excessive potassium can cause cardiac dysrhythmias.

4. A 250 mL bag of 0.9% sodium chloride is ¼ of the solution ordered (1000 mL ÷ 250 mL = 4). Therefore, the nurse should divide the ordered amount of KCl by 4 (20 mEq ÷ 4 = 5 mEq) to determine the amount of KCl to add to a 250 mL bag of solution.

Content Area: Medication Administration
Integrated Processes: Nursing Process: Implementation
Client Need: Physiological Integrity; Pharmacological and Parenteral Therapies
Cognitive Level: Application

42. ANSWER: 4.
Rationale:
Solve the problem by using ratio and proportion.

$$\frac{\text{Desire 60 mg}}{\text{Have 75 mg}} = \frac{x \text{ mL}}{5 \text{ mL}}$$

$$75x = 300$$

$$\frac{75x}{75} = \frac{300}{75}$$

$$x = 300 \div 75$$

$$x = 4 \text{ mL}$$

Content Area: Medication Administration
Integrated Processes: Nursing Process: Planning
Client Need: Physiological Integrity; Pharmacological and Parenteral Therapies
Cognitive Level: Application

43. ANSWER: 3.
Rationales:
1. Placing a plastic cover over the top of the ampule before snapping the constricted neck protects the nurse's hands from injury.
2. The filter needle must be changed to a needle suitable for the injection being given to the patient.
3. Flicking the top of the ampule moves solution in the top of the ampule to below the constricted neck of the ampule. This ensures that the entire dose is in the bottom of the ampule and ready for withdrawal.
4. The use of a filter needle to aspirate solution from an ampule prevents the aspiration of glass particles that may have resulted from snapping the constricted neck of the ampule.

Content Area: Medication Administration
Integrated Processes: Nursing Process: Implementation
Client Need: Physiological Integrity; Pharmacological and Parenteral Therapies
Cognitive Level: Application

44. ANSWER: 2.
Rationales:
1. PRN refers to a medication that is ordered to be administered when a particular situation occurs; for example, morphine sulphate 2 mg IV every 3 hours PRN for moderate incisional pain.
2. The single-dose section is used to document a medication given once. It may be a "STAT" (immediately) dose of a medication given in an emergency, a "one-time only" dose before a diagnostic test or before surgery, or a "now order" when a single dose is given quickly but not as quickly or emergent as a STAT order.
3. The progress note section generally is used to document why a medication was held, the patient's nontherapeutic response to a drug, the reason for a patient refusal, and whether a primary health-care provider was notified.
4. The standing drug section includes medications ordered to be given until they are discontinued or the required number of days has lapsed, such as with antibiotics given for 7 to 14 days.

Content Area: Medication Administration
Integrated Processes: Communication/Documentation; Nursing Process: Implementation
Client Need: Physiological Integrity; Pharmacological and Parenteral Therapies
Cognitive Level: Application

45. ANSWER: 5, 4, 1, 3, 2.
Rationales:
5. The administration of a medication is a dependent function of a nurse. The primary health-care provider's prescription must be verified by the nurse administering the medication.
4. The patient's blood glucose level must be compared to the insulin prescription to determine the exact dose to administer. Doses usually are on a sliding scale with the dose increasing as the patient's blood glucose increases.
1. A nurse must always perform hand hygiene before preparing medication to avoid contaminating the medication cart and other equipment.
3. After completing hand hygiene, the nurse should prepare the medication according to the prescription.
2. A nurse must always wear gloves when there is potential for exposure to a patient's blood or body fluids. An injection pierces the patient's skin, increasing the risk of exposure to the patient's blood or body fluids.
Content Area: Medication Administration
Integrated Processes: Nursing Process: Planning
Client Need: Physiological Integrity; Pharmacological and Parenteral Therapies
Cognitive Level: Analysis

Chapter 15

Pharmacology

KEY TERMS

Adverse effect—Unintended, usually unpredictable harmful response to a medication that is more severe than a side effect.

Allergic reaction—Response of a patient's immune system to the presence of a substance that produces a hypersensitivity reaction.

Biotransformation (metabolism)—Conversion (detoxification) of a medication to a less active form in preparation for excretion.

Idiosyncratic reaction—Resistance, overreaction, or unpredictable reaction to a medication that is different from the expected response.

Peak blood level—Highest blood concentration of a medication.

Pharmacodynamics—Study of the mechanisms of actions of a medication (e.g., biochemical and physiological) and the way in which it achieves its effects in the body.

Pharmacokinetics—Study of the absorption, distribution, biotransformation (metabolism), and excretion of medications.

Potentiation—Interaction of two medications that result in an increase in the action of just one of the medications.

Side effect—Common unintended response to a medication that generally is predictable and well tolerated.

Synergistic effect—Combined effect of two medications is greater than when the effects of each are added together.

Teratogenic effect—Effect of a medication that causes abnormal development of a fetus when taken by a pregnant woman.

Therapeutic range—Maintenance of a blood concentration level of a medication so that the peak blood level and trough blood level fall within the range indicated for medication effectiveness.

Tolerance—Decreased physiological response after repeated exposure to a medication.

Toxic effect—Dangerous, harmful response to a medication.

Trough blood level—Lowest blood concentration of a medication.

I. Introduction to Pharmacology

Medications can be beneficial but also can be harmful if not researched, produced, stored, prescribed, dispensed, and administered appropriately. Federal and state laws have been enacted to protect the public from harm. Nurses can also protect patients from harm by utilizing a variety of resources to become knowledgeable about medications, adhering to nursing standards, and advocating for patients.

A. Laws Related to Pharmacology (Table 15.1)

B. Informational Resources Related to Pharmacology

1. U.S. Pharmacopoeia: Lists medications and standards for their preparation.
2. National Formulary: List of officially recognized medications, including those not listed in the U. S. Pharmacopoeia.
3. U.S. Food and Drug Administration (FDA; www.fda.gov): Disseminates current information about food, medications, medical devices, recalls, medication safety alerts, generic approvals, and other medical information.
4. American Nurses Association (www.nursingworld.org): Publishes standards associated with general and specialty areas of nursing practice.
5. Agency policy and procedure manuals: Provide policies and procedure manuals for nursing practice, pharmacy, and medication therapy.
6. Textbooks: Provide authoritative information about medications. Examples include *Physician's Desk Reference* (PDR), *American Hospital Formulary Service*, and *Davis's Drug Guide for Nurses*.

Table 15.1 Pharmacology-Associated Laws and Related Nursing Responsibilities

Laws	Nursing Responsibilities
Food, Drug, and Cosmetic Act of 1938 • Required medications to be safe and approved by the U.S. Food and Drug Administration (FDA) before marketing. • Established criteria regarding manufacture, distribution, advertising, and labeling of medications.	• Know that this law requires that all medications meet FDA requirements regarding the manufacture, distribution, advertising, and labeling of all medications on the market.
Durham-Humphrey Amendment (1952) • Distinguished the difference between prescription medications (require medical supervision) and nonprescription (over-the-counter [OTC]) medications.	• Know the difference between an OTC medication and a medication that requires a prescription. • Teach the importance of reading packages of OTC medications to avoid an overdose when ingesting different products; for example, some analgesics contain the same active ingredients as cough preparations.
Comprehensive Drug Abuse Prevention and Control Act (1970) • Established controls on the manufacture and distribution of controlled medications and limits on prescription refills. • Identified five categories of controlled substances based on addiction potential. • Established government-funded programs for prevention and treatment of medication dependence.	• Know, understand, and assume accountability for nursing responsibilities associated with criteria established by this law; for example: • Controlled medications must be stored in a double-locked space. • Special inventory forms must be maintained regarding dispensing of controlled substances. • Wasting of controlled medications must be witnessed. • Controlled medications must be counted at the end of every shift.
Food and Drug Administration and Modernization Act (1997) • Allowed more efficient approval of new medications and medical devices, compounding of medications by a pharmacist, and marketing of "off-label" uses of medications to primary health-care providers.	• Access the FDA's official website to learn about new medications and medical devices as well as "off-label" uses of medications. • Verify a new medication with the FDA's official website (www.accessdata.fda.gov/scripts/cder/ob/default.cfm/) before administering it the first time. • Question a primary health-care provider when a medication is prescribed for "off-label" use to ensure that the prescription is appropriate.
Nurse Practice Act • Each state has a nurse practice act that defines the legal scope of nursing practice within the state.	• Know and understand the components of the nurse practice act in the state in which you work. • Always practice nursing within the scope of practice identified by your state nurse practice act. • Seek assistance from a nursing supervisor or nurse educator with questions regarding legal aspects of nursing practice and administration of medications. • Seek legal advice or interpretation of a law from an attorney when necessary. (Institutions generally have legal counsel on retainer for this purpose.)

7. Pharmacists: Have a doctoral degree in pharmacy (Pharm.D.) and are excellent resources for obtaining information about medications and medication therapy.
8. Nursing supervisors and nurse educators: Are excellent resources when faced with questions regarding nursing responsibilities about standards of nursing practice and medications.

II. Pharmacodynamics

Pharmacodynamics is the study of how medications achieve their effects in the body. It takes into consideration how medication molecules interact with cells and tissues of the body as well as their biological responses, which influence the selection of specific medications for a therapeutic regimen. Medications have a variety of names, are classified by their characteristics, and have a primary reason for being administered (therapeutic effect). Because of the numerous medications available for use and their complexity of action, primary and secondary effects, and potential for interactions, nurses must know not only the commonly prescribed medications but also how to access information based on a medication's name or classification.

A. Medication Names
   1. **Chemical.**
      a. Describes a medication's chemical and molecular structure.

Medications and Their Effects on the Body

Medication molecules bind with cellular receptors within the body, thereby exerting their action (pharmacodynamics). Once a medication molecule binds with a site receptor, a pharmacological response occurs. A medication receptor complex can activate a further cellular reaction that promotes or hinders normal cellular function by such actions as altering intracellular enzymes, increasing or decreasing cellular metabolism, altering permeability of cell membranes, and liberating or deactivating neurohormones that influence physiological processes. The specific characteristics of a medication's constituents and receptor site characteristics influence the degree of medication action in the body. Nurses should understand how medications work in the body to better understand their resulting therapeutic and nontherapeutic effects.

  b. Example: *2-(4-isobutylpheny)propionic acid*: ibuprofen (Motrin, Advil).
2. **Generic** (nonproprietary, official).
   a. Simple name that is easier to pronounce.
   b. Begins with a lowercase letter.
   c. Example: 2-(4-isobutylpheny)propionic acid: *ibuprofen* (Motrin, Advil).
3. **Trade** (brand, proprietary).
   a. Usually short and easy to recall.
   b. Begins with a capital letter.
   c. Registered by the U.S. Patent Office and approved by the FDA.
   d. Example: 2-(4-isobutylpheny)propionic acid: ibuprofen (*Motrin, Advil*).
B. **Medication Classifications**
   1. Medications are grouped together based on common characteristics.
   2. Ways to classify medications.
      a. Effect on the body, such as central nervous system depressants.
      b. Therapeutic use, such as anticoagulants.
      c. Chemical characteristics, such as beta-adrenergic blocking agents.
   3. Medications may fit into more than one classification because they have a broad range of effects.
C. **Primary Effects of Medications (Therapeutic Effects) and Related Nursing Care**
   1. **Symptomatic** (palliative).
      a. Used to relieve signs or symptoms of disease, not the disease itself.
      b. Example: Acetaminophen relieves fever.
   2. **Preventive**.
      a. Used to avoid disease.
      b. Example: Measles vaccine prevents measles.

3. **Diagnostic**.
   a. Used to help diagnose the presence of disease.
   b. Example: Radiopaque dye outlines internal body structures.
4. **Curative** (chemotherapeutic).
   a. Used to eradicate a disease or destroy disease-producing pathogens or body cells.
   b. Examples: Antibiotics such as azithromycin (Zithromax) destroy bacteria and antineoplastics such as cisplatin destroy cancer cells.
5. **Health maintenance** (substitutive).
   a. Used to support normal body function.
   b. Examples: Regular insulin (Novolin R) lowers serum glucose level in patients with diabetes; levothyroxine (Synthroid) replaces thyroid hormones in patients with hypothyroidism.
6. **Contraceptive**.
   a. Used to prevent pregnancy.
   b. Example: Combined oral contraceptives (estrogen and progestin) and progestin-only pills are prescribed to prevent pregnancy.
7. **Antidote**.
   a. Used to reverse the toxic effect of another medication.
   b. Examples: Vitamin K limits bleeding due to warfarin (Coumadin) and naloxone (Narcan) limits central nervous system depression due to opioids.
D. **Secondary Effects of Medications (Unintended Effects) and Related Nursing Care**
   1. **Side effect**.
      a. Common unintended response to a medication that generally is predictable and well tolerated.
      b. Examples: Dry mouth, anorexia.
      c. Nursing care.
         (1) Implement palliative independent and dependent measures to address side effects that are not serious.
         (2) Examples: Offering frequent mouth care for a patient experiencing dry mouth; providing food preferences for a patient with anorexia.
   2. **Adverse effect**.
      a. Unintended, usually unpredictable harmful response to a medication that is more severe than a side effect.
      b. Example: Bone marrow depression.
      c. Nursing care.
         (1) Notify the primary health-care provider of the patient's status.
         (2) Discontinue the medication per the primary health-care provider's orders (cessation of the medication generally is indicated).
   3. **Toxic effect**.
      a. Dangerous, harmful response to a medication.
      b. May result from a medication overdose, accumulation of a medication's ingredients due

to impaired biotransformation or excretion (cumulative effect), or the body's abnormal sensitivity to a medication.

c. Examples: Liver damage (hepatotoxicity), kidney damage (nephrotoxicity).

d. Nursing care.

(1) Assess the type and amount of OTC medications the patient is using.

(2) Teach patients how to examine medication labels to identify ingredients in OTC medications that can cause a cumulative effect when taken with another medication with the same ingredient. (e.g., acetaminophen [Tylenol] for pain and an OTC cold remedy that contains acetaminophen taken together may exceed the recommended dose limit for acetaminophen).

(!) (3) Hold the medication and notify the primary health-care provider if the patient exhibits a toxic reaction to a medication.

4. **Allergic reaction.**

a. Response of a patient's immune system to the presence of a substance that produces a hypersensitivity reaction (e.g., medication).

b. Certain classifications of medications frequently cause allergic reactions. (Box 15.1)

c. Example: Rash, breathing difficulty, circulatory collapse (anaphylaxis).

d. Nursing care.

(1) Collect information from the patient and primary health-care provider about a history of medication and food allergies before administering prescribed medications.

(2) Document the presence of allergies according to agency policy and procedure (e.g., on a patient's wrist band, in the nursing history and physical, on the medication administration record, and on the medication reconciliation form).

(3) Secure an allergy alert band to the patient's wrist to alert health-care team members of the patient's history of allergies.

(4) Check the patient's clinical record, medication administration record, and wrist band

---

Box 15.1 Medications That Commonly Cause Allergic Reactions

- Analgesics: Codeine, morphine.
- Antiseizure medications: Phenytoin.
- Antibiotics: Penicillin.
- Iodinated contrast dye.
- Biologic agents: Vaccines.
- Other medications: Quinidine, iodines, phenothiazines.

---

to ensure that the patient has no allergies before administering medications.

(5) Ensure that medication products that a patient is susceptible to are not contained in a prescribed or OTC medications that the patient will be taking.

(6) Assess for clinical manifestations of an allergic response to medications, especially when administering a medication for the first time.

(!) (7) Implement emergency measures if a patient experiences an anaphylactic response to a medication (e.g., initiate the rapid response team and prepare medications that may be prescribed to support the patient such as epinephrine).

(8) Teach a patient who has a medication allergy how to examine medication labels to ensure that OTC medications do not contain offending allergens.

5. **Idiosyncratic reaction.**

a. Resistance, overreaction, or unpredictable reaction that is different from the expected response to a medication.

b. Example: An older adult becomes agitated or restless after receiving a sedative.

c. Nursing care.

(1) Notify the primary health-care provider of the patient's status.

(2) Discontinue the medication per the primary health-care provider's orders; cessation of the medication generally is indicated.

6. **Tolerance.**

a. Decreased physiological response after repeated exposure to a medication.

b. Example: A patient receiving an opioid no longer experiences relief from pain.

c. Nursing care.

(1) Notify the primary health-care provider if tolerance occurs.

(2) Implement the primary health-care provider's orders, which may include discontinuation of the medication, an increase in the medication dose, or replacement of the medication with a different medication.

7. **Teratogenic effect.**

a. Effect that causes abnormal development of a fetus when taken by a pregnant woman, especially during the first trimester of pregnancy, when the organs of the fetus are developing (**organogenesis**).

b. Medications are classified from category A (no risk to fetus) and progressively escalate in level of risk to category D (evidence of fetal risk but potential benefit to the mother may be acceptable).

c. A separate category identified as X classifies medications that cause fetal abnormalities; for example, isotretinoin (Claravis) for severe acne and acitretin (Soriatane) for severe psoriasis.

d. Examples: Classifications include diuretics, antiepileptics, analgesics, antihistamines, antibiotics, and antiemetics.

e. Nursing care.

(1) Ensure that the patient is not pregnant when a medication that is teratogenic is prescribed.

(2) Teach the patient to abstain from sexual intercourse or use more than one contraceptive method during the course of therapy.

E. Medication Interactions

1. **Synergistic effect.**

a. The combined effect of two medications is greater than when the effects of each are added together.

b. Example: Administration of either a diuretic or an antihypertensive to treat hypertension may decrease the patient's blood pressure by 10 percent; however, when administered together, the drugs may have a synergistic effect that exceeds the combined effect of 20 percent and may decrease the patient's blood pressure by 30 percent.

c. Nursing care.

(1) Assess resources to identify whether medications being administered concurrently have the potential for precipitating a synergistic effect.

(2) Assess for clinical manifestations of an excessive response. If one occurs, hold the next dose and notify the primary healthcare provider of the patient's status.

2. **Potentiation.**

a. The interaction of two medications that results in an increase in the action of just one of the medications.

b. Example: Probenecid blocks the excretion of penicillin, increasing the blood level of penicillin and, therefore, its effectiveness.

c. Nursing care.

(1) Assess resources to identify whether medications being administered concurrently have the ability to precipitate a potentiation effect.

(2) Assess for clinical manifestations of the expected therapeutic effects, particularly those related to the medication that is being maximized by the interaction of the two medications.

3. **Physical or chemical incompatibilities.**

a. **Antagonistic relationship.**

(1) One medication decreases the therapeutic effect of another medication.

(2) Example: Loop diuretics can decrease the effects of nonsteroidal anti-inflammatory medications.

b. **Chemical incompatibility.**

(1) Two medications when combined can cause chemical deterioration of one or both medications (usually due to acid-base incompatibility), resulting in precipitate formation, color change, or gas development.

(2) Example: Famotidine (Pepcid) and azithromycin (Zithromax) cannot be combined in one solution.

c. Nursing care.

(1) Assess resources to identify whether medications being administered concurrently are compatible or incompatible.

(2) Administer incompatible intravenous medications separately to maintain the integrity of each medication.

(3) Check mixed solutions before administration for changes in appearance that indicate a medication interaction (e.g., precipitate, color change, or gas development).

III. Pharmacokinetics

Pharmacokinetics is the study of the absorption, distribution, biotransformation (metabolism), and excretion of medications. Each of these factors is related to the concentration of the medication in the body and can be viewed in relation to a time frame associated with the medication's pharmacological effects. (Fig. 15.1) Nurses should understand these concepts as well as the factors that affect pharmacokinetics and related nursing care.

A. Elements of Pharmacokinetics

1. **Absorption.**

a. Process of movement of a medication into the bloodstream.

b. Rate of absorption depends on a number of factors.

(1) Route of administration: Oral route requires time for medication absorption versus the intravenous route, which is distributed immediately.

(2) Presence or absence of food in the stomach: Food in the stomach can delay absorption of medications and lengthen the time it takes for a medication to reach the small intestines, where most medications are absorbed.

2. **Distribution.**

a. Transport of a medication from the site of absorption to the site of medication action.

b. Affected by such factors as degree of membrane permeability; protein binding capacity of the medication; and interruption in arterial blood

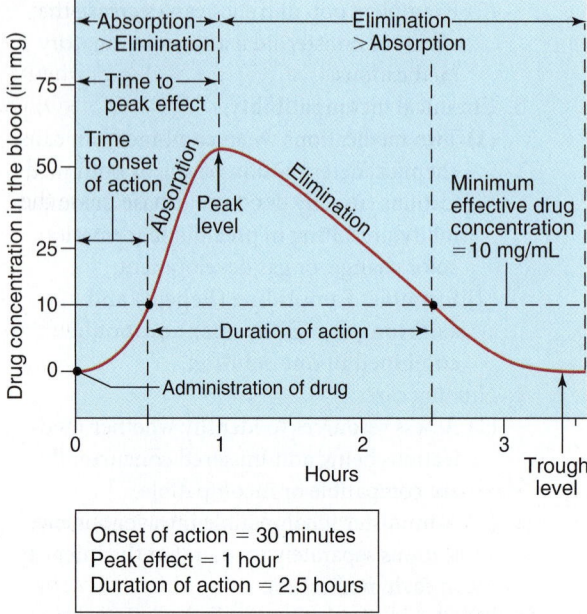

Onset of action = 30 minutes
Peak effect = 1 hour
Duration of action = 2.5 hours

Fig 15.1 Medication concentrations in the blood. (From Vallerand, Sanoski, & Deglin [2013]. *Davis's drug guide for nurses,* 13th ed. Philadelphia: F. A. Davis Company, with permission.)

supply to a tissue, organ, or extremity that limits delivery of a medication to the target site.
  (1) Tightly packed endothelial cells prevent some medications from being distributed to the brain (blood-brain barrier).
  (2) Only medications that are lipid soluble and are more loosely bound to plasma proteins can pass through the blood-brain barrier.

  3. **Biotransformation** (metabolism).
    a. Conversion of a medication to a less active form (**detoxification**) in preparation for excretion.
    b. Occurs mainly in the liver but also can occur in the kidneys, intestinal mucosa, lungs, or blood plasma.
    c. Can be affected by disease states.

  4. **Excretion.**
    a. Elimination of medications by the body.
    b. Occurs primarily via the kidneys, where medications are eliminated from the body via urine but also can occur via feces, perspiration, saliva, breath, and breast milk.
    c. Ability to excrete medications decreases with age, placing older adults at risk for medication accumulation and toxicity.
    d. Kidney disease can interfere with excretion, thereby causing medication accumulation and toxicity.

B. **Concepts Related to Medication Effectiveness**
  1. **Duration.**
    a. Length of time a therapeutic blood concentration of a medication is maintained.

    b. Nursing care.
      (1) Assess the patient's response, considering the medications expected duration of action.
      (2) Notify the primary health-care provider if an unexpected response occurs.
      (3) Example: A patient receiving a sedative is lethargic long after the effect of the medication should have dissipated, requiring a decrease in the dosage of the medication or discontinuation of the medication.

  2. **Half-life.**
    a. Time needed to metabolize or inactivate one-half the amount of a medication.
    b. Nursing care.
      (1) Assess the patient's response, considering the medication's half-life.
      (2) Notify the primary health-care provider if an unexpected response occurs.
      (3) Example: A patient has pain before the next scheduled dose of an analgesic, indicating that the dose should be increased or the time between doses shortened.

  3. **Onset.**
    a. Length of time it takes the body to respond to a medication.
    b. Nursing care.
      (1) Assess the patient's response to a medication at the time of the medication's expected onset.
      (2) Example: Most oral analgesics have an onset of 20 to 30 minutes.

  4. **Peak blood level.**
    a. Highest blood concentration of a medication (see Fig. 15.1).
    b. Nursing care.
      (1) Arrange for the patient's blood to be drawn for a peak plasma level 30 to 60 minutes after medication administration.
      (2) Hold the medication and inform the primary health-care provider if the patient's peak plasma level is higher than the established parameter for a peak plasma level. A decrease in the frequency or dose usually is required.

  5. **Trough blood level.**
    a. Lowest blood concentration of a medication (see Fig. 15.1).
    b. Nursing care.
      (1) Arrange for the patient's blood to be drawn for a trough level just before the next scheduled dose.
      (2) Inform the primary health-care provider if the patient's trough plasma level is lower than the established parameter for a trough level and seek an order for an increase in the prescribed dose and/or frequency.

6. **Therapeutic range**.
   a. Maintenance of a blood concentration level of a medication so that the peak blood level and trough blood level fall within the range indicated for medication effectiveness.
   b. Nursing care.
      (1) Monitor serum peak and trough levels to ensure that levels fall within the established therapeutic window for the medication.
      (2) Example: The peak level for gentamicin should not exceed 10 mcg/mL and trough levels should not be below 2 mcg/mL).

C. **Factors Affecting Pharmacokinetics and Related Nursing Care**
1. **Age**.
   a. Infants have immature body systems and are small in size.
   b. Older adults experience decreased multi-organ functioning, which increases medication absorption and decreases biotransformation and excretion.
   c. Nursing care.
      (1) Ensure that medication doses are appropriate for body weight of infants and children.
      (2) Assess infants, children, and older adults for clinical manifestations of medication toxicity. Patients may require a lower dose of the medication.
2. **Body mass**.
   a. A person with a larger body mass may require a larger dose.
   b. A person with a smaller body mass may require a lower dose.
   c. Nursing care.
      (1) Evaluate the response of obese patients to medications to ensure that a therapeutic response is achieved with the prescribed dose.
      (2) Evaluate the response of a patient with a small body mass to ensure that the dose prescribed is not excessive.
3. **Diet**.
   a. The presence of food can delay the absorption of some medications.
   b. Some medications can cause gastric irritation when not taken with food.
   c. Some foods can alter the action of medications.
      (1) Foods high in vitamin K should be consistently limited in patients receiving the anticoagulant warfarin (Coumadin) because vitamin K is the antidote for warfarin toxicity; in addition, inconsistent intake of vitamin K causes fluctuating prothrombin times and International Normalized Ratio levels.

      (2) Tyramine-rich foods, such as aged cheese, pickled herring, yogurt, raisins, chicken liver, dried sausage, and sauerkraut, when taken with a monoamine oxidase (MAO) inhibitor can precipitate a hypertensive crisis, intracranial bleeding, and death.
      (3) Calcium in milk products can decrease the absorption of some antibiotics, such as tetracycline.
   d. Nursing care.
      (1) Teach patients when a medication should be given with or without food.

🛑 (2) Teach patients about foods to ingest or avoid to prevent nontherapeutic effects of medications.

4. **Environment**.
   a. Hot environments cause peripheral vasodilation, intensifying the action of vasodilators.
   b. Cold environments cause peripheral vasoconstriction, inhibiting the action of vasodilators while increasing the action of vasoconstrictors.
   c. Noisy environments can interfere with the therapeutic effects of sedatives and analgesics.
   d. Nursing care.
      (1) Ensure a temperate (moderate, not excessive) environmental temperature when a patient is receiving a vasodilator or vasoconstrictor.
      (2) Ensure a quiet environment when a patient is receiving a sedative or analgesic.
5. **Gender**.
   a. Medication response discrepancies in men and women are attributable to body fat distribution, percentage of body fluid differences, and hormonal differences that affect medication absorption.
   b. The majority of medication research is based on studies involving men; responses of women may be different than what is documented in medication literature.
   c. Nursing care.
      (1) Understand that manufacturer-provided information about a medication may be based primarily on research using male subjects; data may not be consistent for women.
      (2) Assess for therapeutic and nontherapeutic responses in women.
6. **Genetic, ethnic, and cultural factors**.
   a. Genes can cause liver metabolism to be slow or rapid, influencing medication metabolism.
   b. Research demonstrates that a dose of medication may be therapeutic for individuals in a specific ethnic group and toxic for those in another group (e.g., opioids are metabolized at a slower rate by individuals of Asian descent).

c. Nursing care.
(1) Identify patients who are at risk for nontherapeutic effects of medication therapy because of genetic, ethnic, and cultural factors.
(2) Assess patients of Asian descent who are prescribed opioids for clinical manifestations of medication toxicity.

7. **Illness and disease**.
a. Impaired gastrointestinal, liver, kidney, or cardiovascular function can alter a patient's response to a medication because of altered absorption, transport, biotransformation, or excretion.
b. Nursing care.
(1) Assess patients with impaired gastrointestinal, liver, kidney, or cardiovascular function for nontherapeutic effects as a result of altered medication biotransformation, transport, or excretion.
(2) Example: Assess older adults taking digoxin for toxicity because older adults experience reduced kidney function secondary to aging.

8. **Psychological factors**.
a. If a patient believes that a medication will work, the patient often has a more favorable therapeutic response.
b. If a patient mistrusts the value of a medication, this belief can interfere with the medication's effectiveness.
c. Anxiety can interfere with the therapeutic effect of central nervous system depressants.
d. Nursing care.
(1) Explore the patient's beliefs about the value of a medication regimen.
(2) Clarify the patient's misunderstandings about a medication to increase trust in the value of the regimen.
(3) Employ nursing measures to reduce anxiety when a patient is receiving central nervous system depressants.

9. **Route of administration**.
a. The route influences the volume of medication absorbed into the circulation and its transport to the target site (e.g., oral medications require time to be absorbed and transported, whereas those administered via the intravenous route produce an immediate response).
b. Nursing care.
(1) Ensure that the route is appropriate for the patient's situation. For example, if the patient has gastric surgery, the oral route may not be appropriate; if the patient is confused, the patient may not understand that a troche should be held in the buccal cavity until dissolved.
(2) Assess the patient's response to medication based on the expected onset associated with the route used.

D. **Nursing Care Related to the Potential for Nontherapeutic Reponses to Medications**
1. Check medication compatibility charts before administering medications being given concurrently to ensure that they are compatible.
2. Assess for therapeutic and nontherapeutic clinical manifestations of medication therapy.

🛑 3. Hold a medication when a patient demonstrates a sign or symptom that is more serious than a side effect or if a medication-medication interaction occurs and report the finding to the primary health-care provider.

4. Teach the patient about the medication regimen.
a. The action of and rationale for the prescribed medication.
b. Pertinent information regarding safe administration.
c. Actions to take if a dose is accidentally omitted.
d. Assessments to make to evaluate responses to the medication.
e. Actions to take in the event of a nontherapeutic response.
5. Document consultation with the primary health-care provider regarding a patient's nontherapeutic response to medication therapy and resulting interventions.
6. Document all information associated with medication administration and patient responses to therapy.
7. Implement emergency actions to support a patient who has a serious nontherapeutic response until a primary health-care provider assumes responsibility for prescribing medical interventions; for example, administer oxygen, elevate the head of the bed, and prepare for intubation and mechanical ventilation if a patient is having difficulty breathing.
8. Implement measures based on standing orders; for example, administer an antidote for an overdose or epinephrine for an anaphylactic reaction.

IV. Medication Misuse and Abuse

Many medications, particularly central nervous system stimulants and depressants, have a narrow therapeutic window. When medications are misused or abused, the therapeutic window may be exceeded, resulting in numerous negative physiological and psychological consequences, including death. Nurses must teach patients how to use medications responsibly, assess patients for the clinical manifestations of medication misuse or abuse, and intervene to help patients who are struggling with the negative consequences of medication misuse or abuse.

A. **Terminology Related to Medication Misuse and Abuse**
1. **Abuse:** Continual or periodic maladaptive use of a medication different from the recommended

prescribed pattern, causing physical and/or emotional harm with a risk of disturbance of daily life.

2. **Addiction:** Psychological or physiological dependence on a medication, such as morphine, cocaine, alcohol, or nicotine.
3. **Craving:** Subjective desire for a medication.
4. **Habituation:** Repeated abuse that causes a person to feel better than when not using the medication; the person generally can discontinue use without severe psychological or physical effects.
5. **Illicit medications (street medications):** Medications that are sold illegally.
6. **Physiological dependence:** Need for a medication to avoid physical manifestations of withdrawal.
7. **Psychological dependence:** Emotional need for a medication to maintain a feeling of well-being, satisfaction, or pleasure.
8. **Tolerance:** Condition in which the body becomes accustomed to a medication and needs a larger dose to attain the desired effect or to prevent clinical manifestations of withdrawal.
9. **Withdrawal syndrome:** Presence of specific physical and/or psychological signs and symptoms associated with cessation of a particular medication on which the patient is dependent.

B. Nursing Care Related to Medication Misuse and Abuse
1. Assess for clinical manifestations of physiological dependence on a medication (e.g., signs and symptoms of withdrawal when the medication is not taken).
   a. Stimulants: Pressured speech, hyperactivity or hypoactivity, signs of central nervous system stimulation or depression, and requests for analgesics before the next scheduled dose.
   b. Opioids: Watery eyes, runny nose, dilated pupils, tremors, chills, fever, yawning, diaphoresis, nausea, vomiting, diarrhea, and abdominal cramps.
2. Assess for clinical manifestations of psychological dependence on a medication (e.g., signs and symptoms of anxiety when the medication is not taken, compulsive behaviors associated with procuring and using a medication).
3. Assess for clinical manifestations of tolerance to a medication (e.g., request for a medication before the next scheduled dose, nonachievement of a therapeutic effect after receiving what is considered to be an adequate dose).
4. Assess for clinical manifestations of habituation to a medication (e.g., taking a laxative every day, using an antihistamine to promote sleep).
5. Use interviewing skills to determine insight into personal problems resulting from medication misuse or abuse and explore patient concerns.
6. Teach nonpharmacological strategies to manage stress and anxiety.

7. Teach pregnant women to avoid unnecessary medications, alcohol, and nicotine because of the risk of fetal harm.

8. Reinforce efforts by the patient toward stopping medication misuse or abuse.
9. Provide information about referrals to professionals or agencies that can assist the patient with withdrawal.

V. Herbal Supplements

Herbal supplements are plants used for medicinal purposes. Many people take them to promote health and wellness, increase energy and performance, prevent and treat illnesses, or relieve depression. The use of herbal supplements has increased concurrent with the expanding interest in alternative therapies, as people seek more "natural" therapies. Unfortunately, many people are misinformed of the facts about herbal supplements. Nurses must educate patients so that patients can make informed decisions about the use of herbal supplements.

A. Factual Information About Herbal Supplements
1. Some herbal supplements may prevent, treat, and cure some illnesses through the use of plant substances.
2. Some manufacturers of herbal supplements claim benefits that are unproven.

DID YOU KNOW?
Many people believe that supplements are safe because they are advertised as being "natural." However, this is not necessarily the case. Also, herbal supplements are not regulated by the FDA for safety and efficacy, even though they are chemicals that have an influence on the body.

3. Some herbal supplements, when taken with prescribed or OTC medications, can cause serious medication-medication interactions or nontherapeutic responses.
4. Some patients do not share information regarding self-medication with herbal supplements because either they do not realize the importance of this information or they are embarrassed that they are self-medicating.
5. Information and research about herbal supplements can be obtained from a variety of sources.
   a. FDA official web site (www.fda.gov).
   b. Herb Research Foundation (www.herbs.org).
   c. American Botanical Council (www.abc. herbalgram.org).
   d. WebMD (www.webmd.com).

B. Nursing Care Related to Herbal Supplements
1. Know and understand information related to the most common herbal supplements.
2. Collect data about herbal supplement intake (including the name of each supplement and the

amount, frequency, and reasons for its use), and share this information with patients' primary health-care providers. Also include this information on medication reconciliation forms.

3. Explore each patient's understanding about herbal supplements being taken.

4. Assess for signs and symptoms of adverse reactions to herbal supplements.

5. Teach patients that herbal supplements can increase or decrease the effects of other medications and therefore must be avoided when taking certain prescribed or OTC medications.

6. Teach patients to avoid the ingestion of alcohol with many herbal supplements because of the risk of nontherapeutic interactions.

7. Teach patients about the risk of having an allergic reaction to herbal supplements and instruct them to discontinue intake if signs and symptoms occur.

8. Encourage patients to discuss benefits and risks of taking herbal supplements with their primary health-care providers.

🛑 9. Teach patients to stop the use of herbal supplements that have antiplatelet properties, such as garlic and gingko biloba, when scheduled for dental intervention or surgery.

🛑 10. Encourage women who are pregnant or trying to become pregnant to avoid all herbal supplements because little is known regarding teratogenic effects.

🛑 11. Encourage women who are breast-feeding to avoid taking herbal supplements because of unknown effects on infants.

12. Refer patients to reliable sources of information about herbal supplements.

13. See also Table 15.2 for nursing care related to specific herbal supplements.

Table 15.2 Common Herbal Supplements and Related Nursing Care

Specific Herbs	Effect	Nursing Care
Echinacea	• Believed to increase white blood cells, spleen cells, and the activity of granulocytes, helper T cells, and cytokines. • Used for immune-enhancing properties to prevent and treat upper respiratory infections and the flu. • May decrease the effectiveness of immunosuppressants.	1. Encourage the patient to avoid taking echinacea when receiving an immunosuppressant. 2. Teach the patient to seek a primary health-care provider's attention when no improvement is noted after a few days of treating an upper respiratory infection or flu with echinacea.
Garlic (allium sativum)	• Contains the amino acid *allicin,* which has antibacterial qualities. • Possesses antimicrobial, antitumor, antilipidemic, and antithrombolytic properties. • Used to prevent hypertension, hyperlipidemia, and cardiovascular disease. • Increases antiplatelet action in patients receiving an anticoagulant. • Decreases the effectiveness of antihypertensives. • Allergic reactions are common, such as contact dermatitis, asthma, rash, and diaphoresis. • Chronic use decreases hemoglobin level and causes lysis of red blood cells.	1. Monitor blood pressure if a patient is concurrently taking an antihypertensive to ensure its effectiveness. 2. Assess a patient who is concurrently taking an anticoagulant for bruising or bleeding. 3. Instruct the patient to inform the primary health-care provider of the chronic use of garlic so that hemoglobin and red blood cell levels are monitored.
Gingko Biloba	• Believed to increase cerebral and peripheral blood flow. • Used for memory impairment, dementia, tinnitus, leg cramping, pain caused by walking (intermittent claudication), vertigo, and impotence. • Can increase antiplatelet action of anticoagulants. • Can cause cerebral bleeding.	1. Teach the patient to avoid taking gingko biloba when also taking an anticoagulant. 2. Assess a patient who insists on concurrently taking an anticoagulant for bruising and bleeding.
Ginseng	• Research demonstrates anti-inflammatory, antioxidant, analgesic, diuretic, and anticancer effects. • Used for improving a feeling of well-being, stamina, appetite, sleep pattern, memory, concentration, and energy. • Has nontherapeutic herb-medication interactions with MAO inhibitors, caffeine, and glaucoma medications. • American ginseng increases hepatic lipogenesis and storage of glycogen. • *Panax ginseng* has serious adverse effects.	1. Assess for signs and symptoms of ginseng toxicity: diarrhea, restlessness, nausea, vomiting, and headache. 2. If the patient insists on taking ginseng, encourage taking American ginseng with meals to prevent inadvertent hypoglycemia in people who are not diabetic. 3. Assess a patient who is diabetic more frequently for hypoglycemia until the response is determined.

Table 15.2 **Common Herbal Supplements and Related Nursing Care—cont'd**

Specific Herbs	Effect	Nursing Care
	• Should not be taken by patients with cardiovascular disease, hypertension, or hypotension and those who are receiving steroid therapy because of herb-medication interactions with medications prescribed for these conditions.	4. Encourage a patient taking an MAO inhibitor, glaucoma medication, or any form of caffeine to avoid ginseng because of nontherapeutic herb-medication interactions. 5. Encourage the patient to avoid *panax ginseng* because of adverse effects. 6. Instruct patients with hypertension or hypotension, those receiving steroids, and those with cardiovascular disease to discontinue ginseng due to interactions with medications prescribed for these conditions.
Saw Palmetto	• Has antiandrogenic, anti-inflammatory, and antiproliferative properties in prostate tissue. • Used to reduce the frequency of urination, urgency, hesitancy, and nocturia associated with benign prostatic hyperplasia. • Contraindicated during pregnancy and breastfeeding. • May decrease prostate-specific antigen (PSA) levels, delaying prostate cancer diagnosis.	1. Assess urinary function, such as force of urinary stream, dribbling, straining, urgency, hesitancy, feeling of incomplete bladder emptying, and dysuria. 2. Encourage the patient to consult with a urologist to monitor the size and status of the prostate gland. 3. Instruct a woman who anticipates pregnancy or breastfeeding to discontinue saw palmetto.
St. John's Wort	• Believed to selectively inhibit serotonin, dopamine, and norepinephrine reuptake in the central nervous system. • Used for mild to moderate depression and sleep disorders. • Is safe if used alone. • Reduces therapeutic levels of oral contraceptives, anticoagulants, and antivirals. • Can cause photosensitivity.	1. Teach the patient to avoid taking St. John's Wort when receiving an anticoagulant, antiviral, or oral contraceptive because it increases elimination of these medications. 2. Encourage the patient to reduce sun exposure and teach the patient to use sunscreen to protect from photosensitivity reactions.

CASE STUDY: Putting It All Together

A nurse is caring for a patient with a diagnosis of ovarian cancer who is to receive intravenous CISplatin, a chemotherapeutic medication. The nurse is not familiar with this medication and wants to know important information about the medication, such as how it works in the body, the therapeutic and adverse effects for which the patient should be monitored, and any special nursing implications for which the nurse should be aware.

Case Study Questions

A. List three reputable resources that the nurse can access that will provide accurate information about CISplatin.

1. _____

2. _____

3. _____

Continued

Davis's Drug Guide for Nurses, 13th edition, CISplatin

HIGH ALERT

CISplatin (sis-pla-tin)
Platinol

Classification
Therapeutic: antineoplastics
Pharmacologic: alkylating agents

Pregnancy Category D

Indications
Metastatic testicular and ovarian carcinoma. Advanced bladder cancer. Head and neck cancer. Cervical cancer. Lung cancer. Other tumors.

Action
Inhibits DNA synthesis by producing cross-linking of parent DNA strands (cell-cycle phase–nonspecific). **Therapeutic Effects:** Death of rapidly replicating cells, particularly malignant ones.

Pharmacokinetics
Absorption: IV administration results in complete bioavailability.
Distribution: Widely distributed; accumulates for months; enters breast milk.
Metabolism and Excretion: Excreted mainly by the kidneys.
Half-life: 30–100 hr.

TIME/ACTION PROFILE (effects on blood counts)

ROUTE	ONSET	PEAK	DURATION
IV	unknown	18–23 days	39 days

Contraindications/Precautions
Contraindicated in: Hypersensitivity; OB, Lactation: Pregnancy or lactation.
Use Cautiously in: Hearing loss; Renal impairment (dosage ↓ recommended); HF; Electrolyte abnormalities; Active infections; Bone marrow depression; Geri: ↑ risk of nephrotoxicity and peripheral neuropathy; Chronic debilitating illnesses; Patients with childbearing potential.

Adverse Reactions/Side Effects
CNS: REVERSIBLE POSTERIOR LEUKOENCEPHALOPATHY SYNDROME, SEIZURES, malaise, weakness. **EENT:** ototoxicity, tinnitus. **GI:** severe nausea, vomiting, diarrhea, hepatotoxicity. **GU:** nephrotoxicity, sterility. **Derm:** alopecia. **F and E:** hypocalcemia, hypokalemia, hypomagnesemia. **Hemat:** LEUKOPENIA, THROMBOCYTOPENIA, anemia. **Local:** phlebitis at IV site. **Metab:** hyperuricemia. **Neuro:** peripheral neuropathy. **Misc:** anaphylactoid reactions.

Interactions
Drug-Drug: ↑ risk of nephrotoxicity and ototoxicity with other **nephrotoxic** and **ototoxic drugs (aminoglycosides, loop diuretics)**. ↑ risk of hypokalemia and hypomagnesemia with **loop diuretics** and **amphotericin B**. May ↓ **phenytoin** levels. ↑ bone marrow depression with other **antineoplastics** or **radiation therapy**. May ↓ antibody response to **live-virus vaccines** and ↑ adverse reactions.

Route/Dosage
Other regimens are used.
IV (Adults): *Metastatic testicular tumors*—20 mg/m² daily for 5 days repeated q 3–4 wk. *Metastatic ovarian cancer*—75–100 mg/m², repeat q 4 wk in combination with cyclophosphamide *or* 100 mg/m² q 3 wk if used as a single agent. *Advanced bladder cancer*—50–70 mg/m² q 3–4 wk as a single agent.

Availability (generic available)
Powder for injection: 50 mg/vial. **Injection:** 1 mg/mL.

NURSING IMPLICATIONS

Assessment
- Monitor vital signs frequently during administration. Report significant changes.
- Monitor intake and output and specific gravity frequently during therapy. Report discrepancies immediately. To reduce the risk of nephrotoxicity, maintain a urinary output of at least 100 mL/hr for 4 hr before initiating and for at least 24 hr after administration.
- Encourage patient to drink 2000–3000 mL/day to promote excretion of uric acid. Allopurinol and alkalinization of the urine may be used to help prevent uric acid nephropathy.
- Assess patency of IV site frequently during therapy. Cisplatin may cause severe irritation and necrosis of tissue if extravasation occurs. If a large amount of highly concentrated cisplatin solution extravasates, mix 4 mL of 10% sodium thiosulfate with 6 mL of sterile water or 1.6 mL of 25% sodium thiosulfate with 8.4 mL of sterile water and inject 1–4 mL (1 mL for each mL extravasated) through existing line or cannula. Inject subcut if needle has been removed. Sodium thiosulfate inactivates cisplatin.
- Severe and protracted nausea and vomiting usually occur 1–4 hr after a dose; vomiting may last for 24 hr. Administer parenteral antiemetic agents 30–45 min before therapy and routinely around the clock for the next 24 hr. Monitor amount of emesis and notify health care professional if emesis exceeds guidelines to prevent dehydration. Nausea and anorexia may persist for up to 1 wk.
- Monitor for bone marrow depression. Assess for bleeding (bleeding gums, bruising, petechiae, stools, urine, and emesis) and avoid IM injections and taking rectal temperatures if platelet count is low. Apply pressure to venipuncture sites for 10 min. Assess for signs of infection during neutropenia. Anemia may occur. Monitor for increased fatigue, dyspnea, and orthostatic hypotension.
- Monitor for signs of anaphylaxis (facial edema, wheezing, dizziness, fainting, tachycardia, hypotension). Discontinue medication immediately and report symptoms. Epinephrine and resuscitation equipment should be readily available.
- Medication may cause ototoxicity and neurotoxicity. Assess patient frequently for dizziness, tinnitus, hearing loss, loss of coordination, loss of taste, or numbness and tingling of extremities; may be irreversible. Notify health care professional promptly if these occur. Audiometry should be performed before initiation of therapy and before subsequent doses. Hearing loss is more frequent with children and usually occurs first with high frequencies and may be unilateral or bilateral.
- Monitor for inadvertent cisplatin overdose. Doses >100 mg/m²/cycle once every 3–4 wk are rarely used. Differentiate daily doses from total dose/cycle. Symptoms of high cumulative doses include muscle cramps (localized, painful involuntary skeletal muscle contractions of sudden onset and short duration) and are usually associated with advanced stages of peripheral neuropathy.
- Monitor for signs of RPLS (headache, seizure, lethargy, confusion, blindness). Hypertension may or may not be present. May occur within 16 hr to 1 yr of initiation of therapy. Treat hypertension if present and discontinue cisplatin therapy. Symptoms usually resolve within days.

🍁 = Canadian drug name. ✖ = Genetic implication. S̶t̶r̶i̶k̶e̶t̶h̶r̶o̶u̶g̶h̶ = Discontinued.
*CAPITALS indicates life-threatening; underlines indicate most frequent.

CASE STUDY: Putting It All Together   *cont'd*

_____ **Case Study Questions** _____

B. Answer the following 3 questions by referring to *Davis's Drug Guide for Nurses,* CISplatin.

   1. Identify one trade name for CISplatin.

     _____

   2. Identify the two classifications of CISplatin.

     _____

   3. Identify the pregnancy category of CISplatin.

     _____

C. What are the action and therapeutic effects of CISplatin, as indicated in *Davis's Drug Guide for Nurses?*

   1. _____

   2. _____

D. Identify the four most serious adverse reactions and side effects, as indicated in *Davis's Drug Guide for Nurses,* for which the nurse should monitor a patient receiving CISplatin.

   1. _____

   2. _____

   3. _____

   4. _____

E. Identify the two most important responses for which the nurse should monitor the patient receiving CISplatin and list the related nursing care.

   1. _____

     a. _____

     b. _____

     c. _____

     d. _____

     e. _____

   2. _____

     a. _____

     b. _____

     c. _____

REVIEW QUESTIONS

1. Which is the **best** resource when a nurse requires information concerning recall of a medication, safety alerts, new medications, and generic approvals?
   1. U.S. Food and Drug Administration
   2. American Nurses Association
   3. U.S. Pharmacopoeia
   4. National Formulary

2. Which law should a nurse review if the nurse wants to ensure that the policy and procedures employed in the agency in which he or she works meet requirements regarding controlled medication?
   1. Food, Drug, and Cosmetic Act (1938)
   2. Durham-Humphrey Amendment (1952)
   3. Food and Drug Administration Modernization Act (1997)
   4. Comprehensive Drug Abuse Prevention and Control Act (1970)

3. A patient is receiving a narcotic analgesic for pain associated with cancer of the pancreas. Several weeks after initiation of therapy, the patient says to a nurse, "The medication does not control the pain as much as it did several weeks ago." What response to the medication should the nurse conclude this patient is experiencing?
   1. Tolerance
   2. Potentiation
   3. Adverse effect
   4. Idiosyncratic reaction

4. A nurse is administering an antibiotic to a patient who has an infected leg wound and a history of impaired peripheral circulation to the lower extremities. Which is the nurse's **most** important concern about this patient's status when evaluating a response to the antibiotic?
   1. Competence to biotransform the medication
   2. Ability to move the medication around the body
   3. Potential to excrete the medication from the body
   4. Capacity to absorb the medication into the blood stream

5. A nurse is caring for a patient who has impaired kidney function. For which process associated with pharmacokinetics should the nurse be **most** concerned about when evaluating this patient's response to a medication regimen?
   1. Biotransformation
   2. Distribution
   3. Absorption
   4. Excretion

6. A nurse is caring for a patient who has a prescription for an opioid for pain every 4 hours prn. The patient asks, "How long will it take for the medication to relieve my pain after I take the pill?" Which concept is **most** important for the nurse to explain to the patient?
   1. Peak plasma level
   2. Duration
   3. Half-life
   4. Onset

7. A nurse is caring for a patient who reports taking multiple over-the-counter herbal supplements. Which information about supplements should the nurse include when teaching this patient about supplements? **Select all that apply.**
   1. _____ Herbal supplements are safe to take.
   2. _____ Herbal supplements are regulated by the FDA.
   3. _____ Manufacturers' advertising of benefits are not supported with evidence.
   4. _____ Some patients do not realize the importance of reporting supplement use.
   5. _____ Alcohol should not be ingested with herbal supplements because of the risk of nontherapeutic interactions.

8. A nurse is explaining to a patient the need to perform blood tests to determine if a medication the patient is receiving is in the therapeutic range. Which statement is **most** important for the nurse to include in the discussion?
   1. "We need to draw your blood at the medication's half-life to determine if the dose needs to be adjusted."
   2. "We need to draw your blood just before the next dose to identify the lowest level of the medication in your blood."
   3. "We need to draw your blood two hours after administering the medication to determine the peak plasma level of the drug."
   4. "We need to draw your blood hourly to determine the duration of the therapeutic concentration of the medication in your blood."

9. A nurse is caring for a patient who is receiving an antibiotic intravenously. The patient asks, "Why are you drawing my blood so many times since I've started getting my antibiotic?" Which response by the nurse **best** answers the patient's question?
   1. "We want to ensure that the dose is not too strong that it causes toxicity."
   2. "The results will reflect if the dose is being absorbed appropriately by your body."
   3. "We want to determine if the medication gets into your blood within thirty minutes."
   4. "The results will reveal if the blood level of the medication is being maintained within the therapeutic range."

10. A nurse is caring for a patient who has a prescription for 500 mg of azithromycin (Zithromax). It is available in 250 mg tablets. How many tablets should the nurse administer to the patient? Record your answer using a whole number.

   Answer: _____ tablets

11. A nurse is unfamiliar with a new medication and reviews information about it in *Davis's Drug Guide*. Which information will help the nurse identify the generic name of the medication?
   1. The chemical structure is described.
   2. The name begins with a lowercase letter.
   3. The name is easier to recall than other names.
   4. The medication is registered by the United States Patent Office.

12. A nurse is evaluating a patient's response to a medication. Which is **most** important for the nurse to recall about factors that impact on the efficacy of a medication?
   1. Environment has little effect on responses to medications.
   2. Most medications are best absorbed on a stomach that is empty.
   3. Medication response discrepancies occur between men and woman.
   4. Infants experience multi-organ slowdown, increasing the risk of medication toxicity.

13. A nurse who just came on duty is assigned to care for an older adult male who is receiving chemotherapy for cancer.

Patient's Clinical Record

Primary Health-Care Provider's Orders

CBC, basic metabolic panel daily.
Lasix 40 mg IV push once daily in a.m. Hold Lasix for systolic blood pressure ≤90 mm Hg and inform primary health-care provider.
Discontinue chemotherapy.
Strict I&O.
2 g Na, low-protein, low-potassium diet.
Daily weight.

Laboratory Results

BUN: 60 mg/dL.
Creatinine: 4.1 mg/dL.
Hb: 14.8 g/dL.
WBC: 5,500/mm³.
Platelets: 200,000/mm³.

Progress Notes

The patient states feeling fatigued and drowsy. Pulse 88 beats/minute bounding; respirations 22 breaths/minute, bibasilar crackles; temperature 97.8°F; blood pressure 160/90 mm Hg. 1+ sacral edema noted. Intake last 24 hours: 2,400 mL IV and 800 mL PO. Urine output: 1,000 mL. Jugular venous distention noted. IV site dry, intact, free from signs and symptoms of infiltration and thrombophlebitis.

For which priority concern should the nurse assess the patient for clinical indicators?
   1. Infection
   2. Hemorrhage
   3. Medication toxicity
   4. Deficient fluid volume

14. A nurse is evaluating a patient's response to a medication and identifies a predictable, secondary effect of the medication. Which terminology should the nurse use when documenting the patient's response?
   1. Idiosyncratic reaction
   2. Allergic reaction
   3. Adverse effect
   4. Side effect

15. A patient in the emergency department tells the nurse, "I am allergic to penicillin." What should the nurse do **next**?
   1. Ask the patient about what kind of responses occurred.
   2. Ask the patient about the presence of other types of allergies.
   3. List the allergy on an allergy alert band on the patient's wrist.
   4. List the allergy in the patient's medication administration record.

16. A nurse is caring for a patient with a diagnosis of deep vein thrombosis who is receiving warfarin (Coumadin). Place the following statements in order based on the steps of the nursing process.
    1. Administer 10 mg of Coumadin as prescribed by the primary health-care provider.
    2. The risk of hemorrhage is related to the effects of the anticoagulant Coumadin.
    3. The INR level is 2.5, which is safely within the expected range of 2.0 to 3.0.
    4. The patient will not experience bleeding while receiving Coumadin.
    5. Left calf is pale, cool, and edematous.
    Answer: _____

17. A nurse is caring for a patient diagnosed with diabetes and who is receiving insulin. Which medication use category should the nurse include when discussing insulin with this patient?
    1. Curative
    2. Preventive
    3. Maintenance
    4. Contraceptive

18. A nurse is concerned about a patient's ability to metabolize a newly prescribed medication. Laboratory tests associated with which part of the body should the nurse monitor for functional performance because it is mainly associated with biotransformation of medication?
    1. Liver
    2. Lungs
    3. Kidneys
    4. Intestines

19. A nurse is caring for a middle-aged adult newly admitted to the hospital who has prescriptions for six different medications. Which nursing action is the priority before administering these medications to the patient?
    1. Verify that the medications are compatible.
    2. Have the antidotes for medications easily available.
    3. Teach the patient the therapeutic action of the medications.
    4. Ensure that these medications are included on the medication reconciliation form.

20. A nurse is caring for a patient who is receiving a monoamine oxidase (MAO) inhibitor. Which food should the nurse teach the patient to avoid when receiving this medication? **Select all that apply.**
    1. _____ Yogurt
    2. _____ Sausage
    3. _____ Chocolate
    4. _____ Chicken liver
    5. _____ Cream cheese

REVIEW ANSWERS

1. **ANSWER: 1.**
   Rationales:
   1. The U.S. Food and Drug Administration is the best source of information regarding information about medications, medical devices, and food.
   2. The American Nurses Association is not the best source for information about medications. However, it does publish standards of nursing practice regarding pharmacy and medication therapy.
   3. Although the U.S. Pharmacopoeia lists medications and standards for their preparation, it is not the best all-inclusive source regarding recall of medications, safety alerts, new medications, and generic approvals.
   4. Although the National Formulary lists officially recognized medications, including those not listed in the U.S. Pharmacopoeia, it is not the best source regarding recall of medications, safety alerts, new medications, and generic approvals.
   TEST-TAKING TIP: Identify the word in the stem that sets a priority. The word *best* in the stem sets a priority.
   Content Area: *Pharmacology*
   Integrated Processes: *Nursing Process: Analysis*
   Client Need: *Physiological Integrity; Pharmacological and Parenteral Therapies*
   Cognitive Level: *Comprehension*

2. **ANSWER: 4.**
   Rationales:
   1. The Food, Drug, and Cosmetic Act of 1938 is not related to regulations regarding controlled medications. This act required medications to be safe and approved by the Food and Drug Administration before marketing. Also, it established criteria regarding the manufacture, distribution, advertising, and labeling of medications.
   2. The Durham-Humphrey Amendment (1952) distinguished differences between prescription medications (require medical supervision) and nonprescription medications (over-the-counter).
   3. The Food and Drug Administration Modernization Act (1997) allowed more efficient approval of new medications and medical devices, compounding of medications by a pharmacist, and marketing "off-label" use of medications to primary health-care providers.
   4. The Comprehensive Drug Abuse Prevention and Control Act (1970) not only established controls on the manufacture and distribution of controlled medication, it set limits on prescription refills. Also, it identified 5 categories of controlled substances based on addiction potential and established government funded programs for the prevention and treatment of medication dependence.
   TEST-TAKING TIP: Identify the clang association. The word *controlled* in the stem and the word *control* in option 4 is a clang association. Examine option 4 carefully.
   Content Area: *Pharmacology*
   Integrated Processes: *Nursing Process: Analysis*
   Client Need: *Physiological Integrity; Pharmacological and Parenteral Therapies*
   Cognitive Domain: *Comprehension*

3. **ANSWER: 1.**
   Rationales:
   1. Tolerance is indicated by a decreased physiological response to a medication after repeated exposure to the medication.
   2. Potentiation occurs when an interaction between two medications results in an increase in the action of just one of the medications.
   3. An adverse effect is an unintended, usually unpredictable, harmful response to a medication that is more severe than a side effect.
   4. An idiosyncratic reaction happens when resistance, an overreaction, or an unpredictable reaction to a medication occurs that is different from the expected response.
   Content Area: *Pharmacology*
   Integrated Processes: *Communication/Documentation; Nursing Process: Evaluation*
   Client Need: *Physiological Integrity; Pharmacological and Parenteral Therapies*
   Cognitive Level: *Analysis*

4. **ANSWER: 2.**
   Rationales:
   1. There are no data in the question that indicate a problem with the liver, which mainly detoxifies a medication to a less active form in preparation for excretion. Also, the question does not indicate that this patient is an older adult who may have decreased liver function associated with aging.
   2. The adequacy of the circulation to transport the medication to the target site is essential for eventual medication utilization. The question states that this patient has "a history of impaired peripheral circulation to the lower extremities."
   3. Most antibiotics are excreted via the kidneys. There are no data that indicate that this patient has a problem with renal function. Also, the question does not indicate that this patient is an older adult who may have decreased ability to excrete medication by-products because of reduced kidney function associated with aging.
   4. There are no data in the question that indicate a problem with the ability to absorb medication, such as the presence of or lack of food in the stomach or any gastrointestinal problem that can interfere with absorption. Also, the question does not indicate that this patient is an older adult who may have decreased gastrointestinal function associated with aging.
   TEST-TAKING TIP: Identify the word in the stem that sets a priority. The word *most* in the stem sets a priority.
   Content Area: *Pharmacology*
   Integrated Processes: *Nursing Process: Evaluation*
   Client Need: *Physiological Integrity; Pharmacological and Parenteral Therapies*
   Cognitive Level: *Application*

5. **ANSWER: 4.**
   Rationales:
   1. Biotransformation (metabolism) mainly takes place in the liver, where medications are detoxified into less active forms in preparation for excretion. There is no information in the question that indicates that this patient has impaired liver function.

2. Distribution is involved with the transport of a medication from the absorption site to the site of medication action. There are no data in the question that indicate that this patient is experiencing a problem with cardiovascular function.

3. Absorption is associated with the process of movement of a medication into the blood stream. There is no information in the question that indicates that this patient is having a problem with the gastrointestinal tract.

4. **Most medications are excreted from the body in urine via the kidneys. Kidney disease can interfere with medication excretion, thereby causing medication accumulation. The nurse should be most concerned about the potential for medication toxicity.**

TEST-TAKING TIP: Identify the word in the stem that sets a priority. The word *most* in the stem sets a priority. Identify the obscure clang association. The words *kidney function* in the stem and *excretion* in option 4 is an obscure clang association.

Content Area: *Pharmacology*
Integrated Processes: *Nursing Process: Evaluation*
Client Need: *Physiological Integrity; Pharmacological and Parenteral Therapies*
Cognitive Level: *Comprehension*

6. **ANSWER: 4.**
Rationales:
1. A peak plasma level is associated with the highest blood concentration of a single medication dose, not how fast a person can anticipate pain relief after receiving an opioid.

2. Duration is associated with the length of time a therapeutic blood concentration of the medication is maintained, not how fast a person can anticipate pain relief after receiving an opioid.

3. Half-life is associated with the time needed to metabolize or inactivate one-half the amount of a medication, not how fast a person can anticipate pain relief after receiving an opioid.

4. **Onset is associated with the time it takes for the body to respond to a medication—in other words, how fast a person can anticipate pain relief after receiving an opioid.**

TEST-TAKING TIP: Identify the word in the stem that sets a priority. The word *most* in the stem sets a priority.

Content Area: *Pharmacology*
Integrated Processes: *Communication/Documentation; Nursing Process: Implementation*
Client Need: *Physiological Integrity; Pharmacological and Parenteral Therapies*
Cognitive Level: *Application*

7. **ANSWER: 3, 4, 5.**
Rationales:
1. Herbal supplements are unsafe to take unless the primary health-care provider states that it is safe to take the supplements. Herbal supplements have active ingredients that can cause serious medication interactions with prescribed medications as well as cause serious nontherapeutic effects.

2. Herbal supplements are not regulated by the FDA for safety and efficacy. However, the FDA has an Office of Special Nutritionals in its Center for Food Safety and Applied Nutrition that documents herbal products' adverse effects reported to the FDA.

3. **There are no regulations to hold manufacturers of herbal supplements accountable for the claimed benefits of their supplements.**

4. **Some patients do not report their use of supplements because they are embarrassed that they are self-medicating or do not realize the importance of potential medication-supplement interactions.**

5. **An increased risk of nontherapeutic interactions is associated with alcohol ingestion.**

Content Area: *Pharmacology*
Integrated Processes: *Teaching/Learning; Nursing Process: Planning*
Client Need: *Physiological Integrity; Pharmacological and Parenteral Therapies*
Cognitive Level: *Comprehension*

8. **ANSWER: 2.**
Rationales:
1. This will provide no significant information concerning the therapeutic level of a medication.

2. **This describes the protocol for the determination of the lowest level (trough level) of a medication in the blood. The trough level of a medication should be at or more than the lowest value in the identified blood therapeutic range of the medication.**

3. A peak plasma level is the concentration of a medication in a blood specimen drawn 30 to 60 minutes, not 2 hours, after the administration of a medication.

4. Blood specimens do not have to be drawn hourly to determine the therapeutic concentration of a medication in the blood.

TEST-TAKING TIP: Identify the word in the stem that sets a priority. The word *most* in the stem sets a priority. Identify the options that are opposites. Options 2 and 3 are opposites. Option 2 is associated with a time frame before administration of the medication and option 3 is associated with a time frame after administration of the medication. Review these options carefully.

Content Area: *Pharmacology*
Integrated Processes: *Communication/Documentation; Nursing Process: Implementation*
Client Need: *Physiological Integrity; Pharmacological and Parenteral Therapies*
Cognitive Level: *Application*

9. **ANSWER: 4.**
Rationales:
1. Although this is one of the reasons why a peak plasma level is monitored, an explanation including the words "too strong" and "causes toxicity" may cause anxiety. Another option answers the patient's question is a more positive and less threatening tone.

2. Absorption is not a concern because the medication was administered directly into the intravascular compartment.

3. This is inaccurate information. A medication that is administered via an intravenous line is immediately introduced into the blood, not 30 minutes later.

4. **This response best describes the purpose of the blood test, without using words that may precipitate anxiety.**

TEST-TAKING TIP: Identify the word in the stem that sets a priority. The word *best* in the stem sets a priority. Identify

the global option. Option 4 is the global option. The concept of therapeutic range includes peak and trough levels.
Content Area: Pharmacology
Integrated Processes: Communication/Documentation; Nursing Process: Implementation
Client Need: Physiological Integrity; Pharmacological and Parenteral Therapies
Cognitive Level: Application

10. ANSWER: 2.
Rationale:
Solve the problem by using the formula for ratio and proportion.

$$\frac{\text{Desire } 500 \text{ mg}}{\text{Have } 250 \text{ mg}} = \frac{\text{x tablets}}{1 \text{ tablet}}$$

$$250x = 500 \times 1$$
$$250x = 500$$
$$x = 500 \div 250$$
$$x = 2 \text{ tablets}$$

Content Area: Medication Administration
Integrated Processes: Nursing Process: Planning
Client Need: Physiological Integrity; Pharmacological and Parenteral Therapies
Cognitive Level: Application

11. ANSWER: 2.
Rationales:
1. The chemical, not generic, name describes the chemical and molecular structure of a medication.
2. The generic name begins with a lowercase letter and is easier to pronounce than the chemical name.
3. The trade, not generic, name usually is short and easy to recall.
4. The trade, not generic, name of a medication is registered by the U.S. Patent Office and approved by the U.S. Food and Drug Administration.
TEST-TAKING TIP: Identify the clang associations. The word *name* in the stem and in options 2 and 3 are clang associations. Examine options 2 and 3 carefully.
Content Area: Pharmacology
Integrated Processes: Nursing Process: Implementation
Client Need: Physiological Integrity; Pharmacological and Parenteral Therapies
Cognitive Level: Comprehension

12. ANSWER: 3.
Rationales:
1. The environment may affect the body's response to medications. A hot environment will intensify the action of vasodilators; a cold environment will inhibit the action of vasodilators, while increasing the action of vasoconstrictors; and a noisy environment may interfere with the therapeutic effect of a sedative or analgesic.
2. This is not an accurate statement. Many medications can irritate the gastrointestinal tract and should be taken with food.
3. Medication response discrepancies in men and women are attributable to body fat distribution as well as fluid and hormonal differences, which affect medication absorption. Also, the majority of medication research is

based on studies involving men; responses of women may be different than what is documented in medication literature.
4. Older adults, not infants, experience multiorgan slowdown or impairment, causing greater medication absorption and decreased excretion, which increases the risk of medication toxicity.
TEST-TAKING TIP: Identify the word in the stem that sets a priority. The word *most* in the stem sets a priority.
Content Area: Pharmacology
Integrated Processes: Nursing Process: Evaluation
Client Need: Physiological Integrity; Pharmacological and Parenteral Therapies
Cognitive Level: Comprehension

13. ANSWER: 3.
Rationales:
1. The patient's white blood cell count is within the expected range of 4,500 to 11,000/mm³, indicating that the patient has an adequate volume of white blood cells to protect the body from invading pathogens.
2. The patient's platelet count is within the expected range of 150,000 to 350,000/mm³, indicating that the patient will not hemorrhage due to a platelet deficiency.
3. The patient is at risk for drug toxicity due to impaired renal function, resulting in an inability to excrete toxic substances from the body. Impaired renal function is indicated by a BUN count increased beyond the expected range of 8 to 21 mg/dL and a creatinine count increased beyond the expected range of 0.6 to 1.2 mg/dL. A BUN level higher than 100 mg/dL and a creatinine level higher than 7.4 mg/dL are critical findings.
4. The patient is experiencing excess, not deficient, fluid volume. The BUN and creatinine levels are elevated indicating impaired kidney function. Clinical indicators of excess fluid volume include a fluid intake greater than urine output, an elevated pulse rate, bounding pulse, bibasilar crackles, jugular venous distention, elevated systolic and diastolic blood pressures, and sacral edema.
TEST-TAKING TIP: Identify the word in the stem that sets a priority. The word *priority* in the stem sets a priority.
Content Area: Pharmacology
Integrated Processes: Nursing Process: Evaluation
Client Need: Physiological Integrity; Pharmacological and Parenteral Therapies
Cognitive Level: Analysis

14. ANSWER: 4.
Rationales:
1. An *idiosyncratic reaction* is not a predictable, secondary effect to a medication. An idiosyncratic reaction is a resistance, overreaction, or unpredictable reaction that is different from the expected response.
2. An *allergic reaction* is not a predictable, secondary effect to a medication. An allergic reaction is a patient's immune system response to the presence of a medication.
3. An *adverse effect* is not a predictable, secondary effect to a medication. An adverse effect is an unintended, usually unpredictable harmful effect that is more severe than a side effect.

4. A *side effect* is a predictable, secondary effect to a medication. It is unintended, but is generally well tolerated because the benefit is greater than the inconvenience of the side effect (e.g., drowsiness, dry mouth).

TEST-TAKING TIP: Identify the clang associations. The word *effect* in the stem and in options 3 and 4 are clang associations. Examine options 3 and 4 closely. More often than not, an option with a clang association is the correct answer.

Content Area: Pharmacology
Integrated Processes: Communication/Documentation; Nursing Process: Evaluation
Client Need: Safe and Effective Care Environment; Management of Care
Cognitive Level: Knowledge

15. ANSWER: 1.
Rationales:
1. This information relates to the specific allergy identified by the patient. The specific reaction to each allergy should also be determined as each allergy is identified.
2. This is premature; it ignores the need for further exploration of the patient's statement.
3. This is premature; additional allergies may need to be included.
4. This intervention is premature; additional information should be obtained from the patient.

TEST-TAKING TIP: Identify options that are equally plausible. Options 3 and 4 are equally plausible. Both alert other health team members to the presence of the patient's allergy to penicillin. Option 3 is no better than option 4. Eliminate both options from consideration.

Content Area: Safety
Integrated Processes: Communication/Documentation; Nursing Process: Implementation
Client Need: Safe and Effective Care Environment; Safety and Infection Control
Cognitive Level: Application

16. ANSWER: 5, 2, 4, 1, 3.
Rationales:
5. The first step of the nursing process is assessment. "Left calf is pale, cool, and edematous" are three classic clinical indicators of deep vein thrombosis.
2. The second step of the nursing process is analysis. The patient is receiving Coumadin and therefore there is a risk of hemorrhage related to the effects of the anticoagulant Coumadin.
4. Planning is the third step of the nursing process. It involves identifying an expected outcome. The patient will not experience bleeding while receiving Coumadin is a measurable and realistic outcome. The second half of the planning step is identifying planned interventions. In this situation, the primary health-care provider has prescribed Coumadin, which the nurse plans to implement as prescribed.
1. The fourth step of the nursing process is implementation. Administering Coumadin as prescribed by the primary health-care provider is implementation of a planned intervention.
3. The fifth step of the nursing process is evaluation. In this situation, the nurse must monitor the patient's INR

level to ensure that it remains within the therapeutic range of 2.0 to 3.0 times the control.

Content Area: Pharmacology
Integrated Processes: Nursing Process: Analysis
Client Need: Physiological Integrity; Pharmacological and Parenteral Therapies
Cognitive Level: Analysis

17. ANSWER: 3.
Rationales:
1. Insulin does not cure diabetes. An antibiotic is an example of a medication that eradicates a disease-producing pathogen.
2. Insulin does not prevent diabetes. A vaccine such as the measles vaccine prevents measles.
3. Insulin is considered a health maintenance medication. It supports normal body function and is prescribed to maintain health.
4. Insulin does not prevent conception. A medication, such as an oral contraceptive with estrogen and progestin, is commonly prescribed to prevent pregnancy.

Content Area: Pharmacology
Integrated Processes: Teaching/Learning; Nursing Process: Planning
Client Need: Physiological Integrity; Pharmacological and Parenteral Therapies
Cognitive Level: Application

18. ANSWER: 1.
Rationales:
1. Metabolism (biotransformation) of medications occurs mainly in the liver.
2. Although metabolism of some medications may occur in the lungs, biotransformation mainly occurs in another organ of the body.
3. The kidneys are associated primarily with excretion, not metabolism, of medications in the body. Although metabolism of some medications may occur in the kidneys, biotransformation mainly occurs in another organ of the body.
4. Although metabolism of some medications may occur in the intestinal mucosa, biotransformation mainly occurs in another organ of the body. The intestines are more readily associated with excretion of medication via feces, although excretion of medications mainly is associated with the kidneys.

TEST-TAKING TIP: Identify the word in the stem that sets a priority. The word *mainly* in the stem sets a priority. Identify the unique option. Option 1 is unique because the liver is one organ. There are two lungs, two kidneys, and small and large intestines.

Content Area: Pharmacology
Integrated Processes: Nursing Process: Assessment
Client Need: Physiological Integrity; Pharmacological and Parenteral Therapies
Cognitive Level: Comprehension

19. ANSWER: 1.
Rationales:
1. The priority is to ensure that the six medications are compatible. Medications when combined can cause

chemical deterioration of one or more of the medications (usually due to acid-base incompatibility), resulting in precipitate formation, color change, or gas development. Also, one medication may interfere with the functioning of another medication by increasing or decreasing its effectiveness.

2. Although this may be done, it is not the priority. Also, not all medications have an antidote.

3. Although this may be done, it is not the priority.

4. Although this may be done, it is not the priority.

Content Area: Pharmacology
Integrated Processes: Nursing Process: Planning
Client Need: Physiological Integrity; Pharmacological and Parenteral Therapies
Cognitive Level: Application

20. ANSWER: 1, 2, 3, 4.
    Rationales:
    1. Yogurt contains a significant amount of tyramine and should be avoided by a patient receiving an MAO

inhibitor. An MAO inhibitor prevents the breakdown of tyramine. Too much tyramine leads to excessive epinephrine, causing a hypertensive crisis, which can precipitate an intracranial hemorrhage.

2. Sausage is high in tyramine and should be avoided by a patient receiving an MAO inhibitor.

3. Chocolate is high in tyramine and should be avoided by a patient receiving an MAO inhibitor.

4. Chicken liver is high in tyramine and should be avoided by a patient receiving an MAO inhibitor.

5. Cream cheese and cottage cheese are two types of cheese permitted on a tyramine-restricted diet for a patient receiving an MAO inhibitor because they are not high in tyramine.

Content Area: Pharmacology
Integrated Processes: Teaching/Learning; Nursing Process: Implementation
Client Need: Physiological Integrity; Pharmacological and Parenteral Therapies
Cognitive Level: Analysis

Basic Human Needs and Related Nursing Care

Chapter 16

Hygiene

KEY TERMS

Bulla—Elevated, fluid-filled vesicle more than 1 cm in size.

Crust—Dried residue from serum, blood, or pus.

Cyanosis—Bluish gray color of the skin.

Cyst—Mass of fluid-filled tissue that extends to the subcutaneous tissues or dermis and is more than 1 cm in size.

Ecchymosis—Blue-purple area that progresses to green-yellow caused by shallow bleeding under the skin or mucous membrane.

Erosion—Nonbleeding loss of superficial epidermis.

Erythema—Redness of the skin due to congestion of the capillaries.

Fissure—Linear crack in the skin.

Flushed—Redness of the skin due to dilated capillaries.

Jaundice—Yellow-orange cast to the skin, mucous membranes, and sclerae caused by deposition of bile salts.

Keloid—Raised, irregular scar due to excess collagen formation (hypertrophic scar).

Macule—Flat, circumscribed area from 1 to several centimeters in size.

Nodule—Raised solid mass that extends into the dermis and is 1 to 2 cm in size.

Pallor—Decrease in skin color or ashen gray appearance in dark-skinned people.

Papule—Raised, circumscribed area less than 1 cm in size due to superficial thickening in the epidermis.

Petechiae—Small, red-purple spots caused by intradermal or submucosal hemorrhaging.

Prepuce (foreskin)—Loose skin covering the end of the penis.

Pustule—Vesicle or bulla filled with pus that is more than 1 cm in size.

Scale—Exfoliation (shedding) of dead skin cells.

Scar—Formation of replacement connective tissue and fibrotic changes following healing of a wound.

Smegma—Thick, cheesy, odoriferous secretion from sebaceous glands found under the labia minor and around the clitoris in the female and under the foreskin in the male.

Ulcer—Irregularly shaped loss of skin, extending into or through the dermis.

Vesicle—Raised collection of fluid less than 1 cm in size.

Wheal—Round, raised superficial collection of fluid due to dermal edema and surrounding capillary dilation, extending 1 mm to several cm in size.

I. Providing Hygiene Within the Patient's Environment

When providing care to meet a patient's hygiene needs, the nurse must enter the patient's surrounding environment and invade the patient's personal space. Measures must consider the patient's right to be treated respectfully, such as asking permission to enter the patient's territory (e.g., room, bedside unit, and closet), ensuring that privacy needs are met (e.g., close doors and pull curtains around the bed), and providing a safe and comfortable environment (e.g., bed in the lowest position, clutter minimized, and comfortable room temperature for the patient).

A. **Bedside Unit**
1. Includes the bed, overbed table, and nightstand; access to a telephone, television, bathroom, and individual closet; and a call bell to summon assistance, which should always be in easy reach (e.g., clipped to the pillow case, tied to the bedrail).
2. Nightstand.
   a. Part of the patient's personal space, so the caregiver should always ask for permission to enter it.

   b. Contents.
     (1) The top drawer of the nightstand is for personal items, such as eyeglasses, written material, and clothing.
     (2) The middle drawer generally stores a wash basin, emesis basin, and toiletries.
     (3) The bottom drawer stores the bedpan and urinal.
 3. Overbed table on wheels.
   a. Provides a flat surface to hold such items as a pitcher of water, glass, and tissues.
   b. Often contains a drawer that has an adjustable mirror and a place to store small items, such as a tooth brush and razor.
   c. Also used to position a meal tray in front of the patient.
   d. Should not be used as a side rail or for support because it has wheels and is not stationary and, therefore, could cause a fall.

B. Bed
 1. Height from the floor can be raised or lowered, head can be raised, and foot can be adjusted to raise the knees; teach patients how to use the buttons that regulate the bed to promote independence and support comfort.

🛑 2. Should be lowered to the lowest height when care is not being provided to ensure ease in exiting and entering the bed and provide for patient safety.

 3. Most have four side rails.
   a. The two closest to the head of the bed should be raised at all times to facilitate turning from side to side and promote safety.
   b. Avoid raising all four side rails on a bed.
     (1) Considered a restraint, which requires a primary health-care provider's order.
     (2) Unnecessary use is considered false imprisonment unless their use is the patient's preference.

🛑 4. Keep wheels of bed locked at all times, particularly when a patient is entering or exiting the bed, to prevent falls.

 5. Most have built-in scales to facilitate obtaining daily weights.
 6. Have mattresses and pillows that are covered in a water-repellent material that can be cleaned with a bactericidal solution between patients to prevent cross contamination.
 7. Therapeutic mattresses.
   a. Spread weight over a larger surface area, reducing the intensity of pressure on bony prominences.
   b. Used for patients at risk for skin breakdown.
   c. Examples: Air and egg crate mattresses and air-flotation beds.

C. Environmental Factors
 1. Room temperature: Room temperature can be adjusted according to the patient's preference; generally room temperature ranges from 68°F to 74°F.
 2. Lighting: Each unit has a light on the wall over the head of the bed that generally throws light upward the ceiling and/or down over the head of the bed. Also there generally is a light in the ceiling and a small night light over or under the sink area to facilitate vision at night. Windows have either curtains or blinds so that daylight entering the room can be adjusted. Bed curtains also can be drawn around the bed to decrease light from a window or the hall.
 3. Noise: Televisions have handheld controllers that project sound and can be positioned near the ear so as not to inconvenience a roommate with excess noise. Patients have the option of closing the door to their rooms to reduce hallway noise. Nurses, especially those on the evening and night shift, should make an effort to minimize unnecessary noise so that patients can rest and sleep.
 4. Ventilation and odors: Some rooms have windows that open that can be adjusted to the patient's preference. Room deodorizers and environmental sprays may be used to eliminate or disguise odors.

II. Skin

Providing for a patient's hygiene needs includes not just care of the skin but also care of the mucous membranes, hair, and nails. To better provide appropriate nursing care, the nurse must first understand the functions of these structures, expected assessment findings, and potential variations and the potential implications of these variations.

A. Functions
 1. Largest organ of the body, the condition of which reflects the effects of the body's metabolism and nutritional status.
 2. Protects the body.
   a. Acts as a barrier between the internal and external environments.
   b. Prevents injury to underlying structures.
   c. Provides protection from microorganisms; "acid mantle" (pH between 4 and 5.5).
 3. Regulates body temperature.
   a. Dilates blood vessels and activates sweat glands to cool the body via processes of perspiration, evaporation, conduction, and radiation.
   b. Constricts blood vessels and inactivates sweat glands to conserve heat.
 4. Receives sensations of heat, cold, touch, pressure, and pain via nerve receptors.
 5. Produces vitamin D when skin is exposed to ultraviolet light from the sun.

6. Secretes sebum from sebaceous glands, which lubricates skin and hair; reduces heat loss from skin because of its oily nature; and reduces bacterial growth.

7. Excretes water, sodium chloride, and nitrogenous waste via perspiration.

B. Principles of Assessment of the Skin

1. Obtain the patient's permission for assessment because it invades the patient's personal space.

2. Ensure adequate lighting and that the color of curtains and wall paint does not influence assessments.

3. Use inspection before palpation; rub hands to warm them before placing them on the patient's skin.

4. Consider the mucous membranes, hair, and nails extensions of the skin.

C. Assessment of Skin

1. Skin color.
   a. Recognize that skin color varies according to age and race and that exposed areas are darker than unexposed areas; palms of the hands, soles of the feet, and nail beds are the lightest areas.
   b. Note variations in skin color.
      (1) **Cyanosis:** Bluish-gray color of the skin; may appear ashen gray in dark-skinned people; more obvious in the conjunctivae, tongue, buccal mucosa, palms of the hands, and soles of the feet; associated with hypoxia or exposure to extreme cold.
      (2) **Ecchymosis:** Blue-purple area larger than petechiae that progresses to green-yellow; commonly called a *bruise*; due to shallow bleeding under the skin or mucous membrane; associated with blunt trauma.
      (3) **Erythema:** Redness of the skin due to congestion of the capillaries; associated with inflammation, vasodilation, prolonged pressure, and application of heat or cold.
      (4) **Flushed:** Redness of the skin due to dilated capillaries; most commonly associated with increased body temperature.
      (5) **Jaundice:** Yellow-orange cast to the skin caused by deposition of bile salts; most obvious in sclerae of the eyes, mucous membranes, palms of the hands, and soles of the feet; associated with liver or biliary impairment.
      (6) **Pallor:** Pale skin or ashen gray appearance in dark-skinned people; more obvious in oral mucous membranes, conjunctivae, nail beds, palms of the hands, and soles of the feet; associated with anemia and malnutrition.
      (7) **Petechiae:** Small, red-purple spots caused by intradermal or submucosal hemorrhaging; associated with thrombocytopenia and some febrile illnesses.

2. Skin temperature.
   a. Use the back of the hand or fingers to assess skin temperature (see Fig. 11.16, page 263.); skin should feel warm to touch.
   b. Assess extremities bilaterally and compare for symmetry.
   c. Assess a patient with excessively warm skin further because this finding may indicate a fever; obtain body temperature to verify.
   d. Assess a patient with excessively cool skin further because it may indicate conditions such as impaired circulation, shock, or hypothyroidism.

3. Skin moisture.
   a. Assess by inspection and palpation; skin usually is warm and dry.
   b. Assess a patient with excessively moist skin (profuse diaphoresis) further because this finding may indicate conditions such as hyperthermia, anxiety, exposure to hot environment, or hyperthyroidism.
   c. Assess a patient with excessively dry skin further because this finding may indicate conditions such as dehydration, excessive exposure to the sun, overzealous bathing, or hypothyroidism.
   d. Assess a patient with oily skin further because this finding may be due to excessive sebaceous gland secretion or sebaceous gland inflammation (acne), commonly associated with adolescence.
   e. Assess skin turgor to determine elasticity of the skin, which reflects hydration status; pinch skin on anterior chest below the clavicle, sternum, forehead, or inner thigh and note how long it takes to return to its original position (see Fig. 21.7, page 653.).
      (1) Prolonged tenting (longer than 2 to 3 seconds) is associated with dehydration and aging.
      (2) Resistance to pinching is associated with edema; patient may report that the skin "feels tight" or that rings and shoes do not fit. (For additional information, see the section "Fluid Volume Excess" in Chapter 21, "Fluid and Electrolytes," page 653.)

4. Skin texture.
   a. Recognize that skin texture varies according to age and the area being assessed.
      (1) Exposed areas and elbows and knees tend to be drier and coarser that unexposed areas.
      (2) Skin of infants and children is softer and smoother than that of adults because of lack of exposure to the environment and extent of hydration of tissues.
   b. Identify changes in skin texture related to impaired circulation.
      (1) Peripheral arterial insufficiency is associated with smooth, thin, shiny skin that has little or no hair.

(2) Peripheral venous insufficiency is associated with thick, rough skin that frequently is hyperpigmented.

5. Skin lesions.
   a. Use standard precautions when assessing skin lesions.
      (1) Wash hands before and after.
      (2) Wear gloves.
   b. Identify the type of lesion.
      (1) Primary lesions occur in response to a change in the internal or external environment of the skin due to a disease process (Table 16.1).
      (2) Secondary lesions occur as a result of changes in a primary lesion due to trauma, scratching, or infection (Table 16.2).
   c. Identify the size and shape of the lesion.
      (1) Note size in millimeters.
      (2) Identify whether the lesion is circumscribed or diffuse, round or oval.
      (3) Identify the depth of the lesion.
   d. Identify the texture of the lesion: Depressed, flat, or elevated; hard, solid, or soft; rough or thickened; fluid filled or flakey.
   e. Identify the presence and characteristics (e.g., color, odor) of exudate.

Table 16.1 Primary Skin Lesions

Type of Lesion	Depiction of Lesion
Bulla • Elevated, fluid-filled vesicle more than 1 cm in size (A). • Examples include blister (B), deep partial-thickness burn, and contact dermatitis.	A B
Cyst • Mass of fluid-filled tissue that extends to the subcutaneous tissues or dermis and is more than 1 cm in size (A). • Examples include epidermoid cysts (B) and sebaceous cyst.	A B
Macule • Flat, circumscribed area from 1 to several centimeters in size (A). • Examples include cherry angioma (B), freckles, flat pigmented moles, and measles.	A B
Nodule • Raised solid mass that extends into the dermis and is 1 to 2 cm in size (A). • Examples include pigmented nevus (B) and fibroma.	A B
Papule • Raised, circumscribed area less than 1 cm in size due to superficial thickening in the epidermis (A). • Examples include raised mole (B), ringworm, and wart.	A B

Table 16.1 **Primary Skin Lesions—cont'd**

Type of Lesion	Depiction of Lesion
Pustule • Vesicle or bulla filled with pus that is more than 1 cm in size (A). • Examples include acne vulgaris (B) and impetigo.	
Vesicle • Raised collection of fluid less than 1 cm in size (A). • Examples include herpes simplex (B), chickenpox, and poison ivy.	
Wheal • Round, raised superficial collection of fluid due to dermal edema and surrounding capillary dilation, extending 1 mm to several cm in size (A). • Examples include hives, also known as urticaria (B), and mosquito bites.	

Figures from Dillon (2007). *Nursing health assessment,* 2nd ed. Philadelphia: F. A. Davis Company, with permission.

Table 16.2 **Secondary Skin Lesions**

Type of Lesion	Depiction of Lesion
Crust • Dried residue from serum, blood, or pus (A). • Examples include dried herpes simplex (B) and impetigo.	
Erosion • Nonbleeding loss of superficial epidermis (A). • Examples include candidiasis (B) and chickenpox rupture.	

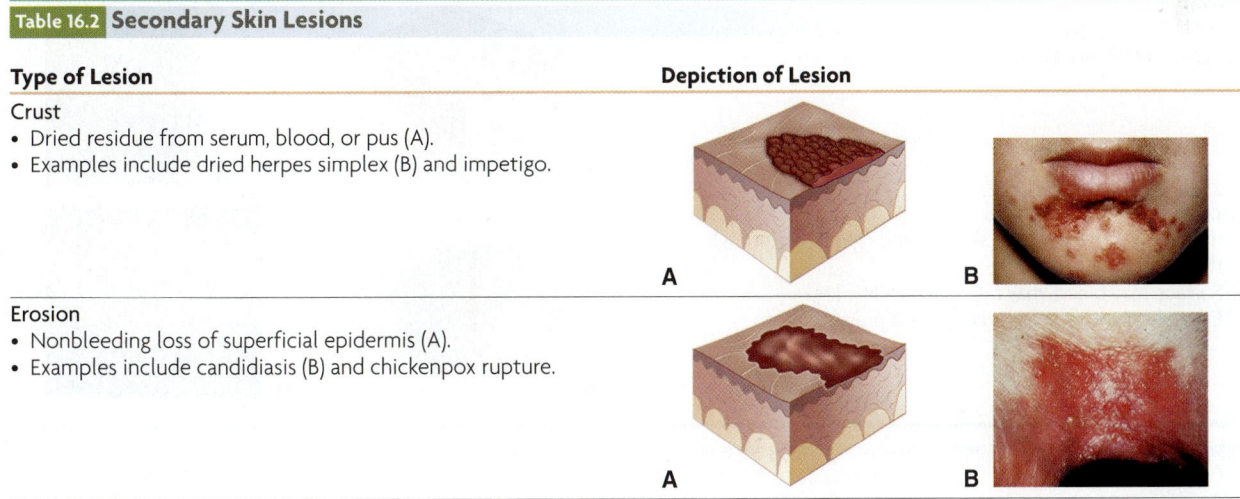

Continued

Table 16.2 Secondary Skin Lesions—cont'd

Type of Lesion	Depiction of Lesion
Fissure • Linear crack in the skin (A). • Examples include cheilitis (B) and athlete's foot.	
Keloid • Raised, irregular scar due to excess collagen formation (hypertrophic scar) (A). • Examples of common sites include surgical incisions (B), ear piercings, and tattoos.	
Scale • Exfoliation (shedding) of dead skin cells. May be dry or oily, loose or adherent, and vary in color (A). • Examples include psoriasis (B) and dandruff.	
Scar • Formation of replacement connective tissue and fibrotic changes following healing of a wound (A). • Examples of common sites include surgical incisions (B) and cuts.	
Ulcer • Irregularly shaped loss of skin, extending into or through the dermis. • Surface may bleed, may become necrotic (A). • Examples include stasis ulcer (B) and pressure ulcer.	

Figures not supplied by the authors are from Dillon (2007). *Nursing health assessment*, 2nd ed. Philadelphia: F. A. Davis Company, with permission.

f. Identify the color of lesion: May have no color, one discrete color, or several colors; color may be red, brown, black, blue, purple, or yellow.

g. Identify the distribution of lesions: Document the location of the lesion(s); symmetry or asymmetry of lesions.

h. Identify the pattern (configuration) of lesions: Arrangement of lesions in relation to each other, such as circular, linear, clustered, arcing, merged together, or following the course of cutaneous nerves.

D. Assessment of Mucous Membranes

1. Consist of an epithelial membrane that lines body surfaces, opening directly to the exterior of the body (e.g., oral cavity, rectum, nose, and urethra) and the entire GI tract from the mouth to the anus.

2. Condition of the mucous membranes is influenced by changes in oxygenation, circulation, nutrition, and hydration.

3. Assessment should reveal membranes that are pink, moist, and intact. See the section "Integumentary System" in Chapter 11, "Physical Assessment," for details concerning assessment of the mucous membranes, page 269.

E. Assessment of Hair

1. Develops in epidermal structures called *follicles.*

2. Shaft is produced in the matrix at the base of the hair root.

3. Distribution is affected by gender, genetics, and age.

4. Functions of hair.
   a. On the head, arms, and legs, provides thermal insulation.
   b. In the nostrils, filters air entering the nasal cavities.
   c. On the face (eyelashes and eyebrows), keeps sweat and debris out of the eyes.

5. Characteristics of hair.
   a. Color: Black, brown, blond, red, gray, or white; loss of pigment as one ages results in gray or white hair.
   b. Quantity: Thick, thin, sparse, none; abnormal hairiness (**hirsutism**); amount of hair may decrease on the lower extremities, pubic and axillary areas, and head as one ages, as the result of chemotherapy, and thyroid disease.
   c. Distribution: Symmetrical; hair in expected or unexpected areas; multiple bald spots; male pattern baldness; male pattern of hair distribution in women is associated with endocrine disorders and steroid medications; lack of hair on distal extremities may indicate inadequate peripheral circulation.
   d. Texture: Coarse or fine; straight, wavy, or curly; oily or dry; dry hair is associated with malnutrition, aging, and hypothyroidism; fine, silky hair is associated with hyperthyroidism; hair return

after chemotherapy may have a different color and/or texture.

e. General condition of hair: Clean and combed; dirty, unkempt, and matted.

f. Condition of scalp: Should be shiny, smooth, mobile, and nontender.

g. Presence of infection or infestations: Wash hands before and after donning clean gloves; systematically part hair in multiple sections, particularly behind the ears and at the nape of the neck, to assess for sores, lice, nits (lice eggs), ringworm (*tinea capitis*), dry flakes (dandruff), or oily scales (seborrhea).

F. Assessment of Nails

1. Found at the ends of the fingers and toes; new cells that contain keratin are produced at the nail root and visible nails result when these cells die.

2. Condition of nails influenced by local problems, systemic problems, and aging.

3. Functions of nails.
   a. Protect the fingers and toes from mechanical injury.
   b. Assist in picking up small objects.

4. Characteristics of nails.
   a. Color: Usually pink or light brown.
      (1) Yellow nails are related to cigarette smoking, fungal infections, or psoriasis.
      (2) Blue nails are related to peripheral disease or hypoxia.
      (3) White nails are related to trauma and liver or renal disease.
      (4) Black nails are related to trauma; color due to accumulation of blood under the nail.
   b. Shape and nail plate angle: Convex curve expected with an angle of 160° between the fingernail and nail bed. (Fig. 16.1a)
      (1) Angle equal to or greater than 180° (clubbing) is related to long-term lack of oxygen. (Fig. 16.1b)
      (2) Spoon-shaped nail is related to iron-deficiency anemia.
   c. Texture: Smooth surface expected.
      (1) Excessively thick nails are related to impaired circulation, chronic fungal infection, and aging.
      (2) Excessively thin nails or the presence of grooves or furrows are related to iron-deficiency anemia.
      (3) Brittle nails are related to malnutrition, calcium, and iron deficiency.
      (4) Longitudinal ridges are related to arterial insufficiency.
   d. Cuticle and surrounding tissue: Smooth intact epidermis expected. Edema, erythema, or exudate indicates inflammation or infection.

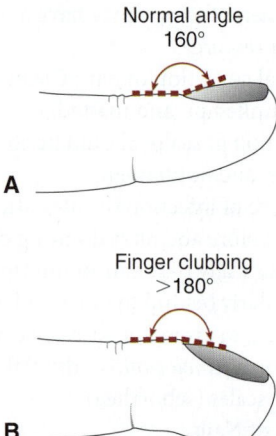

Fig 1.1 Nail plate angle (normal, clubbing). (From Dillon [2007]. *Nursing health assessment,* 2nd ed. Philadelphia: F. A. Davis Company, with permission.)

   e. Capillary refill: Compression of the nail produces blanching and color returns in less than 3 seconds after pressure is released (blanch test); 3 seconds or more indicates cardiopulmonary problems or anemia.

III. Risk Factors for Impaired Skin Integrity and Related Nursing Care

The integrity of the skin must be maintained to preserve one of the first protective lines of defense of the body. Factors such as moisture, excessive or inadequate hydration of the skin, inadequate nutrition, prolonged pressure, and shearing forces can compromise the skin's integrity. Nurses must have a thorough understanding of these factors as they relate to skin breakdown because many of them can be prevented or minimized by nurses when caring for patients.

A. Moisture
1. Incontinence and perspiration because of fever in response to disease or illness can cause prolonged dampness, which softens skin (maceration).
2. Feces and gastric tube drainage that contain digestive enzymes and urine that contains urea can cause loss of superficial layers of the skin (excoriation, denuded skin).
3. Abdominal and perineal skin folds and under the breasts are particularly at risk because these touching skin surfaces confine moisture and are warm, dark, moist places that facilitate growth of bacteria and fungi.
4. Nursing care.
   a. Keep the patient clean and dry, especially skinfolds for a patient who is obese, perspiring, incontinent of urine or stool, or has a gastric or urinary tube.

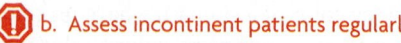 b. Assess incontinent patients regularly.

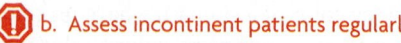 c. Change wet clothing and linens immediately.

   d. Provide a skin barrier to the perineal area or around the entry of a gastrostomy or urostomy tube as ordered; many facilities have standing orders that permit the nurse to use professional judgment concerning the application of products such as A&D ointment.
   e. Engage in a bowel or bladder training program if the patient is a candidate.
   f. Implement a toileting schedule to reduce episodes of incontinence; assist with toileting before and after meals to take advantage of the gastrocolic reflex (food/fluid entering an empty stomach stimulates peristalsis), when awakening in the morning and when going to bed at night, and every 2 hours.

B. Dehydration and Edema
1. Fluid loss due to fever, diarrhea, or vomiting or inadequate fluid intake contributes to dry, cracking skin and mucous membranes.
2. Excessive fluid in interstitial tissue (**edema**) decreases elasticity and flexibility of skin and interferes with oxygenation and clearing of waste from cells, increasing the risk of tissue breakdown.
3. Nursing care.

   a. Ensure that the patient has adequate fluid intake (1,500–2,500 mL/day) to maintain body function.
     (1) Administer IV fluids as ordered.
     (2) Provide fresh water and preferred fluids and assist a patient who is unable to acquire fluid, such as by offering sips of water whenever passing the patient's room.
   b. Maintain fluid restriction as ordered.
   c. Provide pressure relief devices to protect skin surfaces.
   d. Elevate the legs of a patient with dependent edema as long as the patient has no acute cardiac insufficiency.
     (See also the sections "Fluid Volume Deficit" and "Fluid Volume Excess" in Chapter 21, "Fluid and Electrolytes," page 652–653.)

C. Inadequate Nutrition
1. Insufficient protein, carbohydrates, and vitamin C contribute to muscle wasting, insufficient subcutaneous tissue, and weight loss.
2. Insufficient protective cushioning of bony prominences by adequate tissue layers increases the risk of skin breakdown due to pressure.
3. Nursing care.
   a. Assess self-feeding ability; condition of oral cavity, such as lesions, stomatitis, and problems with dentures; current weight; and weight history.

b. Ensure that the patient receives adequate nutrition; evaluate and document the percentage of each meal ingested; avoid using relative terms such as "good" and "poor" to describe intake.

🛑 c. Assist a patient with meals as needed and encourage intake of foods high in calories, protein, and vitamin C to maintain weight and facilitate wound healing.

d. Conduct a calorie count when ordered to evaluate the patient's nutritional intake.

D. Prolonged Immobility

1. When pressure exceeds 15 to 32 mm Hg (capillary occlusion pressure) due to tissue compression between a bony prominence and a hard surface, such as a bed or chair, tissue ischemia occurs, contributing to cell death.

2. Three factors are a concern.
   a. Intensity of pressure.
   b. Duration of pressure.
   c. Degree of tissue tolerance to the pressure due to a concurrent problem.

3. Concurrent problems that contribute to prolonged pressure and skin breakdown include presence of edema, inadequate nutrition, moisture, dehydration, reduced sensation, and impaired cognition that influences the ability to move.

4. Nursing care.
   a. Encourage independence but assist with activities that the patient cannot complete or care for areas that the patient cannot reach.

   🛑 b. Turn and reposition the patient every 2 hours and document on a turning and positioning flow sheet; may be done hourly for patients at risk for skin breakdown.

   c. Teach the patient how to weight shift frequently to reduce the duration of pressure.
   d. Use pressure-relief devices, such as gel cushions, an air mattress, pillows, and elbow and heel pads to distribute weight over a greater area, thereby decreasing the intensity of pressure.
   e. Provide massage, skin care, and range of motion every time a patient's position is changed to increase local circulation and prevent contractures. See the section "Range-of-Motion (ROM) Exercises" in Chapter 17, "Mobility," page 480.

E. Shearing Force

1. Shearing force occurs when gravity pulls down on deep body structures and frictional resistance occurs between the skin and a firm surface.
2. The epidermal layer slides over the dermis and underlying tissue layers.
3. Shearing and frictional forces damage the vascular bed of skin and superficial tissue.
4. Capillary occlusion pressure is significantly reduced when shearing occurs; the combination of pressure and shearing dramatically increases the risk of skin breakdown.

5. Nursing care.
   a. Use a pull sheet to move a patient up in bed.
   b. Avoid using a high- or semi-Fowler position or limit the use of this position to alternating 2-hour intervals.
   c. Use a sliding board when transferring a patient from a bed to a stretcher and back.
   d. Use a mechanical lift to transfer a patient from a bed to a chair and back if the patient is unable to move independently.

IV. Factors Affecting Hygiene Practices and Related Nursing Care

Personal hygiene consists of activities that maintain body cleanliness, promoting physical and psychological well-being. It is highly individualized and determined by numerous personal, cultural, religious, socioeconomic, environmental, and physical factors. Nurses must have a comprehensive understanding of these factors to aid in the assessment of patients and in the planning of nursing interventions that are specific for each patient.

A. Personal Preferences

1. Some people prefer to take a shower versus a bath, bathe in the morning versus the evening, and have specific opinions about the type of products they desire.
2. Personal habits develop based on factors such as culture, home environment, family patterns, and economic circumstances.
3. Nursing care.
   a. Ask about preferences regarding hygiene and grooming activities.
   b. Accept hygiene practices nonjudgmentally.
   c. Support hygiene routines whenever possible using products preferred by the patient.

B. Culture and Religion

1. Maintaining personal cleanliness is not as important in some cultures as in others; North Americans commonly bathe daily and those in other cultures may bathe only once a week.
2. Some cultures expect a person to use deodorant and others believe that it is unnecessary.
3. Different cultures have different beliefs about nudity and privacy; North Americans generally bathe in private and people in other cultures may bathe communally (Box 16.1).
4. Nursing care.
   a. Identify and meet specific preferences based on cultural and religious customs.

   🛑 b. Provide privacy for hygiene and grooming activities; expose only the area of the body being washed.

Box 16.1 **Examples of Cultural and Religious Bathing Preferences**

- Orthodox Jewish women engage in a ritual bath after each menstruation and after childbirth.
- In some cultures, family members provide hygiene and grooming care for ill relatives.
- Muslim women receive personal care only from another woman.
- Muslims use the left hand for cleaning and the right hand for eating and praying.
- In some cultures, family members may perform religious ceremonial washing when a patient dies.

 c. Assign a gender-specific caregiver to a patient when touching between unrelated males and females is forbidden in the patient's culture.

   d. Include a family member in meeting hygiene needs if it is the patient's preference.
   e. Support ceremonial washing of a patient by family members when requested.
C. Developmental Level
   1. Common nursing care.
      a. Encourage patients to provide for their own hygiene needs as independently as possible within developmental, physical, emotional, and mental abilities.
      b. Provide or assist with bathing activities when a patient is unable to reach body parts or when cognitively immature or impaired.
      c. Use hygiene products that are the patient's preference and/or that are designed for a specific developmental age, such as gentle soaps or soap substitutes for infants and older adults.
      d. Use protective skin barrier ointments in the perineal area when a patient is not toilet trained or is incontinent.

 e. Test the temperature of bath water before use, including a bath or shower.

   2. Infants and children.
      a. Have fragile, easily injured skin.
      b. Are incontinent of urine and feces that promote skin breakdown.
      c. Have hygiene activities provided for by parents and caregivers.
      d. Progressively assume more self-care activities as they grow older.
      e. Eventually provide self-care independently.
      f. Specific nursing care.
         (1) Change diaper as soon as soiled.
         (2) Allow children to engage in self-care as gross and fine motor skills develop.

   3. Adolescents.
      a. Have increased sebaceous gland growth and secretion, which makes the skin more oily and susceptible to acne.
      b. May shower several times a day as they become more concerned about personal appearance.
      c. Specific nursing care.
         (1) Support adolescents nonjudgmentally as they engage in meeting hygiene needs to enhance their self-esteem.
         (2) Support use of prescribed acne medications.
   4. Older adults.
      a. Have many integumentary changes that result in fragile, easily injured skin (Fig. 16.2).
      b. May need assistance with hygiene because of problems such as physical limitations, incontinence, cognitive impairments, and reduced sensation, resulting in an inability to sense pressure, heat, cold, and friction or chemical irritants.

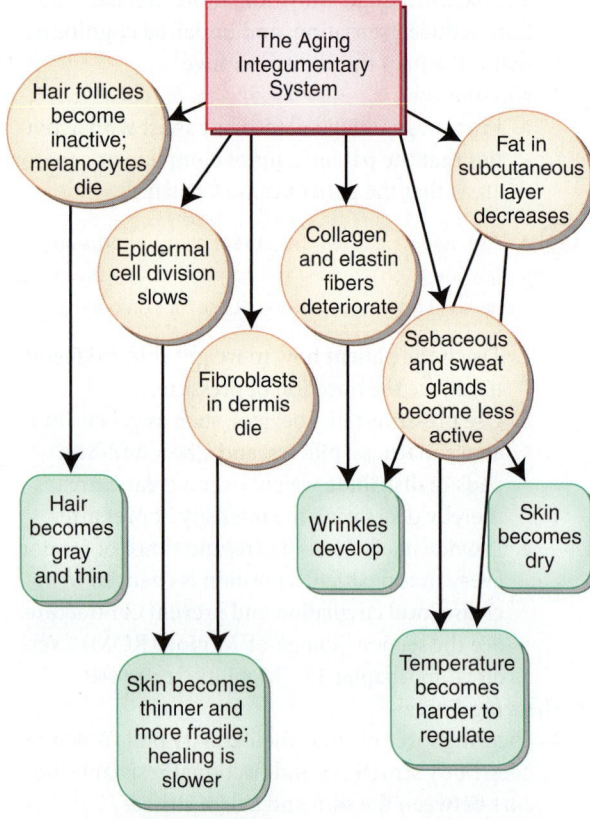

Fig 16.2 The aging integumentary system. Note: Circles indicate physiologic changes; squares indicate observable results of physiologic changes. (From Williams & Hopper [2011]. *Understanding medical surgical nursing,* 4th ed. Philadelphia: F. A. Davis, with permission.)

c. May be reluctant to seek assistance because of fear that they will be viewed as unable to cope.

d. Specific nursing care.

   (1) Provide a complete bath less frequently according to a patient's preference to avoid drying the skin.

   (2) Use mild cleansing products to maintain pH balance of skin and prevent removal of natural moisturizers and lipids that protect the skin.

   (3) Use a soft cloth and pat skin surfaces dry to avoid damage by abrasion.

   (4) Apply a moisturizer/emollient after bathing and at least twice a day to make skin supple and less dry; ensure safety precautions because these products can be slippery.

   (5) Teach the patient to assess all body surfaces, especially bony prominences, daily using a mirror, if needed, to identify tissue trauma.

D. Knowledge, Values, Beliefs, and Motivation

1. Knowledge alone may not precipitate healthful behaviors.

2. Values (an opinion about the worth of something) and beliefs (thoughts that a person considers to be true, which may or may not be based on fact) influence personal hygiene behaviors.

3. Changes in behavior related to health beliefs are based on the patient's perception of these factors:

   (1) Seriousness of the illness.

   (2) Personal risk of developing the illness.

   (3) Personal benefit of the actions to be taken.

4. Motivation (desire or incentive to learn) influences whether a behavior is instituted and/or sustained. (For more information, see the section "Motivation Facilitates Learning" in Chapter 9, "Teaching and Learning," page 193.)

5. Nursing care.

   a. Identify the patient's values and beliefs in relation to hygiene.

   b. Identify the patient's understanding of actions and inactions that impact personal hygiene and bodily functions.

   c. Teach principles associated with hygiene and that are within the patient's values and beliefs.

   d. Help the patient to set goals and outcomes and assist patients to meet these goals and outcomes.

E. Socioeconomic Status and Personal Environment

1. Inadequate income influences the environment in which one lives and the ability to afford hygiene products.

2. A person renting a room or living in a rooming house may not have easy access to bathing facilities.

3. Homeless people carry all belongings with them and may bathe in a sink in a public bathroom.

4. Attaining food, clothing, and shelter may be more important than bathing to people who live in poverty.

5. Nursing care.

   a. Be sensitive to an inability to provide for personal cleanliness due to poverty or homelessness.

   🛑 b. Advocate for the patient and initiate contact with an appropriate social service agency that can address the multiple physical and emotional needs of the patient.

   c. Direct the patient to a food bank that provides hygiene products or a shelter that provides facilities in which to bathe.

   d. Direct the patient to community agencies that help acquire funding for people living in poverty.

F. Health Status and Energy

1. Patients challenged with physical, physiological, emotional, mental, or cognitive problems may not have the physical strength, dexterity, endurance, or psychic energy to provide for their own hygiene needs safely.

2. Common health issues that impact the self-performance of hygiene.

   a. Pain due to problems such as surgery, trauma, and acute or chronic health problems.

   b. Impaired mobility due to problems such as Parkinson's disease, multiple sclerosis, spinal cord injury, or brain attack.

   c. Sensory deficits, such as impaired vision or hearing and neuropathies.

   d. Cognitive deficits, such as delirium, dementia, traumatic brain injury, or lowered level of unconsciousness.

   e. Emotional, mental, or cognitive issues, such as an altered reality state, severe anxiety, or depression.

3. Assess the level of patient assistance needed to meet hygiene needs.

   a. Independent: Patient is able to provide total self-care without assistance.

   b. Set-up with partial assistance: Patient can physically and mentally bathe most body parts when equipment is positioned in easy reach; caregiver assists with body parts that the patient is unable to reach, such as lower legs and feet, back, and buttocks.

   c. Supervision: Patient can physically provide self-care but, because of a mental or emotional impairment, needs coaching to stay focused or complete the steps in a task.

   d. Complete assistance: Patient is physically, emotionally, or mentally incapable of providing self-care; all hygiene and grooming tasks are implemented by the caregiver.

4. Nursing care.
   a. Complete a nursing history and physical and identify factors that may interfere with a patient's ability to provide self-care.
   b. Identify the patient's level of ability to participate in self-care.
   c. Plan and implement a plan of care that addresses hygiene and grooming needs.
   d. For nursing care for patients with specific needs associated with an impaired ability to meet personal hygiene and grooming needs, see Section VI, "Providing Hygiene for Patients With Special Needs," page 460.

V. Providing Personal Care

Activities of daily living related to personal care generally include bathing, perineal care, foot care, oral care, hair care, nail care, and shaving. They also include insertion, removal, and storage of hearing aids and dentures. Each of these activities includes specific nursing interventions that incorporate the principles of medical asepsis and patient safety. Nurses must understand not only what should be done but also the rationale for each of these interventions.

A. Purposes
1. Cleanses the skin by minimizing microorganisms and removing secretions, excretions, and debris from the skin; removes and inhibits unpleasant body odors.
2. Increases circulation by bringing oxygen and nutrients to the cells of the skin and removing cellular waste.
3. Promotes a sense of well-being and fosters relaxation and comfort.

B. Scheduled Hygiene
1. Hourly.
   a. Rounding hourly is also known as "comfort or safety rounds."
   b. Ensures patient's comfort, positioning, and toileting needs are met in a timely manner.
2. Upon awakening.
   a. Also known as "early morning care."
   b. Patient is toileted upon awakening, hands and face are washed, and oral care and comfort interventions (e.g., positioning, medications) are performed in preparation for breakfast and diagnostic testing.
3. Morning care.
   a. Also known as "a.m. care."
   b. After breakfast, patients are assisted with hygiene and grooming activities, such as toileting, bathing, oral care, skin care, shaving if desired, dressing, and positioning in a chair. At this time, linens are generally changed and the room is organized and cleaned.

4. Afternoon care.
   a. Sometime after lunch, patients may be assisted with toileting and returned to bed for rest.
   b. Care may also include performing hand hygiene, providing oral care, repositioning, straightening linens, and providing comfort measures, such as medication for pain.
5. Hour of sleep care.
   a. Also known as "p.m. care."
   b. Includes the same care as afternoon care; in addition, a back massage should be performed to promote relaxation.
   c. The television and lights should be turned off and the door closed, per the patient's preferences. See also Box 16.2.

C. Bathing
1. Commonalities of nursing care for all types of bathing methods.
   a. Explain what is going to be done and why to meet the patient's right to know and promote motivation and participation.
   b. Ask the patient about his or her usual routine and provide for preferences.
   c. Complete hand hygiene to minimize cross-contamination, and collect all equipment to avoid interrupting the bath.
   d. Close the door, pull the curtain, and close all windows to provide privacy and reduce heat loss via convection.
   e. Offer to toilet the patient. Doing so addresses the urge to void that might be stimulated by bathing.
   f. Position a bath blanket over the patient, and remove the top linen from under the bath blanket. Expose only those areas being washed, rinsed, or dried. Doing so provides privacy, comfort, and warmth.
   g. Encourage independence but assist the patient as needed. Self-care supports self-esteem and increases circulation and range of motion.
   h. Use warm, not hot, water to promote vasodilation and prevent dry skin caused by hot water, which excessively removes sebum.
   i. Change water when cool, soiled, or soapy. Doing so promotes vasodilation, supports comfort, and minimizes contamination.

Box 16.2 Safety and Comfort Measures Implemented After Hygiene Care

- Leave the bed in the lowest position.
- Position the call bell within the patient's reach.
- Place the overbed table within easy reach with fresh water, tissues, and other desired items.
- Provide additional blankets if desired by the patient.

j. Make a bath mitt with a washcloth by laying a hand on the washcloth, folding one side over the hand then the other, folding the top down across the hand, and tucking it under the folded edge at the wrist (Fig. 16.3). Doing so retains water and heat and prevents the ends from being tossed about, contaminating the environment.

k. Wash (softens dirt and debris), rinse (removes debris and soap), and dry (removes moisture that supports microbial growth) each part of the body.

l. Reposition the patient in functional alignment to support comfort and reduce stress and strain on bones, joints, muscles, ligaments, and tendons.

m. Discard soiled towels, washcloths, and bath water; clean the basin and return it to the patient's bedside table. Doing so maintains medical aseptic technique and prepares equipment for future use.

n. Evaluate and document the patient's outcomes and tolerance of the activity. Doing so ensures that the patient's status is evaluated and information is communicated to other health-care team members.

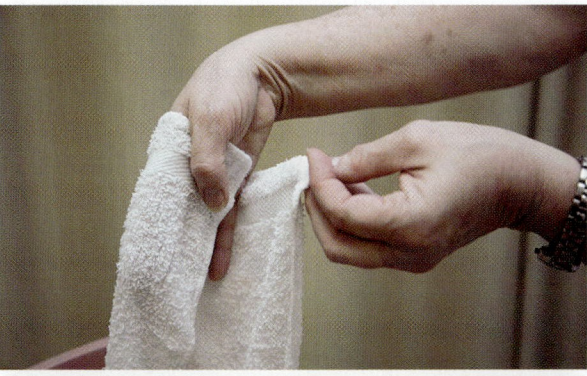
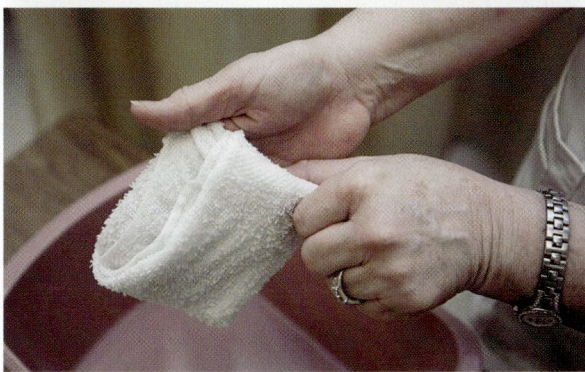

Fig 16.3 Bath mitt. (From Burton and Ludwig [2011]. *Fundamentals of nursing care: Concepts, connections & skills.* Philadelphia: F. A. Davis Company, with permission.)

MAKING THE CONNECTION

Providing Hygiene Care and Making Nursing Assessments

There is no better time to assess body systems than during the administration of a bath. During this activity, the nurse not only has an opportunity to assess the patient's skin, mucous membranes, hair, and nails, but the nurse may be directed to a more focused assessment in response to an unexpected observation. For example, the nurse may identify an impairment in cognition (e.g., altered level of consciousness, impaired problem-solving ability, inability to follow directions), mobility impairment (e.g., inability to turn and move as expected, presence of fatigue, or weakness), or altered respiratory status (e.g., shortness of breath on exertion, activity intolerance). After identifying an unexpected response, the nurse should make a more detailed assessment of the related system. In addition to the opportunity to make focused assessments, the time spent performing personal care also affords patients the opportunity to share emotions and concerns that they might not have expressed otherwise. Lastly, it is an ideal time to establish a professional rapport with the patient and support the development of trust in the caregiver.

2. Bathing methods and related nursing care.
   a. Complete bed bath: Involves washing, rinsing, and drying a patient's entire body; may be performed independently or with some or total assistance from a caregiver (who addresses areas that the patient cannot reach, such as the back and feet).
      (1) Start at the head and work down the body; moves from clean to dirty.
      (2) Cleanse the far side of the body first, then the near side; prevents contamination of the clean side of the body by a dripping washcloth.
      (3) Wash the face with plain water, beginning with the eyes from inner to outer canthus; avoids soap, which has a drying effect and can irritate the eyes, and minimizes secretions entering lacrimal duct by moving from inner to outer canthus.
      (4) Use a different side of the washcloth for each eye to reduce the risk of transferring microorganisms from one eye to the other.
      (5) Wash, rinse, and dry the face, ears, and neck.
      (6) Place a towel under one upper extremity and wash, rinse, and dry the arm, axillae, and hand; stroke from distal to proximal (Fig. 16.4). Repeat for the other arm. Use of a towel keeps the bed dry and stroking from distal to proximal promotes venous blood return.

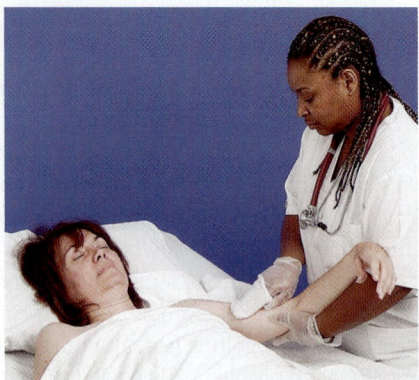

Fig 16.4 Washing an upper extremity distal to proximal. (From Burton and Ludwig [2011]. *Fundamentals of nursing care: Concepts, connections & skills.* Philadelphia: F. A. Davis Company, with permission.)

(7) Rest the patient's hand in the washbasin if hand or nails are excessively soiled to loosen dirt.

(8) Apply deodorant or antiperspirant per patient preference to reduce the risk of body odor.

(9) Wash, rinse, and dry the chest and then abdomen while exposing only the area being bathed.

(10) Clean and dry under the breasts of women or men with enlarged breasts due to obesity or gynecomastia to minimize risk of odor and skin irritation.

(11) Place a towel under a lower extremity and wash, rinse, and dry, stroking from distal to proximal. Repeat for the other leg and foot.

(12) Rest the patient's foot in the washbasin if foot or toenails are excessively soiled to loosen dirt. (Fig. 16.5)

(13) Change the water and provide perineal care. See the section "Perineal Care" later in this chapter, page 453.

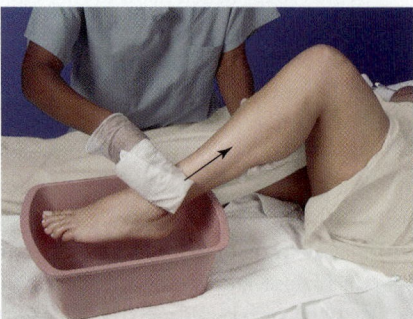

Fig 16.5 Washing the feet. (From Burton and Ludwig [2011]. *Fundamentals of nursing care: Concepts, connections & skills.* Philadelphia: F. A. Davis Company, with permission.)

(14) Change the water before moving to the patient's back. Doing so ensures clean, warm water and prevents contamination.

(15) Turn the patient on the side and place a towel on the bed along back and buttocks.

(16) Wash, rinse, and dry the back and then the buttocks; moves from clean to dirty.

(17) Provide a backrub if not contraindicated. See the section "Back Rub" in Chapter 23, "Pain, Comfort, Rest, and Sleep," page 729. Doing so increases local circulation, promotes relaxation, and supports comfort.

(18) Assist the patient with grooming (e.g., oral care, shaving, hair care).

(19) Put a clean gown on the patient, and make the bed with clean linens; remove the bath blanket from under the clean top sheet.

b. Partial bed bath: Generally includes body areas that have secretions or excretions, cause an odor, are at risk for skin breakdown and infection, or need to be freshened for the day.

(1) Wash the patient's face, hands, axillae, back, perineal area, and under the breasts (for women and men with enlarged breasts). Doing so cleanses essential areas of the body while conserving the patient's energy.

(2) Follow the progression indicated in a complete bed bath to adhere to the principle of clean to dirty.

c. Bath-in-a-bag: Includes a package of 8 to 10 disposable washcloths premoistened with a no-rinse surfactant, diluent substance to trap moisture (humectant), and an emollient; proven to reduce overall skin dryness, skin flaking, and scaling; preferred in critical care and long-term care settings because it is less physically stressful for patients.

(1) Use a microwave or warming unit to warm washcloths to 105°F, following the manufacturer directions.

🛑 (2) Ensure that washcloths are not too hot before use to prevent unintentional burns.

(3) Use one washcloth for each area of the body to follow the concept of clean to dirty, which prevents cross-contamination.

(4) Do not rinse to prevent removal of the emollient.

(5) Allow each area to air dry to ensure that the emollient and skin protectant remain on the skin surface.

d. Blanket/towel bath: Involves placing a bath blanket, towel, and washcloth in a plastic bag and saturating them with a commercially prepared solution of disinfectant, nonrinse cleaning agent, moisturizer, and water and then warming according to manufacturer's directions; proven to provide patient satisfaction and takes less time than a traditional bath; commonly a method of choice for patients with mild to moderate impaired skin integrity, activity intolerance, or cognitive impairment.

(1) Follow agency procedure or manufacturer's directions for the amount of water and products to add to the bag with the bath blanket, towel, and washcloth and warm according to the directions. Doing so ensures that appropriate products and equipment are added, avoids excessive suds, and ensures that the temperature is not too warm.

(2) Place a dry bath blanket over the patient to provide for privacy and protect the patient from drafts.

(3) Replace the dry blanket with the fan-folded wet blanket. Starting at the neck, move the dry blanket down while unfolding the fan-folded wet blanket until the patient is completely covered from the neck to the feet with the wet blanket.

(4) Wash the patient with the wet blanket, moving progressively from the feet to the legs, abdomen, and chest. Fold up the wet blanket as you move from the feet toward the chest and replace it with the dry blanket as you work. Doing so ensures that the principle of clean to dirty is maintained because different parts of the wet blanket are used for each body part and the wet blanket is folded and replaced with the dry blanket as the bath progresses.

(5) Wash the face with plain water, beginning with the eyes from inner to outer canthus. This avoids soap, which has a drying affect and can irritate the eyes; minimizes secretions from entering lacrimal duct by moving from inner to outer canthus.

(6) Use a different side of the washcloth for each eye to reduce the risk of transferring microorganisms from one eye to the other.

(7) Wash, rinse, and dry the face, ears, and neck.

(8) Don gloves to protect self from the patient's blood or body fluids.

(9) Turn the patient on his or her side, unfold the wet bath towel over the patient's back and buttocks, and wash the back and buttocks.

(10) Remove gloves, wash hands, don clean gloves, reposition the patient, and then provide perineal care. For more information, see the section "Perineal Care" on this page.

e. Shower and tub baths: Require an order because the extent of exposure to warm water causes vasodilation and requires more patient effort and energy than other bathing methods; may be ordered as therapeutic baths, such as oatmeal baths, for patients with skin conditions or hydrotherapy-type baths after a burn injury.

(1) Shower: Patient stands or sits on a shower chair under a continuous flow of water.

(2) Tub bath: Involves immersion in a tub of water; provides more thorough washing and rinsing than other types of baths; generally requires a transfer in a chair lift or bathing stretcher to the tub.

(3) Nursing care.

(a) Ensure that the shower or tub is clean before and after use to prevent cross-contamination.

(b) Ensure a nonskid area around the tub or shower, such as by not using a towel on the floor, to promote safety and prevent a fall.

(c) Hang an "in-use" sign outside the tub or shower room to support privacy.

(d) Explain to the patient the steps in the transfer procedure to reduce anxiety and support a sense of control.

(e) Use a shower chair if the patient has activity intolerance. Secure the patient in a transfer chair or stretcher to ensure a safe transfer.

(f) Assist the patient in entering and exiting the shower or tub. Doing so widens the base of support to help prevent a fall.

(g) Encourage the use of handrails and grab bars to facilitate movement and help prevent a fall.

(h) Ensure that the water temperature is no higher than 115°F to avoid unintentional burns.

🛑 (i) Stay with the patient or wait on the other side of a curtain throughout the shower or bath, depending on the patient's ability to be independent and safe.

(j) Limit a bath to 20 minutes to prevent prolonged exposure to warm water, which can cause vasodilation and dizziness, precipitating a fall.

D. Perineal Care (Female and Male)

1. Involves washing the area from the symphysis pubis to the anus.

2. Performed a minimum of once daily, usually as part of a complete or partial bed bath.

3. Performed as often as necessary because of incontinence of urine or feces, profuse diaphoresis, or urethral, vaginal, or rectal discharge.
4. Requires use of a firm but gentle touch to minimize stimulation.
5. Nursing care.
   a. Gather clean, warm water; a towel; and a washcloth to prevent having to interrupt the procedure later to gather additional equipment.
   b. Explain what is to be done and close the door and curtain around the patient's bed. Doing so provides information and maintains the patient's privacy.
   🛑 c. **Don clean gloves to protect self from the patient's body fluids.**
   d. Position the patient for the procedure to access the site that requires hygiene care.
      (1) Female: Place the patient in the supine position with the knees bent and the feet flat on the bed.
      (2) Male: Place the patient in the supine position with the hips and knees extended.
   e. Drape the patient for the procedure to provide for warmth, comfort, and privacy.
      (1) Female: Arrange a bath blanket over the patient in a diamond position with one point at the head, one at the feet, and one point at each side; wrap a side point of the bath blanket around each leg and foot; then drape the point at the feet over the perineal area, where it can be lifted up and folded back (Fig. 16.6).
      (2) Male: Position the bath blanket above the patient's waist and the bed linens over the legs from the thighs to the feet.
   f. Cleanse the perineal area with soap and water using a different side of the wash cloth for each

stroke and cleaning the area of the urinary meatus first and then progressing to more soiled perineal areas. Doing so prevents contamination of clean areas with a soiled part of the washcloth and adheres to the principle of clean to dirty. Soap and water removes thick, cheesy odoriferous secretion of sebaceous glands, desquamated epithelial cells, and mucus (**smegma**), under the loose skin at the end of the penis (**foreskin, prepuce**) of a male or under the labia minora and around the clitoris of the female and minimizes bacterial growth.
(1) Female.
   (a) Spread the labia with one hand and wash the far side, near side, and then down the middle of the vulva from the urinary meatus to the anus, using a separate part of the wash cloth for each stroke (Fig. 16.7); repeat until clean.
   (b) Rinse the vulva using the same principles of clean to dirty.
   (c) Pat dry with a clean towel.
(2) Male.
   (a) Begin with the penile head; retract the foreskin (if uncircumcised) and wash in a circular motion around the tip of the penis and glans and then working down the shaft toward the suprapubic area (Fig. 16.8); repeat until clean.
   (b) Rinse the penis using the same principles of clean to dirty.
   (c) Pat dry with a clean towel.
   🛑 (d) Return the foreskin to its natural position over the glans penis if the patient is uncircumcised to prevent constriction of blood flow that may precipitate edema, pain, and even necrosis of the glans penis.
   (e) Spread the patient's legs and gently wash, rinse, and pat dry the scrotum.

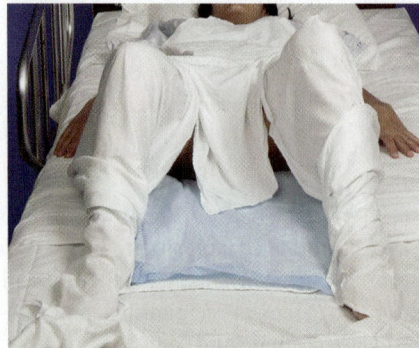

Fig 16.6 Draping a female patient for perineal care. (From Burton and Ludwig [2011]. *Fundamentals of nursing care: Concepts, connections & skills.* Philadelphia: F. A. Davis Company, with permission.)

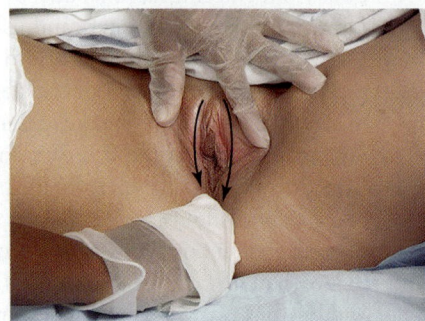

Fig 16.7 Cleansing the labia. (From Burton and Ludwig [2011]. *Fundamentals of nursing care: concepts, Connections & skills.* Philadelphia: F. A. Davis Company, with permission.)

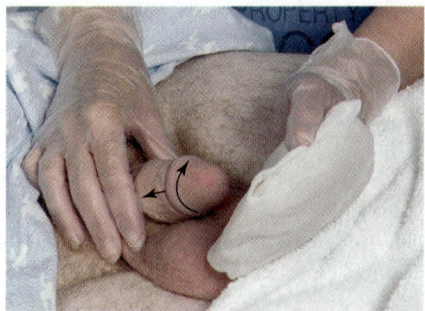

Fig 16.8 Male perineal care. (From Burton and Ludwig [2011]. *Fundamentals of nursing care: Concepts, connections & skills.* Philadelphia: F. A. Davis Company, with permission.)

f. Turn the patient on the side and wash, rinse, and dry the buttocks and then the anus; work from the urinary meatus toward the anus; this follows the principle of clean to dirty.

g. Assess the area for skin breakdown due to contact with urine and feces.

h. Clean a urinary retention catheter if present.

(1) Hold the catheter with one hand close to the urinary meatus and wash with soap and water down the tubing in a circular motion away from the meatus toward the distal end of the catheter; repeat until clean. Doing so avoids traction on the catheter, preventing trauma to the urethra, and follows the principle of clean to dirty.

(2) Rinse and dry tubing to remove moisture minimizes the growth of microorganisms.

i. Continue with the rest of the bath if perineal care is part of a complete bed bath.

E. Foot Care

1. Involves cleaning the feet from the ankles to the toes.

2. Performed as part of a complete bed bath.

3. The feet should be assessed before and reassessed after care; compare assessments for symmetry.

a. Bilateral dorsalis pedis pulses.

b. Temperature and color of skin and toenails.

c. Capillary refill.

d. Movement and sensation.

4. Nursing care.

a. Maintain standard precautions because of the potential to be exposed to impaired skin, particularly if the patient has health problems such as peripheral vascular disease or diabetes.

b. Position the patient in a sitting position in bed or a chair; soak each foot for 5 to 10 minutes at a time in a basin of warm water (105°F to 110°F) that is positioned on a waterproof pad. Do not soak the feet of a patient with peripheral vascular disease or diabetes. Warm water softens dirt and promotes circulation and relaxation. However, it

also removes natural oils, promoting drying and cracking of the skin.

c. Wash, rinse, and dry each foot gently and thoroughly, especially between the toes, and then place feet on a clean pad or towel. Doing so cleanses the skin, removes irritating soap, and prevents skin maceration. A clean surface provides a safe place on which to provide additional foot care.

d. Apply lotion to the feet but avoid areas between the toes and excessive amounts of lotion. Doing so lubricates the skin, but excessive amounts can cause skin maceration, especially if applied between the toes.

e. Provide a bed cradle if the patient has a foot problem to raise linens off the legs and feet, relieving pressure and supporting comfort.

f. Teach the patient precautions to protect the feet.

(1) Assess the feet daily using a mirror, visit a podiatrist routinely, and notify a primary health-care provider if a problem is identified.

(2) Wear well-supporting shoes when out of bed, and ensure that linings and surfaces of shoes are smooth and intact.

(3) Wear socks without seams.

(4) Avoid excessively soaking the feet and dry between the toes well.

(5) Have toenails cut by a podiatrist to ensure professional assessment and care.

(6) Avoid self-treatment of corns, calluses, and other problems with over-the-counter remedies.

F. Oral Care

1. Involves maintaining the integrity of a patient's oral mucous membranes, teeth, gums, tongue, and lips. Includes caring for dentures if present.

2. Performed as part of a partial or complete bed bath, before and after meals, and in the a.m. and p.m.

3. Provided more frequently for patients who are on nothing-by-mouth (NPO) status, mouth breathing, receiving oxygen, or have a nasogastric tube because these situations contribute to dry mucous membranes and collection of bacteria and thick, sticky secretions on the tongue, teeth, and lips (**sordes**).

4. The oral mucosa, teeth, gums, and lips should be assessed for color (pink), extent of tissue hydration (moist), and presence of lesions (absence of lesions).

5. Products based on the patient's preference should be used (e.g., toothbrush, toothpaste, mouthwash, and floss).

6. Oral care for a conscious patient.

a. Wash hands, and then don clean gloves. Doing so minimizes microorganisms on the hands and protects the caregiver from the patient's body fluids.

b. Place the patient in the Fowler's position to minimize the risk of aspiration.

c. Place a towel under the chin and across the patient's chest.

d. Apply a small amount of toothpaste on a moistened tooth brush to avoid excessive foaming and have the patient brush his or her own teeth if able; if unable, complete the procedure for the patient.

e. Instruct the patient to hold the brush at a 45-degree angle and brush the base of the teeth at the gum line with short, vibrating, circular motions; repeat for all surfaces where teeth contact gums. This dislodges plaque that adheres at the base of the tooth.

f. Instruct the patient to brush back and forth over biting surfaces as well as the tongue to dislodge food debris, plaque, and sordes from crevices of teeth and on the tongue.

g. Instruct the patient to rinse the mouth with water or mouthwash and spit (expectorate) it into an emesis basin.

h. Floss the teeth by stretching the floss between the fingers and sliding the floss between two teeth down to the gum line; then move the floss with an up and down motion several times. Use a systematic progression to include all teeth. Doing so loosens and removes debris between teeth and helps prevent the development of plaque.

i. Wipe the patient's mouth with a towel; clean the equipment and return it to the patient's bedside table.

j. Remove gloves and dispose in an appropriate trash container; wash hands.

7. Oral care for an unconscious patient.

a. Position the patient in the side-lying position with the head turned to the side to facilitate drainage of secretions and fluids used in oral care via gravity, which minimizes the risk of aspiration.

b. Place a towel under the patient's chin and across the pillow and mattress; position an emesis basin slightly under the patient's chin.

c. Wear gloves and a gown and face shield if splashing is likely to protect self from contact with the patient's body fluids.

d. Dip a gauze-covered tongue blade or sponge swab in half water and half mouthwash; swab the tongue, teeth, hard palate, and inside of the cheeks and the lips (Fig. 16.9). Gentle friction helps to loosen debris.

🛑 e. Avoid swabbing the last third of the back of the tongue to prevent stimulation of the gag reflex.

f. Rinse the oral cavity using a clean gauze-covered tongue blade or sponge swab.

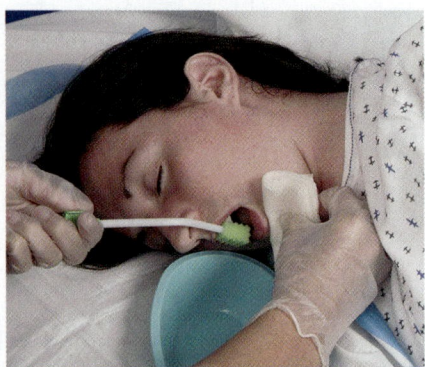

Fig 16.9 Oral care for an unconscious patient. (From Wilkinson and Treas [2011]. *Fundamentals of nursing*, Vol. 2, 2nd ed. Philadelphia: F. A. Davis Company, with permission.)

g. Do not leave the patient until all cleaning solution has drained from the patient's mouth to prevent aspiration.

🛑 h. Stop the procedure and suction the patient if the patient coughs or demonstrates signs of choking; do not leave the patient until the patient's respirations return to the patient's normal rate and rhythm. Doing so minimizes aspiration of solution into breathing passages and provides for patient safety.

8. Care of a patient with dentures.

a. Dentures should be removed and cleaned according to the patient's usual routine; usually removed, cleaned, and stored when sleeping and reinserted in the beginning of the day.

b. Dentures should be inspected for integrity and not be used if cracks or rough edges are present.

c. The mouth, especially the gums under dentures, should be assessed for redness, irritation, lesions, or signs of infection. Ensure that dentures are not loose or tight. Seek an order for a dental consult if there is a concern.

d. Removal of dentures.

(1) Encourage the patient to remove the dentures or remove the dentures for the patient if necessary.

(2) Remove the top denture before the bottom denture to ease removal of the larger top denture.

(3) With a gauze pad, grasp the upper denture with a thumb and forefinger and move the denture up and down to release suction. (Fig. 16.10)

(4) Use your thumbs to push up gently on the bottom denture at the gum line to release suction.

(5) Tilt the dentures vertically slightly when removing them from the mouth to avoid stretching the patient's lips.

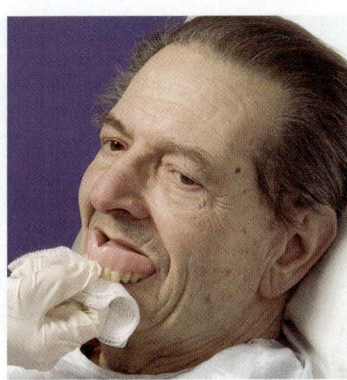

Fig 16.10 Removal of an upper denture. (From Wilkinson and Treas [2011]. *Fundamentals of nursing,* Vol. 2, 2nd ed. Philadelphia: F. A. Davis Company, with permission.)

e. Cleaning of dentures.
   (1) Transport dentures in an emesis basin or denture cup and wash them in a sink padded with a towel. Doing so minimizes risk of breaking the dentures if dropped.
   (2) Use denture cleaner, a soft toothbrush, and warm, not hot, water to clean dentures. Regular toothpaste and a firm toothbrush may be too abrasive. Denture material can warp or become sticky when exposed to hot water.
   (3) Brush gums and tongue with a soft toothbrush; assist to rinse mouth with water or dilute mouthwash.

f. Storage of dentures.
   (1) Soak dentures overnight in a labeled (patient's name and other identifying information) denture cup with dental cleanser and cool water per the patient's preference. This keeps dentures clean and white and prevents warping when stored in cool water.
   (2) Place the denture cup in the bedside table to help prevent loss.

g. Insertion of dentures.
   (1) Apply denture adhesive to the underside of the top denture if preferred by the patient to securely seal the denture to the hard palate and upper gum.
   (2) Tilt the top denture at a slight angle to ease insertion and press into place with a thumb on the palate to promote adherence.
   (3) Repeat with the bottom denture; press gently downward into place. This securely seals the bottom denture to the bottom gum.

G. Hair Care

1. Condition of hair can be a measure of physical and emotional health. See "Assessment of Hair" earlier in this chapter, page 445.

2. The scalp perspires and secretes oils, and hair is a perfect environment for the collection of secretions and dirt.

3. Hair care should include brushing/combing daily and shampooing weekly.

4. Nursing care.
   a. Brushing or combing hair.
      (1) Place a towel over the patient's shoulders.
      (2) Position the patient in the sitting position if able or, if not, the side-lying position.
      (3) Brush or comb hair beginning from distal ends in small sections moving up toward the scalp every 2 to 3 inches as tangles are removed. This removes tangles and stimulates scalp circulation. Attending to small sections and lengths at a time avoids scalp trauma and pain.
      (4) Style hair according to patient's preference; use hair clips or braid long hair per the patient's preference. Avoid inappropriate styles, such as pigtails for older adults. Hair clips or braiding helps prevent matting and facilitates movement in bed when a patient has long hair. Instituting patient preferences supports self-esteem, dignity, and a sense of control.
      (5) Provide additional interventions for hair that is dry, course, curly, or kinky in texture.
         (a) Apply mineral oil or a moisturizing hair cream before combing to lubricate hair and scalp, which limits tangles and matting.
         (b) Use a wide-tooth comb when combing hair to minimize breakage of hair.
      (6) Clean the brush or comb and store it in the bedside table; fold the towel into itself and place it in a linen hamper.
   b. Shampooing hair.
      (1) Comb or brush the hair to remove tangles before shampooing.
      (2) Place the patient in the supine position.
      (3) Place a waterproof pad or plastic garbage bag on the bed, position a shampoo cradle under the patient's head, and place a towel around the patient's neck.
      (4) Position a trough over the side of the bed to a collection receptacle to direct water off the bed and contain it in a collection receptacle.
      (5) Have the patient protect the eyes by holding a towel over the eyes if able and wet the hair with warm water using a water pitcher.
      (6) Apply shampoo and then wash the hair, using products per the patient's preference.
      (7) Cover hair styled in cornrows or braids with a stocking cap and shampoo through the cap.

This cleans the hair while preserving the hair style.

(8) Massage the scalp with the fingertips to stimulate scalp circulation and promote relaxation.

(9) Double-rinse with warm water, and then apply a cream rinse per the patient's preference. Doing so removes shampoo, which may irritate and dry the scalp, causing itching.

(10) Dry hair well using a hair dryer if available.

(11) Comb hair and style according to the patient's preference to support self-esteem, a sense of control, and dignity.

(12) Replace soiled linens with clean linens; dispose of soiled linens in a linen hamper.

(13) Clean equipment and return to storage areas.

H. Shaving

1. Total or partial removal of hair from the face of a man is a personal preference.

   a. Some men consider it an important daily grooming measure.

   b. Some men do not shave because it is forbidden in their culture.

2. Grooming the hair on the face involves its removal or washing, combing, and trimming a beard or mustache.

3. The face and neck should be assessed for skin lesions, eczema, or ingrown hairs because these areas should be avoided during shaving or may be a contraindication for shaving.

4. Nursing care.

   a. Identify the type of razor to use; when possible, defer to the patient's preference.

   🛑 b. **Use an electric shaver if the patient is receiving an anticoagulant or has a low platelet count. Doing so prevents breaks in the skin that can result in excessive bleeding.**

   c. Don gloves to protect self from the patient's blood if shaving breaks the patient's skin.

   d. Use a disposable safety razor.

   (1) Position a warm washcloth on the beard for a few minutes to soften and lift whiskers.

   (2) Spread shaving cream over the beard and mustache area liberally to reduce skin irritation.

   (3) Hold the skin taut and shave in the direction that hair grows (Fig. 16.11). Doing so helps maintain the 45-degree angle of a safety razor blade to the skin, thereby preventing the blade from irritating the skin. This prevents irritation and ingrown hairs.

   (a) Shave cheeks down toward the ridge of the chin.

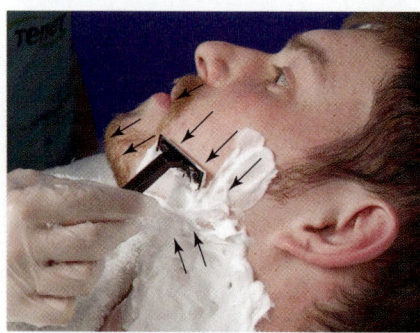

Fig 16.11 Shaving a patient. (From Wilkinson and Treas [2011]. *Fundamentals of nursing*, Vol. 2, 2nd ed. Philadelphia: F. A. Davis Company, with permission.)

   (b) Instruct the patient to position the upper lip over the teeth to increase access to the skin under the nose.

   (c) Shave down from nose to upper lip.

   (d) Shave down from lower lip to chin.

   (e) Shave neck upward to chin.

   (4) Shave the ridge of the chin carefully to minimize the potential for a cut because of its contour.

   (5) Place the disposable razor in a sharps container to reduce the risk of injury.

   (6) Wash the face with a washcloth to remove shaving cream and debris and then pat dry.

   (7) Apply aftershave lotion per the patient's preference to soothe irritated skin.

   e. Use an electric razor.

   (1) Apply preshave lotion to the beard and mustache area to soften and raise whiskers.

   (2) Hold skin taut and shave in the direction that hair grows to prevent ingrown hairs and skin irritation.

   (a) Use a circular motion to shave the cheeks.

   (b) Shave the mustache area in a downward motion.

   (c) Shave the neck in an upward circular motion.

   (3) Apply aftershave lotion per the patient's preference to soothe irritated skin.

   (4) Clean the razor: Remove the head, brush out debris with the small brush provided with the razor, replace the head, and return it to its storage container in the middle draw of the bedside table. Doing so minimizes growth of microorganisms and protects the razor from damage or loss.

   f. Care of a mustache and/or beard.

   (1) Ask the patient's permission to trim a beard or mustache and identify the extent of trimming according to the patient's preference. Doing so supports the patient's preference

and avoids removing too much of the mustache or beard.

(2) Secure signed consent if the patient wants a mustache or beard removed. This protects the caregiver if the patient should regret the change and blames the caregiver.

(3) Use a scissor or razor (disposable or electric) to trim a beard.

(a) Comb a mustache straight down and trim the length just above the upper lip.

(b) Trim the line of a beard so that it is clearly defined.

I. Nail Care

1. Nails are hardened, horny cutaneous plates overlying the dorsal surface of the ends of fingers and toes.
2. Nails grow continuously and should be groomed during a complete bed bath.
3. Nails should be assessed for splitting, cracking, thickening, discoloration, presence of ingrown nails, and clinical manifestations of inflammation or infection around the nail.
4. Nursing care.
   a. Soak the patient's hands or feet in a basin of warm water for 5 minutes to soften nails and cuticles.
   b. Dry hands and feet well, especially between digits to prevent skin maceration and infection.
   c. Use a washcloth or the flat end of an orange stick to gently push back the cuticle; use the pointed end to gently clean under the nails.
   d. Use an emery board to gently file nail edges if permitted by agency policy and procedure. Doing so removes sharp edges, which prevents scratches (Fig. 16.12).
   e. Apply moisturizing lotion to the hands and feet but not between toes. Lotion makes skin soft and supple and avoiding between toes prevents skin maceration and infection.
   f. Seek a referral for a podiatrist for care of toenails, especially for people who have diabetes or vascular occlusive disease. Doing so avoids causing a break in the skin or an ingrown toenail if toenails are clipped too short, which could precipitate an injury or foot ulcer.

J. Care of a Patient With a Hearing Aid

1. A hearing aid is a device that is placed in the external auditory canal; it magnifies sound to improve hearing.
2. The type of hearing aid used by a patient must be identified (Fig. 16.13).
3. Hearing aids should be inspected for cracks, broken cords, or torn ear molds; a device should not be reinserted if it is not intact.
4. Removal of a hearing aid.
   a. Turn off the hearing aid and remove it from the patient's ear.
   b. Wipe the hearing aid with a damp cloth and dry well.
   c. Remove earwax that may be in the small opening in the ear piece using the cleaning instrument provided by the manufacturer. If the device has a screen or filter to block earwax, gently tap the aid against a clean cloth on a table to remove earwax.
   d. Separate the ear mold from the hearing aid if possible; clean the ear mold with mild, warm,

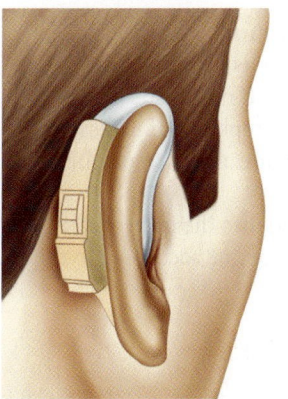
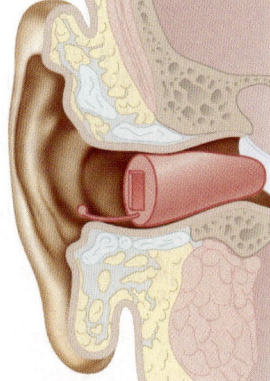

Behind the ear   **A**   In the ear canal   **B**

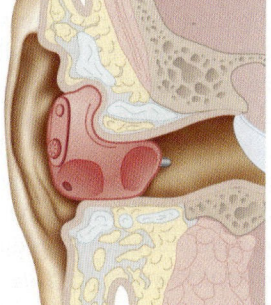

In the ear   **C**

Fig 16.13 Types of Hearing Aids. (A) Behind the ear. (B) In the ear canal. (C) In the ear. (From Burton and Ludwig [2011]. *Fundamentals of nursing care: Concepts, connections & skills.* Philadelphia: F. A. Davis Company, with permission.)

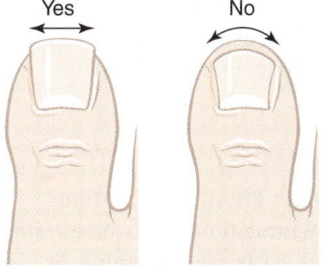

Yes   No

Fig 16.12 Filing nails. (From Wilkinson and Treas [2011]. *Fundamentals of nursing,* Vol. 2, 2nd ed. Philadelphia: F. A. Davis Company, with permission.)

soapy water and then dry it well to minimize the risk of an ear infection.

e. Clean the external auditory canal with a washcloth wrapped around a finger; rinse and dry well.

f. Inspect the ear for any signs or symptoms of irritation, infection, sores, or drainage; notify the primary health-care provider if any are present and do not reinsert the ear mold or hearing aid until the patient is assessed by the primary health-care provider.

5. Storage of a hearing aid.
   a. Remove the battery and store the hearing aid it in its case, which generally is a labeled, moisture-control container. This prolongs battery life.
   b. Place the case in the patient's bedside drawer to protect it from moisture, damage, or loss.
   c. Avoid contact with moisture to prevent impaired functioning of the hearing aid.

6. Insertion of a hearing aid.
   a. Identify whether the hearing aid or mold is labeled right or left to ensure that the correct hearing aid or ear mold is inserted into the correct ear.
   b. Check the battery by turning on the device, turning the volume to its highest capacity, and listening for a whistle. If no whistle occurs, check the battery and replace it if necessary.
   c. Turn down the volume and turn off the hearing aid.
   d. Insert the hearing aid into the correct ear; turn it on and adjust the volume according to the patient's preference.

VI. Providing Hygiene for Patients With Special Needs

Nurses should provide hygiene to or assist all patients with hygiene-related activities every day and whenever needed. The challenges of these activities increase when patients have issues that interfere with understanding what is being done, are unable to participate with the activities, or have unique physical or physiological needs.

A. Patients With Impaired Cognitive Ability

1. May be unaware of the need for hygiene care, unable to remember how to bathe and groom oneself, or unable able to follow directions.
2. Includes unconscious patients.
3. Nursing care.
   a. Assess the patient's ability to comprehend what is to be done and the ability to participate in care.
   b. Teach the benefits and risks of hygiene and grooming activities if the patient is receptive to teaching.

c. Administer prescribed analgesic or anxiolytics to promote relaxation.

d. Postpone bathing if the patient is agitated to prevent escalation of the agitation.

e. Use a bath-in-bag product if available. Doing so limits the perception that interventions are threatening and is quicker to use than a traditional bath.

f. Use simple commands in short phrases and avoid multiple or complicated directions to support understanding.

g. Avoid using mouthwash to prevent it from being swallowed.

🛑 h. Avoid putting hands in the patient's mouth to reduce the risk of caregiver injury.

🛑 i. Apply an eye lubricant and tape the eyes closed or apply an eye shield for an unconscious patient or for a patient who has an absent blink reflex when preparing for sleep. Eye care should be provided every 2 to 4 hours and when necessary. Doing so protects the cornea and delicate mucous membranes of the eye from becoming dry.

B. Patients With Physiological Impairments

1. Causes of impairments.
   a. Physiological problems that affect the neuro-musculoskeletal system, such as immobility due to a brain attack or multiple sclerosis.
   b. Lack of energy due to anemia or a chronic debilitating disease, such as chronic obstructive pulmonary disease.
   c. Pain from surgery or disease processes that impair ability to move.

2. Nursing care.
   a. Assess the patient's overall strength, hand grasp strength, balance, flexibility, coordination, ability to sit unsupported, range of motion, dexterity, and activity tolerance. This assessment helps to determine which aspects of care can be implemented independently and which require assistance.
   b. Encourage independence but provide assistance to complete tasks the patient is unable to complete; provide assistive devices, such as a padded handle on a brush, as indicated to promote independence and support self-esteem.
   c. Provide prescribed pain medication if indicated to reduce pain, which will enable the patient to participate in the activities.

🛑 d. Pace care and provide rest periods to conserve energy and prevent activity intolerance.

C. Patients With Physical Limitations

1. Physical limitations, such as restraints; casts; traction; nasogastric, gastrostomy, or urinary retention catheters; and surgical drains, may interfere with a patient's ability to provide self-care.

2. Nursing care.
   a. Identify the presence of equipment and how it interferes with independence. This assessment determines what activities may require adjustments to meet the patient's hygiene needs without interrupting a therapeutic modality.
   b. Identify the number of caregivers necessary to provide required care to ensure that the safety of the patient and caregivers is maintained.
   c. Provide specific interventions depending on the physical limitation.
      (1) Casts: Protect cast edges with plastic wrap to keep the cast from getting wet during a bath.
      (2) Restraints: Remove only one wrist or mitt restraint at a time while providing care to prevent the patient from injuring self or caregivers.
      (3) Traction.
         🛑 (a) Do not release weights because weights maintain the pull of traction and therefore alignment of the bone.

         (b) Instruct the patient to sit forward to provide access to the patient's back for administering care.
         (c) Instruct the patient to use the trapeze to lift the body off the mattress to provide access to the patient's buttocks for administering care.

D. Patients With Impaired Vision
   1. A visually impaired patient may be challenged when managing the environment and providing for self-care safely.
   2. Nursing care.
      a. Determine the extent of the patient's visual impairment and how it impacts on self-care. Assessment allows for appropriate planning of care.
      b. Describe the location of items in the environment, especially the bedside call bell and nurse alert cord in the bathroom to reduce anxiety and support safety.
      c. Describe the location of items on the overbed table using the numbers on a clock to support independence which promotes self-esteem.
      d. Remain nearby when the patient is providing self-care to support safety.
      e. Assist with activities that the patient is unable to complete.

E. Patients With Impaired Mental Health
   1. Patients with mental illness may be unaware of the need for hygiene; lack the energy to engage in hygiene activities (e.g., with depression); or not take the time to engage in hygiene activities (e.g., with bipolar disorder, manic episode).

2. A person with a mental illness may experience an altered state of reality, such as delusions or hallucinations; paranoia; inability to make decisions; or moderate or severe anxiety that interferes with the ability to provide for one's own hygiene and grooming.
3. Nursing care.
   a. Assess the patient's feelings, mood, and behavior and how they may impact on the performance of hygiene activities. Assessment allows for appropriate planning of care.
   b. Administer prescribed analgesics or anxiolytics before starting care to minimize the patient's anxiety.
   c. Speak calmly using a soft tone; use unhurried, slow motions to limit the perception that actions are threatening.
   d. Provide a bath-in-a-bag or towel bath. Doing so minimizes stress of the procedure, is less threatening, and is quicker to use than a traditional bath.

   🛑 e. Postpone activities if the patient is agitated to prevent escalation of the agitation.

   🛑 f. Avoid touching an angry, hostile, or paranoid patient to provide hygiene care. Doing so prevents an escalation of the patient's feelings or behavior because touching the patient may be perceived as a threat.

F. Patients Who Are Older Adults
   1. A decline in physical mobility and a natural tendency toward thin, dryer skin are common with aging. (See Fig. 16.2., page 448.)
   2. Nursing care.
      a. Assess patient's ability to perform hygiene activities. Assessment allows for appropriate planning of care.
      b. Assess indicators of skin breakdown daily to ensure early identification and intervention.
      c. Bathe less often than every day unless absolutely necessary to limit drying skin.
      d. Use a bath-in-a-bag or towel bath. Doing so limits drying skin because these methods are gentler than washing with soap and water and usually contain an emollient.
      e. Pat rather than rub skin dry to avoid abrasions and skin tears.
      f. Apply moisturizer/emollients to make skin supple and less dry.
      g. Allow the patient to progress at own pace due to developmental decline in mobility. Doing so reduces stress, conserves the patient's energy, and prevents activity intolerance.

G. Patients With Body Piercings
   1. Body piercing is the insertion of barbells, rings, or precious stones in a setting into skin or mucous membranes.

2. Piercings can be found in such areas as around the eyebrow, external ear, nose, lip, umbilicus, tongue, and genitalia.
3. Nursing care.
   a. Assess the sites of piercings for clinical manifestations of inflammation or infection, such as redness, discomfort, swelling, and drainage. Assessment provides for early identification of a problem.
   b. Identify the way in which the patient usually provides self-care; refer to the agency's procedure manual for details (generally, soap and water or alcohol is used to cleanse sites). Doing so limits microorganisms at the site of piercing, preventing infection.

DID YOU KNOW?

Piercings have to be removed because they can interfere with magnetic resonance imaging (MRI) and surgery (e.g., a tongue barbell may interfere with the insertion of an endotracheal tube). Most piercings have at least one end that can be unscrewed to allow removal. These sites close in a few days; therefore, piercings must be reinserted as soon as possible.

VII. Bedmaking

A bed is the patient's most immediate environment. The linens on the bed usually are changed daily as part of morning care or as needed if they become wet or soiled. The pillow and draw sheet should be changed daily, even if the other linens are not because they are a reservoir for microorganisms. Linens include flat sheets or fitted sheets. Flat sheets require specific techniques to secure them to the mattress and limit wrinkles and are discussed in this section.

A. Making an Unoccupied Bed

1. Wear gloves if the risk of exposure to blood or body fluids is present.
2. Loosen tucked-in linen and fold it into itself; carry it positioned away from the body, and place it in a linen hamper. These actions contain soiled linen while avoiding contaminating the caregiver's uniform.
3. Place a clean bottom sheet on the bed and unfold it lengthwise so the center crease is along the center of the bed to ensure that enough clean linen will be available to cover the sides of the bed.
4. Avoid shaking or fluffing linens to avoid raising microorganisms into air currents unnecessarily.
5. Line up the edge of the bottom sheet at the edge of the mattress at the foot of the bed to allow more linen to be tucked in at the head of the bed.
6. Tuck the bottom sheet at the top of the bed under the mattress. This secures the sheet making it less likely to be displaced when the head of the bed is raised.

7. Make mitered corners on the bottom sheet at the head of the bed. Securing the bottom sheet helps to eliminate wrinkles, which can cause pressure, injuring skin, and be uncomfortable.
   a. Pick up the top edge of the sheet or spread about 12 to 18 inches from the end of the bed; lift it on top of the mattress (Fig. 16.14a).
   b. Tuck the sheet hanging below the mattress under the mattress (Fig. 16.14b).
   c. Lift the sheet off the top of the mattress and let it hang free on the side of the bed if it is a top sheet or spread (Fig. 16.14c); tuck in under the mattress along the entire side of the bed if it is a bottom sheet.
8. Spread a draw sheet across the center of the bed and secure it tightly under the mattress on both sides of the bed to help secure the bottom sheet in place.
9. Unfold the top sheet 4 inches down from the head of the bed with the center fold in the center of the bed; open up the sheet and let it hang free over the sides and bottom of the bed. This ensures that there is enough linen on each side and bottom of the bed.

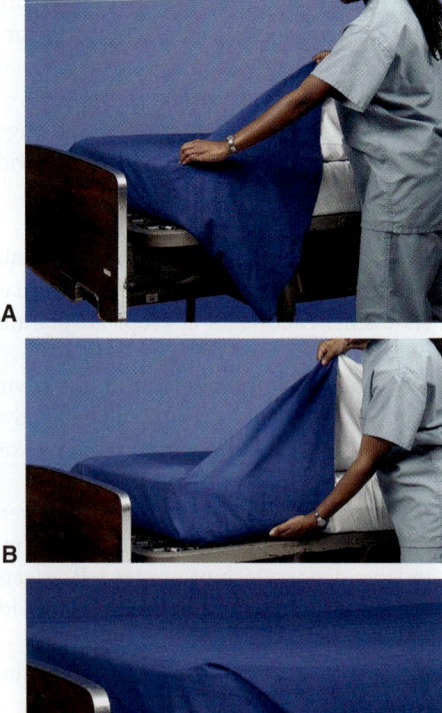

Fig 16.14 Mitered corner. (From Burton and Ludwig [2011]. *Fundamentals of nursing care: Concepts, connections & skills.* Philadelphia: F. A. Davis Company, with permission.)

10. Unfold a spread with the center fold in the center of the bed; position it 8 inches from the top of the top sheet; open up the spread and let it hang free over the sides and bottom of the bed; fold the top sheet over the top edge of the spread.

11. Tuck both the top sheet and spread under the mattress at the foot of the bed on each side of the bed. Make a mitered corner with the top sheet and blanket or spread on both sides at the bottom of the bed; do not tuck it in as with the bottom sheet, but let it hang free (modified mitered corner) (Fig. 16.14c).

12. Make a toe pleat by raising the top linen and making a 2-inch fold down by the feet (Fig. 16.15). Doing so allows for movement of the patient's feet and prevents tight fitting linens from causing footdrop or pressure sores on the toes or heels.

13. Put on a pillowcase: Grasp the closed end of the pillowcase and turn the pillowcase inside out over the same hand holding it; with the same hand gasp the pillow in the middle of one end and slide the pillowcase down over the pillow with the other hand. Position the pillow at the head of the bed. Pillow cases generally harbor the most microorganisms because of the secretions of the nose and mouth.

B. Making an Occupied Bed

1. Raise the side rail on the nonworking side of the bed to prevent the patient from rolling off the bed.

2. Turn the patient toward the nonworking side of the bed.

3. Position the pillow under the patient's head to support functional alignment and prevents unnecessary strain on the neck muscles.

4. Unfold a bath blanket over the patient and remove the top linens from under the bath blanket. Doing so provides for privacy and supports comfort and warmth.

5. Loosen the soiled bottom linen and fan-fold it toward the patient, tucking it just under the legs, buttocks, back, and shoulders (Fig. 16.16).

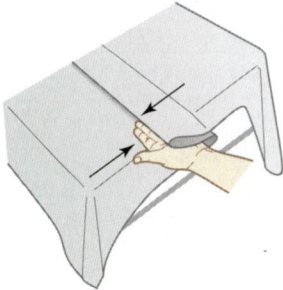

Fig 16.15 Toe pleat. (From Wilkinson and Treas [2011]. *Fundamentals of nursing*, Vol. 2, 2nd ed. Philadelphia: F. A. Davis Company, with permission.)

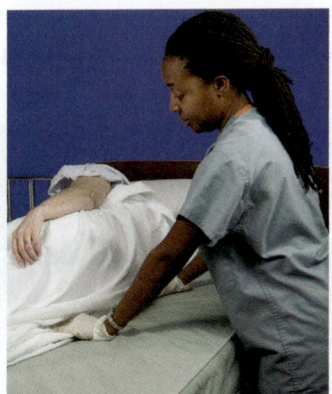

Fig 16.16 Fan-folding dirty linen. (From Wilkinson and Treas [2011]. *Fundamentals of nursing*, Vol. 2, 2nd ed. Philadelphia: F. A. Davis Company, with permission.)

6. Fanfold the clean linen up to just short of the edge of the soiled linen; it may be necessary to position a towel or pad between the soiled linen and clean linen (Fig. 16.17).

7. Raise the side rail and assist the patient to turn to the other side of the bed; explain that it may feel like rolling over a "hump;" position the pillow under the patient's head. This informs the patient about what to expect and maintains the patient's head in functional alignment.

8. Go to the other side of the bed, lower the rail and remove the soiled linen by rolling it up into itself, hold it away from the body, and dispose of it in a soiled hamper or laundry bag; do not put it on the floor or a chair. Doing so contains soiled linen and avoids contaminating the caregiver or the environment.

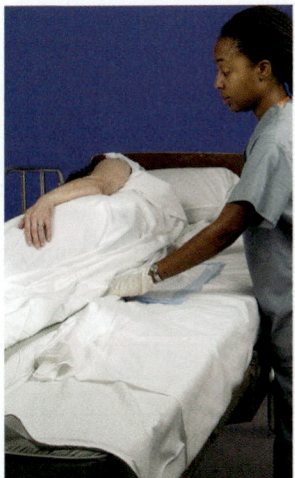

Fig 16.17 Fan-folding clean linen. (From Wilkinson and Treas [2011]. *Fundamentals of nursing*, Vol. 2, 2nd ed. Philadelphia: F. A. Davis Company, with permission.)

9. Pull through the clean linen from under the patient and finish making the bed (Fig. 16.18).

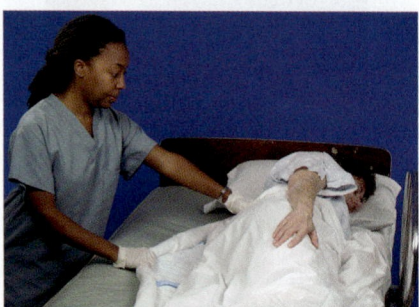

Fig 16.18 Pulling through clean linen. (From Wilkinson and Treas [2011]. *Fundamentals of nursing,* Vol. 2, 2nd ed. Philadelphia: F. A. Davis Company, with permission.)

10. Assist the patient to the supine position in the middle of the bed and then reposition the pillow under the patient's head.
11. Position the top sheet and spread over the bath blanket and remove the bath blanket from underneath.
12. Make the top of the bed and change the pillowcase as indicated in the procedure for an unoccupied bed.

CASE STUDY: Putting It All Together

A female primary nurse is admitting a 70-year-old Muslim woman to a medical unit at a local hospital after the patient was transferred from a nursing home to the emergency department. The patient states that she has chronic back pain as a result of an automobile accident 6 months ago and is unable to care for herself. She spends a lot of time in bed or in a wheelchair and says, "If I don't move much, the pain is tolerable, but if I move even just a little bit, the pain becomes unbearable." The patient was admitted for treatment of a large lesion at the base of the sacrum with exudate that has a foul odor and for pain management. The patient states, "I avoid using a bedpan because it is so uncomfortable to use so I wet myself. I am embarrassed to call for help, so I just stay wet."

Case Study Questions

A. What are the three most important things that the nurse should tell the patient when orienting the patient to her room and the hospital environment?

1. _____
2. _____
3. _____

B. Considering that the patient is a Muslim woman, what information is important to determine when assigning caregivers to this patient?

_____

C. List four components of a thorough assessment of the patient's sacral lesion.

1. _____
2. _____
3. _____
4. _____

CASE STUDY: Putting It All Together   *cont'd*

_____ **Case Study Questions** _____

D. List at least three concerns the nurse may have because of the patient's age and data.

1. _____

2. _____

3. _____

E. Identify at least four actions the nurse should implement when providing for this patient's hygiene needs.

1. _____

2. _____

3. _____

4. _____

REVIEW QUESTIONS

1. A nurse teaches a new nursing assistant to give a partial bed bath. The nurse identifies that the teaching is understood when the nursing assistant says, "When giving a partial bed bath, I should:
   1. help the patient to wash the face, hands, underarms, back, and perineal area."
   2. direct the patient to wash as much as possible and assist with the rest."
   3. instruct the patient to wash the face, hands, and perineal area."
   4. assist the patient to wash only one part of the body at a time."

2. A nurse educator is teaching a class about patient hygiene and grooming to nursing assistants. What problem can be prevented by daily brushing of the patient's hair that the nurse needs to include in the teaching?
   1. Pediculosis
   2. Dandruff
   3. Alopecia
   4. Tangles

3. A nurse is assessing a patient's ability to perform activities of daily living. Place the following classifications of self-care abilities in order from the most independent to the most dependent.
   1. Requires help from another person for assistance or supervision
   2. Requires help from another person and equipment or device
   3. Totally dependent; does not participate in activity
   4. Requires use of equipment or device
   5. Completely independent
   Answer: _____

4. A nurse finishes assisting a patient with a complete bed bath. What is **most** important for the nurse to do before leaving the patient's room, besides moving the bed to its lowest position?
   1. Secure the call bell within easy reach.
   2. Place the overbed table next to the bed.
   3. Leave the door to the patient's room open.
   4. Pull all the side rails up on both sides of the patient's bed.

5. A nurse is caring for a patient whose hair is dry and has a course texture with tight little curls. Which hair care implement is **most** appropriate to use when grooming this patient's hair?

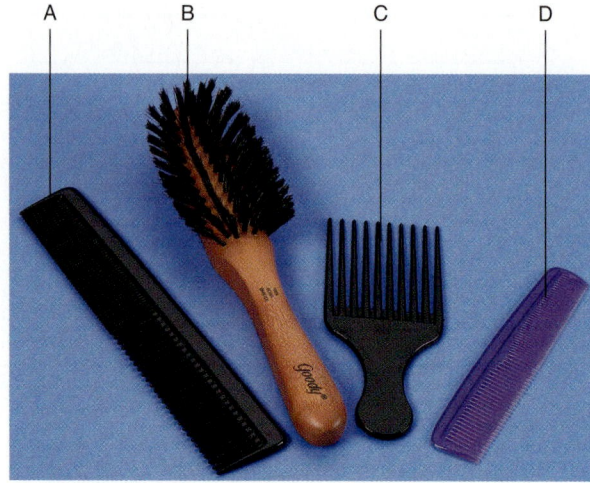

   1. A
   2. B
   3. C
   4. D

6. A nurse identifies clubbing when assessing a patient's hands. Which conclusion can the nurse make concerning this observation?
   1. The patient has liver disease.
   2. The patient has diabetes mellitus.
   3. The patient has a nutritional deficiency.
   4. The patient has a long-term oxygen deficit.

7. An adolescent with the diagnosis of severe nodular acne vulgaris is unresponsive to conventional therapy. The patient is registered in the government regulated iPledge program and the primary health-care provider prescribes isotretinoin (Claravis) 0.5 mg/kg PO daily divided into two doses. The adolescent weighs 132 lb. How many milligrams should the nurse administer for each dose?
   Answer: _____ mg

8. What action should the nurse include in the plan of care that is a common hygiene need of all older adults?
   1. Remove the bottom denture first.
   2. Assist with daily bathing.
   3. Apply a skin moisturizer.
   4. Use deodorant soap.

9. Which actions should be implemented when bathing a patient? **Select all that apply.**
    1. _____ Bathe head to toe.
    2. _____ Bathe clean to dirty.
    3. _____ Use contact precautions.
    4. _____ Use warm water for bathing.
    5. _____ Wash from proximal to distal for extremities.
    6. _____ Change the water after perineal care, not before.

10. Which is the **most** important nursing action when making an occupied bed?
    1. Change all of the linens on the bed.
    2. Make just one side of the bed at a time.
    3. Put the side rail up on the nonworking side of the bed.
    4. Lower the head of the bed until the patient is in the supine position.

11. How can a nurse **best** prevent footdrop in a patient when making an occupied bed?
    1. Tuck the top sheet in loosely.
    2. Make a toe pleat in the top linens.
    3. Place the pillow under the patient's ankles.
    4. Make a square corner when securing the patient's bottom sheet.

12. A nurse is providing oral care for a patient who is wearing full dentures. Which actions should the nurse implement when providing care for this patient? **Select all that apply.**
    1. _____ Clean dentures with cool water using a firm toothbrush and toothpaste.
    2. _____ Use thumbs to push up gently on the bottom denture at the gum line to release the suction.
    3. _____ Soak dentures overnight in a commercial dental cleanser if this is the preference of the patient.
    4. _____ Store dentures in a labeled dry denture cup in the bedside drawer if the patient does not want to wear them.
    5. _____ With a gauze pad, grasp the upper denture with the thumb and forefinger and move the denture up and down to release the suction.

13. Which should the nurse do **first** before initiating a.m. care with a patient?
    1. Ask the patient about preferences.
    2. Raise the bed to working height.
    3. Change the linens on the bed.
    4. Feed the patient breakfast.

14. An unconscious patient's mouth is dry and coated with sticky mucous from mouth breathing. Which actions are essential to prevent aspiration when providing oral care? **Select all that apply.**
    1. _____ Insert 30 mL of diluted mouthwash with a syringe into the side of the mouth to remove toothpaste.
    2. _____ Brush inner and outer teeth surfaces and the gum line with short circular motions.
    3. _____ Use a moderate amount of toothpaste to cleanse the teeth and gums.
    4. _____ Use a padded tongue blade to access various sections of the mouth.
    5. _____ Use an unpadded tongue blade to scrap debris from the tongue.

15. A nurse washes a bedbound patient's entire body without assistance from the patient. The nurse uses a washcloth, several basins of warm water, gentle soap, and a towel to dry the skin. What type of bath should the nurse record in the progress notes of the patient's clinical record?
    1. Complete bath
    2. Partial bath
    3. Towel bath
    4. Bag bath

16. A nurse is providing morning care for a patient with a hearing aid. What should the nurse do when preparing to insert a hearing aid into a patient's ear?
    1. Adjust the volume according to the patient's preference.
    2. Ensure the patient's hearing aid is turned off.
    3. Turn the hearing aid on.
    4. Clean the ear mold.

17. A nurse, caring for a patient with type I diabetes, includes foot care in the patient's plan of care. What actions should be included in the plan? **Select all that apply.**
    1. _____ Assess bilateral dorsalis pedis pulses daily.
    2. _____ Use an antifungal powder liberally between the toes.
    3. _____ Apply moisturizing lotion sparingly to the feet, avoiding between the toes.
    4. _____ Trim the toenails straight across and smooth the edges with an emery board.
    5. _____ Teach the patient to inspect feet daily and use a mirror to see the soles of the feet.
    6. _____ Soak the feet in a basin of warm water for half an hour before trimming toenails if they appear brittle.

18. A nurse performs a physical assessment of an older adult. Which observation does the nurse conclude is unrelated to the aging process?
1. Dry, thin skin
2. Thick toenails
3. Fine, silky hair
4. Sparse pubic hair

19. A nurse identifies the condition below when assessing a patient. Which should the nurse document on the patient's physical assessment form?

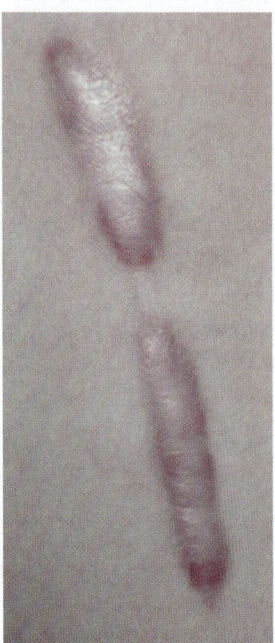

1. Macule
2. Fissure
3. Keloid
4. Scar

20. A nurse identifies that an older adult has long, torturous, yellow toenails. What should the nurse do?
1. File the patient's toenails with an emery board.
2. Cut the toenails straight across with a nail clipper.
3. Soak the patient's feet in hot water to soften the toenails.
4. Have the primary health-care provider write a referral to a podiatrist to trim the toenails.

21. A nurse is preparing a class for adolescents about the common causes of problems with the teeth. Which problems should the nurse include? **Select all that apply.**
1. _____ Periodontal disease
2. _____ Dental caries
3. _____ Stomatitis
4. _____ Cheilosis
5. _____ Halitosis

22. A nurse is caring for a comatose patient. Which intervention is essential when providing eye care for this patient?
1. Apply a protective eye shield to keep the eyes closed.
2. Place a folded washcloth over the eyes to block the light.
3. Administer antibiotic eyedrops daily to lubricate the eyes.
4. Wash the eyes from the inner to outer canthus every eight hours.

23. A nurse is assessing skin turgor in an older adult. Which site should the nurse use to assess for tenting?
1. Hand
2. Ankle
3. Forearm
4. Sternum

24. Which is **most** important to do, as evident in the photograph, when cleaning a patient's dentures?

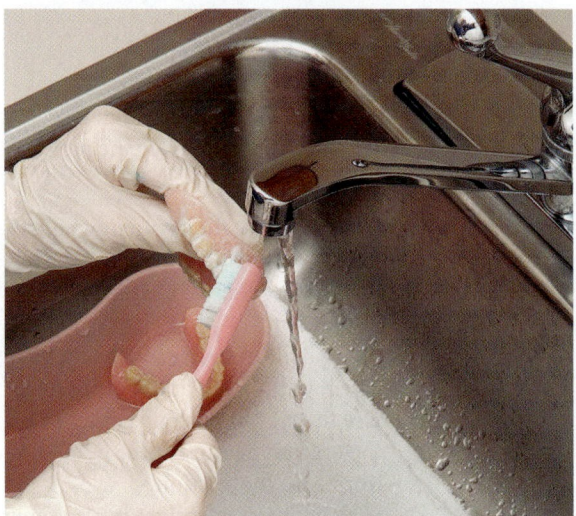

1. Place a washcloth in the bottom of the sink.
2. Ensure a continuous flow of water.
3. Brush the upper appliance first.
4. Wear sterile gloves.

25. What should the nurse do if a patient with a urinary retention catheter experiences a urethral discharge?
1. Increase oral fluid intake.
2. Provide more frequent catheter care.
3. Replace the catheter with a larger size.
4. Apply an antibiotic ointment to the perineal area.

26. A nurse is caring for several patients. Which patient is at greatest risk for skin breakdown?
1. Patient who is dehydrated
2. Patient who has diaphoresis
3. Patient who is incontinent of feces
4. Patient who has difficulty moving up in bed

27. A nurse is assessing a patient with a history of liver disease. Which part of the eye is the **best** site to assess for jaundice?

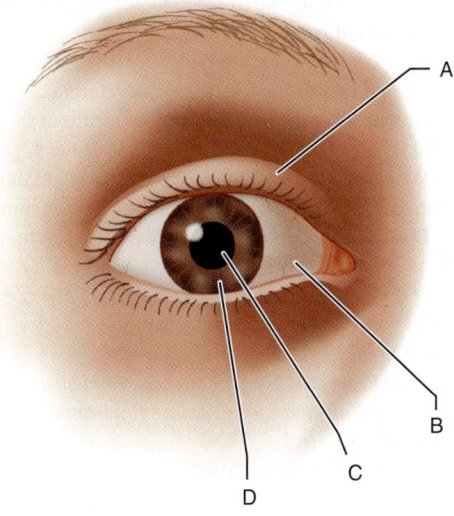

1. A
2. B
3. C
4. D

28. Which outcome associated with physical hygiene is appropriate and should be included in a patient's plan of care?
   1. Will comb hair unassisted
   2. Offer pain medication before providing a bath
   3. Provide clothing with Velcro fasteners instead of buttons
   4. Verbalizes satisfaction with body cleanliness after morning care

29. A nurse is planning nursing care for an older adult who was admitted to the hospital with a diagnosis of brain attack (cerebrovascular accident, stroke).

Patient's Clinical Record

Vital Signs

Temperature: 97.8°F orally.
Pulse: 98 beats/minute.
Respirations: 23 breaths/minute, shallow.
Blood pressure: 160/86 mm Hg.
Oxygen saturation: 95% on room air while resting

Nurse's Progress Note

Patient admitted 9 days ago with a diagnosis of brain attack. The patient has half strength of the right upper and lower extremities. Patient occasionally is incontinent of stool. States that the perineal area is tender; slight perianal erythema identified; skin barrier applied as per standing protocol. Able to turn on right side unassisted but needs assistance to turn on left side. High-top sneakers to prevent foot drop utilized at all times except when bathing. Measured for hand/wrist and leg splint. Social worker visit to discuss posthospital rehabilitation plan of care.

After reviewing the patient's clinical record, which of the following should the nurse identify as **most** important when providing for this patient's hygiene and grooming needs?
   1. Providing a complete bed bath daily
   2. Pacing care to avoid activity intolerance
   3. Asking the patient to choose personal bath products
   4. Implementing range-of-motion exercises during the bath

30. A patient with which condition should the nurse anticipate will need assistance in making decisions regarding hygiene care?
   1. Moderate pain
   2. Altered reality
   3. Sensory deficit
   4. Limited mobility

REVIEW ANSWERS

1. ANSWER: 1.

Rationales:

1. The face, hands, underarms, back, and perineal area should be washed daily because they harbor the most microorganisms.

2. Directing the patient to wash as much as possible and assist with the rest is considered a complete bed bath with assistance, not a partial bed bath.

3. The axillary areas and the back must also be washed along with the areas presented in option 3 in a partial bed bath.

4. Assisting the patient to wash only one part of the body at a time is considered a complete bed bath with assistance.

TEST-TAKING TIP: Identify the option with a specific determiner. Option 4 contains the word *only,* which is a specific determiner.

Content Area: Hygiene

Integrated Processes: Teaching/Learning; Nursing Process: Evaluation

Client Need: Physiological Integrity; Basic Care and Comfort

Cognitive Level: Application

2. ANSWER: 4.

Rationales:

1. Pediculosis is caused by direct contact with lice or their eggs (nits); brushing the hair will not prevent head lice.

2. Shampooing the hair and rubbing the scalp help to limit dandruff.

3. Loss of hair (alopecia) may be caused by nutritional, emotional, iatrogenic, and genetic factors; it is not prevented by brushing.

4. Brushing separates tangles and evenly distributes secretions and oils down the hair shafts.

Content Area: Hygiene

Integrated Processes: Teaching/Learning; Nursing Process: Planning

Client Need: Physiological Integrity; Basic Care and Comfort

Cognitive Level: Application

3. ANSWER: 5, 4, 1, 2, 3.

Rationales:

5. A person who is able to provide complete self-care is the most independent.

4. A person who is completely independent but uses equipment or a device to provide self-care is the second most independent person of the options offered.

1. A person who requires some assistance or supervision from another person is the third most independent person of the options offered.

2. A person who needs help from another person and equipment is more in need of help than a person who only needs assistance or supervision from another person.

3. A person who is totally dependent and is unable to participate in activities is the most dependent person of the options offered.

Content Area: Hygiene

Integrated Processes: Nursing Process: Analysis

Client Need: Safe and Effective Care Environment; Management of Care

Cognitive Level: Analysis

4. ANSWER: 1.

Rationales:

1. It is most important that a patient have the ability to call for help when needed. It is a major safety issue.

2. Although moving the overbed table next to the patient's bed is helpful, it is not essential.

3. The patient may prefer to have the door closed. The nurse should determine the patient's preference.

4. Pulling up all of the side rails of a bed without the patient's consent is considered a restraint. A nurse can engage all of the side rails of a bed if it is necessary to maintain the safety of the patient, but the need for their use must be documented.

TEST-TAKING TIP: Identify the word in the stem that sets a priority. The word *most* in the stem sets a priority. Identify the option with a specific determiner. Option 4 contains the word *all* which is a specific determiner.

Content Area: Hygiene

Integrated Processes: Nursing Process: Implementation

Client Need: Safe and Effective Care Environment; Safety and Infection Control

Cognitive Level: Application

5. ANSWER: 3.

Rationales:

1. This is a regular tooth comb for hair that is straight, relaxed, or slightly curly and has a regular or fine texture. A regular tooth comb can be used on curly hair if used gently.

2. This is a brush that helps to remove tangles, massage the scalp, which increases circulation, and move oil down the hair shafts proximal to distal. It is used for hair that is straight or curly and has a regular or fine texture.

3. A wide-tooth comb is used for hair that is dry and has a course texture to limit hair breakage. Applying mineral oil or moisturizing hair cream before combing also helps to minimize hair breakage.

4. This is a fine-tooth comb mainly used to remove head lice eggs (nits) after the scalp and hair is treated with an antiparasitic agent.

TEST-TAKING TIP: Identify the word in the stem that sets a priority. The word *most* in the stem sets a priority.

Content Area: Hygiene

Integrated Processes: Nursing Process: Implementation

Client Need: Physiological Integrity; Basic Care and Comfort

Cognitive Level: Analysis

6. ANSWER: 4.

Rationales:

1. Clubbing is unrelated to liver disease. Jaundice is related to diseases of the liver.

2. Clubbing is unrelated to diabetes mellitus. Hyperglycemia and complications, such as peripheral vascular disease, kidney disease, and eye problems, are related to diabetes mellitus.

3. Spoon-shaped nails are related to iron-deficiency anemia.

4. A long-term oxygen deficit results in the proliferation of the soft tissues in the terminal phalanges of the fingers; this increases the angle between the fingernail and nail bed beyond 160°.

Content Area: Hygiene

Integrated Processes: Nursing Process: Analysis

Client Need: Physiological Integrity; Physiological Adaptation

Cognitive Level: Analysis

7. ANSWER: 15.

Rationale:

First convert the patient's weight in pounds to kilograms by using ratio and proportion.

$$\frac{\text{Desire 132 lb}}{\text{Have 2.2 lb}} = \frac{x \text{ kg}}{1 \text{ kg}}$$

$$2.2x = 132$$
$$x = 132 \div 2.2$$
$$x = 60 \text{ kg}$$

Now determine the total daily dose by multiplying the patient's weight in kilograms by the prescribed dose of 0.5 mg/kg.

60 kg × 0.5 mg = 30 mg daily.

Now determine the dose to be administered twice a day by dividing the total daily dose by 2.

30 mg ÷ 2 = 15 mg.

Content Area: Medication Administration
Integrated Processes: Nursing Process: Planning
Client Need: Physiological Integrity; Physiological Adaptation
Cognitive Level: Application

8 ANSWER: 3.

Rationales:

1. Dentures are not common to all older adults. In addition, the top denture should be removed and reinserted before the bottom denture because it is larger.

2. A daily bath is not necessary because oil producing sebaceous glands are less active in older adults, making skin drier. Frequent bathing dries skin even further.

3. Applying moisturizer to the skin of an older adult will make skin supple and less dry. The skin of older adults generally is drier because the oil-producing sebaceous glands are less active.

4. Older adults should not use deodorant soap because it dries already-dry skin.

Content Area: Hygiene
Integrated Processes: Nursing Process: Planning
Client Need: Physiological Integrity; Basic Care and Comfort
Cognitive Level: Application

9. ANSWER: 1, 2, 4.

Rationales:

1. The head and upper body generally is less soiled than the lower body. This supports the concept of moving from *clean to dirty*.

2. Washing, rinsing, and drying clean areas first avoids contamination with debris and microorganisms from a dirty area, thereby reducing the risk of infection.

3. Standard, not contact, precautions are necessary to protect the nurse from the patient's blood and body fluids.

4. Warm water is preferable because hot water may cause a burn. In addition, hot water removes protective oils contributing to dry skin.

5. When bathing extremities, move from distal to proximal, not proximal to distal. Washing, rinsing, and drying strokes that move from distal to proximal areas of a limb facilitate venous return.

6. Water should be changed before perineal care because the urinary meatus should not be exposed to soiled, soapy water that may increase the risk of a urinary tract infection. In addition, the perineum should not be exposed to excessive amounts of soap because soap can irritate delicate perineal tissue.

TEST-TAKING TIP: Identify the clang associations. The words *bathing* in the stem and *bathe* in options 1 and 2 and *bathing* in option 4 are clang associations. Carefully examine options with clang associations.

Content Area: Hygiene
Integrated Processes: Nursing Process: Implementation
Client Need: Physiological Integrity; Basic Care and Comfort
Cognitive Level: Application

10. ANSWER: 3.

Rationales:

1. All linens do not have to be changed every time a bed is made. Just the draw sheet and pillowcase need to be changed if the linens are not soiled.

2. This is not an essential action when making an occupied bed. Making just one side of the bed at a time conserves both nurse and patient energy.

3. Putting the side rail up on the nonworking side of the bed is an essential safety measure. It provides a barrier that prevents the patient from falling out of bed.

4. Although lowering the head of the bed until it is flat facilitates making the bed, not all patients can tolerate this position. In addition, patients should be positioned in the lateral, not supine, position.

TEST-TAKING TIP: Identify the word in the stem that sets a priority. The word *most* in the stem sets a priority. Identify the options that contain specific determiners. Option 1 contains the word *all* and option 2 contains the word *just;* these words are specific determiners. Options with specific determiners often are incorrect options.

Content Area: Hygiene
Integrated Processes: Nursing Process: Implementation
Client Need: Safe and Effective Care Environment; Safety and Infection Control
Cognitive Level: Application

11. ANSWER: 2.

Rationales:

1. Although tucking the top sheet in loosely is helpful, it may not provide enough space between the toes and the sheet to minimize tension on the feet that causes plantar flexion and subsequent footdrop.

2. A toe pleat creates enough space between the sheet and the patient's feet to minimize tension on the feet, preventing plantar flexion. Prolonged plantar flexion of the feet results in fibular or tibial nerve injury, causing paralysis of the anterior muscles of the lower extremities.

3. Placing a pillow under the ankles lifts the heels of the feet off the bed, minimizing the development of pressure ulcers on the heels of the feet, not footdrop.

4. No matter how bottom sheets are secured, they will not cause footdrop. Square corners on top linens will tightly secure the linens to the bed, compressing the feet and promoting the development of footdrop.

TEST-TAKING TIP: Identify the word in the stem that sets a priority. The word *best* in the stem sets a priority.
Content Area: Hygiene
Integrated Processes: Nursing Process: Implementation
Client Need: Safe and Effective Care Environment; Safety and Infection Control
Cognitive Level: Application

12. ANSWER: 2, 3, 5.
Rationales:
1. Denture cleaner and a soft toothbrush should be used because regular toothpaste and a firm toothbrush may be too abrasive for dentures.
2. This is the correct way to release the suction of lower dentures.
3. This is a patient-centered intervention.
4. Storing dentures dry can cause them to warp. Dentures should always be covered with cool water when stored in a denture cup.
5. This is the correct way to release the suction of upper dentures.
TEST-TAKING TIP: Identify the option that is patient centered. Option 3 is patient centered because it takes into consideration a patient's preference. Identify the options that are opposites. Options 3 and 4 are opposites. Often times one of the opposites is the correct answer. Consider these options carefully.
Content Area: Hygiene
Integrated Processes: Nursing Process: Implementation
Client Need: Physiological Integrity; Basic Care and Comfort
Cognitive Level: Application

13. ANSWER: 1.
Rationales:
1. **Asking about the patient's personal preferences allows the nurse to individualize the patient's care. Personalizing a patient's care demonstrates respect and caring.**
2. This is premature. Raising the height of the bed may not be necessary if the patient can provide hygiene care independently.
3. The linens should be changed after hygiene care because they can get wet and soiled during care.
4. It is not necessary to eat breakfast before a.m. care. Breakfast can be eaten before or after a.m. care depending on the patient's preference.
TEST-TAKING TIP: Identify the word in the stem that sets a priority. The word *first* in the stem sets a priority. Identify the unique option. Option 1 is unique; it is the only option that addresses the patient's psychological needs. Identify the patient centered option. Option 1 is patient centered.
Content Area: Hygiene
Integrated Processes: Communication/Documentation; Caring; Nursing Process: Implementation
Client Need: Physiological Integrity
Cognitive Level: Application

14. ANSWER: 2, 4.
Rationales:
1. Ten mL or less should be used to rinse the mouth of toothpaste and debris. Larger amounts of fluid increase the risk of aspiration.

2. Short circular motions are the most effective way to brush the teeth of an unconscious patient. Long strokes may precipitate the gag reflex.
3. A small amount of toothpaste is sufficient to cleanse the mouth. Excess foamy toothpaste requires multiple rinses, which increase the risk of aspiration.
4. A padded tongue blade helps to keep the mouth open as well as cleanse all areas of the mouth. In addition, a nurse should never insert fingers in a patient's mouth because the patient may bite down and injure the nurse.
5. The tongue should not be scraped with an unpadded tongue blade because it may injure the tongue. A padded tongue blade may be used to gently swab oral surfaces. Multiple clean swabs should be used, one for each section of the mouth.
Content Area: Hygiene
Integrated Processes: Nursing Process: Implementation
Client Need: Physiological Integrity; Basic Care and Comfort
Cognitive Level: Application

15. ANSWER: 1.
Rationales:
1. **The bath described in the stem is a complete bath because all body surfaces were washed.**
2. A partial bath generally includes those body parts that cause odor (e.g., axillae, perineum), are at risk for skin breakdown (e.g., back and under the breasts), and areas to *freshen* the patient for the day (e.g., face and hands).
3. A towel bath involves saturating a towel and bath blanket in a plastic bag with a commercially prepared solution of disinfectant, nonrinse cleaning agent, moisturizer, and water and then warming the bag in a microwave. There is no need to towel dry the patient because the solution dries quickly. Research demonstrates that patients are satisfied with this type of bath and it takes less time than a traditional bath. Often, it is a method of choice for patients with mild to moderate impaired skin integrity, activity intolerance, or cognitive impairment.
4. A bag bath refers to bathing a patient with premoistened, disposable washcloths. This product generally contains a no-rinse surfactant, a diluent substance to trap moisture (humectant), and an emollient. Research demonstrates that this type of bathing system reduces overall skin dryness, skin flaking, and scaling. It is preferred in critical care and long-term care settings for patients who are unable to bathe themselves. The package of 8 to 10 disposable washcloths is warmed in a microwave in preparation for use.
TEST-TAKING TIP: Identify the obscure clang association. The word *entire* in the stem and the word *complete* in option 1 is an obscure clang association. Both words indicate the concept of total, whole, or all-inclusive.
Content Area: Hygiene
Integrated Processes: Communication/Documentation; Nursing Process: Implementation
Client Need: Physiological Integrity; Basic Care and Comfort
Cognitive Level: Application

16. ANSWER: 2.
Rationales:
1. Although this appears to be a patient-centered option, it violates a basic concept about care of a patient with a hearing aid.

2. A hearing aid should be off during insertion. Once inserted, the hearing aid should be turned on and the volume adjusted from the lowest setting to a setting of the patient's preference. This provides for patient comfort.
3. The hearing aid should be off, not on, when inserted to prevent patient distress and promote patient comfort.
4. The ear mold should be cleaned immediately after it is removed from the ear.
TEST-TAKING TIP: Identify the options with clang associations. The words *hearing aid* in the stem and in options 2 and 3 are clang associations. Examine options 2 and 3 carefully. Identify the options that are opposites. Options 2 and 3 are opposites.
Content Area: Hygiene;
Integrated Processes: Nursing Process: Implementation
Client Need: Physiological Integrity; Basic Care and Comfort
Cognitive Level: Application

17. **ANSWER: 1, 3, 5.**
Rationales:
1. Decreased circulation to the feet is a complication of diabetes because the basement membrane of capillaries becomes impaired. Assessing the dorsalis pedis pulses daily monitors the quality of peripheral circulation and is considered part of care of the feet.
2. Antifungal powder should be applied only if prescribed by a primary health-care provider for athlete's foot; if prescribed, it should be used sparingly, not liberally. An excessive amount of a powdered substance, when moistened, becomes sandpaper-like, which can contribute to further skin breakdown.
3. This is an appropriate nursing action. Excessive moisturizing lotion, especially between the toes, may cause skin maceration or a fungal infection.
4. A podiatrist, not a nurse, should trim the toenails of a patient who has diabetes. An emery board should be avoided because, if not used properly, it can cause an abrasion and foot related complications. Breaks in the skin of the feet of a patient who has diabetes may not heal, become gangrenous, and lead to an amputation.
5. It is important that a patient who has diabetes inspect the feet thoroughly every day. Early recognition and treatment of a problem may prevent a more serious complication.
6. Soaking the feet of a patient who has diabetes should be avoided because it removes natural oils, causing skin cracks. Also, the appropriate temperature for foot soaks (e.g., 105° to 110°F) may cause burns in a patient who has diabetes. Foot soaks for individuals without foot problems should last only 5 to 10 minutes because it removes natural oils, causing skin cracks.
TEST-TAKING TIP: Identify the slightly obscure clang associations. The word *foot* in the stem and the word *feet* in options 3, 5, and 6 are clang associations. Examine these options carefully. Options 3 and 5 are correct answers. Option 6 is a distractor.
Content Area: Hygiene
Integrated Processes: Communication/Documentation; Nursing Process: Planning
Client Need: Physiological Integrity; Reduction of Risk Potential
Cognitive Level: Application

18. **ANSWER: 3.**
Rationales:
1. Dry, thin skin is associated with aging. The skin is dry because sebaceous and sweat glands are less active. The skin appears thinner because of the loss of dermis and subcutaneous fat.
2. Thick toenails are associated with slow nail growth related to aging.
3. Fine, silky hair is not a result of aging. Fine, silky hair is associated with hyperthyroidism. Thin, dry, graying hair is associated with aging. Graying hair occurs as the number of pigment cells in hair bulbs (melanocytes) decrease, causing darker hair to be replaced with nonpigmented hair. A reduction in thyroid hormone production can cause the hair to have a course texture and slower rate of growth as well as increase hair loss. Thyroid hormone affects cell division at the hair follicle.
4. Sparse pubic hair is associated with hormone decline that occurs with aging. Overall hair loss is specifically linked with a decrease in testosterone and thyroid hormone levels.
TEST-TAKING TIP: Identify the word in the stem that indicates negative polarity. The word *unrelated* is the word in the stem that indicates negative polarity. The question is asking, "What clinical manifestation is not caused by aging?"
Content Area: Hygiene
Integrated Processes: Nursing Process: Analysis
Client Need: Physiological Integrity; Basic Care and Comfort
Cognitive Level: Application

19. **ANSWER: 3.**
Rationales:
1. A macule is a flat, circumscribed area from 1 to several centimeters in size. Examples include cherry angioma, freckles, flat pigmented moles, and measles.
2. A fissure is a linear crack in the skin. Examples include cheilitis and athlete's foot.
3. A keloid is a raised, irregular scar due to excess collagen formation (hypertrophic scar). Examples of common sites include surgical incisions, body piercings, and tattoos.
4. A scar is the formation of replacement connective tissue and fibrotic changes following healing of a wound. Examples of common sites include surgical incisions and cuts.
Content Area: Hygiene
Integrated Processes: Nursing Process: Analysis
Client Need: Physiological Integrity; Physiological Adaptation
Cognitive Level: Analysis

20. **ANSWER: 4.**
Rationales:
1. This is unsafe and may injure already impaired tissues.
2. This is unsafe and may injure already impaired tissues. Patients with normal nails may provide self-care in the home by cutting the toenails straight across. This technique prevents ingrown toenails.
3. Yellow toenails indicate that the patient may have inadequate perfusion to the distal extremities. Often, this is accompanied by altered sensation in the extremities. Warm, not hot, water should be used to wash the feet to prevent injury to impaired tissues. A podiatrist may order

that the feet be soaked prior to clipping because it can soften the toenails.

4. Long, torturous, yellow toenails often are associated with problems such as impaired arterial circulation to the feet or a fungal infection. The nails usually are thick, brittle, and difficult to trim. These toenails should be cut by an appropriate practitioner.

TEST-TAKING TIP: Identify the option that is unique. Option 4 is unique. It is the only option that does not provide direct care to the patient's feet or toenails.

Content Area: Hygiene

Integrated Processes: Nursing Process: Implementation

Client Need: Safe and Effective Care Environment; Management of Care

Cognitive Level: Application

21. **ANSWER: 1, 2.**

Rationales:

1. Periodontal disease (pyorrhea) is one of the most common causes of tooth loss. Bleeding and receding gums and destruction of adjacent bone structures lead to infected gums and loosening of teeth that may require their removal.

2. Dental caries (cavities) generally are caused by failure to remove an invisible, destructive bacterial coating that builds up on teeth and destroys the enamel. The nurse should teach people to avoid refined sugars, to floss and brush the teeth at least 3 times during the day, and to consult a dentist at least 2 times a year for an oral assessment and appropriate intervention, including plaque removal.

3. Stomatitis, an inflammation of the oral mucosa, is not one of the two most common causes of problems with the teeth. Stomatitis is caused by mechanical trauma, irritants, nutritional deficiencies, and systemic infection.

4. Cheilosis is a cracking and ulceration seen as reddened fissures at the angles of the mouth, generally caused by vitamin B-complex deficiencies.

5. Halitosis, or bad breath, is not a cause of problems with the teeth. It is a sign of inadequate oral hygiene; dental caries; infection of the mouth; tobacco use; systemic disease, such as liver disease or diabetes; and the eating of such foods as garlic and onions.

Content Area: Hygiene

Integrated Processes: Teaching/Learning; Nursing Process: Planning

Client Need: Health Promotion and Maintenance

Cognitive Level: Application

22. **ANSWER: 1.**

Rationales:

1. A protective eye shield keeps the eyes of a comatose person closed, which prevents the eyes from becoming dry because of a lost blink reflex.

2. A folded washcloth over the eyes may damage the patient's corneas.

3. Antibiotic eye drops treat an eye infection; they are not used to lubricate the eyes of a comatose patient. Saline eye drops or artificial tears may be used to lubricate the eyes.

Also, the primary health-care provider may prescribe a lubricating ointment to protect the eyes from becoming dry.

4. Eight hours is too long a time period between cleansing the eyes of a comatose patient. The patient should have eye care every 2 to 4 hours and whenever necessary. It is correct technique to wash the eyes from the inner to outer canthus to minimize contamination of the lacrimal duct with debris from the eye.

Content Area: Hygiene

Integrated Processes: Nursing Process: Implementation

Client Need: Physiological Integrity; Reduction of Risk Potential

Cognitive Level: Application

23. **ANSWER: 4.**

Rationales:

1. The hands in older adults have a decrease in subcutaneous tissue resulting in numerous wrinkles that interfere with assessment of skin turgor.

2. Many older adults have less efficient venous return or cardiac disease that results in dependent edema. Edema interferes with assessment of skin turgor.

3. The forearms in older adults have a decrease in subcutaneous tissue resulting in numerous wrinkles that interfere with assessment of skin turgor.

4. Pinching the skin over the sternum, anterior chest below the clavicle, or forehead are the preferred sites for assessing tenting. These sites are less likely to have wrinkles or edema that interferes with assessment of skin turgor.

Content Area: Hygiene

Integrated Processes: Nursing Process: Assessment

Client Need: Physiological Integrity; Basic Care and Comfort

Cognitive Level: Application

24. **ANSWER: 1.**

Rationales:

1. Of the four options presented, the placement of a washcloth in the bottom of the sink is the most important action. This minimizes the risk of damaging the denture if the nurse should accidentally drop the denture in the sink.

2. The flow of water does not have to be continuous; it has to flow only when rinsing the denture cleanser off the denture after being cleaned.

3. It does not matter which denture is cleansed first.

4. Clean, not sterile, gloves are necessary to protect the nurse from the patient's oral secretions when cleaning a patient's dentures.

TEST-TAKING TIP: Identify the word in the stem that sets a priority. The word *most* in the stem sets a priority.

Content Area: Hygiene

Integrated Processes: Nursing Process: Implementation

Client Need: Physiological Integrity; Basic Care and Comfort

Cognitive Level: Analysis

25. **ANSWER: 2.**

Rationales:

1. Increasing oral fluids will not decrease the urethral discharge.

2. More frequent catheter care will remove secretions, reducing the risk of skin breakdown and infection. The nurse should notify the primary health-care provider of the urethral discharge. It may be due to just irritation from the catheter but it could also be a sign of an infectious process requiring medical intervention.

3. A larger catheter is indicated if urine leakage occurs around a catheter, not the presence of a urethral discharge.

4. Application of an antibiotic ointment is a dependent function of the nurse and requires a prescription by a primary health-care provider.

TEST-TAKING TIP: Identify the options with a clang association. The stem and options 2 and 3 contain the word *catheter,* which are clang associations.

Content Area: Hygiene
Integrated Processes: Nursing Process: Implementation
Client Need: Physiological Integrity; Reduction of Risk Potential
Cognitive Level: Application

26. **ANSWER: 3.**
Rationales:

1. Although a decrease in interstitial fluid is a risk factor for skin breakdown, it is not as great a risk factor as excretions.

2. Although the secretions of sweat glands (perspiration) increase moisture on the skin causing maceration of skin, perspiration is not as destructive as excretions.

3. Feces contain fluid and digestive enzymes that injure the skin if not removed immediately. In addition, urine contains urea and is acidic. Urine and feces can cause loss of superficial layers of the skin (excoriation, denuded skin).

4. Although people who have difficulty moving up in bed may slide up in bed, exerting a frictional resistance between the skin and the bed (shearing force), they can be taught to use an overbed trapeze that eliminates this problem.

TEST-TAKING TIP: Identify the word in the stem that sets a priority. The word *greatest* in the stem sets a priority.

Content Area: Hygiene
Integrated Processes: Nursing Process: Analysis
Client Need: Physiological Integrity; Basic Care and Comfort
Cognitive Level: Analysis

27. **ANSWER: 2.**
Rationales:

1. The upper eyelid is not the site to assess for the presence of jaundice.

2. The sclera of the eyes, mucous membranes of the oral cavity, and skin are the common sites to assess for the presence of jaundice. The yellow appearance of the sclera, mucous membranes, and skin is caused by deposition of bile pigments (jaundice, icterus).

3. The pupil is not the site to assess for the presence of jaundice.

4. The iris is not the site to assess for the presence of jaundice.

Content Area: Physical Assessment
Integrated Processes: Nursing Process: Assessment
Client Need: Physiological Integrity; Physiological Adaptation
Cognitive Level: Analysis

28. **ANSWER: 4.**
Rationales:

1. This is an incomplete outcome statement because it does not establish a time frame when it should be achieved.

2. This is a nursing intervention, not a patient-centered goal.

3. This is a nursing intervention, not a patient-centered goal.

4. This is an appropriate outcome. It objectively establishes the criteria for achievement, *verbalizes satisfaction with body cleanliness,* and it establishes a time frame in which it should be achieved, *after morning care.*

Content Area: Hygiene
Integrated Processes: Communication/Documentation; Nursing Process: Planning
Client Need: Safe and Effective Care Environment; Management of Care
Cognitive Level: Application

29. **ANSWER: 2.**
Rationales:

1. A complete bath generally is unnecessary for a patient who is an older adult because of decreased sebaceous gland activity and increased drying of skin associated with aging. A complete bath twice a week and partial baths and perineal care provided when necessary is most appropriate when meeting the hygiene needs of an older adult.

2. Providing for the patient's hygiene needs without causing activity intolerance is the most important action presented. Older adults experience a decrease in lung expansion and reduced vital capacity due to weakened thoracic muscles and calcification of costal cartilage associated with aging. Also, older adults have a decreased ability to deliver and diffuse oxygen to cells due to changes in respiratory and vascular tissues secondary to the aging process. This patient's respiratory status (increased respiratory rate, shallow respirations, and an oxygen saturation at the lower range of normal) indicates impaired respiratory functioning. The nurse should avoid unnecessarily straining the patient physically.

3. Although it is important to provide the patient with the opportunity to participate in care by making choices because they support a sense of control, it is not the most important action of the options presented.

4. Although range-of-motion exercises should be implemented when providing care to this patient, it is not the most important action of the options presented.

TEST-TAKING TIP: Identify the word in the stem that sets a priority. The word *most* in the stem sets a priority. Identify the option that is unique. Option 2 is the only option that contains a rationale. Examine option 2 carefully. Use Maslow's hierarchy of needs and Airway, Breathing, and Circulation to help establish the priority. Meeting a patient's need for oxygen is a first level need according to Maslow, and breathing according to the ABCs is essential for life. Preventing activity intolerance is the most important option of the options presented.

Content Area: *Hygiene*
Integrated Processes: *Nursing Process: Planning*
Client Need: *Physiological Integrity; Basic Care and Comfort*
Cognitive Level: *Analysis*

30. **ANSWER: 2.**
    Rationales:
    1. Pain may limit a person's ability to participate in hygiene care but should not impair one's ability to make independent decisions regarding care.
    2. **Altered reality related to delusions, hallucinations, or impaired cognition may impair a person's ability to make personal care decisions.**
    3. Sensory deficits may interfere with a patient's ability to perform hygiene care independently; however, it should not interfere with the person's ability to make independent decisions regarding care.
    4. Limited mobility may interfere with a patient's ability to perform hygiene care independently; however, it should not interfere with the person's ability to make independent decisions regarding care.

    TEST-TAKING TIP: Identify the unique option. Options 1, 3, and 4 are all associated with physical stresses. Option 2 is unique because it is associated with a psychological stress.

    Content Area: *Hygiene*
    Integrated Processes: *Caring; Nursing Process: Planning*
    Client Need: *Physiological Integrity; Basic Care and Comfort*
    Cognitive Level: *Application*

Chapter 17

Mobility

KEY TERMS

Anabolism—Synthesis of protein from amino acids.

Base of support—Points of the body that are touching the ground.

Bones—Rigid connective tissue composed mostly of calcium salts.

Cartilage—Supportive connective tissue.

Catabolism—Protein breakdown.

Center of gravity—Point within the body where the greatest mass of the body exists.

Contracture—Rigidity of a joint due to permanent shortening of a muscle, tendons, and ligaments.

Embolus—Mass consisting of blood cells and cellular debris that blocks a blood vessel.

Gait—Manner in which a person walks.

Joints—Connections between bones.

Ligaments—Bind joints together and connect bones and cartilages.

Line of gravity—Line that is drawn from the top of the head through the individual's center of greatest mass.

Metabolic rate—Minimal energy expended to maintain the body's physical and chemical processes.

Negative nitrogen balance—State caused by inadequate intake of protein to meet body needs, resulting in muscle breakdown that releases nitrogen from muscle cells.

Orthostatic hypotension—Decrease in blood pressure when moving from a recumbent to a sitting or standing position resulting in dizziness.

Range of motion (ROM)—Maximum extent of movement by a joint through sagittal, frontal, and transverse planes.

Tendons—Connect muscle to bone.

Thrombus—Formation of a blood clot within the vascular system.

Valsalva maneuver—Forceful exhalation against a closed glottis, resulting in increased intrathoracic and venous pressures, bradycardia, and decreased blood return to the heart.

I. Foundations of Mobility

Movement requires the interaction of the skeletal system, nervous system, and muscles. The way in which the body moves (body mechanics) involves balance, body alignment, coordination, joint mobility, and gait. Effective body mechanics facilitate the use of muscle groups to limit the amount of stress on body structures, reduce the amount of energy required for an activity, and decrease the risk of injury to both the patient and nurse. Nurses should integrate principles of body mechanics when performing nursing activities to care for patients effectively and safely as well as reduce the risk of occupational injuries.

A. Anatomy Related to Movement
1. Skeletal system.
    a. Components of the skeletal system.
        (1) **Bones:** Rigid connective tissue composed mostly of calcium salts.

(2) **Joints:** Connections between bones.
    (a) Ball and socket: Rounded head of one bone fits into a cuplike structure of another bone; moves in all planes of range of motion (ROM) as well as rotation. Examples include the joints of the shoulders (scapula and humerus) and hips (pelvic bone and femur).
    (b) Condyloid: One oval-shaped bone fits into an elliptical cavity of another bone; moves in one plane with some lateral movement. Examples include the wrists (radius and carpal bones).
    (c) Gliding: Flat plane of the surface of one bone moves past the flat plane of another bone; moves from side to side. Examples include small bones of the wrists and ankles.

(d) Hinge: Convex surface of one bone fits into the cavity of another bone; moves in one plane, flexion and extension. Examples include elbow (humerus, ulna, and radius) and knee (femur, patella, and tibia).

(e) Pivot: Projection of one bone articulates with a ring or notch of another bone; moves by rotating around a single point. An example is the neck (atlas and axis).

(f) Saddle: Concave surface of one bone fits into the convex surface of another bone; moves in several planes. Examples include the thumbs (thumb's metacarpal bone and wrist's carpal bone).

(3) **Cartilage:** Supportive connective tissue.

(4) **Ligaments:** Bind joints together and connect bones and cartilages.

(5) **Tendons:** Connect muscle to bone.

b. Bones serve as levers, and joints serve as fulcrums; a *lever* is a fixed bar that moves about a fixed point known as a *fulcrum*.

2. Nervous system.

a. Autonomic nervous system: Innervates involuntary muscles, such as the heart, blood vessels, and glands.

b. Somatic nervous system: Innervates voluntary skeletal muscles.

c. The motor areas of the frontal lobes of the cerebrum generate the electrochemical impulses that initiate voluntary skeletal muscle contraction.

d. The cerebellum coordinates the muscles involved in voluntary movement.

3. Muscles.

a. Skeletal muscles consist of muscle fibers that can contract (shorten) or extend (stretch), thus moving a joint.

b. Muscle attaches to bone at two points.
(1) Origin: More stationary bone.
(2) Insertion: More moveable bone.

c. Muscle pairs act antagonistic to each other—when one contracts, the other relaxes; permanent

---

MAKING THE CONNECTION

Anatomical Structures and Body Movement

Electrochemical impulses that initiate voluntary motor activity originate in the motor areas of the cerebrum. The cerebellum modifies these impulses, which progress to skeletal muscles, stimulating them to respond. The skeletal muscles respond to these modified impulses by contracting (shorten), which pulls on bones, producing body movement. Skeletal muscles also can extend (lengthen), which allows the muscle to return to its resting length after contraction. For movement to be exact, coordinated, smooth, and efficient, the nervous and skeletal systems and muscles must work together to produce a result not independently obtainable.

---

shortening of a muscle decreases the angle of the joint (contracture) (Fig. 17.1).

B. Body Mechanics

1. Balance.

a. Center of gravity: The point within the body where the greatest mass of the body exists; usually is below the umbilicus to the top of the pelvis.

b. Line of gravity: The line that is drawn from the top of the head through the individual's center of greatest mass.

c. Base of support.
(1) The points of the body that are touching the ground.
(2) Factors that increase the stability of the base of support (Fig. 17.2).
   (a) The center of gravity is between what holds the body up.
   (b) The wider the base of support, the more stable the body.

2. Body alignment.

a. Proper posture places the spine in a neutral position where the line of gravity passes through the center of gravity (alignment).

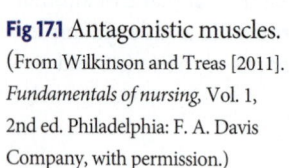

Fig 17.1 Antagonistic muscles. (From Wilkinson and Treas [2011]. *Fundamentals of nursing*, Vol. 1, 2nd ed. Philadelphia: F. A. Davis Company, with permission.)

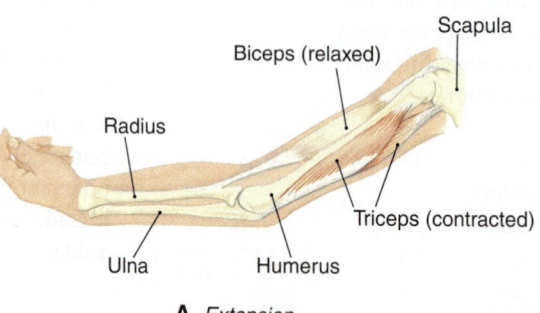

A. *Extension*

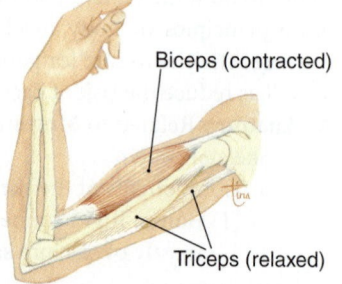

B. *Flexion*

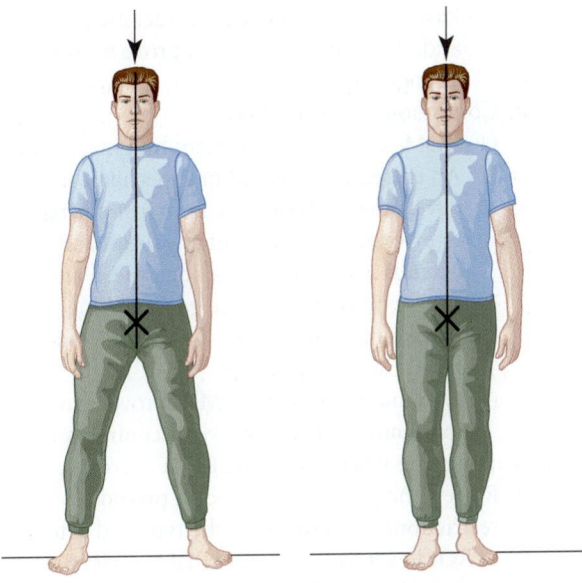

A   **B**

Fig 17.2 Center of gravity. (A) With a wide stance, the center of gravity (X) is closer to the base of support. (B) With a narrow stance, the body is less stable. (From Wilkinson and Treas [2011]. *Fundamentals of nursing*, Vol. 1, 2nd ed. Philadelphia: F. A. Davis Company, with permission.)

b. Body alignment permits muscles, joints, and ligaments to function efficiently.
3. Coordination.
   a. Movement is initiated in the cerebral cortex.
   b. Movement is coordinated by the cerebellum because of an awareness of posture, movement, and position sense (proprioception).
4. Joint mobility.
   a. Joint movement permits the performance of such activities as sitting, standing, bending, and walking.
   b. ROM is the maximum extent of movement by a joint through the sagittal, frontal, and transverse planes.
5. Gait.
   a. Refers to the manner in which a person walks.
   b. Includes such factors as posture, steadiness or unsteadiness, narrow or wide stance, extent of swing through of leg, and extent of arm movement.
   c. Abnormal gaits.
      (1) **Waddling:** Rolling motion in which the opposite hip drops when taking a stride, such as with developmental dysplasia of the hip and pregnancy.
      (2) **Propulsive (festinating, cogwheel):** Small, shuffling steps with involuntary accelerations, such as with Parkinson's disease.

(3) **Spastic:** Stiff, foot-dragging walk, such as with cerebral palsy.
(4) **Steppage:** Exaggerated lifting of the leg to avoid dragging the toes, such as with foot-drop and Guillain-Barré syndrome.
6. Nursing care related to body mechanics.
   a. Raise the bed and overbed table to waist level when providing care to a patient in bed to prevent stress and strain on the nurse's anatomical structures.
   b. Use a wide base of support by spreading the feet apart or placing one in front of the other. The wider the base of support, the more stable the person or object.

DID YOU KNOW?

The risk of falls and musculoskeletal injuries increases when the center of gravity is outside the base of support.

   c. Push, pull, or roll heavy objects when possible rather than lifting to minimize strain because pulling is less strenuous than pushing.
   d. Use gravity to facilitate movements. Doing so allows the patient's weight to promote movement by moving from a higher to lower plane and reduces stress and strain on the nurse and patient.
   e. Contract gluteal, abdominal, leg, and arm muscles before the actual move to prepare muscles for action.
   f. Keep the neck, back, pelvis, and feet in alignment to avoid twisting, which reduces stress and strain on the nurse's anatomical structure.
   g. Squat to lift objects off the floor. The lower the center of gravity, the more stable the body.
   h. Use leg muscles and flex the knees, hips, and ankles when lifting. Doing so permits larger muscles of the body to provide the power and decreases strain on back muscles.
   i. Use both hands and arms with elbows flexed when lifting objects because elbows act as fulcrums while the arms act as levers.
   j. Keep an object close to the body when lifting or carrying it. The closer an object is to the center of gravity, the more stable the body and less strain on the muscles of the back.

II. Exercise

Exercise requires a patient to perform repetitive actions that actively contract and relax muscles. It is an activity that is planned and structured to promote muscle strength, maintain joint flexibility, and/or improve respiratory and cardiovascular status. ROM exercises are designed to prevent contractures and can be performed independently or with assistance or can be received passively when a nurse or other practitioner puts a patient's joints through their full planes of movement. Nurses must understand the types of exercises, their advantages, and examples of activities associated with each type to assist patients with the performance of exercises. Nurses also must understand the principles associated with the provision of ROM exercises to administer these interventions effectively and safely.

A. Types of Exercise
1. Exercises are classified based on the type of muscle contraction (e.g., isotonic, isometric, or isokinetic) and the source of energy (e.g., aerobic) (Table 17.1).

B. Range-of-Motion (ROM) Exercises
1. Movements to maintain joint mobility and function.
2. Help prevent permanent shortening of muscle, tendons, and ligaments that ultimately limits joint mobility (contracture).
3. Applying heat before ROM may relax muscles and increase contractility; however, be aware that the application of heat requires an order from a primary health-care provider.
4. Types of ROM exercise.
   a. Active ROM.
      (1) ROM performed by a patient.
      (2) Requires muscle contraction that improves muscle strength.
   b. Active-assistive ROM.
      (1) ROM initiated by a patient that is completed by another.
      (2) Requires some muscle contraction that eventually improves muscle strength.
   c. Passive ROM.
      (1) ROM performed for a patient by another person.
      (2) Passive ROM does not contract muscles and, therefore, does not improve muscle strength.
   d. Continuous-passive ROM.
      (1) ROM achieved for a patient by a machine.
      (2) An extremity is placed in a mechanical device that supports the limb from distal to proximal and sequentially flexes and extends a joint at a prescribed speed and degree of joint flexion (e.g., a machine placed under the upper thigh to the foot flexes the knee and hip).
      (3) Continuous-passive ROM improves extent of joint movement and prevents contractures.
5. Nursing care when providing ROM exercises.
   a. Review the primary health-care provider's restrictions and orders for the type and extent of ROM exercises to ensure that the exercises are permitted and not contraindicated.
   b. Schedule ROM exercises to permit adequate time to complete the planned routine or complete during another activity, such as a bed bath. Doing so ensures that ROM exercises are performed and do not physically tax the patient.
   c. Wash your hands, identify the patient, introduce yourself, explain the procedure to the patient, and provide privacy.
   d. Assess the patient's status, such as presence of joint stiffness, swelling, or pain; physical ability to perform or assist with exercises; level of motivation; and cognitive ability to follow instructions. Doing so provides data that influence the extent to which ROM exercises should be performed.

Table 17.1 Types of Exercises		
Type	**Advantages**	**Examples**
Isotonic • Muscle shortens to produce muscle contraction and movement.	• Increases muscle tone, mass, and strength. • Promotes joint mobility. • Increases heart rate and circulation.	• Walking. • Swimming. • Calisthenics. • Lifting self with a trapeze. • Performing active range of motion (ROM) and activities of daily living.
Isometric • Change in muscle tension occurs without change in muscle length or joint movement.	• Strengthens muscles. • Increases heart rate and cardiac output slightly but not circulation.	• Tensing muscles, such as muscles of an extremity within a cast. • Exerting pressure against an immovable object.
Aerobic • Amount of oxygen meets or exceeds amount of oxygen needed for the activity.	• Strengthens skeletal muscles. • Increases heart and respiratory rates.	• Rapid, intense exercise, such as brisk walking, jogging, and cycling.
Isokinetic • Activity that includes a variable resistance to movement.	• Combines the best features of isotonic and isometric exercise.	• Activities with specialized machines that provide resistance at a constant, preset speed while muscle moves through full ROM.

e. Encourage the patient to perform active ROM exercises to the extent that the patient's health and mobility permit; assist the patient with those exercises that cannot be performed independently. This promotes independence and assistance ensures that the exercises are performed.

f. Begin each movement with the extremity in functional alignment to prevent strain and injury to the patient's body structures.

g. Assess the patient's response to ensure that ROM exercises do not cause pain. Doing so prevents the joint from being moved beyond its ability to be moved.

h. Put each joint through ROM, moving the body part to the point of resistance and applying slow, gentle pressure if rigidity or a contracture is present. Doing so ensures that the joint is put through the fullest range possible and stretches muscle fibers (Table 17.2).

i. Place hands distal and proximal to the joint (Fig. 17.3) or support the joint with one hand while cradling the distal portion of the extremity with the forearm to support the joint while it is being put through ROM.

Table 17.2 **Performing Range-of-Motion Exercises**	
Range of Motion	**Illustration**
Neck: Pivotal joint	
Flexion: Move head from upright midline position forward, ending with chin on chest. Extension: Move head from flexed position to upright midline position. Hyperextension: Move head from upright midline position backward.	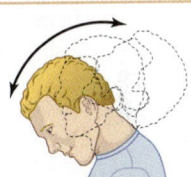
Lateral flexion: Tilt head to side from midline position toward each shoulder.	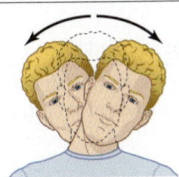
Rotation: Move head in circular motion as far to right or left as possible.	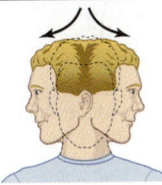
Elbow: Hinge joint	
Flexion: Bend elbow to move forearm toward shoulder. Extension: Straighten arm to bring forearm forward and down.	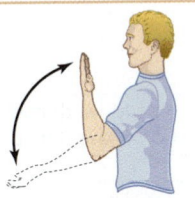
Supination: With elbow flexed at 90°, rotate hand and forearm so that palm is facing toward the floor. Pronation: With elbow flexed at 90°, rotate hand and forearm so that palm is facing toward the ceiling.	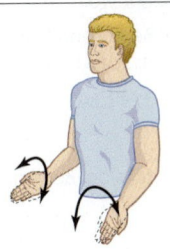

Continued

Table 17.2 Performing Range-of-Motion Exercises—cont'd

Range of Motion	Illustration
Knee: Hinge joint	
Flexion: Bend knee to bring heel toward buttocks. Extension: Straighten knee to move heel away from buttocks.	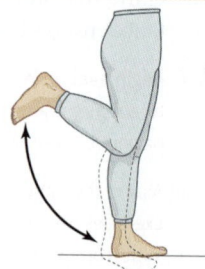
Hands and Fingers: Condyloid joints and hinge joints (interphalangeal joints)	
Flexion: Form a fist with fingers. Extension: Straighten fingers. Hyperextension: Bend fingers back toward outer aspect of forearm.	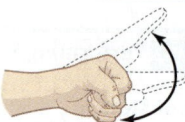
Abduction: Spread fingers apart. Adduction: Move fingers together.	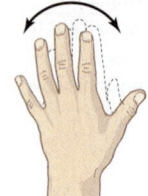
Thumb: Saddle joint	
Flexion: Move thumb across palm toward fifth finger. Extension: Move thumb latterly away from fingers.	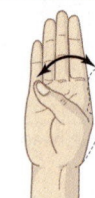
Opposition: Move thumb to tip of each finger.	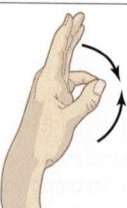
Abduction: Move thumb away from hand. Adduction: Move thumb toward hand.	(See illustration of abduction and adduction under Hands and Fingers above.)
Wrist: Condyloid joint	
Flexion: Bend hand toward inner aspect of forearm. Extension: Straighten wrist in same plane as forearm.	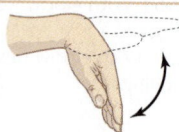
Hyperextension: Bend hand toward outer aspect of forearm.	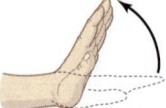

Table 17.2 Performing Range-of-Motion Exercises—cont'd

Range of Motion	Illustration
Abduction (radial flexion): Bend hand toward thumb side. Adduction (ulnar flexion): Bend hand toward fifth finger side	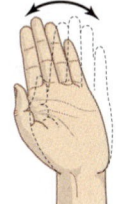
Ankle: Hinge joint	
Flexion (dorsiflexion): Move toes and foot upward toward abdomen. Extension (plantar flexion): Move toes and foot downward away from abdomen.	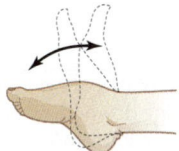
Foot: Gliding joint	
Eversion: Turn sole of foot outward, laterally. Inversion: Turn sole of foot inward, medially.	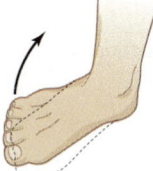
Toes: Hinge joints; intertarsal joints are gliding joints	
Flexion: Curl toes downward. Extension: Straighten toes.	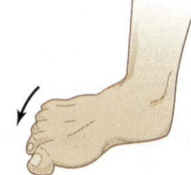
Abduction: Spread toes apart. Adduction: Bring toes together.	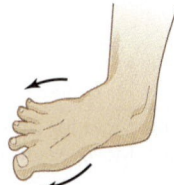
Shoulder: Ball-and-socket joint	
Flexion: Beginning with arm at side of body, raise arm forward and upward to alongside head. Extension: Move arm to side of body. Hyperextension: Beginning with arm at side of body, move arm straight backward.	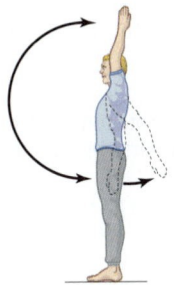

Continued

Table 17.2 Performing Range-of-Motion Exercises—cont'd	

Range of Motion	**Illustration**
Shoulder: Ball-and-socket joint—cont'd	
Abduction: Raise arm laterally with elbow straight to side of head with palm facing outward. Adduction: Move straight arm from side of body to across front midline of body.	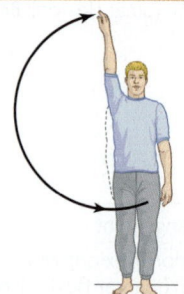
External rotation: Begin with upper arm out to side at shoulder level and elbow bent with fingers pointing downward; then move arm upward until fingers are higher than shoulder. Internal rotation: Move arm forward and downward until fingers are again pointing down below shoulder.	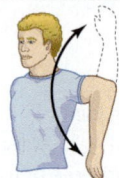
Circumduction: Make a circle with the arm from the shoulder.	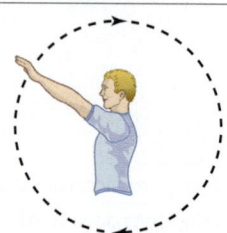
Hip: Ball-and-socket joint	
Flexion: Move leg up and forward. Extension: Move leg down and back beside the other. Hyperextension: Move leg back behind body.	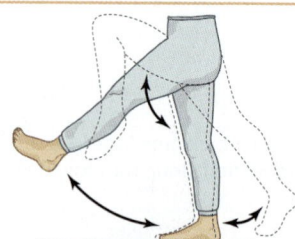
Abduction: Move leg laterally away from body. Adduction: Move leg inward across front midline of body.	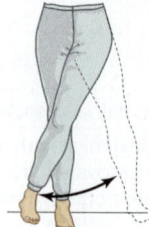
External rotation: Turn leg and foot so they point outward away from other leg. Internal rotation: Turn leg and foot so they point inward toward other leg.	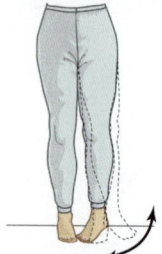

Table 17.2 **Performing Range-of-Motion Exercises—cont'd**	
Range of Motion	**Illustration**
Hip: Ball-and-socket joint—cont'd	
Circumduction: Make a circle with the leg from the hip.	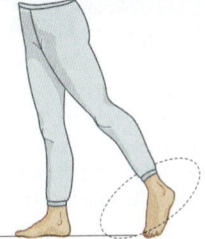

Figure credits: Wilkinson and Treas (2011). *Fundamentals of nursing,* Vol. 2, 2nd ed. Philadelphia: F. A. Davis Company, with permission.

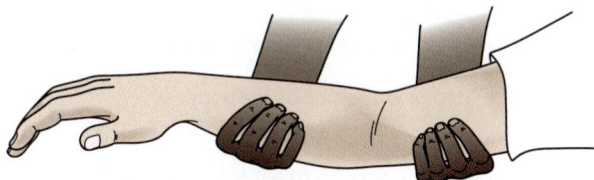

Fig 17.3 Supporting a limb during ROM.

j. Implement ROM slowly, smoothly, and rhythmically to limit stress on the patient's anatomical structures; repeat each movement three to five times to stretch muscle fibers.

k. Monitor the patient's physical, verbal, and nonverbal responses to interventions to provide data that influence continuation of or future implementation of ROM.

l. Use the opportunity to perform other assessments, such as the condition of the skin.

m. Document interventions, extent of mobility of joints, and patient's responses. Doing so documents that the nursing care was provided and communicates information to other members of the health team.

III. Positioning Patients

Clinicians use various positions to maintain patients in functional body alignment with the goal of placing the least stress and strain on the body. Patients generally reposition themselves regularly and move to positions of comfort. However, patients who are physically compromised (e.g., paralyzed, unconscious, or frail), experiencing pain, or cognitively impaired require assistance to change positions. Frequent change in position (every 1 to 2 hours) helps maintain muscle tone and stimulates postural reflexes; it also helps prevent muscle discomfort, compression of blood vessels, damage to superficial nerves, and contractures.

A. Positions

1. Specific positions are used for a variety of reasons, such as patient comfort, prevention of pressure, or access during a procedure (Table 17.3).

2. Each position has its advantages and requires the nurse to place the patient's body, head, and extremities in specific arrangements to maintain body alignment.

B. Commonalities of Nursing Care When Positioning Patients

1. Review the primary health-care provider's activity order and implement the order accordingly (e.g., bedrest, out of bed in a chair for 2 hours twice a day, out of bed). The patient's level of activity requires an order and is a dependent function of the nurse.

2. Assess factors that may influence mobility, such as age, weight, pain, stiffness, contractures, hemiparesis, paraplegia, and mental status. Assessment ensures that nursing care is individualized according to the patient's status and needs.

3. Assess the task to be performed and the patient's status to determine the need for environmental alterations, assistive devices, and additional staff members.

4. Use appropriate assistive devices to move or transfer patients (e.g., pull sheet, gait belt, transfer roller sheets, sit-to-stand lift, and mechanical lift); ensure that all devices are in working order and that wheels on all devices and the patient's bed are locked. Doing so ensures safety of the patient and health team members. (See Chapter 13, "Safety," for additional considerations.)

Table 17.3 **Common Patient Positions**

Position	Nursing Care
Supine 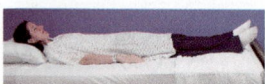 *Advantages:* • Promotes comfort. • Facilitates assessment of the abdomen, breasts, extremities, and pulses. • Prevents headache after spinal anesthesia.	• Keep the head of the bed flat. • Position the patient in the flat, back-lying position with the legs extended. • Place a pillow behind the head and shoulders to prevent hyperextension of the neck. • Keep the arms at the patient's sides. Note: Supported supine position • Elevate the forearms on pillows. • Position a small pillow under the lumbar curvature to limit lordosis. • Place a pillow under the legs from below the knees to above the ankles to keep the heels off the bed. • Place a trochanter roll lateral to each thigh to prevent external rotation. • Use high-top sneakers to support dorsiflexion if ordered.
Dorsal recumbent 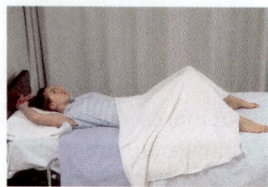 *Advantages:* • Reduces tension on abdominal muscles. • Facilitates assessment of the abdomen, breasts, extremities, pulses, and pelvis.	• Keep the head of the bed flat. • Position the patient in the flat, back-lying position. • Place a pillow behind the head and shoulders to prevent hyperextension of the neck. • Position the patient with the hips and knees slightly flexed and the feet flat on the bed. • Place a pillow under the thighs to support flexion of the knees if necessary. • Place the arms over the head or at the side of the body.
Prone 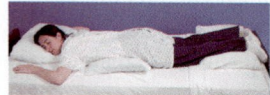 *Advantages:* • Allows full extension of the hips and knees. • Promotes drainage of secretions from the mouth, which helps prevent aspiration. • Relieves pressure on the sacrum and greater trochanter.	• Position the patient on the abdomen. • Turn head to the side on a small pillow to prevent lateral flexion of the neck. • Flex one or both arms. • Change the position in 1 hour or less because the weight of the body on the chest impedes breathing and exerts pressure on the breasts and male genitalia. Note: Supported prone position • Place a small pillow under the abdomen to prevent hyperextension of the lumbar curvature. • Place a small pillow under the lower legs to limit plantar flexion.
Lateral (Side Lying) 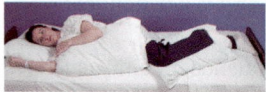 *Advantages:* • Relieves pressure on the sacrum and heels. • Facilitates assessment of the back and perianal areas. • Permits access to the anus to provide perineal care, obtain a rectal temperature, permit insertion of a suppository, or perform an enema. • Promotes rest and sleep.	• Position the patient on a side with a small pillow under the head to prevent lateral flexion of the neck. • Keep lower hip and knee extended to promote functional alignment. • Flex upper hip and knee in front of the body on pillows to prevent adduction and lordosis, promote back alignment, and provide a wider triangular base of support. • Place a pillow behind the back to maintain the lateral position.

Table 17.3 Common Patient Positions—cont'd

Position	Nursing Care
Sims' (Semiprone) 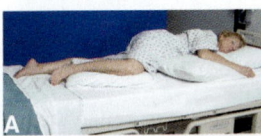 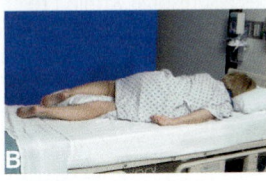 *Advantages* • Facilitates drainage of secretions from the mouth, which helps prevent aspiration. • Relieves pressure on the sacrum, greater trochanter, and heels. • Allows access for perineal assessment or suppository insertion.	• Position the patient halfway between the lateral and prone positions. • Place a small pillow under the head to prevent lateral flexion of the neck. • Keep the lower arm extended behind the body with the palm facing the ceiling and the upper arm in front of the body with the shoulder and elbow flexed on a pillow to prevent internal rotation. • Keep the lower hip and knee extended and the upper hip and knee flexed in front of the body on a pillow to prevent adduction and keep the foot off the mattress.
Fowler 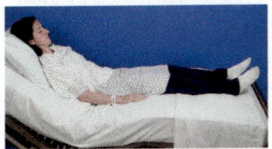 *Advantages:* • Promotes lung expansion. • Limits risk of aspiration associated with gastric feedings and nasotracheal suctioning. • Facilitates intake of oral feedings.	• Position the patient in the back-lying position with the head elevated. Low-Fowler: Head and trunk raised to 15°. Semi-Fowler: Head and trunk raised 16° to 45°. High-Fowler: Head and trunk raised 46° to 90°. • Place a pillow under the head and shoulders to prevent neck flexion and under both arms to limit tension on the shoulders. • Use high-top sneakers to support dorsiflexion if ordered.
Orthopneic 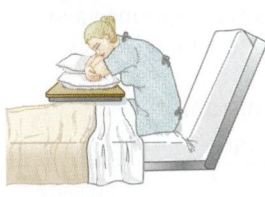 *Advantages:* • Permits maximum lung expansion. • Facilitates exhalation.	• Raise the head of the bed to the high-Fowler position. • Place the patient in the sitting position with a pillow behind the back and leaning on a pillow on an overbed table. • Raise the side rails that do not interfere with placement of the overbed table. • Place patient in a chair leaning forward on a pillow on an overbed table if permitted.
Lithotomy 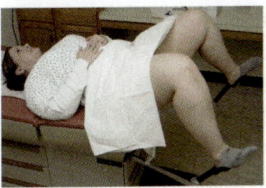 *Advantages:* • Permits access to female perineal area for visual inspection, pelvic examination, perineal hygiene, and vaginal birth. • Facilitates insertion of vaginal suppositories or administration of a douche.	• Position the patient in the back-lying position with the head of the bed flat. • Assist patient with lifting both legs at the same time while placing them in stirrups to limit strain on pelvic structures or place the feet flat on the bed close to the buttocks with the knees flexed and spread apart. • Drape the patient as much as possible to provide for privacy. • Support the legs during the procedure to help a frail patient to maintain the position.

Continued

Table 17.3	Common Patient Positions—cont'd	

Position	Nursing Care
Sitting 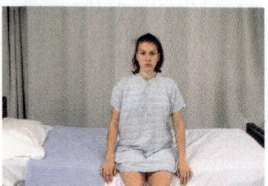 *Advantages:* • Permits assessment of anterior and posterior chest. • Permits assessment of heart and lung sounds. • Promotes function of body systems, especially cardiopulmonary and urinary systems.	• Assist the patient to move from the lying to the sitting position on the side of the bed. • Stand in front of the patient with one foot placed forward between the patient's feet and the other foot placed backward toward the chair to provide a wide base of support. • Ask whether the patient feels lightheaded or dizzy and, if so, return the patient to the lying position if the sensation does not resolve within 1 to 2 minutes. • Ensure that patient's hips and knees are at a 90° angle and that the feet are flat on the floor with foot coverings. • Patient may be assisted to stand and transferred to a chair or wheelchair.

Figure credits: Wilkinson and Treas (2011). *Fundamentals of nursing*, Vol. 2, 2nd ed. Philadelphia: F. A. Davis Company, with permission.)

5. Encourage the patient to assist within the limits of his or her physical status to promote independence and limit muscle atrophy. For example, encourage use of the side rails and trapeze bar to facilitate movement.

6. Follow all the principles of body mechanics.

 a. Ensure that a patient is in functional alignment before changing the patient's position to prevent strain or injury to the patient's body structures.

b. Use a wide base of support. For example, place one foot 8 inches to 10 inches to the side and in front of the other; open the lower support bars of a mechanical lift. Doing so provides a wider base that supports stability.

c. Push, pull, or roll heavy objects when possible rather than lifting to limit the energy and stress required to accomplish the task.

d. Use gravity to facilitate movements because doing so uses the patient's weight and gravity to accomplish the movement and requires less energy to perform the activity. For example, position a bed higher than a chair when getting a patient out of bed and lower the head of the bed before moving a patient up in bed.

e. Use a patient's body mass to help turn the patient. For example, place the patient's arm and leg across the body in the direction the patient is going to turn.

f. Use own body mass and move in the direction the patient is being moved to enhance the power of muscles. For example, rock your body forward when moving patients away from you or backward when moving patients toward you.

g. Allow the person with the heaviest load to coordinate movements when two or more health team members are involved in moving a patient. Doing so ensures coordination of the actions of all health team members involved. Synchronized, smooth movements reduce patient and occupational injuries. For example, direct the movement to begin on the count of three.

h. Turn a patient as a unit (log roll) using 2 to 3 caregivers to maintain spinal alignment following trauma or neuro/orthopedic procedures.

7. Assess the patient's reaction to the activity and record it in the patient's clinical record. Doing so documents that the activity was performed and communicates the reaction to team members.

IV. Negative Effects of Immobility and Related Nursing Care

Immobility is a decrease in the amount and control of movement. It can have major negative effects on many body systems. The longer the inactivity, the greater the risk of the development of a complication of immobility. Nurses can implement a variety of dependent and independent interventions to prevent the negative consequences of immobility. Some of these nursing interventions are general in nature and affect several body systems (Box 17.1) and others are related to specific body systems.

A. **Musculoskeletal System**
   1. Disuse atrophy.
      a. Muscles that are not used decrease in size and physiological ability (**atrophy**).
      b. Muscle begins to lose contractile strength after 24 to 36 hours of inactivity.
      c. Inactivity or bedrest can lead to 7 to 10 percent loss of muscle strength in 1 week.

> **Box 17.1 General Nursing Care for Patients With Limited Mobility**
>
> - Encourage the patient to be as independent as possible.
> - Ensure that immobility is not maintained beyond that which is necessary.
> - Encourage the patient to change position or change a patient's position every 1 to 2 hours, particularly from horizontal to vertical, such as high-Fowler position and out of bed in a chair.
> - Encourage fluid intake (2 to 3 L daily) if not restricted to help prevent responses, such as dehydration, hypercoagulability, thickened respiratory secretions, and constipation.
> - Maintain patient safety at all times, such as by using side rails on the bed, positioning the bed in the lowest position, locking wheels on moveable objects, assisting with ambulation, and encouraging the use of the bathroom and corridor hand rails.
> - Coordinate and support activities performed by other health team members, such as physical, respiratory, and occupational therapists.

2. Contractures.
   a. When a muscle does not contract and relax, it eventually permanently shortens (**contracture**).
   b. Contractures limit joint mobility.
3. Joint stiffness and pain.
   a. Inactive muscles cause connective tissue at joints to become permanently immobile (**ankylosis**).
   b. Demineralization of bone (**osteoporosis**) occurs because of lack of weight bearing.
   c. As bones demineralize, calcium deposits in joints contribute to stiffness and pain.
   d. Demineralized bones may become deformed or fracture easily.
4. Nursing care.
   a. Encourage active ROM or perform passive ROM exercises to maintain joint mobility.
   b. Encourage weight-bearing exercise, such as lifting small handheld weights or using a tilt table, if permitted.
   c. Support joints and limbs when moving patients.
   d. Use assistive devices to maintain body alignment (e.g., trochanter roll, sand bag) or ordered position (e.g., pillow between the legs after hip surgery to keep the legs apart [**abduction**]).
   e. Apply splints or braces as ordered to maintain functional alignment and prevent contracture formation.
   f. Encourage and assist with ambulation if the patient has an order for out of bed.

B. Cardiovascular System
1. Orthostatic hypotension.
   a. Deterioration of the autonomic nervous system results in an inability to equalize blood pressure when moving from a recumbent to a sitting or standing position, causing syncope.
   b. Venous blood pools in the lower extremities because of a decrease in the vasopressor mechanism that normally causes muscle contractions that exert pressure on the veins, promoting venous return.
   c. Orthostatic neurovascular reflex control of blood vessels decreases because of habituation to the lower pressure, higher flow, and increased diameter of vessels in the recumbent position.
2. Increased workload of the heart.
   a. The heart works harder when a person is in the supine position than in an erect position.
   b. Decreased gravity pressure redistributes blood from the legs to other parts of the body, resulting in an increased heart rate, stroke volume, and cardiac output.
   c. Release of the Valsalva maneuver (breath pressed forcibly against a closed glottis) causes a surge of blood to enter the heart that can cause tachycardia and cardiac arrest.
3. Thrombus formation.
   a. Virchow's triad (stasis, activation of clotting, and vessel injury lead to clot formation [thrombus]) can occur.
   b. Venous stasis results from a lack of muscle contraction that promotes venous return.
   c. Hypercoagulability results from an increased concentration of formed elements in blood, a decreased blood volume related to dehydration that often accompanies immobility, and an increased blood calcium level.
   d. Pressure on blood vessels from bed-bound or sitting positions causes intima damage that begins the cascade of clot formation.
   e. A thrombus may move from its place of origin to the lungs (**pulmonary embolus**).
4. Nursing care.
   a. Assess vital signs routinely.
   b. Assess the lower extremities for clinical manifestations of a thrombus, such as localized pain, heat, swelling, and redness.
   c. Teach the patient to avoid performing the Valsalva maneuver, such as by exhaling when attempting a bowel movement or changing positions, because the Valsalva maneuver causes a surge of blood flow when the held breath is released, which can dislodge a thrombus.
   d. Maintain safety due to the potential for orthostatic hypotension.
   e. Apply ordered venous compression devices (e.g., sequential compression devices, antiembolism stockings) that apply pressure to the legs to promote venous return.

⛔ f. Avoid massaging the legs because doing so can cause a thrombus to become a pulmonary embolus.

⛔ g. Encourage intake of 2 to 3 L of fluid daily to prevent dehydration and hypercoagulability.

C. Respiratory System
1. Decreased respiratory movement.
   a. Counterresistance of a bed or chair limits chest movements.
   b. Recumbent positions permit abdominal organs to compress the diaphragm, limiting its usual decent on inspiration.
   c. Muscle disuse or decreased innervation limits the effectiveness of the accessory muscles of respiration.
   d. Medications that act on the central nervous system, such as opioids, anesthesia, and sedatives, may decrease mobility and the rate and depth of respirations.
   e. Decreased lung expansion limits gas exchange.
2. Stasis of respiratory secretions.
   a. Gravity permits secretions to pool in the lungs.
   b. The ability to cough is reduced by a loss of muscle tone and medications that depress the cough reflex.
   c. Patients with mobility problems may have inadequate fluid intake, be dehydrated, or be taking anticholinergic medications that increase the viscosity of secretions.
   d. Secretions may impede exchange of gases between the atmosphere and the lungs and jeopardize a patent airway.
   e. Retained secretions provide a medium for pathogenic microorganisms, resulting in hypostatic pneumonia.
3. Oxygen–carbon dioxide imbalance.
   a. Decreased respiratory movement and stasis of secretions result in deficient ventilation.
   b. Deficient ventilation in conjunction with a decrease in surfactant results in collapse of alveoli (**atelectasis**).
   c. Respiratory acidosis occurs as blood oxygen concentration decreases and carbon dioxide (as hydrogen ions and carbonic acid) increases.
4. Nursing care.
   a. Assess respiratory status, such as rate, regularity, depth (shallow or deep), thoracic or abdominal, easy or labored, length of inhalation and exhalation, productive or nonproductive cough, and oxygen saturation level.
   b. Identify the use of accessory muscles of respiration (e.g., intercostal and sternocleidomastoid muscles).
   c. Assess breath sounds regularly, particularly for crackles and diminished breath sounds.

d. Assess for central nervous system manifestations of hypoxia, such as restlessness, confusion, forgetfulness, and anxiety.

⛔ e. Monitor for clinical manifestations of a pulmonary embolus, such as unilateral chest pain, shortness of breath, dyspnea, tachycardia, tachypnea, and decreased breath sounds on auscultation. These signs and symptoms should be reported to the primary health-care provider immediately.

   f. Maintain semi-Fowler or high-Fowler position if permitted to allow abdominal organs to drop by gravity and promote contraction of the diaphragm.
   g. Encourage the patient to change positions, use an incentive spirometer, and cough every hour to expand the lungs and raise sputum.
   h. Teach the patient to use abdominal muscles to increase the depth of inhalation and prolong exhalation.
   i. Administer oxygen as ordered.
   j. Coordinate activities of the respiratory therapist (e.g., cupping, clapping, postural drainage, nebulizer treatment) if ordered to facilitate mobilization of respiratory secretions.

D. Integumentary System
1. Reduced skin turgor.
   a. Atrophy of skin can occur.
   b. Skin elasticity may decrease because the health of the dermis is affected by fluid shifts between fluid compartments.
2. Skin breakdown.
   a. Decreased circulation as a result of decreased muscle contraction limits the delivery of oxygen and nutrients to cells.
   b. When pressure on a capillary exceeds 15 to 32 mm Hg, its lumen is occluded, resulting in deprivation of oxygen to tissues (**tissue ischemia**) and accumulation of metabolic wastes.
3. Nursing care.
   a. Use predictive measures (such as the Norton Scale [Fig. 17.4]) to assess each patient's risk of pressure ulcer development.
   b. Reposition the patient every 1 to 2 hours to relieve pressure over bony prominences that can lead to pressure ulcers (Fig. 17.5).
   c. Employ actions to avoid shearing, such as using a pull sheet or transfer board and placing the patient in the low-Fowler position.
   d. Use assistive devices to limit the development of pressure ulcers, such as gel pads and an air mattress.
   e. Keep skin clean and dry; use a moisture barrier in the perineal area and implement incontinence management.

Norton Scale for Assessing Risk of Pressure Ulcers

	Physical Condition		Mental Condition		Activity		Mobility		Incontinent		
	Good	4	Alert	4	Ambulant	4	Full	4	Not	4	Total Score
	Fair	3	Apathetic	3	Walk/help	3	Slightly limited	3	Occasional	3	
	Poor	2	Confused	2	Chair-bound	2	Very limited	2	Usually/urine	2	
	Very bad	1	Stupor	1	Bed	1	Immobile	1	Doubly	1	
Name/Date											

The Norton scale uses five criteria to assess patients' risk for pressure ulcers. Scores of 14 or less indicate liability to ulcers; scores of less than 12 indicate very high risk.

Fig 17.4 Norton scale for assessing risk of pressure ulcers. (From Norton, D., McLaren, R., & Exton-Smith, A. N. [1975]. *An investigation of geriatric nursing problems in hospital.* Edinburgh: Churchill Livingstone, with permission.)

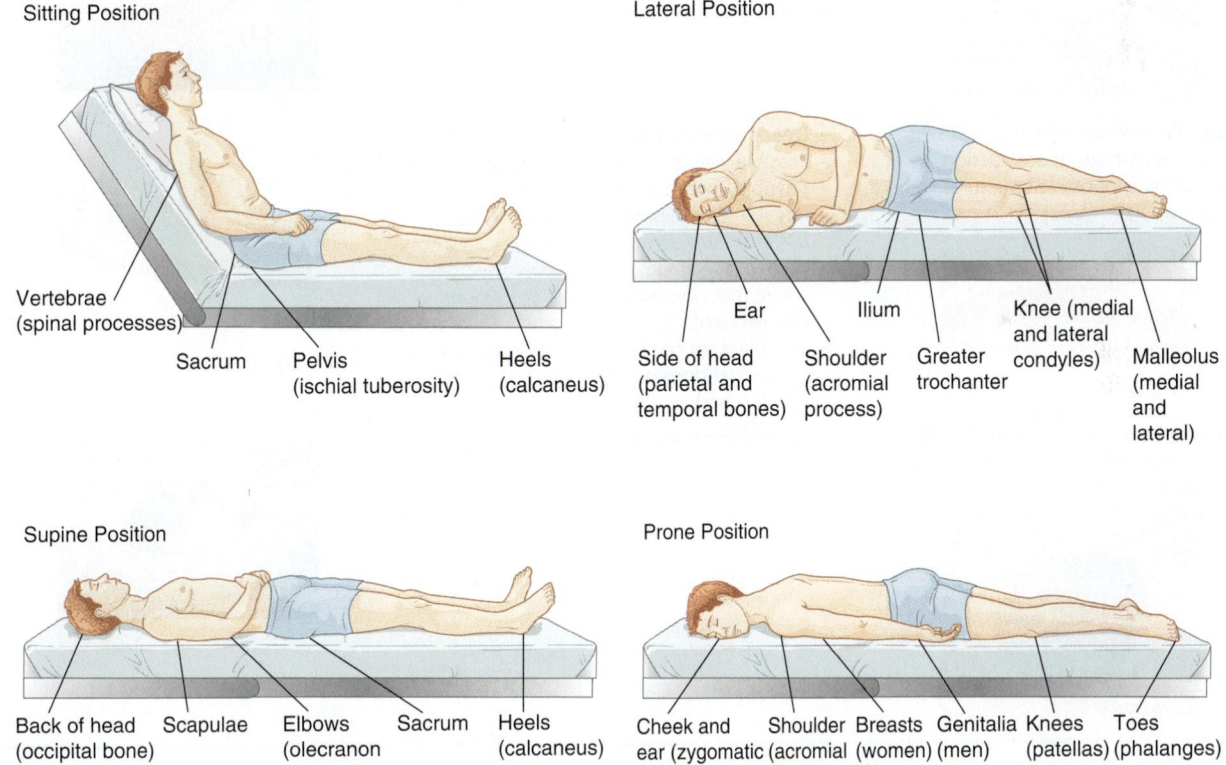

Sitting Position

Vertebrae (spinal processes)
Sacrum
Pelvis (ischial tuberosity)
Heels (calcaneus)

Lateral Position

Ear
Ilium
Knee (medial and lateral condyles)
Side of head (parietal and temporal bones)
Shoulder (acromial process)
Greater trochanter
Malleolus (medial and lateral)

Supine Position

Back of head (occipital bone)
Scapulae
Elbows (olecranon process)
Sacrum
Heels (calcaneus)

Prone Position

Cheek and ear (zygomatic bone)
Shoulder (acromial process)
Breasts (women)
Genitalia (men)
Knees (patellas)
Toes (phalanges)

Fig 17.5 Common sites for pressure ulcer development. (Adapted from *AHRQ clinical practice guidelines,* with permission.)

f. Encourage adequate nutritional and fluid intake, especially foods high in protein and vitamin C.

g. Massage dependent areas to promote circulation.

h. Use dressings (e.g., DuoDERM, transparent adhesives, or films) to protect skin from frictional forces.

i. Assess for the first signs of pressure ulcer development; assess the stage of a pressure ulcer if present. (Table 17.4).

Table 17.4 Pressure Ulcer Stages

Illustration	Nursing Assessment	Photograph
Stage I: Involves only the epidermis. 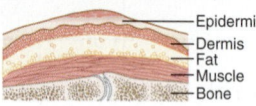	• Erythema that remains for 15 to 30 minutes after release of pressure (**reactive hyperemia**). • Skin that may appear darker than adjacent skin in dark-skinned people. • Lack of blanching when touched with a finger. • Skin that may feel firm, soft, or boggy and warmer or cooler than adjacent tissue. • Tingling or burning at the site.	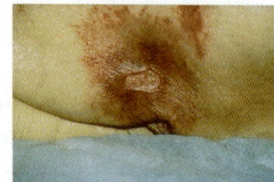
Stage II: Involves the epidermis and partial-thickness loss of the dermis. 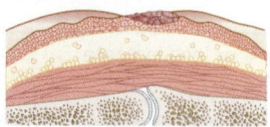	• Serum-filled blister(s) that has ruptured. • Shallow crater that may be pink or red and shiny or dry. • Erythema surrounding skin breakdown that may feel warm to touch.	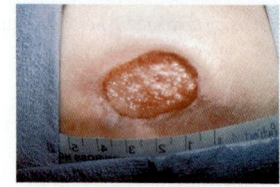
Stage III: Involves the epidermis, full-thickness loss of the dermis, and damage to subcutaneous tissue. 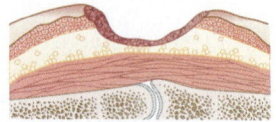	• Deep crater extending down to but not through the fascia. • Damage under outer margins of the ulcer (**undermining**). • Possible presence of exudate.	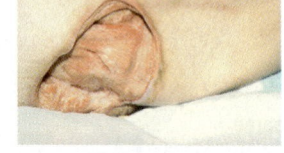
Stage IV: Involves full-thickness skin loss with damage or destruction to muscle, supportive structures, and bone. 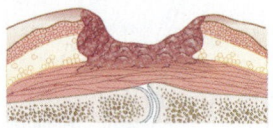	• Deep full-thickness crater. • Possible visible or palpable bone or tendon. • Possible undermining. • Possible development of a sinus tract under the epidermis (**tunneling**). • Tan, yellow, green, gray, or brown necrotic tissue that does not obscure the wound bed (**slough**). • Tan, black, or brown leather-like necrotic tissue that does not obscure the wound bed (**eschar**).	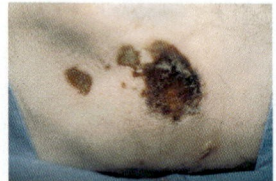
Unstageable: Involves full-thickness skin loss and the base of the wound is obscured by necrotic tissue. 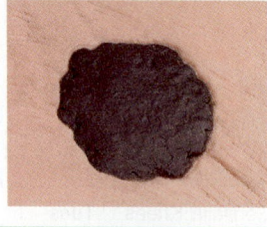	• Base of the wound obscured by slough or eschar.	

The Epidermis, Dermis, Fat, Muscle, and Bone are labeled in the Stage I illustration.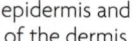

Figure credits: Wilkinson and Treas (2011). *Fundamentals of nursing*, Vol. 2, 2nd ed. Philadelphia: F. A. Davis Company, with permission; and Burton and Ludwig (2011). *Fundamentals of nursing care: Concepts, connections & skills.* Philadelphia: F. A. Davis Company, with permission.

E. Gastrointestinal System
  1. Constipation.
    a. A slowed metabolic rate decreases gastrointestinal motility and delays gastric emptying.
    b. Dehydration, often associated with immobility, results in decreased fluid content in stool.
    c. Ignoring the urge to have a bowel movement may occur due to need to use a bedpan, embarrassment, or inadequate privacy; this weakens the defecation reflex.
    d. Dry, hard stool is more difficult to expel, which may lead to the patient excessively using the Valsalva maneuver.

2. Decreased appetite (**anorexia**).
   a. Appetite diminishes when peristalsis slows, resulting in decreased caloric intake.
   b. Decreased caloric intake results in an inability to meet the body's nutritional needs.
3. Nursing care.
   a. Assess the characteristics of stool, such as frequency, color, and consistency.
   b. Assess the presence and extent of bowel sounds.
   c. Identify the patient's food preferences and incorporate them into the patient's ordered diet when possible.
   d. Encourage the intake of dietary fiber if permitted, such as from whole grains, fruits, and vegetables.
   e. Encourage the patient to assume the sitting position if possible when eating to facilitate the passage of food from the esophagus to the stomach and eventually the intestine.
   f. Teach the patient to respond to the urge to defecate. Toilet a patient immediately when the patient indicates the need to have a bowel movement.
   g. Provide privacy when the patient is attempting to have a bowel movement.
   h. Encourage the patient to use the sitting position for bowel movements, if permitted, to promote gravitational forces and to allow the patient to lean forward to increase intra-abdominal pressure without using the Valsalva maneuver.

F. Metabolic System
1. Decreased metabolic rate.
   a. Metabolic rate, the minimal energy expended to maintain physical and chemical processes, decreases.
   b. Decreased metabolic rate results in a negative nitrogen balance and fatigue.
2. Negative nitrogen balance.
   a. Protein synthesis (**anabolism**) decreases and protein breakdown (**catabolism**) increases.
   b. Catabolized muscles release nitrogen, which is excreted over time; this causes a negative nitrogen balance, which impedes tissue building and wound healing.
   c. Anorexia associated with decreased peristalsis is magnified by the decreased metabolic rate and increased muscle catabolism.
3. Nursing care.
   a. Obtain weekly body weights.
   b. Monitor laboratory values, such as serum albumin and total protein.
   c. Provide preferred foods that are high in protein, such as meat, poultry, fish, eggs, dairy products, and legumes.
   d. Provide small, frequent feedings.

   e. Encourage intake of nutritional supplements (e.g., Boost, Ensure) between meals as ordered.

G. Urinary System
1. Urinary stasis.
   a. When in a horizontal position, urinary stasis occurs due to incomplete emptying of the urinary bladder.
   b. Bladder functioning is further compromised by a decrease in muscle tone.
2. Urinary retention or incontinence.
   a. Urine accumulates in the bladder because of decreased muscle tone.
   b. An inability to relax perineal muscles sufficiently occurs due to unnatural positioning for urination, inadequate privacy, and embarrassment about using a bedpan.
   c. Excessive bladder distention results in involuntary urination (**incontinence**) or involuntary dribbling of urine indicating urinary retention with overflow.
3. Urinary tract infection (UTI).
   a. Demineralization of bone causes hypercalcemia, resulting in urine becoming more alkaline, which supports bacterial growth.
   b. The urinary tract may become contaminated by *Escherichia coli* from inadequate perineal hygiene.
   c. Contaminated urine may back up into the renal pelvis distending the kidneys.
4. Renal calculi.
   a. Demineralization of bone causes hypercalcemia, resulting in calcium salts in urine.
   b. These salts precipitate out as crystals to form renal stones (**calculi**).
5. Nursing care.
   a. Assess the characteristics of the patient's urine, such as color, clarity, and odor.
   b. Assess intake and output.
   c. Encourage the intake of 2 to 3 L of fluid daily if not contraindicated to help flush the kidneys and bladder.
   d. Provide privacy when the patient is urinating.
   e. Encourage assumption of as normal a position as possible when urinating to allow gravity to assist, such as standing for men and sitting for women.
   f. Use techniques to help stimulate urination, such as a warm cloth over the symphysis pubis, hands in a basin of warm water, sound of flowing water from a faucet, and pressure against the suprapubic area with the hands (**Credé's maneuver**).
   g. Assess for clinical manifestations of renal calculi, such as blood in the urine (**hematuria**) and flank pain radiating to the pubic area (**renal colic**).

h. Assess for clinical manifestations of UTI, such as frequency, urgency, hematuria, pus in urine (**pyuria**), and painful urination (**dysuria**).
i. Strain urine if calculi are suspected.
j. Administer prescribed urinary tract analgesics and antibiotics for UTIs.

H. Psychoneurologic System
1. Psychosocial changes.
   a. An inability to fulfill one's role and dependence on others may lower self-esteem and precipitate changes in mood, such as sadness, hostility, and depression.
   b. Narrowed opportunities for socialization may precipitate apathy and withdrawal.
2. Mental changes.
   a. A decrease in a variety of stimuli may precipitate a decreased ability to perceive time accurately, concentrate, problem-solve, and recall sequential events.
   b. A decrease in endorphins, generally released with activity, causes a negative effect on mood.
3. Nursing care.
   a. Assess for clinical indicators of emotional responses associated with limitations in mobility and alterations in body image, such as anxiety, depression, frustration, and anger.
   b. Involve the patient in planning care.
   c. Offer choices whenever possible.
   d. Ensure safety if the patient is cognitively impaired.

VI. Devices Used to Increase Patient Mobility and Related Nursing Care

Patients may present with varying limitations in mobility because of musculoskeletal, neurological, or cardiovascular problems. Devices are available to help patients to maintain independent mobility safely. The nurse should assess each patient to determine the most appropriate device to use because each device serves a purpose and requires specific patient abilities. A major responsibility of the nurse is to assist patients to use these devices safely.

A. Cane
1. A shaft with a handle at one end and one or more points (prongs) that touch the floor.
2. Purposes.
   a. Provides independent mobility.
   b. Limits pressure on weight-bearing joints.
   c. Provides a wide base of support to promote stability.
   d. Promotes walking on flat surfaces as well as using stairs.

3. Nursing care.
   a. Ensure that the patient has the ability to use a cane.
      (1) Ability to bear some weight on both lower extremities.
      (2) Ability to use upper extremity opposite to affected lower extremity.
   b. Ensure appropriate cane length.
      (1) Handle should be level with the greater trochanter.
      (2) Elbow flexed 30° with the wrist extended when holding the handle.
   c. Ensure that the rubber tips on prongs of the cane are intact.
   d. Teach the patient how to use the cane.
      (1) Hold the cane in the hand opposite to the affected lower extremity.
      (2) Distribute weight evenly between the cane and feet.
      (3) Walk erect without leaning forward or toward the cane.
      (4) Advance the cane and the affected lower extremity at the same time and then the other leg.
      (5) Maintain the same length stride with both lower extremities.
      (6) Climb stairs by advancing the unaffected lower extremity and then placing the cane and affected lower extremity on the same step; reverse the procedure when descending the stairs.

B. Walker
1. A U-shaped device with four points that touch the floor; some have two or four wheels and some have a seat.
2. Purposes.
   a. Provides independent mobility.
   b. Limits pressure on weight-bearing joints.
   c. Promotes greater stability by providing a wider base of support than a cane.
   d. Promotes walking on flat surfaces.
   e. Cannot be used on stairs.
3. Nursing care.
   a. Ensure that the patient has the ability to use a walker.
      (1) Ability to bear some weight on both lower extremities.
      (2) Adequate strength in elbow extensors, shoulder depressors, and hand and wrist muscles of both upper extremities to lift and move the walker.
   b. Ensure appropriate walker height.
      (1) Handle should be level with the greater trochanter.

(2) Elbow flexed 30° with the wrist extended when holding the handle.

c. Teach the patient how to use the walker.

   (1) Stand between the back legs of the walker.

   (2) Move the walker forward a short distance.

      (a) Four prong walker: Lift the walker off floor, place all four prongs flat on the floor, and then step between the walker.

      (b) Two-wheeled walker: Lift the back prongs off the floor, roll the walker forward, place the back prongs flat on the floor, and then step between the walker.

      (c) Four-wheeled walker: Push the walker forward and then step between the walker.

C. Crutches

1. A crutch is a shaft that has an axillary bar at the top, a bar for the hands to hold about halfway down the length of the shaft, and one point at the end of the shaft that rests on the floor.

2. Purposes.

   a. Promotes independent ambulation.

   b. Limits or eliminates weight bearing on a lower extremity.

   c. Promotes walking on flat surfaces as well as using stairs.

3. Nursing care.

   a. Ensure that the patient has the ability to use crutches.

     (1) Ability to bear full weight on one leg or partial weight on both legs.

     (2) Adequate strength in the triceps, finger flexors, and wrist and elbow extensors.

   b. Ensure appropriate crutch height.

     (1) Measure the distance from the anterior axillary fold to 6 inches (15 cm) outside of the heel of the foot.

     (2) Allow 2 inches (5 cm) between the axilla and the axillary bar of the crutch.

     (3) Ensure that the hand bar allows extension of the arm with the elbows flexed 30° when weight is placed on the hand.

   c. Ensure that padding on the axillary bars is adequate and the rubber tips on the ends of the crutches are intact.

   d. Teach the patient how to use crutches.

     (1) Use the proper sequence of advancing the crutches and the lower extremities (Table 17.5).

     🛑 (2) Bear weight on the hands, not on the axillae, because bearing weight on the axillae compresses the nerves under the arm, resulting in nerve damage that affects the arms and hands.

     (3) Look forward, not down, when walking to maintain a correct center of gravity; looking down moves the center of gravity forward, jeopardizing stability.

     (4) Maintain balance when using just one lower extremity by keeping the affected lower extremity slightly forward rather

Table 17.5   Crutch-Walking Gaits

Type of Gait	Patient Teaching
Two-point gait • Both lower extremities must be capable of partial weight bearing. • Requires more balance and strength than the 4-point gait. • Maintains 2 points on the floor at all times.	• Move the right crutch and left lower extremity forward simultaneously. • Then move the left crutch and right lower extremity forward simultaneously.
Three-point gait • One lower extremity must be able to support body weight. • Requires more balance and strength in the arms than the 2-point and 4-point gaits.	• Move both crutches and the affected lower extremity forward simultaneously. • Then move the stronger lower extremity forward.
Four-point gait • Both legs must be able to support partial body weight. • Both hands must be able to manipulate crutches. • Maintains 3 points on the floor at all times.	• Move the right crutch forward. • Then move the left lower extremity forward. • Then move the left crutch forward. • Then move the right lower extremity forward.
Swing crutch gaits • Both lower extremities must be able to support partial body weight. • Requires strength in both upper extremities. • Maintains 2 points on the floor at all times.	**Swing-to gait** • Move both crutches forward simultaneously. • Then swing both lower extremities to the level of the crutches. **Swing-through gait** • Move both crutches forward simultaneously. • Then swing both lower extremities slightly past the level of the crutches.

than with the knee flexed; flexing the knee on the affected extremity moves the center of gravity backward, jeopardizing stability.

   (5) Climb stairs by advancing the unaffected lower extremity and then placing the crutches and affected lower extremity on the same step; reverse the procedure when descending the stairs.

D. Wheelchair

1. Wheeled device that consists of a seat with a back, sides to support the arms, foot rests to support the lower extremities, and wheels that allow propulsion by the patient, another person, or a motor.

2. Purposes.
   a. Promotes independent mobility.
   b. Provides mobility for patients who cannot ambulate.
   c. Provides mobility for patients who are too unsteady or frail to use an alternate device.
   d. Eliminates the need to ambulate, thereby decreasing the workload on the heart and oxygen demands of the body.

3. Nursing care.
   a. Maintain safety.
      (1) Ensure that all parts of the wheelchair are in correct working order.
      🛑 (2) Lock the wheels when not moving the wheelchair.
      (3) Keep the wheelchair in close proximity of the bed or chair during a transfer.
      (4) Initiate the transfer by leading from the patient's strongest side.
      (5) Raise the foot rests before transferring the patient to the wheelchair, and place the patient's feet on lowered foot plates after the transfer to the wheelchair.
      (6) Position the patient so that the patient is sitting well back in the wheelchair, with the back of the knees at the edge of but not touching the seat.

🛑 (7) Enter or exit an elevator, maneuver over irregularities in sidewalks, and go down curbs with the large wheels first.

🛑 (8) Place your body between the wheelchair and the lower side of an incline (e.g., push a wheelchair up an incline and back a wheelchair down an incline).

   b. Teach the patient about self-care when using a wheelchair.
   (1) Prevent the development of pressure ulcers over the ischial tuberosities.
      (a) Use a padded cushion or gel pad on the seat to provide a soft surface and distribute body weight more evenly.
      (b) Perform push-ups using the arms of the wheelchair or shift weight side-to-side several times every hour to relieve compression of the capillary beds.
   (2) Prevent hip and knee flexion contractures.
      (a) Avoid sitting in the wheelchair for prolonged periods of time.
      (b) Extend the knees or stand in place if possible every 2 hours to extend the knee and hip joints.
      (c) Assume the prone position when in bed for 20 minutes twice a day to extend the hips and knees.
   (3) Perform assessments to identify early signs of complications.
      (a) Assess the body or have a significant other assess the body routinely to identify early signs of pressure ulcers.
      (b) Identify stiffening of joints that may indicate beginning contractures.
      (c) Notify the primary health-care provider if early signs or symptoms of complications of immobility are identified.
   (4) Inform the patient of the availability of wheelchair accessories (e.g., lap boards, seat belts, removable arms, extended leg panels, motor propulsion).

CASE STUDY: Putting It All Together

An older male patient is admitted to the hospital with a diagnosis of pneumonia and an 8-year history of Parkinson's disease. When transferring the patient from a wheelchair to the bed, a nurse identifies that the patient has stiff joints and is walking with small, shuffling steps with involuntary accelerations. The patient states, "I'm afraid to leave the house because I have difficulty maintaining my balance and I fell twice recently. I hold on to furniture and walls as I walk around my house. Occasionally, I get a little light-headed when I stand up. I really just sit around the house all day because I get too tired and out of breath when I'm more active." When completing a skin check, the nurse identifies in the sacral area several small (1 cm) shallow, red, shiny breaks in the patient's skin that are surrounded by erythema. The nurse also notes rhonchi in the left and right lung fields; heavy, moist cough; occasional expectoration of thick yellow secretions; delayed capillary refill in the toes; respiratory rate of 28/minute and shallow respirations at rest; and dyspnea on exertion. The patient's oxygen saturation is 88 percent on room air and 95 percent with nasal oxygen at 2 L/minute. The primary health-care provider orders passive ROM exercises. Just before leaving the patient's room, the nurse decides to move the patient up in bed.

Case Study Questions

A. Place in order of priority the following concerns identified by the nurse and explain the reasoning behind the sequence identified.

_____ Risk for injury:

_____

_____

_____ Impaired walking:

_____

_____

_____ Ineffective airway clearance:

_____

_____

B. What word(s) should the nurse use when describing the small, shuffling steps with involuntary accelerations?

_____

C. What stage pressure ulcer is associated with several small (1 cm) shallow, red, and shiny breaks in the skin surrounded by erythema?

_____

D. Identify two complications of immobility that affect the cardiovascular system other than orthostatic hypotension, which is already identified in the scenario, and explain why they occur.

1. _____

2. _____

CASE STUDY: Putting It All Together *cont'd*

---- **Case Study Questions** ----

E. Identify six nursing interventions that the nurse should implement to reduce the risk of thrombus formation.

1. _____

2. _____

3. _____

4. _____

5. _____

6. _____

F. Identify seven nursing interventions that the nurse should implement when assisting with or providing ROM exercises.

1. _____

2. _____

3. _____

4. _____

5. _____

6. _____

7. _____

G. Identify ten principles of body mechanics that the nurse should follow when moving a patient up in bed and explain their purposes.

1. _____

2. _____

3. _____

4. _____

5. _____

6. _____

7. _____

8. _____

9. _____

10. _____

REVIEW QUESTIONS

1. Which range-of-motion exercise is being performed when the nurse touches the patient's thumb to the small fifth finger on the same hand?
   1. Extension
   2. Adduction
   3. Opposition
   4. Circumduction

2. What is the cause of pressure (decubitus) ulcers?
   1. Pressure
   2. Desquamation
   3. Skin breakdown
   4. Cellular necrosis

3. Which photograph illustrates the range-of-motion exercise known as supination?
   1.

   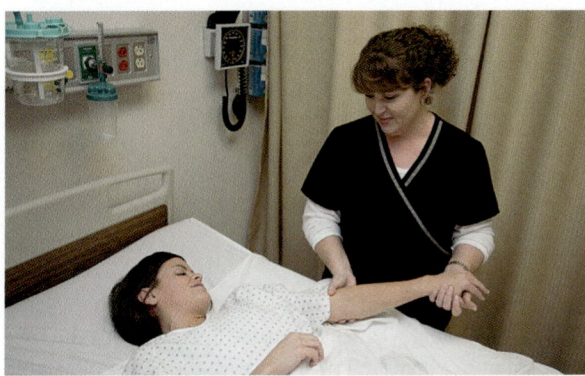

   2.

   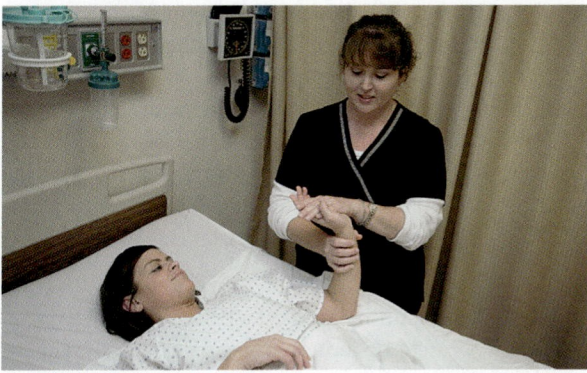

   3.

   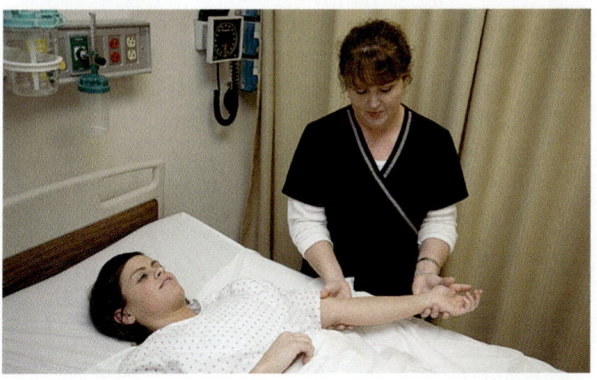

   4.

   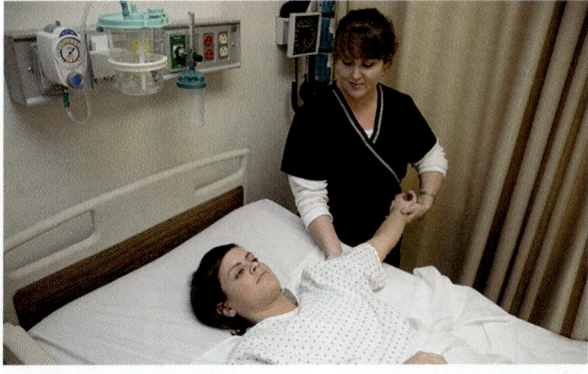

4. A nurse is repositioning a patient in the right Sims' position. What action should the nurse implement when positioning this patient?
   1. Position the left arm behind the body.
   2. Rest the right leg on the top of the left leg.
   3. Flex the right arm and rest it on a pillow.
   4. Turn the body halfway between the lateral and prone position.

5. A nurse teaches the spouse of a patient in a wheelchair how to use a wheelchair safely. Which statement by the spouse indicates that the teaching was effective? **Select all that apply.**
   1. _____ "I will enter an elevator with the wheelchair's big wheels first so that we are facing toward the door."
   2. _____ "I should keep the wheelchair in front of me when going down a steep ramp."
   3. _____ "I can use the footrests of the wheelchair to push a swinging door open."
   4. _____ "I can push the wheelchair in front of me when going up a hill."
   5. _____ "I must lock the brakes when the wheelchair is not moving."

6. A nurse is caring for a patient with a pillow between the legs to prevent adduction of the prosthetic right hip joint. What is wrong with this patient's positioning?

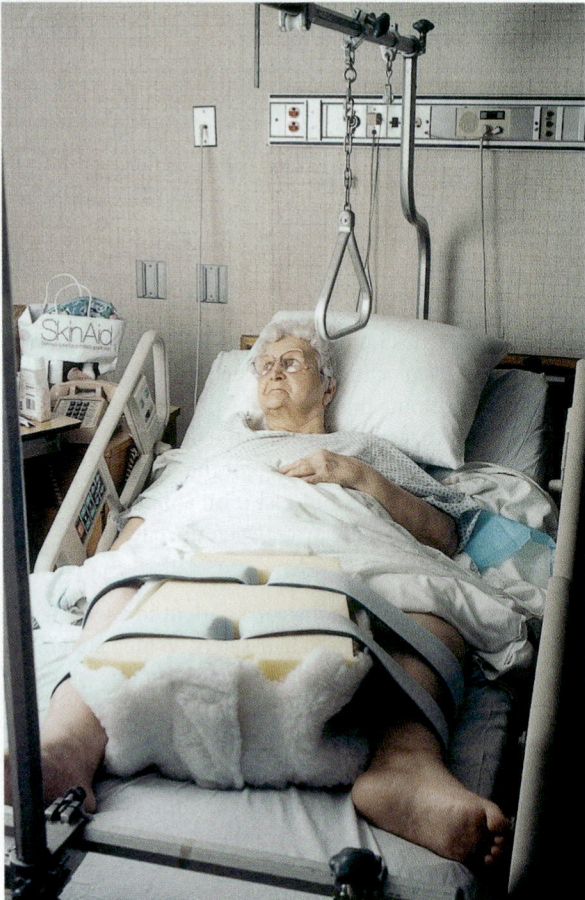

1. The left hip is externally rotated.
2. The left arm should be on a pillow.
3. The trapeze should be closer to the patient.
4. The patient should be in the supine position.

7. A nurse is caring for a patient who recently had spinal surgery requiring the patient to be supine in bed. What dependent nursing action should the nurse implement that will help prevent complications associated with venous stasis?
1. Assess vital signs routinely.
2. Encourage ankle pumping exercises.
3. Apply sequential compression devices.
4. Place in the semi-Fowler position occasionally.

8. A nurse is repositioning a patient in the right lateral position. What action should the nurse implement when positioning this patient?
1. Rest the head on one pillow.
2. Extend the right arm and rest it on a pillow.
3. Support the right hip to the knee with a trochanter roll.
4. Flex the left hip and knee and rest the left leg on the right leg.

9. The primary health-care provider orders the nurse to teach the patient isometric exercises. Which patient activity indicates that the patient understands isometric exercise?
1. Exerts pressure against an immovable object
2. Performs active range-of-motion to joints
3. Walks briskly around the hospital unit
4. Lifts the body using a trapeze

10. A nurse is caring for a patient with pressure ulcers over the right and left ischial tuberosities. In what position should the nurse place the patient to relieve pressure in these areas? **Select all that apply.**
1. _____ Sims'
2. _____ Prone
3. _____ Orthopneic
4. _____ Right lateral
5. _____ High-Fowler

11. A nurse observes a nursing assistant lift a heavy object from the floor. Which action indicates that the nursing assistant is using inappropriate body mechanics?
1. Keeping the back as straight as possible
2. Holding the object away from the body
3. Placing the feet wide apart
4. Bending the knees

12. A nurse is teaching a patient with weakness in the left leg how to use a cane. The nurse first positions the patient in a standing position with the cane in the hand opposite the affected leg. Place the following steps in the order in which they should be implemented.
1. Position the tip of the cane 6 inches in front of the strong foot.
2. Move the affected leg ahead opposite to the cane.
3. Move the cane forward 4 to 6 inches.
4. Move the unaffected leg forward.
5. Put weight on the affected leg.
6. Repeat the sequence of steps.
   Answer: _____

13. A nurse is planning to assist a patient with active assistive range-of-motion exercises. What should the nurse do **first**?
1. Encourage the patient to be as independent as possible when doing range-of-motion exercises.
2. Identify any restrictions regarding the type and extent of range-of-motion exercises.
3. Explain what range-of-motion exercises are and why they are being done.
4. Schedule range-of-motion exercise to occur during the patient's bath.

14. A nurse is completing a head-to-toe assessment of a newly admitted patient. The nurse identifies a lesion that looks like a broken blister over a bony prominence on the patient's foot. Which condition should the nurse conclude the patient is exhibiting?
    1. Pressure ulcer
    2. Plantar wart
    3. Callus
    4. Corn

15. A nurse is positioning a patient in the supported prone position. What action should the nurse implement when positioning this patient?
    1. Put pillows under the patient's thighs.
    2. Place pillows alongside the patient's hips.
    3. Place a large pillow under the patient's head.
    4. Put a small pillow under the patient's abdomen.

16. For which of the following consequences associated with the muscular system should the nurse assess a patient who has been on prolonged bedrest?
    1. Atrophy
    2. Osteoporosis
    3. Pressure ulcers
    4. Skin breakdown

17. Which position is least likely to be used to position a patient with a stage III pressure ulcer of the right greater trochanter?
    1.

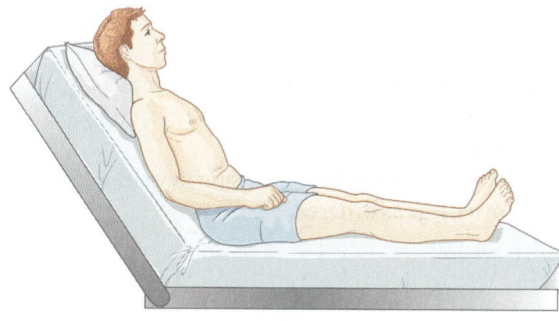

    2.

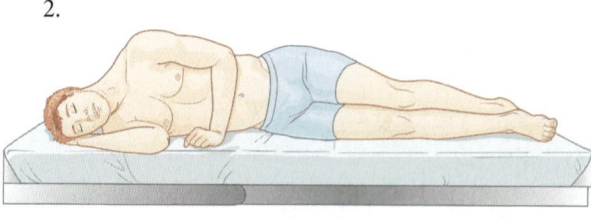

    3.

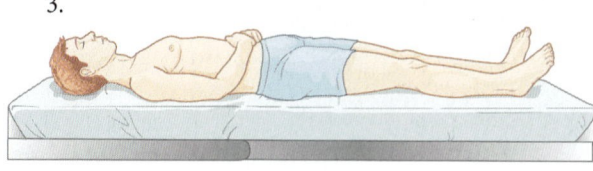

    4.

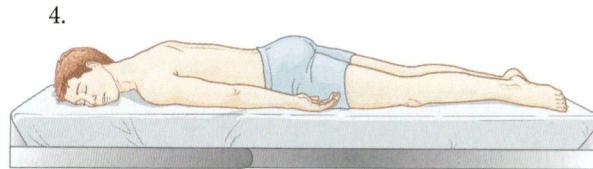

18. A nurse is ambulating a patient in the hall several rooms away from the patient's room. During the walk, the patient states, "I am dizzy and I feel very weak." What action by the nurse is **most** appropriate at this time?
    1. Return the patient to bed.
    2. Lower the patient to the floor gently.
    3. Walk toward the patient's room slowly.
    4. Call another nurse to assist with the patient.

19. A nurse is caring for a bed-bound patient. In which position should the nurse place the patient to prevent a hip flexion contracture?
    1. Prone
    2. Supine
    3. Fowler
    4. Lateral

20. A nurse must transfer a patient from a bed to a wheelchair. Place the following nursing actions in the order that they should be performed.
    1. Lock the brakes on the wheelchair.
    2. Place the wheelchair parallel to the patient's bed.
    3. Stand up and pivot the patient toward the wheelchair.
    4. Inform the patient how the transfer will be performed.
    5. Bend your knees and place your arms under the patient's axillae.
    6. Allow the patient to sit on the side of the bed for several minutes.
       Answer: _____

21. What should the nurse do **first** before moving a patient?
    1. Consider all of the principles of body mechanics that should be followed.
    2. Select assistive devices to support the patient's functional alignment.
    3. Assess for factors that may influence the patient's mobility.
    4. Review the primary health-care provider's activity order.

22. The primary health-care provider writes the following order, "Teach the patient to engage in aerobic exercise." Which exercise should the nurse discuss with the patient?
    1. Tensing and relaxing muscles
    2. Using a machine for resistance while moving a joint
    3. Jogging while progressively increasing the distance over time
    4. Walking around the neighborhood in a gentle but steady pace

23. A nurse is caring for a patient who is comatose and determines that the patient has a stage IV pressure ulcer. Which observations support this conclusion? **Select all that apply.**
   1. _____ Wound obscured with sloughing tissue
   2. _____ Soft tissue over a bony prominence
   3. _____ Deep crater with an intact fascia
   4. _____ Tunneling under the epidermis
   5. _____ Full thickness skin loss

24. A nurse is positioning a patient in the semi-Fowler position. What action should be implemented by the nurse when positioning this patient?
   1. Place 2 pillows under the patient's head.
   2. Raise the head of the patient's bed 15 degrees.
   3. Use pillows to maintain dorsiflexion of the patient's feet.
   4. Put trochanter rolls alongside the patient's knees to the ankles.

25. A primary health-care provider orders active range-of-motion exercises. What nursing action is unique to providing active range-of-motion exercises?
   1. Assisting the patient who is unable to complete the exercises through all planes of movement
   2. Encouraging the patient to perform the exercises independently
   3. Providing a warm bath before the exercises
   4. Demonstrating how to do the exercises

26. Which principle of body mechanics should the nurse implement when providing nursing care?
   1. Hold an object away from the body.
   2. Extend the arms when lifting objects.
   3. Squat when lifting objects off the floor.
   4. Keep feet together when moving an object.

27. A nurse is caring for a patient with a pressure ulcer on the right trochanter. In which position should the nurse place this patient? **Select all that apply.**
   1. _____ Semi-Fowler
   2. _____ Right lateral
   3. _____ Left Sims'
   4. _____ Supine
   5. _____ Prone

28. A nurse is caring for a patient who is at risk for thrombus formation due to decreased mobility. For which clinical manifestation that is the **most** serious should the nurse monitor the patient?
   1. Faint pedal pulse
   2. Edema of the calf
   3. Pain in the lower leg
   4. Unilateral chest pain

29. A nurse is providing passive range-of-motion exercises. Which principle is important?
   1. Increase the speed of the exercises progressively and according to the patient's tolerance.
   2. Assist the patient to complete all planes of movement when the patient is unable to do so.
   3. Support above and below the joint being exercised.
   4. Repeat each movement ten times.

30. Which position requires that the patient be repositioned after only 1 hour, rather than after 2 hours, which is generally the norm?
   1. Sims'
   2. Prone
   3. Lateral
   4. Orthopneic

31. A nurse is caring for a patient who has an order for bedrest. The nurse is concerned about the patient's increased risk for hypostatic pneumonia. Which nursing action should be implemented by the nurse to minimize this risk?
   1. Assess lung sounds for crackles.
   2. Position the patient in a chair for meals.
   3. Encourage the use of an incentive spirometer hourly when awake.
   4. Apply sequential compression devices to the lower legs as ordered.

32. A nurse is caring for a newly admitted patient who has a urinary tract infection and is recovering from a brain attack (cerebrovascular accident, stroke) that left her with mild hemiparesis of the right side. She uses a cane and a lower right leg brace to enable her to walk more normally without having to lift her leg and have her foot slap down on the ground due to a slight footdrop. The primary health-care provider orders an IV antibiotic, out of bed to a chair twice a day, and a regular diet. The nurse reviewed the patient's clinical record, interviewed the patient, and completed a brief physical assessment.

Patient's Clinical Record

Laboratory Results: Urinalysis

Cloudy, concentrated.
RBCs greater than 3 (per high-power field).
WBCs greater than 6 (per high-power field).
Specific gravity: 1.023.
pH: 8.5.
Presence of casts.
Culture positive for *Pseudomonas*.

Patient Interview

States that she spends most of her time lying on the couch. She said that she is limiting her fluid intake starting in the early afternoon so that she does not have to get up so much. However, she said, "Lately I feel as though I have to get up all the time to pass my water. I know that it sounds childish, but I have been wearing an adult incontinence pad so that I don't have to get up so much. The doctor ordered an antibiotic because he said that I have a urinary tract infection."

Physical Assessment

Temperature: 102.4°F, oral.
Pulse: 100 beats/minute, occasional missed beat at irregular intervals.
Respirations: 24 breaths/minute, no dyspnea.
Blood pressure: 138/84 mm Hg.
Voiding small amounts of urine frequently, concentrated, cloudy.
Abdomen does not feel distended.
Patient states that it burns when she urinates.
Perineal area appears red and inflamed, but skin is intact.
IVF running at 125 mL per hour as ordered, site dry and intact with no S&S of infection or infiltration.

What should the nurse do **first** based on the collected data?
1. Apply a protective skin ointment to the perineal area.
2. Teach the patient to limit fluid intake after 6:00 p.m.
3. Take the patient's vital signs every 4 hours.
4. Administer the antibiotic.

33. A nurse identifies that a patient is walking with a propulsive cogwheel gait. Which patient behavior observed by the nurse supports this conclusion?
1. Rolling motion in which the opposite hip drops when taking a stride
2. Exaggerated lifting of the leg to avoid dragging the toes
3. Small, shuffling steps with involuntary acceleration
4. Stiff, foot dragging when ambulating

34. A nurse is caring for a patient with a diagnosis of thrombophlebitis of the lower left leg. Which independent nursing action is important for the nurse to implement?
1. Elevate the left leg on a pillow.
2. Apply a warm soak to the left leg twice a day.
3. Massage the legs gently from distal to proximal.
4. Maintain venous compression devices to both legs.

35. A nurse is caring for a patient who recently sustained a brain attack (cerebrovascular accident, stroke), which caused right-sided hemiparesis. The nurse is concerned about the patient developing contractures related to immobility. Which action is important for the nurse to implement?
1. Providing active and passive range-of-motion exercises
2. Turning the patient from side to side every 2 hours
3. Placing the patient on a tilt table 2 times a day
4. Encouraging coughing and deep breathing

36. Which nursing action is effective in minimizing tissue ischemia due to shearing forces?
1. Massaging gently around the patient's boney prominences every two hours
2. Using a transfer board to move a patient from a bed to a stretcher
3. Placing an air mattress on the bed under the patient
4. Positioning the patient in a semi-Fowler position

37. A patient who has been immobile because of a spinal cord injury develops hypercalcemia. The primary health-care provider prescribes hydrochlorothiazide 50 mg twice a day by mouth. The medication is supplied in capsules of 12.5 mg. How many capsules should the nurse administer for each dose? Record your answer using a whole number.

Answer: _____ capsules

38. A nurse is caring for a patient who is ordered OOB in a chair for 1 hour twice a day. The nurse is concerned about the complication of orthostatic hypotension. What nursing action employed by the nurse will help to minimize the risk of orthostatic hypotension?
    1. Encourage use of an incentive spirometer every 2 hours.
    2. Massage the patient's legs gently before moving to a sitting position.
    3. Teach ways to avoid the Valsalva maneuver when changing position.
    4. Dangle the patient on the side of the bed for 1 minute before standing.

39. A nurse is repositioning a patient who is on bedrest to the orthopneic position. What action should the nurse implement when repositioning this patient?
    1. Position trochanter rolls alongside the hips to the knees of both legs.
    2. Elevate the head of the bed to a high-Fowler position.
    3. Help the patient to stand from a sitting position.
    4. Lift both legs into the stirrups at the same time.

40. A nurse is caring for a patient who is on bedrest and is concerned about the risk of urinary stasis. Which nursing action is effective in reducing the risk of complications associated with urinary stasis?
    1. Strain urine if calculi are suspected.
    2. Pour warm water over the symphysis pubis.
    3. Assist the patient to a normal position when voiding.
    4. Encourage the intake of three liters of fluid daily if permitted.

REVIEW ANSWERS

1. ANSWER: 3.
Rationales:
1. Extension is straightening the finger joints.
2. Adduction is bringing the fingers in alignment next to one another.
3. Opposition is the correct term to describe touching the thumb to the tip of each finger of the same hand.
4. Circumduction is a circular motion of the hip or shoulder joint.
Content Area: Mobility
Integrated Processes: Nursing Process: Implementation
Client Need: Physiological Integrity; Basic Care and Comfort
Cognitive Level: Knowledge

2. ANSWER: 1.
Rationales:
1. Pressure ulcers occur when the pressure in the capillaries exceeds that of the arterioles (15 to 32 mm Hg). Pathologic changes begin within 1 to 2 hours when tissues are deprived of oxygen and nutrients. If pressure is not relieved, tissue breakdown and cellular death (necrosis) occur.
2. Desquamation (shedding of the epidermis) is seen in postmature infants. It is not a cause of pressure ulcers.
3. Skin breakdown is the response to pressure, not the cause of a pressure ulcer; also, skin breakdown may be caused by stressors other than pressure.
4. Cellular necrosis is the death of tissues in response to prolonged pressure and oxygen deprivation; cellular necrosis is the response to pressure, not the cause of a pressure ulcer.
TEST-TAKING TIP: Identify the option that is unique. Option 1 is unique because it is not an example of tissue breakdown but rather the cause of deprivation of oxygen to tissue, which can cause death to cells. Identify equally plausible options. Options 2, 3, and 4 are equally plausible. They all are examples of tissue breakdown. Identify the option with the clang association. The word *pressure* in the stem and in option 1 is a clang association.
Content Area: Mobility
Integrated Processes: Nursing Process: Analysis
Client Need: Physiological Integrity; Reduction of Risk Potential
Cognitive Level: Comprehension

3. ANSWER: 3.
Rationales:
1. Turning the patient's arm so that the palm is facing the floor results in pronation, not supination, of the arm.
2. Bending the fingers of a hand back as far as possible so that the nails of the fingers are facing the forearm results in hyperextension of the wrist, not supination of the arm.
3. Turning the patient's arm so that the palm is facing toward the ceiling results in supination of the arm.
4. Moving the arm so that it is 90 degrees away from the side of the body results in abduction of the shoulder, not supination of the arm.

TEST-TAKING TIP: Identify the options that are opposites. Options 1 and 3 are opposites. In option 1, the arm is positioned so that the palm is facing downward toward the floor. In option 3, the arm is positioned so that the palm is facing upward toward the ceiling. More often than not, the correct answer is one of the options that is an opposite. Examine options 1 and 3 carefully.
Content Area: Mobility
Integrated Processes: Nursing Process: Implementation
Client Need: Physiological Integrity; Basic Care and Comfort
Cognitive Level: Analysis

4. ANSWER: 4.
Rationales:
1. The left arm should be positioned in front of the body, not behind the body.
2. Both legs should be slightly flexed in front of the body with the left leg in front of the right leg.
3. The right arm should be positioned behind the body in extension with the palm facing toward the ceiling.
4. This is correct position of the body when a patient is placed in the Sims' position.
TEST-TAKING TIP: Identify the unique option. Option 4 is the only option that does not discuss positioning of the arms or legs. Examine options that are unique carefully.
Content Area: Mobility
Integrated Processes: Nursing Process: Implementation
Client Need: Physiological Integrity; Basic Care and Comfort
Cognitive Level: Application

5. ANSWER: 1, 4, 5.
Rationales:
1. This is an acceptable practice. The patient should be facing out toward the door as other people in the elevator tend to face. In addition, the big wheels rather than the small wheels of the wheelchair will navigate the space between the floor and the elevator with less interference.
2. This is unsafe. Having the wheelchair in front when going down a steep ramp will not prevent it from rolling down the hill in the event the person pushing the wheelchair loses control.
3. This is unsafe. The pressure of the door may injure the patient's feet or break the footrests of the wheelchair.
4. This is a safe practice. Having the wheelchair in front when going up a hill will help prevent the wheelchair from rolling backwards in the event the person pushing the wheelchair loses control. The body of the person pushing the wheelchair will prevent the wheelchair from rolling backward.
5. This is a safe practice. It is important to lock the brakes when a wheelchair is not in motion to prevent it from moving.
Content Area: Mobility
Integrated Processes: Teaching/Learning; Nursing Process: Evaluation
Client Need: Safe and Effective Care Environment; Safety and Infection Control
Cognitive Level: Application

6. **ANSWER: 1.**
   Rationales:
   1. The focus of the abduction pillow is to prevent adduction of the right leg, which can cause dislocation of the prosthesis. However, the other joints in the body should be maintained in functional alignment. Either a trochanter roll should be aligned along the side of the left leg from the hip to the knee or the left leg should be more securely positioned to the abduction pillow to prevent external rotation of the left hip.
   2. The left forearm and hand are positioned across the abdomen, which is acceptable. This position helps prevent dependent edema in the left hand via the principle of gravity.
   3. The trapeze is the correct distance from the patient. If it is too close to the patient, the patient will not have room to lift the upper body off the bed.
   4. The low-Fowler position is acceptable. However, a high-Fowler position is contraindicated. The hip flexion angle should not exceed 90 degrees because this can cause the prosthetic hip to dislocate.
   TEST-TAKING TIP: Identify the word in the stem that indicates negative polarity. The word *wrong* in the stem indicates negative polarity. Identify the clang association. The word *hip* in the stem and in option 1 is a clang association.
   Content Area: Mobility
   Integrated Processes: Nursing Process: Evaluation
   Client Need: Physiological Integrity; Basic Care and Comfort
   Cognitive Level: Analysis

7. **ANSWER: 3.**
   Rationales:
   1. This is an independent, not dependent, action of the nurse. Although taking vital signs routinely will help identify the patient's cardiovascular status, it will not prevent a complication such as thrombophlebitis due to venous stasis.
   2. Encouraging a patient to do ankle pumping exercises is an independent, not dependent, action of the nurse that will help minimize venous stasis due to immobility.
   3. Applying sequential compression devices ordered by a primary health-care provider will help minimize the risk of complications associated with venous stasis. This is a dependent function of the nurse because it must be ordered by the primary health-care provider.
   4. The supine, not semi-Fowler, position is ordered for this patient.
   Content Area: Mobility
   Integrated Processes: Nursing Process: Implementation
   Client Need: Physiological Integrity; Basic Care and Comfort
   Cognitive Level: Application

8. **ANSWER: 1.**
   Rationales:
   1. Resting the head on one pillow prevents right lateral flexion of the neck and positions the patient's head in functional alignment.
   2. The right arm should be flexed at the elbow and the shoulder externally rotated. The right arm should rest on the mattress without a pillow.
   3. A trochanter roll is unnecessary. The right hip and leg are positioned against the mattress. A trochanter roll is used to prevent external rotation of the hip when the patient is in a supine position.
   4. The left hip and knee should be flexed slightly in front of the right leg and positioned on enough pillows to maintain functional alignment of the left hip, knee, and ankle.
   TEST-TAKING TIP: Identify the unique option. Option 1 is the only option that includes the head rather than an extremity.
   Content Area: Mobility
   Integrated Processes: Nursing Process: Implementation
   Client Need: Physiological Integrity; Basic Care and Comfort
   Cognitive Level: Application

9. **ANSWER: 1.**
   Rationales:
   1. This action is an example of isometric exercise. It requires muscle tension with no change in muscle length or movement.
   2. This is an example of isotonic, not isometric, exercise. Isotonic exercise involves a shortening and then lengthening of muscles to produce movement.
   3. Walking briskly is associated with aerobic, not isometric, exercise. Aerobic exercise involves sustained periods of exertion whereby oxygen is metabolized to support energy.
   4. This is an example of isotonic, not isometric, exercise. Isotonic exercise involves a shortening and then lengthening of muscles to produce movement.
   Content Area: Mobility
   Integrated Processes: Nursing Process: Evaluation
   Client Need: Physiological Integrity; Basic Care and Comfort
   Cognitive Level: Application

10. **ANSWER: 1, 2, 4.**
    Rationales:
    1. An ischial tuberosity is a bony prominence located at the base of each ischium bone at the base of the pelvic girdle. No weight is placed on these boney prominences when in the Sims' position.
    2. An ischial tuberosity is a bony prominence located at the base of each ischium bone at the base of the pelvic girdle. No weight is placed on these boney prominences when in the prone position.
    3. The orthopneic position should be avoided. An ischial tuberosity is a bony prominence located at the base of each ischium bone at the base of the pelvic girdle. Body weight rests on these boney prominences when the body is in the sitting position.
    4. An ischial tuberosity is a bony prominence located at the base of each ischium bone at the base of the pelvic girdle. No weight is placed on these boney prominences when in the right lateral position.
    5. The high-Fowler position should be avoided. An ischial tuberosity is located at the base of each ischium bone at the base of the pelvic girdle. Body weight rests on these bones when the body is in the high-Fowler position.
    Content Area: Mobility
    Integrated Processes: Nursing Process: Implementation
    Client Need: Physiological Integrity; Basic Care and Comfort
    Cognitive Level: Application

11. ANSWER: 2.
Rationales:
1. This action prevents injuries to the back and is an acceptable practice. Keeping the back as straight as possible prevents twisting (torsion). Twisting the back puts strain on the vertebrae, muscles, and tendons.
2. Holding the object away from the body is improper body mechanics. It does not keep the weight close to the body's center of gravity, which minimizes stress on the back's vertebrae, muscles, and tendons.
3. Placing the feet wide apart is proper body mechanics because it promotes stability by increasing the base of support.
4. Bending the knees while lifting an object demonstrates proper body mechanics. It allows the larger muscles of the legs to assist with the lift rather than the weaker muscles of the back. If the legs are not bent, the individual will have to bend at the waist and lean over to pick up the object, putting undue strain on the back.
TEST-TAKING TIP: Identify the word in the stem that indicates negative polarity. The word *inappropriate* in the stem indicates negative polarity. The question is asking, "What action by the nursing assistant is wrong and violates the principles of body mechanics?" Identify the option that contains a clang association. The word *object* in the stem and in option 2 is a clang association.
Content Area: Safety
Integrated Processes: Nursing Process: Evaluation
Client Need: Safe and Effective Care Environment; Management of Care
Cognitive Level: Application

12. ANSWER: 1, 3, 2, 5, 4, 6.
Rationales:
1. When a patient is in the standing position, a cane should be placed 6 inches from the front of the unaffected foot. This distance supports balance in the erect position.
3. The cane is moved forward only 4 to 6 inches because this distance keeps the cane within a tolerable distance from the patient's center of gravity.
2. The affected leg is then moved an equal distance forward opposite to the cane. While the affected leg is being moved, the unaffected leg is bearing the weight of the body.
5. When weight is put on the affected leg, the cane shares the body's weight.
4. When the unaffected leg is moved forward, the affected leg and cane share the body's weight.
6. This sequence is repeated as the patient moves forward.
Content Area: Mobility
Integrated Processes: Nursing Process: Planning
Client Need: Physiological Integrity; Basic Care and Comfort
Cognitive Level: Analysis

13. ANSWER: 2.
Rationales:
1. Although this should be done, it is not the first nursing action implemented by the nurse.
2. Assessment is the first step of the nursing process. Before a patient engages in range-of-motion exercises, the nurse should identify any factors that should be taken into consideration before teaching or providing range-of-motion exercises, such as the presence of contractures, pain, weakness, or impaired cognition.
3. Although this should be done, it is not the *first* thing that the nurse should do.
4. Although this may be arranged, it is not the first thing that the nurse should do.
TEST-TAKING TIP: Identify the word in the stem that sets a priority. The word *first* in the stem sets a priority.
Content Area: Mobility
Integrated Processes: Nursing Process: Assessment
Client Need: Physiological Integrity; Basic Care and Comfort
Cognitive Level: Application

14. ANSWER: 1.
Rationales:
1. A blister over a bony prominence is a stage II pressure ulcer.
2. A plantar wart is a painful growth caused by a virus; generally, it occurs on the sole of a foot, not over a bony prominence.
3. Although a callus may be found over a bony prominence, it is hardened skin, not a blister-like lesion. It is similar to a corn but generally covers a larger surface area and patients report that they are not painful.
4. Although a corn may be found over a bony prominence, it is a thickening of the skin caused by pressure or friction; usually it is due to ill-fitting shoes, and patients report that corns are painful.
Content Area: Mobility
Integrated Processes: Nursing Process: Analysis
Client Need: Physiological Integrity; Basic Care and Comfort
Cognitive Level: Analysis

15. ANSWER: 4.
Rationales:
1. Pillows should not be positioned under the thighs. This will result in lordosis, which puts stress on the vertebrae and muscles of the back. A pillow should be placed under the lower legs; this will keep the feet off the bed, minimizing planter flexion (extension of the ankle).
2. Pillows alongside the hips are unnecessary to maintain functional alignment in this position.
3. A small, not large, pillow should be positioned under the patient's head to maintain the head in functional alignment. A large pillow under the head causes lateral flexion of the neck, which may cause stress and strain on the muscles of the neck.
4. This supports functional alignment because it prevents hyperextension of the lumbar curvature. In addition, it minimizes pressure on the genitalia of male patients and pressure on the breasts of female patients.
Content Area: Mobility
Integrated Processes: Nursing Process: Implementation
Client Need: Physiological Integrity; Basic Care and Comfort
Cognitive Level: Application

16. ANSWER: 1.

Rationales:

1. **Lack of contraction of muscles that occurs with immobility results in a decrease in the size of muscles (atrophy). Muscle strength begins to decline within 48 hours of the initiation of bedrest or immobility.**

2. Osteoporosis is the loss of bone mass and is associated with the skeletal system, not muscles. Immobility contributes to bone loss. Weight-bearing exercises, such as walking, are associated with bone buildup.

3. A pressure ulcer is a lesion caused by tissue compression when capillary occlusion pressure exceeds 15 to 32 mm Hg, causing tissue ischemia and eventual cell death. Pressure ulcers most often are associated with the skin (integumentary system).

4. Skin breakdown is associated with pressure ulcers and is associated with the skin (integumentary system).

TEST-TAKING TIP: Identify the options that are equally plausible. Options 3 and 4 are equally plausible. Pressure ulcers are examples of skin breakdown. Option 3 is no better than option 4. Eliminate both options from further consideration because they are distractors.

Content Area: Mobility
Integrated Processes: Nursing Process: Assessment
Client Need: Physiological Integrity; Basic Care and Comfort
Cognitive Level: Application

17. ANSWER: 2.

Rationales:

1. The high-Fowler position does not put pressure on the right greater trochanter. It places pressure on the vertebrae, sacrum, pelvis (ischial tuberosities), and heels (calcaneus).

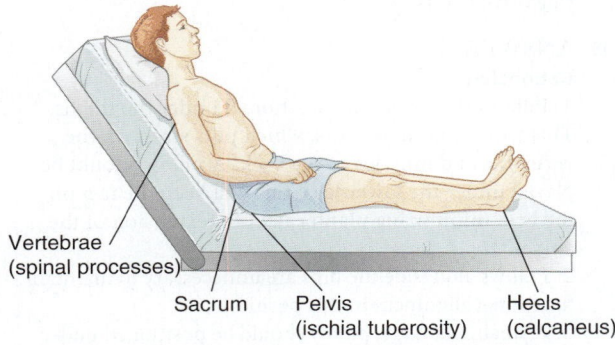

Vertebrae (spinal processes)

Sacrum Pelvis (ischial tuberosity) Heels (calcaneus)

2. **The right side-lying position (right lateral position) places pressure on the right greater trochanter and should be avoided when a patient has a pressure ulcer in this area.** Additional pressure areas associated with the right side-lying position include the side of the head (parietal and temporal bones), ear, shoulder (acromial process), ilium, knee (medial and lateral condyles), and ankle (medial and lateral malleolus).

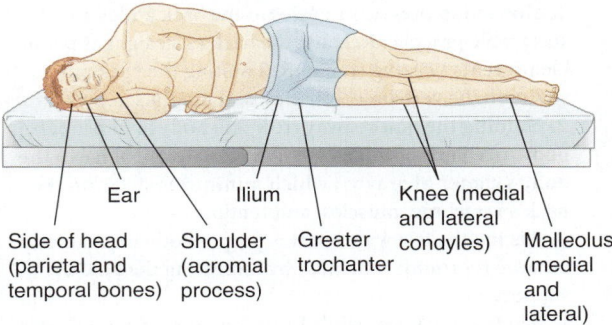

Ear Ilium Knee (medial and lateral condyles)

Side of head (parietal and temporal bones) Shoulder (acromial process) Greater trochanter Malleolus (medial and lateral)

3. The supine position does not put pressure on the right greater trochanter. It places pressure on the back of the head (occipital bone), scapulae, elbows (olecranon process), sacrum, and heels (calcaneus).

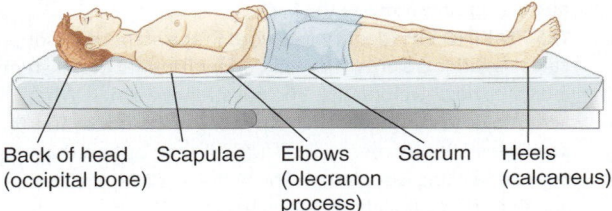

Back of head (occipital bone) Scapulae Elbows (olecranon process) Sacrum Heels (calcaneus)

4. The prone position does not put pressure on the right greater trochanter. It places pressure on the cheek and ear (zygomatic bone), shoulder (acromion process), breasts in women, genitalia in men, and toes (phalanges).

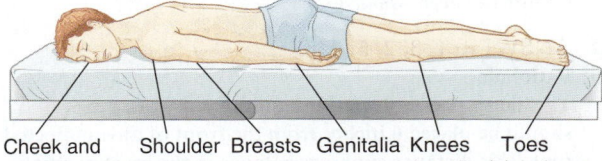

Cheek and ear (zygomatic bone) Shoulder (acromial process) Breasts (women) Genitalia (men) Knees (patellas) Toes (phalanges)

TEST-TAKING TIP: Identify the word in the stem that indicates negative polarity. The word *least* in the stem indicates negative polarity.

Content Area: Mobility
Integrated Processes: Nursing Process: Implementation
Client Need: Physiological Integrity; Basic Care and Comfort
Cognitive Level: Analysis

18. ANSWER: 2.

Rationales:

1. This is inappropriate and unsafe. Rapid movements will exacerbate the patient's feeling dizzy and the patient is feeling weak and will not be able to move quickly.

2. **Lowering the patient to the floor gently allows the nurse to prevent the patient's head from hitting the floor.**

It controls the patient's movement toward the floor, preventing injury to both the patient and nurse.

3. Slowly walking back to the patient's room when the patient feels weak and dizzy may result in the patient falling, injuring both the patient and nurse.

4. Calling for another nurse to assist is an admirable intervention but there may not be enough time for the nurse to arrive to be of assistance.

TEST-TAKING TIP: Identify the word in the stem that sets a priority. The word *most* in the stem sets a priority.

Content Area: Safety
Integrated Processes: Communication/Documentation; Nursing Process: Implementation
Client Need: Safe and Effective Care Environment; Safety and Infection Control
Cognitive Level: Application

19. **ANSWER: 1.**
Rationales:

1. **Placing the patient in the prone position (lying face down on the abdomen) will prevent a hip flexion contracture because the mattress will push against and prevent the hip muscles from contracting. This position should be assumed twice a day for approximately 30 to 60 minutes as long as the patient's respiratory status is adequate.**

2. The supine position will not fully prevent hip flexion contracture because there will be no force to resist hip muscle flexion.

3. The Fowler position may accelerate hip flexion contractures because the hips will be partially flexed and there will be no counter-resistance to prevent contractures.

4. The lateral position will not prevent hip flexion contractures because it will not offer any counter-resistance to natural muscle contraction.

Content Area: Mobility
Integrated Processes: Nursing Process: Implementation
Client Need: Physiological Integrity; Basic Care and Comfort
Cognitive Level: Application

20. **ANSWER: 4, 2, 1, 6, 5, 3.**
Rationales:

4. **Informing the patient about the procedure should be done first to decrease the patient's anxiety and promote teamwork during the transfer.**

2. Placing the wheelchair parallel to the patient's bed minimizes the distance the patient has to transfer and keeps it in the patient's and nurse's line of vision.

1. Locking the brakes of the wheel chair prevents it from moving after it has been placed next to the patient's bed.

6. Prior to transferring the patient, the nurse should let the patient sit on the side of the bed with shoes on and the feet on the floor. This decreases the risk of orthostatic hypotension when the patient stands.

5. Bending your knees and placing your arms under the patient's axillae with the hands supporting the back allows the nurse to control the patient's movement.

3. Standing up assists the patient to an upright position and pivoting, rather than twisting, prevents injury to the patient's and nurse's backs.

Content Area: Mobility
Integrated Processes: Nursing Process: Planning
Client Need: Physiological Integrity; Basic Care and Comfort
Cognitive Level: Planning

21. **ANSWER: 4.**
Rationales:

1. Although this is important, it is not the first thing that the nurse should do before moving a patient.

2. Although this is important, it is not the first thing that the nurse should do before moving a patient.

3. Although identifying factors that may influence a patient's activity, such as age, weight, pain level, presence of contractures, weakness, and mental status, is important, it is not the first action by the nurse.

4. **This is the first nursing action before moving a patient. Maintaining a patient's activity is a dependent nursing action and requires an order by the primary health-care provider.**

TEST-TAKING TIP: Identify the word in the stem that sets a priority. The word *first* in the stem sets a priority. Identify the option with the specific determiner. The word *all* in option 1 is a specific determiner. Rarely is an option with a specific determiner the correct answer. Delete option 1 from further consideration.

Content Area: Mobility
Integrated Processes: Nursing Process: Implementation
Client Need: Safe and Effective Care Environment; Safety and Infection Control
Cognitive Level: Application

22. **ANSWER: 3.**
Rationales:

1. This is an example of isometric, not aerobic, exercise. It requires muscle tension with no change in muscle length or movement.

2. This is an example of isokinetic, not aerobic, exercise.

3. **Jogging is an example of aerobic exercise. It is an intense exercise that metabolizes oxygen to support energy.**

4. Walking at a gentle, steady pace is an example of isotonic, not aerobic, exercise. It involves shortening and lengthening of muscles to produce movement. When done gently at a steady pace, it does not fall into the realm of aerobic exercise.

Content Area: Mobility
Integrated Processes: Teaching/Learning; Nursing Process: Implementation
Client Need: Physiological Integrity; Basic Care and Comfort
Cognitive Level: Application

23. ANSWER: 4, 5.
Rationales:
1. This describes an unstageable pressure ulcer, not a stage IV pressure ulcer. An unstageable pressure ulcer involves full thickness skin loss with the base obscured by necrotic tissue. Slough is necrotic tissue that is tan, yellow, green, gray, or brown in color.
2. Soft, boggy tissue over a bony prominence indicates a stage I, not stage IV, pressure ulcer.
3. A deep crater with an intact fascia indicates a stage III, not stage IV, pressure ulcer. Stage III ulcers extend down to, but not through, the fascia. Undermining and exudate may be present.
4. **Tunneling under the epidermis (sinus tract) occurs because of the deep tissue injury.**
5. **This describes a stage IV pressure ulcer. The pressure ulcer may also have tunneling, undermining, and necrotic tissue that is tan, yellow, green, gray, or brown that does not obscure the wound bed. In addition, a stage IV pressure ulcer may have eschar (tan, black, or brown leathery necrotic tissue) that does not obscure the wound bed.**
Content Area: Mobility
Integrated Processes: Nursing Process: Analysis
Client Need: Physiological Integrity; Basic Care and Comfort
Cognitive Level: Analysis

24. ANSWER: 3.
Rationales:
1. One pillow is sufficient to maintain functional alignment of the head and neck. Two pillows will cause unnecessary flexion of the head, which should be avoided.
2. Raising the head of the bed 15 degrees or less is the low-, not semi-, Fowler position. The semi-Fowler position involves raising the head of the bed 16 to 45 degrees.
3. **Pillows placed against the bottom of the feet support dorsiflexion, which helps prevent footdrop (planter flexion).**
4. Trochanter rolls generally are used to prevent external rotation of the hips when the patient is in the supine position. Trochanter rolls are positioned alongside the hips to the knees, not the knees to the ankles.
Content Area: Mobility
Integrated Processes: Nursing Process: Implementation
Client Need: Physiological Integrity; Basic Care and Comfort
Cognitive Level: Application

25. ANSWER: 2.
Rationales:
1. When a patient needs assistance to complete these exercises, it is called active assistive range-of-motion exercises, not active range-of-motion exercises.
2. **Active range-of-motion exercises require the patient to complete the exercises independently. Active range-of-motion exercises require muscle contraction that eventually improves muscle strength.**
3. Although a warm bath may relax the patient, reducing stiffness, it is not a required or unique action associated with implementing range-of-motion exercises.
4. This is not unique to providing active range-of-motion exercises. Explaining what is to be done and why should be implemented before providing all nursing care.

TEST-TAKING TIP: Identify the option that contains a specific determiner. Option 1 contains the word *all* which is a specific determiner. Identify the options that are opposites. Options 1 and 2 are opposites. Option 1 has the nurse assisting the patient and option 2 encourages the patient to perform the exercises independently. Examine option 1 and 2 carefully. More often than not, an option that is an opposite is the correct answer.
Content Area: Mobility
Integrated Processes: Teaching/Learning; Nursing Process: Implementation
Client Need: Physiological Integrity; Basic Care and Comfort
Cognitive Level: Application

26. ANSWER: 3.
Rationales:
1. Objects should be held close to the body when lifting or carrying an object. The closer the object is to the center of gravity, the more stable the body and less strain on the muscles of the back.
2. Elbows should be flexed when lifting objects; elbows act as fulcrums (the point on which a lever moves).
3. **Squatting uses the stronger muscles of the legs to provide the power when lifting an object, rather than the smaller and weaker muscles of the arms and back. This decreases strain on the weaker muscles.**
4. Feet should be spread wide apart when lifting an object. This provides a wide base of support. The wider the base of support, the more stable the object or person.
Content Area: Mobility
Integrated Processes: Nursing Process: Implementation
Client Need: Physiological Integrity; Basic Care and Comfort
Cognitive Level: Application

27. ANSWER: 1, 3, 4, 5.
Rationales:
1. **There is no pressure on the right trochanter when the patient is positioned in the semi-Fowler position.**
2. The right lateral position should be avoided because it places direct body pressure on the right trochanter.
3. **There is no pressure on the right trochanter when the patient is positioned in the left Sims' position.**
4. **There is no pressure on the right trochanter when the patient is positioned in the supine position.**
5. **There is no pressure on the right trochanter when the patient is positioned in the prone position.**
Content Area: Mobility
Integrated Processes: Nursing Process: Implementation
Client Need: Physiological Integrity; Basic Care and Comfort
Cognitive Level: Application

28. ANSWER: 4.
Rationales:
1. A faint pedal pulse indicates impaired circulation to the foot. Although this is serious, another clinical indicator is life threatening and takes priority.
2. Although edema of the calf indicates the presence of a thrombus in a vein in the calf, it is a localized problem that has not yet become life threatening. Another option is more serious because it is a clinical indicator of a life-threatening event.

3. Although pain in the lower leg may indicate the presence of a thrombus in a vein in the calf, it is a localized problem that has not yet become life threatening. Another option is more serious because it is a clinical indicator of a life-threatening event.

4. Unilateral chest pain that occurs in the presence of a thrombophlebitis indicates that a part of the thrombus has become an embolus that has lodged in the lung. When this occurs, it has the potential to be life threatening.

TEST-TAKING TIP: Identify the word in the stem that sets a priority. The word *most* in the stem sets a priority. Identify the option that is unique. Options 1, 2, and 3 all refer to a lower extremity. Option 4 is unique because it relates to the chest.

Content Area: Mobility
Integrated Processes: Nursing Process: Assessment
Client Need: Safe and Effective Care Environment; Reduction of Risk Potential
Cognitive Level: Application

29. **ANSWER: 3.**
    Rationales:
    1. Each movement should be implemented slowly, smoothly, and rhythmically. This minimizes undue stress and strain on the structures of the joint and adjoining muscles.
    2. With passive range-of-motion exercises, the caregiver moves the patient's joints through their full range to the point of resistance without active participation on the part of the patient.
    3. This is most important because it prevents undue stress, strain, or injury to the muscles, joints, and ligaments that can occur when a joint is unsupported.
    4. Three to five repetitions twice a day is sufficient to maintain full range of motion. Ten repetitions are unnecessary.

    TEST-TAKING TIP: Identify the option with a specific determiner. Option 2 contains the word *all* which is a specific determiner. Identify the options that contain a clang association. The stem contains the word *exercises* and options 1 and 3 contain the words *exercises* and *exercised* respectively. Consider options 1 and 3 carefully because they each contain a clang association.

    Content Area: Mobility
    Integrated Processes: Nursing Process: Implementation
    Client Need: Physiological Integrity; Basic Care and Comfort
    Cognitive Level: Application

30. **ANSWER: 2.**
    Rationales:
    1. The patient can remain in the Sims' position for 2 hours unless circumstances require more frequent repositioning.
    2. Because respiratory exertion is reduced in the prone position due to the pressure of body weight on the chest and because of pressure on the breasts in women and genitalia in men, patients should be repositioned after 1 hour.
    3. The patient can remain in the lateral position for 2 hours, unless circumstances require more frequent repositioning.
    4. The patient can remain in the orthopneic position for 2 hours, unless circumstances require more frequent repositioning.

Content Area: Mobility
Integrated Processes: Nursing Process: Implementation
Client Need: Physiological Integrity; Basic Care and Comfort
Cognitive Level: Application

31. **ANSWER: 3.**
    Rationales:
    1. Assessing a patient for clinical indicators of a hypostatic pneumonia does not lower the risk of hypostatic pneumonia. It only reflects the presence of adventitious breath sounds.
    2. The patient has an order for bedrest. The patient should not be sitting in a chair for meals.
    3. An incentive spirometer helps the patient increase the depth of inhalations, which aerates the lower lobes of the lung; also, it facilitates movement of secretions into upper areas of the lungs whereby coughing may enable expectoration of the secretions. Aeration of the lower lobes of the lungs and expectoration of secretions help reduce stasis of secretions, which can precipitate hypostatic pneumonia.
    4. Sequential compression devices will not reduce the risk of hypostatic pneumonia; they increase peripheral venous return in the legs.

    Content Area: Mobility
    Integrated Processes: Nursing Process: Assessment
    Client Need: Safe and Effective Care Environment; Reduction of Risk Potential
    Cognitive Level: Application

32. **ANSWER: 4.**
    Rationales:
    1. Although this should be done, it is not the priority.
    2. The patient should drink 2 to 3 L of fluid daily to flush the urinary system of invading pathogens; however, it is not the priority.
    3. Although the patient's vital signs should be monitored every 4 hours because the patient has a urinary tract infection, it is not the priority.
    4. A urinary tract infection is a complication associated with urinary stasis as a result of impaired mobility. Administering the antibiotic is the priority as long as the urine specimen has been collected and sent to the laboratory; this is the case in this situation because the laboratory section of the medical record indicates results of a urinalysis and urine culture.

    TEST-TAKING TIP: Identify the word in the stem that sets a priority. The word *first* in the stem sets a priority.

    Content Area: Mobility
    Integrated Processes: Nursing Process: Implementation
    Client Need: Safe and Effective Care Environment; Management of Care
    Cognitive Level: Analysis

33. **ANSWER: 3.**
    Rationales:
    1. This is a waddling gait associated with developmental dysphagia of the hip or due to the enlarged abdomen associated with pregnancy.
    2. This is a steppage gait. It is associated with fooddrop and Guillain-Barré syndrome.

3. This is a propulsive cogwheel gait. It is associated with Parkinson's disease.

4. This is a spastic gait. It is associated with cerebral palsy.

TEST-TAKING TIP: Identify the option with an obscure clang association. The word *propulsive* in the stem and the word *acceleration* in option 3 is an obscure clang association. Both words have the same meaning. Examine options with clang associations carefully. More often than not, an option with a clang association is the correct answer.

Content Area: Mobility
Integrated Processes: Nursing Process: Analysis
Client Need: Physiological Integrity; Basic Care and Comfort
Cognitive Level: Comprehension

34. ANSWER: 1.
Rationales:

1. This is an independent function of the nurse and does not require an order from the primary health-care provider. This action uses the principle of gravity to facilitate venous return and reduce edema in interstitial tissue.

2. Applying heat is a dependent function of the nurse and cannot be implemented without an order from the primary health-care provider. If ordered, the nurse can apply a warm soak to the area. This action causes vasodilation, which increases blood flow to the area.

3. Massaging the legs should be avoided because it can cause a thrombosis to become an embolus, which can travel to a lung, causing a life-threatening situation.

4. Applying a venous compression device to the left leg is contraindicated. This may cause a thrombosis to become an embolus, which can travel to a lung. This is a life-threatening event. In addition, applying venous compression devices requires an order by a primary health-care provider; it is a dependent function of the nurse.

TEST-TAKING TIP: Identify options with a clang association. The words *left leg* in the stem and in options 1 and 2 are clang associations. Examine options 1 and 2 carefully. More often than not, an option with a clang association is the correct answer. Identify equally plausible options. Options 3 and 4 are equally plausible. They both apply external pressure to the legs. Option 3 is no better than option 4. Eliminate options 3 and 4 from further consideration.

Content Area: Mobility
Integrated Processes: Nursing Process: Implementation
Client Need: Physiological Integrity; Physiological Adaptation
Cognitive Level: Application

35. ANSWER: 1.
Rationales:

1. Range-of-motion exercises minimize the formation of contractures. Putting joints through their full range several times daily averts shortening of muscles, which causes contractures.

2. The main purpose of repositioning a patient is to prevent tissue ischemia over boney prominences, which causes pressure ulcers, not to prevent contractures. Also, repositioning can minimize stasis of respiratory secretions, thereby reducing the risk of hypostatic pneumonia.

3. The use of a tilt table will not prevent contractures. A tilt table is used to place weight on the long bones of the body,

helping to reduce bone demineralization. Also, it is used to help the body adapt to changes in circulation when moved from a lying to a standing position.

4. Coughing and deep breathing will not prevent contractures associated with right-sided hemiparesis. Coughing and deep breathing helps to mobilize respiratory secretions, thereby reducing the risk of hypostatic pneumonia.

Content Area: Mobility
Integrated Processes: Nursing Process: Implementation
Client Need: Physiological Integrity; Basic Care and Comfort
Cognitive Level: Application

36. ANSWER: 2.
Rationales:

1. Although massaging around boney prominences every two hours increases circulation in an effort to minimize the risk of a pressure ulcer, it does not prevent shearing.

2. A transfer board helps to prevent shearing forces when moving a patient from a bed to a stretcher. Shearing occurs when the epidermal layer slides over the dermis, causing injury to the vascular bed; in addition, when shearing occurs, it reduces the amount of pressure needed to occlude vessels by half. Shearing often occurs when a patient slides down in bed when the head of the bed is elevated higher than the low-Fowler position and when a patient is dragged across the surface of a mattress when being moved up in bed without the use of a pull sheet.

3. An air mattress helps to distribute body weight over a larger surface area, thereby minimizing the risk of tissue ischemia due to pressure; it does not prevent shearing.

4. A low-, not semi-, Fowler position reduces the risk of shearing forces. Shearing forces occur when the epidermal layer slides over the dermis, causing injury to the vascular bed. Shearing forces occur when the head of a patient's bed is elevated to a semi- or high-Fowler position and the patient slides lower in the bed in response to gravity.

Content Area: Mobility
Integrated Processes: Nursing Process: Implementation
Client Need: Safe and Effective Care Environment; Reduction of Risk Potential
Cognitive Level: Application

37. ANSWER: 4.
Rationale:
Solve the problem by using the formula for ratio and proportion.

$$\frac{\text{Desire } 50 \text{ mg}}{\text{Have } 12.5 \text{ mg}} \times \frac{\text{x capsules}}{1 \text{ capsule}}$$

$$12.5x = 50 \times 1$$

$$12.5x = 50$$

$$x = 50 \div 12.5$$

$$x = 4 \text{ capsules}$$

Content Area: Medication Administration
Integrated Processes: Nursing Process: Planning
Client Need: Physiological Integrity; Pharmacological and Parenteral Therapies
Cognitive Level: Application

38. ANSWER: 4.

Rationales:

1. An incentive spirometer helps minimize the risk of stasis of respiratory secretions, not orthostatic hypotension.

2. The nurse should never massage a patient's legs because doing so could cause a thrombus to become an embolus, which could cause a pulmonary embolus or other life-threatening vascular occlusion.

3. Avoiding the Valsalva maneuver (exhalation pressed forcibly against a closed glottis) causes a surge of blood to enter the heart, which can cause tachycardia and cardiac arrest, not orthostatic hypotension.

4. When moving from a sitting and then to a standing position after being on bedrest, venous blood pools in the lower extremities because of a decrease in the vasopressor mechanism (muscle contraction causing pressure on veins promotes venous return). Having a patient sit for a minute after raising the head of the bed and then having the patient sit on the side of the bed with the legs resting on the floor (dangle) for a minute allows time for the blood pressure to equalize, which minimizes the risk of orthostatic hypotension and a fall.

Content Area: Mobility

Integrated Processes: Nursing Process: Implementation

Client Need: Physiological Integrity; Basic Care and Comfort

Cognitive Level: Application

39. ANSWER: 2.

Rationales:

1. Trochanter rolls are used to prevent external rotation of the hips when a patient is in the supine, not orthopneic, position.

2. This is the correct position of the head of the bed when that patient is in the orthopneic position. Once in the high-Fowler position, a pillow should be placed behind the patient to maintain the patient in a forward leaning position. The orthopneic position allows gravity to move abdominal organs downward away from the thoracic cavity permitting fuller lung expansion.

3. This patient is on bedrest and should not be standing.

4. This action is associated with the lithotomy, not orthopneic, position.

Content Area: Mobility

Integrated Processes: Nursing Process: Implementation

Client Need: Physiological Integrity; Basic Care and Comfort

Cognitive Level: Application

40. ANSWER: 4.

Rationales:

1. Straining urine if calculi are suspected will not prevent them from forming.

2. Although this may be implemented to stimulate voiding, there is no information in the question that indicates that the patient is having difficulty voiding. This will not reduce the risk of complications associated with urinary stasis.

3. Although a sitting position for women and a standing position for men will facilitate voiding, it is not as effective as another option to prevent complications associated with urinary stasis.

4. An increase in fluid intake will help to flush the urinary system of pathogens that invade the urinary tract via the urethra.

Content Area: Mobility

Integrated Processes: Nursing Process: Implementation

Client Need: Health Promotion and Maintenance

Cognitive Level: Application

Chapter 18

Nutrition

KEY TERMS

Cachexia—Extreme loss of lean body mass, marked weakness, muscle wasting, and malnutrition.

Carbohydrate—Organic compound that contains carbon, hydrogen, and oxygen.

Cheilosis—Cracks or lesions at the corners of the mouth.

Complete protein—Nutrient that includes all of the essential amino acids required for protein synthesis.

Enteral nutrition—Administration of a liquid formula via tubing directly into the gastrointestinal tract.

Essential amino acids—Amino acids that cannot be manufactured in the body and must be obtained from food or supplements.

Gingivitis—Inflamed, swollen, spongy gums.

Glossitis—Beefy, red, swollen, sore tongue, indicating inflammation.

Incomplete protein—Nutrient that does not include all of the essential amino acids required for protein synthesis.

Lipid (fat)—Organic compound that contains a carbon chain to which hydrogen, oxygen, and other elements are attached.

Minerals—Inorganic simple elements that have varied roles related to the body's structure and function.

Negative nitrogen balance—State in which nitrogen loss is greater than nitrogen intake.

Nonessential amino acids—Amino acids that can be synthesized by the body and do not need to be obtained from food or supplements.

Obesity—Body mass index more than 30.

Overweight (preobesity)—Body mass index more than 25 but less than 30.

Parenteral nutrition—Administration of nutrients via a catheter directly into the bloodstream.

Protein—Organic compound that contains amino acids linked by peptide bonds.

Stomatitis—Sores on the lips or in the mouth, indicating inflammation

Underweight—Body mass index less than 18.5.

Vitamins—Organic compounds necessary to catalyze metabolic processes in the body.

I. Structures and Functions of the Gastrointestinal System

The structures and functions of the gastrointestinal (GI) system are associated with the ingestion of food and elimination of the waste products of digestion in the form of feces. Nurses must know the basic anatomy and physiology of the GI system when providing care to patients with alterations in nutrition. The anatomy and physiology of the GI system provides the foundation for understanding how essential nutrients are utilized in the body, assessing a patient's nutritional status, implementing nursing care to support a patient's nutritional status, and administering enteral and parenteral nutrition. (See Chapter 22, "Gastrointestinal," for details concerning the structures and functions of the GI system and see Fig. 22.1 "The Gastrointestinal System.")

II. Essential Nutrients

Food contains chemical compounds and elements that provide the nutrients the body requires for the maintenance of life. The **essential nutrients** include macronutrients (e.g., carbohydrates, proteins, and lipids) and micronutrients (e.g., vitamins and minerals). Each nutrient has several types and specific functions and is digested via a process specific to the nutrient. This information is the foundation for understanding the role of nutrition in the promotion of health, prevention of disease, and recovery from illness.

A. Carbohydrates
1. Provides 4 kilocalories per gram.
2. Composed of carbon, hydrogen, and oxygen.
3. Functions.
   a. Primary source of energy for muscle and organ function.

b. Facilitates insulin secretion.
c. Supports a feeling of fullness.
d. Enhances absorption of sodium and excretion of calcium.

4. Types of carbohydrates.
  a. Simple carbohydrates.
    (1) Contain saccharide units (sugar); for example, monosaccharides (contain one saccharide unit) and disaccharides (contain two saccharide units).
    (2) Found in honey, table sugar, milk, sugar cane, molasses, sugar beets, corn syrup, and fruits.
  b. Complex carbohydrates.
    (1) Contain multiple chains of saccharide units; for example, polysaccharides.
    (2) Fiber: Consists of complex carbohydrates found in plants, such as grains, vegetables, and legumes; provides bulk to the diet, which facilitates elimination of waste and fulfills the appetite.
    (3) Starches: Consist of insoluble, nonsweet forms of complex carbohydrates; exist in plants (e.g., grains, potatoes, legumes) and are in processed foods (e.g., bread, flour, and cereal).

5. Digestion.
  a. Starts in the mouth with salivary amylase.
  b. Continues in the small intestine with pancreatic amylase and intestinal sucrase, maltase, and lactase.
  c. Leads to excess carbohydrate compounds being converted to glycogen and stored in the liver or converted to adipose tissue.

B. Protein
1. Provides 4 kilocalories per gram.
2. Composed of amino acids.
  a. **Essential amino acids:** Cannot be manufactured in the body and must be obtained from food or supplements.
  b. **Nonessential amino acids:** Can be synthesized by the body and do not need to be obtained from food or supplements.
3. Functions.
  a. Necessary for tissue growth, maintenance, and repair.
  b. Necessary for production of digestive enzymes, hormones, lymphocytes, and antibodies.
  c. Facilitates fluid and acid-base balance.
  d. Serves as an energy source when carbohydrates and fats are insufficient to meet energy needs.
4. Types of protein.
  a. **Complete protein:** Nutrient that includes all of the essential amino acids required for protein synthesis; for example, eggs, cheese, and milk.

b. **Incomplete protein:** Nutrient that does not include all of the essential amino acids required for protein synthesis; for example, nuts, corn, wheat, beans, seeds, and brown rice.
  c. A complete protein can be made by combining two incomplete proteins, such as red beans and brown rice or peanut butter and whole-grain bread.
5. Digestion.
  a. Starts in the mouth with pepsin.
  b. Continues in the small intestine by the pancreatic enzymes trypsin, chymotrypsin, and carboxypeptidase and the enzymes aminopeptidase and dipeptidase, which are secreted by glands in the intestinal wall.
6. Nitrogen balance.
  a. Reflects the extent of protein anabolism and catabolism in the body.
  b. A **negative nitrogen balance** occurs when nitrogen loss is greater than intake, such as with burns and malnutrition.
  c. A **positive nitrogen balance** occurs when nitrogen intake is greater than loss.

C. Lipids (Fats)
1. Provides 9 kilocalories per gram.
2. Composed of a carbon chain to which hydrogen, oxygen, and other elements are attached; insoluble in water.
3. Functions.
  a. Main source of fuel for the body.
  b. Assist in the absorption of the fat-soluble vitamins A, D, E, and K.
  c. Provide satiety.
  d. Enhance the flavor of food.
  e. Contribute to the formation of adipose tissue, which cushions vital organs and aids thermoregulation by protecting the body from temperature extremes.
  f. Lubricates the skin via secretion of oil from sebaceous glands.
  g. Is an essential constituent of cell membranes and cellular function.
4. Types of lipids.
  a. Glycerides.
    (1) Consist of one molecule of glycerol attached to various length fatty-acid chains.
    (2) Types.
      (a) Monoglyceride: One glycerol molecule and one fatty-acid chain.
      (b) Diglyceride: One glycerol molecule and two fatty-acid chains.
      (c) Triglyceride: One glycerol molecule and three fatty-acid chains.

b. Sterols.
  (1) Consist of rings of carbon and hydrogen.
  (2) Necessary for the development of cell membranes, vitamin D, testosterone, and estrogen.
  (3) Cholesterol: Most important sterol; liver synthesizes 75 percent of body cholesterol and 25 percent is provided from dietary sources, such as beef and pork (particularly the liver and heart), fish, poultry, dairy products, and egg yolk.
c. Phospholipids.
  (1) Consist of two fatty-acid chains attached to a glycerol molecule and one fatty-acid chain attached to a phosphate group.
  (2) Important element of lipoproteins that transport lipids throughout the body.
    (a) Low-density lipoproteins (LDLs): "Bad cholesterol"; saturated fats in the diet increase LDLs in the blood-stream, causing fatty deposits on vessel walls, contributing to cardiovascular disease.
    (b) High-density lipoproteins (HDLs): "Good cholesterol"; moves cholesterol from the bloodstream to the liver where it is used in bile or excreted.
5. Types of dietary lipids.
a. Made up of oxygen, carbon chains, and hydrogen.
b. Categorized by the number of hydrogen atoms.
  (1) Saturated fat.
    (a) Food lipid in which all carbon ions are filled to capacity with hydrogen.
    (b) Found in whole milk, butter, cheese, ice cream, red meat, coconut products, lard, chocolate, palm oil, and cocoa butter.
  (2) Monounsaturated fat.
    (a) Food lipid in which one hydrogen space is unfilled.
    (b) Found in olive, canola, and peanut oils; nuts, such as cashews, almonds, and peanuts; and avocados.
  (3) Polyunsaturated fat.
    (a) Food lipid in which two or more hydrogen spaces are unfilled.
    (b) Found in corn, safflower, soybean, sesame, and cottonseed oils; nuts and seeds; and fish.
  (4) Trans fat.
    (a) Saturated fat produced when a manufacturer adds hydrogen to polyunsaturated plant oils (hydrogenation) to extend

shelf life; intake increases low-density lipoprotein (LDL) cholesterol.
    (b) Found in vegetable shortening, most commercial baked goods, deep-fried chips, fast foods, and most margarines.
6. Digestion.
a. Occurs in the small intestine by a variety of actions.
  (1) Lipids in the duodenum stimulate the release of cholecystokinin by glands in the wall of the intestine, which stimulates the contraction of the gallbladder.
  (2) Contraction of the gallbladder releases bile into the duodenum where bile emulsifies lipids and prepares them for further digestion.
  (3) Pancreatic enzymes act in the small intestine.
    (a) Lipase breaks down lipids, releasing the final products to be absorbed (e.g., fatty acids, diglycerides, monoglycerides, and glycerol).
    (b) Cholesterol esterase combines free cholesterol and fatty acids to form cholesterol esters in preparation for absorption.
  (4) Lecithinase, an intestinal enzyme, acts on lecithin, a phospholipid, to prepare it for absorption.

D. Vitamins
  1. Organic compounds necessary to catalyze metabolic processes.
  2. Essential for growth and development and act as coenzymes in enzymatic systems.
  3. Supplied by the ingestion of plants and animals because they are not made by the body.
  4. Fat-soluble vitamins.
    a. Include vitamins A, D, E, and K (Table 18.1).
    b. Are absorbed from the intestines like fats and primarily are stored in the liver and adipose tissue.
    c. Excessive intake can cause toxicity.
    d. Deficiency occurs with inadequate intake or diseases that inhibit fat digestion and absorption.
  5. Water-soluble vitamins.
    a. Include vitamin C, thiamin, riboflavin, niacin, vitamin B_6, folic acid, vitamin B_{12}, pantothenic acid, and biotin (Table 18.2).
    b. Are required daily because the body eliminates excesses in urine, which may result in deficiencies.
E. Minerals and Electrolytes
  1. **Minerals:** Inorganic simple elements that have varied roles related to structure (e.g., calcium and phosphorous give strength to bones) and function (e.g., sodium and potassium help regulate fluid balance) in the body.

Table 18.1 Fat-Soluble Vitamins

Functions	Sources	Deficiency	Excess
Vitamin A			
• Important for night vision. • Promotes cellular growth and maturity. • Supports growth of bone and teeth. • Maintenance of healthy skin and mucous membranes. • Regulates energy. • Can be converted from beta carotene, a yellow-red pigment in some foods, in the gastric mucosa and act as an antioxidant.	• Pumpkin, sweet potatoes, carrots, spinach, collards, broccoli, cabbage, squash. • Apricots, cantaloupe. • Liver. • Fortified milk, butter, cream, egg yolk.	**Mild:** Night blindness, diarrhea, impaired vision, skin lesions, sore throat, mouth lesions, intestinal infections. **Severe:** Thickening and drying of the outer surface of the eye, leading to blindness and inflammation of the eyes.	**Mild:** Gastrointestinal disturbances, blurred vision, impaired muscle coordination, fetal defects, yellow skin (carotenemia). **Severe:** Bone pain, reports of increased pressure in the skull, other signs and symptoms similar to a brain tumor.
Vitamin D			
• Essential for growth of bone and teeth. • Promotes absorption of calcium.	• Fortified dairy products and egg yolk. • Fatty fish and fish oils. • Synthesized by sunlight.	**Severe:** *Adults:* Osteomalacia (soft, fragile bones of the pelvis, spine, and legs). *Children:* Rickets (impaired growth plates, soft and fragile bones, growth retardation, bowlegs, and knock-knees).	**Mild:** Anorexia, nausea and vomiting, polyuria, weakness, and constipation. **Severe:** Calcium deposits in heart, brain, and kidneys; mental and physical growth retardation.
Vitamin E			
• Functions as an antioxidant. • Protects vitamin A and unsaturated fatty acids from oxidation.	• Wheat and rice germ. • Milk, butter, margarine, vegetable oils, shortening. • Nuts. • Eggs and fish. • Dark green, leafy vegetables.	• Uncommon. • Myopathy, hyporeflexia, and ataxia. • Anemia in premature infants.	• Generally nontoxic. • Large supplemental doses for a year can cause excessive bleeding, impaired healing, depression, nausea, and impaired digestion.
Vitamin K			
• Important for blood clotting factors. • Necessary for bone development.	• Green leafy vegetables (e.g., kale, turnip greens, spinach, and collards). • Liver. • Made by bacteria in the intestine.	• Related to drug therapy, such as antibiotics that eliminate bacteria in the intestine or diseases that impair fat metabolism, which impedes vitamin K absorption.	*Adults:* No clinical indicators of toxicity reported. *Infants:* May cause hemolytic anemia or hyperbilirubinemia, leading to brain damage.

Table 18.2 Water-Soluble Vitamins

Functions	Sources	Deficiency	Excess
Thiamin (B₁)			
• Coenzyme for carbohydrate metabolism. • Needed to convert tryptophan to niacin. • Promotes nervous system functioning.	• Cooked dry beans. • Soy milk. • Whole-grain enriched bread and cereal. • Beef, liver, pork. • Nuts and peas.	**Beriberi** **Mild:** Anorexia, indigestion, constipation. **Severe:** Peripheral paralysis, fatigue, apathy, muscle weakness, cardiovascular problems, and alcoholism related Wernicke-Korsakoff syndrome.	• No clinical indicators of toxicity reported.

Table 18.2 Water-Soluble Vitamins—cont'd

Functions	Sources	Deficiency	Excess
Riboflavin (B₂)			
• Important in energy metabolism. • Assists in red blood cell production.	• Enriched breads and cereals. • Pork, liver, beef. • Eggs, milk, soft cheeses, such as ricotta and cottage cheese. • Mushrooms, soybeans, and spinach.	• Uncommon. • Lesions in the mouth and on the lips; swollen tongue; sore throat. • Facial dermatitis. • Vulval and scrotal skin changes. • Normocytic anemia.	• No clinical indicators of toxicity reported.
Niacin (B₃)			
• Needed for synthesis of fatty acids. • Important in maintaining muscle tone and function of the nervous system. • Coenzyme in creating energy from glucose.	• Enriched bread and cereal. • Chicken breast, liver. • Pickled herring, tuna. • Dairy products, peanuts, and coffee.	**Pellagra** Diarrhea, dermatitis, dementia, weakness, anorexia, and indigestion.	• Itching, facial flushing. • Nausea and vomiting, gastric ulcers, and liver damage.
Pantothenic acid (B₅)			
• Important in metabolism of fat, carbohydrates, and protein. • Needed in synthesis of acetylcholine, a neurotransmitter.	• In most foods. • Best sources: Meats, liver, kidney, whole-grain cereals and bread, sweet potatoes, egg yolks, tomatoes, and legumes.	• No known deficiency.	• No clinical indicators of toxicity.
Pyridoxine (B₆)			
• Needed for amino acid synthesis and catabolism. • Related to metabolism of 60+ enzymes. • Coenzyme for dopamine and serotonin. • Role in production of antibodies. • Aids in amino acid transport.	• Meats, poultry, fish. • Nuts and seeds. • Milk and dairy products. • Whole grains and enriched cereals, wheat germ. • Bananas. • Potatoes and legumes.	• Uncommon. • Dermatitis. • Glossitis and stomatitis. • Depression and confusion. • Linked to 2- to 3-year use of oral contraceptives; infants of mothers who received oral contraceptives for greater than 30 months before pregnancy.	• Due to self-prescribed megadoses. • Neuropathy, such as sensory loss in hands and feet, causing ataxia and problems with walking.
Cyanocobalamin (B₁₂)			
• Necessary for hemoglobin synthesis. • Helps maintain myelin sheath. • Essential in metabolic reactions.	• Meat, poultry, fish, shellfish. • Milk, dairy products, and eggs.	• Numbness and tingling of hands and feet. • Impaired red blood cells. • Depression, confusion, dementia, delusions. • Unrestorable nerve damage and death. **Pernicious anemia** Inadequate intrinsic factor, a protein-binding factor secreted by gastric mucosal cells, causing inadequate absorption of vitamin B₁₂.	• No clinical indicators of toxicity.
Vitamin C			
• Promotes collagen synthesis. • Promotes healing of wounds and fractures. • Is an antioxidant. • Needed for adrenal gland function. • Facilitates iron absorption. • Converts folic acid to active form. • Plays a role in immune function.	• Citrus fruits, such as oranges, grapefruits, and lemons. • Apricot nectar and strawberries. • Green peppers, broccoli, and tomatoes.	**Scurvy** **Mild:** Tender, sore gums; weak blood vessels, causing small skin hemorrhages. **Severe:** Skin changes, impaired wound healing, softening of ends of bones, tooth loss, hemorrhage in joints and around heart and stomach.	• Gastrointestinal disturbances, such as abdominal cramping, diarrhea, and nausea.

Continued

Table 18.2 Water-Soluble Vitamins—cont'd			
Functions	**Sources**	**Deficiency**	**Excess**
Folic acid			
• Needed for deoxyribonucleic acid (DNA). • Role in cellular metabolism and cell renewal. • Needed for hemoglobin formation.	• Liver. • Spinach, asparagus, broccoli, beans, turnip greens. • Oranges and cantaloupe. • Eggs. • Enriched cereals, yeast.	• Megaloblastic anemia. • Link between deficiency and neural tube defect in neonates. • Related to malabsorption, gastrointestinal problems, and illnesses that increase metabolic rate, such as infections, hyperthyroidism, cancer, serious burns, and hemorrhage. • Reduced cell division and protein synthesis, causing red, swollen tongue; heartburn; diarrhea; fatigue; and hypotension.	• Toxicity is rare. • Hives, rashes, pruritus. • Respiratory problems. • Seizures.

2. **Electrolytes:** Chemical elements that when in solution dissociates as ions carrying either a positive or negative charge.
3. Some minerals are electrolytes and others are not; the major minerals in the body that are electrolytes are calcium, sodium, potassium, magnesium, chloride, and phosphorus. (For more information about these electrolytes, see the section "Common Electrolytes" in Chapter 21, "Fluids and Electrolytes," page 655.)

III. Factors That Affect Nutrition

Although food choices should be made based on the essential nutrients in food, usually these choices are dramatically influenced by non-nutritional factors. Physical, developmental, psychosociocultural, individual issues, and medical therapies all impact a person's nutritional intake. Understanding these factors can aid nurses in assessing patients, maintaining a nonjudgmental attitude when working with diverse individuals and populations, and planning individualized approaches to nursing care.

A. **Advertising**
   1. Television commercials have a significant impact on the choices people make regarding food and beverages. Fast food establishments and advertisements for new food products, herbs, and supplements present information in a manner that communicates that these products are safe and fun to eat or drink.
   2. Nursing care.
      a. Encourage people to be cautious and examine the true facts associated with products being advertised.
      b. Encourage patients to review caloric and nutritive value of meals when eating in restaurants.
B. **Alcohol Intake**
   1. Excessive alcohol intake contributes to inadequate nutrition in various ways; for example, alcohol is

high in calories leading to weight gain, it substitutes food in the diet, decreases appetite, and increases the demand for vitamin B because this vitamin is used to metabolize alcohol.
   2. Nursing care.
      a. Encourage judicious intake of alcohol.
      b. Refer patients to Alcoholics Anonymous for help with cessation if alcohol intake is a problem.
C. **Beliefs About Food**
   1. If a person learns that foods high in animal fat are unhealthy and increase the risk of heart disease and brain attack, the person may be motivated to eat foods that have less animal fat.
   2. Some people consume certain foods or fluids because they are believed to be aphrodisiacs, impede aging, or prevent urinary tract infection.
   3. Nursing care.
      a. Determine a person's beliefs regarding nutrition and food.
      b. Identify and correct misconceptions.
D. **Culture and Ethnicity**
   1. Most cultures have certain foods that are traditional, such as Italian people prefer pasta, Asian people prefer rice, Latino people prefer rice and beans, and Indian people prefer food spiced with curry.
   2. Events are commonly accompanied by traditional meals or feasts. For example, when the Amish build a barn, the men build and the women provide a communal meal to celebrate the accomplishment.
   3. Nursing care.
      a. Identify cultural and ethnic influenced food preferences.
      b. Customize food choices when a person receives a therapeutic diet to best address nutritional needs within the patient's cultural and ethnic food preferences. (See Table 18.3 for common food preferences of selected cultural groups.)

Table 18.3 Common Food Preferences of Selected Cultural Groups and Related Nursing Care

Group and Preferences	Nursing Care
Asians Rice, noodles, bread, dumplings, Chinese greens, bean sprouts, mushrooms, bamboo, bok choy, beef, poultry, pork, seafood, eggs, tofu, soybeans, and all fruits	• Encourage steamed rather than fried dumplings, fish, vegetables, and rice. • Discourage fried noodles, rice, eggrolls, tempura battered and fried foods, and spareribs to decrease fat intake.
Cubans Rice, onions, tomatoes, green peppers, black beans, pork, and chorizo (sausage)	• Encourage meals with chicken or beans with rice to reduce fat intake. • Encourage use of salsa to add spice to food. • Encourage substitution of low-fat cheese for cheese high in fat.
Mexicans Tortillas; corn and corn products; chili peppers; tomatoes; onions; beets; cabbage; meat; poultry; eggs; pinto, calico, and garbanzo beans; and cheese	• Discourage intake of refried beans, fried tortillas, and deep fried foods. • Discourage intake of high-fat cheese and sour cream.
Puerto Ricans Red kidney beans, eggs, pork, chicken, fish, garbanzo beans, plantains, Puerto Rican bread, rice and starchy vegetables, and guava and other fruits	
Italians Pasta; pasta sauce with meat; pasta dishes made with cheese, butter, and cream; cheese; bread; salad with olive oil and vinegar dressing; vegetables high in starch; breaded and fried vegetables and meats; numerous types of sausage and seafood; green peppers; onions; and tomatoes	• Encourage grilled meats and seafood, non-fat salad dressing, pasta sauce without meat (substitute with clams). • Discourage fried foods; use of cream, butter and cheese in pasta dishes; and sausage and fatty meats to decrease fat intake.
South African Americans Biscuits; grits; cornbread; white bread; rice; corn; sweet potatoes; yams; collard greens; okra; tomatoes; squash; cabbage; fried meat, pork, chicken, and catfish; black-eyed peas; beans; buttermilk; ice cream; melons; peaches; and bananas	• Encourage substitution of grilled or steamed rather than fried fish, chicken, and vegetables. • Discourage use of lard and bacon grease when cooking; encourage use of fat-free cooking sprays and various spices for flavoring food to decrease fat intake.
Middle Eastern Europeans Rice, pita bread, couscous, feta cheese, yogurt, figs, dates, peaches, grape leaves, tomatoes, onions, peppers, squash, okra, peas, legumes, fennel, lamb, goat, chicken, and fish	• Encourage the intake of grilled or baked meats, vegetables, legumes, dates, figs, citrus fruits, and yogurt for salad dressings to decrease fat intake. • Discourage fried foods, casseroles, sour cream, and excessive butter when making a recipe with filo (flakey pastry dough).
Native Americans Corn, wild rice and oats, Indian biscuits, choke-cherries, black cherries, crab apples, wild mushrooms, root vegetables, wild game, seafood, and nuts	• Encourage the removal of fat from game meats; broil, bake, or grill meats. • Discourage fried foods and use of lard in cooking.
Northern Europeans Dark breads, potatoes, beef, pork, poultry, fish, shellfish, sausage, eggs, all chesses, milk and milk products, fruits, and vegetables	• Encourage use of poached, baked, or steamed lean meats, tomato-based sauces, and consommé. • Discourage use of sausage, fried potatoes, creamed soups and sauces, sour cream, whole milk, and whole-milk products.

E. Economics
1. People living in poverty have fewer food choices because meat and fresh vegetables generally are more expensive than food items such as pasta, rice, and beans.
2. People with adequate financial income generally eat more protein and fats.
3. People who are homeless have a limited ability to purchase, prepare, or store food and, therefore, generally eat an inadequate diet.

4. Nursing care.
   a. Suggest substituting beans and rice for meat.
   b. Encourage buying seasonal foods because they usually are less expensive.
   c. Teach the patient to avoid prepared convenience foods because they are more expensive.
F. Lifestyle
1. Families often do not share meals because children are engaged in multiple sports and social activities, requiring a reliance on fast foods or eating "on the

run"; fast food is high in carbohydrates and salt and usually does not contain the essential nutrients of a balanced diet.

2. Single-parent families and families in which both parents work commonly rely on convenience foods and processed and prepared foods that are quick to make; the majority of these foods are high in carbohydrates and salt.

3. A family may more likely be exposed to a greater variety of food experiences if a parent enjoys cooking.

4. Nursing care.
   a. Encourage making several healthy meals that can be frozen for use in the future when time is limited.
   b. Encourage parents to establish a mealtime that all or most members of the family can attend.

G. Medications and Therapy

1. Antineoplastics can cause such problems as stomatitis, anorexia, nausea, vomiting, and diarrhea and diminish energy, which negatively affects nutritional intake.

2. Drug and food interactions may require a person to avoid certain foods; for example, patients taking warfarin (Coumadin) should avoid foods high in vitamin K because it decreases the effectiveness of the drug.

3. Certain medications (e.g., aspirin) should be taken with food because they are irritating to the stomach lining; levothyroxine (Synthroid) should be taken on an empty stomach because doing so helps the drug to be absorbed better than it would be if it were taken with food.

4. Some medications can damage the liver (hepatotoxicity) or kidney (nephrotoxicity) if intake exceeds the recommended daily dose; for example, exceeding the adult dose of 4g of acetaminophen daily can cause nephrotoxicity.

5. Radiation therapy can affect nutrition; for example, radiation for head and neck cancers can cause dysphagia, altered taste, and decreased salivation; anorexia and fatigue are common side effects of radiation therapy that can significantly interfere with a person's ability to maintain an adequate diet.

6. Nursing care.
   a. Identify the medications and therapies that the patient is receiving and the ways in which they affect the patient's nutrition.
   b. Teach the patient ways to improve nutritional intake in relation to the medications and therapies the patient is receiving.

H. Personal Preferences

1. Food has different meanings to people; some people live to eat and others eat to live.

2. Food preferences are commonly related to childhood experiences. For example, a person may like a certain food because it is associated with happy visits to a loved grandparent or dislike a food that is associated with an unhappy experience.

3. Foods have different tastes, smells, and flavors that affect what a person likes or dislikes. Color, texture, and spices have a significant impact on what people prefer to eat; for example, some people like crisp vegetables and others prefer them to be cooked until soft. Some people do not like the texture of mussels and clams or the flavor of garlic, spices (e.g., curry), or herbs (e.g., cilantro).

4. Some people are willing to try new foods and some prefer to eat the same foods with little variety.

5. Some people prefer a vegetarian diet that includes grains, nuts, vegetables, and fruit and eliminates meat or animal flesh and their by-products; some vegetarian diets are even more selective.

DID YOU KNOW?

The various types of vegetarians are classified according to the variety of foods they are willing to eat or eliminate from the diet. For example,

- **Ovolactovegetarians:** Ingest eggs and dairy products but avoid meat, fish, and poultry.
- **Ovovegetarians:** Ingest eggs but avoid dairy products, meat, fish, and poultry.
- **Lactovegetarians:** Ingest dairy products but avoid eggs, meat, fish, and poultry.
- **Vegans:** Generally ingest brown rice, other grains, and herbal teas and avoid all food of animal origin.
- **Fruitarians:** Ingest only fruits, nuts, honey, and vegetable oils.

6. Nursing care.
   a. Identify a patient's food preferences and collaborate with the patient and dietician so that preferences are provided in the ordered diet when possible; this is essential for vegetarians.
   b. Encourage people to try different foods to expand their palate; teach parents to encourage their children to try different foods appropriate for their developmental level.
   c. Teach the patient who is a vegetarian to follow healthy practices.
      (1) Select foods and plan meals carefully so that adequate nutrition is achieved.
      (2) Combine grains and legumes to provide different amino acids that will form proteins in the body.
      (3) Understand that processed soybeans, soy milk, processed protein products, and tofu enrich the nutritive value of a vegetarian diet and have equal protein value as animal-derived protein; this instruction is not recommended for fruitarians.

(4) Consider taking vitamin and mineral supplements, such as vitamin B_{12}, vitamin D, calcium, iron, and zinc, and protein under the care of a dietician or primary healthcare provider to ensure an adequate intake of essential elements.

🛑 (5) Understand that children who follow a vegetarian diet are at risk for protein and vitamin deficiencies, such as vitamin B_{12} deficiency, if these needs are not adequately addressed.

I. Physical Health

1. Lack of teeth; difficulty or pain on swallowing; inability to adequately digest food; lack of energy for eating; and presence of nausea, vomiting, and diarrhea can interfere with nutrition.
2. Some people have food allergies or are gluten or lactose intolerant, which limits the foods that a person can ingest and/or digest.
3. Factors that increase the basal metabolic rate (BMR) increase the demand for calories and fluids—for example, fever, growth periods, cold environment, prolonged physical exertion, and disease processes, such as hyperthyroidism, cancer, cardiac failure, severe burns, and trauma.
4. Traumatic injuries and large draining wounds increase the demand for protein and vitamin C needed for healing.
5. Illnesses, such as diabetes, cancer, heart disease, and GI disorders, affect nutritional health by interfering with digestion, absorption, metabolism, transport, and utilization of nutrients and excretion of the by-products of nutrition.
6. Nursing care.
   a. Identify a patient's risk factors or health problems that may interfere with nutritional status.
   b. Collaborate with the primary health-care provider, dietician, and patient to ensure that the diet meets the patient's physical needs and preferences.

J. Religious Observances

1. Nutritional practices are closely associated with religious customs and traditions; for example, Catholic people do not eat meat on Fridays during Lent and fast on Good Friday; some Jewish people follow many dietary laws, such as animals must be killed in a certain way, all blood must be drained from meat, pork is forbidden, and dairy products and meat cannot be eaten at the same meal; Native American ceremonies are celebrated with specific foods.
2. For additional information about religious and cultural beliefs related to food and nursing care, refer to the section "Cultural Nursing Care" in Chapter 8, "Psychosocial and Cultural Nursing," page 169.

K. Developmental Level

1. Nutritional needs vary across the life span.
2. Nursing care: Care should be based on a patient's developmental level (Table 18.4).

Table 18.4 **Nutritional Variations Across the Life Span and Related Nursing Care**

Age Group	Developmental Considerations	Nursing Care
Birth to 1 Year	• Most rapid growth period; weight doubles in 6 months and triples by 1 year. • Breastfeeding reduces food allergies and intolerances; is easier to digest than formula; is convenient and economical. • Breastfeeding and formula feeding are recommended until age 1 year. • Eruption of baby teeth begins. • Infant can begin to eat solid food at age 6 months. • Infant begins to self-feed table food by age 1 year.	• Explain the value of breastfeeding or support the need to provide formula to meet growth needs. • Explain that cow's milk increases the risk of an allergic reaction; it is too concentrated for an infant's kidneys to manage, is a poor source of iron and vitamins C and E; and may cause gastrointestinal bleeding. *Teach the parents to:* • Provide finger foods, such as bananas and crackers, and to avoid foods that are choking hazards, such as hot dogs and apples.
Toddlers and Preschoolers	• They strive for autonomy. • Coordination increases, improving the ability to self-feed and use a spoon and folk effectively. • Appetite may be irregular and variable. • They begin to develop likes and dislikes and varied attitudes toward food. • They may use food to manipulate parents. • Milk anemia can occur if toddlers consume 24 or more ounces of milk daily because milk is an inadequate source of iron.	*Teach the parents to:* • Encourage self-feeding and to avoid feeding a child because it is faster and less messy. • Provide opportunities to explore foods with different tastes and textures. • Avoid the use of food to motivate, bribe, or punish the child because doing so may cause inappropriate food attitudes. • Cut food into small pieces. • Avoid foods that can cause an airway obstruction, such as peanuts, gum, popcorn, nuts, peanut butter, hard candy, and grapes.

Continued

Table 18.4 Nutritional Variations Across the Life Span and Related Nursing Care—cont'd

Age Group	Developmental Considerations	Nursing Care
School-Aged Children (6 to 12 years)	• They have an uneven growth pattern. • Permanent teeth replace baby teeth. • Activity increases energy requirements. • They socialize more and become more independent. • Obesity is increasing in this age group.	*Teach the parents to:* • Educate their children about a healthy diet, foods that are important, and foods that should be avoided to prevent obesity. • Provide foods with a high-nutritive value; provide nutritious snacks. • Encourage physical activity, such as participation in active sports.
Adolescents	• Adolescents experience an increase in physical, psychosocial, and sexual development. • The need for calories, protein, calcium, vitamins D and B, and iron increases to sustain growth. • Males increase in muscle, bone, and lean body tissue; females increase in fat deposition and begin menstruating. • Peer pressure influences food choices and eating habits. • Adolescents eat more calorie-dense foods, such as fast foods, donuts, chips, soda, and ice cream. • Adolescents eat more meals outside the home because of sports and social activities. • Deficient food intake, extreme weight loss, muscle wasting, and arrested sexual development is a serious eating disorder (**anorexia nervosa**) of adolescence; more common in females. • Gorging followed by self-induced vomiting and the use of diuretics and laxatives to purge is another serious eating disorder (**bulimia nervosa**) of adolescence. • Depression may develop if an adolescent has a negative body-image related to being underweight or overweight.	*Teach parents to:* • Educate their adolescents, especially those who are active in sports, to learn about foods that support their increased caloric requirements. • Encourage their adolescents who are concerned about gaining weight to learn positive strategies to maintain a healthy weight. • Discourage the use of fad diets that are detrimental to health. • Avoid negative statements about an adolescent's weight because this decreases self-esteem. • Encourage healthy snacks, such as fruits and raw vegetables, instead of junk food that is high in carbohydrates and contains little nutritive value. • Avoid keeping unhealthy foods in the home. • Make a determined effort to schedule meals so that family members eat together; this fosters more regular eating habits. • Avoid conflicts that relate to food because adolescents need to develop responsibility for a healthy diet. • Seek professional help for an adolescent exhibiting clinical indicators of depression, anorexia nervosa, or bulimia nervosa.
Adults	• Growth and development ceases. • Basal metabolic rate decreases with each decade; weight gain and obesity may become a problem. • Activity generally decreases due to stress of work and family responsibilities, which can lead to weight gain. • Postmenopausal women have an increased need for calcium because of the increased risk of osteoporosis.	• Teach about the decrease in metabolic rate and the need to decrease caloric intake and increase exercise to avoid weight gain. • Teach that obesity contributes to chronic illnesses, such as diabetes, hypertension, and mobility problems. • Encourage postmenopausal women to increase calcium and vitamin D intake to reduce the risk of osteoporosis.
Pregnant Women	• Nutrition needs increase due to the growth of maternal tissue, placenta, and fetus, especially in the second and third trimesters. • Essential nutrients needed are protein, iron, folic acid, calcium, and iodine. • Inadequate nutrition can cause impaired growth and development of the fetus. • An enlarging uterus places pressure on the gastrointestinal tract and may cause nausea, vomiting, heartburn, and constipation, which influence nutrition. • Alcohol intake can cause fetal alcohol syndrome. • Fish commonly contains mercury and other toxic substances that should be avoided.	*Teach the woman to:* • Receive ongoing prenatal care. • Take prescribed vitamins and supplements. • Ingest 400 mcg of folic acid daily when trying to conceive and throughout pregnancy to reduce the risk of neural tube defect in the fetus. • Follow a prescribed diet for total weight gain based on prepregnancy body mass index. • Ingest small frequent meals and avoid spicy foods or other foods that contribute to heartburn and other gastrointestinal disturbances. • Avoid alcohol. • Avoid fish such as swordfish, shark, king mackerel, and tile fish; limit fish to 6 ounces of well cooked fish weekly.

Table 18.4 Nutritional Variations Across the Life Span and Related Nursing Care—cont'd

Age Group	Developmental Considerations	Nursing Care
Lactating Women	• Lactating women require 500 additional calories daily. • Inadequate nutrition affects breast milk; it is maintained at the expense of the woman's nutrition. • Alcohol, caffeine, and medications are transferred into breast milk. • Tobacco use decreases milk production.	*Teach the woman to:* • Ingest healthy foods to meet an increase in caloric intake of 500 calories daily and a balanced diet to meet nutritional needs of both mother and baby. • Avoid alcohol, caffeine, and tobacco while breastfeeding. • Avoid over-the-counter medications unless receiving medical supervision.
Older Adults	• Energy output decreases, contributing to weight gain and obesity. • Periodontal disease, loss of teeth, and poorly fitted dentures may cause difficulty chewing. • Decline in taste and smell reduce appetite. • Reduced thirst sensation causes decreased fluid intake, precipitating dehydration and constipation. • Decrease in digestion, absorption, metabolism, and transport of nutrients causes a decline in nutritional status. • Acute and chronic illnesses may impair the ability to ingest, digest, absorb, metabolize, and/or transport nutrients to meet cellular needs and excrete byproducts of nutrition. • Older adults may have limited financial income, which affects the ability to purchase food. • Older adults may be physically unable to procure food and prepare meals. • Older adults may be isolated at home due to illness or living alone, contributing to depression that decreases the interest in eating.	*Teach the adult to:* • Seek regular dental care and keep dentures in good condition. • Chop food to facilitate eating. • Use spices other than salt to make food more palatable. • Eat calorie-dense foods high in nutritive value first to ensure adequate nutritional intake. • Eat high-fiber foods and drink 2L of fluid daily to avoid constipation and dehydration. • Follow the ordered therapeutic diet to treat medical conditions. • Use money-saving strategies, such as clipping coupons, buying foods on sale or store brands, substituting dairy products and beans for meat, avoiding convenience foods that generally cost more, and seeking assistance, such as food stamps or help from a food bank or Meals-on-Wheels–type program. • Become involved in senior citizen organizations to increase one's social life. • Seek medical intervention for depression.

IV. Nutritional Assessment

A nutritional assessment collects objective and subjective data about a patient's nutritional status. It includes personal factors that influence food choices, a health and dietary history, and a physical assessment. The data collected provides baseline information, identifies patients who are at risk for or are experiencing a form of malnutrition, and forms the foundation for the development of an individualized nutritional regimen.

A. Assess for Factors That Affect Nutrition (See page 520.)

B. Obtain a Health History
1. Ask about acute or chronic illnesses, such as allergies; infection; diabetes; cancer; gastroesophageal reflux disease (GERD); and cardiac, renal, GI, or liver disease.
2. Ask about pathology associated with the tongue, gums and teeth, hard or soft palate, and nasopharynx.
3. Ask about oral problems, such as difficulty chewing, ill-fitting dentures, and stomatitis.
4. Ask about the use of medications, such as steroids, antineoplastics, antihypertensives, diuretics, antacids, proton-pump inhibitors, laxatives, antidepressants, and potassium chloride.
5. Ask about a history of such therapies as radiation, total parenteral nutrition, and GI feedings.
6. Ask about drug abuse, excessive alcohol intake, and smoking history.

C. Obtain a Dietary History
1. Have the patient complete a food diary for 3 to 5 days including all food and fluids consumed.
2. Identify foods that the patient states are tolerated and those that cause problems.
3. Identify how many meals a day the patient ingests and at what time they are ingested.
4. Identify food habits, such as preferences, types of snacks, and times meals are eaten.
5. Identify whether the patient has been following a fad diet or taking supplements or health foods.
6. Identify clinical indicators of an eating disorder, such as excessive amount of food intake in a short period of time, induced vomiting after meals,

multiple dental caries and eroded tooth enamel (associated with frequent vomiting), and excessive use of laxatives, diuretics, or weight loss medication.

D. Perform a Physical Assessment.

1. Weight.
   a. **Underweight:** Body mass index (BMI) less than 18.5.
   b. **Cachexia:** Extreme loss of lean body mass, marked weakness, muscle wasting, and malnutrition.
   c. **Overweight:** BMI more than 25 but less than 30.
   d. **Obese:** BMI of 30 or more.
   e. **Onset of change in weight:** Sudden or gradual.
   f. **Duration of change in weight:** Weight history, such as a 3-month, 6-month, or 1-year pattern of losing or gaining weight.
   g. Actions taken to promote weight loss or weight gain.
2. Skin.
   a. Dry, flaky: Aging, dehydration.
   b. Scaly: Vitamin A excess or deficiency, zinc deficiency, essential fatty acid deficiency.
   c. Petechiae or bruises: Vitamin C deficiency.
   d. Transparent: Protein deficiency.
   e. Purpura: Vitamin C deficiency, vitamin K deficiency.
   f. Edema: Protein deficiency, thiamin deficiency.
   g. Nonhealing wounds or lesions: Vitamin C deficiency, zinc deficiency, protein deficiency.
   h. Poor skin turgor: Dehydration.
3. Hair.
   a. Dry, dull, brittle hair: Protein deficiency.
   b. Hair loss: Protein deficiency.
4. Eyes.
   a. Red or pale conjunctivae; dry, soft, dull corneas; dark skin under the eyes: Malnutrition, dehydration.
   b. Night blindness: Vitamin A deficiency.
5. Nails.
   a. Pale, brittle, ridged: Protein deficiency.
   b. Spoon shaped: Iron deficiency.
6. Lips.
   a. Cracks or lesions at the corners of the mouth (**cheilosis**): Riboflavin or niacin deficiency.
   b. Sores on the lips or in the mouth (**stomatitis**): Chemotherapy, Herpes simplex infection.
7. Tongue.
   a. Inflamed, beefy, red, swollen, sore (**glossitis**): Vitamin B deficiency.
   b. Atrophy: Riboflavin, niacin, vitamin B_{12}, folic acid, protein, or iron deficiency.
8. Teeth.
   a. Cavities or missing teeth, mottled teeth, or pain.
   b. Problems due to malnutrition and deficiencies in vitamin D and calcium.
9. Gums.
   a. Inflamed, swollen, spongy gums (**gingivitis**), receding and bleed easily.
   b. Problems due to vitamin C deficiency.
10. Muscles.
    a. Flaccidity; poor tone; wasted, soft, underdeveloped muscles; weakness; and fatigue.
    b. Problems due to malnutrition and protein deficiency.
11. Nervous system.
    a. Neuropathy, paresthesia of the hands and feet, ataxia, decreased deep tendon reflexes and positional sense: Niacin, pyridoxine, and cyanocobalamin deficiencies.
    b. Tetany and increased deep tendon reflexes: Calcium and magnesium deficiencies.
    c. Confusion and irritability: Dehydration.
    d. Disorientation: Thiamin deficiency.
    e. Drowsiness, lethargy, apathetic: Vitamins A and D excess.
12. Bones.
    a. Observed skeletal malformations and poor posture.
    b. Problems due to vitamin D deficiency.
13. Cardiovascular system.
    a. Tachycardia: Iron deficiency anemia.
    b. Increased blood pressure: Excessive salt intake, cardiovascular disease.
    c. Heart failure: Thiamin, phosphorus, and iron deficiencies.
14. Altered sensation.
    a. Poor sense of taste or bad taste in mouth: Infection, medication side effect.
    b. Deficit in smell: Zinc deficiency.
15. Decreased ability to chew and swallow: Poor dentition; weakness; fatigue; problems with the mouth, nasopharynx, and esophagus; dysphagia; impaired movement of the tongue; local inflammation or infection of the oral cavity.
16. GI system: Anorexia, nausea and vomiting, diarrhea, constipation, epigastric discomfort, and distended abdomen: Related to specific illness or disease.
    a. Onset of GI distress: Sudden or gradual.
    b. Duration of GI distress: Short term or long term.
    c. Pattern of GI distress: Continuous or related to factors such as food intake or response to radiation, antineoplastic drugs, or activity.
    d. Actions taken to relieve the problem.

V. Diagnostic Tests Related to Nutritional Status

Diagnostic procedures are performed to obtain additional information about a patient's nutritional status beyond just a history and physical. Noninvasive measures, such as anthropometry measurements, invasive measures, such as a gastrostomy, and blood tests performed either in the laboratory by technicians or at the patient's bedside by nurses can provide valuable data. Because clinical manifestations of malnutrition take time to become evident, the results of laboratory tests may be the first indicator of a nutritional problem. The results of diagnostic tests related to a patient's nutritional status are not evaluated in isolation but rather in conjunction with each other.

A. Anthropometry Measurements

1. Measurement of size, weight, and proportion of makeup of the body.
2. Obtain height and weight and compare findings to the standard for height and weight relationships; provides a quick estimate of ideal body weight.
3. Calculate BMI by dividing weight in kilograms by height in meters squared.
4. Perform a skinfold measurement using special calipers to measure the thickness of the skinfolds, which indicates the amount of body fat; note that the calipers measure only the subcutaneous tissue, not underlying muscle.
   a. Triceps and subscapular skinfolds are commonly measured (Fig. 18.1).
   b. Mid-upper-arm circumference measures muscle mass and protein reserve; patient flexes the forearm and the circumference of the upper arm is measured at the midpoint.
   c. Abdominal-girth measurement objectively measures abdominal distention; measure abdominal circumference with a measuring tape at a place indicated by an X made with an indelible pen or over the umbilicus; measure at the same time each day.

B. Gastrostomy

1. Tube with fiberoptic capability is inserted into the mouth and advanced through the pharynx, esophagus, and stomach and into the duodenum to observe anatomical structures and check for the presence of polyps, lesions, tumors, and bleeding (Fig. 18.2).

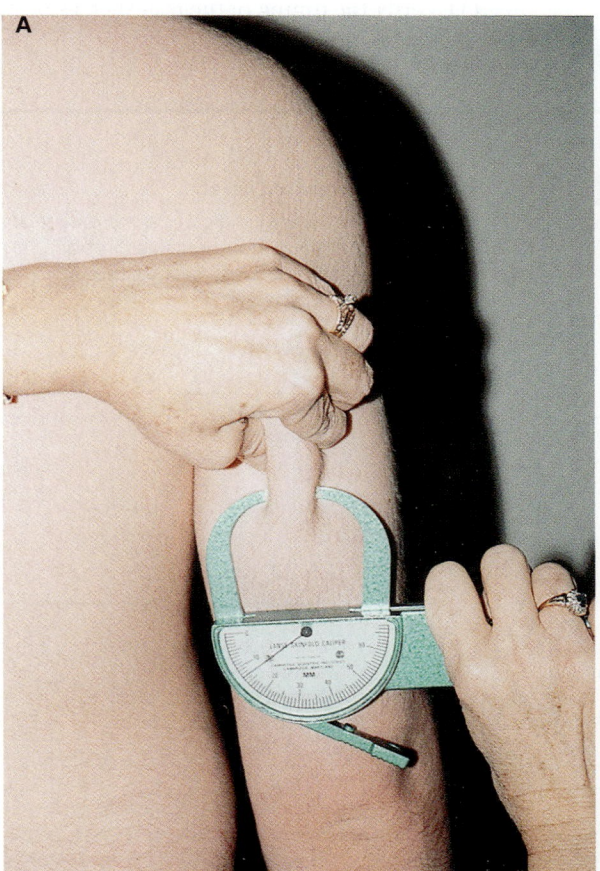
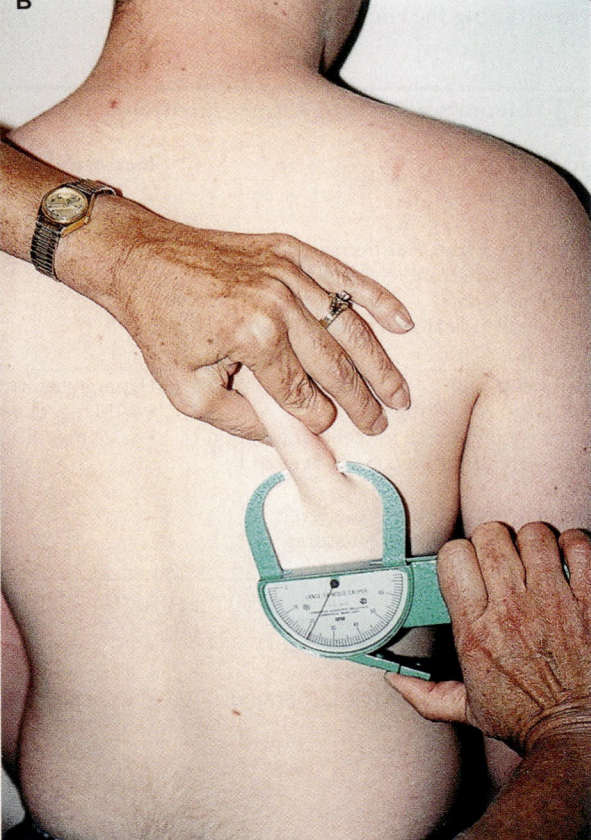

Fig 18.1 Anthropometry measurements: (A) triceps skinfold, (B) subscapular skinfold. (From Wilkinson and Treas [2011]. *Fundamentals of nursing*, Vol. 2, 2nd ed. Philadelphia: F. A. Davis, with permission.)

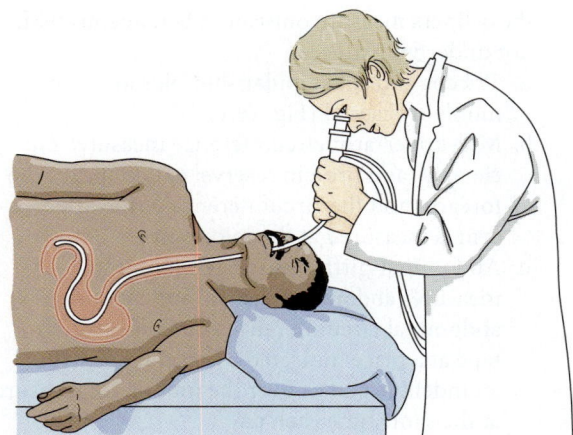

Fig 18.2 Gastroscopy. (From Williams & Hopper [2011]. *Understanding medical surgical nursing,* 4th ed. Philadelphia: F. A. Davis, with permission.)

2. Using this procedure, polyps can be removed, bleeding sites cauterized, and biopsies obtained for diagnostic study.
3. The diagnostic report documents findings and commonly includes photographs taken of pathology during the endoscopy.

C. Laboratory Tests

1. Laboratory tests are used to assess a patient's nutritional status; no one test is used alone; some tests reflect changes within days and some reflect a patient's status over weeks.
2. They assess factors such as fluid balance, hydration, hemorrhage, presence of disease, liver and kidney function, and status of protein and nitrogen balance.
3. See Table 18.5 for a description of laboratory tests commonly used to assess nutritional status.
4. Blood glucose monitoring.
   a. Patients who have diabetes or who are receiving tube feedings or parenteral nutrition require blood glucose monitoring to ensure that blood glucose levels are maintained within the expected range of 70 to 110 mg/dL to avoid complications of hypoglycemia and hyperglycemia.
   b. Blood specimens may be sent to the laboratory for analysis of glucose (e.g., glucose tolerance, 2-hour postprandial, fasting glucose, random glucose) or performed by a nurse at regular and STAT intervals.
   c. Procedure for obtaining a fingerstick (capillary) blood specimen and measuring glucose level.
      (1) Verify the timing of the test, such as before a meal or at bedtime.

Table 18.5 Laboratory Tests to Assess Nutritional Status

Factor	Increased Level	Decreased Level
Albumin *Normal value: 3.5–5 g/dL.* • Synthesized by the liver from amino acids. • Important in fluid and electrolyte balance. • Half-life of 21 days. • Not an ideal indicator of acute protein depletion.	• >5 g/dL. • Dehydration.	• <3.5 g/dL indicates some extent of malnutrition or malabsorption. • Increased loss, such as through a fistula or burns.
Blood glucose *Normal value: 70–110 mg/dL.* • Primary energy source for cellular function. • Excess glucose is stored in the liver and muscles. • Lower than expected glucose levels stimulate metabolism of fat stores.	Hyperglycemia • >110 mg/dL fasting blood sample. • >126 mg/dL random blood sample.	Hypoglycemia • <50 mg/dL.
Blood urea nitrogen *Normal value: 8–21 mg/dL.* • End product of protein metabolism. • Reflects serum protein status. • Reflects balance of urea production and excretion.	• >21 mg/dL. • Acute renal failure. • Excessive protein intake. • Muscle wasting from starvation. • Total parenteral nutrition.	• <8 mg/dL. • Inadequate dietary protein. • Malabsorption. • Pregnancy. • Low-protein diet. • Severe liver disease.
Creatinine *Normal value: 0.5–1.2 mg/dL.* • Released during skeletal muscle metabolism. • Proportion to total body mass.	• >1.2 mg/dL. • Dehydration.	• <0.5 mg/dL. • Reduced total muscle mass. • Severe malnutrition.

Table 18.5 Laboratory Tests to Assess Nutritional Status—cont'd

Factor	Increased Level	Decreased Level
Hemoglobin *Normal value:* *Females:* 12–16 g/dL. *Males:* 14–18 g/dL. • Measures oxygen and iron carrying capacity of blood.	• >16 or 18 g/dL. • Dehydration. • Burns. • Congestive heart failure.	• <12 or 14 g/dL. • Anemia. • Blood loss. • IV overload. • Fluid retention.
Prealbumin *Normal value:* 15–40 mg/dL. • Protein produced by the liver. • Transports thyroxine and triiodothyronine. • Needed to transport vitamin A. • Half-life of 2 to 3 days.	• >40 mg/dL. • Alcoholism. • Steroid therapy. • Chronic renal failure.	• <15 mg/dL indicates mild protein depletion. • <11 mg/dL indicates severe protein depletion. • Malnutrition. • Acute-phase inflammatory response. • Liver disease. • Tissue necrosis.
Total lymphocyte count *Normal values:* 1,000–4,800/mm^3 or 20%–40%. • Lymphocytes decrease as protein decreases. • Important in the immune response.	• >4,800/mm^3 or >40%. • Pathological conditions, such as appendicitis, inflammatory disorders, bone marrow disorders.	• <1,000/mm^3 or <20%. • Decreased nutritional intake. • Anemias. • Malnutrition. • Severe debilitating disease. • Antineoplastic drugs.
Transferrin *Normal value:* 215–380 mg/dL. • Formed in the liver. • Transports up to 70% of the body's iron. • Half-life of 8 days. • Reacts quickly to changes in protein intake.	• >380 mg/dL. • Iron deficiency anemia. • Pregnancy.	• <200 mg/dL indicates moderate protein depletion. • <100 mg/dL indicates severe protein depletion. • Acute or chronic infection. • Excessive protein loss from renal disease. • Malnutrition from cancer.
Lipid profile *Normal values:* LDLs: <100 mg/dL. HDLs: >60 mg/dL. Triglycerides: <150 mg/dL. Total cholesterol: <200 mg/dL. • Used to assess risk of cardiovascular disease.	**Blood Levels Indicating High Risk for Cardiovascular Disease** • LDL: >200 mg/dL. • HDL: <40 mg/dL. • Triglycerides: >160 mg/dL. • Total cholesterol: >240 mg/dL.	

(2) Wash your hands.

(3) Calibrate the glucometer following the manufacturer's directions; ensure that the reagent strip is not expired.

(4) Alternate sites to avoid overuse of one site, which may cause a problem with healing.

(5) Wash the patient's hands with soap and warm water to clean the skin and promote blood flow to the area; dry them well.

(6) Don clean gloves.

(7) Hold the finger in a dependent position to facilitate blood flow to the intended puncture site.

(8) Puncture the side of the finger with a lancet because this area has fewer nerve endings than the fingertip (Fig. 18.3A).

(9) Wipe away the first droplet with sterile gauze.

(10) Position the reagent strip so that it makes contact with the second blood droplet; avoid smearing the blood droplet over the reagent strip (Fig. 18.3B).

(11) Insert the reagent strip into the glucometer and follow the manufacturer's instructions regarding the amount of time to leave the strip in the glucometer.

(12) Apply gentle pressure with a gauze pad over the puncture site.

(13) Dispose of the lancet in a sharps disposal container.

(14) Read the result once it is displayed on the glucometer.

(15) Discard your gloves appropriately and perform hand hygiene.

(16) Document the results in the patient's clinical record.

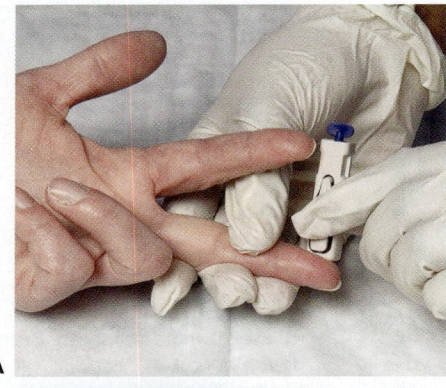

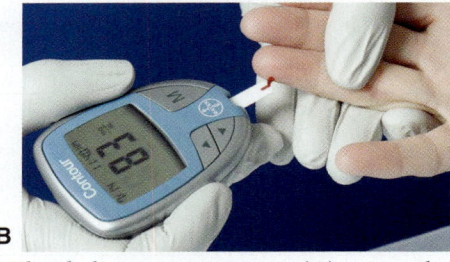

Fig 18.3 Blood glucose monitoring: (A) using a lancet; (B) applying blood to a reagent strip test patch. (From Wilkinson and Treas [2011]. *Fundamentals of nursing*, Vol. 2, 2nd ed. Philadelphia: F. A. Davis, with permission.)

(17) Administer insulin based on the guidelines prescribe by the primary health-care provider if the patient's blood glucose level is elevated.

DID YOU KNOW?

Soap and warm water are sufficient to clean the intended puncture site. If soap and water are unavailable, swipe the site with an alcohol swab but allow the alcohol to dry completely before puncturing the site. Doing so will prevent the alcohol from destroying the substance on the test strip that measures glucose levels. Squeezing or milking the finger of the intended puncture site, particularly after the finger has been punctured, can cause hemolysis and dilution of the blood specimen with fluid from local tissue. Both actions result in false low test results and should be avoided.

VI. Therapeutic Diets and Related Nursing Care

Although most everyone should follow the recommendations of the food guidance system called MyPlate that demonstrates the five food groups that are the foundation of a healthy diet, these guidelines may be inadequate or inappropriate for patients with health problems. The consistency of food, quantity of food, and constituents within foods may have to be altered to maintain health in the presence of physical problems or to promote recovery from an illness. The provision of a diet to a patient is a dependent function of the nurse and requires an order from a primary health-care provider. Details of therapeutic diets can be found in a health-care agency's dietary manual.

A. Commonalities of Diet-Related Nursing Care
1. Verify the diet ordered by the primary health-care provider.
2. Arrange for consult with a dietitian to ensure an individualized assessment and plan.
3. Provide for a patient's personal food preferences as much as possible.
4. Encourage intake of nutrient-dense foods first from the meal tray when the patient is anorexic.
5. Assist the patient with eating as necessary.
6. Document the patient's intake and tolerance objectively in the clinical record.

DID YOU KNOW?

Calorie-dense foods and nutrient-dense foods are often used interchangeably. However, they have very different meaning. Calorie-dense foods provide energy from calories but often have insignificant nutritive value. These foods are appropriate for people who have a high metabolic rate (e.g., patients with cancer or hyperthyroidism, athletes) or are underweight. Calorie-dense foods include foods such as potatoes, rice, beans, fruit juices, snack foods, and fast foods. Nutrient-dense foods provide more nutrients (e.g., protein, carbohydrates, vitamin B, iron, and potassium) than calories. Nutrient-dense foods are appropriate for people who have an inadequate oral intake (e.g., patients with nausea or anorexia) or have increased nutritional needs (e.g., patients who are pregnant or lactating). Nutrient-dense foods include foods such as berries, melons, dark green vegetables, lean meats, nuts, cheese, fish, and whole grains.

B. Nothing By Mouth (Non Per Os [NPO])
1. Restricted oral food and fluid intake.
2. Generally ordered before surgery, procedures, or tests to minimize the risk of aspiration.
3. May be ordered for a patient with a problem, such as undiagnosed abdominal pain or vomiting, until the problem is diagnosed or the nausea and vomiting subside.
4. Nursing care.

   🛑 a. Explain to the patient and family what "NPO" means and why it is ordered; if NPO is violated, it may require postponement of an intervention or aggravate a medical condition.

   b. Remove the patient's water pitcher from the bedside.

c. Ensure that all members of the health-care team are informed of the patient's NPO status; place an "NPO" sign over the patient's bed if permitted by policy.

d. Provide frequent mouth care and instruct the patient not to swallow water or mouthwash during mouth care.

e. Administer intravenous (IV) fluids as ordered.

C. Clear Liquid Diet

1. Provides for hydration and simple carbohydrates to meet a portion of a patient's energy requirement.

2. Prevents dehydration.

3. Generally ordered after surgery or when a patient is recovering from a GI problem, such as vomiting and diarrhea, because it reduces stimulation of the GI mucosa.

4. Allows intake of liquids that are transparent enough to see through, including frozen ice popsicles and gelatin, because they are clear when liquid.

5. Should only be used for a few days because it does not provide adequate protein, calories, or other nutrients necessary for a balanced diet.

6. Once tolerated, a patient is progressed to a full liquid diet.

7. Nursing care.

a. Teach the patient the liquids that are permitted on a clear liquid diet, such as water; clear, fat-free soup (e.g., broth/bouillon); tea; coffee; clear juice (e.g., grape, cranberry, and apple); gelatin; popsicles; clear drinks with electrolytes (e.g., Gatorade, Pedialyte), and carbonated drinks (e.g., nondiet soda).

b. Assess the patient's tolerance, such as free from nausea, vomiting, and epigastric distress.

D. Full Liquid Diet

1. Includes all fluids on a clear fluid diet, fluids that are opaque, or food that becomes liquid at room temperature.

2. Generally ordered as part of a progressive diet from clear to regular.

3. Ordered when a patient is unable to tolerate semisolid or solid food.

4. Is low in calories, protein, and iron.

5. Must be enhanced with a balanced oral supplement (e.g., Ensure, Boost) if the patient is receiving it for more than a few days.

6. Nursing care.

a. Teach the patient that the liquids on a clear liquid diet are also included on a full liquid diet.

b. Teach that additional fluids and foods include milk and milk drinks (e.g., milkshakes); puddings and custards; cream soups; yogurt; ice cream and sherbet; vegetable and fruit juices that are free from pulp; smooth peanut butter; refined cooked cereals (e.g., Cream of Wheat, Cream of Rice); and liquid supplements.

c. Assess the patient's tolerance, such as free from nausea, vomiting, and epigastric distress.

E. Soft Diet

1. Easily chewed, swallowed, and digested foods; promotes the mechanical digestion of food.

2. Includes all foods on a full liquid diet plus soft, chopped, and shredded foods.

3. Ordered for patients with difficulty chewing because of problems with the teeth, gums, jaw, or improperly fitted dentures and those who are weak.

4. Ordered for patients with conditions such as Crohn's disease and ulcerative colitis to reduce stimulation of the GI mucosa.

5. Provides a balanced diet but is low in fiber and may increase the risk of constipation.

6. Nursing care.

a. Teach the patient that the diet includes all clear and full liquids; all soups; chopped or ground meats; well cooked, soft vegetables; cooked or canned fruit without membranes; applesauce; scrambled eggs; bananas; cottage cheese and other soft cheeses; rice; mashed or riced potatoes; pasta; cooked cereal and grits; pancakes; soft bread; bread pudding; and pastry.

b. Encourage the intake of fluid, oatmeal, and cooked and canned fruit to minimize the risk of constipation.

🛑 c. Teach the patient to avoid nuts; foods with seeds, such as tomatoes and berries; raw fruits and vegetables; and whole grains because they are more irritating to the GI mucosa and are high in fiber.

d. Teach the patient to avoid rice, bananas, and other constipating foods.

e. Assess for clinical indicators of constipation.

f. Assess the patient's tolerance, such as free from nausea, vomiting, epigastric distress, constipation, and diarrhea.

F. Pureed Diet

1. Consists of foods that are processed in a blender or food processor so that the consistency is thicker than full liquids but can be served in scooped mounds on a plate.

2. Nursing care.

a. Teach that all food can be included on this diet as long as it is blended to a semisolid consistency.

b. Add a small amount of liquid to food if it is too thick to make it a semisolid consistency that is easy to swallow.

G. Regular Diet

1. Provides a balanced diet of 2,000 calories daily.

2. Ordered for patients with no unique or special nutritional needs.

3. Can be modified to meet specific needs or preferences, such as a kosher or vegetarian diet.
4. Generally avoids fatty, gas-forming, fried, and unpopular foods to appeal to a greater percentage of patients and to promote tolerance.
5. Nursing care.
   a. Teach patients which foods are most important to ingest first from the meal tray.

🛑 b. **Teach patients who have undergone surgery to ingest foods and fluids high in protein and vitamin C to facilitate wound healing.**

H. Antigen-Avoidance Diet
1. Ordered for a patient who is allergic to or has intolerance to a food. The following are examples.
   a. Gluten-free diet: Essential for a person who cannot tolerate gluten because of celiac disease; diet free from grains such as wheat, bran, barley, rye, farina, and semolina.
   b. Lactose-free diet: Essential for a person who cannot tolerate lactose; diet is free from milk and dairy products.
   c. Peanut-free diet: Essential for a person who cannot tolerate peanuts and their products; diet free from peanuts and foods cooked with peanut oil.

DID YOU KNOW?

A patient who cannot eat gluten should avoid foods that contain grains such as pasta, bread, bakery products, cereal, and fillers in processed foods. A patient with lactose intolerance must avoid milk and milk products, such as cheese, bread, cereal, rice, or pasta prepared with milk; vegetables or salad dressings prepared with milk or cheese; cream soups; desert made with cream or milk products, such as sherbet, ice cream, pudding, and cake; anything made with milk solids, curds and whey, or skim milk solids. The nurse should suggest that the patient try, with the primary health-care provider's permission, a nondairy creamer and reduced-lactose milk and cheese products because they may be tolerated. A patient who is allergic to peanuts should avoid foods that contain peanuts or are cooked with peanut oil.

2. Nursing care.
   a. Teach the patient foods to avoid that are high in the offending nutrient.
   b. Teach the patient to investigate ingredients when buying food products or when dining in a restaurant to ensure that the offending nutrient is not used in the recipe.
   c. Identify restaurants that provide menus that address the needs of people with food intolerances and allergies (e.g., the Outback restaurant has extensive choices on a gluten-free menu).

d. Ensure that a child's school has policies in place that protect children with food allergies or intolerances; some schools do not permit any child to bring food into the school that has peanuts or peanut oil in the food.

🛑 e. **Encourage a patient who has a prescription for epinephrine (e.g., Epi-E-Pen, EpiPen Auto-Injector) to keep the device available at all times; teach the patient how to self-administer an epinephrine injection.**

I. Calorie-Restricted Diet
1. Allows a reduced number of calories, such as 1,800; 1,200; or 1,000 calories as ordered.
2. Ordered to facilitate weight loss.
3. Nursing care.
   a. Encourage the patient to participate in a program that provides counseling and support, such as individual counseling, Weight Watchers, or Overeaters Anonymous.
   b. Teach the patient to limit foods that are high in fat and carbohydrates and to substitute foods that are low in calories and carbohydrates.
   c. Use positive, supportive statements to point out success in weight loss.
   d. Avoid negative statements because they can demoralize the patient and negatively affect the nurse-patient relationship.

J. American Diabetes Association (ADA) Diet
1. Maintains acceptable serum glucose levels (premeal level of 70 to 130 mg/dL and postmeal level of less than 180 mg/dL) and reduces lipid levels.
2. Maintaining acceptable serum glucose levels may help minimize the risk of long-term complications of diabetes, such as atherosclerosis, arteriosclerosis, retinopathy, nephropathy, neuropathy, infection, and foot ulcers.
3. Nursing care.
   a. Encourage the patient to seek guidance from a nurse who is a diabetes educator and a dietitian to help design and identify strategies to maintain a nutrition therapy plan.
   b. Encourage the patient to become involved in efforts to reduce the intake of fats and calories to decrease weight and increase exercise because doing so will help reduce blood glucose levels.
   c. Teach the patient high-glycemic foods to avoid because they are high in sugar and carbohydrates, such as pasta, rice, and bread.

K. High Calorie–High Protein Diet
1. Used for patients challenged with increased needs related to wound healing, serious burns, developmental growth, increased metabolism associated with hyperthyroidism, and increased catabolism and wasting related to cancer.

2. Nursing care.
   a. Teach the patient foods that are high in calories and high in protein.
   b. Teach the patient to augment the diet with high-calorie and high-protein supplements.
   c. Add protein powder supplements to soups and liquids as prescribed.

L. High-Fiber Diet
1. Increases the movement of indigestible waste through the large intestines.
2. Minimizes the risk of constipation and is a treatment regimen for diverticulosis.
3. Nursing care.
   a. Teach the patient foods that are high in fiber, such as raw vegetables, whole grains, and raw fruits, such as apples and oranges.
   b. Assess for clinical indicators of constipation and diarrhea.

M. Low-Fat or Fat-Restricted Diet
1. Reduces the total fat ingested and substitutes monounsaturated fats for saturated and polyunsaturated fats.
2. Ordered to promote weight loss or lower cholesterol or triglyceride levels.
3. Ordered for people with atherosclerosis; coronary artery disease; and problems with fat malabsorption related to diseases of the liver, gallbladder, pancreas, lymphatic system, or intestines.
4. Nursing care.
   a. Teach the patient to avoid foods that are high in fat, such as whole-milk products, fried foods, animal fat, gravies, sauces, and chocolate.
   b. Teach the patient to limit use of butter, margarine, mayonnaise, oil, shortening, bacon, cream, and creamed cheese to 1 tablespoon a day or 1 teaspoon per meal.
   c. Encourage intake of fresh fruits and vegetables and fat-free milk and milk products.
   d. Encourage the patient to substitute yogurt for sour cream in recipes.
   e. Teach the patient to limit lean meats to no more than 6 oz daily and eggs to three to four weekly.

N. Low-Residue Diet
1. Contains foods with reduced fiber and cellulose.
2. Decreases GI mucosal irritation.
3. Used for patients with exacerbations of Crohn's disease, ulcerative colitis, and diverticulitis after the acute phase to reduce stimulation of the intestinal mucosa.
4. May be ordered before intestinal surgery.
5. Nursing care.
   a. Teach the patient to avoid foods high in fiber and cellulose, such as raw and dried fruits and vegetables and whole grains.

b. Teach the patient to reduce dairy products to two servings daily.
   c. Teach the patient to avoid nuts and foods with seeds, such as tomatoes and berries (efficacy is controversial).

O. Protein-Restricted Diet
1. Ordered for patients with liver disease to decrease stress on the liver, which metabolizes protein.
2. Ordered for patients with kidney disease because of the need to limit levels of nitrogen, a by-product of protein metabolism.
3. May be accompanied by fluid and sodium restriction.
4. Nursing care.
   a. Teach the patient to limit protein intake to the amount ordered by the health-care provider (e.g., 20 g, 40 g, or 60 g daily).
   b. Teach the patient to limit foods high in protein, such as meat and dairy products.

P. Sodium-Restricted Diet
1. May be restricted to 2,000 mg (mild), 1,000 mg (moderate), 500 mg (strict), or 250 mg (severe).
2. Ordered because salt retains fluid in the body, which contributes to fluid retention.
3. Ordered for patients with hypertension, excess fluid volume, heart failure, and renal failure.
4. Nursing care.
   a. Teach the patient foods to avoid that are high in sodium (Box 18.1).
   b. Teach the patient to substitute foods high in salt with fresh fruit; breads and pasta without salt; low-salt baked goods; low-sodium cheese; and spices, herbs, and vegetables that do not contain salt, such as allspice, almond extract, basil, bay leaves, chili powder, garlic, marjoram,

---

Box 18.1 Foods High in Sodium

- Condiments, such as catsup, mustard, barbecue sauce, and commercial salad dressing.
- Prepared stuffing, cake mixes, and baked goods with baking soda and baking powder.
- Milk from animals; yogurt; and regular cheese and cheese products.
- Treats such as salted pretzels, popcorn, crackers, and chips.
- Instant and prepared rice, pasta, and quick-cooking cereals.
- Bouillon cubes, tenderizers, gravy enhancers, and mixers.
- Canned soups and vegetables, especially sauerkraut.
- Oysters, clams, shrimp, and other shellfish.
- Soy, teriyaki, and Worcestershire sauce.
- Bacon, luncheon meat, and corned beef.
- Salted butter and margarine.
- Olives and pickles.
- Sugar substitutes.
- Egg substitutes.
- Peanut butter.

onion powder, onions, oregano, parsley, pepper, rosemary, sage, tarragon, and thyme.

c. Teach the patient about the Dietary Approaches to Stop Hypertension (DASH) diet, a highly successful diet that emphasizes low sodium intake while increasing fruits, vegetables, and whole gains to reduce blood pressure.

VII. Nutrition Facts Labels

The U.S. Food and Drug Administration requires all packaged foods sold in the United States to have a nutrition facts label. A nutrition facts label provides descriptive information about the food in the package.

A. Purpose of a Nutrition Fact Label
1. Provides information about the amount and nutrient content of the product in addition to other important information.
2. Assists people to make informed choices when purchasing food.
3. Assists people to adhere to a prescribed diet.

B. Includes the Following Sections (Fig. 18.4)
1. Serving size: Identifies the volume of a serving size in household and metric measurements; identifies how many servings are in each package or can.
2. Check calories: Identifies how many calories are contained in one serving.
3. Limit these nutrients: Identifies nutrients that should be limited in a daily diet because they increase the risk of heart disease, some cancers, and hypertension.

MAKING THE CONNECTION

Quantitative Value of Nutrients in a Product and Serving Size

Nurses must teach patients to read nutrition facts labels carefully to determine the total number of nutrients in a package. Many products contain more than one serving per package. For example, a nutrition facts label may indicate that a product contains 100 calories; however, if the product contains three servings and the patient eats the entire package, the total intake of calories is 300. This information is important to teach patients who must limit food intake to the number of calories ordered for a specific diet, such as a 1,200- or 1,800-calorie diet. This concept also applies to the nutrients itemized on the nutrition facts label. A label may identify that the product contains 200 mg of sodium; if the product contains three serving and the patient eats two servings, the total intake of sodium by the patient is 400 mg. This information is important to teach patients who are on sodium-restricted diets.

4. Get enough of these nutrients: Identifies nutrients that should be increased in a daily diet to contribute to good health; for example, increased calcium helps reduce the risk of osteoporosis and increased dietary fiber facilitates bowel function.
5. Footnote: Indicates the percent daily values included on a 2,000 and 2,500 calorie diet for each of the elements indicated.
6. Calories from fat: Identifies how many calories from fat are contained in 1 serving. Total fat calories should be less than 30 percent of calories ingested daily. If a person is on a low-fat diet, knowing the total number of calories from fat in a food enables selection of foods that are low in fat and elimination of those that are high in fat.
7. Quick guide to percent daily value: Identifies what percentage of the recommended daily requirement of the nutrient is provided in one serving related to a 2,000-calorie diet. It can be used to make comparisons among different foods and to help make food substitutions.

VIII. MyPlate

The Center for Nutrition Policy and Promotion, an organization of the U.S. Department of Agriculture, promotes dietary guidelines for Americans as one of its initiatives. The food guidance system, MyPlate, introduced June 2011, provides an easily understood icon to guide people regarding food categories and food choices for a healthier life. This approach to dietary guidance is the successor to MyPyramid. MyPlate demonstrates the five food groups that are the foundation of a healthy diet. It uses a plate divided into four sections—fruits, vegetables, grains, and protein—and the fifth group dairy is represented by a circle that signifies a glass or cup. The plate design is based on the concept that a person should consider what is being put on a plate or in a bowl or cup when selecting foods and fluids in a daily diet (Fig. 18.5).

A. Fruits
1. Should be 25 percent of the plate daily.
2. Includes any fruit that is fresh, canned, or frozen and is whole, cut up, pureed, or 100 percent juice.
3. Examples: Apples, bananas, grapefruit, grapes, oranges, peaches, berries, melons, apricots, kiwi, lemons, limes, mangoes, pears, and papaya.

B. Vegetables
1. Should be 25 percent of the plate daily.
2. Includes any vegetable that is raw, cooked, fresh, frozen, canned, dried, or dehydrated and can be cut-up, mashed, or 100 percent juice.
3. Examples arranged into five categories based on nutritive value.
   a. Dark-green vegetables: Such as broccoli; collard greens; dark-green, leafy lettuce (e.g., romaine lettuce, spinach).

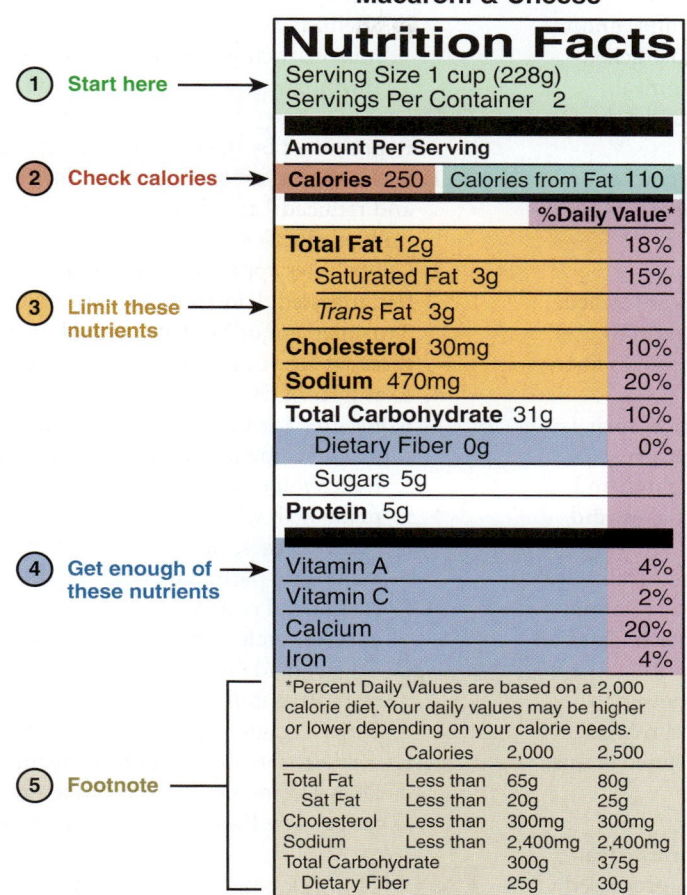

Fig 18.4 Nutrition facts label. (From U.S. Food and Drug Administration, 2004.)

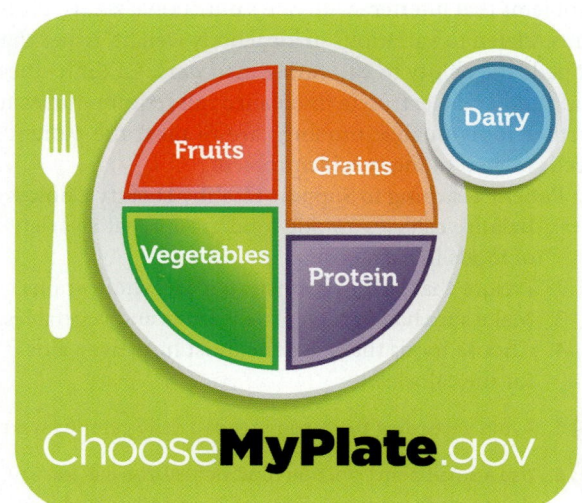

Fig 18.5 MyPlate. (USDA, www.ChooseMyPlate.gov, 2011.)

b. Beans and peas: Beans, such as black, kidney, pinto, white, navy, and soy beans; peas, such as split peas, chickpeas, black-eyed peas; and lentils. Note: Beans and peas also are counted as a subcategory of the protein food group.

c. Starchy vegetables: Such as corn, potatoes, green peas, green lima beans, water chestnuts, green bananas, and plantains.

d. Red and orange vegetables: Such as carrots, sweet potatoes, tomatoes, pumpkin, red peppers, and butternut and acorn squash.

e. Other vegetables: Such as cauliflower, green beans, iceberg lettuce, mushrooms, onions, zucchini, artichokes, asparagus, avocado, beets, bean sprouts, cabbage, celery, cucumbers, eggplant, turnips, and wax beans.

C. Grains

1. Should be 30 percent of the plate daily; half should be whole-grain products.

2. Divided into whole grains and refined grains:
   a. Whole grains.
      (1) Food products made from the entire grain kernel, such as whole-wheat and cracked-wheat flour, oatmeal, whole cornmeal, whole rye, whole-grain barley, millet, buckwheat, and brown rice.
      (2) Examples: Whole-wheat bread, crackers, pasta, tortillas, and cereals; popcorn; wild rice; muesli; and rolled oats.
   b. Refined grains.
      (1) Food products using grains that are milled, which eliminates the bran and germ to make it a finer texture; it also removes fiber, iron, and many B vitamins.
      (2) Examples: White bread; white rice; corn bread and tortillas; flour tortillas; grits; couscous; noodles; pretzels; spaghetti and other macaroni products; corn flakes; and crackers and pitas.
      (3) Some products made with refined grains are enriched with B vitamins, such as thiamin, riboflavin, and niacin; folic acid; iron; and fiber.
3. Products made with grains must be reviewed to identify whether they used whole grains, refined grains, or are a mixture of whole and refined grains.

D. Protein
   1. Should be 20 percent of the plate daily.
   2. Includes foods in the following categories: meat, poultry, seafood, beans and peas, eggs, processed soy, nuts, and seeds.
   3. Lean cuts of meat and poultry should be substituted for fatty cuts of meat and poultry, with all visible fat removed.
   4. Two servings of seafood rich in omega-fatty acids should be included weekly.
   5. Avoid meats, nuts, and seeds with added salt because excessive sodium intake is associated with fluid retention, high blood pressure, and brain attack.
   6. Examples of protein.
      a. Meat such as beef, pork, ham, lamb, veal, bison, rabbit, and venison.
      b. Poultry such as chicken, duck, goose, and turkey.
      c. Beans, peas, lentils, and eggs.
      d. Nuts, such as almonds, cashews, mixed nuts, peanuts and peanut butter, walnuts, filberts, pecans, and pistachios; seeds, such as pumpkin, sesame, and sunflower.
      e. Soy products, such as tofu, tempeh, and texturized vegetable protein.
      f. Fish, such as salmon, catfish, cod, flounder, haddock, halibut, mackerel, porgy, sea bass,

snapper, swordfish, trout, and tuna; canned fish, such as anchovies, tuna, and sardines.
      g. Shellfish, such as clams, crab, crayfish, lobster, mussels, octopus, oysters, scallops, squid, and shrimp.

E. Dairy
   1. Represented by the circle in the MyPlate icon.
   2. Includes not just milk, calcium-fortified soymilk, and reduced-lactose and lactose-free milk, but milk products, such as cheese and yogurt.
   3. Contributes approximately 18 percent of the protein ingested daily in the America diet, which is 3 to 4 percent of MyPlate; should include two or three fat-free or low-fat dairy products daily.
   4. Examples of dairy products.
      a. Fat-free (skim) milk, low-fat milk (1%), and products made with them; fat-free and low-fat milk should replace whole milk and products made with whole milk.
      b. Hard cheeses, such as cheddar, mozzarella, Swiss, and parmesan; soft cheeses, such as ricotta and cottage cheese; and processed cheeses, such as American cheese.
      c. Yogurt made with whole, reduced-fat, low-fat, or fat-free milk.
      d. Deserts made with milk, such as pudding, ice milk, frozen yogurt, and ice cream.
      e. Does not include cream cheese, cream, and butter because these foods contain little calcium.

IX. Nursing Care to Support Nutrition

Nursing responsibilities related to helping patients meet their dietary needs include teaching all patients basic concepts related to making healthy dietary choices, assisting patients who need assistance with feeding themselves, and providing specific nursing interventions related to health problems that interfere with one's nutritional status. Problems related to variations in ideal body weight, issues that impede the ability to eat, eating disorders, GI difficulties, and fluid and electrolyte imbalances all require nurses to further individualize nursing care to meet the patient's needs related to the specific problem.

A. Patient Teaching to Support Healthy Dietary Choices
   1. Balance calories among food groups; eat a variety of foods in each group.
   2. Ensure that half of grains eaten are whole grains.
   3. Make sure half of each plate is fruits and vegetables.
   4. Choose foods that have the most nutritive value for the calories.
   5. Avoid exceeding the recommended daily calorie intake.
   6. Use a small plate, portion food before you eat, eat slowly, and recognize when you have had enough and stop eating to avoid overeating.

7. Replace whole milk and whole-milk products with low-fat milk and low-fat milk products.
8. Reduce the intake of foods high in solid fats, added sugars, and salt, such as ice cream, cake, cookies, candy, sweetened drinks, fried foods, and chips as well as fatty meats, such as sausage, bacon, and hot dogs. Include them once in a while as a treat.

DID YOU KNOW?

Fried foods, such as potato chips and French fries, are unhealthy because they are high in calories, unhealthy fats, and added salt. These foods contain "bad" fat (saturated fat) and increase "bad" cholesterol (LDLs), which stay in the body longer, raising circulating blood triglycerides that decrease "good" cholesterol (HDLs). Foods high in fat and salt are associated with heart disease and stroke (brain attack, cerebrovascular accident) and should be avoided or ingested only occasionally.

9. Reduce sodium intake by comparing nutrition facts labels and selecting low-sodium products, such as those labeled as "no added salt" or "low sodium."
10. Drink 8 glasses of water a day; avoid high-calorie beverages, such as nondiet soda.
11. Balance food intake and physical activity.

B. Commonalities of Nursing Care
1. Before a meal.
   a. Offer to toilet the patient and provide oral care and hand hygiene before meals; if offered by your agency, provide prepackaged wet towels to wash hands before and after meals.
   b. Allow the patient time to engage in religious rituals before a meal, such as saying a prayer.
   c. Ask whether the patient would like to listen to music during the meal to provide a pleasant mealtime environment.
   d. Encourage family members to share mealtimes when able; in residential settings, assist patients to the dining room to support socialization.
   e. Provide a clean and pleasant eating environment.
      (1) Ensure that the patient's room is free from unpleasant odors.
      (2) Remove offensive items from site, such as urinal, toilet paper, emesis basin, and soiled tissues and washcloths.
      (3) Clean the overbed table so that it is ready to receive the patient's meal tray.
   f. Provide privacy during meals if a patient has difficulty eating and is embarrassed.
   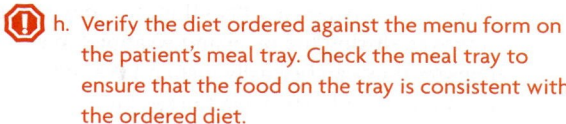 g. If the patient wears dentures, ensure that they are in the patient's mouth; if the patient prefers not to

wear dentures during meals, secure them in a labeled container stored in the patient's bedside table rather than on the patient's tray where they can be accidentally discarded.
   h. Verify the diet ordered against the menu form on the patient's meal tray. Check the meal tray to ensure that the food on the tray is consistent with the ordered diet.

2. During a meal.
   a. Position the patient in an upright sitting position when possible. Have the patient sit in a chair for meals if the patient is able to get out of bed; if the patient is in bed, raise the head of the bed to a comfortable position and place the overbed table over the patient's legs so that the food tray is in easy reach. An upright position uses gravity to facilitate movement of food to the stomach once swallowed.
   b. Encourage self-feeding to support independence.
   c. Use a napkin, not a bib, over clothes to protect them from soiling to support dignity.
   d. Prepare the meal tray: open food and fluid containers; position utensils in easy reach; cut meat; and season food and butter bread, as per the patient's instructions.
   e. Locate food on the tray based on the face of a clock if the patient is visually impaired.
   f. Explain and demonstrate use of assistive devices for eating and drinking when needed to facilitate intake.
   g. Feed a patient who is unable to self-feed.
      (1) Sit at the patient's eye level.
      (2) Ask the patient the order of foods to be presented and whether fluids should be provided after each mouthful.
      (3) Serve small amounts of food at a time because too much food is difficult to manage and may cause aspiration.
      (4) Provide ample time for the patient to chew and swallow food; do not rush the patient.
      (5) Provide finger foods that the patient might be able to manage to self-feed, such as bread, to support independence.
      (6) Provide one food at a time; avoid mixing several foods together, such as mashed potatoes and peas, unless this is the patient's preference. Patients have a right to taste different textures and flavors and serving items individually may be more appetizing to the eye.
      (7) Serve hot foods hot and cold foods cold.
      (8) Have an informal conversation with the patient to create a relaxed mealtime

experience, but do not ask the patient a question while the patient has food or liquid in the mouth to minimize the risk of aspiration.

3. After a meal.
   a. Check the tray for dentures that may have been removed during the meal and wrapped in a napkin; they can be easily lost and are time consuming and expensive to replace.
   b. Assist the patient to wash the hands or to toilet after the meal is completed.
   c. Encourage the patient to remain upright for 40 to 45 minutes after the meal; gravity facilitates movement of food along the GI tract and helps to minimize the risk of aspiration.
   d. Identify and document feeding behaviors and tolerance, such as whether the patient experienced coughing, difficulty swallowing, or dysphagia.

   🛑 e. Record the intake of food as a percentage and fluid in milliliters because these are objective measurements of the patient's intake; avoid using words that are subjective, such as "good," "well," and "poor" to describe the patient's intake.

C. Nursing Care for Patients With Dysphagia and Swallowing Problems
1. Swallowing requires synchronized timing of sensory and motor systems to transport a bolus from the mouth, through the pharynx, and to the esophagus.
2. Conditions that increase the risk of aspiration.
   a. Neuromuscular problems, such as brain attack, Bell's palsy (facial paralysis), cerebral palsy, Parkinson's disease, multiple sclerosis, and myasthenia gravis.
   b. Problems that influence the head, neck, and upper GI tract, such as cancer of the tongue, esophagus, or stomach.
3. Specific nursing care.
   a. Assess for clinical indicators of dysphagia or a swallowing problem, such as statements by the patient about pain, an inability to swallow, or food caught in the back of the mouth; drooling or leaking of liquid or food; pocketing of food; and gagging or coughing when eating food or drinking fluid.
   b. Assess for the presence of cough and gag reflexes, level of consciousness, and swallowing ability.
   c. Inform the primary health-care provider if clinical indicators of dysphagia or a swallowing problem are identified; suggest an order for a swallowing consult by a speech-language pathologist to assess the patient's swallowing ability (generally includes a modified barium

swallow that identifies at what point the complex action of swallowing is impaired).
   d. Learn about the National Dysphagia Diet, which provides guidelines about the use of altering food textures and thickening liquids to facilitate safe swallowing.

   🛑 e. Institute aspiration precautions and communicate this action to all health-care team members in the plan of care and via a notice attached to the front of the patient's clinical record.

   (1) Place the patient in an upright position; instruct the patient to flex the head slightly when swallowing to direct food toward the esophagus rather than the trachea.
   (2) Provide the ordered diet, such as pureed, ground, chopped, and soft food, to facilitate swallowing.
   (3) Introduce food toward the back of the strong side of the mouth because doing so makes it easier to manage and control when swallowing.
   (4) Ensure that all food in the mouth is swallowed before offering the next bite; check the mouth as needed to ensure that food is not *pocketed* between the gums or teeth and cheek.
   (5) Avoid using a straw because fluid is more difficult to control when it enters the middle of the mouth versus directly from a glass or cup.
   (6) Thicken fluids because they are easier to control and swallow than thin fluids. Thickness of fluids progresses from thin, nectar-like, honey-like to pudding-like thickness.
   (7) Teach the patient not to use liquids to promote swallowing unless instructed to do so by the speech-language (swallowing) therapist.
   (8) Avoid serving sticky foods, such as peanut butter and dry mashed potatoes.
   (9) Encourage the patient to dry swallow several times between bites.
   (10) Ensure that a suction machine is accessible if needed to maintain a patent airway.
   f. Collaborate with the primary health-care provider about the potential need for tube feedings if the patient is not ingesting an adequate intake of calories daily.

D. Nursing Care for Patients Who Are Overweight or Obese
1. Overweight and obesity are a national epidemic; more than 68 percent of the population in the United States are overweight or obese (more

than 33.97 percent are obese, and 34.4 percent are overweight).

2. People who are overweight or obese have a greater incidence of chronic illnesses than individuals who are not overweight or obese.

3. Factors that place a patient at risk.
   a. Calorie intake greater than height, weight, activity, and energy requirements; may be due to high-fat diet and inappropriate food choices.
   b. Reduced activity level without concurrent reduction in calorie intake; may be due to impaired mobility.
   c. Cultural influences that support excess weight, such as frequent intake of fried foods or pasta.
   d. Physiological situations, such as an underactive thyroid gland causing a low BMR and subsequent increase in weight.
   e. Psychological factors, such as anxiety, that contribute to inappropriate food choices.

4. Specific nursing care.
   a. Identify factors that place a patient at risk for becoming overweight or obese.
   b. Encourage the patient to use a food diary to help develop insight into eating habits.
   c. Help the patient to identify realistic goals and to review them weekly.
   d. Help the patient understand that healthy eating needs to be an enduring lifestyle change.
   e. Explain how to read a nutrition facts label to identify foods that are high in calories, fat, and carbohydrates that should be avoided in a low-fat, low-calorie diet; this knowledge will empower the patient to have control over food choices.
   f. Teach the patient to avoid shopping for food when hungry to reduce the temptation to buy inappropriate comfort foods.
   g. Identify foods to avoid that are high in fat, such as whole-milk products, fried foods, animal fat, gravies, sauces, nondiet soda, chocolate, and other treats that are high in carbohydrates and sugar.
   h. Teach the patient to limit the use of butter, margarine, mayonnaise, oil, shortening, bacon, cream, cream cheese, and other cheeses to 1 tablespoon a day or 1 teaspoon per meal.
   i. Encourage the patient to eat fresh fruits and vegetables; use fat-free milk and milk products; and substitute yogurt for sour cream in recipes.
   j. Incorporate nutritious morning and afternoon snacks into the meal plan to minimize the desire to graze throughout the day.
   k. Teach the patient to limit lean meats to no more than 6 oz daily and eggs to three or four weekly.
   l. Encourage the patient to serve food on small plates, eat small meals, take small bites, chew food well, eat slowly, and put the eating utensil down between bites.
   m. Encourage the patient to remain in a sitting position for 30 to 45 minutes after meals to use gravity to keep food in the stomach and minimize the risk of reflux and aspiration, which are associated with obesity.
   n. Encourage the patient to participate in counseling and/or a support group, such as Weight Watchers or Overeaters Anonymous.
   o. Encourage the patient to participate in an exercise program to burn calories and increase the BMR; patients should begin with less strenuous exercise at first and build to 40 minutes of exercise 6 days a week.
   p. Encourage adequate sleep because sleep deprivation negatively affects the hormones leptin and ghrelin, which regulate appetite.
   q. Use supportive statements to point out successes in efforts to lose weight; avoid negative statements because they can demoralize the patient and negatively affect the nurse-patient relationship.
   r. Weigh the patient weekly to evaluate progress; a sensible weight loss is approximately 2 lb a week; for a weight loss more than 2 lb a week, the patient should be on a therapeutic weight loss diet and monitored by a primary health-care provider.

E. Nursing Care for Patients Who Have Nausea and Vomiting

1. Factors that place a patient at risk.
   a. Electrolyte imbalances.
   b. Constipation or diarrhea.
   c. Anxiety.
   d. Pain.
   e. Pathological conditions, such as gastric ulcer, pancreatitis, and biliary disease.
   f. Radiation, medications, and/or anesthesia.

2. Specific nursing care.
   a. Monitor intake and output, fluid balance, and electrolyte levels.
   b. Avoid unpleasant procedures before and after meals.
   c. Provide frequent mouth care.
   d. Encourage the wearing of loose clothing to prevent pressure against the epigastric area.
   e. Teach the patient to avoid the use of perfumes and scented hygiene products, such as soaps, aftershave, hairspray, and perfume, that may precipitate nausea.
   f. Provide food that the patient likes, and identify and provide foods that the patient tolerates; dry

foods, such as crackers, breads, potatoes, pasta, and rice, may be better tolerated.

g. Provide small, frequent meals; avoid odorous, high-fat, spicy, and hot food; some patients find that cold food is better tolerated than warm food.

h. Teach the patient to avoid food preparation areas; uncover food plates away from the patient to allow food odors to dissipate somewhat before bringing the tray to the bedside.

i. Remove the meal tray immediately when the patient finishes eating or when the patient is unable to eat because the sight and odor of food can precipitate nausea and vomiting.

j. Encourage the patient to eat slowly, chew food thoroughly, and rest after meals.

🛑 k. Encourage intake of potassium-rich foods, such as orange juice, potatoes, and spinach, if low potassium is a concern with persistent vomiting.

l. Seek a consult by a registered dietitian to address the patient's nutritional needs if nausea or vomiting continues for more than a few days.

F. Nursing Care for Patients Who Are Underweight, Anorexic, or at Risk for Weight Loss
1. Factors that place a patient at risk.
   a. Chemotherapy or radiation therapy.
   b. Weakness or fatigue.
   c. Impaired dentition.
   d. Pain.
   e. Stomatitis or gingivitis.
   f. Impaired swallowing.
   g. Eating disorders, such as anorexia nervosa and bulimia nervosa.
   h. Conditions that increase the metabolic rate, such as hyperthyroidism, cancer, and serious burns.
   i. Conditions that interfere with absorption of nutrients, such as malabsorption syndromes, Crohn's disease, and colitis.
   j. Inadequate income to purchase food.
   k. Inability to shop and prepare meals.
2. Specific nursing care.
   a. Assess for factors that may place a patient at risk for weight loss and for clinical indicators of being underweight or experiencing inadequate nutrition. Complete a 3-day calorie count if ordered.
   b. Employ actions identified in "Nursing Care for Patients Who Have Nausea and Vomiting," page 539.
   c. Administer pain medication before meals to facilitate comfort during meals.
   d. Encourage the patient to eat protein and nutrient-dense foods on the meal tray first; offer milkshakes and other calorie-dense foods and liquids between meals.

e. Provide five or six small meals daily because, over the course of the day, the total calorie intake should be higher than three meals a day and smaller portions are not as overwhelming as three large meals.

f. Secure an order to modify the consistency of food, such as soft, chopped, or pureed, so that it is easier to swallow if swallowing or weakness is a concern.

g. Limit the intake of fluids at meals because they may cause a feeling of fullness, which interferes with food intake.

h. Avoid spicy, acidic, rough, hot, and salty foods for a patient with stomatitis.

🛑 i. Arrange for community services to assist a patient who is unable to procure and prepare meals, such as Meals-on-Wheels, delivery of food from a food bank, application for food stamps, and a home-health aide to cook simple nutritious meals and to assist the patient with eating.

G. Nursing Care for Patients With Cognitive/Mental Impairments
1. Diminished cognitive ability commonly interferes with a person's ability to comprehend the environment, communicate effectively, and eat independently.
2. Factors that place a patient at risk.
   a. Delirium and dementia.
   b. Mental retardation and developmental impairment.
   c. Mental illness, such as depression and bipolar disorder manic episode.
3. Specific nursing care.
   a. Assess the patient's ability to communicate, problem-solve, respond appropriately to stimuli, and self-feed and have an awareness of the need to eat.
   b. Reduce environmental stimuli, such as by turning off the radio or television and discouraging activity around the patient during mealtimes.

🛑 c. Remove unnecessary utensils and items that should not be eaten, such as packages of salt and pepper and container covers, from the food tray; position warm beverages out of reach to avoid a spill that could injure the patient.

d. Use simple phrases to cue the patient, such as "open your mouth," "chew," and "swallow," when feeding the patient.

e. Help the patient to self-feed as appropriate.
   (1) Position a hand over the patient's hand and guide the patient in feeding activities to initiate self-feeding.

(2) Use hand gestures that the patient may recognize and imitate.

(3) Avoid feeding the patient before the patient has had time to self-feed.

(4) Do not rush the patient in self-feeding activities.

f. Provide finger foods for a physically active patient who is unable to sit through a meal.

g. Provide positive reinforcement (e.g., say, "Good job") for efforts at self-feeding.

h. Assist several people positioned at a feeding table (semicircular table generally used in long-term care facilities) for patients who need supervision, prompting to stay focused, or occasional assistance with eating; ensures patient safety, supports socialization, and maximizes the use of a caregiver's time.

🛑 i. Check the patient's mouth for pocketed food after the meal to prevent aspiration.

H. Nursing Care for Patients With Eating Disorders (Anorexia Nervosa, Bulimia Nervosa)

1. Eating disorders are characterized by an impaired relationship with food and body image.

2. Patients perceive that they are overweight, fear obesity, and generally resist treatment.

3. Patients do not see their eating patterns, lack of eating, and/or binging and purging as a problem because of impaired perception.

4. Females are at greater risk for eating disorders, which occur most frequently during adolescence and young adulthood.

5. Eating disorders can be life threatening if intervention is not provided before it is too late to reverse the damage to the body; mortality is as high as 20 percent.

6. Anorexia nervosa.

a. Refusal to maintain body weight equal to or greater than expected weight for age and height; excessive fear of gaining weight or becoming obese even though underweight; disruption in the way one's body weight or contour is experienced; and denial of the gravity of the low body weight.

b. Common clinical physical and physiological indicators include weight loss; muscle wasting; weakness; fatigue; lethargy; brittle hair and nails; lanugo on face; dry, pale, pasty skin; anemia; and amenorrhea. It can lead to severe fluid and electrolyte imbalances, dehydration, impaired sexual development, and death.

c. Common behavioral clinical indicators include avoiding meals; reducing the amount and types of food ingested; compulsively arranging food; cutting food into small pieces; dieting and exercising excessively; denying hunger; wearing baggy clothes; vomiting after ingestion of food is common; and using diuretics and laxatives to reduce weight.

d. Common emotions associated with anorexia nervosa include believing one is fat when really very thin; unhappiness with appearance; irritable; argumentative; overly sensitive to criticism; periods of depression; need for perfection; and low self-esteem.

7. Bulimia nervosa.

a. Characterized by binge eating followed by self-induced vomiting (**purging**) which rids the body of excessive calories and other actions to prevent weight gain; and dissatisfaction with body contour and weight.

b. Clinical physical and physiological indicators associated with binging include dramatic variability in weight; abdominal swelling and pain; edema of the hands, feet and legs; fatigue; nausea; dizziness; and diarrhea from excessive laxative use, leading to dehydration.

c. Clinical indicators of persistent vomiting include hypoglycemia, electrolyte imbalances (especially potassium and sodium); sore throat; excessive dental caries; enamel erosion and staining of the teeth due to contact with gastric acid; and swelling of the salivary glands.

d. Common behavioral clinical indicators include behavior such as avoiding meals; vomiting after meals; evidence of binging, such as large volumes of food missing; hidden food wrappers; laxative, diuretic, and emetic use; stealing food or money to buy food; and night owl behavior so that binging occurs after others have gone to bed.

e. Common emotions associated with bulimia include dissatisfaction with appearance; disinterest in social activities and work; moodiness; depression; irritability; overly sensitive to criticism; and low self-esteem.

8. Specific nursing care.

a. Assess for clinical indicators of the eating disorder; identify verbal and nonverbal responses associated with the patient's perceptions regarding body image.

b. Maintain a consistent, nonjudgmental, nonargumentative, patient-centered approach to support trust and a therapeutic relationship.

c. Maintain a matter-of-fact approach; focus on emotional issues, not food.

d. Assist with designing a contract for a behavior modification program.

e. Monitor weight regularly.

f. Monitor laboratory tests to identify electrolyte imbalances.

g. Support and praise the patient's efforts to control negative behaviors.

h. Provide six small meals that are nutrient dense and several nutritious snacks daily.

🛑 i. Measure oral intake; monitor the patient's behavior for 1 hour after meals to minimize the risk of self-induced vomiting.

j. Support participation in individual, group, and/or family therapy.

k. Assist the patient in identifying and discussing concerns regarding low self-esteem, impaired identity, and family dysfunction.

l. Provide ordered IV therapy to restore electrolyte balance; administer enteral feedings when ordered as a last resort.

I. Nursing Care for Patients With Gastroesophageal Reflux Disease (GERD)

1. Occurs when gastric contents flow up the esophagus.
2. Factors that place a patient at risk.
   a. Conditions that impair the ability of the lower esophageal sphincter to close firmly, such as protrusion of the stomach upward through the esophageal hiatus of the diaphragm (**hiatal hernia**).
   b. Conditions that increase intra-abdominal pressure, such as obesity and pregnancy.
3. Clinical indicators include epigastric discomfort or pain (**heartburn**), dysphagia, regurgitation, aspiration, sore throat, and hoarse voice.
4. Complications include respiratory system problems, such as wheezing, bronchitis, and pneumonia; chronic inflammation of the esophageal mucosa, leading to esophagitis; and epithelial changes known as Barrett's esophagus, a precancerous situation that in turn can lead to esophageal cancer.
5. Specific nursing care.
   a. Encourage the patient to lose weight if overweight or obese.
   b. Teach the patient practices to limit gastroesophageal reflux.
      (1) Use relaxation techniques before and after eating.
      (2) Eat six small meals a day.
      (3) Avoid foods that relax the lower esophageal sphincter, such as those high in fat, chocolate, peppermint, and spearmint; foods that stimulate gastric secretion, such coffee and pepper; and foods that are irritating to the GI mucosa, such as alcohol, spicy foods, citrus fruits and juice, tomatoes, and tomato juice.
      (4) Avoid fluids for a half hour before meals; limit fluids to a half cup with meals; and avoid fluids for 1.5 hours after meals.
      (5) Maintain a sitting position for 2 hours after meals to allow gravity to keep gastric contents from ascending into the esophagus.
      (6) Limit food intake several hours before retiring to minimize the risk of reflux and aspiration.
      (7) Sleep with the head of the bed raised on 6 to 8 inch blocks to minimize gastroesophageal reflux at night.
      (8) Avoid clothing with tight belts to decrease pressure against the epigastric area.
      (9) Take over-the-counter antacids for mild reflux and proton-pump inhibitors or histamine-2 receptor blockers as prescribed.

J. Nursing Care for Patients Who Have or Are at Risk for Osteoporosis

1. Inadequate bone mass that causes fractures in response to mild trauma.
2. Caused by inadequate development of bone mass due to such factors as genetics; inadequate intake of calcium and vitamin D; excessive intake of protein, sodium, and caffeine (impair calcium retention); insufficient exercise; and increased rate of bone loss later in life, especially in response to decreased estrogen in menopausal women.
3. Additional risk factors include reduced mobility, aging process, hyperthyroidism, use of corticosteroids and some antiseizure medications, being small and thin, family history, and intake of alcohol and tobacco.
4. Postmenopausal women are at risk due to the decrease in the protective effects of estrogen on bone; 80 percent of people with osteoporosis are women; 50 percent of women over the age of 50 experience a fracture related to osteoporosis.
5. Clinical indicators include abnormal increased convexity of the curvature of the thoracic spine (**kyphosis**) and loss of height due to vertebral compression fractures; acute or chronic back pain, indicating vertebral facture; pain that limits activities of daily living; and psychological problems, such as impaired body image, fear of falling or fractures, anxiety, and depression.
6. Bone density testing identifies the level of bone density and, when repeated every 1 or 2 years, can identify whether bones are losing density or staying the same; this is helpful in identifying a person's risk for a fracture and can assist in determining a person's treatment regimen.
7. Specific nursing care.
   a. Encourage intake of foods high in calcium, such as milk; cheese; yogurt; salmon; sardines; rainbow trout; oysters; cauliflower; tofu; and green, leafy vegetables, such as spinach, turnip greens, okra, and Chinese cabbage.

b. Encourage exposure to sunlight because the sun's rays stimulate production of vitamin D, which promotes the absorption of calcium.

c. Encourage intake of foods high in vitamin D, such as shiitake and button mushrooms, mackerel, salmon, herring, sardines, catfish, tuna fish, cod liver oil, eggs, and fortified cereals and soy products.

d. Encourage a daily program of weight-bearing exercise, such as walking.

e. Teach the patient about prescribed medications.
   (1) Calcium supplements: 1,000 mg daily for patients 18 to 49 years of age and 1,200 mg daily for patients older than age 50.
   (2) Vitamin D: 1,000 to 5,000 IU daily.
   (3) Bone forming drugs, such as teriparatide (Forteo).
   (4) Antiresorptive medications, such as alendronate (Fosamax) and ibandronate (Boniva).

K. Nursing Care for Patients Who Are Constipated: See "Constipation" in Chapter 22, "Gastrointestinal," page 692.

L. Nursing Care for Patients Experiencing Diarrhea: See "Diarrhea" in Chapter 22, "Gastrointestinal," page 691.

M. Nursing Care for Patients Who Are Dehydrated or Have Fluid Volume Excess: See the section "Nursing Care for Patients With Fluid Imbalances" in Chapter 21, "Fluids and Electrolytes," page 654.

X. Enteral Nutrition

Enteral nutrition is the delivery of liquid formula into the GI tract via a tube that bypasses the mouth, esophagus and, depending on the type of tube, sometimes the stomach. Enteral feedings are designed for patients who have a functioning GI system but have an inability to chew and swallow food, have a high metabolic need, or lack the stamina to eat. Nurses must be proficient in caring for patients with enteral feedings because of the risks associated with this type of therapy.

A. Enteral Nutrition Tubes

1. Nasogastric tube.
   a. Tube inserted via a nostril (**naris**) through the nasopharynx and esophagus into the stomach.
   b. Permits administration of a nutritional formula that enters the stomach (**gavage**), bypassing the mouth and esophagus.
   c. Used when a patient is unable to swallow.
   d. Usually used for less than 4 weeks.
   e. Types.
      (1) Levin: Tube with one unvented lumen.
      (2) Salem sump: Double-lumen tube in which one lumen is used for gavage and the second,

smaller lumen provides an air vent (blue pigtail) that permits inflow of air that keeps the tube from adhering to the stomach mucosa (Fig. 18.6).
      (3) Flexible, small-bore, weighted feeding tube.
         (a) Soft, flexible, small lumen tube inserted through a naris by the use of a wire within the lumen (stylet); stylet is removed when placement is verified.
         (b) Has less risk of mucosal trauma due to having a smaller diameter than other nasogastric tubes.
         (c) Can be used for a longer period of time than other nasogastric tubes.

2. Nasoenteric tube.
   a. Long tube inserted via a naris and advanced further along the GI tract into the intestine.
   b. Permits administration of a nutritional formula directly into the small intestine by bypassing the mouth, esophagus, and stomach.
   c. Decreases the risk of aspiration in patients who have decreased level of consciousness, decreased or absent cough or gag reflex, endotracheal intubation, agitation, GERD, or gastric paresis.
   d. Types.
      (1) Nasoduodenal tube: Inserted via a naris through the nasopharynx, esophagus, and stomach into the duodenum, which extends from the pylorus to the jejunum.
      (2) Jejunostomy tube (J-tube): Inserted via a naris through the nasopharynx, esophagus, stomach, duodenum, and into the jejunum.

3. Surgically implanted GI tubes.
   a. Tube surgically or laparoscopically inserted through the abdominal wall into the stomach or intestine.

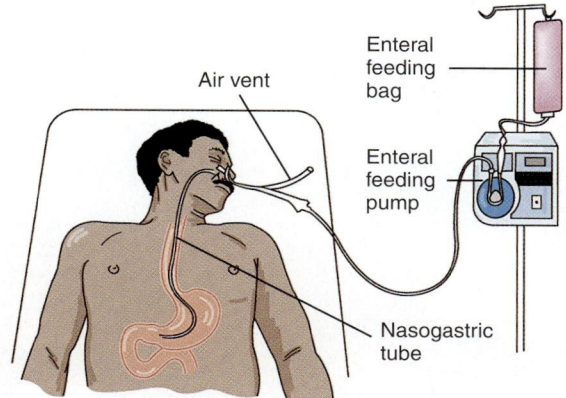

Fig 18.6 Salem sump tube attached to an enteral feeding pump. (From Williams & Hopper [2011]. *Understanding medical surgical nursing*, 4th ed. Philadelphia: F. A. Davis, with permission.)

b. Generally used when nutritional support is required for longer than 4 weeks; however, now also used for short-term nutritional support because of new insertion techniques.

c. Types.
  (1) Percutaneous endoscopic gastrostomy (PEG) tube: Tube inserted through the abdomen into the stomach (Fig. 18.7).
  (2) Percutaneous endoscopic jejunostomy (PEJ) tube: Tube inserted through the abdomen into the jejunum.

d. Advantages.
  (1) Provide reliable access to the GI tract.
  (2) Considered to be the most comfortable feeding tubes.
  (3) PEG tube can be converted to a gastrostomy button (G-button) after the insertion site heals. Button can be capped between feedings and does not protrude from the abdomen (Fig. 18 8).

e. Disadvantages.
  (1) Require surgical or laparoscopic insertion through skin and abdominal wall into stomach or intestine, which increases the risk of infection.
  (2) Insertion site requires surgical asepsis until healed (about 1 month) and then ongoing nursing assessment and meticulous skin care around site.

B. Enteral Nutrition Formulas
1. Formulas include a variety of constituents and caloric values (Table 18.6).
2. Standard formulas require the patient to have adequate digestion and absorption.
3. Special formulas contain constituents to meet a patient's nutritional needs in relation to a specific health problem.

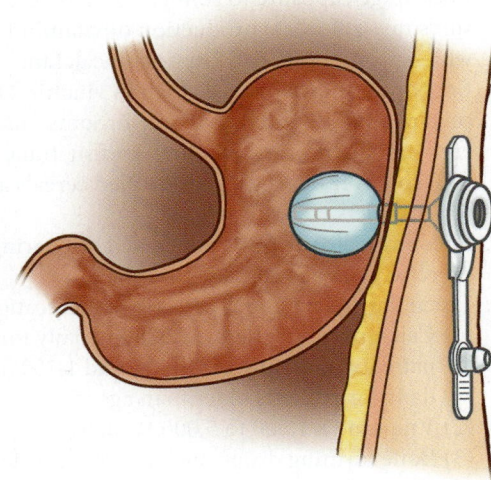

Fig 18.8 Gastrostomy button (G-Button) for gavage. (From Wilkinson and Treas [2011]. *Fundamentals of nursing,* Vol. 1, 2nd ed. Philadelphia: F. A. Davis, with permission.)

C. Nursing Care for Patients Receiving Enteral Nutrition
1. Ensure accurate placement of the tube using several methods.
  a. Obtain x-ray confirmation of placement at the time of insertion per manufacturer or agency policy.
  b. Measure pH of the aspirate; low pH (1 to 5; acidic) indicates the tube is probably in the stomach; high pH (>6; alkaline) indicates the tube is probably in the intestine or respiratory tract.
  c. Inspect the aspirate for amount, color, and consistency.
    (1) Stomach: Greenish/yellow, clear with tan mucus, or brown (digested blood).
    (2) Esophagus: Scant amount, color unreliable.
    (3) Intestine: Yellow to brownish/green.
    (4) Lung: Off-white or tan.
  d. Ensure that the mark made on the tube during placement is just outside the naris.
  e. Instill 5 to 30 mL of air through the tube while auscultating over the epigastric area; "whoosh" sound with gurgling can be heard as air enters the stomach; most unreliable method.
  🛑 f. Notify the primary health-care provider when in doubt to obtain an order for x-ray confirmation of placement.

2. Secure and monitor the tube in the naris.
  a. Secure the tube to the naris if specific placement is to be maintained; use a product designed for this purpose or use tape (Fig. 18.9).

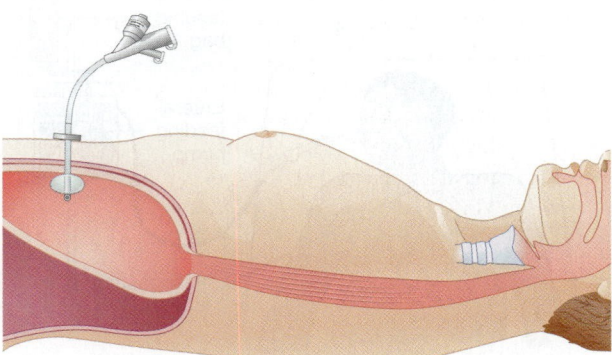

Fig 18.7 Percutaneous gastrostomy (PEG) tube for gavage. (From Wilkinson and Treas [2011]. *Fundamentals of nursing,* Vol. 1, 2nd ed. Philadelphia: F. A. Davis, with permission.)

Table 18.6 Enteral Nutrition Formulas

Formula	Description	Indication for Use
Standard formula		

For example: Nutren, Osmolite.	• Generally provides 1 kcal/mL.
	• Proportionally balanced:
	  • 12–20% protein.
	  • 30–40% fat.
	  • 45– 60% carbohydrates.
	  • Common minerals and vitamins.
	  • Usually lactose free.
		• Patients who are not ingesting adequate nutrients to meet daily energy requirements.
		• Patients with an inability to chew and swallow, but who have no problems with digestion or absorption.

High-protein formula		
For example: Boost High-Protein.	• Additional protein is added to normal nutrients needed daily.	• Patients with large draining wounds, serious burns, or malnutrition.
Hydrolyzed formula (elemental formula)		
For example: Flexical, Peptomen 1.5, Vivonex.	• Contains partially or fully broken down nutritive elements that necessitate minimal digestion. • Fiber free. • Highly osmotic.	• Patients with a disorder that compromises digestion or absorption of nutrients. • Use is controversial.
Renal formula		
For example: Nepro, Suplena	• Contains sodium, potassium, and nitrogen in reduced amounts.	• Patients with renal insufficiency or failure who require tube feedings.
Pulmonary formula		
For example: Pulmocare, NutriVent.	• Contains a higher percentage of fat (e.g., 55%). • As oxygen is consumed, less carbon dioxide is produced.	• Patients with chronic emphysema, asthma, cancer of the lung, and pulmonary fibrosis who require tube feedings.
High-fiber formula		
For example: Jevity, Fibersource HN.	• Contains more fiber than a standard formula.	• Patients with colon cancer, diverticulosis, heart disease, and diabetes. • Patients with reduced activity. • Commonly ordered for patients requiring prolonged enteral feedings.

b. Inspect the site every 2 hours for signs of irritation because pressure and/or friction can cause skin breakdown (Fig. 18.10).

3. Provide PEG or PEJ tube site care; change sterile dressing every 8 hours until healed and then provide meticulous skin care with soap and water.

4. Maintain the head of the bed at a 30° to 45° angle to prevent regurgitation and aspiration.

5. Keep suction equipment at the bedside.

6. Provide frequent oral hygiene to keep mucous membranes moist.

7. Record accurate intake and output; include amount of formula and instillations used to flush the tubing in the intake and subtract instillations used to flush the tubing from the output.

8. Verify tube placement in the stomach before each intermittent feeding and every 4 hours with continuous or cyclic feedings.

9. Maintain tube patency.
   a. Ensure that there are no dependent loops and that nothing is compressing the tube.

b. Flush the tube routinely according to agency policy, usually with 30 mL of water every 4 hours.

c. Ensure that liquid, powdered, and crushable medications are adequately diluted to prevent clogging the tube; flush the tube before and after instillation of medication.

10. Provide specific care when administering an enteral feeding.
   a. Verify the order for the prescribed formula, amount, rate of infusion, and type (continuous, intermittent [bolus], or cyclic [continuous feeding administered for less than 24 hours a day]).
   b. Wash your hands.
   c. Verify the expiration date on the formula and discard the formula if it is expired.
   d. Label the feeding bag with the date, time, formula type, and rate of administration.
   e. Flush the tubing with the formula to remove air before connecting the tubing to the patient's access device and the enteric feeding pump; some pumps automatically purge the tubing.

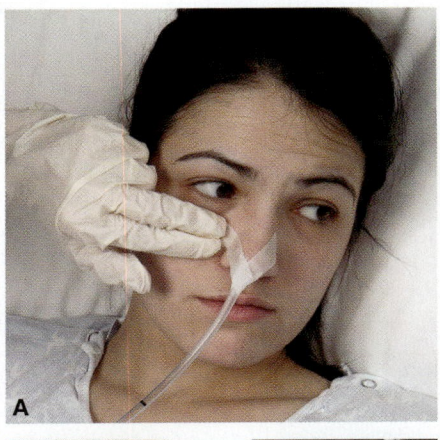

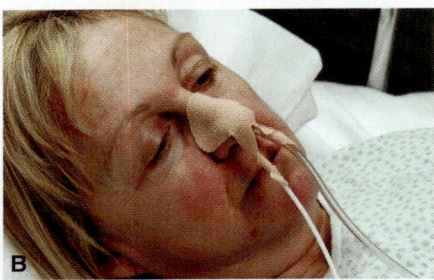

Fig 18.9 Securing a nasogastric tube: (A) with ½-inch tape; (B) with a tube fixation device. (From Wilkinson and Treas [2011]. *Fundamentals of nursing,* Vol. 2, 2nd ed. Philadelphia: F. A. Davis, with permission.)

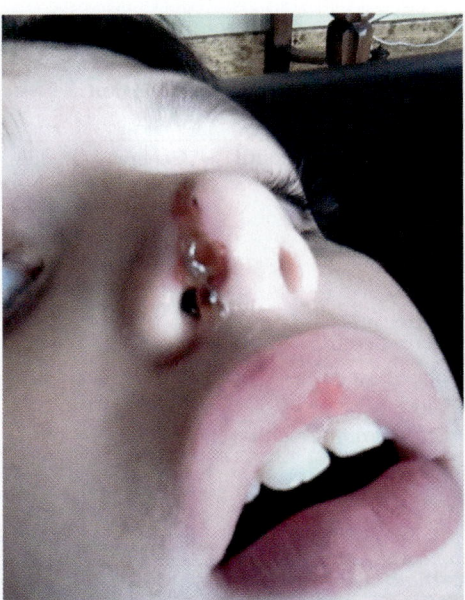

Fig 18.10 Pressure ulcer of a naris: Identified when a nasogastric tube was removed 18 hours after insertion.

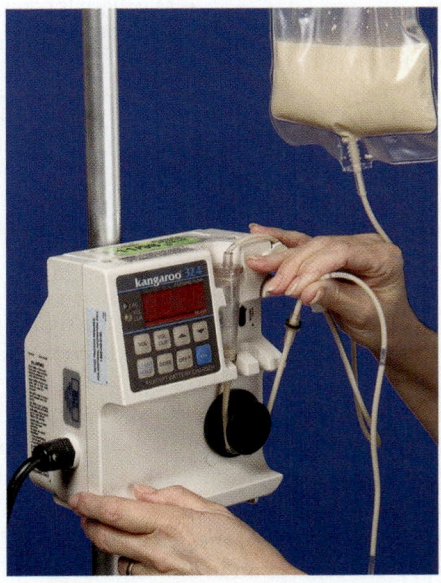

Fig 18.11 Feeding via an infusion pump. (From Wilkinson and Treas [2011]. *Fundamentals of nursing,* Vol. 2, 2nd ed. Philadelphia: F. A. Davis, with permission.)

f. Don clean gloves.

g. Verify placement and measure aspirate before each intermittent or cyclic feeding and every 4 hours with continuous or cyclic feedings; note that measurement of aspirate is not necessary with a PEJ tube because the jejunum is not a reservoir. Hold the next feeding if aspirate exceeds the amount specified by the primary health-care provider or agency policy.

h. Reinstill the aspirate unless it is more than 150 mL or exceeds the flow rate for 1 hour to prevent fluid and electrolyte imbalances.

i. Flush the enteric tube with 30 mL of tap water before the administration of the formula.

j. Administer the feeding as ordered.

(1) Continuous: Formula is administered continuously over 24 hours (Fig. 18.11).

(2) Cyclic: Formula is administered in less than 24 hours; usually given at night when the patient is sleeping.

(3) Intermittent: Formula is administered several times a day via a syringe by gravity (Fig. 18.12). Hold the syringe less than 18 inches above the insertion site to allow the solution to flow slowly and pinch the tubing as the formula reaches the bottom

of the syringe to prevent air from entering the stomach.

k. Flush the enteric tubing with 30 mL of water after completion of an intermittent feeding; flush the tubing of continuous or cyclic feedings with 30 mL of water every 4 hours as ordered; some primary health-care practitioners order a larger volume (e.g., 100 mL) of free water at routine intervals.

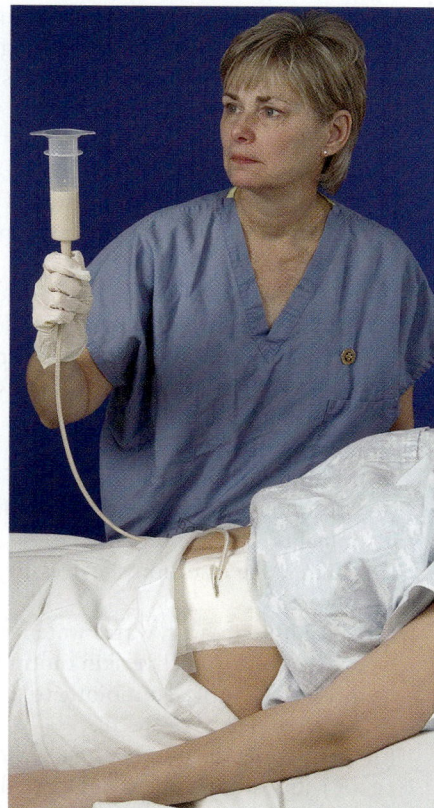

Fig 18.12 Feeding via a syringe by gravity. (From Wilkinson and Treas [2011]. *Fundamentals of nursing*, Vol. 2, 2nd ed. Philadelphia: F. A. Davis, with permission.)

l. Assess the patient's tolerance of feedings: Assess for symptoms of dumping syndrome such as weakness, tachycardia, dizziness, gas, bloating, and cramping abdominal pain,due to hyperpaeristalis, which indicate that the patient is not tolerating the administration of a high-carbohydrate formula.

m. Document the feeding and the patient's response in the patient's clinical record.

n. Notify the primary health-care provider if intolerance or complications occur.

D. Nursing Care Related to Complications of Enteral Nutrition

1. **Aspiration.**

a. Occurs when gastric contents enter the respiratory tract due to gastric reflux or vomiting.

b. Nursing care.

(1) Monitor the patient for clinical indicators of aspiration, such as coughing, shortness of breath, dyspnea, restlessness, tachycardia, tachypnea, and decreased oxygen saturation.

(2) Ensure that suction equipment is readily available.

(3) Ensure that tube placement is radiographically confirmed before use.

(4) Keep the head of the bed (HOB) elevated 30 to 45 degrees throughout feedings; have a patient with an intermittent feeding remain seated or elevate the HOB for 30 to 60 minutes after feedings.

(5) Check for tube placement to ensure that it is in the stomach every 4 hours for continuous feedings and before an intermittent feeding.

(6) Assess for residual volume to ensure that the feeding is being absorbed; every hour initially and then every 4 hours or when administering medication or adding more formula.

(7) Hold a feeding for 30 minutes to 1 hour if gastric residual is higher than the volume indicated by the primary health-care provider or based on policy; usual policy is to recheck the residual in 1 hour and if it is within the prescribed volume, administer the feeding.

(8) Place a continuous feeding pump on hold when administering care that requires the HOB to be lowered; after care is delivered, raise the HOB and reinstitute the feeding. When a patient is receiving an intermittent feeding, provide care that requires the patient's HOB to be lowered before a feeding when possible.

(9) Do not overly sedate a patient because doing so prolongs gastric emptying.

(10) Administer medications that increase gastric motility, such as metoclopramide, as prescribed.

2. **Diarrhea.**

a. Caused by situations such as a hyperosmolar formula, antibiotic therapy, bacterial contamination, and/or malabsorption.

b. Nursing care.

(1) Initiate the flow rate slowly and increase the flow rate after tolerance is determined. Continuous and cyclic feedings are preferred over bolus feedings because they are delivered over a longer period of time and, therefore, their volumes do not overwhelm the GI system.

(2) Prevent contamination of the system.

(a) Change the feeding set every 12 to 24 hours according to agency policy and product recommendations.

(b) Discard a hanging formula after 8 hours if using an open system or after 24 to 48 hours depending on product recommendations if using a closed system.

(3) Administer prescribed medications, such as diphenoxylate/atropine (Lomotil) for diarrhea and Lactinex, a probiotic mixed

culture of *Lactobacillus acidophilus* and *L. bulgaricus,* to restore and maintain normal bacterial balance of the GI tract.

(4) Consult with the primary health-care provider to order a formula that is less hypertonic, fat-free, and/or lactose-free.

3. **Electrolyte imbalances.**
   a. Occur with conditions such as cirrhosis, heart failure, diabetes, and renal insufficiency and excessive GI losses of electrolytes.
   b. Nursing care.
      (1) Monitor electrolyte levels regularly.

   🛑 (2) Reinstill aspirate unless it is more than the recommended volume or exceeds the flow rate for 1 hour.

      (3) Administer prescribed medications, such as potassium.

4. **Dumping syndrome.**
   a. Concentrated formula rapidly enters the intestine, moving water from the bowel wall into the intestinal lumen, causing osmotic diarrhea.
      (1) Occurs 5 to 30 minutes mainly after a bolus enteral feeding.
      (2) Clinical indicators include: Hyperperistalsis, abdominal pain, vomiting, dizziness, weakness, heart palpitations, increased pulse rate, and sweating.
   b. Concentrated formula causes blood glucose to rise and excessive insulin is released in response.
      (1) Occurs approximately 1 to 2 hours mainly after a bolus enteral feeding.
      (2) Clinical indicators include weakness, shakiness, anxiety, confusion, sweating, and tachycardia.
   c. Nursing care.
      (1) Assess for the clinical indicators of dumping syndrome and hyperglycemia.
      (2) Initiate the flow rate slowly and increase the flow rate after tolerance is determined.
      (3) Encourage the patient to rest in the semi-Fowler position for 1 hour after receiving a bolus enteral feeding to delay emptying of the stomach.
      (4) Collaborate with the primary health-care provider to consider changing bolus feedings to a cyclical regimen.

5. **Skin breakdown.**
   a. Caused by gastric secretions leaking around a transabdominal tube site or by unrelieved pressure of an enteral tube taped too tightly to the nose (see Fig. 18.10).
   b. Nursing care.
      (1) Tubes inserted via the nares.
         (a) Monitor the naris every 2 hours for clinical indicators of skin breakdown.

(b) Use a tube fixation device to secure the tube to the patient's nose, making sure to avoid excessive pressure against the naris (see Fig. 18.9).
(c) Change fixation device/tape daily to allow for assessment of the naris.
(d) Clean the nares with a moistened cotton-tipped applicator, dry, and apply a water-soluble lubricant.
(e) Consult with the primary health-care provider regarding using a flexible, small-bore feeding tube or converting to a surgically implanted tube, such as a PEG tube.

(2) Transabdominal tubes.
(a) Monitor for clinical indicators of skin breakdown and local and systemic infection.
(b) Change the insertion site dressing as ordered.
(c) Clean the site with warm water and dry well; apply protective skin ointment or prescribed topical antibiotic to the site or according to protocol.
(d) Ensure that the bumper on a gastrostomy or jejunostomy tube is not too tightly pressed against the abdominal wall.

6. **Hyperglycemia.**
   a. Caused by a formula with high glucose content.
   b. Nursing care.
      (1) Assess for clinical indicators of hyperglycemia, such as weakness, shakiness, anxiety, confusion, sweating, and tachycardia.
      (2) Initiate feedings at a slow rate.
      (3) Monitor blood glucose level every 4 hours.
      (4) Administer hyperglycemia medications as prescribed.
      (5) Consult with the primary health-care provider regarding the use of a low-carbohydrate formula.

7. **Tube obstruction.**
   a. Occurs when tubing is inadequately flushed, crushed medication is not adequately crushed, a feeding is placed on hold to administer nursing care, and when a feeding tube "runs dry;" occurs more frequently with flexible, small-bore tubes.
   b. Nursing care.
      (1) Assess for a slowed or absent flow rate of formula.
      (2) Prevent dependent loops in tubing and ensure that the tubing is not being compressed under the patient.
      (3) Shake cans of formula well before administering.

(4) Flush the tubing with 30 mL of water after completion of an intermittent feeding and after medication administration; flush the tubing of continuous or cyclic feedings with 30 mL of water every 4 hours or as ordered.

(5) Use the liquid form of prescribed medications when possible.

(6) Crush medications if permitted and mix them with water; administer each medication separately and flush the tube with 5 mL of water after each medication.

(7) Reposition the patient and instruct the patient to cough, which may promote a kink in the enteric tube to straighten.

(8) Hold the feeding and notify the primary health-care provider if obstruction or paralytic ileus is a concern.

DID YOU KNOW?

To unclog an enteral nutrition tube, the nurse can employ several interventions that usually are included in agency protocols:

1. First, fill a 60-mL syringe with lukewarm water and attach it to the enteral tube; gently push and pull the plunger of the syringe back and forth several times; clamp the enteral tube for several minutes to allow the warm water to "soak" the internal lumen; gently repeat this action several times until tube patency is reestablished. If this method is unsuccessful, employ one of the following methods.

2. Use a commercially available tube declogger, such as Clog Zapper by CORKAP, a multienzyme cocktail designed to reduce formula clogs; be aware that Clog Zapper generally does not work on clogs caused by medications.

3. Use a cleaning brush, such as a PEG Cleaning Brush by BARD, which can be inserted into the enteral feeding tube using a twisting motion to penetrate and scrape the clog.

4. Use a flexible screw-type device, such as DeCloggers by BIONIX, a soft, flexible threaded device that can be inserted into the enteral tube to clear the clog.

Evidence-based practice results are varied concerning the use of cranberry juice, carbonated beverages, and meat tenderizer to reestablish patency of an enteral nutrition tube. Some findings do not advocate the use of these products because of their acidity or excessive sodium content. Most research demonstrates that gentle irrigation with warm water is most effective.

8. **GI disturbance.**
   a. Occurs with situations such as decreased peristalsis, paralytic ileus, malabsorption problems, hypertonic or cold formulas; cold formulas cause vasoconstriction, which decreases the flow of digestive solutions.
   b. Nursing care.
      (1) Assess for clinical indicators, such as excessive residual, distention, vomiting, diarrhea, reports of gas pains, decreased or increased bowel sounds, nausea, and abdominal cramping.
      (2) Initiate and increase the flow rate slowly as tolerance is determined.
      (3) Administer feedings at room temperature unless otherwise instructed by the manufacturer's directions.
      (4) Assess for residual every hour for the first 4 hours and then every 4 hours, before administering medication, and when adding more formula.
      (5) Administer prescribed medications, such as diphenoxylate/atropine (Lomotil) for diarrhea and Lactinex, a probiotic mixed culture of *Lactobacillus acidophilus* and *L. bulgaricus,* to restore and maintain normal bacterial balance of the GI tract.
      (6) Consult with the primary health-care provider regarding a formula that has less fiber, less fat, and/or is lactose free.
      (7) Hold the feeding and notify the primary health-care provider if obstruction or paralytic ileus is a concern.

9. **Refeeding syndrome.**
   a. Complex metabolic and hormonal changes occur in response to rapid intake of nutrients via the enteral or parenteral route when the patient is nutritionally depleted; can occur after NPO in as little as 14 days.
   b. Related to conditions such as anorexia nervosa, chronic alcoholism, chronic malnutrition, uncontrolled diabetes, and head and neck cancer.
   c. Nursing care.
      (1) Assess for clinical indicators, such as nausea, vomiting, lethargy, and muscle weakness, that may advance to respiratory failure, dysrhythmias, and cardiac arrest.
      (2) Administer specific formula based on a strict refeeding regimen; generally starts with as little as 5 kcal/kg/daily, slowly progressing to 30 kcal/kg/daily by day 10.
      (3) Administer prescribed prophylactic supplements of phosphorous, potassium, and magnesium; restrict sodium to less than 1 mmol/kg/daily and restrict fluids to maintain a zero balance if ordered.
      (4) Monitor tolerance by daily biochemical, electrolyte, and renal and liver function tests.

XI. Parenteral Nutrition (PN)

Parenteral nutrition is the administration of nutrients directly into the bloodstream, bypassing the GI tract. It is used for patients who are incapable of absorbing ample nutrients via the enteral route. Fat or lipid emulsions may be administered weekly to prevent essential fatty acid deficiency or to add calories to the PN regimen. PN solutions are prepared by a pharmacist using a laminar flow hood to reduce the risk of infection and medications are never added to the solution. PN solutions and regimens are specifically designed to meet the individual nutritional needs of patients.

A. Types of PN
1. Total parenteral nutrition (TPN).
   a. For patients with a nonfunctioning GI tract or a high nutritive demand for a long period of time due to severe trauma, burns, infection, or intense cancer therapy.
   b. Administered via a central venous catheter (CVC), which surgically perforates the skin; is inserted into a high-flow vein, such as the subclavian or internal jugular; and is advanced into the superior vena cava (Fig. 18.13).
   c. CVCs have two to four lumens (Fig. 18.14).
   d. Large central veins are used for TPN because the hypertonic solution is diluted quickly due to the high-flow rate of the circulation; TPN solutions are extremely caustic to peripheral veins.
   e. Heparin may be added to the parenteral solution to prevent a blood clot from forming on the tip of the catheter.
   f. Insulin may be added to the parenteral solution because of its high glucose level.
2. Partial parenteral nutrition (PPN).
   a. Administered via a peripherally inserted central catheter (PICC).

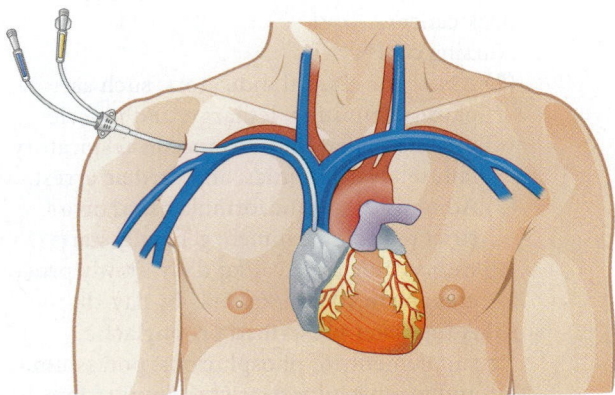

Fig 18.13 Central venous catheter via a subclavian vein for total parenteral nutrition. (From Burton and Ludwig [2011]. *Fundamentals of nursing care: Concepts, connections & skills.* Philadelphia: F. A. Davis, with permission.)

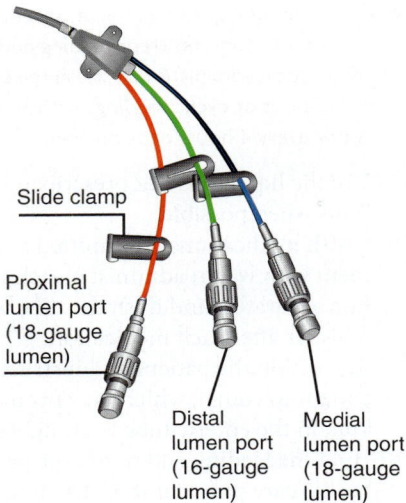

Fig 18.14 Triple-lumen central venous catheter. (From Burton and Ludwig [2011]. *Fundamentals of nursing care: Concepts, connections & skills.* Philadelphia: F. A. Davis, with permission.)

   b. Used for patients who need calories or nutrients beyond what can be taken orally; generally used to supplement oral nutritive intake for a short period of time (generally less than 10 days and for less than 2,000 calories daily).
   c. PPN solution should not exceed 50 percent dextrose and 8.5 percent amino acids at 83 mL/hour.

B. Nursing Care for Patients Receiving PN
1. Commonalities of nursing care.
   a. Ensure PN tube placement is radiographically confirmed before use.
   b. Verify the order (e.g., formula, amount, and rate of infusion), label the PN solution bag (e.g., date, time, and nurse's initials), and verify the expiration date on the formula.
   c. Always use an infusion pump to ensure accuracy; dedicate a port for administration of PN solution.
   d. Refrigerate PN solution until 60 minutes before use.
      (1) Let the solution return to room temperature naturally.
      (2) Cold solutions can cause pain, venous spasm, and hypothermia.
      (3) Do not accelerate warming of a PN solution by placing it in warm water or putting it in a microwave oven because doing so may cause the solution to precipitate, resulting in catheter occlusion or emboli.
   e. Infuse the PN solution as ordered; for example, administer slowly initially and increase the rate in increments of 25 mL/hour until the ordered rate is reached; generally 1 L/day initially and then increased by 1 L/day until the ordered volume is achieved.

f. Monitor for metabolic complications and fluid and electrolyte imbalances because these problems indicate intolerance; the PN may need to be halted, the flow rate decreased, and problems and/or imbalances corrected.

g. Monitor blood glucose levels every 6 hours because PN solutions generally are high in glucose; administer insulin coverage as ordered.

h. Monitor the peripheral site for infiltration, thrombophlebitis, and infection. Monitor vital signs for changes indicating a systemic infection.

i. Weigh the patient weekly; the patient should gain no more than 3 lb/week.

j. Progressively wean the patient off of PN to reduce the risk of metabolic problems, generally over 48 hours. If abruptly discontinuing a PN solution is necessary, replace it with 5 or 10 percent dextrose solution to prevent rebound hypoglycemia until the primary health-care provider is notified and an intervention prescribed.

k. Take steps to minimize the risk of infection.
   (1) Dedicate only one port for PN and do not use the PN port to administer other solutions or medications.
   (2) Ensure that the tubing has an in-line filter because of the high glucose level.
   (3) Do not use a solution if a leak, cloudiness, or floating particles are identified.
   (4) Apply and maintain a sterile transparent occlusive dressing over the insertion site.
   (5) Use 70 percent alcohol pads or chlorhexidine gluconate-based pads to cleanse a port before and after use.
   (6) Change parenteral infusion sets and fat emulsion sets every 24 hours.
   (7) Change the dressing at least every 72 hours. Use meticulous sterile technique, wear a mask, and have the patient not talk and turn the head away from the site when changing the dressing.
   (8) Discard unused parenteral solution in 24 hours after its initiation.
   (9) Document all nursing interventions and the patient's response.

2. Nursing care related to complications of PN.
   a. **Pneumothorax:** Air colleting in the pleural cavity precipitates collapse of the lung; due to a puncture of the pulmonary system, generally during catheter insertion.
      (1) Indicated by sudden severe chest pain, marked dyspnea, reduced oxygen saturation, and absent breath sounds on the side of the chest with the suspected pneumothorax.
      (2) Elevate the head of the bed, administer oxygen, and monitor oxygen saturation.
      (3) Assist with chest tube insertion if necessary to inflate the lung.
   b. **Catheter occlusion:** Blockage of the lumen of the catheter; may be caused by a blood clot at the tip of the catheter.
      (1) Indicated by a sluggish or an absent catheter flow rate.
      (2) Stop the infusion.
      (3) Attempt to relieve the obstruction following the orders of the primary health-care provider or according to agency protocol.
         (a) Flush the catheter with heparin or saline solution.
         (b) If flushing is ineffective, attempt to aspirate the clot.
         (c) If attempts to aspirate the clot are ineffective, follow agency protocol using a thrombolytic agent, such as urokinase.
   c. **Infection:** Entrance of pathogenic microorganisms into the blood via the catheter or catheter insertion site.
      (1) Indicated by elevated vital signs, chills, and positive blood culture.
      (2) Administer prescribed antipyretics and local and/or systemic antibiotics.
   d. **Hyperglycemia and hypoglycemia:** Increased blood glucose level (**hyperglycemia**) or decreased blood glucose level (**hypoglycemia**) due to an excessive or inadequate intake of glucose respectively.
      (1) Hyperglycemia is indicated by polyuria, polydipsia, headache, and lethargy.
      (2) Hypoglycemia is indicated by diaphoresis, shakiness, confusion, and loss of consciousness.
      (3) Initiate and maintain a consistent flow rate as ordered.
      (4) Assess blood glucose level every 6 hours.
      (5) Administer insulin according to the primary health-care provider's prescription if the patient experiences hyperglycemia.
      (6) Administer glucose gel if the patient experiences hypoglycemia.

3. Nursing care for patients receiving lipids.
   a. Review the primary health-care provider's history and physical for information indicating a history or presence of anemia; abnormal liver, biliary, or pancreatic function; or respiratory or coagulation impairments. Collaborate with the primary health-care provider about these conditions

because they are associated with fat emboli and the administration of parenteral lipids.

b. Use a special administration set specific for lipids; use a new administration set for each bottle.

c. Place the patient in the supine position and have the patient perform the Valsalva maneuver when connecting a catheter to the circulatory access to prevent an air embolus.

d. Connect to the port below the filter if lipids are administered concurrently with PN because lipids will not pass through a PN filter due to their large particles.

e. Ensure that the solution is free from froth and separation into layers.

f. Ensure that lipids are at room temperature.

g. Initially infuse 1 mL/minute.

h. Take the vital signs every 10 minutes for 30 minutes and assess for signs and symptoms of intolerance, indicted by fever, chills, flushing, nausea, vomiting, dyspnea, headache, and back pain.

i. If no clinical indicators of intolerance occur, increase the flow rate to the prescribed rate and retake the vital signs every 4 hours.

j. Complete the administration of lipids within 12 hours.

XII. Medications Associated With Nutrition

When a person is diagnosed with a nutritional problem, the primary health-care provider can prescribe a variety of medications depending on the patient's need. The most common medications influencing a patient's nutritional status include antacids, antiemetics, antilipidemics, antisecretory agents, hypoglycemics, and insulin. Nurses should know the mechanisms of action, therapeutic and nontherapeutic effects, and nursing care related to these medications. This information is necessary not only to provide direct patient care but also for patient teaching because these medications are often self-administered over prolonged periods of time.

A. **Antacids:** Decrease gastric acidity, protect stomach mucosa, and reduce epigastric pain (Table 18.7).

B. **Antiemetics:** Decrease nausea and vomiting; prevent and decrease motion sickness (Table 18 8).

C. **Antilipidemics (Lipid-Lowering):** Decrease serum LDH, triglycerides, and total cholesterol levels; increase HDL levels (Table 18.9).

D. **Antisecretory Agents:** Decrease gastric acidity and pain (Table 18.10).

E. **Hypoglycemics (Oral):** Control blood glucose levels in type 2 diabetes (Table 18.11).

F. **Insulins:** Control the blood glucose level in type 1 diabetes (Table 18.12).

Table 18.7 Antacids

Mechanisms of Action	Examples	Nontherapeutic Effects
• Bind with excess acid	• aluminum hydroxide (Amphojel) • magnesium/aluminum hydroxide (Maalox, Mylanta)	• Aluminum salts contribute to constipation and hypophosphatemia

Nursing Care
- Teach the patient to take the medication cautiously with a low-sodium diet because many antacids contain sodium.
- Shake liquids well; give with at least 2 oz of water to promote transit to the stomach.
- Teach the patient to avoid foods that increase epigastric distress, such as spicy foods.
- Encourage the intake of foods high in calcium and iron.
- Assess emesis and feces for obvious and occult blood.
- Monitor serum phosphate and calcium levels with long-term use.
- Encourage the patient to seek a medical evaluation if gastrointestinal signs and symptoms do not subside within 2 weeks.

Table 18.8 Antiemetics

Mechanisms of Action	Examples	Nontherapeutic Effects
Phenothiazines • Inhibit chemoreceptor zone in the central nervous system	• prochlorperazine (Compazine) • promethazine (Phenergan)	• Confusion • Constipation • Photosensitivity • Sedation • Extrapyramidal responses
5-HT$_3$ antagonists • Inhibit serotonin at receptor sites in vagal nerve terminals • Inhibit chemoreceptor zones in the central nervous system	• ondansetron (Zofran)	• Dizziness • Headache • Diarrhea • Constipation

Table 18.8 Antiemetics—cont'd

Mechanisms of Action	Examples	Nontherapeutic Effects
Nonphenothiazines • Inhibit chemoreceptor zones in the central nervous system • Increase gastrointestinal motility and gastric emptying	• metoclopramide (Reglan)	• Restlessness • Sleepiness • Anxiety • Depression • Extrapyramidal responses
Anticholinergics • Correct imbalances of acetylcholine and norepinephrine in the central nervous system that produces motion sickness	• scopolamine (Transderm Scop) • trimethobenzamide (Tigan)	• Sleepiness • *scopolamine:* • Blurred vision • Dry mouth • Tachycardia • Urinary hesitancy • *trimethobenzamide:* • Hypotension • Local irritation

Nursing Care
• Administer before chemotherapy or movement that causes motion sickness.
• Provide for patient safety because of depression of the central nervous system.
• Teach the patient to avoid concomitant use of alcohol and other central nervous system depressants.
• Monitor for the presence of nontherapeutic responses, especially extrapyramidal responses, such as grimacing, rigidity, involuntary movements, and shuffling walk.
Phenothiazines
• Teach the patient to use sunscreen and wear protective clothing.
• Assess for clinical indicators of neuroleptic malignant syndrome, such as hyperthermia, unstable blood pressure, diaphoresis, dyspnea, stupor, muscle rigidity, and urinary incontinence.

Table 18.9 Antilipidemics (Lipid Lowering)

Mechanisms of Action	Examples	Nontherapeutic Effects
HMG-CoA reductase inhibitors • Inhibit the HMG-CoA enzyme, which promotes cholesterol synthesis	• atorvastatin (Lipitor) • rosuvastatin (Crestor) • simvastatin (Zocor)	• Nausea and vomiting • Diarrhea or constipation • Abdominal cramps • Muscle soreness • Hepatoxicity • Decreased absorption of fat-soluble vitamins
Bile acid sequestrants • Bind cholesterol in the GI tract	• cholestyramine (Questran)	
Cholesterol absorption inhibitors • Impede absorption of cholesterol in the small intestine	• ezetimibe (Zetia)	
Fibrates • Impede peripheral lipolysis • Decrease production and synthesis of triglycerides	• fenofibrate (Tricor) • gemfibrozil (Lopid)	
Water-soluble vitamins • Decrease hepatic lipoprotein synthesis • Impede release of free fatty acids from adipose tissue	• niacin	

Nursing Care
• Teach the patient to notify the primary health-care provider of the occurrence of muscle pain, tenderness, weakness, fever, or malaise that may indicate myopathy.
• Encourage the patient to consume a diet low in cholesterol and fat and eat two to three servings of fish high in omega-3 fatty acids weekly.
• Teach the patient to exchange vegetables oils with polyunsaturated fatty acids with those with monounsaturated fatty acids.
• Monitor liver function tests, lipid profile, hemoglobin (Hb) level and red blood cell (RBC) count.
• **Bile acid sequestrants:** Teach the patient to take the medication before meals with 8 oz of water.
• **Cholesterol absorption inhibitors:** Teach the patient to avoid use during pregnancy and lactation.
• **Fibrates:** Teach the patient to notify the primary health-care provider if clinical indicators of bleeding occur with the concurrent use of warfarin (Coumadin).

Table 18.10 Antisecretory Agents

Mechanisms of Action	Examples	Nontherapeutic Effects
H₂ antagonists • Decrease histamine at H₂ receptors in parietal cells, causing a decrease in gastric secretions	• famotidine (Pepcid) • ranitidine (Zantac)	• Decreased RBCs, WBCs, and platelets • Cardiac dysrhythmias • CNS concerns, such as confusion, dizziness, headache, sleepiness • Nephrotoxicity • Hypersensitivity responses
Proton pump inhibitors • Decrease entrance of hydrogen ions into the lumen of the gastrointestinal tract	• esomeprazole (Nexium) • lansoprazole (Prevacid) • omeprazole (Prilosec) • pantoprazole (Protonix)	

Nursing Care
- Teach the patient to notify the primary health-care provider if clinical indicators of bleeding occur with concurrent use of warfarin (Coumadin).
- Be aware that these drugs may be given with an antacid, except ranitidine (Zantac), which must be given 1 to 2 hours before or after an antacid.
- Assess for clinical indicators of altered heart rate and rhythm and frank or occult blood in emesis or feces.
- Monitor complete blood count for signs of blood dyscrasias.
- H₂ antagonists: Teach the patient to avoid smoking because it may inhibit therapeutic action and/or may cause diarrhea.
- Proton pump inhibitors: Teach the patient not to crush or chew the medication; administer 30 minutes to 1 hour before meals depending on the specific drug.

Table 18.11 Hypoglycemics (Oral)

Mechanisms of Action	Examples	Nontherapeutic Effects
Biguanides • Increase sensitivity to insulin • Increase binding of insulin to its receptor	• metformin (Glucophage)	• Hypoglycemia • Lactic acidosis (e.g., sleepiness, dyspnea, malaise, weakness, hyperventilation, brady-cardia, hypotension, myalgia, chills, diarrhea)
Meglitinides • Increase release of insulin from the pancreas	• repaglinide (Prandin)	• Hypoglycemia
Sulfonylureas • Stimulate beta cells to release insulin	• glimepiride (Amaryl) • glipizide (Glucotrol) • glyburide	• Hypoglycemia
Thiazolidinediones • Decrease insulin resistance • Decrease glyconeogenesis	• pioglitazone (Actos) • rosiglitazone (Avandia)	• Upper respiratory tract infection • Edema associated with heart failure (e.g., crackles, dyspnea, peripheral edema, weight gain, jugular vein distension) • Hepatotoxicity (rare)

Nursing Care
- Do not administer these drugs to patients with type 1 diabetes; serious burns or trauma; renal, hepatic, or endocrine disease; and uncontrolled infection or to patients who are pregnant or lactating.
- Teach the patient that therapy controls, not cures, type 2 diabetes; therapy is long term; and the medication regimen should be followed as prescribed.
- Assess for clinical indicators of hyperglycemia, hypoglycemia, and hyperosmolar nonketotic coma.
- Assess blood glucose levels before meals, at bedtime, and whenever necessary if concerned about glucose status.
- Assess for ketones in urine if blood glucose level is 300 mg/dL or higher.
- Encourage the patient to avoid alcohol due to potential for Antabuse-like response.
- Teach the patient not to crush sustained-release tables and to take these medications 30 minutes before meals or according to the primary health-care provider's instructions.
- Thiazolidinediones: Assess the patient who has concurrent heart disease for peripheral edema, crackles, dyspnea, weight gain, and jugular vein distension; assess for clinical indicators of liver impairment, such as nausea, vomiting, abdominal pain, anorexia, fatigue, jaundice, and dark urine.

Table 18.12 Insulins and Their Time Action Profiles

Insulin Type	Examples	Onset	Peak	Duration
Rapid acting	lispro (Humalog)	15–30 min	30 min–1.5 hours	3–4 hours
	aspart (NovoLog)	10–20 min	1–3 hours	3–5 hours
	glulisine (Apidra)	15–30 min	30 min–1.5 hours	3–4 hours
Short acting	regular (Novolin R)	30–60 min	2–5 hours	5–8 hours
	regular (Humulin R)	30–60 min	1–5 hours	6–10 hours
Intermediate acting	NPH (N) Novolin N Humulin N	1.5–4 hours	4–12 hours	18–24 hours
Long acting	glargine (Lantus)	1–1.5 hours	Steadily delivered, no peak action	20–24 hours
	detemir (Levemir)	50 min–2 hours	Unknown	24 hours
Premixed	Novolin 70/30	30 min	2–12 hours	24 hours
	Humulin 70/30	30 min	2–4 hours	14–24 hours
	Novolog Mix 70/30	10–20 min	1–4 hours	24 hours
	Humulin 50/50	30 min	2–5 hours	18–24 hours
	Humalog 75/25	15 min	30 min–2.5 hours	16–20 hours

Nursing Care
- Give only regular insulin IV; rapid-insulin analogs, such as aspart and glulisine, may be given IV in selective situations with medical supervision. Use only a dedicated IV line.
- Roll the vial to mix insulin; do not shake the vial.
- Administer insulin using a calibrated insulin syringe to promote accuracy.
- Administer insulin as prescribed; generally before meals and at hour of sleep.
- Monitor blood glucose levels to determine amount of insulin to administer when providing insulin coverage; note that the primary health-care provider establishes dosages based on glucose levels.
- Monitor for clinical indicators of hyperglycemia and hypoglycemia.

Source: Vitale, B. (2013). *NCLEX-RN Notes: Content review and exam prep* (2nd ed.). Philadelphia: F. A. Davis.

CASE STUDY: Putting It All Together

A public health nurse makes a home visit to an obese woman whose infant son was just discharged from the hospital after a premature birth 1 month ago. The husband is serving in the military and recently left for a 6-month tour of duty on a ship going to the Middle East. In addition to the infant, the mother has another son who is 3 years of age, a 6-year-old daughter, and an adolescent daughter. The mother pumped her breasts and gave the nurses her bottled breast milk when she visited her son every other day while in the hospital. During the visit to the home, the mother asked the nurse, "Can I give my son regular milk now that he is 1 month old?" When the nurse explored the family's diet with the mother, the mother stated, "My three year old only wants to eat hot dogs, french fries, and peanut butter. I tell him that if he eats his vegetables he can have ice cream for dessert. My teenager is constantly on a diet even though she is thin as a rail and says she diets because she doesn't want to get fat like me." The mother voiced a concern about the belief that her adolescent "may have one of those eating problems because she is so thin". Also living in the home is a 75-year-old grandmother who is trying to help the mother with childcare and chores around the house while the mother's husband is deployed. The woman shared that although the grandmother has been helpful around the house, the grandmother has problems with "bad teeth," uses too much salt when she cooks, and constantly depends on her for her social life. The woman's most serious concern about the grandmother is that because of the grandmother's "bad teeth" she has not been eating well and as a result is 20 pounds below her ideal body weight.

Case Study Questions

A. Compose the most appropriate response by the nurse to the mother's question, "Should I continue to breastfeed my infant?"

_____

_____

_____

Continued

CASE STUDY: Putting It All Together

cont'd

Case Study Questions

B. What are three things the nurse should encourage the mother to do to best meet her toddler's nutritional needs?

1. _____

2. _____

3. _____

C. What nine clinical indicators of eating disorders should the nurse teach the mother to observe for when monitoring her adolescent's behavior and physical status?

1. _____

2. _____

3. _____

4. _____

5. _____

6. _____

7. _____

8. _____

9. _____

D. List six nursing interventions that may help the grandmother to meet her nutritional and social needs.

1. _____

2. _____

3. _____

4. _____

5. _____

6. _____

E. What are three important things the nurse should teach the mother about nutrition and breastfeeding?

1. _____

2. _____

3. _____

F. What are at least ten things the nurse should teach the mother to do to achieve a more healthy weight?

1. _____

2. _____

3. _____

4. _____

5. _____

6. _____

7. _____

8. _____

9. _____

10. _____

REVIEW QUESTIONS

1. What should a nurse do to prevent burns during meal-time in patients with mental and physical impairments?
1. Assist patients with warm drinks.
2. Use plastic instead of metal utensils.
3. Serve unsteady patients only cold drinks.
4. Wait until the food is cool before serving.

2. A nurse is caring for a patient who is receiving bolus enteral feedings several times daily. Which nursing intervention is important to help prevent the patient from experiencing diarrhea?
1. Flush the tube after every feeding.
2. Check the residual before each feeding.
3. Elevate the head of the bed during the feeding.
4. Discard the refrigerated opened cans of feeding formula after 24 hours.

3. A nurse is providing dietary teaching about a nutrition facts label to a patient who recently began taking a diuretic daily. What information in the list of nutrients on this nutrition facts label is **most** important for the nurse to include in the teaching plan?
1. A
2. B
3. C
4. D

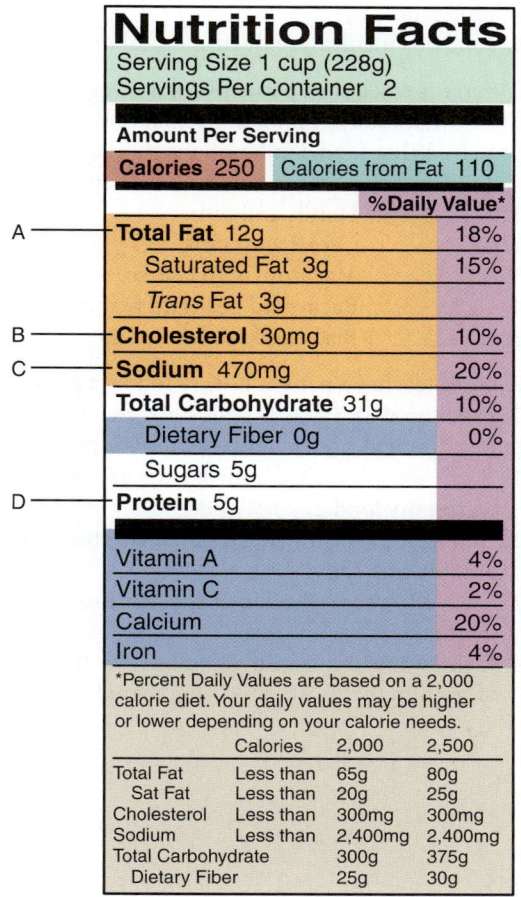

4. A nurse is caring for a patient who is receiving continuous nutritional support via a nasogastric (NG) tube that is regulated by an enteral feeding pump. The nurse identifies that the patient is having difficulty breathing and is restless. What should the nurse do **first**?
1. Use a nasal cannula to provide oxygen.
2. Activate the hold button on the feeding.
3. Raise the bed to the high-Fowler position.
4. Immediately notify the primary health-care provider.

5. A nurse is caring for a patient who is receiving parenteral nutrition. Which nursing actions are essential when providing care for this patient? **Select all that apply.**
1. _____ Use tubing with an in-line filter.
2. _____ Obtain the vital signs every 8 hours.
3. _____ Monitor blood glucose every 4 hours.
4. _____ Compare the patient's daily weight to fluid intake and output.
5. _____ Hang 5% to 10% dextrose solution if the infusion is interrupted.

6. A nurse is caring for a patient who had a large portion of the stomach surgically removed due to stomach cancer and is now experiencing dumping syndrome. For which clinical indicator of dumping syndrome should the nurse assess the patient after the patient completes a meal?
1. Hyperperistalsis
2. Bradycardia
3. Dyspnea
4. Hypoxia

7. A primary health-care provider orders blood glucose monitoring before meals and at bedtime for a patient. Place the following steps in the order in which they should be implemented.
1. Wipe away the first drop of blood.
2. Cleanse the area with alcohol and let it dry thoroughly.
3. Place the hanging drop of blood gently on the end of the test strip.
4. Put the patient's finger in a dependent position in a cup of warm water.
5. Prick the site with the lancet while holding it perpendicular to the patient's finger.
6. Check the code number on the strip and ensure that it compares with the code on the monitor screen.
Answer: _____

8. A nurse is caring for a patient who was admitted to the hospital from home. Family members reported having difficulty getting the patient to eat. Which laboratory test should the nurse monitor because it is the **best** indicator of the patient's nutritional status?
1. Albumin
2. Transferrin
3. Blood urea nitrogen
4. Total lymphocyte count

9. A nurse is caring for a debilitated patient who is on bedrest and has been eating 50 percent of meals. What should the nurse plan to do to stimulate this patient's appetite? **Select all that apply.**
   1. _____ Serve small, frequent meals.
   2. _____ Provide oral care before meals.
   3. _____ Schedule procedures for after meals.
   4. _____ Provide adequate pain medication before meals.
   5. _____ Transfer the patient to a comfortable chair for meals.

10. A nurse is caring for a patient with gastroesophageal reflux disease. What nursing intervention is important?
    1. Instruct the patient to chew food thoroughly.
    2. Serve food that has different textures and aromas.
    3. Offer fluids with food and at a preferred temperature.
    4. Encourage the patient to avoid eating several hours before bedtime.

11. An older frail patient is admitted to the hospital because of malnutrition and an inability to maintain weight. The nurse reviews the results of biochemical laboratory tests. What laboratory results indicate a problem with nutrition? **Select all that apply.**
    1. _____ Hematocrit 42%
    2. _____ Hemoglobin 14 g/dL
    3. _____ Transferrin 190 mg/dL
    4. _____ Serum albumin 2.9 g/dL
    5. _____ Blood urea nitrogen 18 mg/dL

12. A patient is diagnosed with gluten intolerance. What food should the nurse encourage the patient to avoid when eating at restaurants?
    1. White rice
    2. Steamed eggplant
    3. Veal cutlet parmesan
    4. Fruit thickened with tapioca

13. A nurse is providing dietary teaching to a person with a low fixed income. What should the nurse encourage the person to do when making meals on a limited budget? **Select all that apply.**
    1. _____ Substitute eggs and beans for meat.
    2. _____ Purchase luncheon meats for sandwiches.
    3. _____ Buy fresh milk instead of powdered milk.
    4. _____ Read the nutrition facts labels on prepared foods.
    5. _____ Use store brand frozen meals over advertised brands.

14. A nurse is teaching a patient about foods that should be avoided and foods that are acceptable on a lactose-free diet. Which food selected by the patient reflects an understanding of the teaching?
    1. Yogurt
    2. Sherbet
    3. Fruit salad
    4. Rice pudding

15. An older adult who lives alone is experiencing slow but steady weight loss over the past year. What should the nurse encourage the adult to do to address this concern? **Select all that apply.**
    1. _____ Select nutrient-dense foods.
    2. _____ Eat foods high in protein first.
    3. _____ Purchase prepared frozen meals.
    4. _____ Eat an extra meal before bedtime.
    5. _____ Use bullion powder for added flavor.

16. A nurse is planning a teaching program about the medication atorvastatin (Lipitor) for a patient who has high cholesterol. Which information is important for the nurse to emphasize?
    1. Replace oils containing monosaturated fatty acids with oils containing polyunsaturated fatty acids.
    2. Notify the primary health-care provider of muscle pain, weakness, or fever.
    3. Avoid crushing and mixing this medication with applesauce.
    4. Take this medication during a meal or with food.

17. A nurse is teaching a patient who is a vegetarian about what food combinations make a complete protein. What food combinations should the nurse include in the teaching? **Select all that apply.**
    1. _____ Lentils and tofu
    2. _____ Cereal with milk
    3. _____ Macaroni with cheese
    4. _____ Back-eyed peas and rice
    5. _____ Black and red bean soup

18. A nurse teaches a patient how to follow a prescribed 2-g sodium diet. What patient statement indicates that the patient understands the teaching?
    1. "I can use as much salt substitutes as I want to season my food."
    2. "I must limit my intake of salt to two teaspoons of table salt daily."
    3. "I am allowed to drink diet cola because it has less salt than soda with sugar."
    4. "I should read nutrition facts label for the amount of sodium that is in prepackaged foods."

19. A nurse is educating an obese patient who is on a calorie-restricted diet how to analyze a nutrition facts label. Which section of the nutrition facts label on a bag of snack food is **most** important for the obese patient to consider once the number of calories on the label is determined?

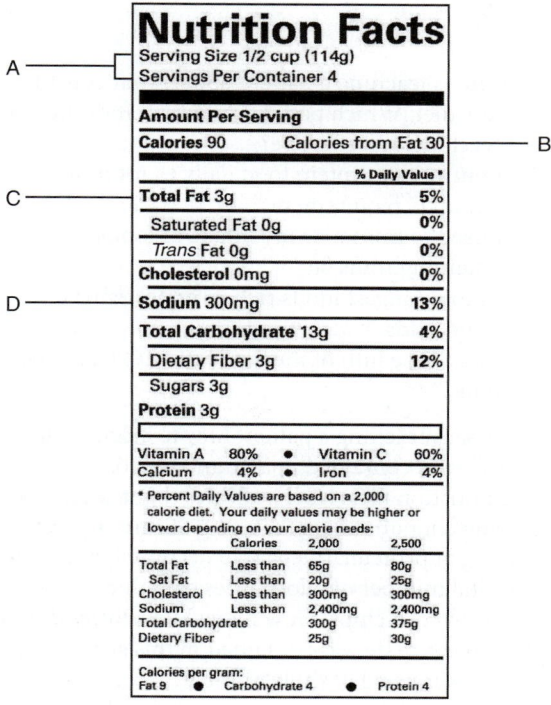

1. A
2. B
3. C
4. D

20. A nurse is providing a class about foods to include and avoid when following a calorie restricted 2-g sodium diet. A patient with which cultural heritage should the nurse be **most** concerned about adjusting to a 2-g sodium diet?
    1. Indian
    2. Chinese
    3. Puerto Rican
    4. Middle Eastern

21. A part-time evening nurse arrives on duty for a 6 p.m. to 12 midnight shift and is assigned to care for a patient receiving peripheral parenteral nutrition (PPN) via a peripheral intravenous catheter inserted at 5 p.m. The nurse reviews the patient's clinical record and completes a blood glucose test before the patient's dinner at 6:10 p.m.

Patient's Clinical Record

Nurse's Progress Note 1500

PPN infusion running as ordered at 83 mL/hour. Slight erythema noted at PPN site. Patient reports some "stinging" at the infusion site. Vital signs stable.

Primary Health-Care Provider's Orders

Peripheral parenteral nutrition: 2,000 mL standard formula with 50% dextrose and 8.5% amino acids at 83 mL/hour.
Weigh weekly.
VS and temperature every 8 hours. If temperature is greater than 100°F, notify primary health-care provider.
Soft diet as tolerated.
BGM a.c. and h.s.; cover as per insulin prescription.
If PPN is interrupted, start 20% dextrose and water at 83 mL/hour and notify the primary health-care provider.
Laboratory tests: Basic metabolic panel, magnesium, and phosphate daily for 3 days then MWF; triglyceride level in a.m. Mondays CBC, INR, triglyceride level, and liver panel.

BGM at 6:10 p.m.

Glucose: 308

In what order should the nurse implement the following interventions?
1. Cover the glucose level with insulin according to the insulin prescription.
2. Discuss the formula order with the primary health-care provider.
3. Hang a bag of 20% dextrose and water and set it at 83 mL/hour.
4. Contact the IV nurse to consider changing the IV site.
5. Discontinue the PPN solution.
   Answer: _____

22. A nurse is preparing to administer a fat emulsion intravenously to an adult. What should the nurse do when administrating this solution?
    1. Run the lipid solution at a rate of 1.0 mL/minute for the first 30 minutes.
    2. Administer the lipid solution within 15 minutes after removal from a refrigerator.
    3. Rotate the lipid solution bottle gently if the solution separates into layers or is cloudy.
    4. Connect the lipid solution infusion set tubing to the port above the filter in the primary infusion line.

23. A nurse is caring for a patient who is receiving a high-calcium diet. Which foods should the nurse teach the patient to include in the diet? **Select all that apply.**
    1. _____ Tuna fish
    2. _____ Prune juice
    3. _____ Whole milk
    4. _____ Pinto beans
    5. _____ Broccoli spears

24. A primary health-care provider prescribes metformin (Glucophage) 500 mg PO bid for a patient newly diagnosed with type 2 diabetes. What should the nurse teach the patient to do when taking this medication?
    1. Increase the intake to three times a day when experiencing stress.
    2. Drink a glass of orange juice if experiencing signs of hyperglycemia.
    3. Be alert for nontherapeutic responses such as sleepiness, myalgia, and hyperventilation.
    4. Explain that it is acceptable to double a dose if a dose is missed, as long as this occurs infrequently.

25. A nurse is caring for a patient who has high cholesterol. Which foods should the nurse teach the patient to avoid? **Select all that apply.**
    1. _____ Eggs
    2. _____ Celery
    3. _____ Asparagus
    4. _____ Calves liver
    5. _____ Baked custard

26. A nurse is caring for a patient who is weak and lethargic. Which action is **most** important when assisting this patient with meals?
    1. Record the intake of food as poor, good, or excellent on the daily activities form.
    2. Ask about preferences regarding the seasoning of food.
    3. Check the mouth for pocketed food after the meal.
    4. Encourage self-feeding.

27. A nurse is caring for a patient who is recovering from abdominal surgery. The patient reports experiencing "gas pains" and asks the nurse what can be done to prevent them in the future. Which should the nurse encourage the patient to avoid until intestinal function fully returns? **Select all that apply.**
    1. _____ Summer squash
    2. _____ Chewing gum
    3. _____ Onions
    4. _____ Lentils
    5. _____ Eggs

28. A primary health-care provider instructs a patient to limit the dietary intake of complex carbohydrates. The intake of which nutrient should the nurse teach the patient to limit?
    1. Milk
    2. Nuts
    3. Eggs
    4. Pasta

29. A nurse is teaching a patient about what constitutes a healthy diet. Which patient statement indicates that the teaching was effective?
    1. "I must eat a protein food daily to meet my vitamin C requirement."
    2. "I need to minimize my intake of foods containing trans fat."
    3. "I should ingest foods rich in nonessential amino acids."
    4. "I want one fifth of the foods on MyPlate to be grains."

30. A nurse is teaching a patient how to calculate the kilocalories contained in an ounce of corn chips. The nutrition facts label indicates that a one ounce serving contains 10 g of fat, 16 g of carbohydrates, and 2 g of protein. The patient accurately calculated the total number of kilocalories contained in one ounce of corn chips. How many kilocalories did the patient calculate was contained in this snack? Record the answer using a whole number.
    Answer: _____ kilocalories

31. A nurse working in a primary care clinic is caring for a patient who was diagnosed with a low vitamin D level. The primary health-care provider prescribes 5,000 units of vitamin D daily and the nurse is teaching the patient foods that are high in vitamin D. The selection of which food by the patient indicates to the nurse that the patient can identify at least one food that is high in vitamin D?
    1. Nuts
    2. Eggs
    3. Liver
    4. Oranges

32. A primary health-care provider prescribes the proton-pump inhibitor omeprazole (Prilosec). The prescription states to take 20 mg once a day. Which instruction should the nurse give the patient regarding this medication?
    1. "Take the capsule several hours before an antacid."
    2. "Sprinkle the capsule contents in applesauce."
    3. "Take the capsule with food."
    4. "Swallow the capsule whole."

33. A nurse is teaching a patient how to calculate the kilocalories contained in one granola bar. The nutrition facts label indicates that one bar contains 1.5 g of fat, 19 g of carbohydrates, and 1 g of protein. How many kilocalories calculated by the patient indicates the correct amount of kilocalories contained in this snack? Record the answer using one decimal place.

    Answer: _____ kilocalories

34. A nurse is teaching a patient about nutrients that will increase the percentage of whole grains ingested daily. Which nutrient selected by the patient indicates that the teaching was effective?
    1. Grits
    2. Noodles
    3. Wild rice
    4. Corn bread

35. Which information is essential for the nurse to include in a program supporting healthy eating habits? **Select all that apply.**
    1. _____ Drink 8 glasses of fluid daily.
    2. _____ Increase the intake of foods high in solid fats.
    3. _____ Make 25% of your plate fruits and vegetables daily.
    4. _____ Cream cheese and butter are included in the dairy circle on MyPlate.
    5. _____ Two servings of seafood rich in omega-fatty acids should be included weekly.

REVIEW ANSWERS

1. ANSWER: 1.
Rationales:
1. Patients with mental and physical deficits need assistance with warm drinks to prevent oral trauma or burns from spills.
2. The use of plastic utensils does not prevent spilling hot liquids.
3. Patients have a right to have a variety of foods presented at different temperatures; serving only cold drinks violates a patient's rights.
4. Warm foods should be served warm and cold foods should be served cold.
TEST-TAKING TIP: Identify the option with the obscure clang association. The word *burns* is a key word in the stem that should direct the test-taker to the word *warm* in option 1. Identify options that deny the patient's rights and that are equally plausible. Options 3 and 4 deny the patient's right to have food and drinks served at warm temperatures and are equally plausible. Identify the option with a specific determiner. Option 3 contains the word *only,* which is a specific determiner. Identify the patient-centered option. Option 1 is patient centered.
Content Area: Nutrition
Integrated Processes: Nursing Process: Implementation
Client Need: Physiological Integrity; Basic Care and Comfort
Cognitive Level: Application

2. ANSWER: 4.
Rationales:
1. Flushing the tube after every feeding moves the formula into the stomach and helps maintain tube patency; it does not reduce the risk of diarrhea.
2. Checking the residual volume informs the nurse about the absorption of the last feeding. This step prevents the addition of more feeding than the patient can digest; it does not prevent diarrhea. Generally, feedings are withheld when a certain residual volume (e.g., half the volume of the last feeding; 150 mL) is identified.
3. Elevating the head of the bed 30° during a feeding helps to keep the formula in the stomach via the principle of gravity and helps to prevent aspiration; it does not prevent diarrhea.
4. Contaminated formula can cause diarrhea. Cans of opened formula support bacterial growth and must be discarded after 24 hours, even when refrigerated.
TEST-TAKING TIP: Identify the unique option. Option 4 is unique. It does not end in the word *feeding* and it is the only option with a number.
Content Area: Nutrition
Integrated Processes: Nursing Process: Implementation
Client Need: Physiological Integrity; Basic Care and Comfort
Cognitive Level: Application

3. ANSWER: 3.
Rationales:
1. The intake of total fat is not as significant to monitor as is another nutrient when a patient is taking a diuretic.

2. The intake of cholesterol is not as significant to monitor as is another nutrient when a patient is taking a diuretic.
3. The patient is taking a diuretic to limit or reduce a fluid volume excess. This patient should avoid excess dietary sodium because sodium helps to retain fluid, which is counterproductive.
4. The intake of protein is not as significant to monitor as is another nutrient when a patient is taking a diuretic.
TEST-TAKING TIP: Identify the word in the stem that sets a priority. The word *most* in the stem sets a priority.
Content Area: Nutrition
Integrated Processes: Teaching/Learning; Nursing Process: Planning
Client Need: Physiological Integrity; Pharmacological and Parenteral Therapies
Cognitive Level: Analysis

4. ANSWER: 2.
Rationales:
1. Oxygen should be initiated after other more important interventions are implemented.
2. The patient's respiratory distress may be due to NG tube migration into the respiratory tract. The feeding should be stopped until this is ruled out.
3. Raising the head of the bed to the high-Fowler position should be done after another more important nursing intervention.
4. The primary health-care provider should be notified of the patient's change in status after emergency nursing actions are initiated.
TEST-TAKING TIP: Identify the word in the stem that sets a priority. The word *first* in the stem sets a priority. Identify the clang association. The word *feeding* in the stem and option 2 is a clang association.
Content Area: Nutrition
Integrated Processes: Nursing Process: Implementation
Client Need: Physiological Integrity; Basic Care and Comfort
Cognitive Level: Application

5. ANSWER: 1, 4, 5.
Rationales:
1. Using tubing with an in-line filter is necessary due to the high glucose concentration of parenteral nutrition solutions.
2. Vital signs should be monitored every 4 hours for signs of infection or sepsis.
3. Blood glucose should be monitored every 6 hours.
4. A weight gain of more than 3 lb weekly indicates fluid retention, which should be addressed.
5. A 5 to 10 percent dextrose solution should be administered when parenteral nutrition is interrupted to prevent hypoglycemia.
TEST-TAKING TIP: Identify the word in the stem that sets a priority. The word *essential* in the stem sets a priority. The question is asking, "What *must* be done when administering parenteral nutrition?"
Content Area: Nutrition
Integrated Processes: Nursing Process: Implementation
Client Need: Physiological Integrity; Pharmacological and Parenteral Therapies
Cognitive Level: Analysis

6. **ANSWER: 1.**
   Rationales:
   1. **Hyperperistalsis occurs when food rapidly enters the intestine and water moves from the bowel wall into the intestinal lumen, causing osmotic diarrhea.**
   2. Tachycardia, not bradycardia, occurs in response to dumping syndrome.
   3. Dyspnea is not associated with dumping syndrome.
   4. Hypoxia is not associated with dumping syndrome.
   TEST-TAKING TIP: Identify the equally plausible options. Options 3 and 4 are equally plausible. Both are concerned with impaired respirations. Neither option is better than the other. Eliminate options 3 and 4 from further consideration.
   Content Area: Nutrition
   Integrated Processes: Nursing Process: Evaluation
   Client Need: Physiological Integrity; Basic Care and Comfort
   Cognitive Level: Application

7. **ANSWER: 6, 4, 2, 5, 1, 3.**
   Rationales:
   6. Checking the code number on the strip and the monitor ensures that the blood glucose monitoring machine is calibrated accurately.
   4. Holding the finger dependent and in warm water increases circulation and dilation of blood vessels at the intended puncture site.
   2. Alcohol cleanses and limits the number of microorganisms at the puncture site limiting the risk of infection. Drying prevents the alcohol from inactivating the substance on the test strip that measures the level of glucose.
   5. Holding the lanced perpendicular to the patient's finger facilitates skin penetration.
   1. Wiping away the first drop of blood reduces the risk of using blood that may be contaminated with a cleaning product, which can alter test results.
   3. Gently placing a droplet of blood on the end of the test strip avoids smearing blood on the test strip which may contribute to an inaccurate test result.
   Content Area: Nutrition
   Integrated Processes: Nursing Process: Planning
   Client Need: Physiological Integrity; Reduction of Risk Potential
   Cognitive Level: Analysis

8. **ANSWER: 2.**
   Rationales:
   1. Although a decreased albumin level is an effective indicator of protein depletion, it is not the first laboratory value to change with protein depletion because its half-life is 21 days.
   2. **A transferrin level is an effective indicator of acute protein depletion because its half-life is only 8 days.**
   3. This is not the best test to assess a patient's nutrition level. Although a blood urea nitrogen level reflects an inadequate intake of dietary protein or malabsorption, it is more often monitored to assess the balance of urea production and excretion.
   4. This is not the best test to assess nutrition level. Although a decreased level may indicate a decreased nutritional intake or malnutrition, it is more often monitored to assess a patient's immune system.

   TEST-TAKING TIP: Identify the word in the stem that sets a priority. The word *best* in the stem sets a priority.
   Content Area: Nutrition
   Integrated Processes: Nursing Process: Assessment
   Client Need: Physiological Integrity; Reduction of Risk Potential
   Cognitive Level: Analysis

9. **ANSWER: 1, 2, 4.**
   Rationales:
   1. **Small, frequent meals are less likely to overwhelm (e.g., physically and visually) a patient than large meals.**
   2. **Oral care cleanses the mouth of debris and odors that can interfere with one's desire to eat.**
   3. Procedures should not be scheduled just after meals because this may cause nausea and vomiting. Procedures just before a meal may inhibit appetite. Procedures should be scheduled as far from meals as possible.
   4. **Adequate pain control will support comfort, which may enhance appetite.**
   5. The patient has an order for bedrest and should not be transferred to a chair for meals.
   Content Area: Nutrition
   Integrated Processes: Nursing Process: Planning
   Client Need: Physiological Integrity; Basic Care and Comfort
   Cognitive Level: Application

10. **ANSWER: 4.**
    Rationales:
    1. Although chewing food thoroughly helps with the digestion of food, it does not help prevent gastroesophageal reflux.
    2. Serving food with different textures and aromas addresses the needs of a patient who has a decrease in the senses of smell and taste; it does not help prevent gastroesophageal reflux.
    3. Fluids with meals will overdistend the stomach, which will increase the risk of gastroesophageal reflux.
    4. **Gastroesophageal reflux is less likely to occur if the stomach is empty when a person is in the supine position, such as when sleeping.**
    TEST-TAKING TIP: Identify the unique option. Option 4 is unique. It is the only option that does not contain the word *food*.
    Content Area: Nutrition
    Integrated Processes: Nursing Process: Implementation
    Client Need: Physiological Integrity; Basic Care and Comfort
    Cognitive Level: Application

11. **ANSWER: 3, 4.**
    Rationales:
    1. A hematocrit level of 42 percent is within the expected range of 40 to 50 percent; a decrease in the hematocrit level indicates anemia.
    2. A hemoglobin level of 14 g/dL is within the expected range of 12 to 16 g/dL for women and 14 to 18 g/dL for men; a decrease in the hemoglobin level indicates anemia.

3. A transferrin level of 190 mg/dL is below the expected range of 215 to 380 mg/dL; a decrease in the transferrin level indicates anemia and protein deficiency.

4. A serum albumin level of 2.9 g/dL is below the expected range of 3.3 to 5 g/dL; a decrease in the albumin level indicates malnutrition or malabsorption.

5. A blood urea nitrogen level of 18 mg/dL is within the expected range of 8 to 21 mg/dL; an increase in blood urea nitrogen level indicates starvation, diarrhea, or a high-protein intake.

Content Area: Nutrition
Integrated Processes: Nursing Process: Analysis
Client Need: Physiological Integrity; Reduction of Risk Potential
Cognitive Level: Analysis

12. **ANSWER: 3.**
    Rationales:
    1. White rice is gluten free.
    2. Steamed eggplant is gluten free.
    3. A veal cutlet is breaded and then fried when preparing veal cutlet parmesan; bread crumbs are made from wheat flour, which contains gluten. Malabsorption occurs in response to the sensitivity to the presence of the gliadin fraction of gluten.
    4. Fruit thickened with tapioca is gluten free.
    TEST-TAKING TIP: Identify the word in the stem that indicates negative polarity. The word *avoid* in the stem indicates negative polarity. This question is asking, "What should the nurse teach the patient *not to eat.*"
    Content Area: Nutrition
    Integrated Processes: Teaching/Learning; Nursing Process: Implementation
    Client Need: Physiological Integrity; Basic Care and Comfort
    Cognitive Level: Analysis

13. **ANSWER: 1, 4.**
    Rationales:
    1. Eggs and beans are less expensive than meat; teach the patient that rice with beans is a complete protein.
    2. Luncheon meats should be avoided because they are expensive and less healthy because of their high sodium levels and the presence of nitrites in cured and smoked meat.
    3. Powdered milk is less expensive than fresh milk.
    4. By reading the nutrition facts label on prepared foods, the patient can ensure the most nutrition for the cost.
    5. Frozen meals should be avoided altogether because they are more expensive than food prepared at home and, generally, they are high in sodium and fat.
    Content Area: Nutrition
    Integrated Processes: Teaching/Learning; Nursing Process: Implementation
    Client Need: Health Promotion and Maintenance
    Cognitive Level: Application

14. **ANSWER: 3.**
    Rationales:
    1. Yogurt is a milk product that contains lactose, which should be avoided.

2. Sherbet is made with milk and milk contains lactose, which should be avoided.

3. Fruit salad is a healthy choice from the menu because fruit does not contain lactose.

4. Rice pudding is made with milk and milk contains lactose, which should be avoided.

Content Area: Nutrition
Integrated Processes: Teaching/Learning; Nursing Process: Evaluation
Client Need: Physiological Integrity; Basic Care and Comfort
Cognitive Level: Analysis

15. **ANSWER: 1, 2.**
    Rationales:
    1. Nutrient-dense foods have a higher nutrient to calorie ratio. A nutrient-dense food provides the most nutrients for the fewest number of calories.
    2. Protein is essential for building and repairing body tissue, regulating body functions, and providing energy when fats and carbohydrates are insufficient. Because of a decreased sense of taste, older adults often prefer concentrated sweets. Once sweets are ingested, older adults no longer feel hungry enough to eat essential nutrients.
    3. Prepared frozen meals should be avoided because they are high in sodium and fat.
    4. Four smaller meals a day may increase caloric intake because one is less overwhelmed and more likely to finish the meal. However, the fourth meal should be no closer than 2 to 3 hours before bedtime; this will reduce the risk of gastroesophageal reflux, which is common with older adults.
    5. Bullion powder is high in sodium and should be avoided. People should be encouraged to use lemon juice, vinegar, herbs, or spices free from sodium to flavor food.
    Content Area: Nutrition
    Integrated Processes: Teaching/Learning; Nursing Process: Implementation
    Client Need: Health Promotion and Maintenance
    Cognitive Level: Application

16. **ANSWER: 2.**
    Rationales:
    1. The opposite is encouraged. Vegetable oils with mono-saturated fatty acids should replace vegetable oils with polyunsaturated fatty acids.
    2. These nontherapeutic side effects, especially if accompanied by fever or malaise, indicate myopathy requiring immediate discontinuation of the medication.
    3. Lipitor is not enteric coated or a time-release capsule; it can be crushed and mixed with applesauce if necessary.
    4. Lipitor can be taken any time of day and can be taken with or without food.
    Content Area: Nutrition
    Integrated Processes: Teaching/Learning; Nursing Process: Planning
    Client Need: Physiological Integrity; Pharmacological and Parenteral Therapies
    Cognitive Level: Application

17. ANSWER: 2, 3, 4.

Rationales:

1. Lentils and tofu are both legumes; legumes must be pared with a grain, nuts, or seeds to make a complete protein.

2. When cereal, which is made from a grain, and milk are served together, they make a complete protein.

3. When macaroni, which is made from a grain, and cheese, which is a milk product, are served together, they make a complete protein.

4. When black-eyed peas, which are a legume, and rice, which is a grain, are served together, they make a complete protein.

5. Black and red beans are both legumes; legumes must be pared with a grain, nuts, or seeds to make a complete protein.

Content Area: Nutrition

Integrated Processes: Teaching/Learning; Nursing Process: Implementation

Client Need: Health Promotion and Maintenance

Cognitive Level: Analysis

18. ANSWER: 4.

Rationales:

1. Salt substitutes are not free from salt; they should be used sparingly because they generally contain half as much salt as regular salt. In addition, large amounts of salt substitutes generally taste bitter rather than salty.

2. Two teaspoons of salt contain 4,000 mg (4 g) of sodium; this exceeds the 2-g sodium diet prescribed by the patient's primary health-care provider.

3. Soda sweetened with aspartame generally has 50 percent more sodium than nonartificially sweetened soda.

4. Patients must learn how to read and interpret nutrition facts labels on prepared foods to ensure that they do not exceed 2,000 mg (2 g) of sodium daily when on a 2-g sodium diet.

TEST-TAKING TIP: Identify the option with a clang association. The word *sodium* in the stem and in option 4 is a clang association.

Content Area: Nutrition

Integrated Processes: Teaching/Learning; Nursing Process: Evaluation

Client Need: Physiological Integrity; Basic Care and Comfort

Cognitive Level: Application

19. ANSWER: 1.

Rationales:

1. Identifying the serving size is critical to determining how many calories are contained in the entire package. This label indicates that there are 4 servings in the product and each serving is 90 calories. When patients ingest the entire product, thinking that they are eating only 90 calories, they are actually ingesting 360 calories.

2. Although it is important to identify the number of calories that are from fat, if patients are unable to identify the serving size and they eat the entire contents in the package, they will be ingesting significantly more fat than they realize. In this instance, 4 servings are in the package, so the total number of fat calories is 120 out of a total of 360 calories if the contents of the entire package are ingested.

3. Although it is important to identify the total grams of fat indicated on the label, if patients are unable to identify the serving size, they could be ingesting significantly more fat than they realize when they eat all of the contents in the package. In this instance, 4 serving are in the package. If the whole bag of snack food is ingested, the total fat intake is 12 g, not just 3 g as indicated on the label.

4. It is important to know how much sodium is indicated on the label because patients who are obese often experience hypertension and are receiving a 2-g sodium diet as well as a calorie-restricted diet. However, it is more important to know how many servings are in a package so that a person can determine how much of the product can be ingested. If the patient ingested the entire package, the patient would take in not just 300 mg of sodium but 1,200 mg of sodium.

TEST-TAKING TIP: Identify the word in the stem that sets a priority. The word *most* in the stem sets a priority.

Content Area: Nutrition

Integrated Processes: Teaching/Learning; Nursing Process: Implementation

Client Need: Physiological Integrity; Basic Care and Comfort

Cognitive Level: Analysis

20. ANSWER: 2.

Rationales:

1. Curry, which is not salty, is very popular in Indian recipes and should not pose a problem with a sodium-restricted diet.

2. Soy sauce, which is very salty, is widely used to season food preferred by people with a Chinese heritage. This may present a problem adjusting to a sodium-restricted diet.

3. People with Puerto Rican heritage often prefer such foods as rice and vegetables, which generally are not seasoned with excessive amounts of salt.

4. People with Middle Eastern heritage usually do not season their food with excessive amounts of salt. Grains, wheat, rice, and chickpeas in the form of hummus are popular.

TEST-TAKING TIP: Identify the word in the stem that sets a priority. The word *most* in the stem sets a priority.

Content Area: Nutrition

Integrated Processes: Teaching/Learning; Nursing Process: Assessment

Client Need: Health Promotion and Maintenance

Cognitive Level: Analysis

21. ANSWER: 5, 3, 1, 2, 4.

Rationales:

5. A PPN formula should not exceed 20 percent dextrose. Dextrose at 50 percent is too high a percentage for dilution by peripheral blood flow.

3. A 20 percent dextrose solution prevents rebound hypoglycemia and follows the primary health-care provider's order for the solution to be hung if the PPN is interrupted.

1. Cover the elevated glucose level with insulin will cause the glucose level to decrease. The objective is to maintain the patient's blood glucose level below 110 mg/dL.

2. The dextrose should be no more than 20 percent when administered in a PPN solution. A dextrose of

10 to 70 percent is permitted when total parenteral nutrition is provided via a central line.

4. Contacting the IV nurse who is an expert regarding IV intervention ensures evaluation of the site. The site may need to be changed given the presence of erythema.

Content Area: Nutrition
Integrated Processes: Nursing Process: Planning
Client Need: Physiological Integrity; Pharmacological and Parenteral Therapies
Cognitive Level: Analysis

22. **ANSWER: 1.**
Rationales:
1. Fat emulsions should be administered slowly over the first 30 minutes to provide time for adjustment to the higher glucose level and allow for observation of an allergic or adverse reaction (e.g., chills, fever, flushing, dyspnea, nausea, and vomiting). If a reaction occurs, the nurse should terminate the infusion and notify the primary health-care provider immediately.
2. Fat emulsions should be administered at room temperature to prevent pain, venous spasms, and hypothermia. It takes approximately 1 hour for the solution to warm to room temperature after removal from a refrigerator.
3. This lipid solution should be discarded. Separation of the emulsion into layers, presence of fat globules, froth, or cloudy solution indicates contamination of the solution and should not be administered.
4. The tubing of the lipid solution infusion set should be inserted into the total parenteral nutrition tubing below the filter because lipid solutions have an increased viscosity that will become trapped in the filter, obstructing the flow of the solution.

Content Area: Nutrition
Integrated Processes: Nursing Process: Implementation
Client Need: Physiological Integrity; Pharmacological and Parenteral Therapies
Cognitive Level: Application

23. **ANSWER: 3, 5.**
Rationales:
1. Three ounces of tuna fish contains 17 mg of calcium; it is not a generous source of calcium.
2. One cup of prune juice contains 700 mg of potassium and only 30 mg of calcium; it is not an adequate source of calcium.
3. One cup of whole milk contains 290 mg of calcium and should be encouraged when a patient is receiving a high-calcium diet.
4. One cup of pinto beans contains approximately 882 mg of potassium and only 86 mg of calcium; they are an excellent source of potassium, not calcium.
5. A broccoli spear contains approximately 205 mg of calcium and should be encouraged when a patient is receiving a high-calcium diet.

Content Area: Nutrition
Integrated Processes: Teaching/Learning; Nursing Process: Implementation
Client Need: Physiological Integrity; Basic Care and Comfort
Cognitive Level: Application

24. **ANSWER: 3.**
Rationales:
1. A patient should never increase the dose or frequency of any medication without being instructed to do so by the primary health-care provider. If the patient is experiencing physical or emotional stress, the patient's pattern of serum glucose levels must be analyzed by the primary health-care provider. Increasing Glucophage alone may not control the patient's glucose level. The patient may need to receive subcutaneously administered insulin temporarily until the stress and glucose levels subside.
2. Orange juice contains sugar and is ingested when a person has hypoglycemia, not hyperglycemia. Ingesting orange juice when experiencing hyperglycemia will cause the glucose level to increase even higher.
3. These responses indicate lactic acidosis, a serious nontherapeutic response to Glucophage, requiring its discontinuation. The risk of lactic acidosis increases with severe infection, dehydration, or severe or continuing diarrhea. Additional clinical indicators of lactic acidosis include chills, diarrhea, bradycardia, low blood pressure, dyspnea, and weakness. The patient should notify the primary health-care provider immediately if any of these signs or symptoms occur.
4. It is never acceptable to double a dose of Glucophage. If a dose is missed it can be taken as long as it is not almost time for the next dose. A double dose can precipitate hypoglycemia.

Content Area: Nutrition
Integrated Processes: Teaching/Learning; Nursing Process: Implementation
Client Need: Physiological Integrity; Pharmacological and Parenteral Therapies
Cognitive Level: Application

25. **ANSWER: 1, 4, 5.**
Rationales:
1. One large egg contains approximately 275 mg of cholesterol and should be avoided when receiving a low-cholesterol diet.
2. One stalk of celery contains approximately 5 mg of cholesterol; celery is permitted on a low-cholesterol diet.
3. Four spears of asparagus contain approximately 3 mg of cholesterol; asparagus is permitted on a low-cholesterol diet.
4. Three ounces of calves liver contains 410 mg of cholesterol and should be avoided when receiving a low-cholesterol diet.
5. One cup of baked custard contains approximately 280 mg of cholesterol and should be avoided when receiving a low-cholesterol diet.
TEST-TAKING TIP: Identify the word in the stem that indicates negative polarity. The word *avoid* in the stem indicates negative polarity.

Content Area: Nutrition
Integrated Processes: Teaching/Learning; Nursing Process: Implementation
Client Need: Physiological Integrity; Basic Care and Comfort
Cognitive Level: Application

26. ANSWER: 3.

Rationales:

1. Food intake should be documented in the percentage of food ingested. The words poor, good, and excellent are relative and subjective.

2. Although asking the patient for preferences is important, it is not the priority of the options presented.

3. This action reduces the risk of food entering the airway. Food pocketed between the gum and cheek increases the risk of aspiration and is the priority of the options presented. A person who is weak and lethargic may have difficulty chewing and swallowing, which increases the risk of pocketing food.

4. Generally, the nurse should encourage a patient to participate in feeding him- or herself; however, in this situation, the patient is weak and lethargic. Feeding the patient helps the patient to conserve energy for chewing, swallowing, and breathing.

TEST-TAKING TIP: Identify the word in the stem that sets a priority. The word *most* in the stem sets a priority.

Content Area: Nutrition

Integrated Processes: Nursing Process: Implementation

Client Need: Physiological Integrity; Safe and Effective Care Environment

Cognitive Level: Application

27. ANSWER: 2, 3, 4.

Rationales:

1. Summer squash is a low carbohydrate food and, therefore, is less likely to produce as much intestinal gas as other vegetables that are high in sugar, starch, or fiber.

2. A person chewing gum will swallow more frequently than when not chewing gum. Swallowed air will increase air in the gastrointestinal tract causing abdominal discomfort.

3. Onions contain fructose, which is a monosaccharide. When not totally digested by the intestinal enzymes sucrase, lactase, and maltase, monosaccharides are acted upon by harmless intestinal bacteria, with gas being a by-product of this bacterial fermentation.

4. Lentils, dried beans, and peas contain carbohydrates that are difficult to digest but are digested by harmless bacteria in the intestine. The harmless bacteria produce hydrogen, carbon dioxide and, in some people, methane, all of which exit the body as flatulence.

5. Eggs are a nongassy protein.

TEST-TAKING TIP: Identify the word in the stem that indicates negative polarity. The word *avoid* in the stem indicates negative polarity.

Content Area: Nutrition

Integrated Processes: Teaching/Learning; Nursing Process: Implementation

Client Need: Physiological Integrity; Basic Care and Comfort

Cognitive Level: Application

28. ANSWER: 4.

Rationales:

1. Milk is a simple sugar, not a complex carbohydrate. A simple sugar contains a single sugar (saccharide) unit called a *monosaccharide*.

2. Nuts are incomplete proteins, not a complex carbohydrate. Incomplete proteins are nutrients that do not include all the essential amino acids required for protein synthesis. A complete protein can be made by combining two incomplete proteins, such as red beans and brown rice or peanut butter with whole-grain bread.

3. Eggs are a complete protein, not a complex carbohydrate. A complete protein is a nutrient that includes all of the essential amino acids required for protein synthesis; additional nutrients that are complete proteins include cheese and milk.

4. Pasta is a complex carbohydrate. Complex carbohydrates consist of long chains of saccharides called polysaccharides. Additional nutrients that are complex carbohydrates include breads, cereals, grains, legumes, and vegetables.

TEST-TAKING TIP: Identify the word in the stem that indicates negative polarity. The word *limit* in the stem indicates negative polarity.

Content Area: Nutrition

Integrated Processes: Teaching/Learning; Nursing Process: Implementation

Client Need: Physiological Integrity; Basic Care and Comfort

Cognitive Level: Application

29. ANSWER: 2.

Rationales:

1. Citrus fruits, such as oranges, grapefruits, and lemons, and green peppers, broccoli, apricot nectar, strawberries, and tomatoes provide vitamin C, not protein foods.

2. Trans fat is a saturated fat that increases the LDH (low-density lipoprotein) level and should be avoided in a healthy diet.

3. Nonessential amino acids can be synthesized by the body and do not need to be obtained from food or supplements.

4. MyPlate guidelines recommend that 30 percent, not 20 percent, of the food a person ingests daily should contain grains. Half of those grains should be whole grains.

TEST-TAKING TIP: Identify the unique option. Option 2 is unique. It is the only option that discusses a nutrient that should be minimized.

Content Area: Nutrition

Integrated Processes: Teaching/Learning; Nursing Process: Evaluation

Client Need: Health Promotion and Maintenance

Cognitive Level: Analysis

30. ANSWER: 162.

Rationale:

Each gram of fat contains 9 kilocalories, each gram of carbohydrate contains 4 kilocalories, and each gram of protein contains 4 kilocalories. Nine kilocalories multiplied by 10 g of fat equals 90 kilocalories, 4 kilocalories multiplied by 16 g of carbohydrates equals 64 kilocalories, and 4 kilocalories multiplied by 2 g of protein equals 8 kilocalories for a grand total of 162 kilocalories.

Content Area: Nutrition

Integrated Processes: Teaching/Learning; Nursing Process: Evaluation

Client Need: Physiological Integrity; Basic Care and Comfort

Cognitive Level: Analysis

31. ANSWER: 2.

Rationales:

1. Nuts are an excellent source of vitamin E, not D. Also, nuts are rich in vitamin B_6, thiamine, and niacin.

2. Eggs are an excellent source of vitamin D and are also rich in vitamin A, vitamin B_{12}, pantothenic acid, biotin, riboflavin, and folic acid.

3. Liver is an excellent source of vitamin K, not vitamin D. Also, liver is rich in vitamin A, folic acid, niacin, biotin, pantothenic acid, riboflavin, and thiamine.

4. Oranges are an excellent source of vitamin C, not D. Also, oranges are rich in folic acid.

Content Area: Nutrition

Integrated Processes: Nursing Process: Evaluation

Client Need: Physiological Integrity; Basic Care and Comfort

Cognitive Level: Analysis

32. ANSWER: 4.

Rationales:

1. Omeprazole (Prilosec) can be taken concurrently with an antacid; no drug-to-drug interaction occurs that interferes with absorption of the medication. Ranitidine (Zantac) should be taken 1 to 2 hours before or after an antacid.

2. A capsule of omeprazole (Prilosec) should not be opened, crushed, or chewed. The pellets in the capsule are designed for delayed absorption.

3. Omeprazole (Prilosec) should be given before food is eaten, preferably breakfast.

4. A capsule of omeprazole (Prilosec) should be swallowed whole and should not be opened, crushed, or chewed. The pellets in the capsule are designed for delayed absorption.

TEST-TAKING TIP: Identify the options that are opposites. Options 2 and 4 are opposites. Examine these options carefully because often times one of the options that is an opposite is the correct answer.

Content Area: Nutrition

Integrated Processes: Communication/Documentation; Teaching/Learning; Nursing Process: Implementation

Client Need: Physiological Integrity; Pharmacological and Parenteral Therapies

Cognitive Level: Application

33. ANSWER: 93.5.

Rationale:

Each gram of fat contains 9 kilocalories, each gram of carbohydrate contains 4 kilocalories, and each gram of protein contains 4 kilocalories. Nine kilocalories multiplied by 1.5 g of fat equals 13.5 kilocalories, 4 kilocalories multiplied by 19 g of carbohydrates equals 76 kilocalories, and 4 kilocalories multiplied by 1 g of protein equals 4 kilocalories for a grand total of 93.5 kilocalories.

Content Area: Nutrition

Integrated Processes: Teaching/Learning; Nursing Process: Evaluation

Client Need: Physiological Integrity; Basic Care and Comfort

Cognitive Level: Analysis

34. ANSWER: 3.

Rationales:

1. Grits are a food product made with refined grains. The milling process eliminates the bran and germ to make a finer texture; it also removes fiber, iron, and many B vitamins.

2. Noodles are made with refined grains. The milling process eliminates the bran and germ to make a finer texture; it also removes fiber, iron, and many B vitamins.

3. Wild rice is a whole-grain food product because it is made from the entire grain kernel.

4. Cornbread is made with refined grains. The milling process eliminates the bran and germ to make a finer texture; it also removes fiber, iron, and many B vitamins.

Content Area: Nutrition

Integrated Processes: Teaching/Learning; Nursing Process: Evaluation

Client Need: Health Promotion and Maintenance

Cognitive Level: Analysis

35. ANSWER: 1, 5.

Rationales:

1. It is recommended that 8 glasses of fluid should be ingested daily. Water is essential because it is a component of circulating blood, is a basic solvent for the body's chemical processes, and helps maintain body temperature.

2. Foods high in solid fats should be reduced, not increased, in a daily diet because they may contribute to atherosclerosis.

3. Fruits should be 25 percent of your plate and vegetables should be another 25 percent of your plate for a total of 50 percent of your plate daily. Fruits and vegetables provide essential nutrients for cellular growth and fiber for intestinal motility.

4. Cream cheese, butter, and cream are not included in the dairy circle because they contain too little calcium.

5. Two servings of seafood rich in omega-fatty acids should be included in the diet weekly. Omega-fatty acids help limit triglycerides, inflammation, hypertension, and cardiovascular and autoimmune diseases.

Content Area: Nutrition

Integrated Processes: Teaching/Learning; Nursing Process: Planning

Client Need: Health Promotion and Maintenance

Cognitive Level: Application

Chapter 19

Oxygenation

KEY TERMS

Accessory muscles of respiration—Use of intercostal, abdominal, and trapezius muscles to help expand the chest cavity.

Aspiration—Breathing foreign matter into the lungs.

Barrel chest—Increase in anteroposterior diameter of the thoracic cavity.

Clubbing—Bulbous swelling of the soft tissue of the end of the phalanx of fingers, causing the nail plates to be equal to or greater than 180°.

Cor pulmonale—Right-sided heart failure.

Diaphragmatic (abdominal) breathing—Expansion of the abdomen on deep inhalation and tightening of the abdominal muscles on exhalation, increasing the amount of air entering and exiting the lungs.

Dyspnea—Difficulty breathing.

Exertional dyspnea—Difficulty breathing with activity.

Expectoration—Coughing up and spitting out of sputum.

Expiratory reserve volume—Maximum amount of air that can be exhaled after exhalation of the tidal volume.

External respiration—Gas exchange at the alveolar-capillary junction.

Exertional dyspnea—Difficulty breathing with activity.

Hypercarbia (hypercapnia)—Increased level of carbon dioxide in the blood.

Hypocarbia (hypocapnia)—Decreased level of carbon dioxide in the blood.

Hypoxemia—Decreased level of oxygen in the blood.

Hypoxia—Inadequate oxygen in organs and tissues.

Inspiratory reserve volume—Maximum amount of air that can be inhaled beyond the tidal volume.

Incentive spirometer—Device that provides a visual goal to increase the volume of breaths.

Internal respiration—Gas exchange at the capillary-tissue junction.

Nasal flaring—Widening of nares during inhalation that reduces resistance to airflow.

Nebulizer—Device with a mouthpiece or mask placed over the nose that produces a medicated aerosol spray that is inhaled.

Orthopnea—Difficulty breathing in the supine position, necessitating an upright position to breathe.

Orthopneic (tripod) position—Forward leaning position utilized while sitting to facilitate breathing.

Oximetry—Identification of the oxygen saturation of arterial blood.

Paroxysmal nocturnal dyspnea—Extreme shortness of breath during sleep that causes an abrupt awakening and immediate need to assume the upright position for relief.

Pneumothorax—Air or gas in the pleural cavity.

Postural drainage—Sequential positioning of a patient in a variety of positions that use gravity to drain secretions from lobes of the lungs.

Preoxygenate—Administration of oxygen before a procedure.

Pursed-lip breathing—Exhalation through the mouth with lips creating a small opening to prolong exhalation, which keeps alveoli open longer for gas exchange.

Residual volume—Amount of air remaining in the lungs after forceful exhalation.

Retractions—Recession of intercostal, supraclavicular, and subcostal tissues during inspiration because of excessive negative pressure required to increase depth of respirations.

Sleep apnea—Transient, brief absences of breathing during sleep.

Sputum—Mucus secretions from the respiratory tract.

Stridor—High-pitched sound heard on inhalation with acute laryngeal obstruction.

Subcutaneous emphysema—Air in tissue beneath the layers of the skin.

Tactile fremitus—Vibration felt on the palmar surface of the hands when the patient vocalizes "99" repeatedly.

Tidal volume—Amount of air moving in and out of the lungs with a normal breath.

Total lung capacity—A combination of the inspiratory capacity and the functional residual capacity.

Vital capacity—Amount of air that is forcefully exhaled after forcefully inhaling with the deepest inspiratory effort possible.

Wheeze—Musical, whistling sound caused when air flows through narrowed airways.

I. The Respiratory System

The exchange of oxygen and carbon dioxide in the body is essential for life. This exchange takes place in the lungs and at the cellular level. The mechanisms of respiration are complex and require an integration of factors involving the nervous system, chemoreceptors in the cardiovascular system, as well as the respiratory system. Knowledge of the anatomy and physiology that influences breathing is the basis for understanding how to best care for patients with oxygenation problems.

A. Structures of the Respiratory System (Fig. 19.1)
1. Airways.
   a. Consist of **upper airways** (located above the larynx; include nasal passages, oral cavity, and pharynx) and **lower airways** (located below the larynx; include trachea, bronchi, and bronchioles).
   b. Humidify the air: Moist mucous membranes add water to the inhaled air.
   c. Warm the air: Heat is transferred from the blood circulating in the capillary beds of the airways to the inhaled air.
   d. Filter the air: Sticky mucus traps debris, and tiny hair-like projections from the walls of the airway (cilia) move debris up and out of the airway.
2. Lungs.
   a. Soft, spongy, cone-shaped organs.
   b. Right lung has three lobes, and left lung has two lobes.
   c. Each lung extends from its top portion (apex), which is just above the clavicle, to its bottom portion (base), which rests on the diaphragm.
   d. Composed of tiny, thin-walled air sacks (**alveoli**) surrounded by an extensive network of capillaries.
   e. Alveoli consist of type I cells that are involved with gas exchange and type II cells that produce a lipoprotein that lowers the surface tension to facilitate alveoli inflation.

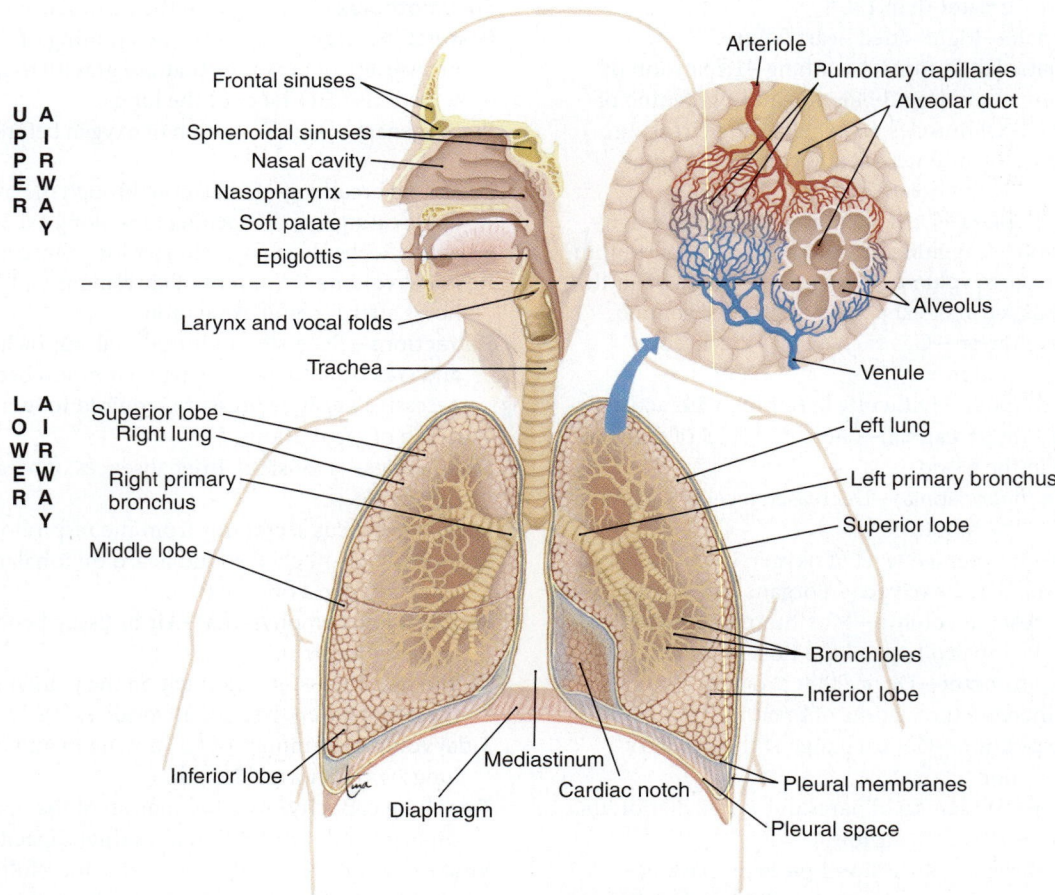

Fig 19.1 Anterior view of the respiratory system. The upper airway lies above the larynx. The lower airway, located below the larynx, is considered sterile. (From Wilkinson and Treas [2011]. *Fundamentals of nursing,* Vol. 1, 2nd ed. Philadelphia: F. A. Davis, with permission.)

B. **Functions of the Respiratory System**
1. Ventilation.
   a. Movement of air into and out of the lungs through the process of breathing.
   b. Involves inhalation and exhalation.
      (1) **Inhalation:** Expansion of the chest cavity and lungs resulting from contraction of the diaphragm that pulls the chest cavity downward and contraction of the intercostal muscles that pulls the ribs outward; lung expansion causes negative pressure that draws air into the respiratory system.
      (2) **Exhalation:** Chest cavity and lungs return to their original size and position when the diaphragm and intercostal muscles relax; this is a passive response that requires no effort.
   c. Factors that affect adequacy of ventilation.
      (1) Respiratory rate and depth: Fast, deep respirations result in hyperventilation; slow, shallow respirations result in hypoventilation.
      (2) Lung compliance: Extent of effort to inflate the lungs; conditions such as pulmonary edema and inadequate surfactant cause reduced lung compliance.
      (3) Airway resistance: Impairment of airflow within the airways; conditions that reduce the diameter of the airways, such as excess respiratory secretions and bronchospasms, cause increased airway resistance.
      (4) Lung elasticity: Ability of elastin fibers to return to their original position during exhalation; conditions that overstretch the alveoli, such as emphysema, result in a reduction of elastic recoil, leaving excess air trapped in the alveoli at the end of exhalation.
2. Respiration.
   a. Exchange of gases that provides oxygenation of blood and body tissues and elimination of carbon dioxide from the lungs.
   b. Occurs at two levels, known as *external* and *internal respiration* (Fig. 19.2).
      (1) **External respiration.**
         (a) Involves alveolar-capillary gas exchange.
         (b) Oxygen diffuses from the alveoli, through the alveolar capillaries, and into the blood.
         (c) Carbon dioxide diffuses out of the blood, through the alveolar capillaries, and into the alveoli.
         (d) Rate of diffusion depends on the thickness of the membranes and extent of lung tissue.
         (e) Conditions that impair external respiration include pleural effusion, pneumothorax, bronchospasm, and excessive secretions.

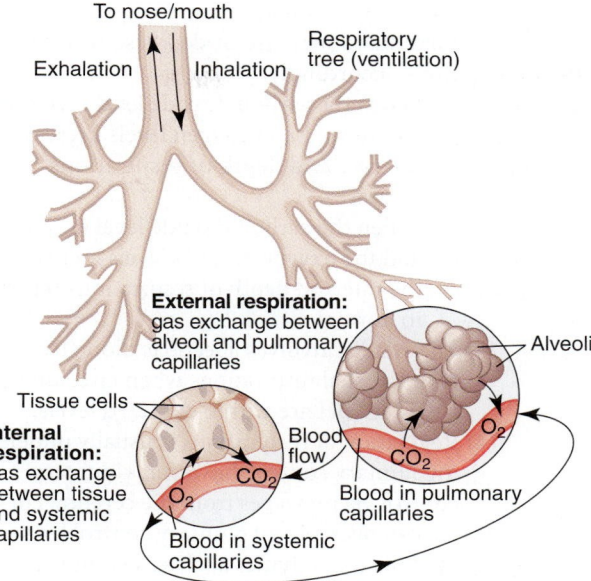

Fig 19.2 External and internal respiration. (From Wilkinson and Treas [2011]. *Fundamentals of nursing,* Vol. 1, 2nd ed. Philadelphia: F. A. Davis, with permission.)

      (2) **Internal respiration.**
         (a) Involves capillary-tissue gas exchange.
         (b) Oxygen diffuses from the blood, through the peripheral capillaries, and into tissue cells; oxygen is used for cellular metabolism.
         (c) Carbon dioxide, which is a waste product of cellular metabolism, diffuses from tissue cells, through the peripheral capillaries, and is transported via the blood to the lungs for exhalation.
         (d) The effectiveness of internal respiration depends on adequate peripheral circulation and external respiration.
         (e) Conditions that impair internal respiration include peripheral arterial and venous occlusive diseases; decreased cardiac output; impaired oxygen-carrying capacity of the blood, such as in anemia; and conditions that increase metabolism, such as fever, cancer, and hyperthyroidism.
   c. Regulated by various mechanisms.
      (1) The respiratory center, located in the medulla oblongata in the brainstem, sends impulses to the phrenic nerve, which precipitate contraction of the muscles of the diaphragm and intercostal muscles.
      (2) Chemoreceptors in the medulla, carotid arteries, and aorta identify changes in the level of circulating carbon dioxide, pH,

and oxygen and send a message to the medulla to increase or decrease respirations accordingly.

(a) When the carbon dioxide level increases and the pH and oxygen levels decrease, the rate and depth of respirations increase.

(b) When the carbon dioxide level decreases and the oxygen and pH levels increase, the rate and depth of respirations return to normal.

(3) The system involves a feedback loop to return to usual respirations when circulating gases and pH are within expected levels.

(4) Regulation of respirations is usually under involuntary control; however, voluntary control via messages from the cerebral cortex can override involuntary control by the medulla for activities such as swimming, talking, swallowing, and whistling.

d. Can be disturbed by problems that affect gas exchange.

(1) **Hypoxemia:** Decreased level of oxygen in the blood due to ineffective external respiration related to lung or pulmonary circulation problems.

(2) **Hypoxia:** Inadequate oxygen in organs and tissues due to hypoxemia or circulatory disorders.

(a) Early clinical indicators: Restlessness, irritability, anxiety, tachypnea, tachycardia, headache, disorientation, and decreased level of consciousness.

(b) Late clinical indicators: Retractions, bradypnea, bradycardia, cardiac dysrhythmias, and cyanosis.

(3) **Hypercarbia (hypercapnia):** Increased level of carbon dioxide in the blood; may be due to an acute problem, such as airway obstruction or drug overdose, or associated with chronic lung diseases.

(4) **Hypocarbia (hypocapnia):** Decreased level of carbon dioxide in the blood due to hyperventilation.

(5) Infections: Conditions include upper respiratory infections, such as colds; conditions that affect the lower respiratory tract, such as bronchitis, pneumonia, and tuberculosis; and conditions that can involve both the upper and lower respiratory tracts, such as influenza.

(6) Conditions that impede inhalation: Includes such conditions as fractured ribs, kyphosis, laryngospasm, and food/foreign body obstruction.

(7) Alveolar-capillary membrane problems: Includes conditions that interfere with the exchange of gases within the alveoli, such as pulmonary edema, emphysema, and pulmonary fibrosis.

(8) Inadequate lung surface for gas exchange: Includes such conditions as alveolar collapse, incomplete expansion of the lung (**atelectasis**), pleural effusion, and pneumothorax.

(9) Pulmonary circulation problems: Includes conditions that interfere with circulation to the alveolar capillary beds; thrombus entry into pulmonary artery (**pulmonary embolus**); and increased pressure within the pulmonary arterial system causing right-sided heart failure (**cor pulmonale**).

II. Factors That Influence Respiratory Functioning

The respiratory system does not function within an enclosed vacuum. It interacts with other physiological processes within the body and with issues external to the body. Factors that influence respiratory functioning include a person's age, multiple environmental stressors, various lifestyle behaviors, and pregnancy. Understanding these factors provides a basis for future nursing assessments and nursing interventions in relation to a patient's respiratory status.

A. Developmental Level

1. Infants (particularly premature infants).
   a. Airways are narrow, small, and immature.
   b. Central nervous system is immature, leading to impaired breathing patterns and periods of apnea.
   c. Small structures and immature immune systems increase the risk of respiratory infections.
   d. Putting small objects in mouth may lead to mechanical obstruction of the airway.
   e. Respiratory distress and sudden infant death syndrome are associated with this age group.

2. Toddlers and preschoolers.
   a. Tonsils and adenoids are large, increasing the risk of tonsillitis.
   b. Putting small objects in the mouth may lead to mechanical obstruction of the airway.
   c. Exposure to children in preschool and transmission of infection via toys increases the risk of upper respiratory infections.
   d. Viral infections, croup, and pneumonia are associated with this age group.

3. School-aged children.
   a. Although the lungs are developed, they are still vulnerable to infections and exercise-induced asthma.

b. Exposure to children in school and after-school activities increases the risk of acquiring a respiratory infection.

4. Adolescents.
   a. Lungs develop adult characteristics.
   b. Vulnerability to peer pressure lead this age group to engage in habits that can impair the lungs, such as smoking and inhaling drugs or toxins.
   c. Although lung diseases generally are uncommon, exercise precipitated asthma continues to be evident.

5. Young and middle-aged adults.
   a. Prior habits that impair the lungs may continue into adulthood.
   b. Subtle progressive respiratory system changes begin in middle adulthood.
   c. Issues such as anesthesia, infections, and diseases may stress the respiratory system, which is becoming less efficient.

6. Older adults.
   a. Reduced lung compliance, increased airway resistance, and decreased lung elasticity impair ventilation.
   b. Drier mucus, fewer cilia, a less effective cough, air trapping in the alveoli, and declining immunity increase the risk of respiratory tract infections.
   c. Problems such as gastroesophageal reflux disease (GERD) and brain attack may result in aspiration, which also can precipitate a respiratory tract infection.

B. Environmental Factors
1. Air quality: Air pollution, such as cigarette smoke, automobile emissions, mold spores, and radon, can precipitate disease in vulnerable people (e.g., infants, toddlers, older adults, people with heart or lung disease).
2. Pulmonary allergens: Allergens, such as dust, animal dander, cockroach particles, environmental grasses, and foods such as peanuts and gluten, can precipitate respiratory hypersensitivity responses and allergies.
3. Altitude: Low oxygen levels place strain on the cardiopulmonary system and lead to increased ventilation, production of red blood cells and hemoglobin, and vascularity of lungs and body tissues.

C. Lifestyle Factors
1. Smoking tobacco and inhaling secondhand smoke.
   a. Tobacco smoke contains tars, toxins, and nicotine; tars and toxins are known to precipitate cancer and nicotine constricts bronchioles.
   b. Smoke also causes mucous membrane inflammation, increases respiratory secretions, breaks down elastin, and decreases the numbers and efficiency of cilia.

c. Prolonged use results in chronic bronchitis, smaller diameter of airways, and loss of alveolar elasticity, leading to emphysema.

2. Improper nutrition: Inappropriate balance of proteins, carbohydrates, and fats may reduce the immune system, impair cellular functioning, impede tissue repair, and cause obesity.
3. Lack of exercise: Sedentary lifestyle results in a depressed metabolic rate and an inability of the cardiopulmonary system to respond when any situation causes an increased metabolic rate; regular exercise increases the heart and respiratory rates, which helps condition the body so that the body can better adapt to physical or emotional stressors.
4. Obesity.
   a. A body mass index more than 30 increases the risk of respiratory infections because excess abdominal adipose tissue limits chest expansion and gas exchange in the alveoli.
   b. **Sleep apnea** occurs due to increased neck girth and fat deposits in the upper airway that obstruct the pharynx.
5. Occupational hazards.
   a. Toxic agents include chemical fumes from cleaning products, carbon monoxide from automobile or machine combustion, particles from construction debris, such as asbestos, and coal dust from coal mines.
   b. Toxic agents can cause chronic inflammation of the mucous membranes of the respiratory system and lung cancer.
6. Substance use or abuse.
   a. Alcohol and medications that depress the respiratory center in the medulla (e.g., opioids, sedatives, anxiolytics, and hypnotics) can cause hypoventilation, aspiration, apnea, and death.
   b. Stimulants, such as amphetamines and cocaine, hallucinogens, and marijuana, also adversely affect lung tissue, increase the risk of aspiration, and depress respirations.

D. Pregnancy
1. Body metabolism increases by 15 percent and oxygen consumption increases by 15 to 25 percent.
2. The enlarging uterus rises into the abdominal cavity, limiting enlargement of the chest cavity and downward movement of the diaphragm.
3. Maternal respiratory rate increases and the mother may experience shortness of breath with activity.

III. Respiratory System Assessment

A respiratory assessment can be performed as part of a comprehensive health assessment or as a focused assessment. It begins with obtaining a health history to identify risk factors for potential respiratory problems. The physical examination includes assessing breathing patterns and breath sounds; determining whether the results of inspection, palpation, and percussion of the thoracic cavity are significant; exploring the characteristics of a cough if present; and examining the characteristics of sputum. Data collected from these assessments help determine whether the patient's respiratory status is functioning adequately or further definitive action is required by the nurse or primary health-care provider.

A. Obtain a Health History to Identify Risk Factors
1. Identify age and assess for developmental stressors and changes.
2. Identify environmental and occupational stressors.
3. Identify lifestyle behaviors that impact the cardiopulmonary system.
4. Obtain list of prescribed, over-the-counter, and "recreational" medications taken by the patient.
5. Assess overall physical and emotional health status and determine whether the patient has any problems that impact the respiratory status.

B. Assess Breathing Patterns
1. Perform assessment of breathing patterns unobtrusively because involuntary breathing efforts are more desirable to assess than voluntary breathing efforts.
2. Note the patient's position.
   a. Sitting allows the chest to expand and the diaphragm to move downward with inspirations.
   b. Difficulty breathing in the supine position (**orthopnea**) may occur because the abdominal organs press against the diaphragm and impede chest expansion.
   c. Leaning forward while sitting (**orthopneic, tripod position**) (Fig. 19.3) increases the thoracic area, allowing for greater chest expansion.
   d. Extreme shortness of breath during sleep that causes an abrupt awakening and immediate need to assume the upright position for relief (**paroxysmal nocturnal dyspnea**).
3. Observe the rate, depth, and rhythm of respirations. (Table 19.1; see also the section "Measurement of Respirations" in Chapter 11, "Physical Assessment," page 255.)
4. Identify the degree of respiratory effort.
   a. Breathing should be effortless.
   b. Difficulty breathing (**dyspnea**) and difficulty breathing with activity (**exertional dyspnea**) occur with inadequate oxygenation.
   c. Shortness of breath and fatigue are subjective symptoms that can be reported only by the patient.
   d. Physical signs usually accompany difficulty breathing.
5. Identify signs of increased respiratory effort.
   a. **Use of accessory muscles of respiration:** Use of intercostal, abdominal, and trapezius muscles to help expand the chest cavity.

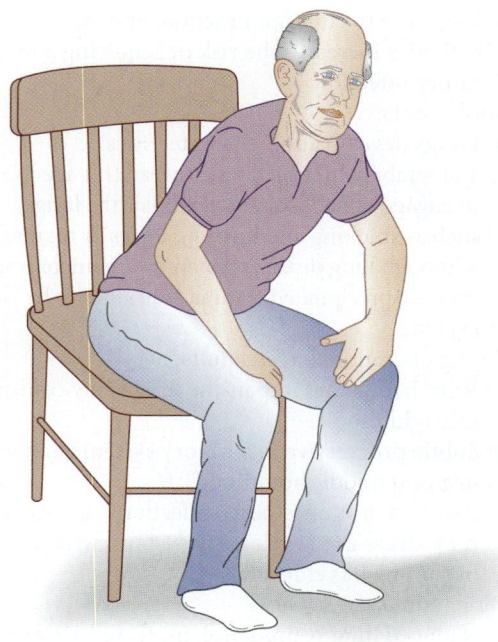

Fig 19.3 Orthopneic or tripod position. (From Williams & Hopper [2011]. *Understanding medical surgical nursing,* 4th ed. Philadelphia: F. A. Davis, with permission.)

   b. **Retractions:** Intercostal, supraclavicular, and subcostal tissues recede during inspiration as a result of excessive negative pressure required to increase the depth of respirations.
   c. **Nasal flaring:** Widening of the nares during inhalation to reduce resistance to airflow; more common in infants and young children.
   d. **Grunting immediately before exhalation:** Closed glottis at the height of inspiration keeps alveoli open to enhance gas exchange; grunt occurs when air is expelled through the larynx.
   e. **Pursed-lip breathing:** Exhalation through the mouth with lips positioned to create a small opening to prolong exhalation; keeps alveoli open longer for gas exchange and more efficiently expels trapped air.

C. Perform Inspection
1. Determine whether the chest expands and recoils with inhalation and exhalation, respectively.
   a. Movement should be symmetrical.
   b. Asymmetrical expansion may indicate a pneumothorax.
2. Measure the chest's anteroposterior-to-lateral ratio, which should be 1:2.
   a. An increase in the anteroposterior diameter (**barrel chest**) is associated with chronic retention of carbon dioxide, which occurs with chronic obstructive pulmonary disease (Fig. 19-4).

Table 19.1 Breathing Patterns

Pattern	Explanation
Eupnea (normal)	• 12 to 20 breaths/minute. • Not too deep or too shallow. • Unlabored. • Regular rhythm.
Bradypnea	• Less than 12 breaths/minute. • Regular rhythm. • Associated with neuromuscular disorders, electrolyte imbalances, and opioid medications.
Tachypnea	• More than 20 breaths/minute. • Regular rhythm. • Associated with physical exertion, anxiety, pain, and central nervous system and metabolic disorders.
Kussmaul	• Increased rate and depth of respirations. • Regular rhythm. • Associated with metabolic acidosis, fear, and panic.
Biot	• Varying depths of respirations (usually shallow), alternating with periods of apnea. • Irregular rhythm. • Associated with severe, persistent increased intracranial pressure and damage to the respiratory center in the medulla.
Cheyne-Stokes (periodic breathing)	• Gradual increase in depth of respirations, followed by a gradual decrease and then a period of apnea. • Regular rhythm. • Associated with increased intracranial pressure, drug poisoning, and damage to the respiratory center in the medulla.
Apnea	• Absence of breathing. • Respiratory arrest. • Requires mechanical ventilation or cardiopulmonary resuscitation.

Figures adapted from Wilkinson and Treas (2011). *Fundamentals of nursing*, Vol. 2, 2nd ed. Philadelphia: F. A. Davis Company, with permission.

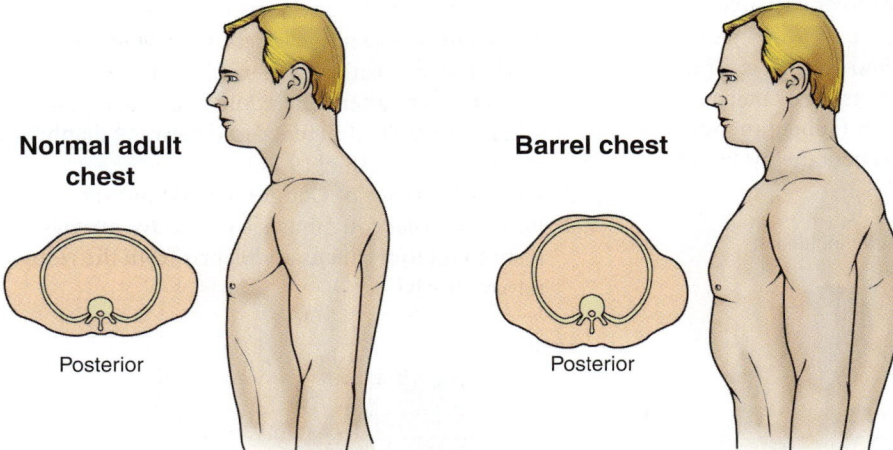

Normal adult chest

Posterior

Barrel chest

Posterior

Fig 19.4 Anteroposterior diameter of chest: Normal adult chest, barrel chest. (From Wilkinson and Treas [2011]. *Fundamentals of nursing*, Vol. 1, 2nd ed. Philadelphia: F. A. Davis, with permission.)

3. Assess the mucous membranes, which should be pink, moist, and intact.
   a. Dry mucous membranes indicate dehydration or a side effect of such medications as anticholinergics.
   b. Pale or bluish color indicates inadequate oxygenation.

4. Assess the lips, which should be slightly lighter or darker than skin color.
   a. Pale lips may indicate anemia or hypoxia.
   b. Cherry-red lips may indicate carbon monoxide poisoning or acidosis.
   c. Pallor around the lips (**circumoral pallor**) may indicate inadequate oxygenation.

5. Assess the fingers and nail plate angles for signs of bulbous swelling of the soft tissue of the end of the phalanx of fingers causing the nail plates to be equal to or greater than 180° (**clubbing**), which indicates prolonged inadequate oxygenation. (see Fig. 16.1)
6. Assess the color of fingers and nails.
   a. Yellow or brown color indicates nicotine stains from a prolonged history of smoking.
   b. Pallor or cyanosis indicates impaired oxygenation.

D. Perform Palpation
1. Follow a sequence similar to that used for auscultation of breath sounds (see page 577).
2. Assess the extent of respiratory excursion: Place your hands on either side of the patient's vertebrae and have the patient inhale (Fig. 19.5); provides a gross measurement of chest expansion on inspiration.
   a. Lack of movement on one side is associated with pneumothorax and lobectomy.
   b. Limited excursion is associated with obstructive airway diseases.
3. Assess tactile fremitus: Place the palmar surface of your hands on the patient's chest wall while keeping the fingers raised off of the chest wall; vibrations should be detected when the patient vocalizes "99" repeatedly (Fig. 19.6).
   a. Increased tactile fremitus is associated with pulmonary edema.
   b. Decreased tactile fremitus is associated with decreased air movement related to obstructive airway diseases.
4. Assess for tenderness, masses, and crackling; air in subcutaneous tissue when compressed by palpation exhibits a crackling sensation (**subcutaneous emphysema**); air leaking into subcutaneous tissue

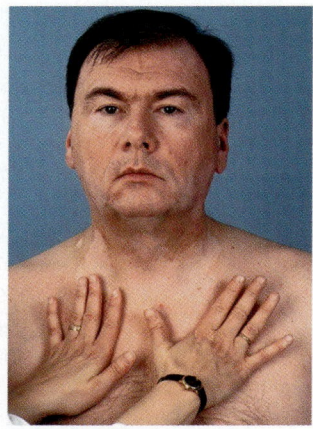

Fig 19.6 Palpation of tactile fremitus. (From Wilkinson and Treas [2011]. *Fundamentals of nursing,* Vol. 1, 2nd ed. Philadelphia: F. A. Davis, with permission.)

usually is due to a pneumothorax or associated with a chest tube site.

E. Perform Percussion
1. Follow a sequence similar to that for auscultation of breath sounds (see page 577).
2. Percuss over the intercostal spaces rather than over the ribs or scapulae.
3. Note whether sounds are drum-like (tympanic), hollow (resonant), hyperresonant (echoing), quiet and thudding (dull), or quiet and flat (flat) to determine whether underlying structures are solid or hollow and contain fluid or air.
4. Assess diaphragmatic excursion: Percuss the base of the lung at the posterior chest while the patient holds a deep breath and then while the patient holds a breath after exhalation; mark each point and measure the difference to determine diaphragmatic excursion (Fig. 19.7).

F. Assess for Presence of Coughing and Sputum
1. Recognize that coughing is a protective mechanism to remove mucus and debris from the respiratory airways.

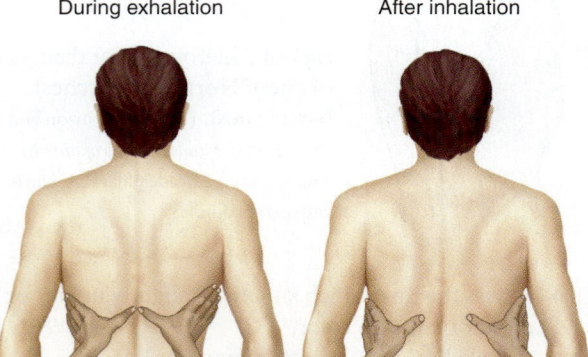

During exhalation   After inhalation

Fig 19.5 Palpation of respiratory excursion: Left, during exhalation; right, after inhalation. (From Williams & Hopper [2011]. *Understanding medical surgical nursing,* 4th ed. Philadelphia: F. A. Davis, with permission.)

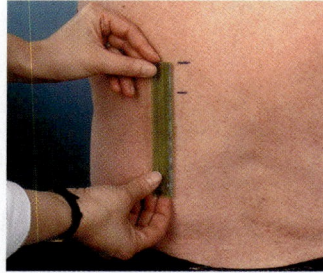

Fig 19.7 Measuring diaphragmatic excursion. (From Wilkinson and Treas [2011]. *Fundamentals of nursing,* Vol. 1, 2nd ed. Philadelphia: F. A. Davis, with permission.)

2. Coughing and sputum can be caused by irritants such as smoke, dust, and chemical fumes; food, fluid, or a foreign object that gets lodged in the respiratory airways; and inflammation associated with respiratory tract infections or tumors.

3. Identify whether mucus is being produced by the mucous membranes of the trachea, bronchi, and lungs (**sputum**).

4. Identify whether coughing is not bringing up sputum (**nonproductive cough**) or bringing up sputum (**productive cough**).

5. Identify the characteristics of sputum.
   a. Amount: From slight to copious.
   b. When produced: From once to continuous; in the a.m.; when lying down; after behaviors such as smoking.
   c. Color.
      (1) Clear/white: Associated with viral infections.
      (2) Yellow/green: Associated with bacterial infection.
      (3) Black: Associated with inhalation of smoke, soot, or coal dust.
      (4) Red/rust colored: Associated with the presence of blood (**hemoptysis**), tuberculosis, and pneumococcal pneumonia.
      (5) Pink/frothy: Associated with pulmonary edema.
   d. Odor: Foul smelling, associated with bacterial infections such as pneumonia and abscesses of the lung.

6. Obtain a sputum specimen for culture and sensitivity (C&S) (see the section "Culture and Sensitivity of Sputum" under "Respiratory System Diagnostic Tests and Related Nursing Care," page 582).

G. Auscultate Breath Sounds

🛑 1. Clean the ear pieces and diaphragm of the stethoscope before and after use; have a dedicated stethoscope for a patient in isolation.

2. Place the patient in a sitting position to provide access to the patient's anterior, posterior, and lateral chest; warm the diaphragm of the stethoscope with your hands before use to promote patient comfort.

3. Place the diaphragm directly on the patient's skin and follow a systematic sequence to ensure all lung fields are assessed (Fig. 19.8).

4. Instruct the patient to breathe deeply through the mouth; provide for a period of regular breathing when necessary to prevent hyperventilation and respiratory alkalosis.

5. Note the duration of inspiration and expiration.

6. Note the pitch, intensity, and other characteristics of sounds; if you hear air moving through fluid,

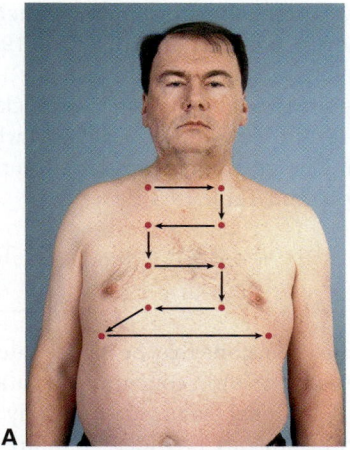

A

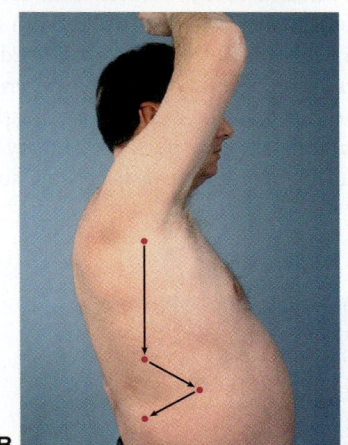

B

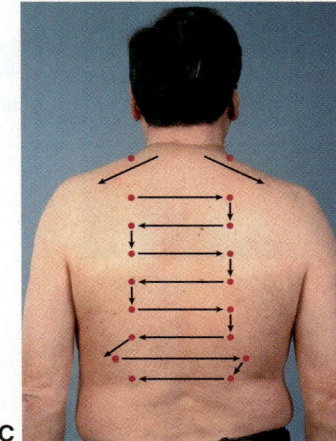

C

Fig. 19.8 Sequence of auscultation of breath sounds. (A) Sequence of anterior auscultation sites. (B) Sequence of lateral auscultation sites for both sides. (C) Sequence of posterior auscultation sites. (From Burton and Ludwig [2011]. *Fundamentals of nursing care: Concepts, connections & skills.* Philadelphia: F. A. Davis, with permission.)

have the patient cough and reassess breath sounds to help distinguish between crackles and rhonchi (coughing will eliminate rhonchi but will not eliminate crackles).

7. Identify expected breath sounds: Bronchial, bronchovesicular, and vesicular (Fig. 19.9 and Table 19.2).
8. Identify abnormal breath sounds: Crackles (rales), rhonchi (sonorous wheezes), **stridor,** wheezes (sibilant wheezes), and pleural friction rub (Fig. 19.10 and Table 19.3).

IV. Respiratory System Diagnostic Tests and Related Nursing Care

Physical examination alone may be inadequate to provide comprehensive information concerning a patient's respiratory status. Additional diagnostic tests may be ordered by the primary health-care provider. Some are essential to arrive at a medical diagnosis (e.g., tuberculin skin testing, sputum C&S), whereas others are employed to identify specific information about a patient's oxygenation status or the extent of functioning of a patient's respiratory system (e.g., pulse oximetry, peek expiratory flow rate). Nurses must understand these tests because some of them are performed by the nurse and all of them require patient teaching.

A. Pulse Oximetry
1. Identifies the percentage of arterial oxygen saturation by assessing the percentage of hemoglobin molecules carrying oxygen (Fig. 19.11). (See the section "Measurement of Arterial Blood Oxygen Saturation" in Chapter 11, "Physical Assessment," page 261.)
2. Can be used intermittently or continuously.
3. Expected value is 95 to 100 percent.
4. Nursing care.
   a. Verify the primary health-care provider's order (e.g., intermittent or continuous assessment; while receiving oxygen or on room air).
   b. Explain to the patient that the test is noninvasive and will cause no discomfort.
   c. Select the site to be used for the sensor, such as a fingertip, toe, ear lobe, or forehead; use the appropriate sensor for the chosen site and patient size.

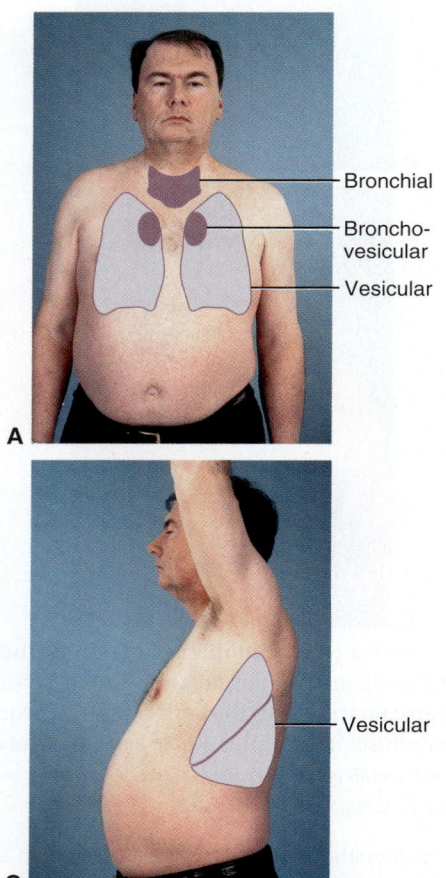

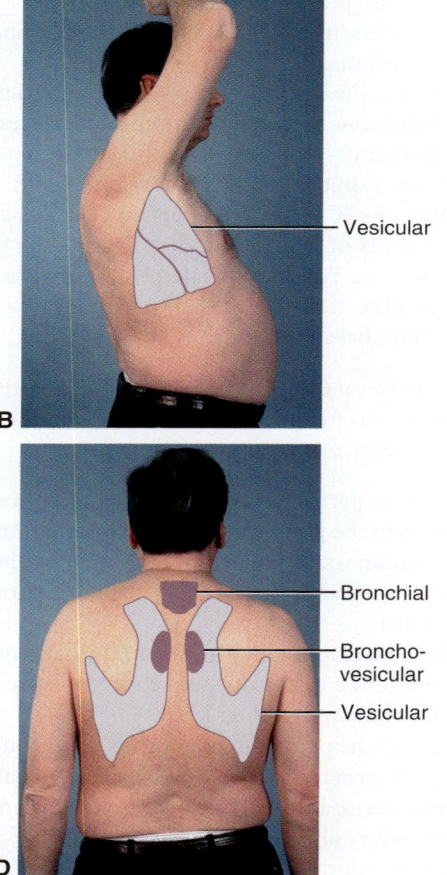

Fig 19.9 Locations of normal breath sounds. (From Wilkinson and Treas [2011]. *Fundamentals of nursing,* Vol. 1, 2nd ed. Philadelphia: F. A. Davis, with permission.)

Table 19.2	**Recognizing Normal Breath Sounds**	
Breath Sound	**Description**	**Location**
Bronchial	• Caused by air moving through the trachea. • Loud, high-pitched, hollow, blowing sound. • Inspiration shorter than expiration.	• Over the trachea anteriorly. • Nape of the neck posteriorly.
Bronchovesicular	• Caused by air moving through large bronchi. • Medium-pitched, medium intensity, blowing sounds. • Inspiration and expiration equal in length.	• Over the first and second intercostal space on either side of the sternum anteriorly. • Between the scapulae posteriorly.
Vesicular	• Caused by air moving through smaller airways of the respiratory tract. • Soft, low-pitched, breezy sounds. • Inspiration is louder, higher pitched, and longer than expiration.	• Over the periphery of the lung.

Figures adapted from Wilkinson and Treas (2011). *Fundamentals of nursing,* Vol. 2, 2nd ed. Philadelphia: F. A. Davis Company, with permission.

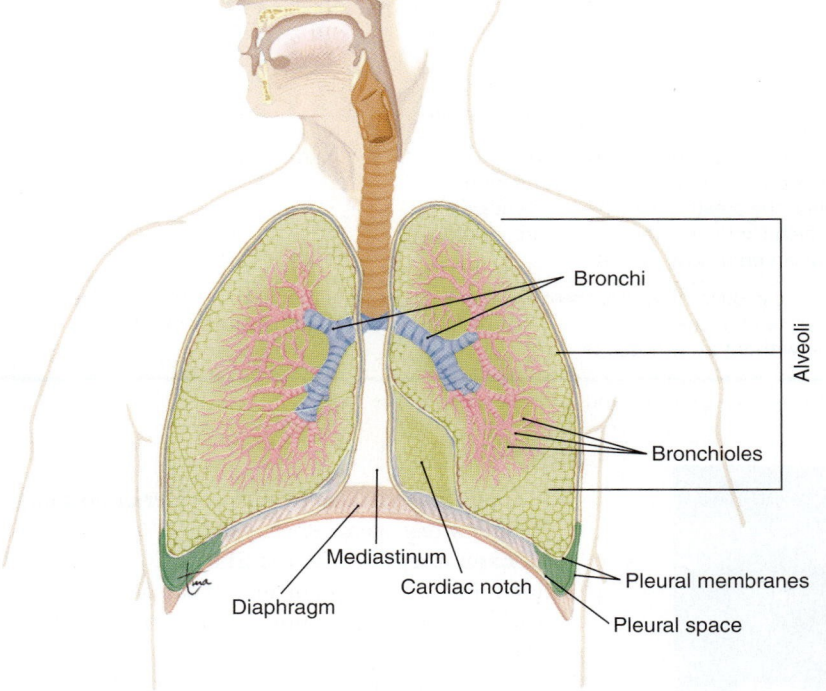

Fig 19.10 Location of abnormal breath sounds: Crackles—yellow; rhonchi—orange and blue; wheeze—pink; pleural friction rub—green. (Adapted from Wilkinson and Treas [2011]. *Fundamentals of nursing,* Vol. 1, 2nd ed. Philadelphia: F. A. Davis, with permission.)

d. Change the pulse oximetry sensor site every 2 hours to prevent tissue necrosis from pressure if monitoring is continuous.

e. Ensure the site is dry, has no dark nail polish or artificial nails, and has adequate circulation as determined by a capillary refill of less than 3 seconds.

f. Document the results in the patient's clinical record, and notify the primary health-care provider if the results are outside the expected

Table 19.3	**Distinguishing Abnormal Breath Sounds**	

Breath Sound	Description and Location	Etiology

Crackles (rales)
 	
I ────── E
 	
Crackles
	• Air bubbling through moisture in the alveoli.
	• Not cleared by coughing.
	• Heard in periphery of lung.
	• Classified as:
	  • **Fine:** Soft, high-pitched crackling sound heard at height of inspiration.
	  • **Medium:** Lower-pitched, popping sound heard during the middle of inspiration.
	  • **Coarse:** Loud, bubbling sound heard throughout inspiration.
		• Inflammation due to pneumonia or bronchitis.
		• Hypervolemia due to congestive heart failure.
		• Alteration in structure or function, such as in emphysema.

Rhonchi (sonorous wheeze) I ────── E Rhonchi	• Mucus accumulated in large bronchi. • Loud, coarse, low-pitched sound heard during inspiration and/or expiration. • May be cleared by coughing. • Heard over larger bronchi.	• Inflammation due to bronchitis. • Narrowed airways. • Alteration in structure or function, such as in emphysema or fibrotic lungs.
Wheeze (sibilant wheeze) I ────── E Mild Wheeze I ────── E Moderate Wheeze I ────── E Severe Wheeze	• Air moving through narrowed airways. • High-pitched, musical sound that may be heard throughout inspiration and expiration; more prominent during expiration. • Heard over bronchi. • May be audible without a stethoscope.	• Narrowing of small airways by spasms, inflammatory process, mucus accumulation, or tumors.
Pleural Friction Rub I ────── E Friction Rub	• Inflamed pleural surfaces rubbing together. • Low-pitched, grating sound during inspiration and/or expiration; more prominent at height of inspiration. • Disappears when the breath is held (versus pericardial friction rub, which continues when the breath is held). • Heard at lateral, anterior, base of lung.	• Inflammation of the pleural membranes (pleurisy).
Stridor	• High-pitched crowing sound; more prominent during inspiration. • Heard over larynx and trachea. • May be audible without a stethoscope.	• Tracheal or laryngeal spasm. • Partial airway obstruction.

Figures from Dillon (2007): *Nursing health assessment: Clinical pocket guide*, 2nd ed. F. A. Davis Company, with permission.

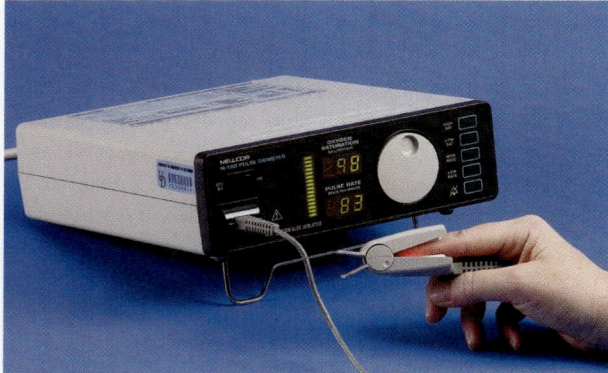

Fig 19.11 Pulse oximetry. (From Wilkinson and Treas [2011]. *Fundamentals of nursing*, Vol. 1, 2nd ed. Philadelphia: F. A. Davis, with permission.)

range, as indicated by the provider or hospital policy (e.g., generally less than 92%).

B. Peak Expiratory Flow Rate (PEFR)

1. Identifies the amount of air that can be exhaled with forcible effort, expressed in liters per minute (Fig. 19.12).
2. Compared to the individual's "personal best" baseline result to determine dosage and effectiveness of respiratory medications.
   a. Green: Peak flow is within 80 to 100 percent of personal best baseline; continue prescriptions as ordered.
   b. Yellow: Peak flow is within 50 to 80 percent of personal best baseline; reflects onset of airway changes that are reducing peak flow by 20 to

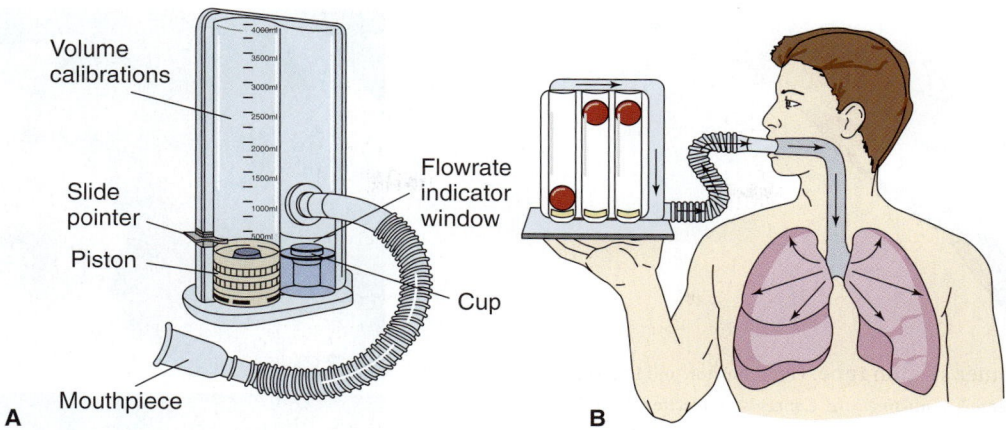

Fig 19.18 Incentive spirometers. (A) Voldyne volumetric deep-breathing exerciser. (B) Triflow II incentive breathing exerciser. (Modified from Barnes, T.A. [1991]. *Respiratory care principles* [p. 434]. Philadelphia: F. A. Davis.)

d. Place the patient in the high-Fowler position for meals; have a nursing team member assist with the entire meal and ensure that patient's mouth is empty of food after the meal.

e. Offer small, frequent meals; alter the consistency of food as indicated, such as mechanical soft, soft, chopped, and pureed; feed slowly.

f. Keep the patient in the semi- or high-Fowler position for at least 30 minutes after meals.

3. Maintain aspiration precautions for patients receiving enteral feedings.

a. Maintain the head of the bed at 30° if the patient is receiving continuous tube feedings.

b. Raise the head of the bed to 45° before the patient receives an intermittent tube feeding; intermittent tube feedings have a larger volume than continuous tube feedings, which increases the risk of aspiration; maintain head elevation for at least 30 minutes after the feeding.

c. Aspirate stomach contents to ensure that the nasogastric tube is in the stomach and to measure residual volume; hold the next feeding if the residual volume exceeds the parameter indicated by the primary health-care provider or facility policy (depends on amount and frequency of feedings).

4. Assess for signs of excessive secretions in the airways, such as rattling sounds in the throat, shortness of breath, ineffective cough, and rhonchi or crackles on auscultation.

🛑 5. Suction the patient if respiratory secretions compromise the airway.

a. **Commonalities of nursing care related to suctioning.**
(1) Wash your hands.
(2) Provide for the patient's privacy.

(3) Assess breath sounds, vital signs, and pulse oximetry before the procedure.

(4) Place the patient in the semi- or high-Fowler position.

(5) Set the wall suction at an appropriate pressure (e.g., 100 to 150 mm Hg for adults, 100 to 120 mm Hg for children, and 50 to 95 mm Hg for infants).

(6) Don a face shield and appropriate gloves.

(7) Begin suctioning.

(8) Reposition the patient and reinstitute the prescribed oxygen therapy after suctioning is completed.

(9) Assess breath sounds, vital signs, pulse oximetry, and the patient's response to the procedure and document these results in the patient's clinical record.

(10) Discard used equipment in appropriate disposal containers.

b. **Oropharyngeal suctioning.**
(1) Don clean gloves.
(2) Obtain equipment.
  (a) Yankauer (tonsil-tip) suction tube (Fig. 19.19) to remove secretions from the oral cavity.
  (b) Suction catheter (e.g., 12 to 18 French for adults, 8 to 10 French for children, and 5 to 8 French for infants) to remove secretions from the oropharyngeal or nasopharyngeal area.
(3) Lubricate the tip of the tube or catheter with sterile normal saline solution.

🛑 (4) Advance the tube or catheter (3 to 4 inches) along the inside of the cheek to the pharyngeal area; avoiding the center of the tongue limits gagging.

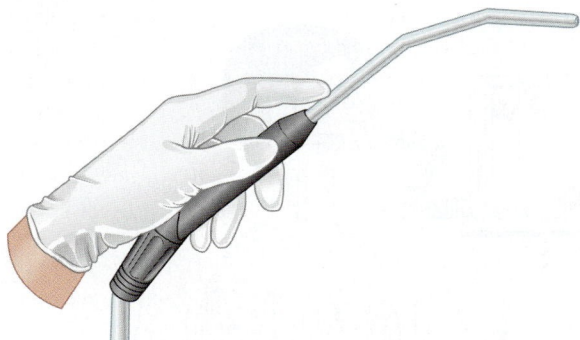

Fig 19.19 Yankauer suction tube. (From Burton and Ludwig [2011]. *Fundamentals of nursing care: Concepts, connections & skills.* Philadelphia: F. A. Davis, with permission.)

🛑 (5) Apply negative pressure for only 10 to 15 seconds to remove secretions and prevent hypoxia.

   (6) Suction the cheek pouches and under the tongue to remove pocketed secretions (Fig. 19.20).

  c. **Nasopharyngeal suctioning.**
    (1) Don clean gloves.
    (2) Measure from the tip of the patient's nose to the tip of the patient's earlobe to determine the extent the catheter should be inserted (Fig. 19.21a).
    (3) Lubricate the tip of the catheter with water-soluble jelly.
    (4) Extend the patient's head and advance the catheter into a naris the predetermined length, usually 5 to 6 inches (Fig. 19.21b).

🛑 (5) Apply intermittent negative pressure for 10 to 15 seconds only when rotating and withdrawing the catheter.

    (6) Suction normal saline solution to clear the catheter of secretions.
    (7) Repeat previous steps alternating nares and waiting 30 seconds between each pass of the catheter to allow the patient time to breathe.

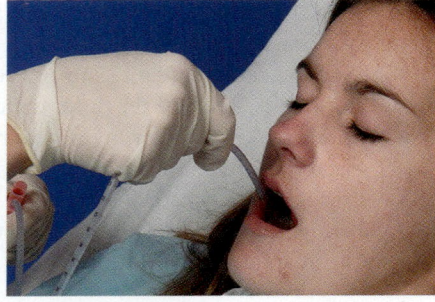

Fig 19.20 Suction cheek pouches and under the tongue. (From Wilkinson and Treas [2011]. *Fundamentals of nursing,* Vol. 1, 2nd ed. Philadelphia: F. A. Davis, with permission.)

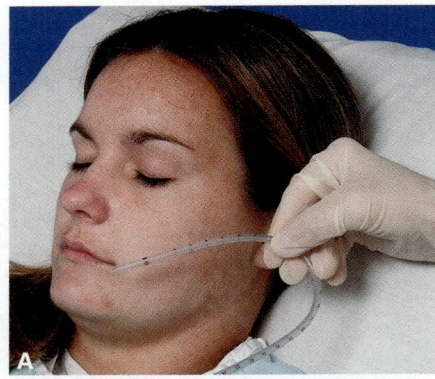

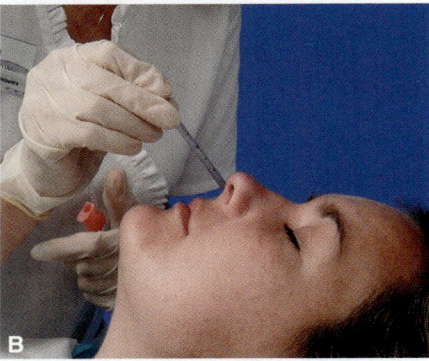

Fig 19.21 Nasopharyngeal suctioning. (A) Measure from the tip of nose to tip of ear lobe. (B) Insert lubricated catheter into naris. (From Wilkinson and Treas [2011]. *Fundamentals of nursing,* Vol. 1, 2nd ed. Philadelphia: F. A. Davis, with permission.)

  d. **Endotracheal and tracheal suctioning.**
    (1) Preoxygenate the patient by using a resuscitation bag connected to an oxygen source; compress the bag 3 to 5 times.

🛑 (2) Do not preoxygenate if the patient has copious secretions because doing so can force secretions deeper into the lung and delay their removal.

    (3) Don sterile gloves.
    (4) Lubricate the tip of the catheter with sterile normal saline solution.
    (5) Advance the catheter without applying negative pressure until resistance is felt (usually just above the bifurcation of the mainstream bronchi; endotracheal tube—usually 5 to 6 inches for an adult; tracheostomy tube—usually 2 to 3 inches for an adult).

🛑 (6) Apply intermittent negative pressure for 10 to 15 seconds only when rotating and withdrawing the catheter (Fig. 19.22).

E. Institute Basic Life Support (Cardiopulmonary Resuscitation [CPR]) (Table 19.4)
  1. Perform external cardiac compression and ventilation to increase blood flow to the heart and brain,

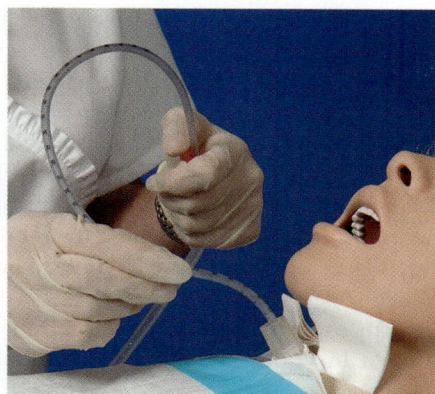

Fig 19.22 Tracheal suctioning. (From Wilkinson and Treas [2011]. *Fundamentals of nursing*, Vol. 1, 2nd ed. Philadelphia: F. A. Davis, with permission.)

following the sequence of Circulation, Airway, Breathing (CAB).

2. Shake the patient by the shoulder and shout, "Are you okay?" to assess level of consciousness.
3. If no response, call for help or activate EMS system to ensure help and the presence of a defibrillator and resuscitative medications.
4. Palpate the carotid pulse for adult or brachial or femoral pulse for an infant or child to assess circulation.
5. Deliver 30 external cardiac compressions to promote cardiac output (ensure victim is on a hard surface in supine position).

6. Assess and establish an airway; open the airway (head tilt–chin lift maneuver or jaw thrust without neck hyperextension if cervical injury is suspected) to listen, look, and feel for air exchange.
7. If the patient is not breathing, give 2 breaths to instill air into the lungs (maintain head-tilt or jaw thrust maneuver while pinching victim's nostrils).
8. Maintain the ratio of compressions to ventilations for 5 cycles and then reassess the pulse.
9. If successful, discontinue CPR and position the victim in a side-lying (recovery) position.
10. If unsuccessful, resume compressions and then ventilations according to appropriate age and number of rescuers ratio; terminate CPR when ordered by the primary health-care provider or when rescuer exhaustion occurs.

F. Prevent and Manage Partial and Total Airway Obstructions

1. Education for family members with small children.
   a. Ensure toys are as large as a clenched fist and inspect toys for small removable parts.
   b. Store plastic bags where they cannot be reached by small children.
   c. Cut food into very small pieces, and avoid foods such as olives, grapes, and frankfurters.
   d. Do not give small children hard candy, nuts, popcorn, marshmallows, chewing gum, or balloons.
   e. Discuss how and when to perform the universal choking sign (Fig. 19.23).

Table 19.4 Performing CPR

CPR	Infant (< 1 year)	Child (> 1 year–adolescent)	Adult
Rate of compressions	• Administer at least 100 compressions per minute. • Rotate health-care providers every 2 minutes. • Keep interruptions to less than 10 seconds.		
Compression landmark	• Identify center of chest below the nipples.	• Identify center of chest between the nipples.	• Identify lower half of the sternum.
Depth of compressions	• Compress the chest about 1.5 inches.	• Compress the chest about 1.5 to 2 inches, depending on the child's size.	• Compress the chest at least 2 inches.
Ratio of compressions to ventilations	• Compress the chest 30 to 2 (1 rescuer). • Compress the chest 15 to 2 (2 rescuers).		• Compress the chest 30 to 2 regardless of whether there are 1 or 2 rescuers.
Compression method "Hard and fast" with complete chest recoil	• Use 2 fingers with 1 rescuer. • Use 2 thumbs with hands encircling chest with 2 rescuers.	• Use the heel of 1 hand. -or- • Use the heel of 1 hand with fingers interlocked with the other.	• Use the heel of 1 hand with fingers interlocked with the other.

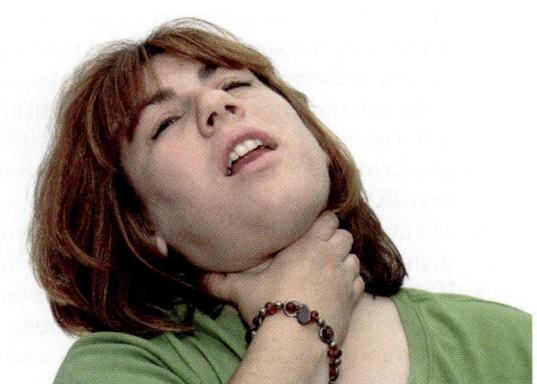

Fig 19.23 Universal sign for choking. (From Wilkinson and Treas [2011]. *Fundamentals of nursing,* Vol. 1, 2nd ed. Philadelphia: F. A. Davis, with permission.)

2. Assess for the presence of partial or total airway obstruction and intervene accordingly (Table 19.5: Airway Obstructions).

G. Administer Oxygen

1. Commonalities of nursing care specific for patients receiving oxygen.

   a. Perform all preliminary nursing interventions, such as verifying the order, washing your hands, collecting appropriate equipment, identifying the patient, providing privacy, and explaining the procedure to the patient.

   b. Obtain vital signs, measure the patient's pulse oximetry level (may not be a reliable indicator for patients with COPD or impaired peripheral circulation), and perform a focused respiratory assessment, including auscultation of breath sounds, before initiation of therapy to have baseline data.

   c. Initiate oxygen flow according to the manufacturer's directions, and place the device on the patient.

   d. Hang an "oxygen in use" sign near the patient's bed, use cotton gowns and linens to prevent static electricity, and prohibit smoking and open flames near the patient because oxygen supports combustion.

   e. Routinely monitor delivery of oxygen, ensuring that all connections are secure.

   f. Assess the patient's skin where elastic straps, the mask, or oxygen tubing may produce pressure or friction that could cause skin trauma (e.g., nares and top of ears with a nasal cannula, ears, bridge of the nose, and zygomatic archs with masks).

Table 19.5 Airway Obstructions

	Infant (< 1 year)	Child/Adolescent (>1 year)	Adult
Assess extent of obstruction	**Partial Obstruction** • Can cough and make sounds. **Total Obstruction** • Cannot cough, make sounds, or speak; has difficulty breathing, pallor, and cyanosis. • In addition, a child or adult may encircle the throat with the hands (universal choking sign). Nurse should ask the victim, "Are you choking?"		
Victim is conscious	**Partial Obstruction** • Continue to monitor; allow the victim's efforts to dislodge the object.		
	Total Obstruction in an Infant • Deliver 5 back blows followed by 5 chest thrusts. • Repeat until object is expelled or victim is unresponsive.	**Total Obstruction in a Child or an Adult** • Activate EMS system. • Ask victim, "Can I help?" • Perform abdominal thrust maneuver until the object is expelled or victim is unresponsive. **How to perform the abdominal thrust maneuver** • Encircle a conscious victim's waist with intertwined clenched fists. • Thrust upward and inward against the victim's diaphragm. • Repeat thrusts until the object is expelled or the victim becomes unresponsive.	
Victim is unconscious	• Head tilt–chin lift maneuver; inspect the mouth; remove the object if present in the pharynx. • Implement cardiopulmonary resuscitation, but inspect the mouth before each two rescue breaths.		

MAKING THE CONNECTION

Avoidance of High Levels of Oxygen Therapy and Patients With Obstructive Respiratory Diseases

The carbon dioxide level in the body is the primary regulator of breathing because increased or decreased levels affect the pH of the blood. Changes in the oxygen level in the blood do not change the blood's pH. Normally, when the carbon dioxide level in the body increases and pH and oxygen levels decrease, the chemoreceptors in the carotid arteries, aorta, and medulla identify these changes and send a message to the medulla to increase respirations accordingly. However, people with obstructive airway disease become accustomed to increased carbon dioxide levels and their stimulus to breathe is no longer increased levels of carbon dioxide but rather low oxygen levels. Therefore, when administering oxygen to people with obstructive airway diseases, the delivery of oxygen should not exceed 2 L/minute. Excessive exogenous oxygen decreases the respiratory drive, resulting in decreased breathing and increased carbon dioxide retention. In addition, the Haldane effect suggests that the adverse effects of increased oxygen are caused by the inability of oxygen-saturated hemoglobin molecules to transport carbon dioxide. Both issues relate to excessive levels of carbon dioxide in the body associated with excessive exogenous oxygen (**CO_2 narcosis**). Patients with obstructive airway diseases who are receiving oxygen should be assessed for the clinical manifestation of CO_2 narcosis, which include decreased rate and depth of respirations, confusion, decreased level of consciousness, tremors, convulsions, and even death.

g. Routinely assess the patient's vital signs, pulse oximetry, breath sounds, and other patient responses, and evaluate data in relation to expected outcomes of interventions.

h. Document the procedure and the patient's response in the patient's clinical record.

2. For nursing care for patients receiving oxygen via specific oxygen delivery systems, see Table 19.6.

3. Care for a patient with an artificial airway.

a. Device used to permit air to enter and exit the lungs, thereby maintaining an open airway.

b. Used for patients who are unconscious, at risk for airway obstruction, or require mechanical ventilation.

c. Should be suctioned only when necessary to maintain an open airway and limit trauma to mucous membranes of the respiratory tract.

d. Nursing care varies by type of device (Table 19.7).

VI. Medications That Affect the Respiratory System

When a person is diagnosed with a respiratory problem, the primary health-care provider can prescribe appropriate medications to dilate the respiratory airways, increase the volume and decrease the viscosity of respiratory secretions, and limit coughing. Nurses should know the mechanisms of action, therapeutic and nontherapeutic effects, and nursing care related to the common bronchodilators, expectorants, and antitussives (Table 19.8).

Table 19.6 | **Oxygen Delivery Systems**

Type	Description	Advantages and Disadvantages	Nursing Care
Simple face mask 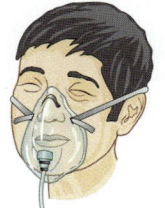	• Delivers oxygen to the nose and mouth via a clear, flexible mask. • *Liter flow:* 5 to 10 L/minute. • *Fraction of inspired oxygen (FIO_2):* 40% to 60%, depending on liter flow.	*Advantages* • Patient may breathe through the nose or mouth. *Disadvantages* • Some patients feel claustrophobic. • Some patients feel hot because the mask retains body heat. • The mask must be removed for eating and drinking. • Speech is muffled.	• Place the mask securely over the nose and mouth with the elastic straps above the ears. • Ensure the flow rate is ≥5 L/minute to prevent carbon dioxide accumulation in the mask. • Switch to a nasal cannula when eating.
Nasal cannula 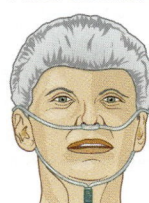	• Delivers oxygen to the nares via clear, flexible prongs. • *Liter flow:* 1 to 6 L/minute. • *FIO_2:* 24% to 44%, depending on liter flow.	*Advantages* • The device is comparatively comfortable. • The patient may eat, drink, and talk unimpeded. *Disadvantages* • It may dry the nasal mucosa and irritate the nares. • Device's effectiveness decreases if the patient breaths through the mouth.	• Place the nasal prongs curved downward into the nares with the elastic straps wrapped around the ears and the slider under the chin. • Assess for dryness of the nasal mucosa. • Humidify oxygen if the flow rate is >3 L/minute.

Continued

Table 19.6 **Oxygen Delivery Systems—cont'd**

Type	Description	Advantages and Disadvantages	Nursing Care
Partial rebreather mask 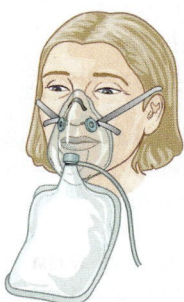	• Delivers oxygen to the nose and mouth via a clear, flexible mask with an attached bag (reservoir). • Some exhaled air is rebreathed; most exhaled air is discharged through ports on the side of the mask. • *Liter flow:* 6 to 15 L/minute. • *FIO_2:* 50% to 90%, depending on liter flow.	*Advantages* • Rebreathing some exhaled carbon dioxide lowers the pH of the gas, which stimulates breathing and helps prevent carbon dioxide narcosis. *Disadvantages* • Some patients feel claustrophobic.	• Flood the reservoir with oxygen before attaching the mask to the patient. • Ensure that the reservoir does not collapse during inhalation; a higher flow rate is required if this occurs.
Nonrebreather mask 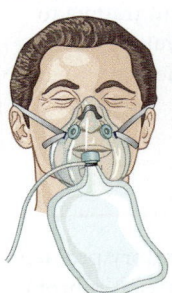	• Delivers oxygen to the nose and mouth via a clear, flexible mask with an attached bag (reservoir). • All exhaled air is discharged through ports on the side of the mask. • *Liter flow:* 6 to 15 L/minute. • *FIO_2:* 70% to 100%, depending on liter flow.	*Advantages* • This is the only oxygen delivery system that can deliver 100% oxygen when liter flow is 15 L/minute. It allows higher FIO_2 levels because the reservoir fills with oxygen; ⅓ of the air in the reservoir is depleted when the patient inhales; the reservoir is then refilled by the oxygen flow. *Disadvantages* • Some patients feel claustrophobic.	• Flood the reservoir with oxygen before attaching the mask to the patient. • Ensure that the reservoir remains half full during inhalation; if not, a higher flow rate is required.
Venturi mask 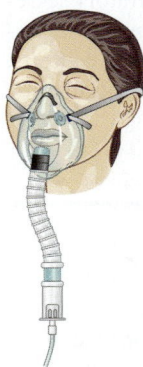	• Delivers oxygen to the nose and mouth via a clear, flexible mask with a valve and tubing attached between the mask and the oxygen tubing. • Interchangeable color-coded valves permit a specific mix of room air and oxygen to deliver a precise percentage of oxygen. • Exhaled air is discharged through ports on the side of the mask to keep carbon dioxide buildup to a minimum. • *Liter flow:* Depends on valve being used. • *FIO_2:* 24% to 60%, depending on color-coded valve used.	*Advantages* • Precise percentages of oxygen can be delivered to individualize therapy to meet specific patient's needs, particularly those with an obstructive respiratory disease. *Disadvantages* • Some patients feel claustrophobic. • Color codes of valves may differ among manufacturers.	• Connect the color-coded valve consistent with the FIO_2 ordered by the primary health-care provider. • Set the oxygen flow rate indicated on the color-coded plastic valve.
Face tent 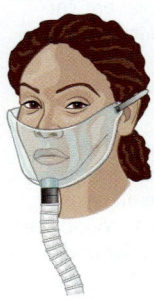	• Delivers oxygen to the nose and mouth via a clear mask that fits under the chin and is open on the top. • *Liter flow:* 8 to 12 L/minute. • *FIO_2:* 30% to 55%.	*Advantages* • Most patients do not feel claustrophobic. • High levels of humidity can be used. *Disadvantages* • Exact levels of oxygen cannot be delivered.	• Monitor pulse oximetry routinely because the percentage of oxygen delivered is not precise.

Figures from Burton and Ludwig (2011). *Fundamentals of nursing care: Concepts, connections & skills.* Philadelphia: F. A. Davis Company, with permission.

Table 19.7 Types of Artificial Airways

Type of Tube	Nursing Care	Illustration
Oropharyngeal • Hard plastic tube that extends from the front of the teeth to the pharynx. • Holds the tongue away from the back of the pharynx. • Used only for patients who are unconscious (often postoperative patients immediately after surgery) because it can precipitate gagging, vomiting, and laryngospasm in conscious patients.	• Begin insertion with the inner curve of the device facing the nose (a). • Rotate the device 180° when the airway reaches the posterior wall of the pharynx (b). • Do not tape the airway in place. • Remove the device as soon as the patient's gag reflex returns.	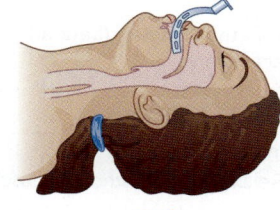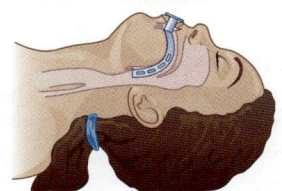
Nasopharyngeal • Flexible tube that extends from the nares to the pharynx. • Provides an avenue for air to enter and exit the lungs. • Used for patients who are semiconscious and at risk for airway obstruction. • Does not stimulate gagging.	• Advance the airway along the floor of the nostril to the posterior pharynx; the outer flange should rest just outside the nostril and the distal tip of the tube in the posterior pharynx, which can be visualized by depressing the patient's tongue with a tongue blade and inspecting the posterior pharynx. • Feel for the passage of air at the outer flange. • Auscultate for bilateral breath sounds. • Remove the tube every 8 hours to assess for mucous membrane irritation and to clean the tube.	
Tracheostomy • Insertion of a tube into the trachea through an incision in the neck. • Provides an airway to bypass an upper airway obstruction. • May be temporary or permanent. • Has three parts: Outer cannula (with or without an inflatable cuff); obturator that fills the blunt end of the outer cannula to promote ease of insertion into the tracheotomy; and inner cannula (disposable or can be cleaned). • Cuff on an outer cannula is inflated to prevent aspiration of fluids or prevent an air leak if the patient is receiving mechanical ventilation; "pillow" expands when cuff is inflated.	• Record the type and size of the tracheostomy tube. • Maintain the outer cannula in place with twill ties or Velcro tracheostomy tube holders. **Tracheostomy Care** • Provide tracheostomy care routinely, at least every 8 hours. • Don clean gloves and remove the dressing under tracheostomy tube and the inner cannula. • Don sterile gloves and replace the inner cannula with a new inner cannula if disposable OR remove the inner cannula and clean with ½ hydrogen peroxide and ½ normal saline solution, rinse with normal saline, and dry the internal lumen with pipe cleaners. • Clean around the stoma with normal saline solution using a cotton-tipped applicator; clean the faceplate of the tracheostomy tube with 4 × 4 gauze dampened with normal saline solution. • Replace the twill ties every 24 hours; do not remove old ties until the new ties are in place. • If the tracheal stoma is permanent, teach the patient to perform self-care, to wear a stoma bib to protect the tracheal opening from debris and warm air, to avoid water-related activities, and to wear a tracheal shield when showering.	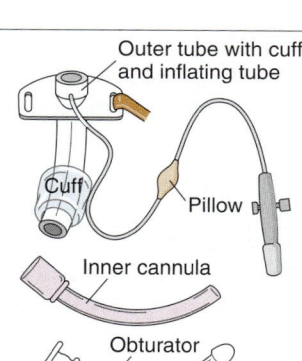 Outer tube with cuff and inflating tube Cuff Pillow Inner cannula Obturator
Endotracheal • Insertion of tube into the trachea through the mouth or nose (intubation). • Provides airway for mechanical ventilation. • Has an inflatable cuff to provide a seal to prevent an air leak when the patient is receiving mechanical ventilation.	• Maintain cuff inflation with minimal occlusive volume to prevent necrosis of the mucous membranes. • Inflate the cuff with the volume of air recommended by the manufacturer; cuff pressure usually is 20 to 25 mm Hg. • Place the stethoscope over the carotid pulse. • Remove 1 mL of air from the cuff at a time until a slight air leak is identified at the height of inhalation. • Reinstill 1 mL of air back into the cuff. • Assess placement of the tube. • Assess for symmetrical chest movements. • Auscultate the bilateral lung fields to ensure the tube has not slipped into the right main bronchus.	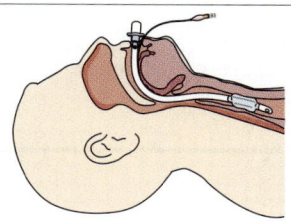

Figures adapted from Wilkinson and Treas (2011). *Fundamentals of nursing*, Vol. 2, 2nd ed. Philadelphia: F. A. Davis Company, with permission; and from Burton and Ludwig (2011). *Fundamentals of nursing care: Concepts, connections & skills*. Philadelphia: F. A. Davis Company, with permission.

Table 19.8 Medications That Affect the Respiratory System

Mechanism of Action	Examples	Nontherapeutic Effects
Bronchodilators		
Sympathomimetics (beta-adrenergic agonists) • Stimulate beta receptors to dilate bronchioles.	• albuterol (Proventil) • metaproterenol	• Tachycardia • Tremors • Anxiety
Xanthines • Relax bronchial smooth muscle.	• aminophylline • theophylline	• Tachycardia • Tremors • Anxiety • Nausea and vomiting
Anticholinergics • Decrease action of acetylcholine receptors in bronchial smooth muscle.	• ipratropium (Atrovent) • tiotropium (Spiriva)	• Dizziness • Headache • Palpitations • Nervousness • Dry mouth • Blurred vision • Urinary retention
Leukotriene receptor antagonists • Inhibit leukotriene synthesis or activity. • Minimize inflammation and edema.	• montelukast (Singulair) • zafirlukast (Accolate) • zileuton (Zyflo)	• Headache • Weakness • Nausea and vomiting
Inhaled and nasal route steroids • Decrease inflammatory response and edema.	• budesonide (Pulmicort) • fluticasone (Flovent) • triamcinolone acetonide (Azmacort)	• Headache • Oropharyngeal fungal infections • Dysphonia • Hoarseness • Flulike syndrome (budesonide)
Mast cell stabilizers • Stabilize mast cells to decrease histamine release.	• cromolyn sodium (Intal) • nedocromil (Tilade)	Uncommon but may include: • Hoarseness • Nausea • Dry, irritated throat • Coughing • Bad taste in mouth
Combination agents • Depends on individual action of agents.	• albuterol and ipratropium (Combivent) • budesonide and formoterol (Symbicort) • fluticasone and salmeterol (Advair)	• Headache • Sore throat • Upper respiratory infection • Additional effects depending on individual agents
Expectorants		
• Increase volume and decrease viscosity of respiratory secretions in trachea and bronchi.	• guaifenesin (Mucinex, Robitussin)	Uncommon but may include: • Nausea and vomiting • Headache • Dizziness • Serious allergic reaction (rare): Itching/swelling of face, throat and tongue, rash, severe dizziness, and difficulty breathing
Antitussives		
• Suppress cough reflex.	• codeine • dextromethorphan (DM suffix in cough preparations)	• Sedation at high doses

CASE STUDY: Putting It All Together

A nurse is admitting a 72-year-old obese woman to a medical unit after the patient was stabilized in and transferred from the emergency department. The patient has a history of obstructive airway disease. In addition, she was a smoker (two packs a day for 30 years) but stopped at age 48, had asthma as a child, and was diagnosed with emphysema at age 68. Last month, the patient had an episode of bronchitis. Today, she was exposed to environmental smoke as a result of a house fire in her neighborhood. She tells the admitting nurse, "After breathing the smoke from the fire, I started wheezing, my voice became hoarse, my chest felt tight, and I could barely catch my breath. I used my rescue inhaler several times, but it didn't help, so I came to the hospital. I feel better since they gave me oxygen, a nebulizer treatment, and medications in the emergency department." The nurse reviews the patient's clinical record from the emergency department.

Patient's Clinical Record

Vital Signs

Temperature:	99.6°F orally.
Respirations:	32 breaths/minute, shallow, labored.
Pulse:	115 beats/minute.
Blood pressure:	170/84 mm Hg.

Primary Health-Care Provider's Orders

High-flow humidified oxygen 100% nonrebreather mask.
Chest x-ray.
Complete blood count.
Basic metabolic panel.
EKG.
Carboxy hemoglobin level (carbon monoxide level in the blood).
Support orthopneic/tripod position.
dexamethasone (Decadron) 10 mg, IVPB, every 8 hours.
IVF: 0.9% Sodium Chloride 100 mL/hour.
Albuterol/Atrovent nebulized solution 1 unit dose each via nebulizer mask every 4 hours.
Albuterol nebulized solution 1 unit dose via nebulizer mask every 2 hours, prn for breakthrough wheezing or respiratory distress.

Assessments on Admission to the Emergency Department

Oxygen saturation 86%.
Patient is restless.
Sitting on the side of the bed, leaning forward, and resting arms on a pillow on the overbed table.
Circumoral pallor; capillary refill of toenails delayed;
    4 seconds.
Reported shortness of breath and fatigue.
Subclavicular retractions noted on inspiration.
Stridor on inspiration.

Continued

CASE STUDY: Putting It All Together *cont'd*

Case Study Questions

A. Which assessment noted on the patient's clinical record from the emergency department should cause the nurse the most concern and why?

_____

B. Identify nine signs and symptoms of impaired respiratory function for which the nurse should assess the patient.

1. _____
2. _____
3. _____
4. _____
5. _____
6. _____
7. _____
8. _____
9. _____

C. Identify five factors that placed this patient at risk for a problem with pulmonary function and explain why.

1. _____
2. _____
3. _____
4. _____
5. _____

D. Identify at least ten independent nursing actions the nurse should implement when caring for this patient.

1. _____
2. _____
3. _____
4. _____
5. _____
6. _____
7. _____
8. _____
9. _____
10. _____

REVIEW QUESTIONS

1. An unconscious patient has excessive oral secretions. In which position should the nurse place the patient to help prevent aspiration?
   1. Sims'
   2. Supine
   3. Fowler
   4. Contour

2. A nurse is to perform a purified protein derivative (PPD) test on a patient who was exposed to a person with the diagnosis of tuberculosis. What are essential nursing interventions related to this test? **Select all that apply.**
   1. _____ Encircle the injection site with an indelible pen.
   2. _____ Identify if the patient is taking an immunosuppressant.
   3. _____ Determine if the patient had a previous positive reaction.
   4. _____ Inject the purified protein derivative via an intradermal injection.
   5. _____ Explain that the results must be evaluated within twenty-four hours.

3. A patient is scheduled to have pulmonary function tests. What should the nurse instruct the patient to do before the test?
   1. Avoid smoking for 6 hours before the test.
   2. Take a bronchodilator 1 hour before the test.
   3. Abstain from food for 2 hours before the test.
   4. Drink 8 oz of water immediately before the test.

4. A nurse documents that a patient is experiencing Kussmaul respirations. What observations about the patient's respirations did the nurse make to come to this conclusion?
   1. More than twenty breaths/minute
   2. Increased rate and depth of respirations
   3. Varying depths of respirations, generally shallow, alternating with periods of apnea
   4. Gradual increase in depth of inhalations, followed by a gradual decrease, and then a period of apnea

5. An older adult patient asks a nurse, "Why am I experiencing more frequent respiratory tract infections now that I am older?" Which information about the aging process should the nurse include in a response to the patient's question? **Select all that apply.**
   1. _____ Thoracic and expiratory muscles are weaker.
   2. _____ There is an increase in the cough and laryngeal reflexes.
   3. _____ Vital capacity increases as the residual volume decreases.
   4. _____ The rib cage becomes more rigid due to calcification of costal cartilage.
   5. _____ Decreased mobility associated with aging causes less effective gas exchange.

6. A nurse is caring for a patient with a bacterial infection of the lungs. What type of sputum should the nurse anticipate the patient to expectorate?
   1. Yellow-green
   2. Clear white
   3. Pink frothy
   4. Red rust

7. A nurse is monitoring a patient's respiratory status. What should the nurse instruct the patient to do when teaching about the use of the device in the photograph?

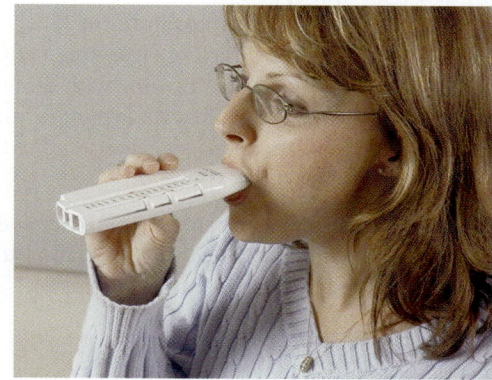

   1. "Inhale and exhale normally."
   2. "Hold the inhalation for several seconds."
   3. "First fully inflate your lungs before you exhale fully."
   4. "Inhale slowly and as deeply as possible through the mouthpiece."

8. A nurse is caring for a patient who is experiencing a laryngeal spasm. For which clinical indicator should the nurse assess the patient?
   1. Stridor
   2. Wheeze
   3. Crackles
   4. Rhonchi

9. Which independent nursing actions are associated with caring for a patient who is experiencing hypoxemia? **Select all that apply.**
   1. _____ Elevate the head of the bed.
   2. _____ Attach a pulse oximeter to the patient's finger.
   3. _____ Remain calm and speak in a normal tone of voice.
   4. _____ Administer oxygen at 4 L/minute via a nonrebreather mask.
   5. _____ Encourage the patient to cough when the patient has secretions.

10. A nurse is caring for a patient requiring continuous pulse oximetry. What should the nurse do when using this monitoring device?
    1. Explain that the test is noninvasive but may cause discomfort.
    2. Dampen the site slightly before applying the sensor.
    3. Ensure that capillary refill is more than 4 seconds.
    4. Change the site of the device every 2 hours.

11. An older adult comes to the clinic reporting shortness of breath and yellow mucus. What factors in the patient's history may have contributed to this situation? **Select all that apply.**
    1. _____ Has a body mass index of 35
    2. _____ Smokes 1 pack of cigarettes a day
    3. _____ Drinks 1 glass of wine with dinner
    4. _____ Takes a 2-mile walk every morning
    5. _____ Reports eating a vegetarian diet for the last 3 years

12. A nurse identifies that a patient is experiencing exertional dyspnea. Difficulty breathing in relation to what behavior led the nurse to this conclusion?
    1. Eating
    2. Exercise
    3. Lying down
    4. Leaning forward while sitting

13. A nurse is teaching a patient how to use a vibratory positive expiratory pressure device to facilitate expectoration of respiratory secretions. What should the nurse teach the patient to do to ensure an expected outcome?
    1. Sit in a chair with the chin tilted slightly toward the chest.
    2. Forcefully inhale 50% of a usual breath and hold it for 3 seconds.
    3. Place the mouthpiece in the mouth with the lips firmly around the stem while keeping the cheeks relaxed.
    4. Complete the procedure with 2 additional breaths using the device but inhale fully and exhale forcefully with each breath.

14. When a nurse is performing a physical assessment, the patient reports feeling short of breath. For what signs of dyspnea should the nurse assess the patient? **Select all that apply.**
    1. _____ Pursed-lip breathing
    2. _____ Supraclavicular retractions
    3. _____ Grunting just before exhaling
    4. _____ Oxygen saturation level of 96%
    5. _____ Respiratory rate of 20 breaths per minute

15. A patient who had been in a house fire is experiencing a productive cough. What color should the nurse expect the patient's sputum to exhibit?
    1. Yellow
    2. White
    3. Black
    4. Red

16. A nurse must obtain a sputum specimen from a patient with an endotracheal tube. Place the following steps in the order in which they should be performed.
    1. Verify the order and wash the hands.
    2. Don a protective eye shield and sterile gloves.
    3. Apply suction when the patient coughs or when meeting resistance.
    4. Lubricate the catheter tip with normal saline and advance it into the endotracheal tube.
    5. Remove the catheter and attach the tubing on the specimen container to the attached adapter.
    Answer: _____

17. A nurse is auscultating a patient's breath sounds. What action should the nurse employ?
    1. Place the patient in the supine position.
    2. Instruct the patient to breathe in through the nose.
    3. Keep the stethoscope at each site for at least one minute.
    4. Identify the breath sound heard before moving to the next site.

18. When auscultating breath sounds the nurse identifies the presence of stridor. What should the nurse do?
    1. Notify the primary health-care provider immediately.
    2. Plan to reassess the patient in one hour.
    3. Implement oropharyngeal suctioning.
    4. Arrange for an x-ray examination.

19. A patient arrives in the emergency department with portable oxygen at 3 liters/minute via nasal cannula. The nurse in the emergency department obtains the patient's health history and vital signs and performs a focused physical assessment.

Patient's Clinical Record

Health History From Spouse

68-year-old man, lives with wife.
60-year history of asthma, 10-year history of emphysema.
Gave up smoking 3 years ago because of progressive shortness of breath.
For years he has been using oxygen 2 liters/minute via nasal cannula whenever the shortness of breath intensifies.
Patient has had a cold for 5 days and has been using the oxygen without relief.
Wife increased the oxygen to 3 L/minute 6 hours ago.
Patient has been lethargic all day; when he had profuse sweating, the wife brought him to the emergency department.

Vital Signs

Temperature: 100.2°F orally.
Pulse: 92 beats/minute, regular.
Respirations: 10 breaths/minute, shallow, regular.
Blood Pressure: 150/88 mm Hg.

Focused Physical Assessment

Reports feeling drowsy and dizzy.
Confused and unable to report recent facts concerning his condition.
Exhibiting fine muscle twitching (fasciculations).
Auscultation reveals bilateral rhonchi and wheezes.
Oxygen saturation: 84%.

What should the nurse do **first** based on this information?
1. Walk the patient from the triage area to a bed.
2. Reduce the oxygen flow rate to 2 liters per minute.
3. Increase the oxygen flow rate to 6 liters per minute.
4. Encourage the patient to perform pursed lip breathing.

20. A nurse is caring for a patient who is to have an oropharyngeal tube in place while recovering from general anesthesia. Which nursing action is associated with this tube?
1. Secure the tube in position by taping it in place.
2. Remove the tube occasionally to assess for irritation of the nose.
3. Begin the tube's insertion with the inner curve facing the tongue.
4. Rotate the tube 180 degrees when it reaches the end wall of the pharynx.

21. A patient with chronic obstructive pulmonary disease (COPD) who is receiving 2 L/minute of oxygen via nasal cannula has dyspnea and is using accessory muscles of respiration to breathe. The patient's oxygen saturation is 88 percent. Place the following actions in order that they should be performed beginning with what the nurse should do **first**.
1. Obtain the patient's vital signs.
2. Teach the patient pursed-lip breathing.
3. Place the patient in the high-Fowler position.
4. Inform the patient's primary health-care provider.
5. Monitor the patient's pulse oximetry level continuously.
Answer: _____

22. A patient is admitted to the emergency department after sustaining injuries in an automobile collision. The patient is semiconscious and the nurse is concerned about maintaining the patient's airway while diagnostic tests are completed. Which should the nurse anticipate will be ordered by the primary health-care provider?
1. Endotracheal tube
2. Tracheostomy tube
3. Oropharyngeal tube
4. Nasopharyngeal tube

23. A primary health-care provider orders 60 percent oxygen for a patient. Which oxygen delivery equipment should the nurse use to administer the oxygen to this patient?
1. Nonrebreather mask
2. Nasal cannula
3. Venturi mask
4. Face tent

24. A nurse must perform nasopharyngeal suctioning. Place the following actions in the order in which they should be performed.
1. Don sterile gloves.
2. Open the suction kit.
3. Lubricate the suction catheter tip.
4. Place the patient in the high-Fowler position.
5. Insert suction catheter into the patient's nasopharynx.
6. Determine the distance between the patient's nose and earlobe with the catheter.
Answer: _____

25. A primary health-care provider orders oxygen 4 L/minute via nasal cannula. What nursing action is essential?
1. Position the prongs in the patient's nares so that they curve upward.
2. Secure elastic straps around the patient's head.
3. Ensure that the oxygen is humidified.
4. Provide oral hygiene every shift.

26. A nurse is caring for a patient receiving intermittent enteral feedings. Which nursing intervention should the nurse implement to reduce the risk of aspiration?
1. Hold the feeding if the residual exceeds the indicated parameter.
2. Keep the head of the bed elevated 30° at all times.
3. Suction the patient before initiating the feeding.
4. Thicken the formula with a thickening solution.

27. A nurse is planning a class for parents about how they can reduce the risk of their toddlers experiencing an airway obstruction. Which information should the nurse include in the program? **Select all that apply.**
1. _____ Cut hot dogs into small pieces.
2. _____ Do not give toddlers marshmallows.
3. _____ Teach a toddler the universal sign for choking.
4. _____ Ensure that toys are larger than a clenched fist.
5. _____ Store plastic bags where they cannot be reached by small children.

28. A nurse is caring for an adult patient with excessive respiratory secretions. What should the nurse do when suctioning this patient?
1. Set the wall pressure at approximately 60 mm Hg.
2. Evaluate breath sounds after the procedure.
3. Place the patient in a lateral position.
4. Use a sterile 8 French catheter.

29. A nurse is caring for a patient with a history of chronic obstructive pulmonary disease. Which is the **most** important nursing action when administering oxygen via a nasal cannula to this patient?
1. Assess the ears for irritation due to the oxygen tubing.
2. Hang an "oxygen in use" sign near the patient's bed.
3. Monitor the patient's oxygen saturation routinely.
4. Limit oxygen flow rate to 2 L/minute.

30. A primary health-care provider orders 100 percent oxygen for a patient experiencing respiratory difficulty. Which type of oxygen mask should the nurse use when implementing this order?
1.

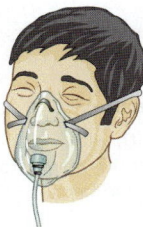

2.

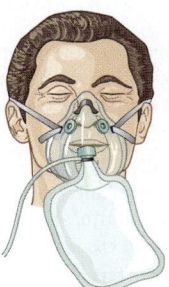

3.

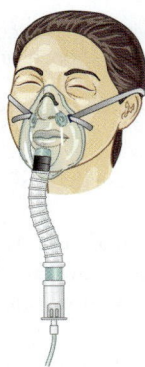

4.

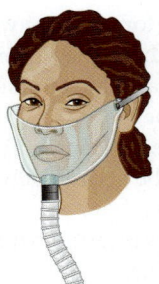

31. A patient has a respiratory rate of 24 breaths/minute and is having shortness of breath. What should the nurse do **first**?
    1. Administer 100% oxygen.
    2. Obtain an oxygen saturation level.
    3. Elevate the head of the patient's bed to a 60-degree angle.
    4. Inform the primary health-care provider of the patient's status.

32. A nurse is admitting a patient to a unit from the emergency department. The nurse reviews the patient's clinical record and assesses the patient.

Patient's Clinical Record

Vital Signs

Temperature: 104°F rectally.
Pulse: 100 beats/minute and regular.
Respirations: 17 breaths/minute and shallow.
Blood pressure: 138/88 mm Hg.

Transfer Nurse's Note 10-9-2013 1330

Patient transferred to room via stretcher from the emergency department with side rails raised. Patient in semi-Fowler position, skin appears flushed and patient is diaphoretic. Patient states that she feels warm, has no pain but is very sleepy. IV in right hand set at ordered rate of 125 mL/hour. IV in left hand is an intravenous lock. Both IVs are dry and intact, no clinical indicators of infiltration or inflammation noted. Patient attempted to void on a bedpan but was unsuccessful. Has not voided since 1030. Oxygen running at 2 L/minute via nasal cannula. Tylenol 650 mg administered at 1300.

Primary Health-Care Provider's Orders 10-9-2013

1. Bedrest.
2. Regular diet.
3. Vital signs every 4 hours.
4. I&O.
5. Tylenol 650 mg PO every 4 hours prn for temperature 101.2°F.
6. IVF 1000 mL 0.45% NaCl with 20 mEq KCl at 125 mL/hour.
7. Oxygen 2 L via nasal cannula.

What concern should be the priority?
1. Urinary retention
2. Respiratory status
3. Increased temperature
4. Potential for dehydration

33. A patient has a respiratory rate of 24 with mild labored breathing. The nurse raises the head of the patient's bed, but the patient's breathing does not improve. What should be the nurse's **next** action?
    1. Perform cupping and clapping on the patient's back.
    2. Call the patient's primary health-care provider.
    3. Obtain a pulse oximetry level and vital signs.
    4. Administer one hundred percent oxygen.

34. A nurse is caring for a patient receiving a steroidal nasal spray. For which nontherapeutic effect should the nurse assess the patient?
    1. Dry mouth
    2. Blurred vision
    3. Urinary retention
    4. Oral fungal infection

35. A patient has a respiratory infection and the primary health-care provider prescribes ciprofloxacin (Cipro) 400 mg IVPB every 8 hours. The vial of ciprofloxacin states that there is 50 mg per mL. How many mL should be obtained to prepare the prescribed IVPB? Record your answer using a whole number.
    Answer: _____ mL

1. ANSWER: 1.
Rationales:
1. The Sims' position is the most effective position to prevent aspiration, particularly in an unconscious patient because excessive oral secretions will drain out of the side of the mouth. In addition, this position will be easy to maintain in a patient who is unconscious.
2. The supine position will not aid in the prevention of aspiration because lying on the back will promote the flow of secretions to the back of the oropharynx and trachea.
3. The Fowler position may assist in the prevention of aspiration but will not be as effective another position. In addition, an unconscious patient may have difficulty maintaining the Fowler position.
4. The contour position will have minimal effect in preventing aspiration because the head will not be elevated enough. In addition, an unconscious patient may have difficulty maintaining this position.
TEST-TAKING TIP: Identify the equally plausible options. Options 3 and 4 are equally plausible because both positions elevate the head of the bed and position the body in a sitting position.
Content Area: Oxygenation
Integrated Processes: Nursing Process: Implementation
Client Need: Physiological Integrity; Physiological Adaptation
Cognitive Level: Application

2. ANSWER: 1, 2, 3, 4.
Rationales:
1. This ensures that the appropriate site is evaluated.
2. Immunosuppressants can cause a false-positive result.
3. A severe reaction may occur when the purified protein derivative (PPD) is injected into a patient who had a previous positive reaction; the patient has been immunosensitized.
4. The intradermal route is used for this test. The allergen is injected just below the epidermis where a reaction will be able to be observed.
5. This will result in an inaccurate evaluation. The site of the intradermal injection of PPD should be evaluated within 48 to 72 hours after the PPD is injected.
TEST-TAKING TIP: Identify the clang association. The words *purified protein derivative* in the stem and in option 4 is a clang association. Examine option 4 carefully because, more often than not, an option with a clang association is a correct answer.
Content Area: Oxygenation
Integrated Processes: Nursing Process: Implementation
Client Need: Physiological Integrity; Reduction of Risk Potential
Cognitive Level: Analysis

3. ANSWER: 1.
Rationales:
1. Smoking constricts the bronchi and bronchioles, which will cause inaccurate test results; therefore, the patient should be instructed to avoid smoking for 6 hours before the test.
2. This should be done when advised to do so only by the primary health-care provider. Medications that influence the respiratory tract may invalidate test results.

3. It is not necessary to abstain from food for any length of time before the test.
4. It is not necessary to drink fluid before the test.
Content Area: Oxygenation
Integrated Processes: Communication/Documentation; Nursing Process: Implementation
Client Need: Physiological Integrity; Reduction of Risk Potential
Cognitive Level: Application

4. ANSWER: 2.
Rationales:
1. This is tachypnea. Respirations should be between 12 to 20 breaths/minute, have a regular rhythm, and be unlabored.
2. This is Kussmaul respirations.
3. This is Biot respirations.
4. This is Cheyne-Stokes respirations.
TEST-TAKING TIP: Identify the clang associations. The word *respirations* in the stem and in options 2 and 3 are clang associations. Examine these options carefully.
Content Area: Oxygenation
Integrated Processes: Communication/Documentation; Nursing Process: Assessment
Client Need: Physiological Integrity; Reduction of Risk Potential
Cognitive Level: Analysis

5. ANSWER: 1, 4, 5.
Rationales:
1. This is true. There is a loss of muscle tone due to a more sedentary life style and an increase in thoracic rigidity as one ages.
2. The opposite is true. As one ages there is an increase in airway resistance, a loss of muscle tone, and a reduced elastic recoil in the lungs and thoracic muscles, which all contribute to a decrease in the cough and laryngeal reflexes.
3. The opposite is true. As the residual volume increases, the vital capacity decreases with aging.
4. This is true. With less lung expansion, the risk of respiratory infection increases. This is due to insufficient lung inflation and decreased ability to expel foreign or accumulated material.
5. This is true. A more sedentary life style associated with aging causes less effective gas exchange and decreased lung inflation, increasing the risk of respiratory infection.
Content Area: Oxygenation
Integrated Processes: Communication/Documentation; Nursing Process: Planning
Client Need: Health Promotion and Maintenance
Cognitive Level: Application

6. ANSWER: 1.
Rationales:
1. Yellow-green colored sputum is associated with bacterial infections. It consists of cellular debris, phagocytic cells, and microorganisms.
2. Clear white colored sputum is associated with viral infections.
3. Frothy sputum is associated with fluid in the lung due to pulmonary edema. The pink color is related to blood in the sputum.

4. Red rust colored sputum is associated with the presence of blood (hemoptysis).
Content Area: Oxygenation
Integrated Processes: Nursing Process: Analysis
Client Need: Physiological Integrity; Reduction of Risk Potential
Cognitive Level: Application

7. **ANSWER: 3**
Rationales:
1. This is not the correct way to use this device.
2. This instruction is associated with a nebulizer treatment, not the device in the photograph. Holding the inhalation for several seconds when using a nebulizer facilitates longer contact of the fine mist of a nebulized drug to be in contact with the alveoli.
3. **This device is used to monitor peak expiratory flow rates. The patient should exhale fully into the peak flowmeter after fully inflating the lungs with a deep breath. It measures in liters per minute the volume of air a person can exhale after fully inflating the lungs.**
4. This instruction is associated with an incentive spirometer, not the device in the photograph. An incentive spirometer promotes deep breathing, stimulates coughing to help remove mucus from the respiratory system, and prevents atelectasis.
TEST-TAKING TIP: Identify the options that are opposites. Options 1 and 3 are opposites. More often than not, an option that is an opposite is the correct answer. Examine these options carefully.
Content Area: Oxygenation
Integrated Processes: Teaching/Learning; Nursing Process: Implementation
Client Need: Physiological Integrity; Physiological Adaptation
Cognitive Level: Analysis

8. **ANSWER: 1.**
Rationales:
1. **Laryngeal spasm is characterized by stridor, which is a high-pitched crowning sound more prominent during expiration; it is caused by constriction of the larynx.**
2. A wheeze is a high-pitched, musical sound that may be heard more prominently during expiration. It is associated with narrowing of small airways by spasms, inflammatory processes, mucus accumulation, or tumors.
3. Crackles, also known as rales, are fine, medium, or coarse sounds caused by air bubbling through moisture in the alveoli. It is associated with inflammation due to such conditions as pneumonia, bronchitis, hypervolemia due to congestive heart failure, or emphysema.
4. Rhonchi, also known as a sonorous wheeze, is a loud, coarse, low-pitched sound heard during inspiration and/or expiration. It may be cleared by coughing. It is associated with inflammation due to bronchitis, narrowed airways, alterations in structure or function associated with emphysema, and fibrotic lungs.
Content Area: Oxygenation
Integrated Processes: Nursing Process: Implementation
Client Need: Physiological Integrity; Reduction of Risk Potential
Cognitive Level: Application

9. **ANSWER: 1, 2, 3, 5.**
Rationales:
1. Elevating the head of the bed is an independent nursing action. It does not require an order from a primary health-care provider. Raising the head of the bed uses gravity to move abdominal organs away from the diaphragm, facilitating respirations.
2. This is an independent function of the nurse. The nurse does not need an order from a primary health-care provider to monitor a patient's oxygen saturation level.
3. These are independent functions of the nurse. Impaired oxygenation is a frightening experience. It is important for the nurse to remain calm and not contribute to the patient's fear and/or anxiety.
4. The nurse can administer 2 L/minute of oxygen by nasal cannula in an emergency without an order from a primary health-care provider. Other oxygen delivery systems, such as a nonrebreather mask or elevating the oxygen level higher than 2 liters per minute, require an order from a primary health-care provider.
5. **Coughing facilitates expulsion of secretions from the respiratory tract. When secretions are cleared from the respiratory tract, more air can be inhaled into the alveoli and carbon dioxide exhaled.**
Content Area: Oxygenation
Integrated Processes: Nursing Process: Implementation
Client Need: Physiological Integrity; Physiological Adaptation
Cognitive Level: Application

10. **ANSWER: 4.**
Rationales:
1. A pulse oximetry sensor does not cause discomfort.
2. The skin should be dry before applying the sensor.
3. Capillary refill should be less than 3 seconds otherwise the test results will not be able to accurately test oxygen saturation because circulation to the area is compromised.
4. **The sensor site should be changed every 2 hours to prevent tissue necrosis from pressure if monitoring is continuous.**
TEST-TAKING TIP: Identify the clang association. The word *device* in the stem and in option 4 is a clang association. Examine option 4 carefully.
Content Area: Oxygenation
Integrated Processes: Nursing Process: Implementation
Client Need: Physiological Integrity; Reduction of Risk Potential
Cognitive Level: Application

11. **ANSWER: 1, 2.**
Rationales:
1. A body mass index more than 30 increases the risk for respiratory problems because abdominal adipose tissue limits chest expansion and gas exchange in the alveoli.
2. Tobacco smoke contains tars, toxins, and nicotine. Tars and toxins irritate the mucous membranes of the respiratory system making them more vulnerable to disease processes. Nicotine constricts blood vessels, which impairs oxygenation of body tissues.
3. One glass of wine has been reported to promote cardiopulmonary functioning. Excessive intake of alcohol may depress the respiratory center, resulting in hypoventilation and aspiration.

4. Exercise increases the metabolic rate and functioning of the heart and lungs; these responses condition the body, which promotes adaptation to physical stressors.

5. A vegetarian diet provides all the basic nutrients required for a healthy diet. An imbalance of proteins, carbohydrates, and fats may reduce the immune system and impair cellular functioning.

Content Area: Oxygenation
Integrated Processes: Communication/Documentation; Nursing Process: Assessment
Client Need: Health Promotion and Maintenance
Cognitive Level: Analysis

12. **ANSWER: 2.**
Rationales:

1. Although a full stomach impedes contraction of the diaphragm and expansion of the thoracic cavity, its relationship to dyspnea is not known as exertional dyspnea.

2. Exercise increases the metabolic rate causing an increase in the heart and respiratory rates. Exertion increases the demand for oxygen; when the body cannot meet the demand for oxygen, difficulty breathing results and is known as exertional dyspnea.

3. Difficulty breathing when lying down necessitating having to sit up to breathe is known as orthopnea.

4. Leaning forward when sitting in an effort to expand the thoracic cavity is a sign of difficulty breathing but is not known as exertional dyspnea; it is known as using the orthopneic or tripod position to facilitate breathing.

TEST-TAKING TIP: Identify the word in the stem that is a clang association. The word *exertional* in the stem and *exercise* in option 2 are associated and is an obscure clang association.

Content Area: Oxygenation
Integrated Processes: Nursing Process: Analysis
Client Need: Physiological Integrity; Reduction of Risk Potential
Cognitive Level: Application

13. **ANSWER: 4.**
Rationales:

1. The patient should sit in a chair with the head slightly tilted upward. This position facilitates movement of gases in and out of the upper airway and pharynx.

2. The patient should slowly, not forcefully, inhale 75 percent, not 50 percent, of a usual breath and then hold the breath for 2 to 3 seconds.

3. Although the lips should be firmly around the stem, the cheeks should be kept stiff because this allows the airways to vibrate rather than the cheeks during the procedure.

4. This is the correct way to end the procedure. This helps to clear the lower airways once the upper airways are treated.

TEST-TAKING TIP: Identify the clang association. The word *device* in the stem and in option 4 is a clang association. Examine option 4 carefully.

Content Area: Oxygenation
Integrated Processes: Teaching/Learning; Nursing Process: Implementation
Client Need: Physiological Integrity; Reduction of Risk Potential
Cognitive Level: Application

14. **ANSWER: 1, 2, 3.**
Rationales:

1. Making the opening to the mouth smaller during exhalation slows the flow of air out of the respiratory tract, which keeps the alveoli open longer for gas exchange and limits the collapse of small air passages that trap air in the respiratory tract.

2. Retractions reflect the use of accessory muscles of respiration, indicating the need for an increased effort to bring air into the respiratory tract.

3. Closing the glottis at the height of inspiration keeps air in the alveoli slightly longer, which promotes gas exchange in the alveolar capillary beds. A grunt results when the glottis opens during exhalation, as air passes through the vocal cords.

4. This value is within expected limits. The expected value for oxygen saturation is 95 to 100 percent.

5. The expected respiratory rate is 12 to 20 breaths/minute; in addition, it should have a regular rhythm and be unlabored.

Content Area: Oxygenation
Integrated Processes: Nursing Process: Assessment
Client Need: Physiological Integrity; Reduction of Risk Potential
Cognitive Level: Application

15. **ANSWER: 3.**
Rationales:

1. Yellow and yellowish-green sputum are associated with bacterial infections.

2. White sputum most often is associated with viral infections.

3. Black sputum is associated with exposure to a fire because of the inhalation of smoke.

4. Red sputum reflects blood in the sputum (hemoptysis), which is associated with conditions such as pneumococcal pneumonia and pulmonary edema.

Content Area: Oxygenation
Integrated Processes: Nursing Process: Analysis
Client Need: Physiological Integrity; Reduction of Risk Potential
Cognitive Level: Application

16. **ANSWER: 1, 2, 4, 3, 5.**
Rationales:

1. Dependent functions of the nurse require an order from an individual with a prescriptive license. Washing the hands limits the transmission of microorganisms.

2. A protective eye shield protects the nurse in the event the splashing of body fluids occurs during the procedure. Wearing sterile gloves maintains the sterility of the catheter that is inserted into the patient's endotracheal tube and the sterility of the specimen.

4. Lubricating the tip of the catheter with normal saline limits friction and trauma to the mucous membranes of the respiratory tract. Inserting the catheter into the endotracheal tube accesses the trachea where sputum can be obtained.

3. The catheter must be advanced to where sputum can be obtained. Coughing mobilizes sputum, facilitating its removal, and resistance indicates that it has reached the carina of the trachea.

5. The catheter should be removed slowly and the tubing secured to seal the specimen in the collection receptacle.

Content Area: Oxygenation
Integrated Processes: Nursing Process: Planning
Client Need: Physiological Integrity; Reduction of Risk Potential
Cognitive Level: Analysis

17. **ANSWER: 4.**
Rationales:
1. The patient should be placed in a sitting position so that the anterior and posterior aspects of the chest are accessible for auscultation.
2. The patient should be instructed to breathe in through the mouth; this reduces the friction associated with air passing through the nasal passages and allows a larger volume of air to enter the lungs.
3. This is not necessary and would prolong the assessment that could result in hyperventilation and fatigue.
4. **Each site should be assessed long enough to detect the presence of expected and abnormal breath sounds. The characteristics of the sounds, such as pitch and presence of fluid, length of inhalation and exhalation, and appropriateness of the sounds heard at the site, should be assessed.**
TEST-TAKING TIP: Identify the clang association. The words *breath sounds* in the stem and *breath sound* in option 4 is a clang association.
Content Area: Oxygenation
Integrated Processes: Nursing Process: Implementation
Client Need: Health Promotion and Maintenance
Cognitive Level: Application

18. **ANSWER: 1.**
Rationales:
1. **Stridor is caused by narrowing of the larynx and/or trachea, which may be life threatening. The patient needs immediate medical supervision.**
2. This will allow the patient's condition to get progressively worse; this intervention does not meet the needs of the patient.
3. Suctioning the patient experiencing laryngospasm is contraindicated. The problem is not excessive secretions. Suctioning a patient experiencing stridor may exacerbate the laryngospasm, precipitating total obstruction of the airway.
4. This will delay medical attention, and the delay may compromise the patient's physical status. Stridor involves narrowing of the larynx, while an x-ray examination focuses on lung tissue.
TEST-TAKING TIP: Identify the options that are opposites. Options 1 and 2 are opposites because option 2 delays doing something for one hour and option 1 does something immediately. Look at these options carefully; more often than not, one of the opposite options is the correct answer.
Content Area: Oxygenation
Integrated Processes: Communication/Documentation; Nursing Process: Implementation
Client Need: Safe and Effective Care Environment; Management of Care
Cognitive Level: Application

19. **ANSWER: 2.**
Rationales:
1. Activity will increase the metabolic rate and the demand for oxygen. The patient should be transferred via a wheelchair. Sitting in a wheelchair promotes thoracic expansion because the diaphragm can expand downward without the abdominal organs compressing against the diaphragm. When transferred to a bed the patient should be maintained in the high-Fowler position.
2. **The patient probably is experiencing carbon dioxide narcosis (CO_2 narcosis). Because a person with emphysema has chronically increased carbon dioxide levels (the usual stimulus to breathe in a healthy person), a person with emphysema responds to decreased oxygen levels as the stimulus to breathe. Therefore, the stimulus to breathe decreases when excessive oxygen is administered to a person with emphysema. In addition, with an increase in exogenous oxygen, there is an increase in the degree to which diseased alveoli are perfused with blood relative to other less diseased alveoli, resulting in a larger fraction of blood passing through parts of the lung that are poorly ventilated, which results in retained carbon dioxide. The primary health-care provider should be notified immediately because arterial blood gases may be drawn and the oxygen level lowered even more until the problem is corrected.**
3. Administering additional oxygen is contraindicated. This will further complicate this patient's problem.
4. Although this should eventually be done, it is not the primary nursing intervention. Exhaling through the mouth with the lips positioned to create a small opening to prolong exhalation (pursed-lip breathing) keeps the alveoli open longer for gas exchange and more efficient exhalation of trapped air.
TEST-TAKING TIP: Identify the word in the stem that sets a priority. The word *first* in the stem sets a priority. Identify the options with a clang association. The word *liters* in the stem and in options 2 and 3 are clang associations. Identify the options that are opposites. Options 2 and 3 are opposites. Consider these options carefully. Often times, one of the opposite options is the correct answer.
Content Area: Oxygenation
Integrated Processes: Nursing Process: Implementation
Client Need: Physiological Integrity; Physiological Adaptation
Cognitive Level: Analysis

20. **ANSWER: 4.**
Rationales:
1. An oropharyngeal tube should not be taped in place. As the gag reflex returns, the patient will attempt to spit out the tube. If it is taped in place and the gag reflex returns, it may cause retching, laryngospasm, vomiting, and aspiration.
2. An oropharyngeal tube is positioned in the mouth, not the nose. A nasopharyngeal tube is inserted in the nose and extends from the nares to the pharynx. A nasopharyngeal tube is used for patients who are semiconscious and are at risk for airway obstruction because it does not stimulate gagging and vomiting.
3. The tube should initially be inserted with the inner curve of the device facing the nose, not the tongue. This

avoids potential occlusion of the airway. If the curve is facing the tongue, it could push the tongue to the rear of the mouth, occluding the airway.

4. The tube should be rotated from the curve facing the nose 180 degrees into place with the curve facing the tongue.

TEST-TAKING TIP: Identify the unique option. Option 4 is unique. It is the only option with a number.

Content Area: Oxygenation
Integrated Processes: Nursing Process: Implementation
Client Need: Physiological Integrity; Physiological Adaptation
Cognitive Level: Application

21. ANSWER: 3, 1, 2, 4, 5.
Rationales:
3. Placing a patient in the high-Fowler position will lower the abdominal viscera, thus allowing the lungs to expand more effectively. Relieving distress is the priority.
1. Obtaining the patients vital signs is important but should be performed after implementing an intervention that may relieve the patient's current distress.
2. Teaching the patient pursed-lip breathing will help the patient exhale more slowly, which will keep the alveoli expanded and prevent collapse of the bronchioles. This is done after an initial intervention to relieve the distress and collect more data. Teaching the patient pursed-lip breathing may take a little time.
4. The patient is the priority. Informing the patient's health-care provider about the patient's status will be necessary after attempts to alleviate the patient's distress are instituted first.
5. The nurse already knows that the patient's oxygen saturation is 88 percent. After performing essential nursing interventions to improve the patient's physical status, the nurse should continue to monitor the patient's oxygen saturation level. This will provide data about the patient's response to care or identify a progressive deterioration of the patient's respiratory status.

Content Area: Oxygenation
Integrated Processes: Nursing Process: Planning
Client Need: Physiological Integrity; Physiological Adaptation
Cognitive Level: Application

22. ANSWER: 4.
Rationales:
1. This tube is inappropriate in this situation. An endotracheal tube has an inflatable cuff to provide a seal, preventing an air leak when a patient is receiving mechanical ventilation.
2. This tube is inappropriate in this situation. A tracheostomy tube is used for a patient with an upper airway obstruction. This tube is surgically inserted and circumvents an obstruction. It can be temporary or permanent.
3. An oropharyngeal tube is contraindicated for a semiconscious patient because it may stimulate gagging, laryngospasm, vomiting, and aspiration.
4. This is the most appropriate tube for the patient in this situation. It maintains the airway without stimulating a gag reflex.

Content Area: Oxygenation
Integrated Processes: Nursing Process: Planning
Client Need: Physiological Integrity; Physiological Adaptation
Cognitive Level: Application

23. ANSWER: 3.
Rationales:
1. This is not the appropriate oxygen delivery system to deliver 60 percent oxygen to the patient. A nonrebreather mask delivers 70 to 100 percent oxygen, depending on the oxygen liter flow rate.
2. This is not the appropriate oxygen delivery system to deliver 60 percent oxygen to the patient. A nasal cannula delivers 24 to 44 percent oxygen, depending on the oxygen liter flow rate.
3. This is the appropriate mask to deliver 60 percent oxygen to a patient. A Venturi mask delivers 24 to 60 percent oxygen, depending on the oxygen liter flow rate and plastic valve used.
4. This is not the appropriate oxygen delivery system to deliver 60 percent oxygen to the patient. A face tent delivers 30 to 55 percent oxygen, depending on the oxygen liter flow rate.

Content Area: Oxygenation
Integrated Processes: Nursing Process: Implementation
Client Need: Physiological Integrity; Physiological Adaptation
Cognitive Level: Analysis

24. ANSWER: 4, 2, 1, 6, 3, 5.
Rationales:
4. Placing the patient in the high-Fowler position will facilitate nasal cannula insertion and allow for thoracic expansion during suctioning. This should be done before donning sterile gloves.
2. Opening the suction kit should be done before donning sterile gloves because the outside of the kit is not sterile.
1. Donning sterile gloves should be done after opening the suction kit to allow the nurse to handle the kit's contents, which are sterile.
6. Determining the distance between the patient's ear and nose with the catheter should be done before lubricating the catheter tip to avoid having the lubricant drip on the patient or the catheter becoming contaminated. This measurement ensures that the catheter will reach the patient's nasopharyngeal area to aspirate secretions.
3. Lubricating the catheter tip must be done to facilitate insertion of the catheter into the patient's nares; it reduces friction and trauma to the mucous membranes.
5. Inserting the suction catheter should be done after the above steps have been completed.

Content Area: Oxygenation
Integrated Processes: Nursing Process: Planning
Client Need: Physiological Integrity; Physiological Adaptation
Cognitive Level: Analysis

25. ANSWER: 3.
Rationales:
1. The curved prongs should be positioned in the nose with the curve facing downward. This follows the natural curve of the internal pathway of the nose.

2. A nasal cannula oxygen delivery system does not include elastic straps. The tubing of a nasal cannula is wrapped around the ears and the slider is positioned under the chin.

3. An oxygen flow rate higher than 3 L/minute can dry the mucous membranes. Humidification of oxygen helps minimize drying of the mucous membranes.

4. Oral care should be provided every 4 hours because oxygen therapy can dry mucous membranes.

TEST-TAKING TIP: Identify the word in the stem that sets a priority. The word *essential* in the stem sets a priority. Identify the clang association. The word *oxygen* in the stem and in option 3 is a clang association.

Content Area: Oxygenation
Integrated Processes: Nursing Process: Implementation
Client Need: Physiological Integrity; Physiological Adaptation
Cognitive Level: Application

26. **ANSWER: 1.**
    Rationales:
    1. If a residual exceeds the ordered parameter, an enteral feeding is held for 1 hour to allow more time for the patient to digest the previous feeding. After 1 hour, the residual should be checked again.
    2. The head of the bed should be raised to 45° during the feeding and for at least 1 hour after the feeding. This uses the principle of gravity to help keep the solution in the stomach, thereby minimizing the risk of regurgitation and aspiration.
    3. Suctioning should be implemented only when a patient is unable to clear respiratory secretions that are threatening the airway.
    4. Enteral feeding formulas should not be thickened because they may clog the feeding tube.
    TEST-TAKING TIP: Identify the specific determiner. The word *all* in option 2 is a specific determiner. Rarely is an option with a specific determiner the correct answer. Identify the clang associations. The word *feeding* in the stem and in options 1 and 3 are clang associations. Examine these options carefully.

    Content Area: Oxygenation
    Integrated Processes: Nursing Process: Implementation
    Client Need: Physiological Integrity; Basic Care and Comfort
    Cognitive Level: Application

27. **ANSWER: 2, 4, 5.**
    Rationales:
    1. Hot dogs should be avoided, not just cut into small pieces, because the casing is difficult to chew and swallow.
    2. Toddlers should not be given marshmallows because they are sticky and difficult for toddlers to chew and swallow. Marshmallows can obstruct the airway.
    3. This is not an age appropriate instruction; this is unrealistic for a toddler to understand.
    4. Toys should be larger than a clenched fist and have no removable parts; these prevent aspiration and an airway obstruction.
    5. Plastic bags and plastic wrap should be stored out of the reach of young children. A plastic bag or plastic wrap can impair a child's ability to breathe by occluding the

airway, causing hypoxia and death. Also, if a plastic bag is placed over the head, it can cause suffocation (asphyxiation).

Content Area: Oxygenation
Integrated Processes: Teaching/Learning; Nursing Process: Planning
Client Need: Health Promotion and Maintenance
Cognitive Level: Application

28. **ANSWER: 2.**
    Rationales:
    1. Wall suction pressure should be set between 100 and 150 mm Hg for adults, 100 and 120 mm Hg for children, and 50 and 95 mm Hg for infants.
    2. The nurse should assess breath sounds after suctioning to ensure that the patient's airway is patent. In addition, pulse oximetry should be assessed before and after suctioning because it is objective data that reflects arterial blood oxygen saturation. After suctioning, a patient's oxygen saturation level should increase.
    3. A patient should be positioned in a semi- or high-Fowler position when being suctioned. These positions use gravity to move abdominal organs away from the thoracic cavity, facilitating lung expansion.
    4. A 12 to 18 French catheter is used when suctioning an adult. An 8 to 10 French catheter is used when suctioning a child and a 5 to 8 French catheter is used when suctioning an infant. The higher the catheter gauge, the larger the lumen.
    TEST-TAKING TIP: Identify the unique option. Option 2 is unique because it is the only option that involves the evaluation step of the nursing process. Options 1, 2, and 4 all involve interventions associated with suctioning.

    Content Area: Oxygenation
    Integrated Processes: Nursing Process: Implementation
    Client Need: Physiological Integrity; Physiological Adaptation
    Cognitive Level: Application

29. **ANSWER: 4.**
    Rationales:
    1. Although this should be done, it is not the priority.
    2. Although hanging an "oxygen in use" sign is important, it is not the priority.
    3. Although this may be done, it is not a reliable indicator for patients with chronic obstruction pulmonary disease or impaired peripheral circulation. The nurse should assess for signs of carbon dioxide narcosis, such as mental confusion and lethargy.
    4. Do not exceed 2 L/minute for patients with chronic obstructive lung disease because their bodies have become accustomed to increased carbon dioxide levels and their stimulus to breathe is a low oxygen level; assess for signs of carbon dioxide narcosis, such as mental confusion and lethargy.
    TEST-TAKING TIP: Identify the word in the stem that sets a priority. The word *most* in the stem sets a priority.

    Content Area: Oxygenation
    Integrated Processes: Nursing Process: Implementation
    Client Need: Physiological Integrity; Physiological Adaptation
    Cognitive Level: Application

30. ANSWER: 2.
Rationales:
1. This mask will not deliver 100 percent oxygen. This is a simple face mask that is set at 5 to 10 L of oxygen and delivers 40 to 60 percent oxygen.
2. This is a nonrebreather mask that is used to deliver 100 percent oxygen. It has one or two side vents that open only when the patient exhales and remains closed on inspiration. This mask prevents mixing of room air with oxygen and does not allow entry of exhaled air. It can deliver 70 to 100 percent oxygen.
3. This mask will not deliver 100 percent oxygen. This is a Venturi mask. This mask allows for an exact mixing of room air and oxygen so that a specific amount of oxygen is delivered. Valves and oxygen flow rates are used to control the specific percentage of oxygen to be delivered.
4. This mask will not deliver 100 percent oxygen. This is a face tent. It does not deliver an exact amount of oxygen because the top is open; however, it does allow for delivery of high amounts of humidity. Because a face tent does not deliver precise amounts of oxygen, it is essential that the patient's oxygen saturation be assessed.
Content Area: Oxygenation
Integrated Processes: Nursing Process: Implementation
Client Need: Physiological Integrity; Physiological Adaptation
Cognitive Level: Analysis

31. ANSWER: 3.
Rationales:
1. Although oxygen may be needed, it is premature to administer oxygen without obtaining more data. In addition, administering oxygen will need a health-care provider's order unless it is an emergency situation.
2. Obtaining a pulse oximetry level will provide useful data, but it will not assist in alleviating the patient's symptoms.
3. Elevating the head of the bed should be the first intervention because it is the least invasive, does not require a health-care provider's order, and may alleviate the problem. Raising the head of the bed allows the abdominal organs to drop by gravity, facilitating expansion of the thoracic cavity during inhalation.
4. Notifying the patient's primary health-care provider may be necessary, but it is premature if done before additional data are collected and other interventions are attempted to alleviate the problem.
TEST-TAKING TIP: Identify the word in the stem that sets a priority. The word *first* in the stem sets a priority.
Content Area: Oxygenation
Integrated Processes: Nursing Process: Implementation
Client Need: Physiological Integrity; Physiological Adaptation
Cognitive Level: Application

32. ANSWER: 2.
Rationales:
1. Although the patient has not voided in 4 hours and 15 minutes and should be encouraged to void, it is not as serious a concern as another option at this time. If the patient has not voided in 8 hours, the patient's primary health-care provider should be informed.

2. Respirations of 17 shallow breaths per minute are a concern. One would expect the respiratory rate to be higher in light of the elevated temperature and concurrent increase in the basal metabolic rate. Also, the patient currently is receiving 2 L per minute of oxygen that obviously is ineffective in improving the patient's respiratory status.
3. Although the temperature is high, the patient was administered Tylenol 650 mg at 1300. Also, the patient may be in the defervescence phase of fever abatement, as indicated by the clinical indicators of flushed appearance, diaphoresis, and reports of feeling warm.
4. Although the patient may have been dehydrated on admission to the emergency department, the patient has been receiving 125 mL per hour of fluid for the past several hours and will continue to receive IV fluid until discontinued by the primary health-care provider.
TEST-TAKING TIP: Identify the word in the stem that sets a priority. The word *priority* in the stem sets a priority.
Content Area: Oxygenation
Integrated Processes: Nursing Process: Analysis
Client Need: Physiological Integrity; Reduction of Risk Potential
Cognitive Level: Analysis

33. ANSWER: 3.
Rationales:
1. Cupping and clapping are unnecessary. There is no indication that the patient is having difficulty mobilizing respiratory secretions.
2. Calling the patient's primary health-care provider at this time is premature. More information is needed regarding the patient's status.
3. Vital signs, including oxygen saturation, are essential pieces of data that should be obtained to provide a better understanding of the patient's cardiorespiratory status. This information will direct future interventions.
4. Administering oxygen may be needed, but it is premature without gathering more information about the patient's status.
TEST-TAKING TIP: Identify the word in the stem that sets a priority. The word *next* in the stem sets a priority.
Content Area: Oxygenation
Integrated Processes: Nursing Process: Implementation
Client Need: Physiological Integrity; Physiological Adaptation
Cognitive Level: Application

34. ANSWER: 4.
Rationales:
1. Dry mouth is associated with an anticholinergic bronchodilator.
2. Blurred vision is associated with an anticholinergic bronchodilator.
3. Urinary retention is associated with an anticholinergic bronchodilator.
4. Steroidal nasal sprays can depress the immune system, which can lead to an oropharyngeal fungal infection.
Content Area: Oxygenation
Integrated Processes: Nursing Process: Implementation
Client Need: Physiological Integrity; Pharmacological and Parenteral Therapies
Cognitive Level: Application

35. ANSWER: 8.

Rationale:

Solve the problem using ratio and proportion.

$$\frac{\text{Desire } 400 \text{ mg}}{\text{Have } 50 \text{ mg}} = \frac{x \text{ mL}}{1 \text{ mL}}$$

$$50x = 400 \times 1$$

$$50x = 400$$

$$x = 400 \div 50$$

$$x = 8 \text{ mL}$$

Content Area: Medication Administration
Integrated Processes: Nursing Process: Planning
Client Need: Physiological Integrity; Pharmacological and Parenteral Therapies
Cognitive Level: Application

Chapter 20

Urinary Elimination

KEY TERMS

Anuria—Absence of urine output or output less than 200 mL daily.

Bladder ultrasound scan—Noninvasive use of sound waves to detect the amount of urine in the bladder.

Blood urea nitrogen (BUN) level—Reflects the blood level of urea, which is a by-product of protein metabolism.

Clean-catch (midstream) specimen—Provides a urine specimen with minimal introduction of microorganisms from the perineal area.

Continuous bladder irrigation—Constant instillation of a genitourinary (GU) irrigant (e.g., normal saline solution) into the bladder via a three-lumen urinary catheter to maintain tube patency when clots and debris are expected after urinary system surgery.

Creatinine level—Amount of creatinine in blood, which is a by-product of muscle catabolism.

Credé maneuver—Application of manual pressure over the bladder to initiate voiding.

Cystoscopy—Insertion of a fiberoptic instrument through the urethra to examine the bladder.

Dysuria—Painful or difficulty voiding.

Enuresis—Involuntary passage of urine when awake.

Glomerulonephritis—Inflammation of the glomeruli.

Hematuria—Blood in the urine.

Hydronephrosis—Stretching of the renal pelvis due to the accumulation of urine as a result of an obstructed ureter.

Ileal conduit—Use of a segment of the ileum as a reservoir in which the ureters are implanted and the end is brought through the abdominal wall to form a stoma from which urine drains continuously.

Incontinence—Involuntary passage of urine.

Intermittent bladder irrigation—Periodic instillation of a solution into the urinary bladder to administer medication, flush the bladder, or to maintain patency of a urinary retention catheter.

Intravenous pyelogram (IVP)—Test in which a radiopaque dye is injected intravenously and concentrates in the urine, facilitating x-ray visualization of the kidneys, ureters, and bladder.

Kock pouch—Pocket formed by connecting the ureters to a reservoir made from a portion of the ileum, which is connected to the skin and emptied via a surgically created nipple valve.

Nephrolithiasis—Kidney stones.

Nephrosis—Degenerative changes in the kidneys, especially in the renal tubules, without the presence of inflammation.

Nephrostomy tube—Tube placed into the pelvis of a kidney to drain urine.

Nocturia—Awakening at night to void.

Nocturnal enuresis—Involuntary passage of urine when sleeping.

Oliguria—Urine output less than 500 mL daily.

Overflow incontinence—Involuntary frequent passage of a small amount of urine in conjunction with a distended bladder.

Polyuria—Abnormally large volume of urine output daily.

Pyelonephritis—Inflammation of the kidney and renal pelvis.

Pyuria—Pus in the urine.

Suprapubic tube—Catheter surgically inserted through a small incision above the symphysis pubis to drain urine from the bladder.

Transurethral resection of the prostate—Surgical removal of prostate gland tissue using an instrument inserted via the urethra.

Urinalysis—Physical, chemical, and microscopic examination of urine to aid in the medical diagnosis of disease.

Urinary frequency—Voiding that occurs more often than usual.

Continued

KEY TERMS—cont'd

Urinary hesitancy—Delay in initiating voiding.
Urinary retention—Accumulation of urine in the bladder.
Urinary urgency—Strong desire to void.
Urine pH—Measure of the kidneys' ability to maintain a balanced hydrogen ion concentration in the blood.

Urine specific gravity—Measure of the kidneys' ability to concentrate urine.
Urodynamic studies—Tests that measure stored urine, its flow and elimination in the lower urinary tract, bladder and urethra pressure, and muscle activity.

I. Structures and Functions of the Urinary System

The ability to produce and eliminate waste in the form of urine is essential for life. The mechanisms of glomerular filtration and the production of urine are complex and require an integration of factors, involving effective functioning of the kidneys, ureters, urinary bladder, and urethra. In addition, elimination of urine in the male is influenced when an enlarged prostate gland causes obstruction of the urethra. Knowledge of anatomy and physiology that influences urinary elimination is the basis for understanding how to best care for patients with urinary elimination problems (Fig. 20.1).

A. Kidneys
1. Filter metabolic waste, excess ions, bacterial toxins, water-soluble drugs, drug metabolites, and water from the blood and excrete them as urine.
2. Form urine by filtration, reabsorption, and secretion.
3. Regulate blood volume, blood pressure (BP), fluid and electrolyte balance, and acid-base balance.
4. Secrete rennin that causes the conversion of angiotensinogen to angiotensin I, which is subsequently converted to angiotensin II, which stimulates the nephrons to promote sodium and water retention.
5. Secrete erythropoietin, which acts on the bone marrow to produce red blood cells.
6. Converts part of calcidiol, a vitamin D metabolite, to calcitriol, the biologically active form of vitamin D, which travels in the blood to control the concentration of calcium and phosphate and promote growth and remodeling of bone.
7. Produce a volume of filtrate in 1 minute (glomerular filtration rate [GFR]).

B. Ureters
1. Transport urine produced by the kidneys to the bladder.
2. Funnel shaped at the renal pelvis.
3. Are 10 to 12 inches (25 to 30 cm) in length.
4. Enter the bladder at the posterior corners of the bladder floor.

MAKING THE CONNECTION

Glomerular Filtration Rate and the Production of Urine

Each kidney contains over a million nephrons. Each nephron has six structures: Glomerulus, Bowman's capsule, proximal convoluted tubule, loop of Henle, distal convoluted tubule, and collecting duct. Each structure has its own role in filtering the blood, removing metabolic waste, and controlling the excretion and retention of fluids and solutes based on the needs of the body. Approximately 1,200 mL of blood is routed through the kidneys every 60 seconds. The amount of glomerular filtrate (a substance with a similar composition to plasma that contains water, electrolytes, glucose, amino acids, and metabolic wastes) formed by the kidneys every minute is called the glomerular filtration rate (GFR). When the kidneys are diseased, the GFR decreases because the ability of the nephrons to produce urine is impaired and metabolic waste, toxins, excess ions, and water accumulate to toxic levels that, in turn, can cause damage to the cells of the body. A GFR below 60 percent indicates impaired kidney function and a decreased ability to produce urine. In addition, the appearance of clinical manifestations of impaired kidney function occur, such as an elevation in blood pressure, presence of blood or protein in the urine, elevation of toxic substances in the blood (e.g., blood urea nitrogen and creatinine), and fluid retention, resulting in edema and weight gain.

C. Bladder
1. Receives urine from the ureters.
2. Stores urine (600 to 1,000 mL) until it is eliminated.
3. Urge to eliminate is stimulated by 200 to 250 mL of urine.

D. Urethra
1. Transports urine from the bladder and semen from the prostate gland in males to outside the body.
2. Is 1.5 to 2 inches long in a female and 8 inches in a male.
3. Opens at the urinary meatus.

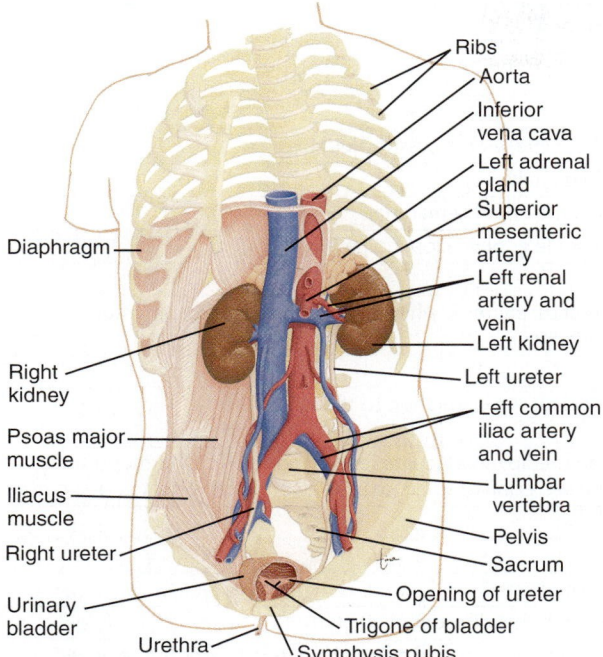

Fig 20.1 Structures of the urinary system. The organs of the urinary system include the kidneys, ureters, bladder, and urethra. (From Wilkinson and Treas [2011]. *Fundamentals of nursing*, Vol. 1, 2nd ed. Philadelphia: F. A. Davis Company, with permission.)

E. **Prostate Gland (in a Male)**
 1. Ring-like gland through which the urethra passes.
 2. Contracts rhythmically and secretes prostatic fluid with male ejaculate, which has an alkaline pH that helps sperm to survive in the acid environment of the female reproductive tract and mobilizes sperm after ejaculation.

II. Urination

After urine is produced, it is stored in the bladder until voiding occurs. The ability to void requires an integrated operative functioning of the bladder, urethra, brain, spinal cord, and peripheral nerves supplying the bladder and urethra. In addition, a person must be able to recognize and respond to the urge to void. A nurse must understand the integrated operative function of urination and identify the expected characteristics of a patient's urine and common problems associated with the urinary system to better meet a patient's urinary elimination needs.

A. **Process of Urination**
 1. Urination (**voiding, micturition**) is the act of emptying the urinary bladder.
 2. The detrusor muscle in the bladder contracts, urging stored urine through the relaxed internal urethral sphincter into the urethra, which results in a conscious urge to void.

 3. The external urethral sphincter inhibits the release of urine until a person is ready to urinate; once ready, the brain signals the external sphincter to relax and further detrusor muscle contraction empties the bladder.
B. **Urine Characteristics**
 1. Color.
   a. Indicates the degree of concentration.
   b. Usually straw colored, pale to amber.
 2. Clarity or turbidity.
   a. Indicates the presence of abnormal constituents.
   b. Usually transparent or translucent.
 3. Amount.
   a. Indicates the volume of production and excretion of urine.
   b. Usually 1,200 to 1,500 mL daily.

DID YOU KNOW?

The body produces approximately 60 mL of urine per hour. Because the bladder stimulates the urge to void every 200 to 250 mL, voiding typically occurs every 3 to 6 hours. In addition, the volume of urinary output should be close to that of fluid intake.

 4. Odor.
   a. Is aromatic.
   b. Can indicate the presence of certain foods and constituents related to infection.
 5. Specific gravity.
   a. Reflects the kidneys' ability to concentrate urine.
   b. Usually 1.001 to 1.029.
 6. pH.
   a. Reflects the kidneys' ability to maintain a balanced hydrogen ion concentration in the blood.
   b. Usually between 4.6 and 8.0; average is 6.0.
 7. Protein.
   a. Exists in molecules that generally are too large to leak into the glomerular filtrate, but leakage can occur in the presence of glomerular damage or impaired tubular reabsorption.
   b. A random urine specimen more than 6 mg/dL when tested with a dip stick indicates renal disease.
   c. The amount in a 24-hour specimen indicates the severity of kidney disease; an expected 24-hour result is 25 to 150 mg.
C. **Abnormal Characteristics of Urine** (See Table 20.1 for abnormal characteristics of urine and their implications.)

III. Factors Affecting Urinary Function

Age, psychosociocultural influences, nutrition, hydration, activity, position, mobility, medical problems, surgical and diagnostic procedures, ability to communicate,

Table 20.1 **Abnormal Characteristics of Urine and Their Implications**

Characteristic	Implication
Color	
Dark amber (concentrated urine).	Related to decreased fluid intake or excessive fluid loss.
Clear color (dilute urine).	Related to excessive fluid intake.
Red, pink, or rusty brown.	Related to blood cells in the urine (hematuria).
Dark orange.	Related to medication use (e.g., phenazopyridine [Pyridium]).
Clarity	
Cloudiness in fresh specimen.	Indicates presence of mucus, bacteria, white blood cells, pus, prostatic fluid, or products of vaginal discharge.
Amount	
Urine output less than 30 mL/hour in absence of obstruction.	Generally indicates a decrease in circulation to the kidneys.
Excessive urine output beyond fluid intake.	Associated with diuretic therapy, inadequate level of antidiuretic hormone, and liquids that increase the secretion of urine, such as alcohol, caffeine, tea, and coffee.
Odor	
Ammonia-like or fetid odor.	Indicates infection.
Sweet odor.	Indicates a high glucose content.
Syrup odor.	Indicates a congenital metabolic disorder.
Other characteristic odors.	Indicates intake of certain foods that can cause characteristic odors (e.g., garlic, asparagus, and onions).
Specific Gravity	
More than 1.029.	Indicates concentrated urine due to decreased fluid intake, dehydration after excess fluid loss, or kidney disease.
Less than 1.001.	Indicates dilute urine usually due to increased fluid intake.
pH	
Less than 4.5 (acidic).	Associated with acidosis, starvation, diarrhea, and a diet high in protein foods or cranberry juice.
More than 8 (alkaline).	Associated with alkalosis, urinary tract infection (UTI), and a high intake of fruits and vegetables (e.g., vegetarian diet).
Other Findings	
Presence of protein: More than 8 mg/dL.	Associated with renal disease, diabetic disease of the kidney, toxemia of pregnancy, inflammation of the glomeruli (glomerulonephritis), and degenerative changes in the kidneys, especially in the renal tubules (nephrosis).
Presence of glucose.	Associated with undiagnosed or uncontrolled diabetes.
Presence of ketone bodies, the end-products of fatty acid breakdown.	Associated with diabetes, fasting/starvation, high-protein diet, vomiting, and being on nothing-by-mouth without nutritional support.
Hemoglobin: Red blood cells via microscopic exam more than 5/higher power field (hpf).	Associated with bleeding from the urinary tract, urinary tract infection, glomerulonephritis, inflammation of the kidney and renal pelvis (pyelonephritis), trauma, kidney stones (nephrolithiasis), or hemolytic reactions.

and medications can dramatically affect urinary function. Understanding these factors will aid nurses in assessing patients, maintaining a nonjudgmental attitude when working with diverse individuals, and planning individualized nursing care.

A. Developmental
1. Infants.
   a. Generally produce 8 to 10 wet diapers daily.
   b. Develop voluntary control at 18 to 24 months of age.
2. Children: May experience involuntary passage of urine when awake (**enuresis**) or when sleeping (**nocturnal enuresis**).
3. Older adults.
   a. Experience a decline in urinary system function.
   b. Are less able to filter waste and maintain acid-base and fluid and electrolyte balance.
   c. Experience a loss of bladder tone, contributing to urgency, frequency, and incomplete emptying of the bladder.

d. Older women: Experience additional weakening of pelvic floor muscles due to childbearing and genitourinary atrophy.

e. Older men: May experience an enlarged prostate, causing urine leakage, awakening at night to void (**nocturia**), and urine retention.

B. Psychosociocultural

1. Lack of privacy or an unfamiliar environment may lead to an inability to void in public (bashful bladder).

2. Loss of dignity related to toileting activities in a health-care environment, especially if the patient is catheterized, can cause emotional distress.

3. Cultural influences may cause a person to insist on a caregiver of the same gender to provide toileting assistance.

C. Nutrition and Hydration

1. As fluid intake increases, a corresponding increase in urine output occurs; as fluid intake decreases, a corresponding decrease in urine output occurs.

2. Some substances increase urine production (e.g., coffee, tea, cola, alcohol, and chocolate) by inhibiting the release of antidiuretic hormone.

3. Sodium intake produces water retention, causing decreased urine production.

D. Activity and Position

1. Exercise maintains detrusor and pelvic floor muscle tone, which helps the bladder to empty completely.

2. Heavy exercise can precipitate dehydration via sweating, causing the kidneys to retain water, reducing urine output.

3. Gravity assists in the flow of urine and the ability to empty the bladder completely; typically, the sitting position is best for women and the standing position is best for men.

4. The bladder may not empty completely when on a bed pan or when using a urinal while lying flat; the side-lying position may facilitate urination for men.

E. Medications and Anesthetic Agents

1. Many classifications of drugs can damage kidney cells (**nephrotoxic**) or cause urinary retention, such as antispasmodics, antihistamines, tricyclic antidepressants, anticholinergics, antihypertensives, antiparkinsonism drugs, and chemotherapeutic agents for cancer.

2. Diuretics cause an increase in urine production; if urine output is excessive in relation to fluid intake, dehydration occurs; urine output decreases when a patient is dehydrated.

3. Some drugs change the color of urine; for example, phenazopyridine (Pyridium) causes the urine to appear reddish orange.

4. Anesthetic agents generally decrease BP and GFR, causing a decrease in urine production; spinal anesthesia reduces the perception of the need to void, leading to bladder distention.

F. Medical Problems

1. Problems can interfere with the production of urine; for example, cardiovascular and metabolic disorders that reduce blood flow through the kidneys (e.g., hypertension, heart failure, shock, and diabetes mellitus).

2. Problems can impair the nervous system that innervates the urinary system; for example, brain attack (stroke) or spinal cord injury.

3. Problems can interfere with the flow of urine; for example, calculi and enlargement of the prostate gland.

4. Problems can cause inflammation of the structures of the urinary system; for example, urinary tract infection (UTI).

5. Impaired cognition (e.g., delirium, dementia) or a mental health/psychiatric problem may alter a person's perception of the need to void.

G. Surgical and Diagnostic Procedures

1. Rectal, vaginal, and pubic surgery and childbirth can result in trauma to and edema of local tissues, causing pressure on the structures of the urinary system and loss of pelvic floor muscle control.

2. Some surgical procedures (e.g., hysterectomy, transurethral resection of the prostate) require insertion of a temporary indwelling urinary catheter postoperatively.

3. Insertion of a fiberoptic instrument (cystoscope) through the urethra to examine the bladder (**cystoscopy**) can cause urethral swelling, obstructing urinary excretion.

H. Communication or Mobility Problems

1. An inability to communicate the need to void can result in what appears to others to be an episode of incontinence when in fact the patient cannot indicate personal needs to others.

2. An inability to engage in toileting activities, such as undressing, can result in episodes of urination before reaching a toilet.

3. An inability to be mobile, such as with patients who are bed- or chair-bound, may prevent a patient from obtaining assistance in time to make it to the bathroom.

IV. Urinary System Assessment

The first step of the nursing process is assessment. When collecting information relative to a patient's urinary function, the nurse obtains a patient history, performs a physical assessment, and assesses the volume and characteristics of urine. Data collected from these assessments help determine whether the patient's urinary system is functioning adequately or further action is required by a nurse or the primary health-care provider.

A. Obtain a Health History

1. Identify any change in urination habits or urine characteristics.
2. Ask questions about the presence of clinical manifestations that indicate infection.
   a. Strong desire to void (**urinary urgency**).
   b. Voiding that occurs more often than usual (**frequency**).
   c. Painful or difficulty voiding (**dysuria**).
   d. Blood in the urine (**hematuria**).
3. Ask questions about the clinical manifestations of obstruction of urine flow.
   a. Delay in initiating voiding (**urinary hesitancy**).
   b. Awakening at night to void (**nocturia**).
   c. Involuntary frequent passage of a small amount of urine in conjunction with a distended bladder (**overflow incontinence**).
4. Ask about daily urine volume.
   a. Urine output less than 500 mL daily (**oliguria**).
   b. Abnormally large volume of urine output daily (**polyuria**).
   c. Absence of urine output or urine output of less than 100 mL daily (**anuria**).
5. Ask about involuntary passage of urine (**incontinence**).
6. Assess for flank pain that indicates a problem with the kidneys.
7. Identify a history of urinary system problems (e.g., infection, kidney or bladder problems, urinary tract surgery or urinary system diagnostic procedures or tests).
8. Assess lifestyle factors that can affect the urinary system (e.g., daily caffeine and fluid intake, smoking history, management of activities of daily living, emotional stress, and access to a bathroom).
9. Identify any medications the patient is currently taking that may impact the urinary system.
10. Ask how long the patient has been experiencing any identified problems; how the patient manages the problem; and what has been done medically to treat the problem.

B. Perform a Physical Assessment

1. Assess the characteristics of urine. (See the section "Urine Characteristics," page 611.)
2. Measure intake and output (I&O).
3. Assess for weight gain and edema.
4. Palpate for enlarged kidneys with the patient in the supine position.
5. Palpate the bladder for distention if the patient is unable to void.
   a. Indicates urine accumulation in the bladder (**urinary retention**); more than 500 mL of urine produces a bulge in the central lower abdomen just above the symphysis pubis when the patient is in the supine position.
   b. May be difficult to identify in an obese patient.
6. Use a bladder ultrasonic scanner to assess for the amount of urine retained in the bladder after voiding; this assessment is more objective than palpation and percussion.
7. Auscultate the abdominal aorta and renal arteries for an adventitious sound of arterial blood flow; presence indicates a vascular problem.
8. Assess perineal skin integrity.
   a. Assess for presence of a perineal rash with macerated skin (ammonia contact dermatitis), which may extend to the thighs and is usually caused by urinary incontinence.
   b. Assess for the presence of a perineal red rash with satellite lesions, which may extend to the thighs and is related to a fungal infection (*Candida* rash).
9. Assess the vaginal vault for clinical manifestations of atrophic vaginitis (e.g., dry, thin mucosa; tenderness; pallor; easy bleeding).
10. Assess the patient's mental status, mobility, dexterity, and visual acuity to determine ability to self-toilet.
11. Assess for the presence of a urinary diversion.

V. Urinary System Diagnostic Tests and Related Nursing Care

A history and physical may need to be supplemented with data collected via diagnostic tests ordered by the primary health-care provider. Some tests are essential to arrive at a medical diagnosis (e.g., urine culture and sensitivity, cystoscopy), whereas others are employed to identify specific information about a patient's urinary function (e.g., blood chemistry tests, urodynamic studies). Nurses must understand these tests because some of them are performed by the nurse, some require specific nursing interventions before and after the test, and all of them require patient teaching.

A. Urine Specimens

1. **Urinalysis.**
   a. Most commonly ordered laboratory test for overall screening and aiding in the medical diagnosis of disease.
   b. Macroscopic and microscopic analysis of urine for normal and abnormal constituents (physical and chemical); includes color, turbidity, pH, specific gravity, protein, glucose, ketones, red

blood cells, white blood cells, bacteria/yeast, and casts (precipitation of protein substances).

c. Commonalities of nursing care when collecting a urine specimen.

(1) Wash your hands and collect the necessary equipment.

(2) Explain the procedure to the patient.

(3) Wear clean gloves to prevent exposure to the patient's body fluids.

(4) Instruct the patient to void into a clean bed pan, urinal, or specimen hat positioned under the toilet seat. For infants, wash the genital area, allow the area to dry, and then place a collection device over the infant's genital area.

(5) Avoid contaminating the specimen with feces, toilet tissue, or menstrual blood; if the patient is menstruating, note it on the laboratory slip.

(6) Pour at least 30 mL of urine into a clean specimen cup or tube.

(7) Label the container with the patient's name, date, and time of collection according to agency policy and place it in a biohazardous bag to reduce the transmission of infection.

(8) Assist the patient with perineal and hand hygiene.

(9) Clean or dispose of supplies.

(10) Remove your gloves and then wash your hands.

(11) Document the procedure in the patient's clinical record.

(12) Send the specimen to the laboratory with the appropriate laboratory slip within 15 minutes; place the specimen in a specimen refrigerator if a delay occurs.

2. **Clean-catch (midstream) specimen.**

a. Provides a urine specimen with minimal introduction of microorganisms from the perineal area.

b. Specific nursing care.

(1) Maintain sterility of the urine specimen cup by turning the inside of the lid of the cup toward the ceiling when placing it on a clean surface, avoiding touching the perineum with the cup, and closing the lid without touching the inside of the cup or lid.

(2) Collect urine or teach the patient how to collect the urine.

(a) For males: Retract the foreskin to expose the urinary meatus if the patient is uncircumcised; clean the urinary meatus in a circular motion with three different swabs; have the patient begin voiding; after some urine is voided, position the sterile container under the stream and collect the specimen; allow the patient to finish voiding; return the foreskin to the expected position if necessary; and close the container without contaminating the inside of the cup or lid.

(b) For females: Separate the labia minora and cleanse the area from the pubis to the rectum with three different swabs; have the patient begin to void while keeping the labia separated; allow urine to flow and then hold the sterile specimen cup under the stream and collect the specimen; remove the container; release the hand from the labia; allow the patient to finish voiding; and close the container without contaminating the inside of the cup or lid.

3. **Twenty-four-hour urine specimen.**

a. Measures kidneys' excretion of substances, such as protein, uric acid, creatinine, selected hormones, urobilinogen, and other substances, that the body does not excrete at an even rate throughout the day.

b. Specific nursing care.

(1) Explain the need to collect all urine for the next 24 hours.

(2) Post reminders for the patient and staff on the bathroom door if permitted by policy.

(3) Check with the laboratory whether the specimen container has a preservative or needs to be kept in a basin of ice.

(4) Begin by having the patient void, discard this urine, and record the time.

(5) Collect all voided urine during the next 24 hours.

(6) Have the patient void at the end of the 24 hours and add this urine to the container.

4. **Culture and sensitivity.**

a. Identifies the causative microorganism and the most effective antibiotic to eradicate the microorganism; takes 24 to 72 hours for organisms to multiply and be identified.

b. Specific nursing care.

(1) Collect a clean-catch urine specimen or a specimen from a urinary catheter.

(2) Maintain surgical asepsis to prevent contamination of the specimen.

🛑 (3) Obtain the urine specimen before the patient takes a prescribed antibiotic.

5. **Dipstick testing of urine.**

a. Provides a quick, bedside assessment of specific constituents of urine (e.g., pH, specific

gravity, protein, glucose, ketones, and occult blood).
b. Specific nursing care.
  (1) Ensure that the correct stick is used and that it has not expired.
  (2) Dip the test strip into the urine, tap the strip to dislodge excess urine, and place the strip horizontally across the top of the urine cup to prevent urine from flowing down the strip or collecting at one site on the strip causing inaccurate results.
  (3) Begin timing according to the manufacturer's directions and at the correct time; compare the results to the color chart on the dipstick bottle.
  (4) Document the results in the patient's clinical record and report any abnormalities to the primary health-care provider.
6. **Collecting a urine specimen from a urinary catheter.**
  a. Specific nursing care when collecting a specimen via a single-lumen catheter.
    (1) Insert a single lumen urinary catheter into the bladder following all the principles associated with surgical asepsis. (See the section "Inserting a Urinary Catheter," page 624.)
    (2) Collect the specimen and then immediately remove the catheter.
  b. Specific nursing care when collecting a specimen from an indwelling urinary catheter (Fig. 20.2).
    (1) Ensure that the drainage tube is free from urine and then clamp it below the level of the specimen port on the drainage tubing

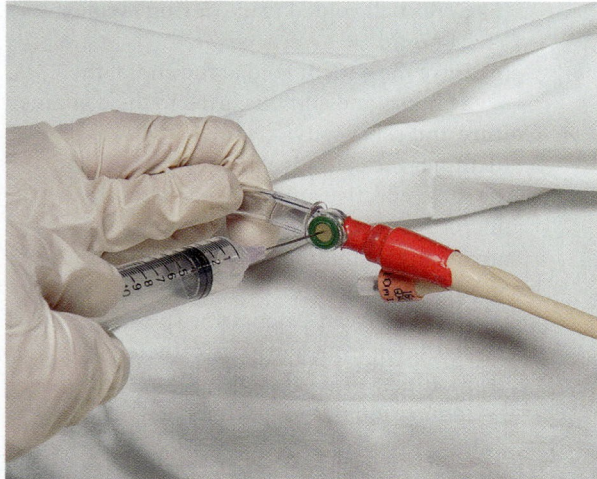

Fig 20.2 Obtaining a specimen from an indwelling urinary catheter. (From Burton and Ludwig [2011]. *Fundamentals of nursing care: Concepts, connections & skills.* Philadelphia: F. A. Davis Company, with permission.)

for 15 to 30 minutes, allowing fresh urine to collect.
  (2) Wash your hands and don clean gloves.
  (3) Clean the specimen port with an alcohol swab.
  (4) Insert the needle of a sterile syringe into the port and aspirate the required amount of urine.
  (5) Transfer the specimen to a sterile specimen cup.
  (6) Discard the needle and syringe into a sharps disposal container.
  (7) Close the lid tightly on the specimen cup without contaminating the inside of the cup or lid.
  🛑 (8) Maintain the closed drainage system; never separate the catheter from the drainage tubing to collect a specimen because it creates a portal of entry for microorganisms, and never collect a specimen from the collection bag because the urine is not fresh.
  🛑 (9) Remove the clamp from the drainage tubing.
B. Blood Chemistry Tests
1. **Blood urea nitrogen (BUN).**
  a. Reflects the level of urea nitrogen, a by-product of protein metabolism, in blood.
  b. Expected level is 10 to 20 mg/dL.
  c. Increased levels.
    (1) Occur in kidney disease because urea excretion is decreased.
    (2) Can also occur due to digested blood from GI bleeding, dehydration, high-protein diet, steroids, strenuous activity, and nephrotoxic drugs.
  d. Decreased levels.
    (1) Generally indicate overhydration.
    (2) Can also be caused by severe liver damage, a low-protein diet, malnutrition, phenothiazine medications, and IV glucose without protein intake.
  e. Specific nursing care.
    (1) Keep the patient on nothing-by-mouth (NPO) status for 8 hours.
    (2) Avoid hemolysis of the specimen (e.g., avoid shaking the specimen tube and send the specimen to the lab immediately).
    (3) Identify drugs the patient is taking that may increase BUN (e.g., antibiotics, diuretics, antihypertensives, nephrotoxic drugs, sulfonamides, morphine, lithium carbonate, and salicylates).
2. **Creatinine level.**
  a. Reflects the level of creatinine, a by-product of muscle catabolism, in blood.
  b. Expected level is 0.5 to 1.5 mg/dL.

c. More than 2.5 mg/dL is indicative of kidney impairment.

d. Is more reliable than BUN in determining kidney function because the level is not affected by diet or fluid intake.

e. Specific nursing care.

(1) Instruct the patient to avoid eating red meat the night before the test.

(2) Identify drugs that the patient is taking that may increase levels (e.g., cefazolin [Ancef], methyldopa [Aldomet], cephalothin [Keflin], gentamicin, methicillin, ascorbic acid, barbiturates, and lithium carbonate).

C. Radiologic Tests

1. Commonalities of nursing care for patients undergoing a radiologic test.

a. Explain the test, including the fact that it will be painless.

b. Obtain a signed consent form.

c. Encourage the patient to void before the examination.

d. Encourage increased fluid intake after the procedure to facilitate excretion of the contrast/radioactive substance.

e. Monitor I&O after the procedure to ensure kidney function.

2. Intravenous pyelogram (IVP).

a. Radiopaque dye injected by IV concentrates in urine.

b. Facilitates x-ray visualization of kidneys, ureters, and bladder.

c. Is risky when a patient has kidney failure because it requires use of a dye.

d. Specific nursing care.

🛑 (1) Ensure that the patient does not have an allergy to iodine because the contrast dye contains iodine and can precipitate anaphylaxis.

DID YOU KNOW?

People who are allergic to shellfish generally are allergic to the protein it contains rather than iodine. People who are allergic to shellfish are at a no greater risk of an allergic reaction to the contrast dye than someone who is not allergic to shellfish.

(2) Explain that the patient may experience a warm, flushed sensation or a salty taste when the dye is injected.

(3) Explain that it takes about 1 hour to complete; x-ray films are taken at various intervals as the dye moves through the urinary system.

(4) Ensure that an enema or a laxative is taken before the procedure, as ordered, to ensure that stool and gas do not interfere with the test.

(5) Withhold food and fluid as ordered.

(6) Assess for reactions to the contrast media (e.g., rash, nausea, and hives) during and after the test.

D. Ultrasound Tests

1. Noninvasive tests using high-frequency sound waves to create an image of the urinary system.

2. Can identify the amount of urine in the bladder, masses, cysts, edema, and stones.

3. Safe for patients with kidney failure because they do not require dye.

4. Commonalities of nursing care for patients having ultrasound tests.

a. Explain the test, including the fact that it will be painless.

b. Provide privacy.

c. Explain that a conductive gel is applied to the skin and that a transducer is moved smoothly back and forth over the gelled site while a machine visualizes structures of the urinary system.

d. Provide hygiene after the test to remove the conductive gel.

5. Bladder ultrasound scan (Fig. 20.3).

a. Noninvasive test using sound waves to detect the amount of urine in the bladder.

b. Provides data for determining the need for catheterization.

c. Can be done at the bedside by trained caregivers.

d. Specific nursing care.

(1) Place the patient in the supine position.

(2) Expose only the lower abdomen and suprapubic area.

(3) Turn the scan device on to female or male; use male if the patient had a hysterectomy.

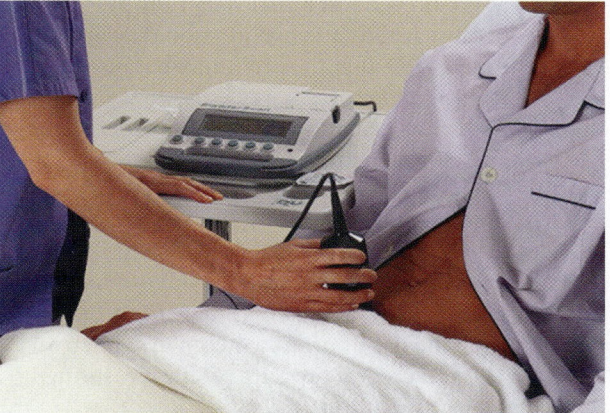

Fig 20.3 Bladder ultrasound scanner. (From Burton and Ludwig [2011]. *Fundamentals of nursing care: Concepts, connections & skills.* Philadelphia: F. A. Davis Company, with permission.)

(4) Use an ultrasound gel pad or 5 mL of conducting gel to improve ultrasound conduction.

(5) Place the scan head approximately 1.5 inches (4 cm) above the pubic bone midline below the umbilicus (symphysis pubis), aiming the scan head toward the patient's coccyx.

(6) Press the scan head button, wait until it beeps, and release the button.

(7) Look for bladder volume to be displayed.

(8) Repeat the measurement because several measurements ensure accuracy.

(9) Press "DONE" and then "PRINT" for a hard copy when the procedure is complete.

(10) Clean the scan head with isopropyl alcohol.

(11) Wash your hands.

(12) Document the results and patient responses in the patient's clinical record.

E. Cystoscopy

1. Insertion of a fiberoptic tube through the urethra to directly visualize the inside of the bladder (**cystoscopy**) to identify stones, lesions, tumors, irritation, or structural problems.

2. Allows specialized instruments to be passed through the tube to take a biopsy or remove small stones or to provide local treatment.

3. Nursing care.
   a. Obtain a signed consent form.
   b. Explain that urine may be pink initially after the procedure because of slight bleeding due to irritation of the mucous membranes of the urinary tract.
   c. Encourage increased fluid intake before and after the procedure.
   d. Administer prescribed antibiotics (e.g., 1 STAT dose after the procedure, 1 day before and 3 days after the procedure).
   e. Maintain bed rest initially after the procedure because orthostatic hypotension may occur.
   f. Assess I&O after the procedure because urinary retention may occur.
   g. Assess for hematuria, dysuria, bladder spasms, and clinical manifestations of infection after the test.

F. Urodynamic Studies

1. Measure stored urine, its flow and elimination in the lower urinary tract, bladder and urethra pressure, and muscle activity.

2. Include the use of uroflowmetry, cystometrograms, and urethra pressure profile measuring devices.

3. Nursing care.
   a. Encourage the patient to drink fluid so that the bladder is full before the test.

b. Explain to the patient that a catheter will be inserted through the urethra into the bladder as part of the test.
c. Encourage the patient to drink 8 to 10 glasses of fluid after the test to flush the urinary structures.
d. Administer the prescribed STAT dose of antibiotic after the test.
e. Teach the patient clinical manifestations of UTI and instruct the patient to notify the primary health-care provider if any occur.

VI. Nursing Care to Assist Patients With Urinary Elimination

Nursing interventions related to the urinary system involve activities concerning the assessment of a patient's urinary status, collection of specimens for diagnostic tests, promotion of efficient urinary functioning, and the prevention and treatment of urinary problems. Many of these interventions are independent functions of the nurse; however, some require a primary health-care provider's order. Nurses must have a thorough understanding of when and how to implement these interventions.

A. Independent Nursing Interventions

1. Assess the patient's urinary functioning and the amount and characteristics of urinary output. (See the section "Urinary System Assessment," page 613.)

2. Encourage the patient to follow consistent daily routines.

3. Encourage the patient to engage in regular exercise to help maintain pelvic floor and bladder muscle tone.

4. Encourage the patent to drink 8 to 10 glasses of fluid daily.
   a. Provide hourly goals for intake.
   b. Keep fluids in easy reach.
   c. Provide fluids that the patient prefers.

5. Assist the patient with toileting as soon as the need to void is indicated by the patient.

6. Provide privacy during toileting.

7. Encourage the patient to void (e.g., when the urge to void is felt; on awakening, after meals, and at bedtime; every 2 hours).

8. Encourage the patient to completely empty the bladder when voiding to prevent urinary stasis.

9. Assist with positioning.
   a. Female: Sitting.
   b. Male: Standing or side lying.

10. Provide a commode at the bedside for patients who are unable to ambulate to a bathroom.

11. Assist bedbound patients to use a bedpan.
    a. Keep the bed in the lowest position.

b. Assist the patient onto the bedpan depending on ability (see Fig. 22.5).
  (1) Roll the patient to one side; with the rounded end toward the back, place the bedpan centered against the buttocks; and roll the patient back to the supine position.
  (2) Have the patient flex the knees and lift the buttocks off the bed; and with the rounded end toward the back, place the bedpan centered against the buttocks
c. Keep the side rails raised during toileting; raise the head of the bed to the low-Fowler position; and have the patient hold onto the side rails for support.
d. Have the patient flex the knees and hips while on the bedpan and place the call bell within easy reach.
e. Transfer a patient off of a bedpan as soon as the patient is done voiding and provide perineal care.

12. Promote urination.
a. Put the patient's hands in warm water.
b. Turn on a sink tap so that the patient can hear the sound of running water.
c. Pour warm water over the patient's perineum.
d. Place a warm moist wash cloth over the patient's perineum.
e. Apply manual pressure over the patient's bladder (**Credé maneuver**).

13. Teach the patient techniques to prevent UTIs. (See the section "Urinary Tract Infection," page 622.)

14. Provide nursing care for patients who are incontinent of urine. (See the section "Urinary Incontinence," this page.)

15. Teach the patient about ordered diagnostic tests and the interventions to self-perform in relation to the test.

B. Dependent Nursing Interventions

1. Implement care that prepares a patient for a test that requires an order or a prescription (e.g., NPO, medications, enema).

2. Obtain urine specimens for ordered diagnostic tests. (See the section "Urinary System Diagnostic Tests and Related Nursing Care," page 614.)

3. Insert and maintain urinary catheters as ordered. (See the section "Urinary Catheters," page 623.)

4. Provide nursing care for patients with a urinary diversion. (See the section "Nursing Care for Patients With a Urinary Diversion," page 627.)

5. Administer prescribed kidney-specific anti-infectives, urinary antispasmodics, and estrogen; teach the patient information about the medications and self-administration of the medication regimen. (See the section "Medications That Affect the Urinary System," page 629.)

VII. Nursing Care for Patients With Urinary System Problems

Urinary incontinence, UTI, nocturnal enuresis, and urinary retention are common problems related to the urinary system. It is essential that nurses understand the clinical manifestations, precipitating factors, and nursing care associated with each problem.

Nursing interventions include activities concerned with promotion of efficient urinary functioning and the prevention and treatment of urinary problems. Many of these interventions are independent functions of the nurse; however, some require a primary health-care provider's order or a standing order.

A. Urinary Incontinence

1. Overview.
a. Inability to control the passage urine.
b. May be acute and reversible (e.g., when due to infection or medication side effect) or chronic and nonreversible (e.g., when due to neurological problems, such as spinal cord injury).

2. Clinical manifestations: See Table 20.2 for types, clinical manifestations, and precipitating factors of urinary incontinence.

3. Commonalities of nursing care for patients with urinary incontinence.
a. Independent nursing care.
  (1) Provide perineal care immediately after voiding or on a regular schedule.
  (2) Encourage the use of/or apply an appropriate incontinence device (e.g., pads, Depends, external condom catheter); avoid the use of the word "diaper."
  (3) Apply an external condom catheter for a male patient.
    (a) Provide perineal care; rinse and dry thoroughly.
    (b) Avoid lubricants or the catheter will slide off.
    (c) Measure the circumference of the penis to ensure correct catheter size.
    (d) Hold the penis and place the condom over and beyond the glans penis (Fig. 20.4a); unroll the condom the full length of the penis, leaving 1 to 2 inches between the glans penis and drainage tubing of the catheter (Fig. 20.4b).
    🛑 (e) Do not retract the foreskin if the patient is uncircumcised.
    (f) Secure the condom: For a condom with internal adhesive, grasp the penis and gently compress so the entire condom comes into contact with the penile shaft; for a condom with an external adhesive

Table 20.2 Types of Urinary Incontinence

Type of Incontinence	Clinical Manifestations	Precipitating Factors
Total Continuous and unpredictable passage of urine.	• Lack of awareness of bladder filling. • Nocturia. • Absence of bladder contraction or distention.	• Neurologic dysfunction causing micturition at unpredictable times. • Diseases or trauma affecting the spinal cord nerves.
Urge Passage of urine after a strong need to void.	• Urgency and frequency more often than every 2 hours. • Inability to reach the bathroom in time to void. • Voiding <100 mL or >550 mL at each voiding. • Bladder spasms. • Nocturia.	• Overactive bladder tone. • Decreased bladder capacity or overdistention of the bladder. • Bladder spasms. • Bladder infection. • Intake of irritating fluids or foods, such as caffeine or alcohol. • History of conditions such as pelvic inflammatory disease, genitourinary atrophy; abdominal surgery; presence of an indwelling urinary catheter.
Stress Passage of urine (<50 mL; dribbling) when intra-abdominal pressure increases.	• Urgency or frequency more often than every 2 hours. • Precipitated by a behavior that increases intra-abdominal pressure.	• Activities that increase intra-abdominal pressure, such as exercise, laughing, coughing, sneezing, bending, and lifting. • Degenerative changes in pelvic muscles and structural supports due to pregnancy, childbirth, aging, or chronic constipation. • Incompetent bladder outlet. • Overdistention between voidings. • Obesity.
Overflow Passage of urine related to a distended bladder.	• Frequent loss of small amounts of urine.	• Urinary retention. • Fecal impaction. • Neurologic disorders. • Prostate enlargement.
Reflex Passage of urine occurring at approximate predictable times when a certain bladder volume is achieved.	• Absence of urge or sense of bladder fullness. • Inability to inhibit or initiate urine flow voluntarily. • Absence of voiding sensation.	• Spinal cord lesion interfering with messages above the level of the sacral reflex arc. • Inflammation of the bladder. • Radical pelvic surgery.
Transient Short-term incontinence precipitated by a situation that, once addressed, will resolve the incontinence spontaneously.	• With diuretics: Urgency, frequency, and large urine volume. • With urinary tract infection: Burning on urination, dysuria, bladder spasms, pyuria, hematuria, foul odor to urine, chills, fever, back pain, nausea, and vomiting.	• Medications, such as diuretics. • Urinary tract infections.

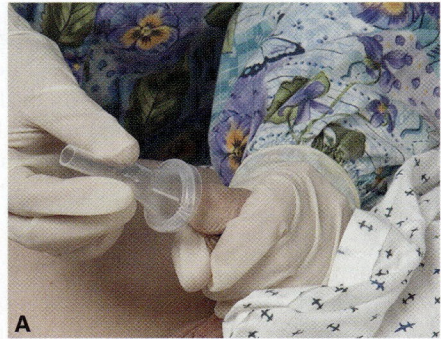 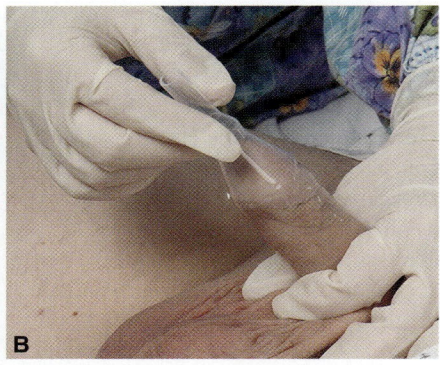

Fig 20.4 Condom catheter. (A) Placing a condom over and beyond the glans penis. (B) Leaving 1 to 2 inches between the glans penis and drainage tubing. (From Wilkinson and Treas [2011]. *Fundamentals of nursing,* Vol. 2, 2nd ed. Philadelphia: F. A. Davis Company, with permission.)

strip, wrap the strip in a spiral along the
shaft but do not overlap the ends or use
surgical tape because these actions can
act as a tourniquet.

(g) Ensure that the condom is not twisted
to prevent trauma (e.g., obstruction of
urine flow, irritation at meatus, skin
breakdown).

(h) Secure the catheter to the thigh to prevent tissue trauma.

(4) Encourage necessary lifestyle changes, such
as cessation of smoking, weight management, and dietary changes.

(5) Assess for clinical manifestations of a vaginal infection or UTI, such as hematuria,
dysuria, and vaginal irritation.

b. Dependent nursing care.

(1) Apply a perineal skin barrier as per agency
policy.

(2) Administer medications as prescribed.

(3) Teach the patient how to use a prescribed
anti-incontinence device (e.g., intravaginal
support [pessary], penis clamp, internal
urethral meatus plug).

4. Specific nursing care for patients with stress and
urge incontinence.

a. Teach the patient to avoid constipation (e.g.,
increase fluid intake, eat high-fiber foods, and
increase activity).

b. Teach the patient to limit activities that
increase intra-abdominal pressure (e.g.,
high-impact exercises, lifting, bending).

c. Encourage the patient to perform Kegel exercises to strengthen the pelvic floor.

(1) Tighten the pelvic muscles as if to stop
urination or passing of gas.

(2) Hold for 5 to 10 seconds and then rest 5 to
10 seconds.

(3) Repeat two to four times a day with 15 repeti-
tions per session.

(4) Explain to the patient that it may take 6 to
12 months for positive results.

d. Teach vaginal weight training to females if
ordered.

(1) Insert a small cone-shaped weight into the
vagina and contract the pelvic floor muscles
to keep it in place.

(2) Keep the cone-shaped weight in the vagina
for 15 minutes twice a day.

e. Employ a bladder retraining program, particularly for patients with urge incontinence (e.g.,
using a voiding diary, holding larger amounts
of urine between voidings; scheduling regular
times for voiding; using distraction and relaxation techniques).

f. Administer prescribed medications to relax the
detrusor muscle and increase bladder capacity
(e.g., anticholinergics, smooth-muscle relaxants, calcium channel blockers, antidepressants) and estrogen for women who have
genital atrophy.

5. Specific nursing care for patients with overflow
incontinence.

a. Identify distension of the urinary bladder (e.g.,
bladder scan indicates urinary volume; palpation reveals smooth, round, tense mass in
suprapubic area).

b. Insert a single-lumen or indwelling urinary
catheter if ordered.

6. Specific nursing care for patients with reflex
incontinence.

a. Precipitate urination (e.g., stroke inner thigh,
pull on pubic hair).

b. Insert a single-lumen urinary catheter if
ordered.

c. Administer prescribed medications to relax the
urinary sphincter (e.g., diazepam [Valium]).

7. Specific nursing care for patients with functional
incontinence.

a. Teach the patient to schedule routine toileting,
especially 15 minutes before the identified
pattern of incontinence.

b. Teach the patient methods to facilitate toileting
(e.g., Velcro clothing closures, bedside commode
or urinal, gait and strength training, raised toilet
seat, and bathroom grab bars).

B. **Urinary Tract Infection (UTI)**

1. Overview.

a. Invasion of the bladder by bacteria, viruses, or
fungi; *Escherichia coli,* which normally resides
in the colon, most commonly invades the urinary tract.

b. May occur in the urethra (**urethritis**), bladder
(**cystitis**), ureters, kidneys (**pyelonephritis**), or
several structures of the urinary system.

2. Clinical manifestations.

a. Burning on urination (**dysuria**).

b. Bladder spasms or back pain.

c. Frequency.

d. Hematuria.

e. Chills; fever.

f. Pus in the urine (**pyuria**).

g. Foul odor to urine.

h. Positive urine culture.

3. Precipitating factors.

a. Sexual activity; use of spermicidal contraceptive gel.

b. Dryness of the mucosa and decrease in normal
flora due to aging.

c. Presence of an indwelling urinary catheter.

d. Illnesses that affect the kidneys (e.g., diabetes mellitus, renal calculi).

e. Conditions that cause urinary stasis (e.g., prostate gland enlargement, hypotonic bladder).

4. Independent nursing care.

a. Teach the patient clinical manifestations of UTI.

b. Provide perineal care immediately after voiding or on a regular schedule.

c. Encourage the use of or apply an incontinence device (e.g., pads, Depends, external condom catheter).

d. Teach the patient preventative measures.

(1) Void every 2 to 4 hours, not just in response to the urge.

(2) Avoid food and beverages that can irritate the bladder (e.g., citrus fruits, caffeinated beverages, alcohol, and some spices).

(3) For women: Wear cotton underwear; void before and after intercourse; avoid bubble and baking soda baths, perineal deodorant sprays, and douches.

(4) Drink at least 24 oz of cranberry juice daily.

5. Dependent nursing care.

a. Collect a urine specimen before initiating antibiotic therapy.

b. Apply a topical barrier to maintain skin integrity per agency protocol.

c. Administer prescribed medications.

(1) Antibiotics, such as cephalexin (Keflex), nitrofurantoin (Macrodantin), and ciprofloxacin (Cipro), to eradicate the causative organism.

(2) Urinary analgesics, such as phenazopyridine (Pyridium), to limit discomfort.

(3) Anticholinergic drugs, such as hyoscyamine (Anaspaz, Cystospaz), to inhibit involuntary bladder contractions.

C. Nocturnal Enuresis

1. Overview.

a. Involuntary passage of urine when asleep.

b. Occurs after voluntary control should have been established.

2. Clinical manifestations.

a. Urinating when asleep.

b. Person fails to awaken when the bladder empties.

3. Precipitating factors.

a. Health problems that interfere with the ability to concentrate urine.

b. Health problems associated with excessive urine output (e.g., diabetes mellitus, diabetes insipidus).

c. UTI.

d. Trauma or diseases of the spinal cord.

e. Structural defects of the urinary tract.

f. Misguided attempts at toilet training.

g. Emotional stressors (e.g., birth of sibling, illness or death in the family, separation from family).

DID YOU KNOW?

Up to 25 percent of 5-year-old children experience nighttime bedwetting. It occurs three times more frequently in males than in females and is more common in first-born children. It decreases to 8 percent of male children and 4 percent of female children by the age of 12, and less than 3 percent of adolescents still experience nighttime bedwetting. To be diagnosed with nocturnal enuresis, a child 5 to 6 years of age must have two or more episodes per month and a child older than 6 years of age must have 1 or more episodes per month. There is no single explanation for nocturnal enuresis; it is believed to be multifactorial, including a familial tendency. Medical causes are ruled out first before addressing psychological factors because they are generally believed to be the result, not the cause, of nocturnal enuresis. In fact, research demonstrates that children with nocturnal enuresis do not have an increased incidence of emotional problems and, for most children, it is not a rebellious act.

4. Independent nursing care.

a. Include the patient in formulating a plan of care; offer hope and encouragement that the plan will work.

b. Train the bladder to hold larger amounts of urine when awake (e.g., gradually increase time between voidings).

MAKING THE CONNECTION

Cranberry Juice and Decreased Incidence of Urinary Tract Infections

Research data indicate that the ingestion of cranberry juice or cranberry extract tablets is related to a significant decrease in the incidence of symptomatic UTIs. Constituents in cranberries prevent bacteria from adhering to a person's cell surface membranes, thereby impairing colonization and subsequent infection, rather than by the historical premise that acidification of urine provides an antibacterial effect. Cranberry intake has been found to be a safe, herbal choice for *preventing* a UTI. However, it should be used cautiously in long-term use for patients who have a propensity to form urinary oxalate stones. Interestingly, conclusions of randomized trials reported no evidence demonstrating that cranberry is effective in *treating* a UTI. Therefore, ingestion of cranberry juice (24 oz daily) or extract tablets (300 to 400 mg twice a day) is recommended in the prophylaxis of a UTI but is not recommended for its treatment.

c. Teach family members not to make the patient feel guilty or ashamed.

d. Encourage the patient to avoid fluid intake after the evening meal.

e. Encourage the patient to empty the bladder just before going to bed.

5. Dependent nursing care.

a. Administer prescribed medications.

(1) Tricyclic antidepressants, such as imipramine (Tofranil); administer at bedtime; ensure monthly blood tests to assess for granulocytosis; question the order if prescribed for a child younger than age 6 years; must be gradually reduced over 6 days to prevent withdrawal.

(2) Anticholinergics, such as oxybutynin (Ditropan); teach parents to assess for clinical manifestations of urinary retention.

b. Teach the patient to use a bed alarm, which awakens the patient when voiding, only if ordered by a primary health-care provider trained in the treatment of enuresis.

D. Urinary Retention

1. Overview.

a. Accumulation of urine in the bladder due to an inability to empty the bladder completely.

b. Excessive distention of the urinary bladder impairs contractility of the detrusor muscle, further impairing urination.

2. Clinical manifestations.

a. Bladder distention.

b. Reported feeling of bladder fullness.

c. Overflow incontinence exhibited as frequent urination of small amounts of urine.

3. Precipitating factors.

a. Factors that cause inflammation and swelling of the genitourinary tract (e.g., infection and pelvic surgery).

b. Neurologic problems that affect the brain, spinal cord, or peripheral nerves (e.g., brain attack, tumors, and blunt trauma to neurological tissue).

c. Infection (e.g., genital herpes).

d. Obstructions (e.g., enlarged prostate, strictures, tumor, urinary calculi, and fecal impaction).

e. Medications (e.g., antihistamines, tricyclic antidepressants, beta-adrenergic blockers, monoamine oxidase inhibitors, antispasmodics, antiparkinsonism medications, and anesthetic agents).

4. Independent nursing care.

a. Monitor I&O.

b. Palpate the suprapubic area for bladder distention.

c. Encourage the patient to use a position that facilitates voiding by the use of gravity.

d. Provide privacy when toileting.

e. Use techniques to encourage voiding.

5. Dependent nursing care.

a. Assist the patient with a warm water bath that exposes just the perineal area to the water (**sitz bath**).

b. Measure postvoiding residual (e.g., catheterization with a single-lumen tube, bladder ultrasound).

c. Insert a single-lumen catheter or indwelling urinary catheter as ordered.

d. Provide preoperative and postoperative care for a patient having surgery to remove an obstruction, such as prostate surgery.

e. Teach intermittent self-catheterization to drain the bladder for patients with spinal cord injuries or neurologic disorders.

VIII. Urinary Catheters

A urinary catheter may be inserted into the urinary bladder via the urethra to collect a specimen, empty the urinary bladder and then be removed, or remain in place to mitigate a problem. The insertion of a urinary catheter is a dependent function of the nurse and requires an order from a primary health-care provider. There are various types of urinary catheters, each with its own distinct purpose. The nurse must know the principles associated with urinary catheter insertion, nursing care common to all types of urinary catheters, and nursing care specific to each type of catheter to ensure that the patient's urinary elimination needs are met based on established standards of nursing practice.

A. Purpose

1. Obtain a sterile specimen.

2. Maintain an empty bladder during diagnostic tests and during or after surgical procedures.

3. Treat or prevent urinary retention.

4. Measure the volume of residual urine.

B. Types (Fig. 20.5)

1. Single-lumen (straight) catheter.

a. Inserted to obtain a sterile urine specimen, to measure residual urine after voiding, or for the immediate relief of urinary retention.

b. Immediately removed after purpose is achieved.

2. Indwelling catheter (retention catheter).

a. Double-lumen tube used for continuous bladder drainage.

b. One lumen to inflate the balloon to keep the tube in place and a second lumen to drain urine.

3. Triple-lumen catheter.

a. Used for continuous bladder irrigation.

b. One lumen to inflate the balloon, second lumen to continuously instill a GU irrigant, and third lumen to drain urine and irrigant into a collection container.

Fig 20.5 Types of urinary catheters. (A) A single-lumen catheter is used to obtain a urine sample or immediately drain the bladder. (B) A double-lumen catheter is the most commonly used indwelling catheter. (C) A triple-lumen catheter is inserted when the patient requires irrigation of the bladder. (From Wilkinson and Treas [2011]. *Fundamentals of nursing*, Vol. 1, 2nd ed. Philadelphia: F. A. Davis Company, with permission.)

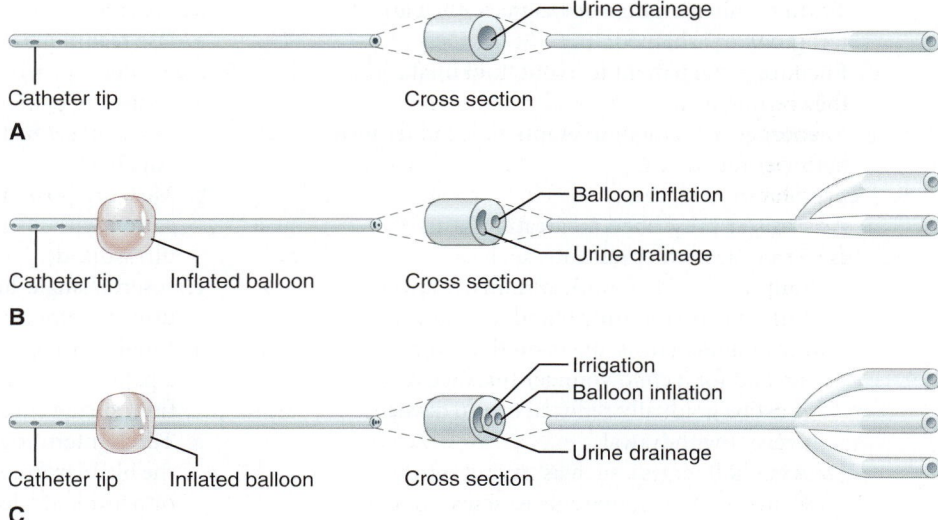

C. Inserting a Urinary Catheter

1. Explain what is going to be done and why, provide privacy, and wash your hands.
2. Position the patient in the supine position, and drape the patient exposing only the perineal area.
   a. *Women:* Flex the knees, and allow the thighs to externally rotate; Sims' position with the upper leg flexed is also acceptable.
   b. *Men:* Slightly separate the legs with the knees and hips extended.
3. Don clean gloves, wash the perineal area, remove your gloves, and wash your hands.
4. Arrange the work area.
   a. Open a sterile catheter kit on a clean bedside table without contaminating the inside.
   b. Arrange a trash receptacle impervious to liquid in easy reach.
5. Don sterile gloves and maintain their sterility throughout the procedure.
6. Place the first sterile drape in position without contaminating the drape.
   a. *Women:* Under the perineal area.
   b. *Men:* Across the thighs.
7. Position the second sterile drape with the opening (fenestrated drape) arranged so that the urinary meatus is visible.
   a. *Women:* Over the perineum with the hole over the labia.
   b. *Men:* Over the thighs with the hole over the penis.
8. Organize the sterile supplies in the catheter kit.
   a. Pour the antiseptic solution over the cotton balls.
   b. Arrange the forceps near the cotton balls.
   c. Squeeze sterile lubricant into the kit tray.
   d. Connect the syringe to the catheter port.
   e. Roll the catheter tip in the lubricant (a length of 2 inches for women and 8 inches for men).

9. Position the catheter kit on the sterile field.
   a. *Women:* Between the patient's legs.
   b. *Men:* On top of the thighs or between the patient's legs.
10. Place the collection bag on the field or nearby if it is preattached to the catheter and tubing.
11. Cleanse the urinary meatus.
    a. *Women:* With one hand, spread and gently pull the labia majora and minora upward, exposing the urinary meatus, and hold this position throughout the procedure (see the black arrow in Fig. 20.6); with the other hand, hold an antiseptic-soaked cotton ball with the forceps and wipe from the pubis to the rectum along the far labia and then discard the cotton ball in the trash receptacle; repeat this along the near labia and then down the middle using a new cotton ball each time (see the red arrows in Fig. 20.6).
    b. *Men:* Reach through the fenestrated drape and grasp the penis (retract the foreskin if the patient

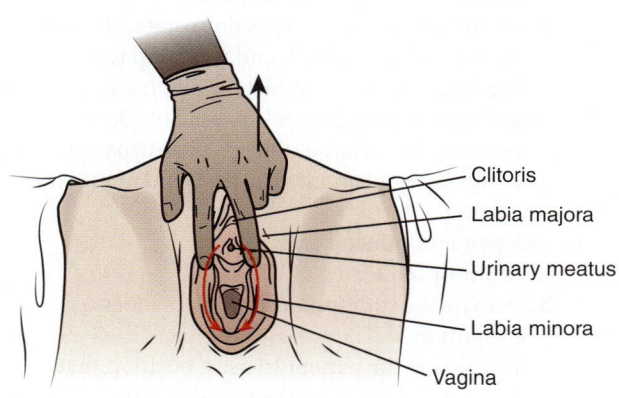

Fig 20.6 Female catheterization.

is uncircumcised) and hold this position throughout the procedure; with the other hand, hold an antiseptic-soaked cotton ball with the forceps and wipe in a circular motion from the center of the urinary meatus outward and down the penis and then discard the cotton ball in the trash receptacle; repeat this two more times using a new cotton ball each time (Fig. 20.7).

12. Insert the catheter.
   a. *Women:* Insert the lubricated end of the catheter 2 to 3 inches into the urinary meatus until urine begins to flow into the tubing and then advance it 1 more inch (this ensures that the catheter has completely passed through the urethra); encourage the patient to take deep breaths to facilitate relaxation; if the catheter touches unsterile linen or the labia or vagina, it is no longer sterile and a new sterile catheter must be used.
   b. *Men:* Insert the lubricated end of the catheter 7 to 9 inches into the urinary meatus until urine begins to flow and then advance 1 more inch to ensure that the catheter has completely passed through the urethra (Fig. 20.8); do not force catheter insertion if resistance is felt; lower the penis when the bladder is empty; replace the foreskin if the patient is uncircumcised.
13. Hold the catheter in place and, with the other hand, inflate the balloon using the attached saline-filled syringe (Fig. 20.9); if the patient complains of discomfort, deflate the balloon,

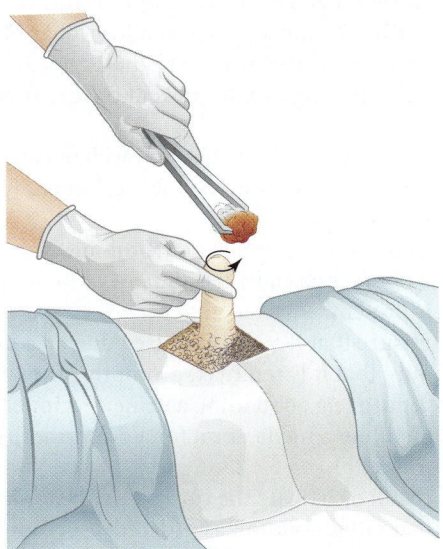

Fig 20.7 Cleansing the male urinary meatus. (From Wilkinson and Treas [2011]. *Fundamentals of nursing,* Vol. 2, 2nd ed. Philadelphia: F. A. Davis Company, with permission.)

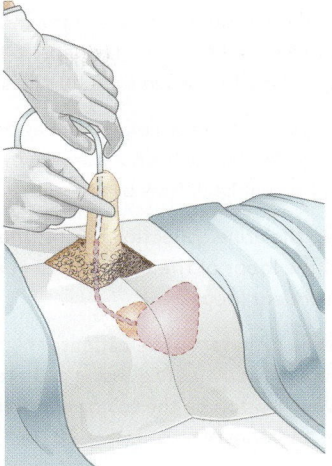

Fig 20.8 Inserting a urinary catheter into the penis. (From Wilkinson and Treas [2011]. *Fundamentals of nursing,* Vol. 2, 2nd ed. Philadelphia: F. A. Davis Company, with permission.)

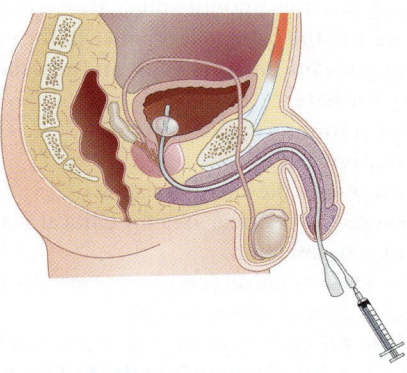

A   Catheter placement, male

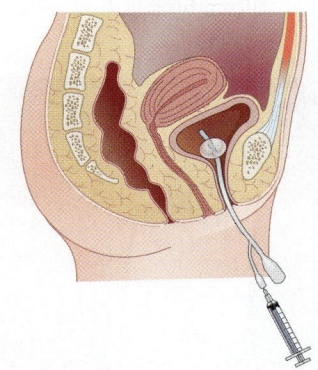

B   Catheter placement, female

Fig 20.9 Catheter placement. (A) Male. (B) Female. (From Wilkinson and Treas [2011]. *Fundamentals of nursing,* Vol. 2, 2nd ed. Philadelphia: F. A. Davis Company, with permission.)

advance the catheter 1 inch, and reinflate the balloon because the catheter may be in the urethra.

14. Discard used supplies, remove your gloves, and wash your hands.

15. Hang the urine collection bag on the bed frame rather than on a side rail to prevent trauma to the urinary meatus and bladder when the side rail is moved.

    a. Always hang a urine collection bag below the level of the bladder to promote urine flow by gravity and prevent back flow of urine into the bladder;

    b. Keep the urine collection bag off the floor and coil the loops of the tubing on the bed to avoid dependent loops.

16. Secure the catheter to the patient's thigh for females or abdomen for males (e.g., using catheter strap, tape) to prevent tension on the tubing and trauma to the bladder and urinary meatus (Fig. 20.10).

17. Don clean gloves, cleanse the perineal area, and remove your gloves.

18. Return the patient to a comfortable position and wash your hands.

19. Document the amount and characteristics of urine and the patient's response to the procedure.

D. Nursing Care for Patients With an Indwelling Urinary Catheter

1. Perform routine assessments.
   a. Monitor I&O.
   b. Monitor urine characteristics.
   c. Assess the perineal area for clinical manifestations of infection.
   d. Assess for clinical manifestations of a UTI.

2. Provide care to prevent a UTI.
   a. Keep the collection bag below the level of the bladder by attaching it to the bed frame and

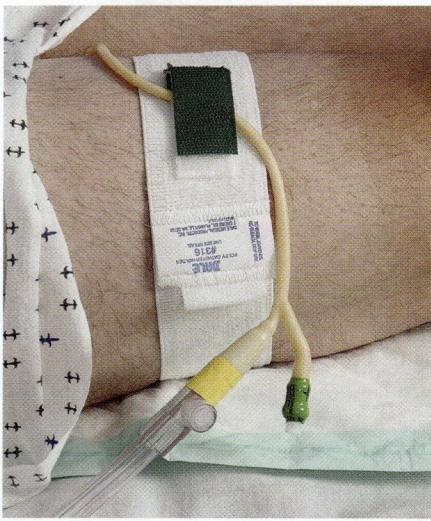

Fig 20.10 Securing a urinary catheter. (From Wilkinson and Treas [2011]. *Fundamentals of nursing*, Vol. 2, 2nd ed. Philadelphia: F. A. Davis Company, with permission.)

coiling the tubing on the bed to prevent dependent loops.

b. Maintain a closed system to prevent the introduction of pathogens by maintaining the integrity of all connections; if the tubing becomes disconnected, wipe both ends of the tubing with an antiseptic solution before reconnecting them.

c. Wash the perineal area and around and down the catheter with mild soap and water and rinse and dry thoroughly every 8 hours; avoid using powders and lotions after perineal care because these products provide a medium for the growth of microorganisms.

d. Encourage ambulation and the upright position to facilitate bladder emptying if permitted.

e. Encourage the intake of 3 L of fluid daily, if permitted, to help flush the urinary tract.

f. Encourage the intake of foods that increase urine acidity (e.g., cranberry juice, eggs, meat, poultry, whole grains, plums, prunes, and tomatoes); acidic urine discourages the growth of microorganisms.

g. Discourage the intake of foods that increase urine alkalinity (e.g., most fruits, vegetables, legumes, milk, and milk products); alkaline urine favors the growth of microorganisms.

h. Maintain aseptic technique when emptying the collection bag (e.g., keep the drainage bag off the floor; ensure the spout does not touch the collection graduate or floor).

i. Teach the patient the importance of meticulous perineal care after a bowel movement.

j. Administer a prescribed oral or intravenous antibiotic and a prescribed topical antibiotic or antifungal ointment to the perineal area.

3. Specific nursing care to prevent obstruction of the catheter.
   a. Ensure the catheter has no mechanical obstructions (e.g., kinks in the tubing, patient lying on the tubing).
   b. Monitor the patency of the tubing every 2 hours, especially if sediment or hematuria is present.
   c. Ensure that if a clamp is used during a procedure that it is removed promptly after the procedure (e.g., obtaining a urine specimen, instilling a medication for a prescribed time frame).
   d. Instill or irrigate the catheter with sterile normal saline solution as ordered, especially if the patient's urine has blood clots or large amounts of sediment.
   e. Change the catheter if drainage is impaired.

4. Removal of an indwelling urinary catheter.
   a. Clamp the drainage tubing distal to the French catheter as ordered by the primary health-care provider (e.g., clamp for 2 hours and release for 15 minutes 3 times a day) to increase bladder tone in preparation for discontinuation of the urinary catheter.

🛑 b. Use a needless syringe to remove the fluid in the balloon before removal of the urinary catheter; never use a scissor to cut a urinary catheter to drain the balloon because it can compress the lumen preventing removal of the fluid.

IX. Urinary Diversions

Because of a disease process or injury to the urethra, bladder, or ureter, a patient may require the creation of a urinary diversion to permit evacuation of urine. An ileal conduit, Kock pouch, nephrostomy tube, suprapubic tube, and ureterostomy tube are types of urinary diversions surgically created for the elimination of urine. To best meet patients' urinary elimination needs, the nurse must understand each type of diversion, including the way in which it is formed and the way in which it works; the general physical and psychological nursing care of a patient with a urinary diversion; and the specific nursing care related to the each type of urinary diversion.

A. **Types**
   1. **Ileal conduit** (Fig. 20.11).
      a. A segment of the ileum is removed and used as a pouch reservoir.
      b. One end is brought through the abdominal wall to form a stoma.
      c. Ureters are implanted into the pouch.
      d. Urine drains continuously.

2. **Kock pouch** (Fig. 20.12).
   a. Portion of the ileum is used to form a pouch reservoir, which is connected to the skin.
   b. Ureters empty into the pouch.
   c. A nipple valve is created surgically and the pouch is emptied by inserting a clean catheter every few hours (continent diversion).
   d. A small dressing is worn over the nipple stoma between emptying.
3. **Nephrostomy tube** (Fig. 20.13).
   a. A tube is placed into the pelvis of a kidney to drain urine into a collection container.

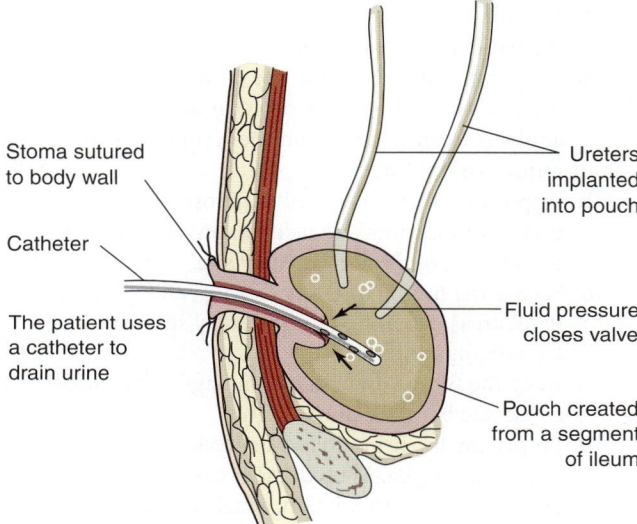

Fig 20.12 Kock pouch. (From Burton and Ludwig [2011]. *Fundamentals of nursing care: Concepts, connections & skills.* Philadelphia: F. A. Davis Company, with permission.)

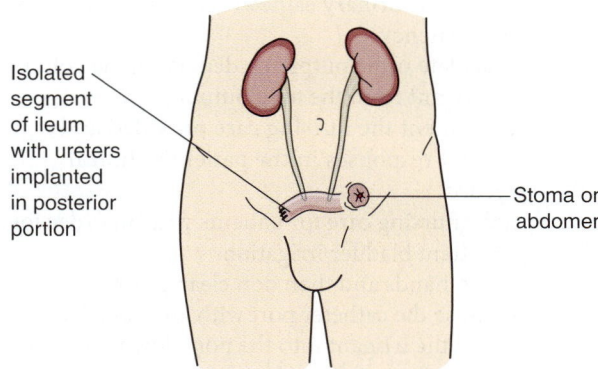

Fig 20.11 Ileal conduit. (From Burton and Ludwig [2011]. *Fundamentals of nursing care: Concepts, connections & skills.* Philadelphia: F. A. Davis Company, with permission.)

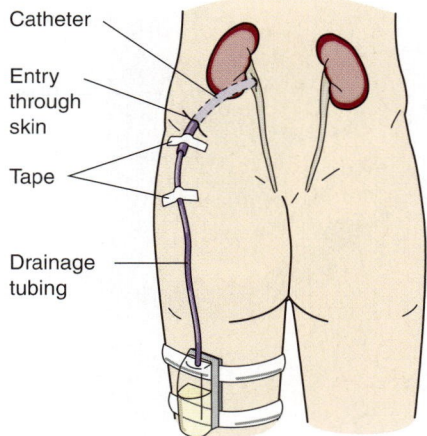

Fig 20.13 Nephrostomy tube with leg bag. (From Williams & Hopper [2011]. *Understanding medical surgical nursing,* 4th ed. Philadelphia: F. A. Davis, with permission.)

b. Prevents accumulation of urine and stretching of the renal pelvis (**hydronephrosis**) due to an obstructed ureter.

4. **Suprapubic tube** (Fig. 20.14).
   a. A catheter is surgically inserted through a small incision above the symphysis pubis to drain urine into a collection container.
   b. It diverts urine when flow of urine through the urethra is impaired.
   c. It may be temporary or permanent.

B. **Nursing Care for Patients With a Urinary Diversion**
   1. Monitor I&O.
   2. Assess site for clinical manifestations of inflammation or infection.
   3. Provide emotional support and teach self-care if the patient is able to learn.
   4. Keep the skin around the site clean and dry, protect it with a moisture-proof skin barrier and apply povidone-iodine ointment if prescribed to reduce risk of infection.
   5. Apply a prescribed topical antibiotic (e.g., bacitracin) or antifungal (e.g., nystatin) ointment on the skin around the tube entry site.
   6. Secure the tubing to the body (e.g., abdomen or flank area) depending on the entry site to reduce tension on the tube.
   7. Keep the tubing and collection bag(s) dependent to the site being drained.
   8. Empty smaller urine collection devices (e.g., leg bag) frequently; leg bag is used under clothing during the day to facilitate ambulation; attach the tubing to a larger collection device when the patient is sleeping.

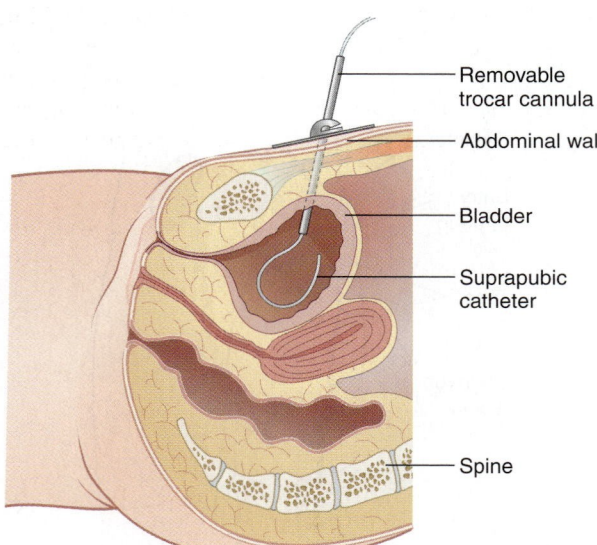

Fig 20.14 Suprapubic tube. (From Burton and Ludwig [2011]. *Fundamentals of nursing care: Concepts, connections & skills.* Philadelphia: F. A. Davis Company, with permission.)

9. Suprapubic tube: In preparation for removal of a temporary tube, clamp the catheter for 3- to 4-hour periods during the day to assess whether the patient is voiding a satisfactory volume through the urethra; residual is measured to determine what is satisfactory.

X. Bladder Irrigations

Instillation of a solution into the urinary bladder may be ordered by the primary health-care provider to flush the bladder, instill medication into the bladder, or maintain patency of a urinary catheter. Instillations may be intermittent or continuous. The nurse must know the principles of and implement actions related to commonalities of nursing care and specific nursing care associated with both intermittent and continuous bladder irrigation to best meet patient's urinary elimination needs.

A. **Types**
   1. Intermittent irrigation.
      a. Used to instill medication.
      b. Used to restore catheter patency.
   2. Continuous irrigation.
      a. Used to maintain catheter patency when hematuria, clots, or debris are anticipated, generally after surgery (e.g.., transurethral resection of the prostate).
      b. Involves use of a triple-lumen catheter: One to inflate the balloon to hold the catheter in the bladder, the second to continuously instill the GU irrigant, and the third to drain urine and irrigant to a collection device.

B. **Nursing Care**
   1. Commonalities of nursing care when implementing a bladder irrigation.
      a. Provide for privacy.
      b. Assess the patient's comfort, including the presence of painful bladder spasms.
      c. Assess the urinary catheter frequently to ensure tube patency.
      d. Calculate urine output by deducting the volume of irrigant from the total output.
      e. Document the nursing care provided and patient responses in the patient's clinical record.
   2. Specific nursing care for patients with an order for intermittent bladder irrigation.
      a. Wash hands and then don clean gloves.
      b. Cleanse the catheter port with an alcohol swab.
      c. Instill the irrigant into the port slowly to facilitate the flow of the irrigant into the bladder and limit trauma to the mucous membranes of the urinary tract (Fig. 20.15).
      d. Allow the solution to return via gravity.

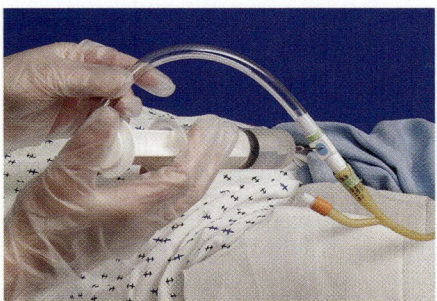

Fig 20.15 Intermittent bladder irrigation. (From Burton and Ludwig [2011]. *Fundamentals of nursing care: Concepts, connections & skills.* Philadelphia: F. A. Davis Company, with permission.)

3. Specific nursing care for patients with an order for continuous bladder irrigation (Fig. 20.16).
   a. Connect a 3-L bag of the ordered solution to the input port of the three-way catheter.
   b. Adjust the flow rate as ordered; a specific rate may be ordered (e.g., 40 to 60 drops per minute) or the rate may be left to the discretion of the nurse to keep the output pink and free from clots.
   c. Assess output every 15 minutes to ensure patency of the tubing; if the tubing becomes occluded, bladder distention and fluid backup can cause distention of the pelvis of the kidney and impede kidney function.
   d. Ensure that the 3-L bag of irrigant is replaced when the previous bag is low on fluid so it does not run out because the flow must be uninterrupted to ensure catheter patency.

XI. Medications That Affect the Urinary System

When a person is diagnosed with a urinary system problem, the primary health-care provider can prescribe medication, such as kidney-specific anti-infectives to treat a UTI; urinary antispasmodics to reduce bladder spasms, increasing bladder capacity and decreasing incontinence;

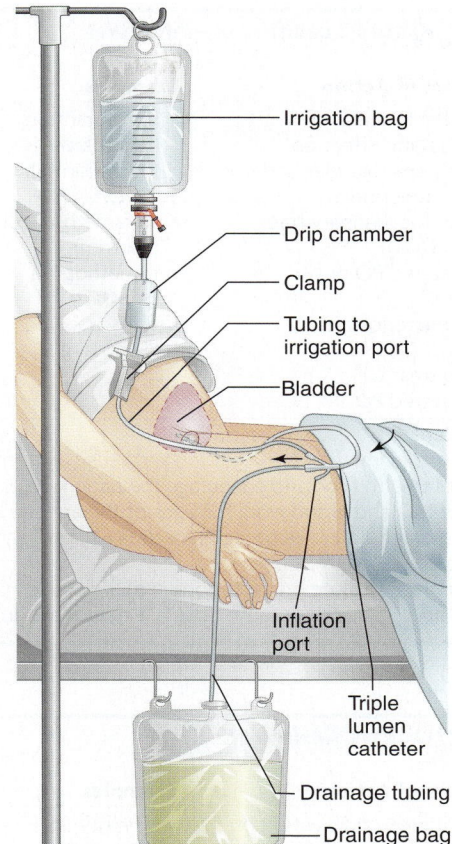

Fig 20.16 Continuous bladder irrigation. (From Burton and Ludwig [2011]. *Fundamentals of nursing care: Concepts, connections & skills.* Philadelphia: F. A. Davis Company, with permission).

or estrogen to decrease vaginal and vulvar itching, inflammation, and dryness, which impact the urinary system. Nurses should know the mechanisms of action, therapeutic and nontherapeutic effects, and nursing care related to the common medications prescribed to treat urinary system problems.
A. **Kidney-Specific Anti-infectives:** Table 20.3.
B. **Urinary Antispasmodics:** Table 20.4.
C. **Estrogen:** Table 20.5.

Table 20.3 Kidney-Specific Anti-infectives

Mechanism of Action	Examples	Nontherapeutic Effects
• Have a bactericidal or bacteriostatic effect on kidney, ureter, bladder, and urethral infections. • Used for local urinary tract infection (UTI). • Administered PO or IV. *Sulfonamides* • Have a bacteriostatic effect. • Used to treat UTI. • Administered PO, IM, IV.	• nitrofurantoin (Macrobid, Macrodantin) *Sulfonamides* • sulfamethoxazole (Bactrim) • trimethoprim (Septra) • sulfisoxazole (Gantrisin)	• Irritation of GI mucosa, such as anorexia, nausea, vomiting, abdominal pain, diarrhea, and pseudomembranous colitis. • Allergic responses, such as skin rash and exfoliative dermatitis. • Neurotoxicity, such as headache and peripheral neuropathy. • Nephrotoxicity. • Decreased white blood cell, red blood cell, and platelet counts. • Photosensitivity. • Staining of teeth. *Sulfonamides* • Same as above plus hepatic necrosis, toxic epidermal necrolysis, agranulocytosis, aplastic anemia, erythema multiforme, and Stevens-Johnson syndrome.

Nursing Care
- Obtain a specimen for urine culture and sensitivity before initiating antibiotics.
- Administer with food and encourage the patient to rinse the mouth to minimize GI irritation.
- Monitor I&O and blood work for signs of therapeutic and nontherapeutic effects.
- Increase oral fluid intake to facilitate drug excretion and minimize risk of toxicity and crystalluria.
- Protect from sunlight.
- *Nitrofurantoin:* Dilute oral solutions in milk or juice, use a straw, and have the patient rinse the mouth to minimize staining of teeth; do not open capsules or crush tablets; explain that urine will be brown or rust in color.

Table 20.4 Urinary Antispasmotics

Mechanism of Action	Examples	Nontherapeutic Effects
• Have antispasmodic action on smooth muscle of the urinary tract. • Increase bladder capacity. • Decrease frequency, urgency, and urge incontinence.	• oxybutynin (Ditropan) • tolterodine (Detrol)	• Anticholinergic effects, such as palpitations, tachycardia, headache, dizziness, dry mouth, urinary retention, allergic reaction, drowsiness, blurred vision, and constipation. • Sedation and weakness in older adults.

Nursing Care
- Monitor I&O and for clinical manifestations of therapeutic and nontherapeutic effects.
- Administer 30 to 60 minutes before meals and at hour of sleep.
- Teach the patient to avoid driving or activities requiring alertness if drowsiness occurs.
- Encourage the patient to chew gum or suck on hard candy or ice chips to relieve dry mouth.
- *Oxybutynin:* Teach the patient to avoid hot environments because the ability to perspire may be impaired.

Table 20.5 Estrogen

Mechanism of Action	Examples	Nontherapeutic Effects
• Decreases vaginal and vulvar itching, inflammation, and dryness. • Used to treat atrophic vaginitis. • Inserted with a vaginal applicator.	• estropipate vaginal cream • estradiol vaginal tablet (Vagifen) • estradiol vaginal ring (Femring, Estring)	• *Femring:* Risk of endometrial carcinoma in patients with an intact uterus.

Nursing Care
- Teach the patient the method for using the vaginal applicator; explain that the dose is marked on the applicator and the patient should wash the applicator with soap and water and dry it after each use.
- Encourage the patient to remain in the supine or recumbent position for 30 minutes after insertion.
- Teach the patient to avoid the use of tampons and to use a sanitary pad to protect clothing.

CASE STUDY: Putting It All Together

A 67-year-old man visits his primary health-care provider because of an inability to urinate and lower abdominal distension. The provider diagnoses urinary retention and sends the patient immediately to the hospital for the insertion of a urinary retention catheter. At the hospital, a urinary retention catheter is inserted and the patient is admitted to a surgical unit for diagnostic tests in preparation for surgery to remove obstructing prostate tissue. The nurse completes an admission interview, identifies the patient's home medications, and reviews the primary health-care provider's orders, which were faxed to the hospital from the provider's office. The nurse read the patient's clinical record.

Patient's Clinical Record

Admission Interview

This 67-year-old male explained that he rents a room in a boarding house and shares a bathroom with three other men. He stated, "I am being treated for heart disease, allergies in the spring, and depression. I smoke two packs of cigarettes a day, love my four cups of coffee in the morning, and enjoy a six-pack of beer and bag of potato chips every night while watching TV. There is not much to do since my third heart attack 10 months ago." He explained that over the past year he had two urinary tract infections and more frequent nighttime awakenings to urinate. He described urinary hesitancy, frequency, a slow urinary stream, and discomfort when urinating. When asked what brought him to his primary health-care provider today, he stated, "For 24 hours, I couldn't urinate. When my lower belly started to get bigger and I felt a lot of pressure down there (pointing to his suprapubic area), I went to the doctor. The doctor said that I had to go to the hospital because I had an enlarged prostate and that I needed surgery."

Primary Health-Care Provider's Orders

2-gram sodium diet.
OOB to chair with assistance.
Vital signs every shift.
Urinary retention catheter to gravity.
I&O.
Pelvic and renal sonogram.
Urinalysis, urine C&S.
CBC, metabolic profile.
tamsulosin (Flomax) 0.4 mg PO every a.m.
IV 0.9% Sodium Chloride 75 mL per hour for 2 L.

Medication Reconciliation Form

Hydrochlorothiazide 50 mg PO daily in a.m.; for hypertension; last taken this a.m.
Loratadine (Claritin) 10 mg PO daily; for seasonal allergies; last taken this a.m.
Sertraline (Zoloft) 50 mg PO a.m.; for depression; last taken this a.m.

Case Study Questions

A. Identify at least eight factors in this scenario may have impacted the patient's urinary elimination and why?

1. _____
2. _____
3. _____
4. _____
5. _____
6. _____
7. _____
8. _____

Continued

CASE STUDY: Putting It All Together   *cont'd*

Case Study Questions

B. Identify at least five additional clinical indicators of urinary retention the nurse should explore with the patient to ensure a complete history.

1. _____

2. _____

3. _____

4. _____

5. _____

C. Which medications that the patient was taking at home may have had an impact on the patient's urinary system and why?

1. _____

2. _____

3. _____

D. After surgery, the patient is expected to have a triple-lumen urinary catheter for continuous bladder irrigation. Identify at least ten nursing interventions that should be implemented for patients with any type of urinary tube, and three nursing interventions that are specific to caring for patients with a triple-lumen urinary catheter for continuous bladder irrigation.

Common principles associated with caring for patients with any type of urinary tube:

1. _____

2. _____

3. _____

4. _____

5. _____

6. _____

7. _____

8. _____

9. _____

10. _____

Specific principles when caring for a patient with a triple-lumen urinary catheter for continuous bladder irrigation:

1. _____

2. _____

3. _____

REVIEW QUESTIONS

1. A hospitalized 70-year-old adult has a computed tomography (CT) scan with contrast at 11 a.m. The patient has an IV running at 125 mL per hour and ingested 50 percent of lunch with a cup of coffee and 4 oz of soup at 12 noon. The nurse is going on a break at 1 p.m. and provides the following information to the nurse accepting responsibility for the patient. Which information about the patient is of **most** concern to the nurse accepting responsibility for the patient?
   1. Urine output - 100 mL
   2. Presence of slight nausea
   3. Medicated for a mild headache
   4. Blood pressure - 150/84 mm Hg

2. A nurse is assisting a female patient who is experiencing numerous daily episodes of urge incontinence to gain better bladder control. Which outcome reflects achievement of a goal associated with this patient's urge incontinence?
   1. Urinates every two hours while remaining dry between voiding
   2. Wears an adult incontinence brief only when venturing outside the home
   3. Empties the bladder every time before leaving the house, limiting incontinence
   4. Uses deep, slow breathing until the sensation to void subsides, increasing intervals between voiding

3. A nurse identifies that a patient may be experiencing urinary retention. Which clinical indicators support this inference? **Select all that apply.**
   1. _____ Voiding small amounts of urine several times hourly
   2. _____ Abdominal palpation indicating bladder distention
   3. _____ Tenderness over the symphysis pubis on palpation
   4. _____ Dysuria on urination
   5. _____ Blood-tinged urine

4. A nurse is caring for an older adult female who says, "Why am I always getting bladder infections?" Which response by the nurse is **most** appropriate?
   1. "Women have a shorter urethra than men do, and that makes women more susceptible than men to bladder infections."
   2. "Older adults may experience retained urine, which becomes more acidic and promotes the development of bladder infections."
   3. "It is hard for women to cleanse the urinary meatus, which increases the risk of bladder infections."
   4. "Infrequent sexual intercourse predisposes women to bladder infections."

5. A nurse is caring for a patient who has a urinary retention catheter. The primary health-care provider orders a urine culture and sensitivity. Which step ensures that the collected specimen is sterile?
   1. Swab the specimen port with an antiseptic swab.
   2. Don sterile gloves when obtaining the specimen.
   3. Use a urinalysis container to collect the specimen.
   4. Collect the specimen early in the morning before breakfast.

6. A primary health-care provider prescribes nitrofurantoin (Macrodantin) 100 mg twice a day by mouth for a patient with a urinary tract infection. The pharmacy sends up unit dose packages labeled 25 mg per capsule. The primary nurse on the 12-hour day shift checks the medication drawer to ensure that there are enough capsules for the next 24 hours. How many tablets should be available for disbursement to the patient?
   Answer: _____ capsules

7. While all of the following clinical manifestations are important to report to a primary health-care provider, which is **most** important?
   1. Anuria
   2. Dysuria
   3. Polyuria
   4. Nocturia

8. A patient reports concern about not having urinated in several hours. The patient reports the sensation of the need to void and has moderate abdominal distention. What should the nurse do **first**?
   1. Encourage the patient to drink more fluid.
   2. Stroke the inner aspect of the patient's thigh.
   3. Pour warm water over the patient's perineal area.
   4. Have the patient assume an upright position for voiding.

9. A patient with a history of urinary tract infections asks the nurse for suggestions to limit their occurrence. Which should the nurse encourage the patient to ingest to inhibit the growth of microorganisms that can cause a bladder infection? **Select all that apply.**
   1. _____ Eggs
   2. _____ Meats
   3. _____ Apple juice
   4. _____ Cranberry juice
   5. _____ Whole-grain breads

10. Which nursing intervention is **most** effective when assisting a patient to completely empty the bladder?
   1. Place the patient's hands in warm water.
   2. Stroke an inner aspect of the patient's thigh.
   3. Encourage the patient to attempt to double void.
   4. Turn a faucet on in the patient's room to produce sounds of flowing water.

11. A patient reports signs and symptoms associated with urge incontinence. Which action should the nurse teach the patient to employ to gain better bladder control?
   1. Avoid lifting heavy objects.
   2. Avoid products with caffeine.
   3. Use the Credé maneuver when voiding.
   4. Respond immediately to the sensation to void.

12. A home-care nurse is caring for a cognitively intact woman who has arthritis that affects her hands and slows her mobility. The patient tells the nurse about having a few episodes of urinary incontinence that were upsetting. The nurse identifies that the patient is experiencing functional incontinence. Which nursing interventions in the plan of care are specific to limiting episodes of incontinence in this patient? **Select all that apply.**
   1. _____ Encourage wearing clothing with Velcro closures instead of buttons and zippers.
   2. _____ Suggest purchasing a lift chair if economics permit.
   3. _____ Encourage avoiding products with caffeine.
   4. _____ Teach to position a commode nearby.
   5. _____ Teach the patient Kegel exercises.
   6. _____ Suggest voiding every 2 hours.

13. A nurse is caring for a female patient who has a history of frequent urinary tract infections. What should the nurse teach the patient to do?
   1. Wear nylon underwear.
   2. Void before having intercourse.
   3. Take a bubble bath rather than showering.
   4. Urinate when the urge to urinate is perceived.

14. A patient has a urinary retention catheter in place. The nurse must obtain a sterile urine specimen for culture and sensitivity. Where should the nurse place the clamp to allow urine to collect in the tubing so that the nurse can collect a specimen?
   1. A
   2. B
   3. C
   4. D

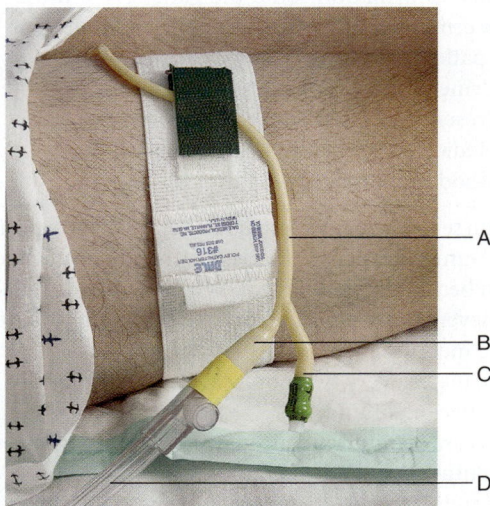

15. A nurse is caring for a group of patients. Which patient should cause the **most** concern about potential urinary retention?
   1. The patient who is immobile in bed
   2. The patient who just had a retention catheter removed
   3. The patient who is disoriented to time, place, and person
   4. The patient who just was placed on a fluid restricted diet

16. A nurse is caring for a postoperative patient with a urinary retention catheter. The nurse reviews the surgeon's orders, reviews the last nursing progress note, and performs a physical assessment of the patient.

Patient's Clinical Record

Surgeon's Postoperative Orders 0900

IVF 0.9% Sodium Chloride at 50 mL/hour.
Full liquid diet progress to 2-g Na diet as tolerated.
I&O.
Ambulate in room this p.m. and progress to 50 feet bid in a.m.
Apply sequential compression devices when in bed.
OOB in chair for meals starting noon tomorrow.
Maintain Foley to bedside collection bag.
Heparin 5,000 units Sub-Q bid.
PCA: Dilaudid 1 mg/hour with 0.2 mg/15-minute lockout, not to exceed 7.2 mg in 4 hours.
Colace 100 mg PO daily.

Progress Notes 0900

Patient received from the PACU at 0900; vital signs stable. Alert to time, place, and person. States that pain is a level 2 and tolerable. Abdominal dressing dry and intact. IVF 0.9% NS in right antecubital space; site dry, and intact; running at 50 mL/hour. PCA infusion site is dry and intact and infusion pump is set at ordered rate. 60 mL noted in hourly urine collection chamber and emptied into the main collection chamber. Urine is straw colored, no sediment noted.

Nurse's Physical Assessment 1000

Patient resting in bed; vital signs stable; patient states pain is tolerable on a level 3 and it was unnecessary to push the PCA pump during the last hour. Dressing dry and intact; 70 mL urine noted in hourly urine chamber. 100 mL oral fluids tolerated. IVF 0.9% NS running at 50 mL/hour. States a desire to engage in ankle pumping exercises.

Which action should the nurse perform **first**?
1. Ambulate the patient in the room.
2. Encourage coughing and deep breathing.
3. Empty the patient's urine collection chamber hourly.
4. Turn off the compression device during ankle pumping exercises.

17. A patient is scheduled for thoracic surgery and is told by the surgeon that after surgery a catheter will be placed in the bladder. After the surgeon leaves, the patient asks the nurse, "Why am I going to have a tube in my bladder when I am having surgery in my chest?" Which response by the nurse is **most** appropriate?
    1. "It is more convenient to control urine flow rather than having to clean a patient after being incontinent."
    2. "We want patients to rest after your type of surgery. You will not be burdened with having to use a bedpan or urinal."
    3. "A urinary catheter enables us to easily secure a urine specimen for laboratory tests that generally are ordered after surgery."
    4. "Hourly urine production is monitored with a urinary catheter. It is an effective way to assess kidney and circulatory function."

18. A nurse is caring for a 3-week-old infant. Which assessment regarding the number of diapers the infant soils daily should cause concern?
    1. 7
    2. 8
    3. 9
    4. 10

19. A nurse is caring for a group of patients with a variety of urinary retention catheters. Which of the following nursing interventions are common to all types of urinary catheters? **Select all that apply.**
    1. _____ Provide perineal care three times a day and whenever necessary.
    2. _____ Position the collection container below the level of the pelvis.
    3. _____ Ensure that the balloon is filled with sterile saline.
    4. _____ Hang the collection bag on the bed frame.
    5. _____ Tape the catheter to the inner thigh.

20. Place these interventions in the order that they should be performed when collecting a urine specimen from an infant.
    1. Wash the hands and don clean gloves.
    2. Apply a collection device over the genitals.
    3. Wash the genital area and allow the area to dry.
    4. Remove the collection bag once the infant urinates.
    5. Send the entire bag in a specimen container to the laboratory.
       Answer: _____

21. Which of the following is essential to ensure reliable bedside dipstick testing of urine? **Select all that apply.**
    1. _____ Use the correct reagent.
    2. _____ Ensure adequate lighting.
    3. _____ Ensure that the kit is not past the expiration date.
    4. _____ Avoid delegating the procedure to another nursing team member.
    5. _____ Read the test results one minute after dipping the test strip in urine.

22. A patient's specific gravity is 1.032. For what additional clinical indicators should the nurse assess the patient? **Select all that apply.**
    1. _____ Presence of thirst
    2. _____ Peripheral edema
    3. _____ Decreased skin turgor
    4. _____ Rapid, weak pulse rate
    5. _____ Decreased blood urea nitrogen

23. A nurse is caring for a patient who is having urine collected for a 24-hour urine test. During the afternoon of the testing period, the patient forgets and accidentally voids into the toilet but tells the nurse right away. What should the nurse do?
    1. Start the test again in the morning.
    2. Identify the time and begin a new test.
    3. Add the time since the previous voiding to the end of the test.
    4. Notify the primary health-care provider about the delay of the test.

24. A nurse is assessing a patient with the diagnosis of urinary tract infection (UTI). Which clinical indicator identified by the nurse supports this medical diagnosis?
    1. Sweet, fruity odor to the urine
    2. Dark amber color of urine
    3. Cloudy urine
    4. Foamy urine

25. A nurse is caring for a patient with a diagnosis of UTI. Which clinical indicators identified during a nursing assessment support the medical diagnosis? **Select all that apply.**
    1. _____ Dysuria
    2. _____ Hematuria
    3. _____ Urinary retention
    4. _____ Urgent sensation to void
    5. _____ Distended suprapubic area

26. A nurse is assessing a patient and is concerned that the patient may be experiencing urinary retention. Which clinical indicators support this conclusion? **Select all that apply.**
    1. _____ Blood-tinged urine
    2. _____ Amber colored urine
    3. _____ Reports of abdominal pressure
    4. _____ Lower abdominal distention on palpation
    5. _____ Voiding small amounts of urine at a time

27. A patient has urinary retention and the primary health-care provider orders a straight catheterization. The draining volume reaches 750 mL without completely emptying the bladder. What alternative does the nurse have to help prevent bladder spasms?
    1. Remove the catheter and reinsert a retention catheter.
    2. Continue the complete emptying of the patient's bladder.
    3. Release the remaining urine in the bladder slowly over 20 minutes.
    4. Take the catheter out and then recatheterize the patient in 20 minutes.

28. A nurse is caring for a patient who has an indwelling urinary catheter. Which nursing actions are important to include in this patient's plan of care? **Select all that apply.**
    1. _____ Obtain the vital signs routinely.
    2. _____ Cleanse the perineal area several times a day.
    3. _____ Monitor the tubing for kinks and obstructions.
    4. _____ Assess the urine for color, cloudiness, and volume.
    5. _____ Attach the drainage collection bag to the bed railing.
    6. _____ Position the drainage bag above the level of the bladder.

29. A nurse receives an order to initiate continuous bladder irrigation. Which catheter should the nurse choose to perform the procedure correctly?
    1. Straight catheter
    2. Indwelling catheter
    3. Triple-lumen catheter
    4. Double-lumen catheter

30. A nurse is to perform a onetime bladder catheterization. The nurse verifies the primary health-care provider's order, washes the hands, and identifies the patient. Place the following steps of the procedure in the order in which they should be performed.
    1. Don sterile gloves.
    2. Lubricate the catheter tip.
    3. Assess the patient for a latex allergy.
    4. Unwrap the catheter kit creating a sterile field.
    5. Advance the catheter 1 inch after urine begins to flow.
    6. Clean the urethral meatus with the solution provided in the kit.
    Answer: _____

31. A postoperative patient has an indwelling catheter that has not drained urine in 3 hours. What should the nurse do **first**?
    1. Ask the primary health-care provider for an order to irrigate the catheter.
    2. Milk the tubing to dislodge any mucus or sediment in the catheter.
    3. Palpate the patient's suprapubic area to assess for distention.
    4. Recognize the patient's status is within expected limits.

32. A nurse is caring for a patient receiving continuous bladder irrigation (CBI). Which nursing action is essential when caring for this patient?
    1. Check the volume of the patient's output every hour to ensure tube patency.
    2. Increase the irrigation solution flow rate until the return flow is pink and free from clots.
    3. Irrigate the double-lumen catheter according to the primary health-care provider's orders.
    4. Turn the patient from side to side to promote output, which minimizes clot formation in the urine.

33. A primary health-care provider orders a 24-hour urine test. Which actions should be implemented by the nurse when conducting this test? **Select all that apply.**
    1. _____ Have the patient void one last time at the end of the 24 hours and add it to the volume being collected.
    2. _____ Have the patient void one last time at the end of the 24 hours and discard the urine.
    3. _____ Collect the first voiding and then add the urine voided for the next 24 hours.
    4. _____ Discard the first voiding and then collect the urine for the next 24 hours.
    5. _____ Store the collected urine for 24 hours in a large collection container.

34. A nurse is caring for a patient with a history of experiencing residual urine after voiding. The nurse uses a bladder ultrasound scanner (BUS) to detect the amount of urine that remains in the bladder after the patient voids. What action should the nurse implement that is essential to this test?
    1. Give perineal hygiene before the procedure is initiated.
    2. Position the patient in the left lateral position for the duration of the procedure.
    3. Explain that no discomfort will be experienced as the transducer is moved on the surface of the skin.
    4. Place the scan head on the abdomen, four inches midline above the pubic bone, aiming the scan head toward the coccyx.

35. A nurse is caring for a patient who is scheduled for a cystoscopy. Which information should the nurse include when teaching the patient about what to expect after the procedure?
    1. Urinary retention may occur after the procedure.
    2. Urine may be dark red initially after the procedure.
    3. Bedrest is necessary for several days after the procedure.
    4. A clear liquid diet generally is ordered for a few days after the procedure.

36. A nurse is applying a condom urinary catheter. Place the following steps in the order in which they should be implemented.
    1. Hold the penis and place the catheter beyond the glans, leaving at least a 1-inch space at the tip of the penis.
    2. Unroll the condom along the full length of the shaft of the penis.
    3. Wrap the external adhesive strip in a spiral along the shaft.
    4. Secure the condom with gentle compression.
    5. Hang the collection bag from the bed frame.
    6. Provide perineal care and dry thoroughly.
    Answer: _____

37. A nurse is obtaining a health history from a patient. The patient states that she is embarrassed about episodes of incontinence when she sneezes or exercises and that she no longer attends an exercise program for this reason. She now walks several miles a day to lose the 50 lb she gained when pregnant with her fifth child. Based on this information, which nursing intervention will **best** help the patient to address the underlying cause of her lack of urine control?
    1. Teach the patient foods to avoid that irritate the bladder mucosa.
    2. Encourage the patient to return to her exercise class.
    3. Engage the patient in a toileting program.
    4. Teach the patient Kegel exercises.

38. The nurse is caring for an older adult who is receiving oxybutynin (Ditropan) to reduce the occurrence of bladder spasms related to a UTI. For which side effect should the nurse assess the patient?
    1. Diaphoresis
    2. Palpitations
    3. Gastric irritation
    4. Orange-colored urine

39. A nurse is caring for a patient with an indwelling urinary retention catheter. The primary health-care provider orders a urine specimen for culture and sensitivity. What should the nurse do when collecting this specimen?
    1. Place the urine specimen in a sterile urine container.
    2. Obtain the urine specimen from the hourly urine chamber of the collection bag.
    3. Collect the urine specimen from the drainage port at the bottom of the collection bag.
    4. Take the urine specimen directly from the distal end of the catheter after separating it from the tubing.

40. A nurse is caring for a 75-year-old male patient with an indwelling catheter. The nurse identifies that the patient has had no additional urine in the bag over a 2-hour period. Place the nurse's actions in the order in which they should be performed.
    1. Obtain an order to irrigate the patient's catheter.
    2. Continue to assess the patient over the next hour.
    3. Encourage the patient to drink fluids.
    4. Palpate over the patient's bladder.
    5. Milk the patient's catheter.
    Answer: _____

REVIEW ANSWERS

1. ANSWER: 1.

Rationales:

1. A urine output of 100 mL is too little output with an intake of 735 mL over 2 hours and may reflect reduced kidney efficiency in reaction to the contrast dye. This is a serious concern and should be reported to the primary health-care provider.

2. Slight nausea is a mild, not critical, reaction to the contrast dye; however, continued monitoring of this symptom should occur.

3. A headache is a mild, not critical, reaction to the contrast dye; however, ongoing monitoring should occur to ensure that the patient obtains relief.

4. A blood pressure of 150/84 mm Hg is within the expected range of 120 to 160 systolic and 80 to 95 diastolic for a patient who is 70 years of age.

TEST-TAKING TIP: Identify the word in the stem that sets a priority. The word *most* in the stem sets a priority. All the options reflect information that should be communicated, but one is *most* essential.

Content Area: Urinary Elimination

Integrated Processes: Communication/Documentation; Nursing Process: Evaluation

Client Need: Safe and Effective Care Environment; Management of Care

Cognitive Level: Application

2. ANSWER: 4.

Rationales:

1. Although scheduled voiding may be done initially, it does not specifically address overcoming the urge to void.

2. Although wearing an incontinence brief may provide a patient with a sense of security, it will not help reduce the urge to void.

3. People with urge incontinence often void every time they leave the house and stay close to a bathroom to minimize the risk of incontinence. While this action may prevent incontinence, it does not help to reduce the urge to void.

4. **Deep, slow breathing helps to progressively relax a person and has proven successful in reducing the urge sensation. Additional interventions include strengthening perineal muscles (Kegel exercises), biofeedback, lifestyle modifications (e.g., avoidance of caffeine, weight reduction, and fluid modifications), and intake of antimuscarinic agents.**

TEST-TAKING TIP: Identify the options with specific determiners. The words *every* in options 1 and 3 and *only* in option 2 are specific determiners. Rarely are options with specific determiners the correct answer. Examine option 4 carefully.

Content Area: Urinary Elimination

Integrated Processes: Nursing Process: Evaluation

Client Need: Physiological Integrity; Basic Care and Comfort

Cognitive Level: Application

3. ANSWER: 1, 2, 3.

Rationales:

1. **Voiding small amounts of urine several times hourly is characteristic of urinary retention. Pressure within the bladder increases as urine collects until the external urethral sphincter is unable to hold back the urine and voiding of small amounts of urine occurs (retention with urinary overflow).**

2. **When the bladder fills to capacity, it rises up out of the pelvis and can be palpated over the symphysis pubis; this is characterized as bladder distention.**

3. **Retained urine causes stretching of the bladder wall which precipitates a feeling of pressure, discomfort, and tenderness over the symphysis pubis.**

4. Dysuria or pain on urination most often is associated with bladder infection, not urinary retention.

5. Blood-tinged urine most often is associated with irritation of or trauma to the bladder and urethral mucosa (e.g., bladder infection, bladder cancer, physical trauma).

Content Area: Urinary Elimination

Integrated Processes: Nursing Process: Assessment

Client Need: Physiological Integrity; Basic Care and Comfort

Cognitive Level: Application

4. ANSWER: 1.

Rationales:

1. **This statement is true. The shorter urethra in woman makes them more susceptible to bladder infections than men who have a longer urethra. Also, the female urinary meatus is close to the anus, which increases the risk of transmission of microorganisms from the intestinal tract to the urinary meatus.**

2. Retained urine associated with aging becomes more alkaline, not acidic, which is an ideal site for bacterial growth.

3. This should not be an issue as long as a woman cleanses the perineal area when bathing daily.

4. Frequent, not infrequent, sexual intercourse predisposes women to bladder infections.

TEST-TAKING TIP: Identify the word in the stem that sets a priority. The word *most* in the stem sets a priority.

Content Area: Urinary Elimination

Integrated Processes: Communication/Documentation; Nursing Process: Implementation

Client Need: Health Promotion and Maintenance

Cognitive Level: Application

5. ANSWER: 1.

Rationales:

1. **Swabbing the specimen port with an antiseptic swab is necessary to remove microorganisms from the port that may contaminate the specimen. In addition, it reduces the risk of introducing microorganisms into the closed urinary retention catheter and collection bag system.**

2. Sterile gloves are not necessary to maintain sterility of the specimen. Clean gloves protect the nurse from the patient's blood and body fluids.

3. The urine collection container must be a sterile urine collection container, not the clean container used for specimens for unsterile urinalysis specimens.

4. The time of day a specimen is collected from a urinary retention catheter will not alter the sterility of the specimen.

Content Area: *Urinary Elimination*
Integrated Processes: *Nursing Process: Implementation*
Client Need: *Physiological Integrity; Reduction of Risk Potential*
Cognitive Level: *Application*

6. **ANSWER: 8.**
Rationale:
Use ratio and proportion to identify the number of capsules required for each dose. Then multiply the product of this calculation by 2 because the prescribed dose is to be administered twice a day.

$$\frac{\text{Desire 100 mg}}{\text{Have 25 mg}} = \frac{\text{x capsules}}{\text{1 capsule}}$$

$$25x = 100 \times 1$$

$$25x = 100$$

$$x = 100 \div 25$$

$$x = 4 \text{ capsules}$$

Multiple 4 capsules by 2 (the number of times the dose is to be administer in a 24-hour period) to arrive at 8 capsules required for the patient in a 24-hour period.
Content Area: *Medication Administration*
Integrated Processes: *Nursing Process: Planning*
Client Need: *Physiological Integrity; Pharmacological and Parenteral Therapies*
Cognitive Level: *Application*

7. **ANSWER: 1.**
Rationales:
1. Anuria describes urine output of less than 100 mL in 24 hours. Anuria is associated with kidney disease or congestive heart failure; both can be life-threatening situations.
2. Dysuria refers to painful or difficult urination. Although this is serious and may be associated with infection or partial obstruction of the urinary tract, generally it is not as critical as another clinical manifestation.
3. Polyuria refers to excessive urination. Although serious and may be caused by excessive hydration, diabetes mellitus, diabetes insipidus, or kidney disease, generally it is not as critical as another clinical manifestation.
4. Nocturia is defined as awakening at night to void. Although a concern because it may be associated with excessive fluid intake and a variety of urinary tract and cardiovascular problems, it generally is not as critical as another clinical manifestation.
TEST-TAKING TIP: Identify the word in the stem that sets a priority. The word *most* in the stem sets a priority.
Content Area: *Urinary Elimination*
Integrated Processes: *Communication/Documentation; Nursing Process: Analysis*

Client Need: *Safe and Effective Care Environment; Management of Care*
Cognitive Level: *Analysis*

8. **ANSWER: 4.**
Rationales:
1. Although encouraging an increase in oral fluid intake may be implemented, it does not immediately address the patient's need to void. Also, the patient's bladder already is moderately distended.
2. Stroking the inner aspect of the patient's thigh may stimulate sensory nerves and promote the micturition reflex. However, this action should not be the first intervention.
3. Although pouring warm water over the perineal area may stimulate voiding, it is not the first action the nurse should take.
4. Assuming an upright position for voiding uses gravity to move urine downward toward the urinary meatus. Also, it is the most common position that people use to urinate. Assuming this position psychologically may facilitate voiding.
TEST-TAKING TIP: Identify the word in the stem that sets a priority. The word *first* in the stem sets a priority. Identify the clang association. The word *void* in the stem and *voiding* in option 4 is a clang association.
Content Area: *Urinary Elimination*
Integrated Processes: *Nursing Process: Implementation*
Client Need: *Physiological Integrity; Basic Care and Comfort*
Cognitive Level: *Application*

9. **ANSWER: 1, 2, 4, 5.**
Rationales:
1. Eggs increase urine acidity, which tends to inhibit the growth of microorganisms.
2. Meats increase urine acidity, which tends to inhibit the growth of microorganisms.
3. Apple juice does not increase urine acidity. Pathogenic microorganisms exist and multiply more readily in alkaline environments.
4. Cranberry juice increases urine acidity, which tends to inhibit the growth of microorganisms.
5. Whole-grain breads increase urine acidity, which tends to inhibit the growth of microorganisms.
Content Area: *Urinary Elimination*
Integrated Processes: *Teaching/Learning; Nursing Process: Implementation*
Client Need: *Health Promotion and Maintenance*
Cognitive Level: *Analysis*

10. **ANSWER: 3.**
Rationales:
1. Although placing a patient's hands in warm water may initiate micturition, it is not the most effective intervention to facilitate complete bladder emptying.
2. Although stroking the inner aspect of a patient's thigh may initiate micturition, it is not the most effective intervention to facilitate complete bladder emptying.
3. Encouraging a patient to wait until urine stops flowing and then attempting to void again (double void) may facilitate complete bladder emptying. A small amount

of urine remains in the bladder after voiding (residual urine), which can support bacterial growth; therefore, complete bladder emptying contributes to a decreased risk of bladder infection.

4. Although sounds of flowing water may initiate micturition, it is not the most effective intervention to facilitate complete bladder emptying.

TEST-TAKING TIP: Identify the word in the stem that sets a priority. The word *most* in the stem sets a priority. Identify the unique option. Option 3 is unique because the actual action used to completely empty the bladder is performed by the patient, not the nurse.

Content Area: Urinary Elimination
Integrated Processes: Nursing Process: Implementation
Client Need: Physiological Integrity; Basic Care and Comfort
Cognitive Level: Application

11. **ANSWER: 2.**
Rationales:

1. Avoiding lifting heavy objects is an intervention to reduce incontinence associated with stress, not urge, incontinence.

2. Caffeine irritates the mucosa of the bladder and should be avoided to reduce bladder irritability and urge incontinence.

3. The Credé maneuver, application of pressure over the bladder, is used to promote emptying of the bladder. It is not used to gain better bladder control as a result of urge incontinence.

4. With urge incontinence, the person should be taught to slowly deep breathe to reduce the sense of urgency so that more time elapses between voidings.

Content Area: Urinary Elimination
Integrated Processes: Teaching/Learning; Nursing Process: Implementation
Client Need: Physiological Integrity; Basic Care and Comfort
Cognitive Level: Analysis

12. **ANSWER: 1, 2, 4, 6.**
Rationales:

1. This patient is experiencing functional incontinence. Functional incontinence involves the inability to get to the bathroom in time because of environmental factors or sensory, cognitive, or mobility issues. This patient has impaired mobility and dexterity of the hands. Velcro closures, instead of buttons and zippers, may facilitate quicker disrobing to urinate.

2. A lift chair will facilitate moving from a sitting to standing position shortening the time it takes to move to a bathroom to void.

3. Avoiding products with caffeine is encouraged to reduce bladder irritability associated with urge, not functional, incontinence.

4. A commode positioned nearby will reduce the distance a person with a mobility problem has to move to get to a toilet.

5. Kegel exercises are recommended to strengthen weak pelvis muscles associated with stress and urge, not functional, incontinence.

6. Voiding at timed intervals avoids waiting until a bladder is full and, as a result, enables more time to move to the bathroom or commode.

Content Area: Urinary Elimination
Integrated Processes: Communication/Documentation; Nursing Process: Planning
Client Need: Physiological Integrity; Basic Care and Comfort
Cognitive Level: Analysis

13. **ANSWER: 4.**
Rationales:

1. Cotton underwear should be worn because nylon prevents evaporation of moisture. Bacteria multiply in a warm, moist, dark environment.

2. The patient should urinate after, not before, intercourse to flush away bacteria that may have entered the urethra during sexual activity.

3. Bubble baths and baking-soda baths should be avoided because they increase the risk of a urinary tract infection.

4. Voiding immediately when the urge is perceived helps to avoid stagnant urine in the bladder. Bacteria multiply in stagnant urine.

TEST-TAKING TIP: Identify the clang association. The word *urinary* in the stem and the word *urinate* in option 4 is a clang association. Examine this option carefully when considering which option is the correct answer.

Content Area: Urinary Elimination
Integrated Processes: Teaching/Learning; Nursing Process: Implementation
Client Need: Health Promotion and Maintenance
Cognitive Level: Application

14. **ANSWER: 4.**
Rationales:

1. Compression here may permanently compromise the patency of the lumen than drains urine from the bladder and the lumen that permits inflation and deflation of the balloon.

2. Compression here may permanently compromise the patency of the lumen that drains urine from the bladder.

3. Compression here may permanently compromise the patency of the lumen that permits inflation and deflation of the balloon.

4. Compression at this site will interrupt the flow of urine from the urinary bladder to the urine collection bag. Urine will collect above the specimen port in the drainage tubing without compromising the integrity of the urinary catheter.

TEST-TAKING TIP: Identify the unique option. Option 4 is unique. Options 1, 2, and 3 are related to the catheter. Option 4 is related to the collection bag tubing. Examine option 4 carefully.

Content Area: Urinary Elimination
Integrated Processes: Nursing Process: Implementation
Client Need: Physiological Integrity; Reduction of Risk Potential
Cognitive Level: Analysis

15. **ANSWER: 2.**
Rationales:

1. Immobility is more likely to contribute to urinary incontinence than urinary retention because of a decrease in bladder tone.

2. The bladder loses tone while a urinary retention catheter is in place. Intake and output should be monitored after its removal because urinary retention is a potential problem. If urinary retention occurs, the primary health-care provider will either order the patient to be straight catheterized and output monitored for another 8 hours or the urinary retention catheter will be reordered.

3. Disorientation to time, place, and person is more likely to contribute to urinary incontinence than urinary retention because of a decreased ability to comprehend and react to the sensation of a full bladder.

4. Urinary retention is not a complication associated with a fluid restricted diet.

TEST-TAKING TIP: Identify the word in the stem that sets a priority. The word *most* in the stem sets a priority. Identify the option with the clang association. The word *retention* in the stem and in option 2 is a clang association. More often than not, an option with a clang association is the correct answer. Examine option 2 carefully.

Content Area: Urinary Elimination
Integrated Processes: Nursing Process: Assessment
Client Need: Physiological Integrity; Reduction of Risk Potential
Cognitive Level: Analysis

16. ANSWER: 3.

Rationales:

1. Ten in the morning is too early to ambulate the patient. The surgeon's orders indicate that the patient should be ambulated around the room during the p.m. hours.

2. Although this is an independent function of the nurse and should be encouraged when caring for postoperative patients, it is not the first thing the nurse should do from among the options presented.

3. It is 1 hour since the last assessment and the hourly urine collection container should be emptied into the large chamber of the collection device. Monitoring hourly urine output helps to assess cardiac and renal status and accuracy is essential.

4. The sequential compression devices should only be turned off and removed when the patient is out of bed.

TEST-TAKING TIP: Identify the word in the stem that sets a priority. The word *first* in the stem sets a priority.

Content Area: Urinary Elimination
Integrated Processes: Nursing Process: Implementation
Client Need: Physiological Integrity; Physiological Adaptation
Cognitive Level: Analysis

17. ANSWER: 4.

Rationales:

1. Urinary retention catheters are not used to make it more convenient for the nursing staff to care for a patient. A urinary retention catheter increases the risk for a bladder infection; therefore, it is used only when absolutely necessary.

2. Urinary retention catheters generally are not used to make it more convenient for the patient. The risk of infection outweighs the benefit to the patient. Exceptions include when a urinary retention catheter is used to protect a patient

from urinary incontinence when a person is actively dying or when a patient has a large sacral pressure ulcer.

3. Urinary retention catheters are never used to make it more convenient for the nursing staff to contain or collect urine.

4. After abdominal or thoracic surgery, assessing hourly urine production is an effective way to assess kidney and circulatory function. Also, hourly urine production may be monitored to assess a nonsurgical patient who is in critical condition.

TEST-TAKING TIP: Identify the word in the stem that sets a priority. The word *most* in the stem sets a priority. Identify the options that are equally plausible. Options 1 and 2 are both concerned with care being more convenient. Option 1 is no better than option 2. Eliminate options 1 and 2 from further consideration. Identify the options with a clang association. The words *urinary* and *catheter* in the stem and in options 3 and 4 are clang associations. Examine options 3 and 4 carefully.

Content Area: Urinary Elimination
Integrated Processes: Communication/Documentation; Nursing Process: Implementation
Client Need: Physiological Integrity; Reduction of Risk Potential
Cognitive Level: Application

18. ANSWER: 1.

Rationales:

1. Seven diapers is too small a number of soiled diapers daily for an infant who is several weeks old.

2. Eight soiled diapers daily is expected for a 3-week-old infant. A well-hydrated infant who is several weeks old produces enough urine to soil 8 to 10 diapers daily.

3. Nine soiled diapers daily is expected for a 3-week-old infant. A well-hydrated infant who is several weeks old produces enough urine to soil 8 to 10 diapers daily.

4. Ten soiled diapers daily is expected for a 3-week-old infant. A well-hydrated infant who is several weeks old produces enough urine to soil 8 to 10 diapers daily.

TEST-TAKING TIP: Identify the words in the stem that establish negative polarity. The words *cause the most concern* asks the test-taker to identify an assessment that is unexpected.

Content Area: Urinary Elimination
Integrated Processes: Nursing Process: Assessment
Client Need: Physiological Integrity; Reduction of Risk Potential
Cognitive Level: Application

19. ANSWER: 1, 2, 4.

Rationales:

1. Perineal care should be provided three times a day and whenever necessary, such as after passing of stool, for all patients with urinary retention catheters.

2. Positioning the collection container below the level of the pelvis is common for all types of urinary retention catheters. This prevents the flow of urine back into the bladder, which can cause an infection.

3. All urinary retention catheter balloons should be filled with sterile water because saline will crystallize, resulting in partial deflation of the balloon when it is removed. A

partially deflated balloon will cause trauma to the urethral mucosa during removal.

4. The collection bag should be hung on the bed frame, not the side rail, for all types of urinary retention catheters. A bed rail should not be used because when the rail is raised it could raise the collection bag higher than the pelvis. When the rail is lowered it could cause strain on the catheter or pull the catheter out, causing trauma to the urethra.

5. A catheter should be taped to the abdomen, not the thigh, of a male patient. A catheter can be taped to the inner thigh of a female patient.

Content Area: Urinary Elimination
Integrated Processes: Nursing Process: Implementation
Client Need: Physiological Integrity; Reduction of Risk Potential
Cognitive Level: Analysis

20. **ANSWER: 1, 3, 2, 4, 5.**

   Rationales:

1. First: Washing the hands limits the presence of microorganisms. The nurse should don clean gloves because they protect the nurse from blood and body fluids.

3. Second: Wash the genital area and allow it to dry to remove soiled matter, prevent specimen contamination, and prepare the skin for adhesion of the collection bag.

2. Third: Apply the collection device to enable the collection of a urine specimen.

4. Fourth: Remove the bag immediately after the infant voids to ensure that a fresh sample of urine is tested.

5. Fifth: The entire bag should be sent to the laboratory because it is difficult to remove urine from an infant collection bag. In addition, it protects the specimen from contamination by environmental elements.

Content Area: Urinary Elimination
Integrated Processes: Nursing Process: Planning
Client Need: Safe and Effective Care Environment; Management of Care
Cognitive Level: Analysis

21. **ANSWER: 1, 2, 3.**

   Rationales:

1. The correct reagent must be used to ensure reliable results.

2. Adequate lighting facilitates accurate interpretation of the color chart with the dipstick.

3. The kit must not be past the expiration date to ensure reliable results.

4. The procedure may be delegated to unlicensed assistive personnel as long as the individual knows how to perform the skill. Have the person report the results, but have the specimen saved in case the urine has to be retested.

5. The strip should be read at the exact time indicated on the bottle label; waiting times may vary depending on the manufacturer's instructions.

Content Area: Urinary Elimination
Integrated Processes: Nursing Process: Implementation
Client Need: Physiological Integrity; Reduction of Risk Potential
Cognitive Level: Application

22. **ANSWER: 1, 3, 4.**

   Rationales:

1. Presence of thirst is the first symptom of fluid volume loss. An elevated specific gravity of 1.032 most commonly indicates a state of fluid volume deficit or dehydration; as the kidneys attempt to conserve water, the urine becomes more concentrated. The expected range of specific gravity is 1.001 to 1.029.

2. Peripheral edema is a sign of fluid volume excess, not a sign of fluid volume deficit.

3. Decreased skin turgor is a sign of fluid volume deficit, as is a specific gravity of 1.032. Fluid is pulled from the intracellular and interstitial spaces into the vascular compartment, causing decreased skin turgor and dry skin and mucous membranes.

4. A rapid, weak pulse is a sign of fluid volume deficit, as is a specific gravity of 1.032. The heart rate increases as blood vessels constrict in response to less fluid in the circulation and in an attempt to meet the body's peripheral cellular needs. The volume of the pulse is weak (thready) because of hypovolemia.

5. A decrease in blood urea nitrogen occurs with fluid volume excess, not deficit. In fluid volume deficit, the blood urea nitrogen level increases because there is less fluid in proportion to the solid substances in the blood.

Content Area: Urinary Elimination
Integrated Processes: Nursing Process: Assessment
Client Need: Physiological Integrity; Reduction of Risk Potential
Cognitive Level: Analysis

23. **ANSWER: 2.**

   Rationales:

1. It is not necessary to wait until the morning to begin the test again.

2. This is the most appropriate action by the nurse. The test is based on urine collected during any 24-hour time period.

3. This action is inappropriate and will cause inaccurate test results.

4. Although the primary health-care provider should be notified of the delay in the test, it is not the priority at this time.

Content Area: Urinary Elimination
Integrated Processes: Nursing Process: Implementation
Client Need: Physiological Integrity; Reduction of Risk Potential
Cognitive Level: Application

24. **ANSWER: 3.**

   Rationales:

1. A sweet, fruity odor to urine is associated with incomplete fat metabolism related to diabetes mellitus or starvation, not a UTI. The sweet, fruity odor is caused by excess glucose in the urine.

2. Dark, amber urine is caused by high levels of bilirubin in the urine associated with liver dysfunction, not a UTI. Urine may also be dark amber if the urine is very concentrated.

3. Cloudy urine is caused by the presence of bacteria, white blood cells, and/or red blood cells associated with a UTI.

4. Foamy urine is caused by protein in the urine and is associated with renal disease, not a UTI.

Content Area: Urinary Elimination
Integrated Processes: Nursing Process: Assessment
Client Need: Physiological Integrity; Physiological Adaptation
Cognitive Level: Application

25. ANSWER: 1, 2, 4.
Rationales:
1. Dysuria (pain or burning on urination) is caused by urine flowing over inflamed mucosal tissue and is associated with a UTI.
2. Hematuria (blood-tinged urine) is caused by irritation of the bladder and urethral mucosa and is associated with a UTI.
3. Urinary frequency, not retention, is associated with a UTI. Urinary retention is associated with the inability of the bladder to empty because of obstruction, inflammation and swelling, neurological problems, anxiety, or an adverse effect of a medication.
4. Urgency (an overwhelming sensation of the need to void) is caused by bladder irritability secondary to a UTI.
5. A distended suprapubic area is associated with urinary retention, not a UTI.
TEST-TAKING TIP: Identify equally plausible options. Options 3 and 5 are equally plausible. The suprapubic area will be distended with urinary retention. These options can be eliminated from consideration.
Content Area: Urinary Elimination
Integrated Processes: Nursing Process: Assessment
Client Need: Physiological Integrity; Physiological Adaptation
Cognitive Level: Application

26. ANSWER: 3, 4, 5.
Rationales:
1. Blood-tinged urine is caused by irritation of the bladder and urethral mucosa associated with a urinary tract infection, not retention.
2. Amber colored urine is associated with concentrated urine related to dehydration or high levels of bilirubin related to liver dysfunction.
3. Abdominal pressure occurs as the bladder fills beyond a comfortable level of stretch, which is associated with urinary retention.
4. When the bladder is distended, it rises up out of the pelvis and is identified when the lower abdomen is palpated.
5. With urinary retention, pressure builds in the bladder to where the external urethral sphincter is unable to maintain closure. It opens temporarily and a small amount of urine escapes until pressure subsides and the sphincter closes. This can happen several times every hour and is a classic sign of urinary retention. It is called urinary retention with overflow.
Content Area: Urinary Elimination
Integrated Processes: Nursing Process: Assessment
Client Need: Physiological Integrity; Basic Care and Comfort
Cognitive Level: Application

27. ANSWER: 3.
Rationales:
1. Removing the catheter and inserting a retention catheter is contraindicated because it increases the risk of a bladder infection. In addition, the retention catheter will continue to empty the bladder which may precipitate bladder spasms.
2. Continuing to empty the patient's bladder after 750 mL has been removed may precipitate bladder spasms.
3. Releasing the urine over 20 minutes decreases irritability as the bladder distention is relieved; this will help reduce bladder spasms.
4. Removing the catheter and recatheterizing the patient is contraindicated because doing so increases the risk of a bladder infection.
TEST-TAKING TIP: Identify equally plausible options. Options 1 and 4 are equally plausible. They both involve inserting a urinary catheter. Identify the options that are opposites. Options 2 and 3 are opposites. Examine options 2 and 3 carefully.
Content Area: Urinary Elimination
Integrated Processes: Nursing Process: Implementation
Client Need: Physiological Integrity; Reduction of Risk Potential
Cognitive Level: Application

28. ANSWER: 1, 2, 3, 4.
Rationales:
1. A foreign body in a body cavity increases the risk for an infection. Vital signs will increase when the patient has an infection.
2. Cleansing the perineal area reduces the risk of a urinary tract infection. It removes debris and microorganisms away from the urinary meatus.
3. When a urinary drainage tube is kinked or compressed, it interferes with drainage of urine and urine will back up into the bladder. Stasis of urine increases the risk of a bladder infection.
4. These assessments are necessary for identifying the presence of a urinary tract infection. Urine that is cloudy or pink may indicate the presence of an infection.
5. Attaching the drainage bag to the bed railing is contraindicated because, if the railing is raised, urine may flow back into the bladder. Also, if the rail is raised or lowered with the bag attached, it may cause trauma to the urinary meatus.
6. Positioning the urinary drainage bag above the bladder is contraindicated; this will cause urine to flow back into the bladder.
Content Area: Urinary Elimination
Integrated Processes: Communication/Documentation; Nursing Process: Planning
Client Need: Physiological Integrity; Reduction of Risk Potential
Cognitive Level: Application

29. ANSWER: 3.
Rationales:
1. A straight catheter has one lumen and is used for one-time bladder drainage.
2. An indwelling catheter is a double-lumen catheter used for ongoing bladder drainage. One lumen permits passage

of sterile water for balloon inflation and the other for urinary drainage.

3. A triple-lumen catheter is used for continuous bladder irrigation. One lumen permits passage of sterile water for balloon inflation, another for instilling a GU irrigant into the bladder, and the third for bladder drainage (combination of urine and GU irrigant).

4. A double-lumen catheter is used as an indwelling catheter.

TEST-TAKING TIP: Identify the options that are equally plausible. Options 2 and 4 are equally plausible because they both have two lumens. These options can be deleted from further consideration.
Content Area: Urinary Elimination
Integrated Processes: Nursing Process: Planning
Client Need: Physiological Integrity; Basic Care and Comfort
Cognitive Level: Application

30. **ANSWER: 3, 4, 1, 6, 2, 5.**
Rationales:
3. Equipment used for a bladder catheterization often contains sterile gloves and catheters that are composed of latex. Latex-free supplies can be obtained if the patient is allergic to latex.
4. The outside of a sterile package is not sterile and can be touched with the hands.
1. After a sterile field is established, sterile gloves must be worn to maintain sterility of the field and the equipment touched during the procedure.
6. Cleaning the urethral meatus with the provided antiseptic removes debris and microorganisms; this limits the risk of a bladder infection.
2. A lubricated catheter tip limits trauma to the urinary meatus and mucous membranes of the urinary tract.
5. Advancing the catheter 1 inch after urine flows ensures that the catheter is past the internal and external urinary sphincters.
Content Area: Urinary Elimination
Integrated Processes: Nursing Process: Planning
Client Need: Physiological Integrity; Reduction of Risk Potential
Cognitive Level: Analysis

31. **ANSWER: 2.**
Rationales:
1. An attempt should be made to reestablish patency of the catheter lumen before obtaining an order for irrigation.
2. Three hours should produce a minimum of 90 mL of urine, even if the patient had no fluid intake. Milking the tubing should be performed first to dislodge sediment or mucus plugs that may be interfering with the flow of urine.
3. Palpating the patient's suprapubic area may not reveal distention because 90 mL is a small fraction of bladder capacity.
4. Some action is required because urine output over three hours should be at least 90 mL (i.e., 30 mL/hour).
TEST-TAKING TIP: Identify the word in the stem that sets a priority. The word *first* in the stem sets a priority. Identify the clang association. The word *catheter* in the stem and in

options 1 and 2 are clang associations. Examine options 1 and 2 carefully. More often than not, an option with a clang association is the correct answer.
Content Area: Urinary Elimination
Integrated Processes: Nursing Process: Implementation
Client Need: Physiological Integrity; Reduction of Risk Potential
Cognitive Level: Application

32. **ANSWER: 2.**
Rationales:
1. One hour is too long a period of time to wait between assessments of tube patency with a CBI. The volume of output should be checked every 15 minutes. The faster the flow rate, the more frequently the nurse should assess the output. If the tube becomes obstructed soon after being checked and it is not reassessed for a long period of time, then a large volume of urine and solution can collect in and distend the bladder; this increases the potential of injury to the operative site as well as result in reflux to the kidneys.
2. Increasing the flow rate of the irrigating solution helps to dilute the effluent from the bladder, thereby minimizing the formation of clots in the urine. A pink effluent, without the presence of clots, is the clinical indicator that indicates that the irrigating solution flow rate is sufficient to maintain patency.
3. A CBI requires a triple-lumen, not double-lumen, urinary retention catheter. One lumen is attached to the urine collection bag, a second lumen is used to inflate the balloon that holds the catheter in the bladder, and a third lumen is attached to the tubing from the irrigation solution bag.
4. A patient may be encouraged to turn from side to side to facilitate respirations, relieve pressure on bony prominences, and promote venous return from the lower extremities, not to promote urinary elimination.
TEST-TAKING TIP: Identify the word in the stem that sets a priority. The word *essential* in the stem sets a priority. Identify the clang association. The word *irrigation* in the stem and in option 2 is a clang association. More often than not, an option with a clang association is the correct answer. Examine option 2 carefully.
Content Area: Urinary Elimination
Integrated Processes: Nursing Process: Implementation
Client Need: Physiological Integrity; Reduction of Risk Potential
Cognitive Level: Application

33. **ANSWER: 1, 4, 5.**
Rationales:
1. Having the patient void one last time at the end of the 24-hour period and adding it to the large collection container completes the test. It accurately includes the urine being produced within the specified 24-hour period.
2. This urine is not discarded but is added to the volume being collected. The urine voided one last time at the end of the 24 hours completes the test.
3. The first voiding is discarded and then all additional urine voided, including the last voiding at 24 hours, is collected.

4. Discarding the first voiding is the correct way to initiate a 24-hour urine test. If the first voiding is included, the urine volume will incorporate more hours of urine produced than what should be included in 24 hours. The test results will be altered by excessive amounts of constituents in the greater volume of urine collected. This test can test for levels of adrenocortical steroids, hormones, protein, and creatinine clearance.
5. All voided urine for 24 hours is collected and then stored in a large collection container.
TEST-TAKING TIP: Identify opposite options. Options 1 and 2 are opposites. One of these options is correct and the other is a distractor. Options 3 and 4 are opposites. One of these options is correct and the other is a distractor.
Content Area: Urinary Elimination
Integrated Processes: Nursing Process: Implementation
Client Need: Physiological Integrity; Reduction of Risk Potential
Cognitive Level: Application

34. ANSWER: 3.
Rationales:
1. Perineal hygiene is not necessary before implementing the procedure. However, washing the conducting gel from the abdomen and suprapubic area is necessary after completing the procedure.
2. The patient is placed in the supine position so that the lower abdomen and suprapubic areas are exposed.
3. **This is accurate information. This is a painless noninvasive procedure that should cause no discomfort.**
4. The transducer is applied 1.5 inches, not 4 inches, midline above the pubic bone, aiming the scan head toward the patient's coccyx for an accurate reading.
TEST-TAKING TIP: Identify the word in the stem that sets a priority. The word *essential* in the stem sets a priority.
Content Area: Urinary Elimination
Integrated Processes: Communication/Documentation; Nursing Process: Implementation
Client Need: Physiological Integrity; Reduction or Risk Potential
Cognitive Level: Application

35. ANSWER: 1.
Rationales:
1. **Urinary retention may occur after the procedure due to urethral edema.**
2. It is not uncommon to experience pink, not red, urine after the procedure. The instrumentation may irritate the mucosal lining of the urinary tract, resulting in minor bleeding.
3. It is not necessary to maintain bedrest for several days after the procedure. Bedrest may be encouraged on the day of the procedure because hypotension may occur immediately after the procedure.
4. The patient can resume a regular diet immediately after the procedure. The patient will be advised to increase fluid intake for several days. A large amount of dilute urine decreases dysuria, prevents stasis, and limits the accumulation of bacteria in the bladder.

Content Area: Urinary Elimination
Integrated Processes: Teaching/Learning; Nursing Process: Planning
Client Need: Physiological Integrity; Reduction of Risk Potential
Cognitive Level: Application

36. ANSWER: 6, 1, 2, 4, 3, 5.
Rationales:
6. The first step is providing perineal hygiene and drying the penis thoroughly. A penis that is clean and free from debris and moisture reduces the risk of infection, skin breakdown, and nonadherence of the condom.
1. The second step ensures that the catheter does not compress the glans and that there is a 1- to 1½-inch distance between the glans penis and the drainage tubing. These actions prevent pressure against the glans and tissue at the distal end of the penis.
2. The third step is applying the condom to the full length of the shaft of the penis. Holding the penis firmly, perpendicular to the abdomen, extends the penis and facilitates the unrolling of the condom down the shaft of the penis.
4. The fourth step is securing the condom to the shaft by grasping the penis and gently compressing it so that the entire condom comes into contact with the penal shaft.
3. The fifth step is taping the external adhesive strip over the condom in a spiral along the length of the shaft. Applying it in a spiral reduces the risk of obstructing circulation, which can occur when it is applied around the condom at the proximal end of the penis.
5. The last step in the procedure is hanging the urine collection bag on the bed frame below the level of the bladder.
Content Area: Urinary Elimination
Integrated Processes: Nursing Process: Planning
Client Need: Safe and Effective Care Environment; Management of Care
Cognitive Level: Analysis

37. ANSWER: 4.
Rationales:
1. An irritated bladder is associated with urge, not stress, incontinence.
2. Returning to her exercise class will help her continue to lose weight because obesity is a contributing factor for stress incontinence; however, the information in another option is a more effective intervention that will improve the underlying cause of her problem.
3. Although a toileting program may help to keep the bladder less full just before exercise or other planned strenuous activity, it will not help prevent the underlying cause of stress incontinence.
4. **The patient is experiencing stress incontinence, most likely due to weakened pelvic floor muscles as result of five pregnancies and obesity. Stress incontinence occurs when intra-abdominal pressure increases related to such activities as exercise, laughing, coughing, sneezing, bending, and lifting. Kegel exercises help to increase pelvic floor muscle tone and should help the patient regain control of urine.**

TEST-TAKING TIP: Identify the word in the stem that sets a priority. The word *best* in the stem sets a priority. Identify the clang associations. The word *exercise* in the stem and in options 2 and 4 are clang associations. Examine options 2 and 4 carefully.
Content Area: Urinary Elimination
Integrated Processes: Teaching/Learning; Nursing Process: Implementation
Client Need: Physiological Integrity; Basic Care and Comfort
Cognitive Level: Analysis

38. ANSWER: 2.
Rationales:
1. Decreased sweating, not diaphoresis, is associated with Ditropan.
2. The patient may experience the side effect of palpitations caused by the anticholinergic effects of Ditropan.
3. Gastric irritation is not associated with Ditropan.
4. Orange-colored urine is associated with the drug phenazopyridine (Pyridium), a urinary tract analgesic, not Ditropan.
TEST-TAKING TIP: Identify words in the stem that indicate negative polarity. The words *side effect* in the stem indicate negative polarity. The question is asking, *"What is not a therapeutic effect of oxybutynin?"*
Content Area: Urinary Elimination
Integrated Processes: Nursing Process: Evaluation
Client Need: Physiological Integrity; Pharmacological and Parenteral Therapies
Cognitive Level: Application

39. ANSWER: 1.
Rationales:
1. The urine specimen should be collected and contained following the principles of sterile technique. A sterile container will not introduce environmental microorganisms into the specimen. This ensures that the results of the culture and sensitivity reflect the microorganisms present in the patient's urinary tract.
2. Urine in this section of the urinary collection device may be as long as 1 hour old and, therefore, not current. The hourly urine section of the collection bag moves collected urine into the main portion of the urine collection container when it is lifted. Generally, it does not have its own port.
3. This is contraindicated because the urine in this section of a urinary collection device may be many hours old.
4. Urinary retention catheters and collection bags generally are designed as closed drainage systems so they cannot be separated; this avoids unnecessary separation of tubing that may permit introduction of pathogenic microorganisms.
TEST-TAKING TIP: Identify the unique option. Option 1 is unique. Options 2, 3, and 4 all relate to the removal of urine from the drainage system. Option 1 is the only option that contains an intervention that is performed after the urine is actually collected.
Content Area: Urinary Elimination
Integrated Processes: Nursing Process: Implementation
Client Need: Physiological Integrity; Reduction of Risk Potential
Cognitive Level: Application

40. ANSWER: 5, 4, 3, 2, 1.
Rationales:
5. Milking the catheter should be performed first after it was observed that the patient did not void over a 2-hour period. This action will push sediment and mucus toward the collection bag and reestablish patency of the tube.
4. Palpating the patient's bladder should be done after establishing patency of the catheter. This will determine if the bladder is distended.
3. Encouraging the patient to drink fluids should be done after essential actions are implemented. Drinking fluids will increase the glomerular filtrate and increase the urinary output.
2. Continuing to observe the patient over the next hour may be done after actions have been taken to rectify the problem. Previous interventions may resolve the problem.
1. An order for irrigation should be obtained after other interventions have been attempted. This is an invasive intervention that should be left to last.
Content Area: Urinary Elimination
Integrated Processes: Nursing Process: Planning
Client Need: Safe and Effective Care Environment; Management of Care
Cognitive Level: Analysis

Chapter 21

Fluids and Electrolytes

KEY TERMS

Active transport—Active process whereby metabolic energy moves substances across a membrane from a less concentrated solution to a more concentrated solution.

Anasarca—Massive generalized edema.

Anions—Ions that have a negative charge.

Buffer—Substance that combines with a strong acid or base to change it to a weaker acid or base.

Cations—Ions that have a positive charge.

Dehydration—Loss of fluid without a significant loss of electrolytes, resulting in a hyperosmolar imbalance.

Diffusion—Passive process whereby molecules move across a membrane from a more concentrated solution to a less concentrated solution.

Drop factor—Number of drops per milliliter that the tubing of an intravenous set delivers.

Edema—Excessive amount of fluid in subcutaneous tissue.

Electrolytes—Chemical substances that dissociate into electrically charged particles (ions) when dissolved in water.

Extracellular fluid (ECF)—Fluid outside of cells, which accounts for about 30 percent of body fluid and is further divided into interstitial fluid (fluid in the spaces between body cells), intravascular fluid (fluid within blood vessels [plasma]), and transcellular fluid (specific fluids, such as lymph, cerebrospinal, and peritoneal).

Filtration—Passive process whereby fluid and smaller molecules move from an area of higher pressure to an area of lower pressure.

Hydrostatic pressure—Pressure exerted by a fluid within a closed system against the walls of the system.

Hypertonic (concentrated)—Small amount of solvent contains a large amount of solute.

Hypervolemia—Excessive amount of fluid and sodium in isotonic proportions.

Hypotonic (dilute)—Large amount of solvent contains a small amount of solute.

Hypovolemia—Loss of both fluids and electrolytes in equal or isotonic proportions.

Insensible fluid loss—Fluid loss that is not perceived or easily measurable.

Isotonic—Osmotic pressures of two liquids are equal.

Intracellular fluid (ICF)—Fluid within cells, which accounts for about 70 percent of body fluid.

Oncotic pressure (osmotic pressure)—Power of a solution to draw water across a semipermeable membrane.

Sensible fluid loss—Fluid loss that is perceived and measurable.

Solute—Dissolved substance.

Solvent—Substance in which a solute is dissolved.

I. Concepts Related to Fluids and Electrolytes

More than 50 percent of the human body is composed of fluid, which is divided between the intracellular compartment and the extracellular compartment; the extracellular compartment is further divided into the intravascular, interstitial, and transcellular compartments. Fluid and electrolytes constantly move among these compartments via osmosis, diffusion, filtration, and active transport. Regulation of the body's fluid balance is more complex than just the amount of fluid taken into the body and the amount of fluid excreted from the body. It involves a variety of internal feedback mechanisms, including the thirst mechanism, antidiuretic hormone, renin-angiotensin-aldosterone system, and atrial natriuretic peptide. These basic concepts provide the foundation for understanding the balance of fluid within the human body.

A. Body Fluids
  1. Definition.
     a. Primarily water.
     b. Contains dissolved substances, such as gases (e.g., oxygen, carbon dioxide), electrolytes, glucose, and urea.

2. Functions.
   a. Maintains blood volume.
   b. Controls body temperature.
   c. Transports substances to and from cells, such as nutrients, gases, and waste products.
   d. Serves as a medium for metabolic reactions within cells.
   e. Assists with digestion of nutrients.
   f. Lubricates joints.
3. Distribution (Fig. 21.1).
   a. Intracellular and extracellular compartments are separated by selectively permeable membranes of cells and capillaries.
   b. Total body fluid.
      (1) Full-term newborn: 70 to 80 percent.
      (2) 1-year-old: 64 percent.
      (3) Adult male: 55 to 60 percent.
      (4) Adult female: 45 to 55 percent.
      (5) Older adult: 45 to 50 percent.
   c. Intracellular (ICF): Fluid within cells; about 70 percent.
   d. Extracellular (ECF): Fluid outside of cells; about 30 percent.
      (1) Interstitial: Fluid in the spaces between body cells; about 22 percent.
      (2) Intravascular: Fluid within blood vessels (plasma); about 6 percent.
      (3) Transcellular: Specific fluids, such as lymph, cerebrospinal, peritoneal, synovial, pleural, intraocular, biliary, and pancreatic; about 2 percent.
   e. Third spacing: Accumulation and sequestration of fluid in extracellular spaces as a result of injury or disease, such as edema, ascites, and pleural effusion.
   f. Injury or inflammation: Increased capillary permeability permits fluid, electrolytes, and proteins to move into ECF compartment due to trauma, burns, and sepsis.

4. Movement of fluid and electrolytes.
   a. Fluid intake.
      (1) Includes oral and intravenous (IV) intake.
      (2) Recommended oral intake.
         (a) 2,200 mL/day for women and 3,000 mL/day for men.
         (b) 80 percent from drinking fluids and 20 percent from food.
   b. Fluid output.
      (1) Sensible fluid loss: Fluid that is perceived and measurable.
         (a) Urine: About 1,500 mL/day; varies based on intake and losses via other routes; at least 30 to 50 mL/hour.
         (b) Feces: 100 to 200 mL/day; soft stools contain more water than hard stools.
      (2) Insensible fluid loss: Fluid not perceived or easily measurable.
         (a) Skin: 300 to 600 mL/day; extent of perspiration depends on body and environmental temperature, extent of muscle contraction, and metabolic activity.
         (b) Lungs: About 300 mL/day; increased respiratory rate increases amount lost.
   c. **Osmosis** (Fig. 21.2).
      (1) Passive process whereby water moves across a membrane from a less concentrated solution to a more concentrated solution.
      (2) **Oncotic pressure (osmotic pressure):** Power of a solution to draw water across a semipermeable membrane.
         (a) For example: Plasma proteins and hypertonic IV solutions increase oncotic pressure because fluid moves from the interstitial compartment into the intravascular compartment.
         (b) For example: Low levels of protein in the blood, usually due to starvation or liver disease, decrease oncotic pressure because fluid moves from the intravascular compartment into the interstitial compartment.

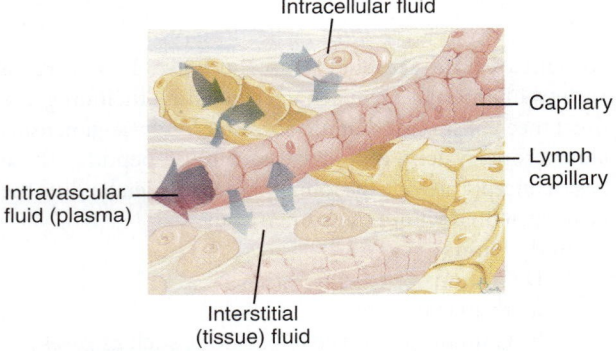

Fig 21.1 Distribution of body fluids. (From Wilkinson and Treas [2011]. *Fundamentals of nursing,* Vol. 1, 2nd ed. Philadelphia: F. A. Davis, with permission.)

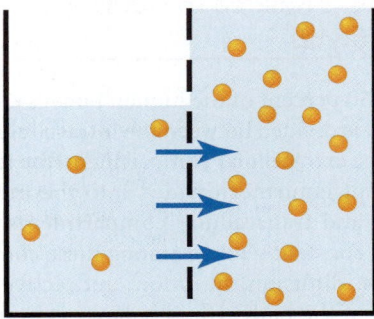

Fig 21.2 Osmosis. (From Wilkinson and Treas [2011]. *Fundamentals of nursing,* Vol. 1, 2nd ed. Philadelphia: F. A. Davis, with permission.)

d. **Diffusion** (Fig. 21.3).
   (1) Passive process whereby molecules move across a membrane from a more concentrated solution to a less concentrated solution.
   (2) For example: Oxygen moves from the alveoli into the pulmonary capillaries and carbon dioxide moves from the pulmonary capillaries into the alveoli.
e. **Filtration** (Fig. 21.4).
   (1) Passive process whereby fluid and smaller molecules move from an area of higher pressure to an area of lower pressure.
   (2) **Hydrostatic pressure:** Pressure exerted by a fluid within a closed system against the walls, such as the force exerted by blood against the vascular walls.
   (3) For example: Increased hydrostatic pressure associated with heart failure or kidney disease promotes movement of fluid out of the intravascular compartment into the interstitial compartment.
f. **Active transport** (Fig. 21.5).
   (1) Active process whereby metabolic energy moves substances across a membrane from a less concentrated solution to a more concentrated solution.

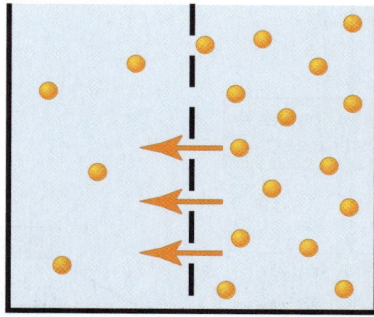

Fig 21.3 Diffusion. (From Wilkinson and Treas [2011]. *Fundamentals of nursing,* Vol. 1, 2nd ed. Philadelphia: F. A. Davis, with permission.)

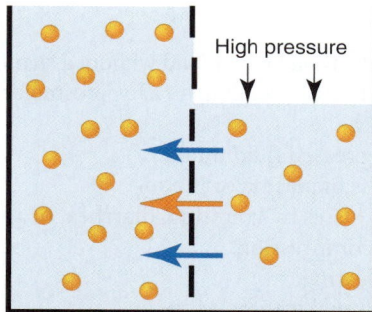

Fig 21.4 Filtration. (From Wilkinson and Treas [2011]. *Fundamentals of nursing,* Vol. 1, 2nd ed. Philadelphia: F. A. Davis, with permission.)

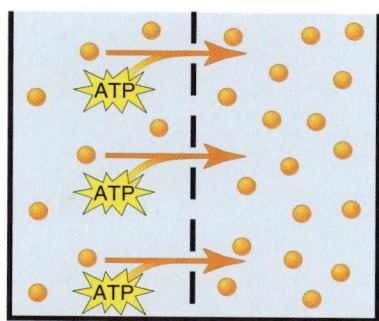

Fig 21.5 Active transport. (From Wilkinson and Treas [2011]. *Fundamentals of nursing,* Vol. 1, 2nd ed. Philadelphia: F. A. Davis, with permission.)

   (2) For example: The sodium-potassium pump moves sodium out of cells and potassium into cells.
B. **Maintenance of Fluid Balance**
   1. Thirst mechanism.
      a. The thirst center in the hypothalamus is stimulated when an increase in the concentration of particles within the intravascular compartment (serum osmolarity) occurs.
      b. An increase in osmolality is caused by a decrease in fluid intake, excessive fluid loss, or excessive sodium intake via the diet or IV fluids.
   2. Antidiuretic hormone (ADH).
      a. ADH causes the kidneys to retain fluid.
      b. Pressure sensors in the vascular system stimulate or inhibit the release of ADH.
   3. Renin-angiotensin-aldosterone system (Fig. 21.6).
      a. Decreased blood flow or decreased blood pressure stimulates the release of renin from the kidneys.
      b. Renin stimulates the conversion of angiotensin I to angiotensin II.
      c. Angiotensin II acts on the kidneys to retain sodium and water and stimulates the adrenal cortex to release aldosterone.
      d. Aldosterone stimulates the kidneys to reabsorb sodium and excrete potassium.
   4. Atrial natriuretic peptide (ANP).
      a. Atrial stretching in the heart stimulates release of ANP.
      b. ANP acts as a diuretic by increasing sodium excretion and inhibiting the thirst mechanism.

II. Alterations in Fluid Balance

Fluid imbalances include an inadequate amount of body fluid (fluid volume deficit) or an excessive amount of body fluid (fluid volume excess). These imbalances arise from a

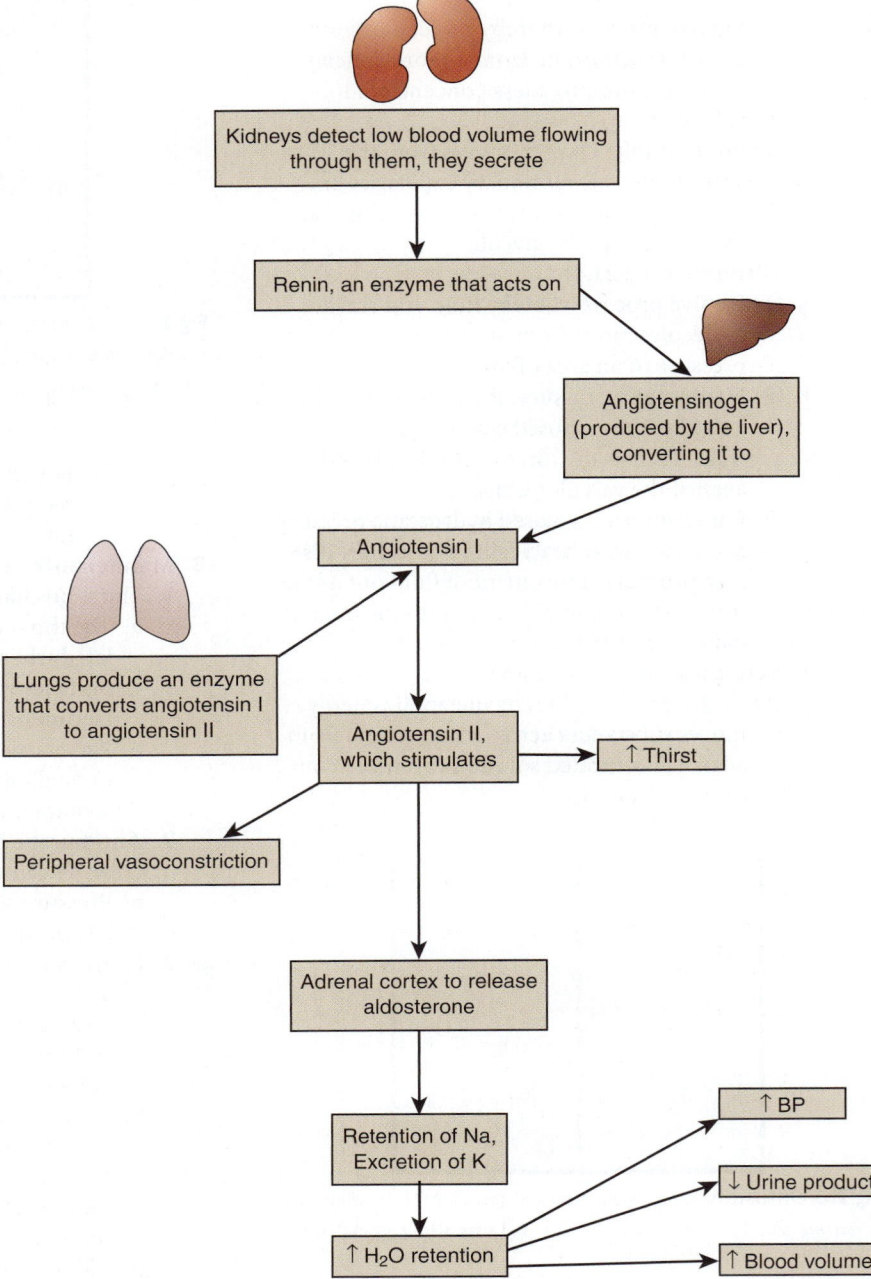

Fig 21.6 Renin-angiotensin-aldosterone system. (From Burton and Ludwig [2011]. *Fundamentals of nursing care: Concepts, connections & skills.* Philadelphia: F. A. Davis, with permission.)

variety of conditions, and each has associated clinical manifestations. Nursing care for patients with alterations in fluid balance include many nursing interventions that pertain to both imbalances. However, some are specific to either fluid volume deficit or fluid volume excess. Nurses must have a thorough knowledge of all this information to provide comprehensive nursing care for patients with alterations in fluid balance.

A. Fluid Volume Deficit (FVD)

1. **Hypovolemia:** Loss of both fluid and electrolytes in equal or isotonic proportions.

2. **Dehydration:** Loss of fluid without a significant loss of electrolytes, resulting in a hyperosmolar imbalance.

3. Causes.
   a. Decreased fluid intake.
   b. Loss of plasma or blood.
   c. GI losses by vomiting, diarrhea, or gastric decompression.
   d. Sweating.
   e. Adrenal insufficiency.
   f. Excessive urination (polyuria), possibly due to diuretics or diabetes.

4. Clinical manifestations.
   a. Weight loss.
   b. Flushed, dry skin and mucous membranes.
   c. Decreased tissue turgor; pinched skin on forehead or over sternum takes several seconds to return to original position (Fig. 21.7).
   d. Thirst.
   e. Low-grade fever.
   f. Sunken eyeballs.
   g. Hypotension, orthostatic hypotension.
   h. Weak, thready, rapid pulse.
   i. Flat neck veins.
   j. Decreased capillary refill.
   k. Atonic muscles.
   l. Lethargy.
   m. Mental confusion.
   n. Decreased urine output (oliguria, anuria).
   o. Hemoconcentration results in increased hematocrit (>50%), blood urea nitrogen (>21 mg/dL), and urine specific gravity (>1.029).

B. Fluid Volume Excess (FVE)
1. **Hypervolemia:** Excessive amount of fluid and sodium in isotonic proportions.
2. Causes.
   a. Excessive sodium intake via diet.
   b. Excessive IV fluids containing sodium.
   c. Congestive heart failure.
   d. Kidney disease.
   e. Cirrhosis of the liver.
   f. Increased aldosterone.
   g. Increased ADH.
3. Clinical manifestations.
   a. Weight gain.
   b. Pale, cool skin.
   c. Edema (dependent, generalized [**anasarca**], periorbital, pulmonary); increased tissue turgor; use scale for objective measurement of edema (Fig. 21.8A and Fig. 21.8B).

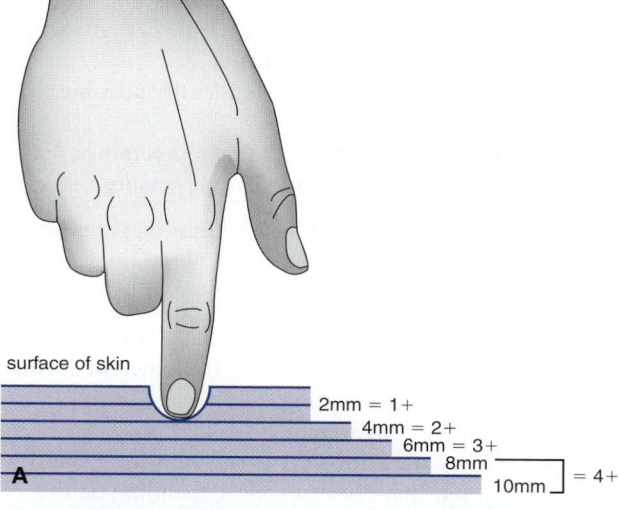

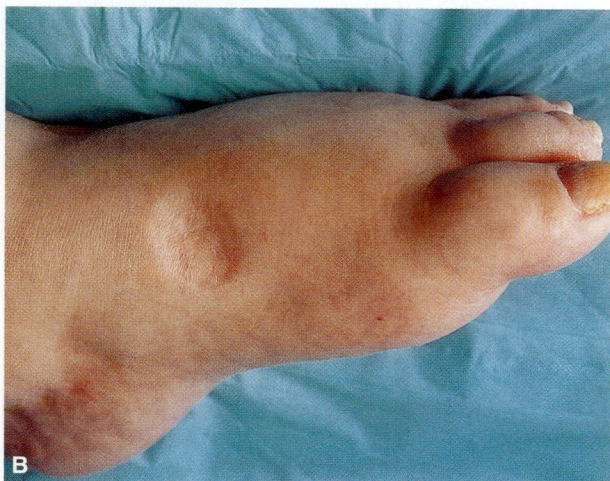

Fig 21.8 (A) Edema scale. (B) Pitting edema. ((A) From Nugent and Vitale [2012]. *Test success,* 6th ed. Philadelphia: F. A. Davis, with permission. (B) From Burton and Ludwig [2011]. *Fundamentals of nursing care: Concepts, connections & skills.* Philadelphia: F. A. Davis, with permission.)

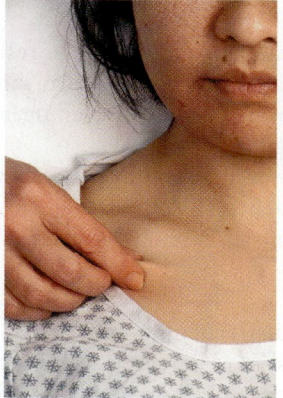

Fig 21.7 Tenting. (From Wilkinson and Treas [2011]. *Fundamentals of nursing,* Vol. 2, 2nd ed. Philadelphia: F. A. Davis, with permission.)

   d. Third heart sound (S_3 gallop) on auscultation of the heart.
   e. Increased, shallow respirations; dyspnea.
   f. Crackles on auscultation of the lungs.
   g. Hypertension.
   h. Full, bounding, rapid pulse.
   i. Distended neck veins.
   j. Muscle weakness, fatigue.
   k. Mental confusion.
   l. Diluted urine, possibly with increased volume.
   m. Hemodilution results in decreased hematocrit (<40%) and blood urea nitrogen (<8 mg/dL).

C. Nursing Care for Patients With Fluid Imbalances

1. **Commonalities of nursing care for patients with a fluid imbalance.**

   a. Obtain a health history to identify possible causes.

   b. Obtain vital signs, including temperature, pulse, respirations, and blood pressure.

   🛑 c. Assess breath sounds and characteristics of breathing; be aware that crackles and dyspnea indicate possible fluid overload.

   d. Assess mucous membranes, presence of thirst, and skin turgor; determine the extent of edema or presence of tenting.

   e. Obtain a daily weight.

      (1) Use the same scale every time; use a standing, chair, or bed scale, depending on the patient's ability to stand, sit, or need to remain in bed.

      (2) Weigh the patient at same time every day, such as before breakfast after the first voiding.

      (3) Weigh the patient each day wearing similar clothes or use similar linens when using a bed scale.

      (4) Notify the primary health-care provider of a change in weight of equal to or more than 2 lb (2.2 lb equal 2,000 mL of fluid) in a day or equal to or more than 5 lb in 1 to 2 weeks.

   f. Monitor intake and output (I&O).

      (1) Institute I&O for patients who are unstable, critically ill, or febrile; are receiving diuretics, continuous or intermittent IV infusions, or tube feedings; have had a procedure; or have fluid restrictions because of conditions such as FVD, FVE, or heart or kidney failure.

      (2) Measure all fluid that goes into the body, such as oral, IV, tube feedings, and instillations into the GI tract or urinary bladder.

      (3) Measure all fluid that exits from the body, such as urine, liquid feces, vomitus, wound drainage, and fluid from gastric decompression; and identify characteristics of output (e.g., color, clarity, and odor).

DID YOU KNOW?

A nurse can delegate the task of measuring amounts of intake and output not requiring a sterile intervention to assistive nursing personnel. However, it is the responsibility of the delegating nurse to ensure that the intervention is within the person's job description and that the person has the knowledge and skill necessary to complete the skill accurately and safely. Tallying the results, determining the significance of the information, and notifying a primary health-care provider of results outside expectations is also the delegating nurse's responsibility.

   (4) Use standard precautions when collecting certain body fluids, such as urine from a urinary retention catheter collection bag or liquid feces; use surgical asepsis when collecting certain body fluids, such as keeping the port of a wound drainage device sterile when collecting wound drainage.

   (5) Measure volume in milliliters with an accurate measuring device and weigh diapers or incontinence pads; do not estimate volume.

   (6) Record solid food that becomes a liquid at room temperature, such as ice cream and gelatin, in its entire volume.

   (7) Record ice chips at half their volume; for example, 4 oz of ice chips equals 2 oz of fluid.

   (8) Document immediately after administration or collection of fluid at the appropriate time on the I&O record (Fig. 21.9).

   (9) Tally volumes of I&O as ordered, such as hourly, at the end of each shift, and at the end of a 24-hour period.

   (10) Teach the patient and family about monitoring fluid intake and output; encourage self-monitoring of I&O if the patient is capable.

   g. Assess level of consciousness, energy level, and changes in behavior.

   h. Monitor laboratory results, such as hematocrit, blood urea nitrogen, serum electrolytes, creatinine clearance, and urine specific gravity.

   i. Provide for safety, such as by assisting the patient with getting out of bed.

   j. Change position and massage dependent areas (except calves) every 2 hours to prevent pressure ulcers.

   k. Facilitate oral fluid intake or restriction: Allot one-half during the day, two-thirds of the remaining fluid in the evening, and the rest during the night.

2. **Specific nursing care for patients with fluid volume deficit (FVD).**

   a. Administer IV fluids as ordered.

   🛑 b. Use an intravenous controller device.

   c. Provide frequent mouth care.

   d. Use assistive devices, such as sheep skin, gel cushion, and elbow and heel pads, to protect the skin over bony prominences.

DAILY INTAKE AND OUTPUT RECORD

DATE JUNE 5

| | INTAKE | | | | | | | OUTPUT | | | |
| | I.V. FLUIDS | | | | | | | | | N.G. | |
Time	Bottle	Amount	Solution	Medication and Dosage	*ABS	⊤LIB	ORAL	URINE	EMESIS	TUBE	HEMOVAC
8	1	1000	NS	20 mEq KCl				650			
8:30							360				
10:00							120				
11:30							240	150			
12:00									160		
1:40									90		60
2:15								250			
3:00						525	475					45
7-3 TOTAL		8-HR TOTAL			525	475	720	1050	250		105
3-11 TOTAL		8-HR TOTAL									
11-7 TOTAL		8-HR TOTAL									
24 HOUR TOTAL											

INTAKE GRAND TOTAL [ ]   OUTPUT GRAND TOTAL [ ]

* ABS. = amount absorbed   ⊤ LIB = Left in bag

Fig 21.9 Daily intake and output record. (From Nugent and Vitale [2012]. *Test success,* 6th ed. Philadelphia: F. A. Davis, with permission.)

e. Facilitate ordered oral fluid intake (oral rehydration therapy).
   (1) Set short-term goals, such as 4 oz/hour.
   (2) Offer preferred fluids.
   (3) Serve fluids at appropriate temperatures, such as cold beverages and hot tea and coffee.
   (4) Encourage intake of foods that become liquid at room temperature, such as ice cream and custard.

3. **Specific nursing care for patients with fluid volume excess (FVE).**
   a. Assess the extent of third spacing by measuring with a centimeter tape over the umbilicus for abdominal girth associated with ascites and circumference of extremity associated with peripheral edema or compartment syndrome (mark the site on the extremity for continuity of assessments).
   b. Maintain the patient in a mid- or high-Fowler position to promote respirations.
   c. Restrict dietary sodium as ordered.
   d. Administer prescribed diuretics.
   e. Facilitate ordered fluid restriction.
      (1) Offer fluids between rather than with meals.
      (2) Offer ice chips to relieve thirst; liquid volume is half frozen volume.
      (3) Use a small container to promote perception of a larger volume when providing fluids.
      (4) Suggest chewing sugarless gum to help keep the oral cavity moist.

III. Electrolytes

Electrolytes are chemical substances that dissociate into electrically charged particles (ions) when dissolved in water. **Cations** (e.g., sodium, potassium, calcium, and magnesium) have a positive charge; **anions** (e.g., chloride, bicarbonate, and phosphate) have a negative charge. Electrolyte balance depends on normal kidney, hypothalamic, adrenocortical, and nervous system functioning. Imbalances can be identified by serum electrolyte levels and clinical manifestations.

A. Common Electrolytes
   1. Sodium (Na^+): Normal serum level = 135 to 145 mEq/L.
      a. Major cation in ECF.
      b. Promotes fluid and acid-base balance, nerve impulse conduction, and cellular chemical reactions.

2. **Potassium** (K+): Normal serum level = 3.5 to 5.0 mEq/L.
   a. Major cation in ICF.
   b. Promotes nerve impulse conduction in cardiac, skeletal, and smooth muscles.
   c. Serves as a cofactor with enzymes in cellular metabolism.
3. **Calcium** (Ca++): Normal serum level = 8.5 to 10.5 mEq/L.
   a. Promotes bone health and cardiac and neuromuscular function.
   b. Serves as a factor in blood clotting.
   c. Has its level controlled by parathyroid gland secretion of parathyroid hormone.
   d. Has a reciprocal relationship with phosphorous; a decrease or increase in one results in the opposite reaction in the other.
4. **Magnesium** (Mg++): Normal serum level = 1.32 to 2.14 mEq/L.
   a. Essential for enzyme and neurochemical activities.
   b. Promotes cardiac and skeletal muscle excitability.
5. **Chloride** (Cl-): Normal serum level = 97 to 107 mEq/L.
   a. Major anion in ECF.
   b. Functions with sodium to regulate serum osmolality and blood volume.
   c. Component of hydrochloric acid (HCl) which is involved with regulating acid-base balance.
6. **Bicarbonate** (HCO_3^-): Normal serum level = 22 to 26 mEq/L.
   a. Most important buffer in ECF.
   b. Helps regulate acid-base balance by neutralizing excess hydrogen ions as part of the carbonic-bicarbonate buffering mechanism.

7. **Phosphate** (PO_4^-): Normal serum level = 2.5 to 4.5 mEq/dL.
   a. Most important buffer in ECF.
   b. Helps regulate acid-base balance by neutralizing excess hydrogen ions as part of the phosphate buffer system.
   c. Essential for functioning of red blood cells, nerves, and muscles.
   d. Involved in metabolism of proteins, carbohydrates, and fats.

B. Electrolyte Imbalances
1. Commonalities of nursing care for patients with electrolyte imbalances.
   a. Perform a history and physical to collect data that may help identify the cause of the imbalance.
   b. Monitor laboratory reports for serum electrolyte levels.
   c. Assess for clinical manifestations of each electrolyte imbalance.
   d. Monitor vital signs.
   e. Monitor cardiopulmonary status, particularly for impaired airway, respiratory depression, and dysrhythmias.
   f. Administer prescribed oral or IV fluids and electrolytes, using a volume controller for IV administration.
   g. Encourage intake or restriction of foods high in the electrolyte of concern, as appropriate.
   h. Maintain safety related to decreased level of consciousness, confusion, muscle weakness, and potential for seizures.
2. Common electrolyte imbalances, their causes, clinical manifestations, and specific nursing care (Table 21.1).

Table 21.1 Common Electrolyte Imbalances

Imbalance	Causes	Clinical Manifestations	Specific Nursing Care
Sodium			
Hypernatremia Serum level >145 mEq/L.	• Increased intake of dietary sodium, such as foods high in salt or sodium bicarbonate. • Excessive IV saline solutions. • Fluid volume deficit. • Increased fluid retention, such as from cardiac, renal, and liver diseases. • Conditions in which fluid loss exceeds sodium loss, such as diaphoresis, diabetes mellitus, and diabetes insipidus.	• Thirst. • Dry, sticky mucous membranes. • Increased temperature, pulse, and blood pressure. • Agitation. • Confusion. • Nausea and vomiting. • Muscle weakness and cramps. • Lethargy.	• Maintain dietary sodium restrictions. • Give prescribed intravenous fluids, such as 5% dextrose in water or a hypotonic solution. • Teach the patient to avoid foods high in sodium, such as cheese, condiments, canned foods, luncheon meat, snacks, and nonsalt substitutes.

Table 21.1 **Common Electrolyte Imbalances—cont'd**

Imbalance	Causes	Clinical Manifestations	Specific Nursing Care
Hyponatremia Serum level <135 mEq/L.	• Low-salt diet. • Excessive sweating. • Gastrointestinal (GI) losses via vomiting, diarrhea, or gastric decompression. • Excessive intake of sodium-free fluids (dilutional hyponatremia). • Burns. • Syndrome of inappropriate antidiuretic hormone (SIADH). • Adrenal insufficiency.	• Headache. • Confusion. • Personality changes. • Nausea and vomiting. • Muscle weakness and cramps. • Lethargy.	• Promote intake of dietary sodium. • Maintain seizure precautions. • Give prescribed IV fluids (e.g., normal saline). • Give prescribed osmotic diuretics if the patient is hypervolemic.
Potassium			
Hyperkalemia Serum level >5.0 mEq/L.	• Fluid volume deficit. • Massive cellular damage, such as burns. • Medications, such as potassium-sparing diuretics. • Excessive intake of potassium supplements. • Acidosis, especially ketoacidosis. • Kidney disease. • Adrenal insufficiency.	• Muscle weakness. • Fatigue. • Flaccid paralysis. • Slow, weak, irregular pulse. • Dysrhythmias. • Peaked T waves, flattened P waves, and wide QRS complexes on electrocardiogram (ECG). • Nausea. • Abdominal cramps. • Diarrhea. • Increased bowel sounds.	• Maintain ordered potassium-restricted diet. • Administer prescribed exchange resin to promote potassium excretion, such as sodium polystyrene sulfonate (Kayexalate) or hypertonic glucose IV solution with insulin to move potassium into cells. • Monitor the heart rate for a dysrhythmia
Hypokalemia Serum level <3.5 mEq/L.	• GI losses via vomiting, diarrhea, or gastric decompression. • Decreased dietary intake of potassium. • Medications, such as laxatives and potassium-wasting diuretics. • Profuse diaphoresis. • Polyuria, diuretic phase of kidney failure.	• Muscle weakness. • Fatigue. • Decreased deep tendon reflexes. • Weak, irregular pulse. • Ventricular dysrhythmias. • Flattened T waves and elevated U waves on ECG. • Nausea and vomiting. • Abdominal distension. • Decreased bowel sounds.	• Ensure adequate urinary output before giving IV potassium supplements. • Assess for signs and symptoms of phlebitis at the infusion site. • Teach the patient about foods high in potassium, such as bananas, cantaloupe, oranges, strawberries, potatoes, carrots, raisins, spinach, fish, pork, veal, and beef. • Monitor the heart rate for a dysrhythmia. • Assess a patient receiving digoxin because hypokalemia increases the risk of digitalis toxicity.
Calcium			
Hypercalcemia Serum level >10.5 mEq/L.	• Prolonged immobility. • Medications, such as thiazide diuretics or lithium. • Excessive intake of antacids, calcium, or vitamin D supplements. • Hyperparathyroidism. • Excessive intake of foods high in calcium. • Cancer of the bone or bone metastasis. • Osteoporosis.	• Deep bone pain. • Flank pain due to renal calculi. • Anorexia. • Nausea and vomiting. • Constipation. • Weak, relaxed muscles. • Lethargy. • Hypoactive reflexes. • Increased urine calcium (Sulkowitch test). • Confusion. • Decreased level of consciousness. • Dysrhythmias. • Shortened QT segment on ECG.	• Encourage fluid intake to prevent renal calculi. • Encourage dietary fiber to prevent constipation. • Teach the patient to avoid foods high in calcium. • Prepare for hemodialysis, if ordered. • Handle the patient gently to prevent a pathologic fracture.

Continued

| Table 21.1 | Common Electrolyte Imbalances—cont'd | | |

Imbalance	Causes	Clinical Manifestations	Specific Nursing Care
Hypocalcemia Serum level <8.5 mEq/L.	• GI disturbances, such as diarrhea or malabsorption. • Inadequate vitamin D intake. • Medications, such as steroids, INH, furosemide, and cisplatin. • Hypoparathyroidism. • Kidney disease due to increased phosphorous.	• Paresthesia. • Hyperactive reflexes. • Muscle cramps. • Tetany. • Seizures. • Facial nerve twitching (Chvostek sign). • Carpopedal spasm (Trousseau sign). • Laryngeal spasms. • Stridor. • Hypotension. • Palpitations. • Dysrhythmias. • Prolonged QT segment on ECG.	• Administer prescribed calcium supplements. • Maintain a patent airway and seizure precautions. • Teach the patient about foods high in calcium, such as dairy products; green, leafy vegetables; salmon; and sardines. • Encourage weight-bearing exercise. • Handle the patient gently to prevent a pathological fracture.
Magnesium			
Hypermagnesemia Serum level >2.14 mEq/L.	• Medications, such as magnesium-containing antacids. • Excessive intake of magnesium supplements. • Kidney disease. • Adrenal insufficiency.	• Drowsiness. • Lethargy. • Hypoactive reflexes. • Muscle weakness. • Bradycardia. • Hypotension. • Flushed, warm skin. • Increased thirst. • Respiratory depression. • Bradypnea.	• Monitor respiratory status and reflexes; notify the primary health-care provider of absent patellar reflexes. • Teach the patient to avoid foods high in magnesium.
Hypomagnesemia Serum level <1.32 mEq/L.	• GI disturbances such as diarrhea, malabsorption, and prolonged gastric decompression. • Medications, such as diuretics and aminoglycoside antibiotics. • Pancreatitis. • Liver cirrhosis. • Hyperparathyroidism.	• Disorientation. • Variability of mood. • Neuromuscular irritability. • Muscle weakness. • Seizures. • Dysrhythmias. • Nystagmus. • Diplopia.	• Teach the patient about foods high in magnesium, such as whole grains; green, leafy vegetables; meat; and seafood. • Maintain seizure precautions. • Assess a patient receiving digoxin because of the risk of digitalis toxicity.

Figures from Wilkinson and Treas (2011). *Fundamentals of nursing,* Vol. 2, 2nd ed. Philadelphia: F. A. Davis, with permission.

IV. Acid-Base Balance

pH reflects the strength of hydrogen ions in a solution. When a state of acid-balance exists in the extracellular compartment, pH is 7.35 to 7.45. A pH less than 7.35 is acidic; greater than 7.45, alkaline. When in balance, body fluid has 27 mEq of bicarbonate (HCO_3^-) per liter and 1.35 mEq of carbonic acid (H_2CO_3) per liter; the bicarbonate-carbonic acid ratio is 20:1 (Fig. 21.10). This balance is fragile and is maintained through a variety of mechanisms.

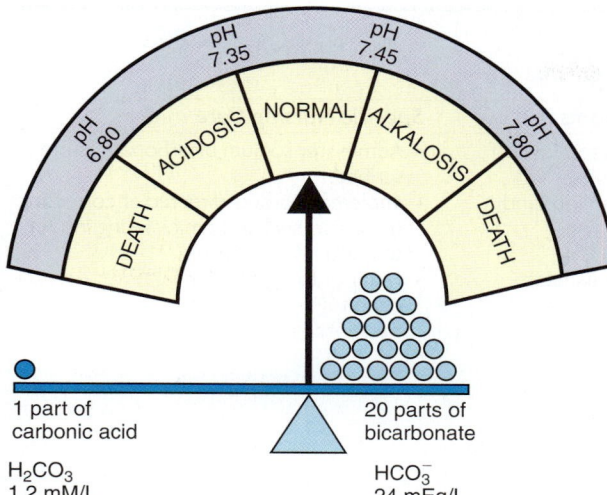

Fig 21.10 Acid-base balance. (From Phillips [2005]. *IV therapy notes,* 1st ed. Philadelphia: F. A. Davis, with permission.)

When this balance is disrupted, acid-base imbalances occur. Carbonic acid imbalances lead to respiratory acidosis or respiratory alkalosis, and bicarbonate and hydrogen imbalances lead to metabolic acidosis or metabolic alkalosis.

A. Components of Acid-Base Balance
  1. Acid.
     a. Substance that has more hydrogen ions than bicarbonate ions.
     b. Yields hydrogen ions in solution.
  2. Base.
     a. Substance that has more bicarbonate ions than hydrogen ions.
     b. Accepts hydrogen ions in solution.
  3. Salt.
     a. Compound that results when an acid and a base are mixed.
     b. The acid releases H^+ ions while the base releases OH^- ions in a process called *hydrolysis*.

B. Mechanisms That Maintain Acid-Base Balance
  1. **Buffer mechanisms:** First line of defense; respond in seconds.
     a. Buffer.
        (1) Substance that combines with a strong acid or base to change it to a weaker acid or base.
        (2) Substance that accepts or releases hydrogen ions to correct an acid-base imbalance.
     b. Bicarbonate buffer system.
        (1) Most important buffer in extracellular fluids (ECF).
        (2) Neutralizes excess hydrogen ions.
     c. Phosphate buffer system.
        (1) Most important buffer in intracellular fluids (ICF).
        (2) Neutralizes excess hydrogen ions.
     d. Plasma protein system.
        (1) Proteins can attract or release hydrogen ions.
        (2) Functions in both ICF and ECF.
     e. Hemoglobin system.
        (1) Chloride shifts into or out of cells, depending on the oxygen level; oxygen is carried in the hemoglobin molecule.
        (2) As chloride shifts into or out of cells, bicarbonate ions move in the opposite direction.
  2. **Respiratory mechanisms:** Second line of defense; respond in minutes.
     a. When carbonic acid reaches the lungs, it breaks down into water (H_2O) and carbon dioxide (CO_2).
     b. Respiratory rate changes depending on the level of carbon dioxide in ECF under control of the medulla oblongata.
        (1) Rate increases with increased carbon dioxide.
        (2) Rate decreases with decreased carbon dioxide.
  3. **Renal mechanisms:** Third line of defense; respond in hours to days.
     a. Kidneys control the buffer sodium bicarbonate ($NaHCO_3$) by excreting or conserving hydrogen ions.
     b. Kidneys also combine ammonia (NaH_3) with hydrochloric acid (HCl) to form ammonium (NH_4Cl), which is then excreted.

C. Acid-Base Imbalances and Related Nursing Care
  1. Commonalities of nursing care for patients with acid-base imbalances.
     a. Perform a history and physical examination to collect data that may help identify the cause.
     b. Obtain vital signs.
     c. Assess for and maintain a patent airway.
     d. Monitor cardiopulmonary status for respiratory impairment or dysrhythmias.
     e. Monitor laboratory results for arterial blood gas and serum electrolyte levels.
     f. Administer ordered oral and IV fluids and electrolyte supplements.
     g. Maintain patient safety; institute seizure precautions when necessary.
     h. Monitor intake and output.
  2. Common acid-base imbalances, related blood tests, their causes, compensatory mechanisms, clinical manifestations, and specific nursing care (Table 21.2, page 660).

V. Administration of IV Solutions

Sometimes, oral rehydration therapy is not enough to correct a fluid volume deficit. In these cases, administration of IV fluids may be necessary to correct the imbalance. A variety of solutions (e.g., isotonic, hypotonic, or hypertonic) might be ordered, depending on the cause

Table 21.2 Common Acid-Base Imbalances

Metabolic Acidosis

Related Blood Tests	Compensatory Mechanisms	Specific Nursing Care
• pH <7.35. • HCO$_3$ <22mEq/L. **Causes** • Base bicarbonate deficit due to severe diarrhea. • Increased acids resulting from lactic acidosis, ketoacidosis, aspirin poisoning, starvation, kidney disease, and terminal cancer.	• Hyperventilation occurs to blow off carbon dioxide. • Kidneys excrete hydrogen ions and retain bicarbonate. **Clinical Manifestations** • Deep, rapid breathing (Kussmaul respirations). • Headache. • Confusion. • Coma. • Fruity odor to breath. • Nausea, vomiting, or diarrhea. • Weakness or drowsiness. • Hypotension. • Dysrhythmias. • Warm, flushed skin due to vasodilation.	• Administer sodium bicarbonate as prescribed. • Implement orders directed at correcting the cause, such as administering insulin to correct ketoacidosis. • Monitor for hypokalemia because, as the condition resolves, potassium moves back into cells.

Respiratory Acidosis

Related Blood Tests	Compensatory Mechanisms	Specific Nursing Care
• pH <7.35. • PaCO$_2$ >42 mm Hg. **Causes** • Impaired gas exchange at the alveolar-capillary membrane due to conditions such as pneumonia, pulmonary edema, and emphysema. • Respiratory obstructions such as: *Mechanical:* For example, tumors and foreign objects. *Functional:* For example, cystic fibrosis and asthma. • Medications that depress respirations, such as opioids and anesthesia. • Neuromuscular impairment, such as trauma to the medulla oblongata, spinal cord injury, and myasthenia gravis.	• Respirations increase in rate and depth. • Kidneys excrete hydrogen ions. • Kidneys retain sodium to increase sodium bicarbonate. **Clinical Manifestations** • Increased rate and depth of respirations. • Use of accessory muscles of respiration. • Dyspnea, shortness of breath. • Tachycardia. • Hypotension. • Warm, flushed skin due to vasodilation. • Restlessness. • Irritability. • Headache. • Disorientation. • Coma.	• Assess for signs of respiratory distress. • Maintain a patent airway, such as by administering prescribed bronchodilators and suctioning the airway. • Maintain semi- to high-Fowler position. • Encourage the patient to turn, cough, and deep breathe. • Encourage oral fluid intake as ordered, usually 2 to 3 L/day to thin respiratory secretions. • Perform chest physiotherapy as ordered, such as postural drainage and percussion. • Prepare for endotracheal intubation if ordered.

Metabolic Alkalosis

Related Blood Tests	Compensatory Mechanisms	Specific Nursing Care
• pH >7.45. • HCO$_3$ >26 mEq/L. **Causes** • Loss of acid gastric secretions due to vomiting, gastric decompression, and lavage. • Medications, such as thiazide and loop diuretics and antacids with sodium bicarbonate.	• The rate and depth of respirations decrease. • Kidneys excrete excess sodium bicarbonate and retain hydrogen ions. **Clinical Manifestations** • Paresthesia, tremors, and muscle hypertonicity. • Bradypnea. • Tachycardia. • Hypotension. • Dysrhythmias. • Dizziness. • Confusion. • Coma. • Decreased GI motility. • Hypotonic bowel sounds. • Decreased serum potassium.	• Administer prescribed IV fluids, such as sodium chloride. • Monitor serum potassium levels. • Implement orders that address the underlying cause, such as discontinuing mediations or correcting hypokalemia.

Table 21.2	Common Acid-Base Imbalances—cont'd

Respiratory Alkalosis

Related Blood Tests	*Compensatory Mechanisms*	*Specific Nursing Care*
• pH >7.45. • $PaCO_2$ <38 mm Hg. **Causes** • Hyperventilation due to anxiety or aggressive mechanical ventilation. • Fever. • Pain. • Hypoxia.	• Kidneys excrete excess bicarbonate. • Kidneys retain hydrogen ions. **Clinical Manifestations** • Tachypnea. • Light-headedness, dizziness, confusion, and decreased level of consciousness. • Paresthesia. • Hyperreflexia. • Tetany. • Seizures. • Nausea and vomiting. • Epigastric pain. • Dysrhythmias related to hypokalemia.	• Stay with the patient during an anxiety attack. • Encourage the use of appropriate breathing techniques, such as breathing more slowly. • Change the settings on the mechanical ventilator as ordered, such as decreased rate or depth settings.

of the imbalance and the patient's status. Nurses must be familiar not only with these solutions but also with the tubing used to administer IV fluids, the sites appropriate for insertion of IV access devices, and the various devices that control the flow of solution. Nurses must continuously assess and reassess patients for the desired outcomes of therapy as well as implement nursing care to prevent or treat the complications associated with the administration of IV fluids.

A. Solutions
   1. Liquids that contain a dissolved substance.
      a. **Solute:** Dissolved substance.
      b. **Solvent:** Substance in which a solute is dissolved.
   2. Concentration of solutions.
      a. **Isotonic.**
         (1) Osmotic pressures of two liquids are equal.
         (2) Solutions that have the same concentration of solutes as blood plasma, such as 0.9 percent sodium chloride, 5 percent dextrose in water (D_5W), and lactated Ringer's solution.
         (3) When infused, these solutions remain inside the intravascular compartment.
      b. **Hypotonic (dilute).**
         (1) Large amount of solvent contains a small amount of solute.
         (2) Solutions that have a lesser concentration of solutes than blood plasma, such as 0.45 percent sodium chloride and 0.33 percent sodium chloride.
         (3) When infused, these solutions pull body water from the intravascular compartment into the interstitial fluid compartment.
      c. **Hypertonic (concentrated).**
         (1) Small amount of solvent contains a large amount of solute.

      (2) Solutions that have a greater concentration of solutes than blood plasma, such as 5 percent dextrose in sodium chloride (D_5NS), 5 percent dextrose in 0.45 percent sodium chloride ($D_5\frac{1}{2}NS$), and 5 percent dextrose in lactated Ringer's solution (D_5LR).
      (3) When infused, these solutions move fluid from the interstitial compartment to the intravascular compartment.

B. **Venipuncture Sites for Administration of IV Infusions**
   1. Selected based on the patient's needs and the primary health-care provider's order.
   2. Depends on a multiplicity of factors.
      a. Age.
         (1) Adults: Use veins in hands and arms (Fig. 21.11).
         (2) Infants: Use veins in scalp and dorsal foot.
      b. Type of solution: Large veins are used for parenteral nutrition and hypertonic, viscous, or irritating solutions because the infused solution is diluted faster than in small veins.
      c. Rate of volume to be infused: Large veins can accommodate a larger volume of fluid and a faster rate of fluid administration than small veins can.
      d. Duration of infusion therapy.
         (1) Intermittent or short-term continuous infusions: Use metacarpal, basilic, and cephalic veins (Fig. 21.12A).
         (2) Long-term therapy using a central venous catheter: Use subclavian, jugular, or femoral veins (Fig. 21.12B).
         (3) Long-term therapy using a peripherally inserted central venous catheter (PICC): Use basilic or cephalic vein (Fig. 21.13).

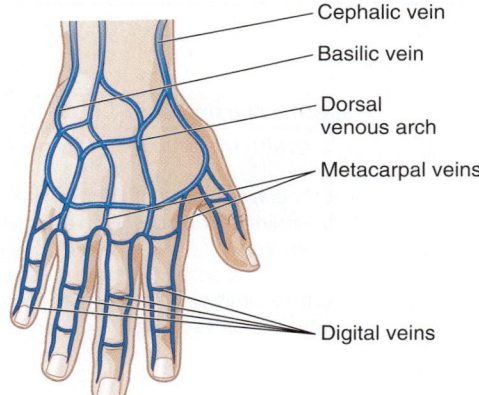

A **Superficial veins of the hand**

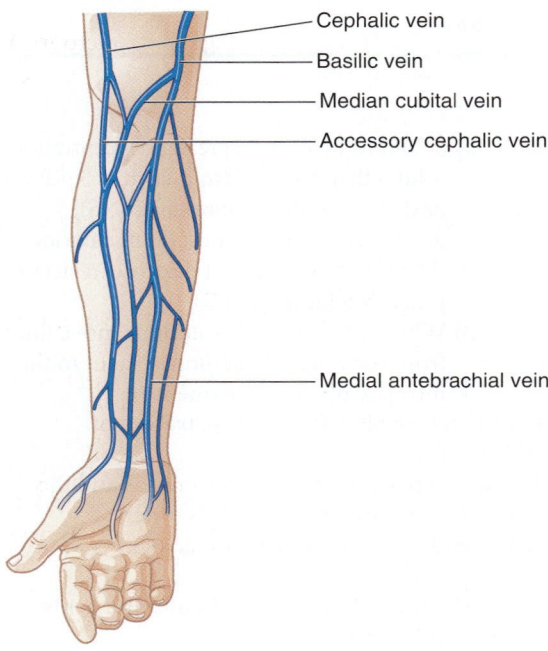

B **Superficial veins of the forearm**

Fig 21.11 Common venipuncture sites. (From Wilkinson and Treas [2011]. *Fundamentals of nursing,* Vol. 1, 2nd ed. Philadelphia: F. A. Davis, with permission.)

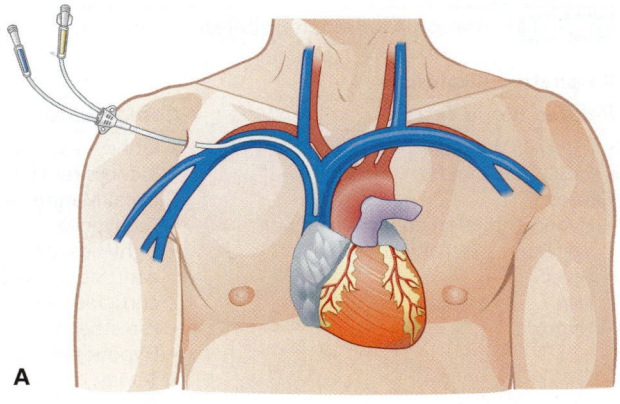

A

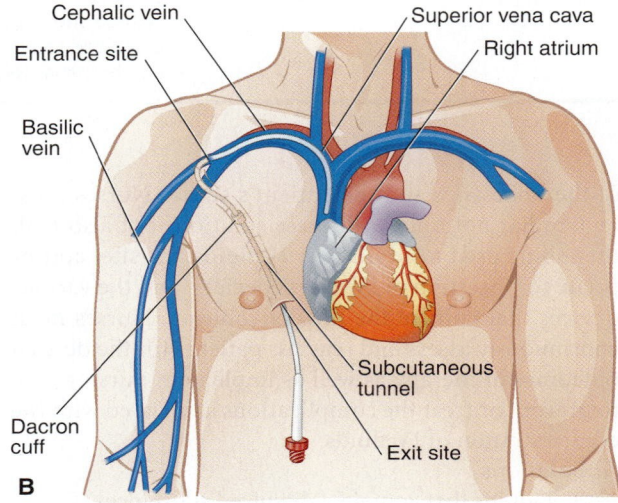

B

Fig 21.12 Central venous catheters. (A) Nontunneled central venous catheters are inserted into the jugular, subclavian, and, occasionally, femoral veins. (B) Tunneled central venous catheter is inserted through subcutaneous tissue in the chest wall into the jugular or subclavian vein. (From Wilkinson and Treas [2011]. *Fundamentals of nursing,* Vol. 1, 2nd ed. Philadelphia: F. A. Davis, with permission.)

(4) Long-term therapy using an implanted venous access port: Use subclavian or jugular vein (Fig. 21.14).

C. Devices Used for Administration of IV Infusions
   1. **Gravity flow infusion sets.**
      a. Used when a machine to control the flow of solution is unavailable or when a patient is stable.
      b. Has tubing that connects an IV solution bag at one end to a patient's venous access device.
         (1) Primary administration set: Has a backcheck valve and two or more injection ports (Fig. 21.15A).

(a) The port most distal from the patient is used for insertion of a secondary line to administer an intermittent infusion (intravenous piggyback [IVPB]).
(b) The port closest to the patient is used for the administration of IV push medication.
   (2) Secondary administration set: Shorter tubing than a primary administration set and has no ports or check valve; connects a small volume intermittent infusion to the primary tubing (Fig. 21.15B).
   c. Flow regulated at drops per minute; a roller clamp or inline dial-a-flow device in a primary administration set is used to compress tubing to attain the prescribed rate.

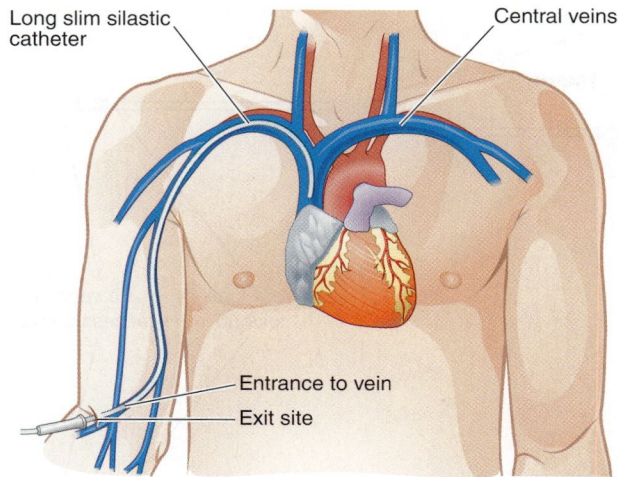

Fig 21.13 Peripherally inserted central venous catheter (PICC). A PICC line is a long, soft, flexible catheter inserted through a vein in the arm and threaded into a central vessel. (From Wilkinson and Treas [2011]. *Fundamentals of nursing*, Vol. 1, 2nd ed. Philadelphia: F. A. Davis, with permission.)

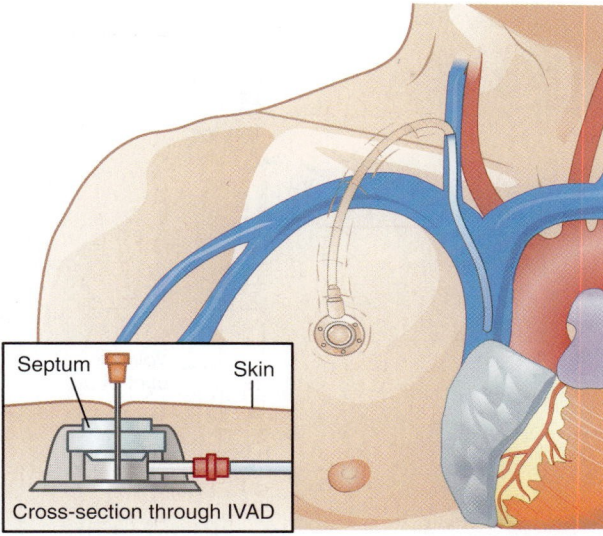

Fig 21.14 Implanted venous access port: A central venous access device that enters the subclavian or jugular vein and is tunneled to a completely implanted subcutaneous reservoir (port) in the upper chest. (From Wilkinson and Treas [2011]. *Fundamentals of nursing*, Vol. 1, 2nd ed. Philadelphia: F. A. Davis, with permission.)

   d. **Drop factor:** Determined by the number of drops per mL that the tubing delivers; usually 10, 15, or 60 drops per milliliter.

   e. Calculate flow rate using the following formula:

$$\text{drops per minute} = \frac{\text{total mLs to be infused} \times \text{drop factor}}{\text{total time in minutes (hours} \times \text{60 minutes)}}$$

2. **Electronic infusion device (EID)** (Fig. 21.16).
   a. Use when a patient is physiologically fragile or a solution must be strictly controlled.
   b. Delivers a solution at a preset rate by exerting positive pressure.
   c. Has alarms that can detect factors such as an empty solution container, tube obstruction, air in the tubing, infiltration, or low battery.
   d. Set at mL/hour, using the following formula:

$$\text{mL/hour} = \frac{\text{total mLs to be infused}}{\text{total time to be infused in hours}}$$

3. **Volume control device** (e.g., Volutrol, Buretrol, Soluset) (Fig. 21.17).
   a. Used for infants and children.
   b. Works on the principle of gravity.
   c. Drop factor usually is 60 gtt/mL (microdrip).
   d. Volume equal to the prescribed hourly rate is drained into the volume-control chamber; ensures excess fluid does not infuse.
   e. Permits medication to be added by syringe to the chamber of the volume control device.

D. **Nursing Care Related to Administration of IV Infusions**
  1. Verify the primary health-care provider's order.
  2. Perform hand hygiene and then collect appropriate equipment.
  3. Identify the patient and yourself, and explain the procedure.
  4. Obtain the patient's vital signs and assess status for selection of the insertion site and the presence of risk factors that may precipitate a complication, such as age, physical instability, restlessness, and altered mental status.
  5. Hang the prescribed solution. Apply a time tape to the IV solution container; attach a label with the date and time and your initials.
  6. Prime the tubing to remove air and fill the drip chamber to half full.
  7. Attach the IV administration tubing to the equipment accessing the patient's vein (e.g., venous catheter or peripheral IV lock) while wearing clean gloves following agency procedure.
  8. Secure the tubing with a transparent dressing and regulate the flow rate (Fig. 21.18A).
  9. Label the equipment and dressing with the date and time and your initials and, on the dressing, add the venous access type and size (Fig. 21.18B).

🛑 10. Set parameters for alarms when using an electronic infusion device and ensure that alarms are activated (do not shut off alarms); respond to alarms immediately.

🛑 11. Promote patency and integrity of the line by coiling the tubing on the bed; avoiding dependent loops; keeping the tubing over rails, not through them; and

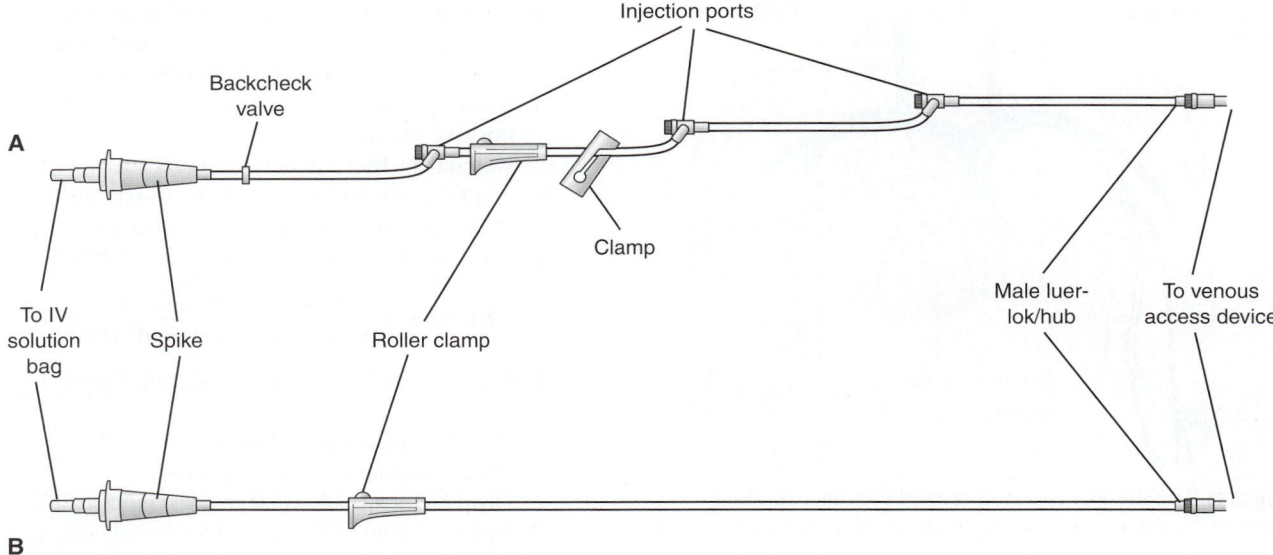

Fig 21.15 Intravenous administration sets. Intravenous administration sets: (A) Primary administration set; (B) Secondary administration set.

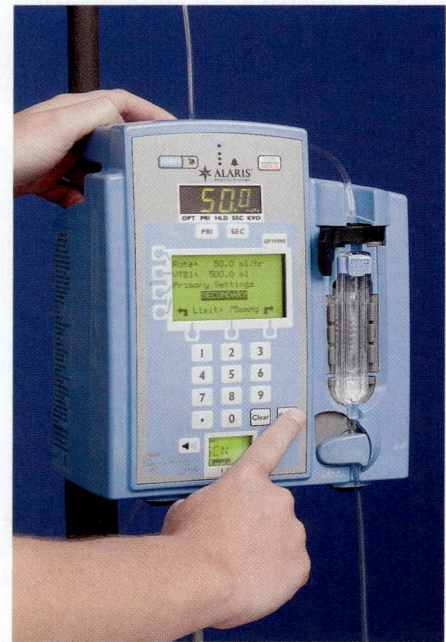

Fig 21.16 Electronic infusion device (pump). (From Wilkinson and Treas [2011]. *Fundamentals of nursing,* Vol. 2, 2nd ed. Philadelphia: F. A. Davis, with permission.)

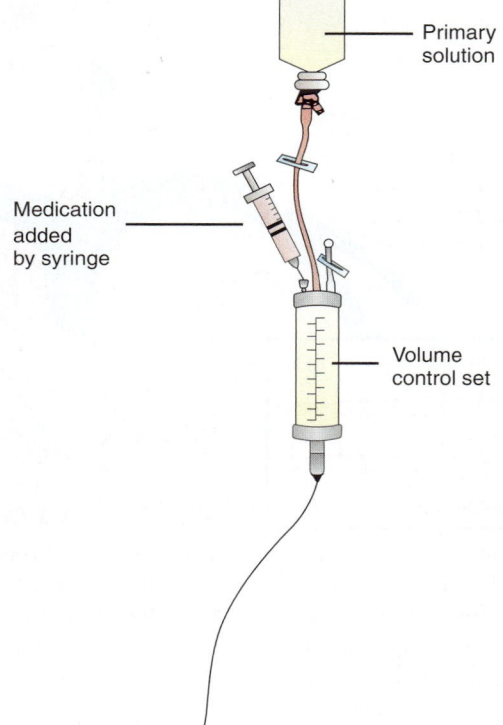

Fig 21.17 Volume control device. (From Phillips [2005]. *IV therapy notes,* 1st ed. Philadelphia: F. A. Davis, with permission.)

ensuring the patient is not lying on the tubing or excessively moving the involved extremity.

12. Monitor every hour or less; monitor more frequently if the solution contains a medication, such as potassium.
13. Change the IV solution bag, tubing, and dressing over the site according to agency protocols; for

example, the solution is changed every 24 hours and the tubing and dressing are changed every 72 hours.
14. Assess the patient's response to the infusion, such as vital signs.

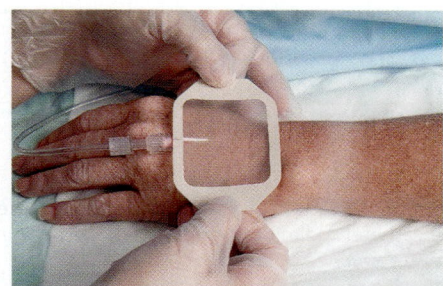

A

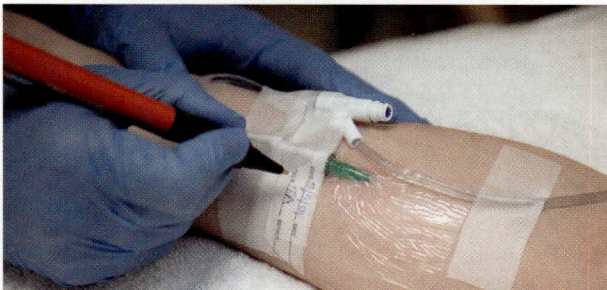

B

Fig 21.18 (A) Applying a transparent occlusive dressing to an IV site. (B) Documenting important information on an IV site label. (From Burton and Ludwig [2011]. *Fundamentals of nursing care: Concepts, connections & skills.* Philadelphia: F. A. Davis, with permission.)

15. Assess for signs of complications as a result of the administration of an IV solution.
16. Document the specific fluid and amount absorbed on the I&O record.
17. Document the patient's response in the clinical record.

E. Complications Associated With IV Solutions.
1. Complications of IV therapy can be local or systemic and can cause minor discomfort or be life threatening.
2. Common complications associated with IV solution administrations, their causes, clinical manifestations, and related nursing care (Table 21.3).

VI. Medications That Affect Fluid Volume Excess

The human body has compensatory mechanisms that help maintain fluid balance. However, when these mechanisms are inefficient or overwhelmed, the nurse can implement interventions ordered by a primary health-care provider. When patients have a fluid volume deficit, oral rehydration fluids or IV fluids are usually prescribed because there are no medications that can promote fluid intake. When patients have a FVE, medications can be prescribed that directly increase the excretion of urine (diuretics) or indirectly increase the excretion of urine by increasing cardiac output and interrupting the angiotensin I-angiotensin II cascade (cardiac medications).

A. Diuretics
1. Increase excretion of urine.
2. Examples: Table 21.4
B. Cardiac Medications That Affect Fluid Volume Excess
1. Improved cardiac functioning increases renal blood flow, which increases fluid and electrolyte excretion and inhibits release of renin (precursor to the angiotensin I-angiotensin II cascade).
2. Examples: Table 21.5.

Table 21.3 Complications of IV Therapy and Related Nursing Care

Complication	Clinical Manifestations	Nursing Care
Fluid Overload		
• Excessive fluid within the intravascular compartment. **Causes** • Fluid is infused too rapidly. • Excess amount of fluid is infused. • IV volume overwhelms patient's status.	• Weight gain. • Edema. • Distended neck veins. • Hypertension. • Tachycardia. • Shortness of breath.	**Prevention** • Use an infusion device to regulate the flow rate. • Monitor the patient and infusion frequently (e.g., every 30 to 60 minutes). **Intervention** • Decrease the flow rate of the infusion to keep the vein open while awaiting medical orders. • Place the patient in the high-Fowler position. • Obtain and monitor the vital signs. • Administer oxygen. • Document the patient's status and notify the primary health-care provider.
Infiltration		
• IV fluid accidentally leaks into the interstitial compartment. **Causes** • IV catheter tip is displaced outside of the vein.	• Decreased flow rate. • Cessation of flow. • Coolness, pallor, swelling, and tenderness at site.	**Prevention** • Secure the catheter to limit movement in the vein. • Instruct the patient to minimize flexion of the involved extremity. **Intervention** • Remove the catheter and restart one at another site. • Elevate the affected arm on a pillow. • Document the event.

Continued

Table 21.3 Complications of IV Therapy and Related Nursing Care—cont'd

Complication	Clinical Manifestations	Nursing Care
Phlebitis		
• Inflammation of a vein. **Causes** • Mechanical irritation. • Caustic solution, such as potassium chloride, antibiotics, and vitamin C. • Infection.	• Redness, warmth, swelling, and pain at site. • Decreased flow rate. • Palpable erythematous cord along vein.	**Prevention** • Use the smallest catheter practical. • Use a polyurethane catheter instead of a Teflon catheter. • Secure the catheter to limit movement in the vein. • Rotate the site every 72 hours. **Intervention** • Remove the catheter and restart one at another site. • Elevate the affected arm on a pillow. • Follow agency protocol (e.g., apply cold compress initially, apply warm compress every 4 to 6 hours for 20 minutes). • Document patient's status and notify the primary health-care provider if erythema or streaking is present.
Infection		
• Invasion and multiplication of a pathogenic organism within the IV site. **Causes** *Local* • The cannula or IV site is contaminated. *Systemic* • Pathogens or their toxic products enter the intravascular compartment.	*Local* • Redness, swelling, warmth, and exudate at site. *Systemic* • Fluctuating fever. • Tachycardia. • Hypotension. • Chills. • Altered mental status. • Increased white blood cell count.	**Prevention** • Use sterile technique to insert and maintain integrity of the catheter and site. • Use sterile technique when changing IV solution bags and tubing. • Change the solution bag every 24 hours. • Change the tubing per agency protocol (e.g., every 48 to 72 hours); rotate site every 72 hours. • Examine the solution for clarity and presence of particulate matter; if present, discard. **Intervention** • Remove the catheter, apply a sterile dressing, and restart one at another site. • Notify the primary health-care provider of the patient's status. • Prepare to obtain a specimen for culture and sensitivity testing. • Administer antibiotics as prescribed.
Extravasation		
• Vesicant leaks into the interstitial compartment causing tissue damage. *Note:* A vesicant is an irritating solution that causes tissue to blister, slough, and become necrotic. **Causes** • IV catheter tip is displaced outside of the vein.	• Decreased flow rate. • Cessation of flow. • Pallor, coolness, swelling, and pain at the site. • Blanching and coolness of the surrounding skin. • Blistering of the skin. • Necrosis of the dermis.	**Prevention** • Use an infusion device to regulate flow. • Secure the catheter to limit movement in the vein. • Instruct the patient to minimize flexion of the involved extremity; secure an arm or hand to a flat board to minimize movement. **Intervention** • Stop the infusion immediately. • Follow agency protocol (e.g., elevate involved extremity on a pillow, apply cool or warm compresses). • Document the patient's status and notify the primary health-care provider immediately. • Administer prescribed antidotes to alter the pH, alter DNA binding, and/or dilute or neutralize the drug.

Table 21.4 Diuretics That Affect Fluid Balance

Mechanism of Action	Examples	Nontherapeutic Effects
Thiazide and Thiazide-Like Diuretics • Promote excretion of sodium, potassium, and chloride in distal renal tubules.	• hydrochlorothiazide (HydroDIURIL) • chlorothiazide (Diuril) • chlorthalidone • metolazone (Zaroxolyn)	• Dehydration • Hypokalemia • Hyponatremia • Hypomagnesemia • Possible hyperglycemia in patients with diabetes. • Furosemide: Hearing problems if administered rapidly; aspirin toxicity if taken concurrently.
Loop Diuretics • Inhibit reabsorption of sodium and chloride in the ascending loop of Henle and distal renal tubules. • Promote renal excretion of water, sodium, chloride, potassium, calcium, and magnesium.	• bumetanide (Bumex) • ethacrynic acid (Edecrin) • furosemide (Lasix) • torsemide (Demadex)	

Table 21.4 **Diuretics That Affect Fluid Balance—cont'd**

Mechanism of Action	Examples	Nontherapeutic Effects
Potassium-Sparing Diuretics • Inhibit sodium reabsorption in the distal tubules and collecting ducts. • Promote renal excretion of water and sodium, leading to potassium retention.	• amiloride (Midamor) • eplerenone (Inspra) • triamterene (Dyrenium) • spironolactone (Aldactone)	• Hyperkalemia • Hypocalcemia • Hypomagnesemia

Table 21.5 **Cardiac Medications That Affect Fluid Balance**

Mechanism of Action	Examples	Nontherapeutic Effects
Angiotensin-Converting Enzyme Inhibiters (ACEIs) • Block conversion of angiotensin I to angiotensin II. • Used for patients with hypertension.	• captopril (Capoten) • enalapril (Vasotec) • lisinopril (Prinivil) • quinapril (Accupril)	• Orthostatic hypotension • Dizziness • Headache • Diarrhea • Hyperkalemia • Alterations in heart rate • Teratogenic • Erectile or ejaculation dysfunction. • ACEIs: Possible dry cough and angioedema • Captopril: Possible agranulocytosis or neutropenia.
Angiotensin II Receptor Blockers (ARBs) • Block vasoconstriction and aldosterone-secreting effects of angiotensin II. • Used for patients with hypertension.	• candesartan (Atacand) • eprosartan (Teveten) • losartan (Cozaar) • valsartan (Divan)	
Cardiac glycoside • Inhibits ATPase, which increases intracellular calcium that ultimately slows and strengthens cardiac contractions.	• digoxin (Lanoxin)	• GI irritation • Bradycardia • Fatigue • Weakness • Toxicity: Anorexia, nausea, vomiting, diarrhea, yellow vision around lights, diplopia, abdominal distress, headache, dysrhythmias, disorientation. *Note:* Hypercalcemia and hypokalemia increase risk of toxicity.

C. **Nursing Care for Patients Receiving Medications That Affect Fluid Volume Excess**

1. Monitor I&O and daily weight.
2. Monitor vital signs routinely, particularly for irregular heart rate; volume of pulse, such as bounding or thready; blood pressure, such as hypotension-hypovolemia or hypertension-hypervolemia.
3. Obtain vital signs before and after medication administration.
   a. Digoxin: Apical rate.
   b. ACEIs and ARBs: Blood pressure and heart rate and rhythm; notify the primary healthcare provider or follow agency protocol if results are outside predetermined parameters; for example, hold drug if apical rate is <50 or >110 beats/minute; hold drug if systolic BP is <100 mm Hg.
4. Assess skin turgor, location, and extent of edema.
5. Assess for clinical manifestations of electrolyte imbalances, particularly hypokalemia and hyperkalemia.
6. Monitor serum electrolyte and blood glucose levels.
7. Encourage dietary intake of foods high in potassium, calcium, and magnesium, except if the patient is taking a potassium-sparing diuretic.
8. Administer diuretics in the morning so their effects occur during waking hours; if needed, administer the second dose in early afternoon.
9. Maintain patient safety, such as by teaching the patient to rise slowly and teaching the patient signs and symptoms of nontherapeutic drug effects.
10. Digoxin (Lanoxin): Monitor blood levels of the drug, which should remain between 0.9 and 2.0 ng/mL; have digoxin immune Fab, the antidote for digoxin toxicity, readily available.
11. Monitor for therapeutic and nontherapeutic effects of medications.
12. Document medication administration and the patient's response.

CASE STUDY: Putting It All Together

A 76-year-old man who lives alone since his wife died 6 months ago is admitted to the hospital from the emergency department with a 3-day history of nausea, vomiting, and diarrhea that the patient attributes to a stomach virus. He states, "I feel weak and dizzy when I stand up and I can't seem to keep anything down." He is currently receiving hydrochlorothiazide (HCTZ) daily for hypertension. When his symptoms did not subside after 3 days and he progressively "felt worse," he went to his primary health-care provider, who sent him to the emergency department for admission to the hospital.

Patient's Clinical Record

Nursing Assessment

Sticky, dry oral mucosa.
Cracked lips.
Flushed face.
Tenting over the sternum.
50 mL of dark amber urine.
Weight loss of 5 lb from regular weight of 1 week ago.
Unsteadiness when transferring from chair to bed.

Vital Signs

Temperature: 99°F orally.
Blood pressure: 98/64 mm Hg; orthostatic hypotension identified.
Heart rate: 126 beats/minute, thready, regular rhythm.
Respiratory rate: 26 breaths/minute, regular rhythm.

Primary Health-Care Provider's Orders

NPO.
Out of bed to chair for 1 hour twice daily.
Culture and sensitivity of stool and urine.
CBC, basic metabolic panel (BMP), and urinalysis.
IVF 1,000 mL 0.45% NaCl with 20 mEq KCl at 125 mL/hour.
I&O, daily weight.
Vital signs every 4 hours.
Discontinue hydrochlorothiazide (HCTZ).
Tylenol 650 mg every 4 hours for temperature more than 101°F prn.
Zofran 4 mg every 4 hours IVPB for nausea prn.

Case Study Questions

A. Identify a cluster of subjective information that supports a concern about the patient's fluid balance.

1. _____
2. _____
3. _____
4. _____

B. Identify a cluster of objective information that supports a concern about the patient's fluid balance.

1. _____
2. _____
3. _____
4. _____
5. _____
6. _____

CASE STUDY: Putting It All Together   *cont'd*

Case Study Questions

C. What human response is the patient exhibiting based on the nurse's initial collection of data?

_____

D. The following list includes the significant data collected by the nurse. How is each abnormal clinical indicator related to dehydration?

1. Temperature of 99°F

_____

2. Weak, thready pulse of 126 beats/minute with a regular rhythm

_____

3. Blood pressure of 98/64 mm Hg; orthostatic hypotension when moving from sitting to standing position

_____

4. Respirations of 26 breaths/minute with a regular rhythm

_____

5. Cracked lips, sticky and dry oral mucosa, and tenting (decreased turgor)

_____

6. Fatigue and weakness

_____

7. Unsteadiness when transferring from chair to bed

_____

8. Oliguria and concentrated urine

_____

9. 5-lb weight loss in less than 1 week

_____

E. The following laboratory results support the nurse's conclusion that the patient is dehydrated. What is the relationship of each of the abnormal findings to dehydration?

1. Elevated serum Na^+

_____

2. Elevated blood urea nitrogen

_____

3. Elevated urine specific gravity

_____

4. Elevated serum creatinine

_____

5. Elevated hemoglobin

_____

Continued

CASE STUDY: Putting It All Together *cont'd*

_____ **Case Study Questions** _____

6. Elevated hematocrit

_____

7. Decreased serum K⁺

_____

F. What independent and dependent nursing interventions should the nurse implement for this patient in relation to the following areas?

1. Vital signs

_____

2. Diagnostic tests

_____

3. Nutrition

_____

4. Activity

_____

5. Hydration

_____

6. Hygiene

_____

7. Prescribed medications

_____

8. Health teaching

_____

G. Discuss the patient's status associated with the following areas when evaluating the effectiveness of nursing care.

1. Vital signs

_____

2. Laboratory results

_____

3. Intake and output

_____

4. Complications of fluid overload

_____

REVIEW QUESTIONS

1. How much fluid should a nurse teach a female patient to consume during 24 hours to maintain normal fluid balance?
   1. 500 mL
   2. 1,00 mL
   3. 1,500 mL
   4. 2,200 mL

2. A patient who is scheduled for chemotherapy is receiving 1 L of fluid over a 2-hour period before receiving nephrotoxic chemotherapy. The nurse assesses the patient frequently for hypervolemia during this 2-hour period. For what early sign of hypervolemia should the nurse assess the patient?
   1. Poor skin turgor
   2. Crackles in the lungs
   3. Jugular vein distention
   4. Increased urinary output

3. A nurse is caring for a patient who is receiving a low-potassium diet. Which food should the nurse teach the patient to avoid? **Select all that apply.**
   1. _____ Chicken liver
   2. _____ Tomato soup
   3. _____ Lima beans
   4. _____ Spinach
   5. _____ Carrots

4. A patient receiving Lasix daily is admitted with a diagnosis of dehydration and hypokalemia. The patient's IV fluid is 1,000 mL 0.9 percent normal saline with 20 mEq of potassium chloride infusing at 125 mL/hour. What is **most** important for the nurse to assess?
   1. Food intake
   2. Intravenous site
   3. Intake and output
   4. Pulse and respirations

5. A nurse is completing a patient's intake and output form for May 6. What is the total fluid intake for May 6?
   Answer: _____ mL

Intake and Output

INTAKE	11-7	7-3	3-11	24 HR	11-
Oral/Tube	150	450	400		
Blood/Plasma					
I.V.	650	650	650		
Other					
Other					
TOTAL					
OUTPUT	11-7	7-3	3-11	24 HR	11-
Liquid Stool					
Urine					
G.I. Suction					
Emesis					
Bowel Movement					
Other					
TOTAL					
INITIALS					

6. A nurse is monitoring the most recent laboratory results for a group of patients. Which result should cause the **most** concern?
   1. Serum potassium of 5.8 mEq/L for a patient after cardiac surgery
   2. Hemoglobin level of 10 mg/dL for a patient with a history of anemia
   3. Blood glucose of 124 mg/dL for a patient with a history of type 1 diabetes
   4. White blood cell count of 10,000/mm³ for a patient who had a colon resection 3 days ago

7. A nurse in the emergency department is caring for a variety of patients. Which patients should the nurse identify are at risk for a fluid volume deficit? **Select all that apply.**
   1. _____ Man with chronic kidney disease
   2. _____ Older adult with perfuse diaphoresis
   3. _____ Adolescent experiencing ketoacidosis
   4. _____ Infant experiencing diarrhea for 12 hours
   5. _____ Woman who is in the 8th month of gestation

8. A nurse is caring for a patient who is experiencing fluid volume excess evidenced by significant dependent edema. The primary health-care provider orders a 1,000 mL fluid restriction. Which nursing intervention is **most** important?
   1. Offer ice chips frequently.
   2. Provide frequent mouth care.
   3. Assess extent of edema daily.
   4. Keep the legs lower than the heart.

9. A nurse is assessing a patient for fluid volume excess. What questions should the nurse ask the patient to obtain information concerning this problem? **Select all that apply.**
1. _____ "Do your rings feel tighter lately?"
2. _____ "How often do you need to urinate?"
3. _____ "How much water do you drink a day?"
4. _____ "Have you noticed an increase in thirst?"
5. _____ "Did you gain weight in the last few days?"

10. A nurse is caring for a patient with a serum calcium level of 7.5 mEq/L. What nursing intervention is important when caring for this patient?
1. Give the patient the prescribed calcium supplement.
2. Teach the patient to avoid foods high in calcium.
3. Assess the patient for hypoactive reflexes.
4. Prepare the patient for hemodialysis.

11. A patient is receiving an intravenous infusion of 0.9 percent sodium chloride (NaCl) at 75 mL/hour. At 10 a.m. the patient received an antibiotic diluted in 100 mL of NaCl; this solution was infused over 1 hour. At 2 p.m. the patient received an antiemetic diluted in 50 mL of sterile water; this solution was infused over 30 minutes. Both medications were hung as IVPB infusions through a secondary line that interrupted the primary infusion of NaCl. How much intravenous solution did the patient receive between 8 a.m. and 8 p.m.? Record your answer using a whole number.
Answer: _____ mL

12. A nurse is caring for a patient admitted to the hospital with a diagnosis of congestive heart failure and is retaining fluid. For what clinical indicator should the nurse assess the patient that supports the presence of this condition?
1. Weight loss
2. Hypotension
3. Bounding pulse
4. Hemoconcentration

13. A primary health-care provider orders 0.9 percent sodium chloride with 10 mEq of potassium chloride to be infused at 40 mL/hour. The nurse has intravenous tubing with a drop factor of 60 gtt/mL. How many drops per minute should the nurse administer to deliver the ordered amount of solution? Record your answer using a whole number.
Answer: _____ drops/minute

14. A nurse is caring for a patient who reports having severe diarrhea and vomiting for the last few days. The patient's laboratory results indicate that the patient has a serum sodium level of 146 mEq/L. For which clinical indicator unique to this serum sodium level should the nurse assess the patient?
1. Confusion
2. Headache
3. Agitation
4. Thirst

15. A nurse is monitoring several patients for clinical manifestations of either hyperkalemia or hypokalemia. What clinical manifestations can occur with both imbalances? **Select all that apply.**
1. _____ Irregular pulse
2. _____ Muscle weakness
3. _____ Facial nerve twitching
4. _____ Increased bowel sounds
5. _____ Flattened T wave on an electrocardiogram tracing

16. A nurse is obtaining a health history from a patient who is has a serum potassium level of 3.2 mEq. What patient statement indicates a potential precipitating cause of this clinical manifestation?
1. "I've had diarrhea for several days."
2. "We eat a lot of green leafy vegetables in our house."
3. "I take electrolyte supplements because I'm on a diuretic."
4. "My blood glucose has been very high lately because I have diabetes."

17. A nurse is assessing a patient with a diagnosis of hypocalcemia. Which patient clinical manifestation supports this diagnosis?
1. Hypoactive reflexes
2. Relaxed muscles
3. Deep bone pain
4. Muscle cramps

18. A nurse is caring for a patient who is experiencing impaired venous return secondary to immobility. The primary health-care provider prescribes furosemide (Lasix) 40 mg PO daily. Place the following statements in order of application of the nursing process.
1. Excess fluid volume is related to impaired venous return secondary to immobility.
2. The patient's potassium level remains within the expected range.
3. The patient has 2+ edema of the lower extremities.
4. Administer furosemide (Lasix) 40 mg PO daily.
5. The patient will lose 1.5 lb daily.
Answer: _____

19. A nurse is caring for a patient who has a cardiac monitor. The patient's serum potassium level is 5.9 mEq/L. The nurse should check the cardiac monitor for the presence of which altered cardiac tracing related to this patient's potassium level?
1. Peaked P wave
2. Peaked T wave
3. Elevated U wave
4. Narrow QRS complex

20. A nurse working on the 8 a.m. to 4 p.m. shift is monitoring the intake and output of a patient. In the morning, the patient voids 640 mL, drinks 4 oz of orange juice and 6 oz of coffee, and consumes 6 oz of milk in cereal. For lunch, the patient has 3 oz of cream of chicken soup, a chicken breast with a portion of rice, and a 12-oz can of ginger ale. After lunch, the patient reports feeling nauseated and ultimately vomits 280 mL of greenish yellow fluid containing food particles from lunch. The primary health-care provider orders NPO with ice chips to help relieve thirst. The nurse gives the patient an 8-oz cup of ice chips that the patient consumes by the end of the shift. The patient voids 320 mL at 3 p.m. The patient vomits another 130 mL of fluid just before the end of the shift. What is the patient's intake for the 8 a.m. to 4 p.m. shift?

Answer: _____ mL

21. A nurse is caring for two patients, one with a diagnosis of fluid volume excess and one with fluid volume deficit. Which nursing intervention is unique to fluid volume excess, which is unrelated to fluid volume deficit?
1. Obtain a daily weight.
2. Record intake and output.
3. Place the patient in the mid-Fowler position.
4. Monitor laboratory values for renal function and electrolytes.

22. A nurse is caring for a patient receiving digoxin (Lanoxin) to improve cardiac function. For the past few days, the patient has been experiencing diarrhea and vomiting due to a gastrointestinal infection. For which clinical manifestation should the nurse assess the patient?
1. Orthostatic hypotension
2. Visual disturbances
3. Increased pulse
4. Muscle cramps

23. An older adult is admitted to the hospital via the emergency department for unexplained episodes of fainting. When the patient arrives on the unit, the nurse reviews the primary health-care provider's orders, obtains the patient's vital signs, and performs a physical assessment.

Patient's Clinical Record

Vital Signs

Temperature: 99.9°F, temporal.
Pulse: 104 beats/minute.
Respirations: 16 breaths/minute, regular rhythm.
Blood pressure: 96/64 mm Hg.

Primary Health-Care Provider's Orders

Regular diet.
Encourage PO fluids.
OOB to a chair with assist.
Vital signs every 8 hours.
Intake and output.
Daily weight.
Urinalysis.
IVF 1,000 mL 0.9% normal saline bolus × 1.

Physical Assessment

Voiding dark amber urine.
Tenting of skin over sternum.
Weight is 116 lb. Patient states a loss of 3 lb in the last 2 days.

What should the nurse do based on this information?
1. Offer a variety of fluids to keep at the patient's bedside.
2. Hold the lunch tray until the patient talks with the dietitian.
3. Teach the patient how to collect a midstream urine specimen.
4. Have the patient sit on the side of the bed for a minute before standing.

24. A patient is receiving a potassium-sparing diuretic. For which nontherapeutic effect should the nurse assess the patient?
1. Muscle weakness
2. Hypoactive reflexes
3. Respiratory depression
4. Dry sticky mucous membranes

25. A patient is admitted to the hospital after several days of diarrhea, nausea, and vomiting. Which clinical indicator should the nurse expect to identify when completing an admission nursing assessment?
1. Adventitious breath sounds
2. Nonelastic skin turgor
3. Frothy sputum
4. Weight gain

26. A nurse is caring for an older adult and suspects that the patient may be experiencing hypovolemia. For which clinical indicator should the nurse assess the patient that supports this conclusion?
    1. Distended neck veins
    2. Bradycardia
    3. Dilute urine
    4. Weak pulse

27. Which independent nursing actions are associated with a patient with fluid volume deficit? **Select all that apply.**
    1. _____ Lubricating the lips
    2. _____ Assessing skin turgor
    3. _____ Discontinuing diuretics
    4. _____ Increasing oral fluid intake
    5. _____ Providing intravenous fluids

28. A nurse is caring for a patient who has orders for an oral fluid restriction of 1400 mL in 24 hours. The patient is receiving medication in a 50 mL IVPB four times a day. How much fluid should the nurse allocate for oral intake during the day?
    1. 400 mL
    2. 800 mL
    3. 1,000 mL
    4. 1,300 mL

29. A patient is admitted to the hospital with a diagnosis of dehydration. Which type of IV fluid should the nurse expect the primary health-care provider to order?
    1. 5% dextrose in water
    2. 0.45% sodium chloride
    3. 0.9% sodium chloride
    4. $D_5\frac{1}{2}NS$

30. A nurse is caring for a patient who is receiving a 2-g sodium diet. Which food should the nurse teach the patient to avoid? **Select all that apply.**
    1. _____ Processed cheese
    2. _____ Canned soup
    3. _____ Tomatoes
    4. _____ Bananas
    5. _____ Eggs

31. A nurse is caring for a patient who is hyperventilating. What should the nurse do **first** to reduce the risk of respiratory alkalosis?
    1. Teach the patient breathing techniques.
    2. Have the patient breathe into a paper bag.
    3. Encourage the patient to try to remain calm.
    4. Position the patient in a high-Fowler position.

32. A nurse is caring for a patient who reports having an "upset stomach" with vomiting and a low-grade fever for several days. The nurse collects the following vital signs: Blood pressure 100/72 mm Hg, pulse 92 beats/minute and thready, respirations 24 breaths/minute, and temperature 100.6°F. Which additional clinical indicator supports the nurse's conclusion about the patient's problem?
    1. Peripheral edema
    2. Jugular vein distension
    3. Red tongue with furrows
    4. Decreased blood urea nitrogen

33. A 58-year-old woman comes to the emergency department reporting multiple vague discomforts. The nurse obtains the patient's history and performs an intake interview. The primary health-care provider performs a physical assessment and orders x-rays, an electrocardiogram, a complete blood count, a urinalysis, and a metabolic panel.

▌ Patient's Clinical Record

Medical/Surgical History

Patient is a 58-year-old woman who was diagnosed with cancer of the breast 8 years ago. Initially had a mastectomy, radiation, and chemotherapy. Had a hysterectomy 10 years ago for multiple fibroids.

Patient Interview

Patient reports experiencing a decreased appetite and chronic constipation. States she has been feeling very tired, weak, and achy all over for several weeks. A family member states that the patient has become a little confused lately.

Physical Assessment

Temperature: 99.4°F, oral.
Pulse: 88 beats/minute, irregular rhythm.
Respirations: 22 breaths/minute.
Deep tendon reflexes: Hypoactive.
Movement of extremities through range of motion increases achy feeling.

What is the **most** important nursing intervention while caring for this patient?
1. Encouraging the patient to increase fiber in her diet
2. Handling the patient carefully when completing the ordered tests
3. Obtaining the blood specimens before sending the patient for x-rays
4. Performing the electrocardiogram after determining if the patient has a pacemaker

34. A nurse in the emergency room is caring for a patient with a diagnosis of respiratory acidosis due to an asthma attack. Which medication should the nurse anticipate that the primary health-care provider **most** likely will prescribe?
1. Diuretic
2. Bronchodilator
3. Sodium chloride
4. Sodium bicarbonate

35. A nurse is taking a patient's blood pressure. After the blood pressure cuff was inflated above the patient's systolic pressure, the patient's hand and wrist appeared as in the illustration. For which additional clinical indicator should the nurse assess the patient?

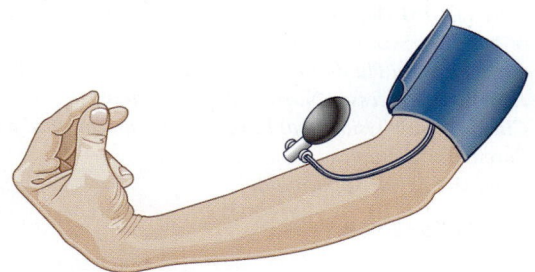

1. Irregular heart rate
2. Nonelastic skin turgor
3. Sticky mucous membranes
4. Decreased deep tendon reflexes

36. A patient is receiving hydrochlorothiazide (HydroDIURIL). When evaluating the patient's response to HydroDIURIL, which nontherapeutic response is **most** important for the nurse to monitor?
1. Dysrhythmias
2. Impaired airway
3. Elevated glucose
4. Elevated blood pressure

37. A nurse is inserting a catheter to provide short-term intravenous therapy. Which site should the nurse use that is appropriate for short-term therapy but is not appropriate for long-term therapy?
1. Basilic vein
2. Cephalic vein
3. Subclavian vein
4. Metacarpal vein

38. A nurse is preparing a class for a group of patients about what foods to eat when receiving a diuretic. Which foods should the nurse discuss in the class? **Select all that apply.**
1. _____ Potatoes
2. _____ Skim milk
3. _____ Nonfat yogurt
4. _____ Cranberry juice
5. _____ Salad dressings

39. A nurse is caring for a patient who is receiving an intravenous piggyback medication intermittently via a primary intravenous infusion line. Which nursing intervention is **most** important to prevent infection associated with this therapy?
1. Wipe the port on the primary intravenous set with an alcohol sponge before connecting the intravenous piggyback.
2. Prime the tubing of an intravenous piggyback until a drop of solution appears at the distal end of the tubing.
3. Set the alarm on the electronic infusion device to alert the nurse if the tubing becomes obstructed.
4. Wear sterile gloves when preparing and administering parenteral solutions.

40. A nurse monitors the laboratory reports of a patient with a fluid and electrolyte imbalance. Which laboratory value indicating hypernatremia should the nurse report to the primary health-care provider?
1. 3.2 mEq/L potassium
2. 5.6 mEq/L potassium
3. 128 mEq/L sodium
4. 158 mEq/L sodium

1. ANSWER: 4.
Rationales:
1. 500 mL is an inadequate amount of intake to maintain normal fluid balance.
2. 1,000 mL is an inadequate amount of intake to maintain normal fluid balance.
3. 1,500 mL is an inadequate amount of intake to maintain normal fluid balance.
4. **2,200 mL is an average daily intake necessary for a female to maintain fluid balance.**
Content Area: Fluids and Electrolytes
Integrated Processes: Teaching/Learning; Nursing Process: Implementation
Client Need: Physiological Integrity; Basic Care and Comfort
Cognitive Level: Knowledge

2. ANSWER: 2.
Rationales:
1. Assessing skin turgor does not provide critical information regarding a patient's hypervolemic status; it is a better indicator of dehydration.
2. **The patient's respiratory status is the best indicator of the patient's tolerance for a large amount of fluid given intravenously. Crackles in the lungs usually are the first sign of hypervolemia because fluid leaves the low-pressure pulmonary system and moves into the lungs.**
3. Jugular vein distention is a later sign of hypervolemia.
4. An increase in urinary output is an expected response to an increase in fluid intake.
Content Area: Fluids and Electrolytes
Integrated Processes: Nursing Process: Evaluation
Client Need: Physiological Integrity; Pharmacological and Parenteral Therapies
Cognitive Level: Application

3. ANSWER: 2, 3, 4.
Rationales:
1. Three chicken livers contain approximately 90 mg of potassium.
2. One cup of canned tomato soup contains approximately 450 mg of potassium and should be avoided when receiving a low-potassium diet.
3. A half cup of lima beans contains 550 mg of potassium and should be avoided when receiving a low-potassium diet.
4. A half cup of cooked spinach contains approximately 420 mg of potassium and should be avoided when receiving a low-potassium diet.
5. A half cup of cooked frozen carrots contains approximately 115 mg of potassium.
TEST-TAKING TIP: Identify the word in the stem that indicates negative polarity. The word *avoid* in the stem indicates negative polarity. The question is asking, "Which foods should a patient *not eat* when receiving a low potassium diet?"
Content Area: Fluids and Electrolytes
Integrated Processes: Teaching/Learning; Nursing Process: Implementation
Client Need: Physiological Integrity; Basic Care and Comfort
Cognitive Level: Application

4. ANSWER: 3.
Rationales:
1. Although monitoring how much high-potassium food the patient is ingesting is important, it is not as important as another option.
2. Although monitoring the IV site for infiltration or irritation is important, it is not as critical as another option.
3. **Measuring the intake and output is essential when administering IV potassium because hyperkalemia can occur rapidly. Hyperkalemia can cause cardiac dysrhythmias.**
4. Although monitoring the pulse and respirations will reflect tolerance of IV fluid intake, it is not as significant as another option. Fluid intake of 125 mL/hour intravenously is appropriate for a patient who is dehydrated and is unlikely to cause hypervolemia early in treatment.
TEST-TAKING TIP: Identify the word in the stem that sets a priority. The word *most* in the stem sets a priority.
Content Area: Fluids and Electrolytes
Integrated Processes: Nursing Process: Evaluation
Client Need: Physiological Integrity; Pharmacological and Parenteral Therapies
Cognitive Level: Application

5. ANSWER: 2,950.
Rationale:
The nurse should total the oral/tube intake for 11 to 7, 7 to 3, and 3 to 11 for a total of 1,000 mL and then total the IV intake for 11 to 7, 7 to 3, and 3 to 11 for a total of 1,950 mL. The total oral/tube intake (1,000) should be added to the total IV intake (1,950) for a grand total of 2,950 mL.
Content Area: Fluids and Electrolytes

Intake and Output

INTAKE	11-7	7-3	3-11	24 HR	11-
Oral/Tube	150	450	400	1000	
Blood/Plasma					
I.V.	650	650	650	1950	
Other					
Other					
TOTAL	800	1100	1050	**2950**	
OUTPUT	11-7	7-3	3-11	24 HR	11-
Liquid Stool					
Urine					
G.I. Suction					
Emesis					
Bowel Movement					
Other					
TOTAL					
INITIALS					

Integrated Processes: Nursing Process: Assessment
Client Need: Physiological Integrity; Basic Care and Comfort
Cognitive Level: Analysis

6. ANSWER: 1.
Rationales:
1. A serum potassium level of 5.8 mEq/L is higher than the expected range of 3.5 to 5.0 mEq/L and should be reported to the primary health-care provider immediately. A high serum potassium level can cause dysrhythmias and cardiac arrest.
2. A hemoglobin level (Hb) of 10 g/dL for a patient with anemia is not unexpected. The expected range for a male is 14 to 18 g/dL and for a female 12 to 16 g/dL.
3. A serum glucose level of 124 mEq/dL is close to the expected range of 70 to 100 mg/dL. It is not unusual for a patient with diabetes to have a slightly elevated serum glucose level.
4. A white blood cell count of 10,000/mm³ is within the expected range of 4,500 to 10,000/mm³.
TEST-TAKING TIP: Identify the word in the stem that sets a priority. The word *most* in the stem sets a priority.
Content Area: Fluids and Electrolytes
Integrated Processes: Communication/Documentation; Nursing Process: Assessment
Client Need: Physiological Integrity; Reduction of Risk Potential
Cognitive Level: Analysis

7. ANSWER: 2, 3, 4.
Rationales:
1. People with chronic kidney problems usually experience fluid volume excess, not fluid volume deficit.
2. Physiological responses to alterations in fluid balance, such as the thirst mechanism, in older adults are diminished; these diminished responses increase the risk of fluid volume deficit in older adults.
3. The passage of a large volume of urine in a short period of time (polyuria) and insensible fluid loss related to the deep, rapid respirations associated with ketoacidosis will precipitate a fluid volume deficit.
4. A large volume of fluid can be lost with frequent watery stools (diarrhea); infants are particularly vulnerable to fluid balance problems because 65 to 80 percent of their body weight is related to fluid.
5. Fluid volume deficit usually is not associated with pregnancy. Toward the latter part of pregnancy, women may experience dependent edema at the end of the day because pressure of the gravid uterus impedes venous return.
Content Area: Fluids and Electrolytes
Integrated Processes: Nursing Process: Assessment
Client Need: Physiological Integrity; Physiological Adaptation
Cognitive Level: Analysis

8. ANSWER: 3.
Rationales:
1. This is a dependent function of the nurse. If the patient is receiving a restricted fluid intake, the order should include if and how often ice chips can be given to the patient to keep the mucous membranes of the mouth moist.
2. Although this is important when a patient has a fluid restriction, it is not the priority.

3. The nurse should assess the extent of edema daily by using an objective measure, such as a 1+, 2+, 3+ and 4+ scale or, if the edema is extending up the legs, measure the circumference of the calves at the same place daily. In addition, a daily weight is an objective measure of fluid retained in the body. A 2.2 lb weight gain is equal to 1 L of fluid.
4. Keeping the legs lower than the heart inhibits venous return, which will promote venous stasis and exacerbate the dependent edema in the legs.
TEST-TAKING TIP: Identify the word in the stem that sets a priority. The word *most* in the stem sets a priority. Identify the equally plausible options. Options 1 and 2 are associated with keeping the mucous membranes of the mouth moist. One of these is no better than the other. Eliminate options 1 and 2 from further consideration. Identify the clang association. The word *edema* in the stem and in option 3 is a clang association. Examine option 3 carefully.
Content Area: Fluids and Electrolytes
Integrated Processes: Nursing Process: Assessment
Client Need: Physiological Integrity; Physiological Adaptation
Cognitive Level: Application

9. ANSWER: 1,5.
Rationales:
1. Fluid retention results in an increase in interstitial fluid; swelling in the hands and feet can result in rings and shoes feeling tighter.
2. The volume of urine excreted a day is more important than the number of times a person urinates. An increase in the number of times a person urinates (frequency) is related to a urinary tract infection or retention with overflow.
3. This information by itself is useless. Fluid balance is assessed by comparing the amount of fluid taken into the body and the amount of fluid exiting the body.
4. Thirst is associated with fluid volume deficit, not fluid volume excess.
5. One liter of fluid is equal to 2.2 lb. Retained fluid will cause weight gain.
Content Area: Fluids and Electrolytes
Integrated Processes: Communication/Documentation; Nursing Process: Assessment
Client Need: Physiological Integrity; Physiological Adaptation
Cognitive Level: Analysis

10. ANSWER: 1.
Rationales:
1. The patient is experiencing hypocalcemia because the patient's serum calcium level is less than the expected range of 8.5 to 10.5 mEq/L. Calcium supplements are necessary to prevent cardiac dysrhythmias, a major concern with hypocalcemia.
2. The patient should be ingesting, not avoiding, foods high in calcium.
3. Hypoactive reflexes are related to hypercalcemia. The patient's serum calcium level of 7.5 mEq/L indicates hypocalcemia.
4. A patient with hypercalcemia, not hypocalcemia, may receive hemodialysis.

TEST-TAKING TIP: Identify the clang associations. The word *calcium* in the stem and in options 1 and 2 are clang associations. Examine these options carefully. Identify the options that are opposites. Options 1 and 2 are opposites. Option 1 addresses increasing calcium intake, and option 2 addresses avoiding foods high in calcium. Examine options 1 and 2 carefully because, more often than not, an option that is an opposite is the correct answer.
Content Area: Fluids and Electrolytes
Integrated Processes: Nursing Process: Implementation
Client Need: Physiological Integrity; Reduction of Risk Potential
Cognitive Level: Application

11. **ANSWER: 638.**
    Rationale:
    For 6 hours, the patient received the ordered infusion of NaCl, which totaled 450 mL. The antibiotic infusion interrupted the primary infusion of NaCl; therefore, 100 mL of NaCl containing the antibiotic infused over 1 hour. The antiemetic interrupted the primary infusion of NaCl for half an hour; therefore, 50 mL of sterile water containing the antiemetic infused for half an hour and the original infusion of NaCl infused for half an hour. The total amount of intravenous solution that infused was 450 + 100 + 50 + 38 (half of 75 is 37.5, but it must be rounded up to 38) = 638 mL.
    Content Area: Fluids and Electrolytes
    Integrated Processes: Nursing Process: Evaluation
    Client Need: Physiological Integrity; Pharmacological and Parenteral Therapies
    Cognitive Level: Analysis

12. **ANSWER: 3.**
    Rationales:
    1. Weight loss is associated with fluid volume deficit, not fluid volume excess. Congestive heart failure is associated with excess fluid volume (hypervolemia).
    2. Hypotension is associated with fluid volume deficit, not fluid volume excess. Congestive heart failure is associated with excess fluid volume (hypervolemia).
    3. A bounding pulse is associated with fluid volume excess. Congestive heart failure is associated with excessive fluid volume (hypervolemia).
    4. Hemoconcentration is associated with fluid volume deficit, not fluid volume excess. Congestive heart failure is associated with excess fluid volume (hypervolemia).
    TEST-TAKING TIP: Identify the equally plausible options. Options 1, 2, and 4 are all associated with hypovolemia. One of these options is no better than another. Option 3 is unique because it is the only option related to hypervolemia, which is associated with congestive heart failure.
    Content Area: Fluids and Electrolytes
    Integrated Processes: Nursing Process: Assessment
    Client Need: Physiological Integrity; Physiological Adaptation
    Cognitive Level: Application

13. **ANSWER: 40.**
    Rationale:
    The drops per minute are determined by multiplying the total number of milliliters ordered by the drop factor divided by 60 minutes.

    $$\text{Drops per minute} = \frac{40\ (\text{mL})\ (\times 60\ (\text{gtt}))}{60\ \text{minutes}} = \frac{2400}{60} = 40\ \text{drops/minute}$$

    Content Area: Fluids and Electrolytes
    Integrated Processes: Nursing Process: Planning
    Client Need: Physiological Integrity; Pharmacological and Parenteral Therapies
    Cognitive Level: Application

14. **ANSWER: 4.**
    Rationales:
    1. Increased and decreased serum sodium levels can cause confusion because of interference with nerve impulse conduction and cellular chemical reactions.
    2. The patient's serum sodium level is higher than the expected range of 135 to 145 mEq/L. Decreased, not increased, serum sodium levels cause a headache due to cerebral edema.
    3. Decreased and increased serum sodium levels can cause agitation because of interference with nerve impulse conduction and cellular chemical reactions.
    4. The sensation of thirst is triggered when plasma osmolarity increases due to inadequate fluid intake in the presence of excessive fluid loss.
    TEST-TAKING TIP: Identify the equally plausible options. Options 1 and 3 are equally plausible. One is no better than the other. Eliminate both from further consideration.
    Content Area: Fluids and Electrolytes
    Integrated Processes: Nursing Process: Assessment
    Client Need: Physiological Integrity; Physiological Adaptation
    Cognitive Level: Analysis

15. **ANSWER: 1, 2.**
    Rationales:
    1. Potassium is a component of the sodium-potassium pump that is involved with muscle contraction. The heart is a muscle; therefore, an increase or decrease in serum potassium will result in dysrhythmias and abnormalities evident on an electrocardiogram.
    2. Potassium is a component of the sodium-potassium pump that is involved with muscle contraction. An increase or decrease in serum potassium will result in muscle weakness and fatigue.
    3. Facial nerve twitching (Chvostek sign) is associated with hypocalcemia, not hyperkalemia.
    4. Increased bowel sounds, diarrhea, and abdominal cramps are associated with hyperkalemia. Abdominal distention, decreased bowel sounds, and constipation are associated with loss of muscle tone related to hypokalemia.
    5. On an electrocardiogram tracing, the T wave will be flattened with hypokalemia (due to delayed repolarization) and peaked with hyperkalemia (due to rapid repolarization).

Content Area: Fluids and Electrolytes
Integrated Processes: Nursing Process: Assessment
Client Need: Physiological Integrity; Physiological Adaptation
Cognitive Level: Analysis

16. **ANSWER: 1.**
    Rationales:
    1. The expected serum potassium level is 3.5 to 5.0 mEq; a level of 3.2 mEq indicates hypokalemia. Potassium is an ion found in gastrointestinal fluids; vomiting, gastric decompression, and diarrhea all can result in hypokalemia.
    2. This should not result in hypokalemia. Green leafy vegetables, such as spinach, contain potassium.
    3. Excessive intake of potassium chloride can result in hyperkalemia, not hypokalemia.
    4. Diabetic ketoacidosis precipitates hyperkalemia; potassium, an intracellular ion, is released when cells break down to meet energy needs.
    Content Area: Fluids and Electrolytes
    Integrated Processes: Communication/Documentation; Nursing Process: Analysis
    Client Need: Physiological Integrity; Physiological Adaptation
    Cognitive Level: Analysis

17. **ANSWER: 4.**
    Rationales:
    1. Hypoactive reflexes are associated with hypercalcemia because of loss of cell membrane excitability.
    2. Weak, relaxed muscles and hypoactive reflexes are associated with hypercalcemia.
    3. Deep bone pain is associated with hypercalcemia as calcium moves out of bones and into the intravascular compartment.
    4. Calcium is involved with neuromuscular functioning; therefore, a decrease in serum calcium results in muscle cramps, hyperactive reflexes, and paresthesia.
    TEST-TAKING TIP: Identify options that are opposites. Options 2 and 4 are opposites. Consider these options carefully. Identify equally plausible options. Options 1 and 2 are equally plausible. One of these options is no better than the other. Eliminate both from consideration.
    Content Area: Fluids and Electrolytes
    Integrated Processes: Nursing Process: Analysis
    Client Need: Physiological Integrity; Physiological Adaptation
    Cognitive Level: Application

18. **ANSWER: 3, 1, 5, 4, 2.**
    Rationales:
    3. This is a nursing assessment and is the first step of the nursing process.
    1. This is the identification of the patient's problem and is the second step of the nursing process.
    5. This is an expected outcome and is the first part of the third step of the nursing process, planning. The second half of the planning step involves identifying planned nursing interventions.

4. This is an intervention implemented by the nurse in relation to the data in this scenario. Implementation of a planned nursing intervention is the fourth step of the nursing process.
2. When evaluating outcomes associated with administration of Lasix, it is not only weight loss and a decrease in blood pressure that is expected, but that the potassium level will remain within the expected range.
Patients receiving Lasix are at risk for hypokalemia. Therefore, monitoring serum potassium levels is important when a patient is receiving Lasix.
Content Area: Fluids and Electrolytes
Integrated Processes: Nursing Process: Analysis
Client Need: Safe and Effective Care Environment; Management of Care
Cognitive Level: Analysis

19. **ANSWER: 2.**
    Rationales:
    1. A P wave is flattened, not peaked, with hyperkalemia.
    2. A peaked T wave is associated with an elevated serum potassium level higher than 5.0 mEq/L.
    3. An elevated U wave is associated with hypokalemia, not hyperkalemia.
    4. A QRS complex is widened with hyperkalemia.
    Content Area: Fluids and Electrolytes
    Integrated Processes: Nursing Process: Assessment
    Client Need: Physiological Integrity; Physiological Adaptation
    Cognitive Level: Application

20. **ANSWER: 1,050.**
    Rationale:
    120 mL (4 oz of orange juice); 180 mL (6 oz of coffee); 180 mL (6 oz of milk); 90 mL (3 oz of soup); 360 mL (12 oz of ginger ale); 120 (ice chips; liquid volume of ice chips is equal to half the volume of the frozen volume of ice chips). The total oral intake is 1,050 mL.
    Content Area: Fluids and Electrolytes
    Integrated Processes: Nursing Process: Assessment
    Client Need: Physiological Integrity; Basic Care and Comfort
    Cognitive Level: Application

21. **ANSWER: 3.**
    Rationales:
    1. This assessment provides valuable information whether the patient has a fluid volume excess (FVE) or fluid volume deficit (FVD). Weight loss or gain is an objective measure of fluid loss or fluid gain. One liter of fluid is equal to 2.2 lb.
    2. Monitoring intake and output should be done for patients with a FVE or a FVD. The intake and output should be relatively balanced. If the intake is greater than the output the patient may develop FVE. If the output is greater than the intake the patient may develop FVD.
    3. A patient with FVE should be positioned with the head of the bed elevated. This minimizes the movement of fluid from the vascular system to the lungs, which is a low pressure system. A mid-Fowler position is not

necessary for patients with a diagnosis of FVD because this would place excess pressure on the sacral area, which should be avoided. The integrity of the skin is compromised in a person with dehydration, which increases the risk of pressure ulcers.

4. These results will reflect the physiological status of patients whether they are experiencing FVD or FVE.

Content Area: Fluids and Electrolytes
Integrated Processes: Nursing Process: Implementation
Client Need: Physiological Integrity; Physiological Adaptation
Cognitive Level: Analysis

22. ANSWER: 2.

Rationales:

1. Orthostatic hypotension is a side effect of diuretics, angiotensin-converting enzyme inhibitors, and angiotensin II receptor blockers, not digoxin.

2. Yellow vision around lights and diplopia are classic signs of digoxin toxicity. Hypokalemia caused by vomiting and diarrhea increases the risk of digoxin toxicity.

3. An increased pulse rate is associated with hypernatremia, not digoxin toxicity. Bradycardia, not tachycardia, is a nontherapeutic response to digoxin.

4. Muscle cramps are associated with hypocalcemia, not digoxin toxicity.

Content Area: Fluids and Electrolytes
Integrated Processes: Nursing Process: Evaluation
Client Need: Physiological Integrity; Pharmacological and Parenteral Therapies
Cognitive Level: Application

23. ANSWER: 4.

Rationales:

1. Although this should be done, it is not the priority. Because the patient is receiving a 1,000 mL bolus of IV fluid, the oral intake at this time is not as critical as the action in another option.

2. There is no indication to hold the patient's lunch.

3. Although a urine sample should be collected because it is ordered by the primary health-care provider, the nurse should collect the specimen and not expect an older adult with a history of fainting to collect the specimen independently.

4. Safely moving the patient out of bed to a chair is the priority. The patient who is dehydrated generally is hypovolemic, which can precipitate orthostatic hypotension. Having a patient sit for a minute after raising the head of the bed and then having the patient sit on the side of the bed with the legs resting on the floor (dangle) for a minute allows time for the blood pressure to equalize, which minimizes the risk of orthostatic hypotension and a fall.

Content Area: Fluids and Electrolytes
Integrated Processes: Nursing Process: Implementation
Client Need: Physiological Integrity; Physiological Adaptation
Cognitive Level: Analysis

24. ANSWER: 1.

Rationales:

1. Muscle weakness is a classic nontherapeutic response to a potassium-sparing diuretic that indicates hyperkalemia. The amount of potassium accumulating in the blood eventually causes hyperkalemia.

2. Hypoactive reflexes indicate hypercalcemia. Hypocalcemia, not hypercalcemia, is a nontherapeutic response to a potassium-sparing diuretic.

3. Respiratory depression indicates hypermagnesemia. Hypomagnesemia, not hypermagnesemia, is a nontherapeutic response to a potassium-sparing diuretic.

4. Dry sticky mucous membranes indicate hypernatremia, which is not a nontherapeutic response to a potassium-sparing diuretic.

TEST-TAKING TIP: Identify the word in the stem that indicates negative polarity. The word *nontherapeutic* in the stem indicates negative polarity. The question is asking, "What effect is not a therapeutic response to the drug."

Content Area: Fluids and Electrolytes
Integrated Processes: Nursing Process: Evaluation
Client Need: Physiological Integrity; Pharmacological and Parenteral Therapies
Cognitive Level: Application

25. ANSWER: 2.

Rationales:

1. Adventitious breath sounds, such as moist crackles, are associated with fluid volume excess (FVE), not fluid volume deficit (FVD).

2. Nonelastic skin turgor occurs with hypovolemia because fluid has moved from the interstitial spaces into the intravascular system; the pinch of skin does not return to its original position in less than 2 to 3 seconds.

3. Frothy sputum is associated with FVE, not FVD; the elevated blood pressure associated with hypervolemia can cause movement of fluid into the lung (pleural effusion), resulting in frothy sputum.

4. Weight loss, not weight gain, is associated with FVD. Every liter of fluid is equal to 2.2 lb.

Content Area: Fluids and Electrolytes
Integrated Processes: Nursing Process: Assessment
Client Need: Physiological Integrity; Basic Care and Comfort
Cognitive Level: Application

26. ANSWER: 4.

Rationales:

1. Distended neck veins are associated with hypervolemia, not hypovolemia. Flat neck veins are associated with hypovolemia due to the decrease in intravascular fluid volume.

2. Tachycardia (more than 100 beats/minute), not bradycardia (less than 60 beats/minute), is associated with hypovolemia. Heart rate increases to more quickly transport oxygen to body cells.

3. Dilute urine is associated with hypervolemia, not hypovolemia. With hypovolemia, urine is concentrated and amber in color as the body attempts to retain fluid.

4. A weak pulse is associated with hypovolemia because of the decrease in intravascular fluid volume; it is referred to as a weak, thready pulse.
TEST-TAKING TIP: Identify the options that are opposites. Options 1 and 4 are opposites. They are both related to the volume of fluid within a vein. A weak pulse occurs with hypovolemia, and distended neck veins occur with hypervolemia. Examine options 1 and 4 carefully.
Content Area: Fluids and Electrolytes
Integrated Processes: Nursing Process: Assessment
Client Need: Physiological Integrity; Basic Care and Comfort
Cognitive Level: Analysis

27. **ANSWER: 1, 2.**
Rationales:
1. Lubricating the lips of a patient is an independent nursing action because a nurse has a license to treat human responses. It does not require an order from a primary health-care provider.
2. Assessing skin turgor is an independent nursing action. It does not require an order from a primary health-care provider.
3. Discontinuing a drug is a dependent function of the nurse. It requires an order from a primary health-care provider.
4. This is a dependent function of the nurse. The nurse must have a diet order with no fluid restriction before encouraging an increase in oral fluid intake.
5. This is a dependent function of the nurse. Providing intravenous fluids requires an order from a primary health-care provider.
Content Area: Fluids and Electrolytes
Integrated Processes: Nursing Process: Implementation
Client Need: Physiological Integrity; Physiological Adaptation
Cognitive Level: Analysis

28. **ANSWER: 2.**
Rationales:
1. Although at first it may seem appropriate to divide fluid intake equally over the entire course of the day, it is inappropriate. Less fluid is needed at night when the patient generally is sleeping.
2. Fluids administered intravenously must be accounted for in a restricted fluid diet. Therefore, 200 mL should be subtracted from the 1,400 allocated for fluid intake before dividing the remaining fluid across 24 hours. Eight hundred mL allocated for the daylight hours with 300 mL for evenings and 100 mL for nights is an appropriate division of 1,200 mL of fluid over 24 hours. More fluid should be allocated in the daylight hours because the patient is awake.
3. This is too large an amount of fluid to be allocated to the daylight hours. One thousand mL of fluid during the day leaves only 200 mL to be divided between the evening and night hours, which is too small a volume for these time frames.
4. Oral fluid in the daylight hours of 1,300 mL, in addition to the 200 mL for the 4 intravenous piggybacks, total

1,500 mL in 24 hours; this exceeds the 1,400 mL of fluid restriction.
Content Area: Fluids and Electrolytes
Integrated Processes: Nursing Process: Planning
Client Need: Physiological Integrity; Pharmacological and Parenteral Therapies
Cognitive Level: Analysis

29. **ANSWER: 3.**
Rationales:
1. This is inappropriate for dehydration. Five percent dextrose in water is hypotonic and, when infused, pulls water from the intravascular compartment into the interstitial fluid compartment. This is used for hyperglycemia.
2. This is inappropriate for dehydration. 0.45% sodium chloride is hypotonic and, when infused, pulls water from the intravascular compartment into the interstitial fluid compartment. This is used for hyperglycemia.
3. This fluid commonly is ordered to treat dehydration. 0.9% sodium chloride is isotonic and remains in the blood stream (intravascular compartment) when infused.
4. This fluid is hypertonic and generally is used to stabilize blood pressure, increase urine output, and reduce edema, not to treat dehydration.
Content Area: Fluids and Electrolytes
Integrated Processes: Nursing Process: Planning
Client Need: Physiological Integrity; Pharmacological and Parenteral Therapies
Cognitive Level: Analysis

30. **ANSWER: 1, 2.**
Rationales:
1. One slice (1 oz) of processed cheese has 380 to 400 mg of sodium and should be avoided when receiving a 2-g sodium diet.
2. One cup of canned soup on average contains 900 to 1,000 mg of sodium and should be avoided when receiving a 2-g sodium diet.
3. One tomato contains approximately 10 mg of sodium.
4. One banana has 1 mg of sodium.
5. One large egg contains 69 mg of sodium.
TEST-TAKING TIP: Identify the word in the stem that indicates negative polarity. The word *avoid* in the stem indicates negative polarity. The question is asking "What food should the patient *not eat* when receiving a 2-g sodium diet?"
Content Area: Fluids and Electrolytes
Integrated Processes: Teaching/Learning; Nursing Process: Implementation
Client Need: Physiological Integrity; Basic Care and Comfort
Cognitive Level: Application

31. **ANSWER: 1.**
Rationales:
1. Breathing techniques help to rebalance the oxygen and carbon dioxide levels in the blood. Breathing techniques involve slowing the rate of respirations. For example, inhale slowly using abdominal breathing for 5 seconds, hold the breath for 2 seconds and then exhale

slowly over 5 seconds, repeat for 2 cycles and then breathe regularly for 5 cycles and then repeat. This engages the patient in focusing on the breathing and relaxing.

2. Breathing into a paper bag is controversial and should be avoided. While it may not hurt a person who is hyperventilating due to a panic attack, it has not proven to be that beneficial. However, if the hyperventilation is due to an underlying medical problem, such as asthma or cardiac ischemia, breathing into a paper bag can make the condition worse and may even be fatal.

3. Telling the patient to remain calm in the mists of an episode of hyperventilation is inappropriate. This is not patient centered.

4. Although the high-Fowler position may be comfortable for a patient experiencing hyperventilation, it generally is used to facilitate respiratory excursion when experiencing respiratory acidosis.

TEST-TAKING TIP: Identify the obscure clang association. The word *hyperventilating* in the stem and the word *breathing* in option 1 is an obscure clang association. Examine option 1 carefully. Identify the option that denies the patient's feelings and concerns. Option 3 denies the patient's feelings and concerns.
Content Area: Fluids and Electrolytes
Integrated Processes: Nursing Process: Implementation
Client Need: Physiological Integrity; Physiological Adaptation
Cognitive Level: Application

32. **ANSWER: 3.**
Rationales:
1. Peripheral edema is related to fluid volume excess (FVE), which is not the patient's problem.
2. Jugular vein distension indicates hypervolemia and FVE, which is not consistent with the vital signs identified in the stem.
3. **The cluster of data in the stem indicates that the patient is experiencing a fluid volume deficit. A red tongue with furrows supports the conclusion that the patient is dehydrated; fluid from the intracellular and interstitial compartments moves to the intravascular compartment in an attempt to maintain the circulating blood volume.**
4. The blood urea nitrogen will be increased, not decreased, with the patient's problem.
Content Area: Fluids and Electrolytes
Integrated Processes: Nursing Process: Assessment
Client Need: Physiological Integrity; Basic Care and Comfort
Cognitive Level: Analysis

33. **ANSWER: 2.**
Rationales:
1. Although this may be done eventually, it is not the priority at this time.
2. **The patient's clinical manifestations (e.g., anorexia, constipation, fatigue, weakness, confusion, and depressed deep tendon reflexes) are consistent with the signs and symptoms of hypercalcemia. Metastasis to the bone precipitates hypercalcemia. The demineralization of bone,** resulting in osteoporosis, causes achy bone pain. This patient is at high risk for pathologic fractures. Extreme caution should be used when moving the patient and the extremities should be supported above and below joints.
3. This is not necessary.
4. Although this may be done as part of the patient's assessment, it is not the priority at this time.
TEST-TAKING TIP: Identify the word in the stem that sets a priority. The word *most* in the stem sets a priority.
Content Area: Fluids and Electrolytes
Integrated Processes: Nursing Process: Implementation
Client Need: Safe and Effective Care Environment; Safety and Infection Control
Cognitive Level: Analysis

34. **ANSWER: 2.**
Rationales:
1. Diuretics cause diuresis of excess fluid in the body. Excess fluid in the body is not the cause of respiratory acidosis in a patient with asthma.
2. **Asthma causes airway obstruction due to inflammation of the respiratory passages. A bronchodilator offers some relief of the clinical manifestations of acute asthma by quickly dilating and opening respiratory passages. Improved breathing will bring more oxygen into the alveoli and subsequently the circulation resolving the respiratory acidosis.**
3. Administration of sodium chloride is associated with the treatment of metabolic alkalosis.
4. Administration of sodium bicarbonate is associated with the treatment of metabolic acidosis, not respiratory acidosis.
TEST-TAKING TIP: Identify the word in the stem that sets a priority. The word *most* in the stem sets a priority.
Content Area: Fluids and Electrolytes
Integrated Processes: Nursing Process: Planning
Client Need: Physiological Integrity; Pharmacological and Parenteral Therapies
Cognitive Level: Application

35. **ANSWER: 1.**
Rationales:
1. **Flexion of the wrist and hand when a blood pressure cuff is inflated above the patient's systolic level (Trousseau's sign) indicates hypocalcemia. Cardiac irregularity is a serious consequence of a decrease in serum calcium (hypocalcemia).**
2. Nonelastic skin turgor is not associated with the problem related to the patient's manifestation in the illustration.
3. Sticky mucous membranes are associated with an increase in serum sodium (hypernatremia). The clinical manifestation reflected in the illustration is not related to hyponatremia.
4. Deep tendon reflexes increase, not decrease, with the patient's physical problem. A decrease in deep tendon reflexes occurs with a decrease in serum potassium (hypokalemia) and with an increase in serum calcium (hypercalcemia).

Content Area: Fluids and Electrolytes
Integrated Processes: Nursing Process: Assessment
Client Need: Physiological Integrity; Physiological Adaptation
Cognitive Level: Analysis

36. ANSWER: 1.
Rationales:
1. A dysrhythmia is a serious nontherapeutic effect associated with hydrochlorothiazide therapy. It indicates a low-potassium level (hypokalemia).
2. An impaired airway is unrelated to hydrochlorothiazide therapy.
3. An elevated glucose level is unrelated to hydrochlorothiazide therapy.
4. A decreased, not increased, blood pressure is related to hypovolemia, which is a nontherapeutic response to diuretic therapy.
TEST-TAKING TIP: Identify the word in the stem that sets a priority. The word *most* in the stem sets a priority. Identify the word in the stem that indicates negative polarity. The word *nontherapeutic* in the stem indicates negative polarity.
Content Area: Fluids and Electrolytes
Integrated Processes: Nursing Process: Implementation
Client Need: Physiological Integrity; Pharmacological and Parenteral Therapies
Cognitive Level: Application

37. ANSWER: 4.
Rationales:
1. A basilica vein is a larger vein used for long-term therapy. Larger veins accommodate hypertonic, viscous, or irritating solutions because the infused solution is diluted by a greater volume of blood than in smaller veins. Also, larger veins can accommodate a larger volume of fluid and at a faster rate than fluid administered via a small vein.
2. A cephalic vein is a large vein used for long-term therapy. Larger veins accommodate hypertonic, viscous, or irritating solutions because the infused solution is diluted by a greater volume of blood than in smaller veins. Also, larger veins can accommodate a larger volume of fluid and at a faster rate than fluid administered via a small vein.
3. A subclavian vein is a large vein used for long-term therapy. Larger veins accommodate hypertonic, viscous, or irritating solutions because the infused solution is diluted by a greater volume of blood than in smaller veins. Also, larger veins can accommodate a larger volume of fluid and at a faster rate than fluid administered via a small vein.
4. A metacarpal vein is a small vein that can be used for short-term intravenous therapy.
Content Area: Fluids and Electrolytes
Integrated Processes: Nursing Process: Planning
Client Need: Physiological Integrity; Pharmacological and Parenteral Therapies
Cognitive Level: Application

38. ANSWER: 1, 2, 3.
Rationales:
1. One baked potato with the skin contains approximately 845 mg of potassium, which, if ingested, can replace potassium lost because of the diuretic.
2. One cup of skim milk contains approximately 400 mg of potassium, which, if ingested, can replace potassium lost because of the diuretic.
3. Eight ounces of nonfat yogurt contains approximately 580 mg of potassium, which, if ingested, can replace potassium lost because of the diuretic.
4. One cup of cranberry juice contains approximately 60 mg of potassium and is not a good source of potassium in the diet.
5. One tablespoon of salad dressing contains 2 to 20 mg of potassium and is not a generous source of potassium in the diet.
Content Area: Fluids and Electrolytes
Integrated Processes: Teaching/Learning; Nursing Process: Planning
Client Need: Physiological Integrity; Pharmacological and Parenteral Therapies
Cognitive Level: Application

39. ANSWER: 1.
Rationales:
1. This is essential to prevent the introduction of pathogens into an intravenous line.
2. Priming the tubing of the intravenous piggyback set prevents air from entering the primary intravenous line.
3. Although this may be done, it alerts the nurse of an obstruction, not the presence of infection.
4. Sterile gloves are not necessary to maintain sterility of equipment when preparing and attaching an IVPB to a primary intravenous infusion line. If there is a risk of coming into contact with a patient's blood or body fluids, the nurse should wear clean gloves.
TEST-TAKING TIP: Identify the word in the stem that sets a priority. The word *most* in the stem sets a priority. Identify the clang associations. The words *intravenous piggyback* in the stem and in options 1 and option 2 are clang associations. Examine options 1 and 2 carefully.
Content Area: Fluids and Electrolytes
Integrated Processes: Nursing Process: Implementation
Client Need: Physiological Integrity; Reduction of Risk Potential
Cognitive Level: Application

40. ANSWER: 4.
Rationales:
1. A serum potassium level of 3.2 mEq/L indicates hypokalemia.
2. A serum potassium level of 5.6 mEq/L indicates hyperkalemia.
3. A serum sodium level of 128 mEq/L indicates hyponatremia.
4. A serum sodium level of 158 mEq/L is above the expected range of 136 to 148 mEq/L, indicating hypernatremia.
Content Area: Fluids and Electrolytes
Integrated Processes: Nursing Process: Assessment
Client Need: Physiological Integrity; Reduction of Risk Potential
Cognitive Level: Application

Gastrointestinal System

Chapter 22

KEY TERMS

Anabolism—Synthesis of larger compounds from smaller compounds.

Bolus—Rounded mass of food and saliva.

Catabolism—The breakdown of complex compounds into simple compounds, releasing energy for other body processes.

Colostomy—Formation of an opening (stoma) between the colon and the surface of the abdomen to permit feces to exit the body.

Constipation—Intestinal hypomotility that precipitates two or less stools a week and hard, dry feces.

Diarrhea—Intestinal hypermotility that precipitates passage of fluid and unformed stool three or more times a day.

Enema—Instillation of solution into the intestine via the anus and rectum.

Fecal impaction—Hard, dry stool firmly wedged in the rectal vault that cannot be passed.

Fecal incontinence—Involuntary passage of feces and flatus from the anus.

Flatulence—Excessive gas in the stomach and intestines that leads to distention of these organs precipitating physical discomfort.

Flatus—Gas in the stomach and intestines as a natural by-product of digestion.

Gluconeogenesis—The conversion of protein or fat into glucose by the liver.

Glycogenolysis—The breakdown of glycogen from the liver when the blood glucose decreases, releasing glucose.

Glycogenesis—The conversion of excess glucose to glycogen, which is stored in the liver.

Hemorrhoid—Engorged, painful, bleeding vein in the lining of the rectum or anus.

Hydrolysis—Splitting of a compound into small segments in preparation for GI absorption and metabolism.

Ileostomy—Formation of an opening (stoma) between the ileum and the surface of the abdomen to permit feces to exit the body.

Mastication—Process of chewing.

Obstipation—Intractable constipation.

Perceived constipation—Self-diagnosed constipation.

I. Structures and Functions of the Gastrointestinal (GI) System

The structures and functions of the GI system are associated with the ingestion of food and elimination of the waste products of digestion in the form of feces. Many factors can affect a person's bowel elimination, including developmental level, emotional and cultural factors, dietary and fluid intake, activity, medications, perioperative issues, and medical problems. Nurses must understand the basic anatomy and physiology of the GI system and the issues that impact a patient's bowel elimination to better meet patients' nursing needs.

A. Structures of the GI System (Fig. 22.1)
1. Mouth.
   a. Includes lips, cheeks, hard and soft palates, gums, tongue, tonsils, and salivary glands.
   b. Structures move in concert to chew food (**mastication**), mix food with saliva to form a rounded mass of food (**bolus**), and move the bolus toward the posterior pharynx where it is swallowed.

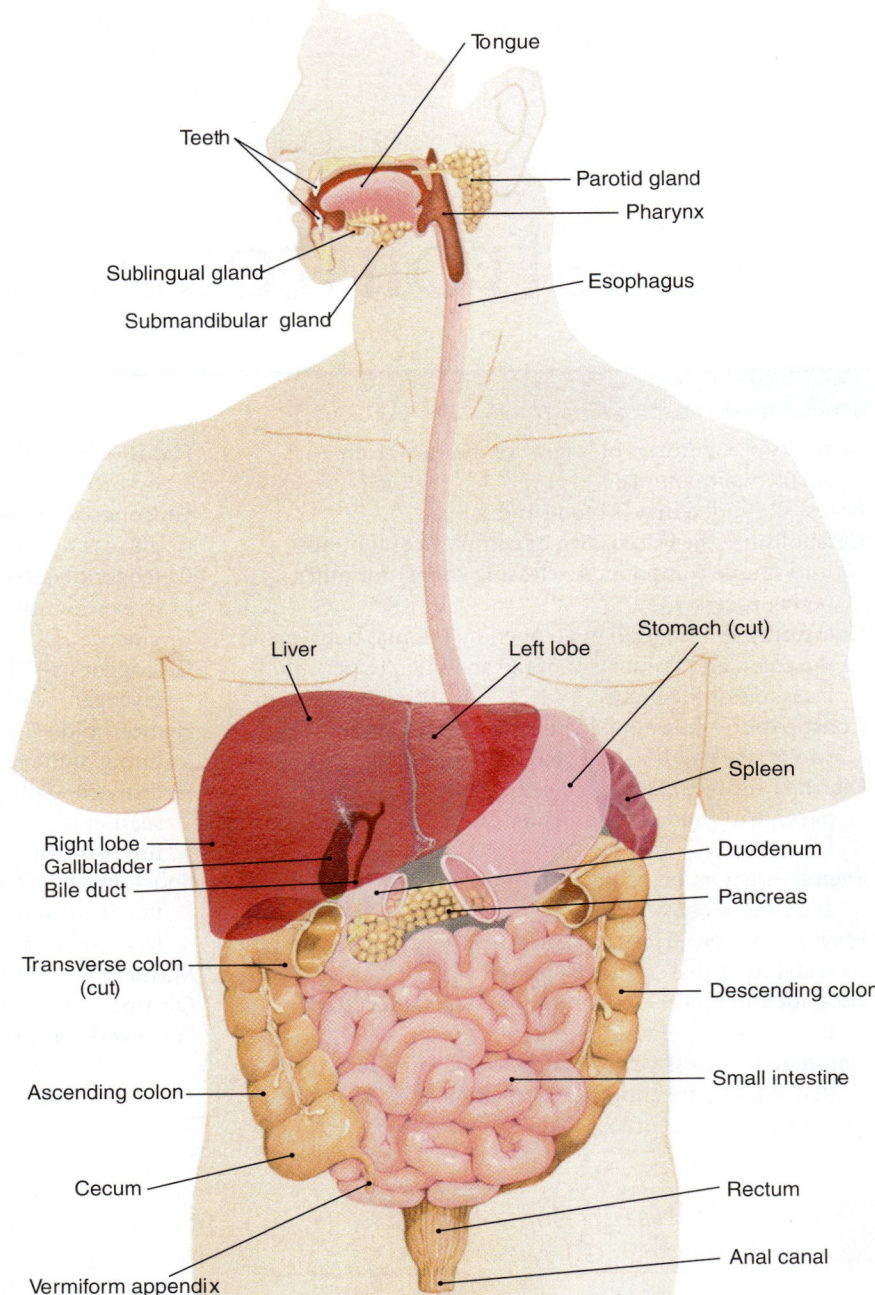

Fig 22.1 Structures of the gastrointestinal system. The digestive organs shown in anterior view of the trunk and left-lateral view of the head. (The spleen is not a digestive organ but is included to show its location relative to the stomach, pancreas, and colon.) (From Scanlon [2011]. *Essentials of anatomy and physiology,* 6th ed. Philadelphia: F. A. Davis, with permission.)

2. Esophagus.
   a. Collapsible muscular tube that extends from the posterior pharynx, through an opening in the diaphragm, to the stomach.
   b. Secretes mucus and facilitates movement of food from the mouth to the stomach.
3. Stomach.
   a. Elongated C-shaped pouch mainly in the epigastric area of the abdomen. The cardiac sphincter is at the connection between the esophagus and the upper portion of the stomach; the pyloric sphincter is at the connection between the duodenum and the lower portion of the stomach.
   b. Stores and liquefies food.
   c. Secretes gastric juices (e.g., gastrin, pepsin, hydrochloric acid, intrinsic factor, and mucin).

4. Small intestine.
   a. Tubular structure approximately 1 inch in diameter and 28 feet long that progresses from the duodenum, to the jejunum, to the ileum.
   b. Involved with digestion and absorption of nutrients.
   c. Secretes the enzymes sucrose, lactase, and maltase.
   d. Secretes cholecystokinin, which stimulates the gallbladder to release bile.
   e. Receives secretions from the liver, gallbladder, and pancreas.
5. Large intestine.
   a. Tubular structure approximately 2.5 inches in diameter and 5.5 feet long that progresses from the cecum, to the ascending colon, transverse colon, descending colon, sigmoid colon, rectum, and anus.
   b. Absorbs water and sodium ions and temporarily stores feces.
   c. Produces mixing movements and wave-like movements (**peristalsis**) that create a fecal mass, move waste product toward the anus, and promote defecation.
6. Vermiform appendix.
   a. Blind-end small tubular structure at the cecum beyond the ileocecal valve.
   b. Part of the immune system.
7. Liver.
   a. Large structure located in the upper right quadrant of the abdomen that consists of thousands of lobules that drain bile through the hepatic duct.
   b. Involved in protein, carbohydrate, and fat metabolism; secretes bile, which emulsifies fats, acts as a vehicle for excretion of bile pigments and cholesterol, and facilitates the absorption of the fat-soluble vitamins A, D, E, and K.
8. Gallbladder.
   a. Small sac that lies underneath the liver; the cystic duct exists the gallbladder and connects with the hepatic duct; the cystic and hepatic ducts unite and form the common bile duct, which drains bile through the sphincter of Oddi into the duodenum.
   b. Concentrates and stores bile.
9. Pancreas.
   a. Comma-shaped structure that extends from the duodenal curve to the spleen in the epigastric and upper left areas of the abdomen.
   b. Secretes the enzymes trypsin, lipase, and amylase, which are transported to the duodenum via the pancreatic duct.
   c. Contains Islets of Langerhans.
      (1) Alpha cells secrete the hormone glucagon, which promotes an increase in the amount of blood glucose.

(2) Beta cells secrete insulin, which decreases the amount of blood glucose and facilitates the metabolism of carbohydrates, proteins, and fats.

B. Functions of the GI System
1. **Digestion.**
   a. Mechanical digestion: Changes the consistency of food by mastication and mixing it with saliva and moves it through the GI system by swallowing and peristalsis.
   b. Chemical digestion: Splits compounds into small segments (e.g., hydroxyl group into one fragment and the hydrogen atom into another) in preparation for absorption and metabolism (**hydrolysis**). (See the section "Essential Nutrients" in Chapter 18, "Nutrition," for a discussion of the digestion of carbohydrates, proteins, and fats, page 515.)
2. **Absorption.**
   a. Small molecules that result from hydrolysis move against a concentration gradient (active transport) through the intestinal mucosa into the circulatory system.
   b. Most nutrients are absorbed in the small intestine; most water is absorbed in the large intestine.
3. **Metabolism.**
   a. Includes all the chemical reactions involved in energy production and expenditure.
      (1) **Anabolism:** Synthesis of larger compounds from smaller compounds.
      (2) **Catabolism:** Complex compounds are broken down into simple compounds releasing energy for further body processes (e.g., muscle contraction, heat production).
   b. Metabolism requires energy.
      (1) Carbohydrates are the preferred source of fuel for energy; cells catabolize glucose first, sparing proteins and fats; most cells catabolize fats next, sparing protein (amino acids).
      (2) Excess glucose is converted to glycogen and stored in the liver (**glycogenesis**).
      (3) The liver converts protein or fat into glucose (**gluconeogenesis**).
      (4) When blood glucose decreases, gluconeogenesis increases and glycogen from the liver breaks down releasing glucose (**glycogenolysis**).

C. Factors Affecting Bowel Elimination
1. Developmental level.
   a. Toddlers: Develop intestinal control at about 2 to 3 years of age.
   b. Pregnant women: Enlarged uterus imposes on intestinal structures, resulting in decreased peristalsis.
   c. Older adults: Experience decreased peristalsis.

2. Emotional and cultural factors.
   a. Lack of privacy: Some cultures are open and others prefer privacy when attending to bodily functions.
   b. Inadequate amount of time to defecate.
   c. Embarrassment: Fecal elimination is often associated with sights and odors that may be offensive to others and make the patient self-conscious.
3. Nutrition.
   a. Lack of fiber and excessive milk: Results in a decrease in peristalsis.
   b. Irregular eating patterns: Can interfere with regularity of bowel movements or decrease peristalsis.
   c. Caffeine and fiber promote peristalsis.
4. Fluid intake.
   a. Need 6 to 8 glasses of water daily.
   b. Decreased fluid intake causes constipation.
5. Activity.
   a. Activity increases muscle tone and stimulates peristalsis.
   b. Inactivity contributes to decreased muscle tone and constipation.
6. Medications.
   a. Antibiotics destroy normal intestinal flora.
   b. Antacids often slow peristalsis.
   c. Iron causes constipation.
   d. Analgesics, opioids, and antimotility drugs slow peristalsis.
   e. Laxatives and cathartics increase peristalsis.
7. Perioperative issues: Anesthesia and handling of the bowel during surgery may slow motility and cause cessation of peristalsis (**adynamic ileus, postoperative ileus, paralytic ileus**).
8. Medical problems: Common problems include GI infections, food allergies, cancer, diverticulosis and diverticulitis, irritable bowel syndrome, and malabsorption syndromes.

II. Nursing Assessment of the GI System

The first step of the nursing process is assessment. When collecting information relative to a patient's GI status, the nurse obtains a patient history, performs a physical assessment and assesses the characteristics of stool. This section provides guidelines to facilitate a comprehensive assessment of a patient's GI status.

A. Obtain a Patient History
1. Ask about usual elimination pattern and any changes in pattern or bowel habits.
2. Determine the patient's dietary habits, use of supplements, change in appetite, and daily fluid intake.
3. Ask about level of activity, mobility, and exercise.
4. Ask about ability to self-toilet.
5. Determine whether the patient has been experiencing any pain or discomfort.
6. Ask about past and present illnesses, injury, and surgery that might affect GI function.
7. Ask whether the patient is using any medications that can affect GI function, such as antibiotics, iron, laxatives, cathartics, antacids, and analgesics.
8. Assess the patient's emotional status and current stressors.
9. Take a social history (e.g., number of people using one bathroom, cultural background).

B. Perform a Physical Assessment
1. Inspect the contour, shape, and symmetry of the abdomen. (See the section "Inspect the Abdomen" in Chapter 11, "Physical Assessment," page 271.)
2. Inspect the anus and perianal area.
3. Auscultate bowel sounds in all four quadrants, listening for 1 minute in each quadrant; usual is 3 to 35 gurgles per minute. (See the section "Auscultate the Abdomen" in Chapter 11, "Physical Assessment," page 272.)
   a. Hyperactive: High pitched and more than 35 gurgles per minute.
   b. Hypoactive: Low pitched, quiet, infrequent, or absent gurgles.
4. Percuss the abdomen to detect dullness, indicating fluid, gas, or a mass in the abdomen. (See the section "Percuss the Abdomen" in Chapter 11, "Physical Assessment," page 272.)
5. Palpate the abdomen, which should be soft, firm, and tender. (See the section "Palpate the Abdomen" in Chapter 11, "Physical Assessment," page 273.)

C. Assess Characteristics of Stool
1. Characteristics of stool are influenced by factors such as dietary and fluid intake, exercise, medications, and disease processes.
2. Characteristics of stool include color, consistency, quantity, shape, odor, and constituents (Table 22.1).

III. GI System Diagnostic Tests and Related Nursing Care

Diagnostic tests may be ordered by the primary health-care provider to provide information regarding a patient's GI functioning. The tests presented mainly are ordered to support a medical diagnosis. Nurses must understand these tests because some of them require the nurse to collect a specimen, others require nursing interventions before and after the test, and all of them require patient teaching.

A. Stool Examination
1. **Commonalities of nursing care for obtaining stool specimens.**
   a. Perform hand hygiene, and wear clean gloves.
   b. Instruct the patient to defecate in a clean, dry bedpan or container under the toilet seat.

Table 22.1 Characteristics of Normal and Abnormal Stool	
Expected Features	**Abnormal Features and Precipitating Factors**
Color • Adult: Brown. • Infant: Yellow.	• Clay colored: Lack of bile due to biliary obstruction; barium used for diagnostic tests. • White: Undigested fat (**steatorrhea**); barium used for intestinal diagnostic tests. • Red: Lower GI bleeding; foods such as beets. • Black, tarry: Digested blood from upper GI tract; stool darkened by blood pigments (**melena**). • Pale brown: Malabsorption; diet high in milk or low in meat. • Green: Intestinal infection, such as *C. difficile*.
Consistency • Formed, soft, moist, liquid.	• Unformed, liquid: Increased intestinal motility (See "Diarrhea," page 691). • Hard, dry: Decreased intestinal motility (See "Constipation," page 692).
Quantity • 100 to 400 g produced daily, evacuated every 1 to 3 days. • Amount depends on intake.	• Excessive: Excessive intake of high-fiber foods, diarrhea. • Absent or small amount: Inadequate intake of food, especially foods high in fiber; GI obstruction; constipation.
Shape • Tubular, about 1 inch in diameter.	• Pencil shaped: Inflamed mucosa. • Ribbon shaped: Intestinal obstruction.
Odor • Aromatic; depends on foods eaten and patient's intestinal flora.	• Pungent: Intestinal infection; blood in stool.
Constituents • Undigested roughage, epithelial cells, protein, bile pigments, inorganic matter, dead bacteria.	• Mucus: Intestinal inflammation. • Pus: Bacterial infection. • Blood (GI bleeding): Black—upper GI bleeding; red—lower GI bleeding. • Fat in large amounts: Malabsorption syndrome, enteritis, pancreatic disease.

c. Use medical aseptic technique to collect 1 inch of formed stool or 15 to 30 mL of liquid stool.

d. Ensure that the specimen is not contaminated with urine, water, or toilet paper.

e. Place the labeled container with the specimen into a biohazard, fluid-impervious bag; include appropriate label and laboratory forms.

f. Use a preservative if required.

g. Note on the label if the patient is menstruating.

h. Send the specimen to the laboratory promptly because bacteriological changes may alter test results if testing is delayed.

2. **Gross and microscopic stool examination in the laboratory.**

a. Gross examination: Assesses stool for consistency, color, presence of blood, mucus, excess fat, and pus.

b. Microscopic examination: Identifies constituents, such as WBCs, unabsorbed fat, and parasites.

3. **Culture and sensitivity.**

a. Culture assesses stool for presence of pathogens.

b. Sensitivity identifies the most effective antibiotics.

c. Obtain a specimen using sterile technique.

d. Place the specimen in a sterile container.

4. **Occult blood (guaiac, Hemoccult).**

a. Assesses stool for microscopic amounts of blood in feces.

b. Teach the patient to avoid red meat, poultry, fish, vitamin C, aspirin, and nonsteroidal anti-inflammatory drugs before the test because these substances can cause false-positive results.

c. Ensure that the specimen is not contaminated with menstrual blood.

d. Use a commercial kit.

(1) Apply a thin smear of stool on the designated window of the test packet.

(2) Apply a reagent on the area following the specific times indicated by the manufacturer.

(3) Note that a blue color in response to the reagent indicates the presence of occult blood.

(4) Repeat the test for three consecutive defecations of stool.

5. **Ova and parasites.**

a. Assessment via a stool specimen.

(1) Assesses stool for the presence of parasites and their eggs.

(2) Collect several specimens from various sections of the stool.

(3) Transport the specimen to the laboratory while still warm to maintain viability of the parasites and eggs.

b. Assessment via tape test for intestinal parasites.

(1) Assesses for pinworm eggs from around the anus.

(2) Wear clean gloves to protect self from the patient's body fluids.

(3) Collect the specimen in the morning as soon as the patient awakens.

(4) Spread the buttocks, press clear cellophane tape against the skin surrounding the anal opening, remove tape immediately, and place it on a slide.

DID YOU KNOW?

Pinworms migrate at night from the rectum to the perianal area to deposit eggs and then return to the rectum before the morning. This is the reason why test tape specimens should be performed in the morning before the patient has a bowel movement or performs perineal hygiene.

B. Barium Studies

1. **Commonalities of nursing care for patients having barium studies.**

   a. Teach the patient about the procedure and secure consent for the procedure.

   b. Encourage increased fluid intake for 24 hours after the procedure to facilitate defecation of barium.

   c. Administer laxatives or cathartics as prescribed to facilitate expulsion of the barium.

2. **Upper GI series.**

   a. Radiologic examination in which the patient drinks contrast medium and films are taken every 20 minutes until the medium reaches the terminal ileum.

   b. Teach about and maintain dietary restrictions, such as providing a low-residue diet for 48 hours before the test and withholding of food for 8 hours and fluid for 4 hours before the test.

   c. Teach about or implement bowel prep, such as tap water enema and/or cathartic the evening before the test.

   d. Instruct the patient to drink barium.

   e. Monitor stool, which will be chalky white for 72 hours or until the barium is completely evacuated.

3. **Lower GI series (barium enema).**

   a. Fluoroscopic radiologic examination of the colon after a contrast medium is instilled rectally.

   b. Teach about and maintain dietary restrictions, such as providing a clear liquid diet for 24 hours before the test and maintaining nothing-by-mouth (NPO) status for 8 hours before the test.

   c. Teach about and/or implement bowel prep, such as a laxative, enema, or suppository, the evening before and/or the morning of the test.

   d. Instill barium through the tube inserted into the rectum.

   e. Position the patient on left side, back, and then prone during the test; fluoroscope follows the progress of the barium and x-rays are taken.

f. Monitor stool, which will be chalky white for 24 to 48 hours or until the barium is completely evacuated.

C. Endoscopy

1. **Commonalities of nursing care for an endoscopy.**

   a. Teach the patient about the procedure, and secure consent for the procedure.

   b. Instruct the patient to arrange transportation home after the procedure and to avoid driving for 24 hours because conscious sedation is used.

   c. Ensure that a crash cart is readily available.

   d. Administer prescribed medications, such as a sedative or anxiolytic, before the procedure.

   e. Monitor the patient's airway, vital signs, and pulse oximetry every 15 minutes during and after the procedure when the patient is receiving conscious sedation and opioids.

2. **Upper GI endoscopy (esophagogastroduodenoscopy).**

   a. Insertion of a flexible endoscope through the mouth to visualize the mucous membrane lining of the esophagus, stomach, and duodenum.

   b. Explain that a scope will be inserted through the mouth into the esophagus, stomach, and duodenum and that material will be suctioned, polyps excised, and a biopsy taken.

   c. Withhold food and fluids for 6 to 8 hours before the procedure or as ordered.

   d. Remove any dental appliances and eyewear.

   e. Explain that the patient may experience mild bloating, belching, or flatulence after the procedure.

   f. Teach that drinking and eating is permitted after the gag reflex and ability to swallow return.

   g. Teach the patient to notify the primary health-care provider immediately if any of the following occur: Difficulty swallowing; epigastric, substernal, or shoulder pain; black, tarry stools; vomiting of blood; or fever.

3. **Colonoscopy.**

   a. Insertion of a flexible endoscope through the anus to visualize the entire colon.

   b. Teach the patient about and implement bowel prep, such as medications, cathartics, and enemas the day before and morning of the procedure to cleanse the bowel.

   c. Teach about or maintain a clear liquid diet for 48 hours before and NPO after midnight the night before the procedure.

   d. Explain that the scope will be inserted through the anus into the colon and that polyps may be excised, feces suctioned, and a biopsy taken.

e. Explain to the patient that increased flatus may occur after the test because air is inflated into the bowel during the test to promote visualization.

f. Instruct the patient to notify the primary health-care provider if abdominal pain, fever, chills, mucopurulent discharge, or rectal bleeding occur after the test because these signs may indicate bowel perforation, hemorrhage, or infection.

g. Instruct the patient to avoid heavy lifting for a week and high-fiber foods for 48 hours if a polyp was excised or biopsy was taken during the procedure.

4. **Sigmoidoscopy.**

a. Insertion of a tubular speculum for examination of the sigmoid colon and rectum.

b. Teach the patient about and maintain a clear liquid or light diet the day before the test.

c. Position the patient in the knee chest position or on the left side.

d. Encourage the patient to take deep breaths to reduce discomfort and relax muscles.

e. Sit the patient up slowly to avoid hypotension after the procedure.

D. X-ray

1. Radiographic views of the abdomen, such as abdominal flat plate, anterior, and posterior views; can identify impaction or distended bowel.

2. Assist with positioning the patient for the x-ray.

3. Assist the patient to a comfortable position after the x-ray.

IV. Common Human Responses Related to the GI System and Nursing Care

Diarrhea, constipation, fecal incontinence, hemorrhoids, and flatulence are common human responses related to the GI system. It is essential that the nurse understand the clinical manifestations, precipitating factors, and nursing care associated with each human response to better meet patients' needs associated with each of these responses.

A. Diarrhea

1. Description.

a. Intestinal hypermotility that precipitates passage of fluid and unformed stool.

b. Frequency of stool occurs three or more times a day.

2. Clinical manifestations.

a. Frequent loose stools.

b. Abdominal cramps, pain, or urgency.

c. Abdominal distention.

d. Hyperactive bowel sounds or flatus.

e. Anorexia, nausea, and vomiting.

f. Blood in the stool (frank, occult).

g. Clinical manifestations of fluid volume deficit, such as weight loss; thready pulse; hypotension; decreased tissue turgor; furrows of the tongue; flushed, dry skin and mucous membranes; sunken eyeballs; decreased urine output; atonic muscles; and mental confusion.

h. Electrolyte imbalances, such as hyponatremia and hypokalemia.

i. Stool possibly positive for causative pathogen or helminthic.

j. With *Clostridium difficile,* characteristic odor and green-colored stool.

3. Precipitating factors.

a. Viral, bacterial, or parasitic gastroenteritis.

b. Spicy or greasy food.

c. Raw seafood.

d. Contaminated food and water.

e. Excessive dietary fiber.

f. Anxiety or other emotional disturbance.

g. Drug side effects: Antibiotics suppress normal GI flora; antineoplastics and laxatives irritate the mucous membranes of the intestines increasing peristalsis.

h. Enteral nutrition (nasogastric or gastrostomy); hypertonic formula or too-rapid administration precipitates peristalsis. (For additional information about enteral nutrition, see the section "Enteral Nutrition" in Chapter 18, page 543.)

i. Health problems, such as lactose intolerance, irritable bowel syndrome, malabsorption syndrome, and celiac disease.

j. Ingestion of heavy metals, such as lead or mercury.

k. Inflammatory bowel diseases, such as ulcerative colitis or Crohn's disease.

4. Nursing care for patients who have diarrhea.

a. Assess the patient.

(1) Stool frequency, amount, and characteristics, such as consistency, color, and odor.

(2) Signs and symptoms of FVD and electrolyte imbalances.

(3) Recent foreign travel and dietary intake.

b. Obtain a stool specimen (e.g., culture and sensitivity, ova and parasite).

🛑 c. Maintain standard precautions, such as frequent hand hygiene and gloves for perineal care, when assisting with fecal elimination. Institute contact precautions if diarrhea is caused by infection or infestation; wear a gown and gloves.

d. Assist with elimination, such as providing privacy and transferring the patient to the toilet, commode, or bed pan; use air fresheners discretely.

e. Provide perineal care, such as assessing skin for breakdown and using a protective skin barrier or emollient.

f. Maintain the prescribed diet, such as NPO, clear liquid, full liquid, bland, low fiber, or dairy- or gluten-free.

g. Increase oral fluid intake gradually because a large amount can precipitate peristalsis.

h. Administer prescribed medications, such as antibiotics, antidiarrheals, antihelminthics, enteric bacterial replacements, and electrolytes.

i. Administer ordered IV fluids.

j. Provide health teaching.

(1) Discourage intake of spicy and fatty foods; caffeine; and high-fiber foods, such as whole grains, raw fruits and vegetables, figs, and prunes.

(2) Discourage intake of hot and cold fluids because they stimulate peristalsis.

(3) Encourage foods high in sodium, such as tomatoes and bullion, and potassium, such as bananas, oranges, apricots, and potatoes.

(4) Teach correct handling and refrigeration of food.

(a) Clean surfaces with hot water and soap after preparing raw chicken.

(b) Provide adequate refrigeration of perishable foods, such as milk and dairy products and foods containing mayonnaise.

k. Document assessments, interventions, and patient responses.

B. Constipation

1. Description.

a. **Constipation:** Intestinal hypomotility that precipitates two or less stools a week and hard, dry feces.

b. **Obstipation:** Intractable constipation.

c. **Perceived constipation:** Self-diagnosed constipation.

d. **Fecal impaction:** Hard, dry stool firmly wedged in the rectal vault that cannot be passed.

2. Clinical manifestations.

a. Hypoactive bowel sounds.

b. Distended abdomen.

c. Rectal pressure or back pain.

d. Straining at stool.

e. Anorexia.

f. Blood-streaked stool.

g. Possible fluid and electrolyte imbalances.

h. For fecal impaction: Oozing diarrhea around an impaction; fecal mass confirmed by digital examination.

3. Precipitating factors.

a. Elimination habits.

(1) Laxative or enema abuse.

(2) Urge ignored because of inaccessible bathroom or anticipation of pain because of hemorrhoids, rectal or anal fissures, or other rectal or anal problems.

b. Inadequate fluid intake (less than 2 L/day).

c. Inadequate intake of fiber (e.g., whole grains, fruits, vegetables) in diet.

d. Side effects of opioids, iron, or anesthesia.

e. Developmental level.

(1) Child: Stool withholding behavior.

(2) Pregnant woman: Uterine compression of intestine, decreasing peristalsis.

(3) Older adult: Decreased peristalsis.

f. Inadequate physical activity.

g. Presence of mechanical obstruction or anal lesion.

h. Weak abdominal muscles; pelvic floor dysfunction or damage.

i. Anxiety or other emotional disturbance.

j. Cultural and family health beliefs, such as daily use of a laxative or cathartic.

4. Nursing care for patients who have constipation.

a. Assess stool for frequency, amount, color (e.g., greenish black due to iron intake), and shape (e.g., ribbon shape due to obstruction, pencil shape due to mucosal inflammation).

b. Maintain standard precautions, such as performing frequent hand hygiene and wearing gloves when providing perineal care and assisting with fecal elimination.

c. Assist with elimination, such as providing privacy and encouraging the patient to sit in an upright position, lean forward at the hips, apply manual pressure over the abdomen, and bear down while exhaling to prevent straining.

🛑 d. Encourage toileting after meals or offer a warm drink before a patient's attempt to defecate to take advantage of the gastrocolic reflex. The gastrocolic reflex is the initiation of peristaltic waves when food enters the stomach, particularly when the stomach is empty.

e. Administer prescribed medications, such as laxatives and cathartics.

f. Administer ordered enemas, such as oil retention, small volume hypertonic solution, tap water or soapsuds.

g. Provide or assist with manual (digital) removal of feces.

h. Provide health teaching.

(1) Encourage intake of high-fiber foods, such as whole grains, fruits, and vegetables.

(2) Discourage intake of binding foods, such as bananas and rice.

(3) Encourage increased fluid intake, activity, and exercise.

(4) Encourage consistent bowel habits, and teach the patient to respond to the urge to defecate.

i. Provide perioperative nursing care if surgery is necessary to remove a fecal impaction.

j. Document assessments, interventions, and patient responses.

C. Fecal Incontinence

1. Description.
   a. Involuntary passage of feces and flatus from the anus.
   b. Extent of incontinence ranges from partial (e.g., occasional episodes of seepage of stool) to total (e.g., complete loss of control of bowel movements) loss of control of the passage of stool.

2. Clinical manifestations.
   a. Inability to control exit of feces from the body.
   b. Embarrassment due to soiling.

3. Precipitating factors.
   a. Inability to recognize the urge to defecate or the presence of rectal fullness due to altered thought processes.
   b. Impaired anal sphincter control or its nerve supply (e.g., brain attack and spinal cord damage).
   c. Decreased muscle tone.
   d. Diarrhea.

4. Nursing care for patients who have fecal incontinence.

   🛑 a. Maintain a nonjudgmental environment; understand that incontinence may be viewed by the patient as regression.

   b. Provide privacy and positive reinforcement.
   c. Provide prompt hygiene care.
   d. Use an incontinence device, such as Depends; avoid using the word "diaper," which is demeaning.
   e. Encourage attempts to defecate (e.g., in the morning, evening, and after meals to take advantage of the gastrocolic reflex).
   f. Implement and teach the patient about a bowel retraining program.
      (1) Follow the patient's usual pattern.
      (2) Follow the schedule exactly.
      (3) Increase fiber in the diet gradually.
      (4) Encourage the intake of 8 or more glasses of water daily.
      (5) Administer a prescribed suppository or cleansing enema to empty the bowel to help promote eventual regularity.

D. Hemorrhoids

1. Description.
   a. Engorged, painful, bleeding veins in the lining of the rectum and anus.
   b. Can be internal or external.

2. Clinical manifestations.
   a. Rectal pressure, burning, and pain.
   b. Frank red blood from the anus.

3. Precipitating factors.
   a. Constipation or straining on defecation.
   b. Situations that increase venous pressure, such as pregnancy, weightlifting, standing for long periods of time, heart failure, and chronic liver disease.

4. Nursing care for patients who have hemorrhoids.
   a. Assess the anal area for the extent of swelling.
   b. Assess levels of rectal pain.
   c. Provide meticulous perianal hygiene, especially after defecation.
   d. Administer prescribed medications, such as stool softeners, local anesthetics, and anal lubricants.
   e. Administer ordered thermal therapy to the perianal area, such as cold (e.g., cold packs) or heat (e.g., compresses, warm sitz baths).
   f. Provide health teaching.
      (1) Encourage the intake of high-fiber foods after acute episodes have subsided.
      (2) Encourage the intake of at least 2 L of fluid daily.
      (3) Teach the patient to avoid standing or sitting for long periods.
   g. Provide care related to band ligation, hemorrhoidectomy, sclerotherapy, cryosurgery, infrared photocoagulation, or laser surgery.

MAKING THE CONNECTION

Heat and Cold Therapy and the Length of Application

Heat or cold can be applied to areas of the body for 20 to 30 minutes every 2 to 6 hours to achieve a local effect. When heat is applied, the blood vessels dilate, bringing more plasma, oxygen-carrying red blood cells, white blood cells, and nutrients to the treated area. When cold is applied, vasoconstriction occurs, which decreases blood flow to the area, resulting in reduced edema, discomfort and pain, muscle spasm, and a numbing sensation. However, when heat or cold is applied longer than 30 minutes, a rebound phenomenon occurs, causing an opposite effect. When heat therapy is applied too long, vasoconstriction occurs for unknown reasons, which then prevents the dissipation of the applied heat and in turn may cause a burn or worsen the condition. When cold therapy is applied too long, vasoconstriction initially persists, denying cells of oxygen and nutrients; when the local temperature decreases below 60°F, vasodilation occurs as a protective mechanism. These responses can worsen the condition and cause tissue injury and even tissue necrosis. To prevent tissue injury, nurses must understand, as well as teach patients about, the rebound phenomenon related to heat and cold therapy.

E. Flatulence
1. Description.
   a. **Flatus:** Gas in the stomach and intestines as a natural by-product of digestion; expelled through the anus.
   b. **Flatulence:** Excessive gas in the stomach and intestines that leads to distention of these organs precipitating physical discomfort.
2. Clinical manifestations of flatulence.
   a. Hyperactive bowel sounds.
   b. Cramping and/or abdominal pain.
   c. Abdominal distention.
3. Precipitating factors.
   a. Absent or decreased GI motility due to such factors as inadequate fiber in the diet, immobility, anesthesia, and opioids.
   b. Gas-forming foods and fluids, such as beans, peas, cabbage, onions, cauliflower, highly spicy foods, milk and milk products, and carbonated beverages.
   c. Swallowing of air that accompanies the intake of food and fluid.
4. Nursing care for patients who have flatulence.
   a. Inspect the abdomen for abdominal distention
   b. Auscultate bowel sounds for hypoactivity or hyperactivity; be aware that the absence of bowel sounds may indicate cessation of peristalsis (such as from adynamic ileus, postoperative ileus or paralytic ileus).
   c. Encourage activity.
      (1) Encourage in-bed activity when on bed rest, such as turning from side to side.
      (2) Increase ambulation; progressive ambulation after surgery.
   d. Administer prescribed medications, such as antiflatulents or bulk cathartics.
   e. Insert a lubricated rectal tube as ordered (4 to 5 inches for 15 to 20 minutes every 3 to 4 hours).
   f. Administer a return-flow enema (Harris flush).
   g. Teach the patient to avoid gas-forming foods and fluids.

V. Enemas

An **enema** is the instillation of solution into the intestine via the rectum. The administration of an enema is a dependent function of the nurse that requires an order from a primary health-care provider. There are various types of enemas, each with its own distinct purpose because of the way in which it precipitates a response in the body. Commonalities of nursing care for patients receiving an enema are presented here as well as nursing care specific to each type of enema.

A. Commonalities of Nursing Care for Patients Receiving an Enema
1. Maintain standard precautions, such as performing hand hygiene and wearing gloves.
2. Explain the procedure to the patient.
3. Prepare the equipment.
   a. Fill the enema container with solution that is 105°F or obtain a prefilled hypertonic enema kit.
   b. Flush the tubing or nozzle to remove air.
   c. Lubricate the tip of the tube or nozzle with water-soluble jelly.
4. Provide privacy, such as by closing the door, pulling the curtain, draping the patient, and ensuring that the bathroom is accessible and reserved.
5. Place the patient in left-lateral or left Sims' position to allow the solution to flow by gravity along the natural curve of the sigmoid.
   a. For small volume enemas (e.g., hypertonic, oil retention): Insert the probe attached to the container its full length into the anus slowly (Fig. 22.2).
   b. Large volume enemas (e.g., tap water, soapsuds): Insert the rectal tube into the anus slowly, 3 to 4 inches for an adult (Fig. 22.3).
6. Interrupt the flow of solution if abdominal pain or cramping occurs; resume the flow when the patient states the feeling has subsided.
7. Encourage the patient to retain the fluid as long as possible to promote maximum evacuation.
8. Assist the patient to a commode or toilet or assist the patient onto a bedpan (regular or fracture bedpan [Fig. 22.4]) when a patient is on bed rest or is unable to exit the bed (Fig. 22.5).
   a. Begin with the patient in the supine position.

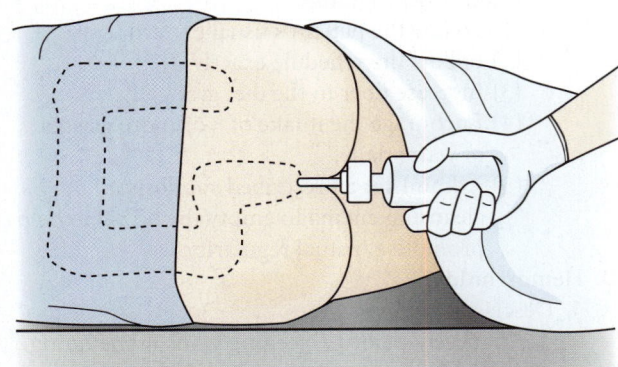

Fig 22.2 Patient position for an enema. (From Burton and Ludwig [2011]. *Fundamentals of nursing care: Concepts, connections & skills.* Philadelphia: F. A. Davis, with permission.)

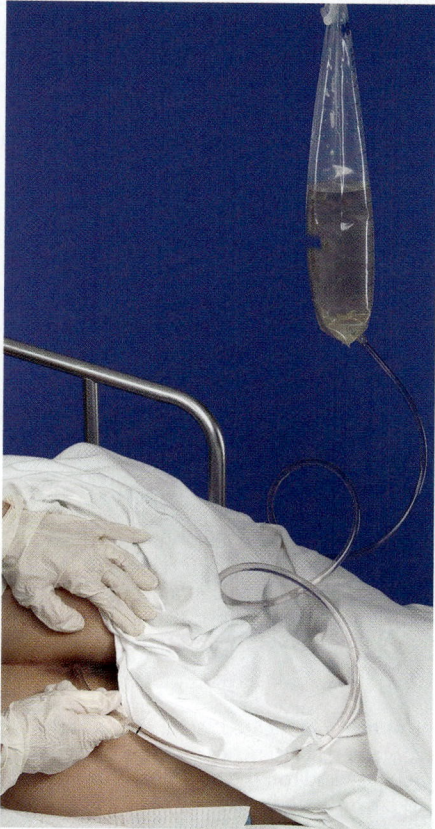

Fig 22.3 Tap-water enema. (From Wilkinson and Treas [2011]. *Fundamentals of nursing,* Vol. 2, 2nd ed. Philadelphia: F. A. Davis, with permission.)

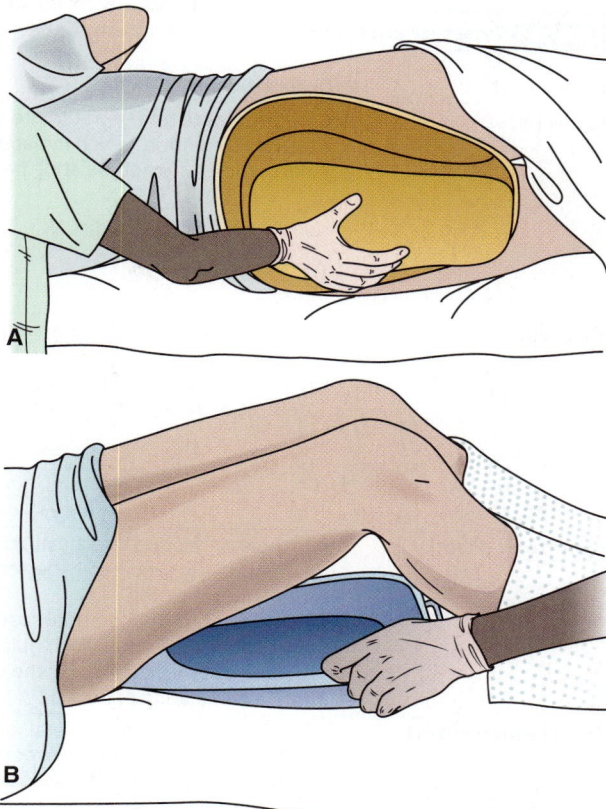

Fig 22.5 Placing a patient on a bedpan: (A) Regular bedpan. (B) Fracture bedpan.

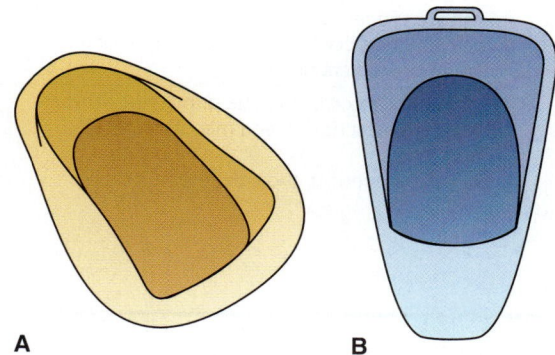

Fig 22.4 Types of bedpans: (a) Regular. (b) Fracture.

   b. Turn the patient on the side or have the patient flex the hips and knees and lift the pelvis up off the bed.
   c. Position the closed end of a regular bedpan or the closed, flat end of a fracture bedpan against the buttocks.

   d. Assist the patient to return to the supine position while the nurse holds the bedpan in place.
   e. Raise the side rails.
   f. Raise the head of the bed to a comfortable height for the patient.
   g. Position a call bell within easy reach.
 9. Remain close to the patient during evacuation because it may cause dizziness, which is a safety concern.
10. Provide perineal hygiene care after the procedure.
11. Monitor for therapeutic effect (fecal returns) and untoward results (distension, bleeding); notify the primary health-care provider if untoward effects occur.
12. Document patient responses.
 B. **Types of Enemas and Specific Nursing Care** (Table 22.2)

VI. Bowel Diversions

Because of a disease process or injury to the bowel, a patient may require partial or total surgical removal of the bowel and the creation of a bowel diversion to permit

Table 22.2 Types of Enemas and Related Nursing Care

Type	Description	Specific Nursing Care
Tap water.	• Involves induction of water into the colon. • Causes distention, which initiates the defecation reflex, stimulating peristalsis.	• Use 500 to 1,000 mL of tap water. • Raise the bag 12 inches above the anus or 18 inches above the anus for a "high" enema. • Assess for signs and symptoms of water toxicity or circulatory overload, such as hypertension, bounding pulse, tachycardia, and tachypnea; may progress to restlessness, anxiety, moist breath sounds, crackles, and dyspnea.
Soapsuds.	• Involves induction of soapy water into the colon. • Irritates the bowel, which initiates the defecation reflex, stimulating peristalsis.	• Use 500 to 1,000 mL of solution. • Raise the bag 12 inches above the anus or 18 inches above the anus for a "high" enema. • Give a maximum of three times when order includes "enemas until clear." • Use only the liquid castile soap included in the enema kit because other soaps and detergents can cause bowel irritation and damage.
Hypertonic (Fleet).	• Involves induction of a small volume of commercially prepared hypertonic solution into the colon. • Pulls fluid out of interstitial spaces via osmosis filling the colon with fluid. • Causes distention initiating the defecation reflex stimulating peristalsis.	• Insert prelubricated rectal tube of the 4 to 6 ounce container 3 to 4 inches into rectum. • Squeeze and roll the container slowly from distal to proximal end until empty. • Assess for signs and symptoms of dehydration and electrolyte imbalances.
Oil-retention enema.	• Involves induction of mineral oil into the colon, which lubricates the rectum and sigmoid colon and softens stool. • A tap water or soapsuds enema often follows an oil-retention enema according to manufacturer's directions.	• Insert a prelubricated rectal tube of the 30 to 60 mL container 3 to 4 inches into the rectum. • Squeeze and roll the container slowly from the distal to proximal end until empty. • Encourage retention for as long as possible for best results.
Return-flow enema (Harris flush, Harris drip).	• Involves slow induction and exit of solution to facilitate expulsion of flatus. • Commonly used after surgery to relieve flatulence. • Reduces abdominal distention.	• Instill 100 to 200 mL of solution slowly into the colon. • Lower the solution container slightly below the anus to withdraw fluid and gas into the collection container via the same tubing. • Repeat the raising and lowering process five or six times. • Evaluate the results, such as bubbles returning into the collection container and reduction of abdominal distention and cramping.
Medicated enemas.	• Involves instillation of a solution containing a drug to achieve a specific action. *Sodium polystyrene sulfonate (Kayexalate)* • Exchanges sodium ions for potassium ions, promoting the excretion of potassium. *Antibiotic solution (e.g., neomycin)* • Reduces bacteria in the colon before bowel surgery to decrease the risk of infection.	• Administer according to the primary health-care provider's prescription and manufacturer's directions. • Evaluate the results and side effects of the medication.

evacuation of intestinal wastes. There are many commonalities of nursing care for patients with bowel diversions, but specific nursing care relates to the differences in the consistency of the fecal discharge (effluent), the type of appliance required, and factors that determine the need for intestinal irrigation.

A. Types (Fig. 22.6)

   1. Colostomy.

     a. Formation of an opening (stoma) between the colon and the surface of the abdomen to permit feces to exit the body.

     b. Stoma in ascending colon: Liquid stool collected in an appliance.

     c. Stoma in transverse colon: Semisolid stool collected in an appliance.

     d. Stoma in descending colon: Solid stool collected in an appliance; may be controlled by daily irrigations with effluent eliminated in the toilet.

     e. Stoma in sigmoid colon: Solid stool controlled by daily intestinal irrigations, with effluent eliminated in the toilet.

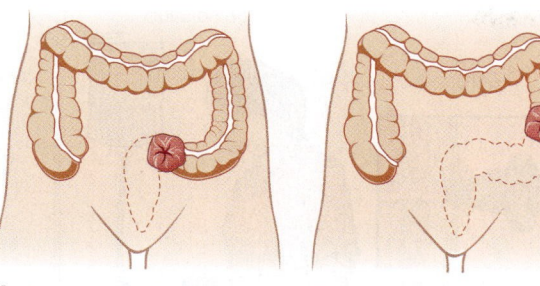

A. Sigmoid colostomy   **B.** Descending colostomy

C. Transverse colostomy, double-barreled   **D.** Ascending colostomy

E. Ileostomy

Fig 22.6 Location of various bowel diversion ostomies. Shaded areas indicate sections of the bowel that are removed or being "rested." The closer the colostomy is to the ascending colon ("higher"), the more liquid and continuous the drainage will be. (From Wilkinson and Treas [2011]. *Fundamentals of nursing,* Vol. 1, 2nd ed. Philadelphia: F. A. Davis, with permission.)

2. **Ileostomy**
   a. Formation of an opening (stoma) between the ileum and the surface of the abdomen to permit feces to exit the body.
   b. Typical ileostomy: Liquid stool collected in an appliance.
   c. Continent Kock pouch: Tube inserted into an external stoma empties an internal reservoir of liquid stool; external pouch unnecessary.
   d. Ileal-anal anastomosis: Procedure that preserves evacuation through the anus, but evacuation is spontaneous rather than voluntary; liquid stool.

B. **Nursing Care for Patients With a Bowel Diversion**
   1. Assess the stoma, which should be deep pink or brick red, shiny, and moist (Fig. 22.7); a pale,

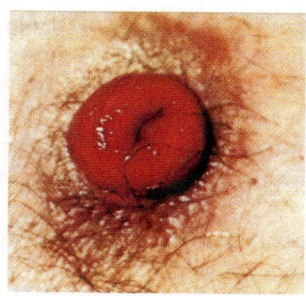

Fig 22.7 Healthy stoma. (From Wilkinson and Treas [2011]. *Fundamentals of nursing,* Vol. 1, 2nd ed. Philadelphia: F. A. Davis, with permission.)

purple, or black stoma indicates ischemia and the primary health-care provider should be notified immediately.

2. Assess for bowel sounds and the presence of distention; motility generally returns 3 to 6 days after surgery.
3. Assess the amount, consistency, and characteristics of stool.
4. Change the appliance every 3 to 5 days or as needed; note that many ostomy supplies are available on the market (Fig. 22.8).
   a. Clean the area with soap and water.
   b. Use a protective barrier on the skin under the appliance.
   c. Apply an antifungal agent on the skin under the appliance if prescribed.

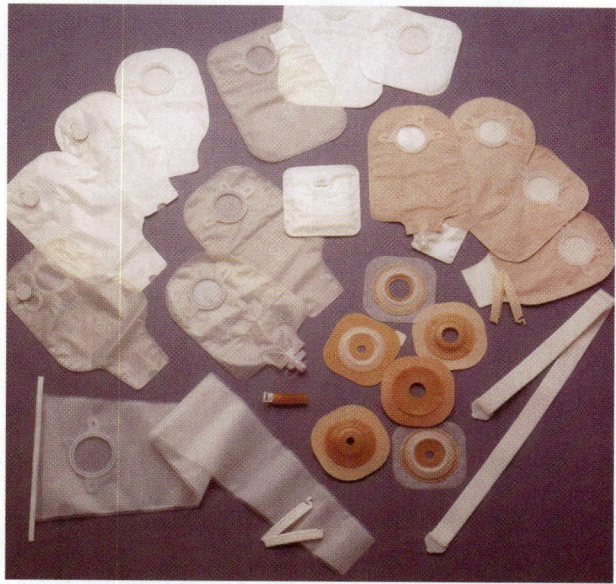

Fig 22.8 Ostomy supplies. (From Burton and Ludwig [2011]. *Fundamentals of nursing care: Concepts, connections & skills.* Philadelphia: F. A. Davis, with permission.)

d. Measure and then apply the appliance with a ⅛-inch clearance to avoid stoma damage or skin exposure to stool (Fig. 22.9A and Fig. 22.9B).

5. Empty the bag when it is half full to avoid excessive tension on the appliance interfering with the integrity of the adhesive resulting in leakage of stool.

6. Refer the patient to the United Ostomy Association or an enterostomal therapist.

7. Irrigate a distal colostomy (Fig. 22.10).
   a. Irrigate at the same time every day; note that the procedure may take as long as 60 minutes.
   b. Ensure privacy and adequate access to the bathroom.
   c. Prepare the irrigating bag with 300 to 1,000 mL of irrigating solution, as prescribed.
   d. Ensure the irrigating solution is at or slightly above body temperature.
   e. Flush the solution through the tubing to expel air (priming).

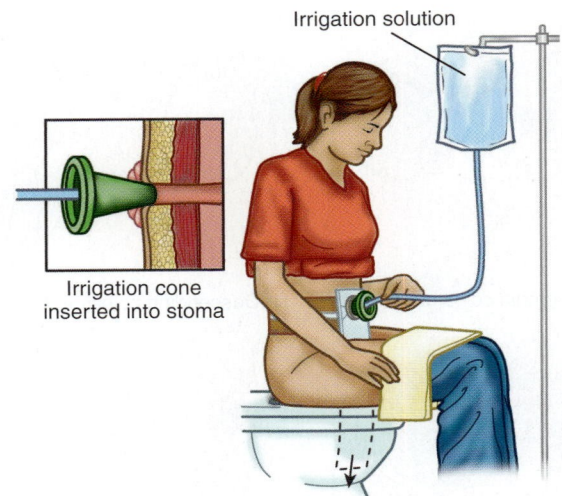

Fig 22.10 Colostomy irrigation. (From Wilkinson and Treas [2011]. *Fundamentals of nursing,* Vol. 2, 2nd ed. Philadelphia: F. A. Davis, with permission.)

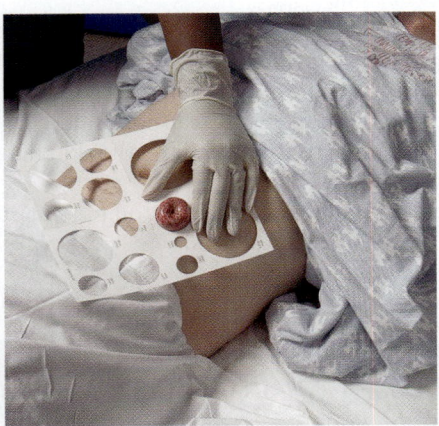

A Measuring stoma size

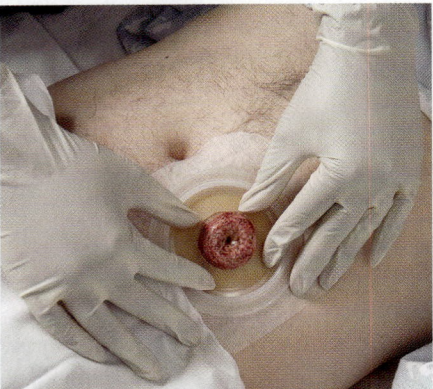

B Applying a stoma appliance

Fig 22.9 (A) Measuring stoma size. (B) Applying a stoma appliance. (From Burton and Ludwig [2011]. *Fundamentals of nursing care: Concepts, connections & skills.* Philadelphia: F. A. Davis, with permission.)

f. Lubricate the cone at the end of the tubing.
g. Position the patient on a toilet or in a side-lying position in bed.
h. Place the irrigating sleeve over the stoma.
i. Insert the lubricated cone through the opening of the sleeve gently into the stoma in the direction of the lumen; hold the cone in place during the inflow of solution.

🛑 j. Stop the procedure and notify the primary health-care provider if resistance occurs when inserting the cone.

🛑 k. Shut off the flow of solution if the patient experiences cramping; restart the flow once cramping subsides.

l. Remove the cone and tubing when the inflow of solution is complete; allow at least 30 minutes for evacuation through the sleeve into the toilet or bedpan.
m. Provide hygiene.
n. Apply an appliance.
o. Document the results and the patient's response.

VII. Medications That Affect the GI Tract

When a person is diagnosed with a GI problem, the primary health-care provider can prescribe appropriate medications, depending on the patient's need. The most common medications affecting fecal elimination include antidiarrheals, cathartics and laxatives, and antiflatulents. Additional medications, such as antacids, antiemetics, and antisecretory agents, usually are prescribed for problems interfering with nutrition, but they indirectly influence the GI tract. Nurses should know the mechanisms of action, therapeutic and nontherapeutic effects, and nursing care related to the common medications that are specifically designed to address a patient's GI needs.

A. Antidiarrheals: Decrease Diarrhea and Increase the Production of Formed Stool (Table 22.3).

B. Laxatives and Cathartics: Prevent or Treat Constipation; Evacuate the Bowel for Diagnostic Tests or Surgery (Table 22.4).

C. Antiflatulents: Decrease the Amount of Intestinal Gas (Flatus) (Table 22.5).

D. Antacids, Antiemetics, and Antisecretory Agents: See Chapter 18, "Nutrition," pages 552–554 for Information and Nursing Care Related to these agents.

Table 22.3 Antidiarrheals

Mechanism of Action	Examples	Nontherapeutic Effects
Motility Suppressants • Inhibit mucosal receptors responsible for peristalsis.	• diphenoxylate HCl with atropine sulfate (Lomotil) • loperamide (Imodium)	• Tachycardia. • Respiratory depression. • Ileus. • Urinary retention. • Dry mouth. • Sedation, lethargy, and drowsiness. • Dizziness and weakness.
Enteric Bacterial Replacement • Reestablishes the intestinal flora.	• *lactobacillus acidophilus* (Bacid)	• Abdominal cramps. • Increased flatulence.

Nursing Care
- Assess for frequency of bowel movements and the color and characteristics of stool.
- Auscultate bowel sounds for a decrease in intestinal hypermotility, indicating a therapeutic effect.
- Monitor for signs and symptoms of fluid and electrolyte imbalances, such as fluid volume deficit, hypokalemia, and hyponatremia.
- Encourage increased fluid intake.
- Assess for therapeutic and nontherapeutic effects.
- Diphenoxylate HCl with atropine sulfate: Encourage the patient to suck on hard candy to stimulate salivation associated with dry mucous membranes.

Table 22.4 Laxatives and Cathartics

Mechanism of Action	Examples	Nontherapeutic Effects
Bulk Forming • Increases bulk to stimulate peristalsis.	• methylcellulose (Citrucel) • psyllium (Metamucil)	• Diarrhea. • Fluid passed with feces.
Stool Softeners • Promote entry of water and fat into feces to soften and decrease drying of stool. • May take several days to act.	• docusate sodium (Colace)	
Stimulants and Irritants • Irritate bowel, causing propulsion of contents out of the body. • Are rapid acting.	• bisacodyl (Dulcolax) • cascara/senna (Senokot, Ex-Lax)	
Lubricants • Soften feces.	• mineral oil	• Diarrhea. • Decreased absorption of fat-soluble vitamins.
Saline Osmotics • Draws water into intestinal lumen, distending the bowel and stimulating peristalsis.	• magnesium salts (Milk of Magnesia) • sodium phosphate (Fleet Phospho-Soda)	• Diarrhea. • Dehydration. • Hypernatremia. • Decreased absorption of fat-soluble vitamins.

Nursing Care
- Assess frequency of bowel movements and color and characteristics of stool.
- Identify situations when these medications are contraindicated (e.g., in the presence of nausea and vomiting, abdominal pain, or additional signs and symptoms of acute abdomen because these may indicate bowel obstruction).
- Avoid administering saline osmotics to older adults or children because of the risk of fluid and electrolyte imbalances.
- Administer at bedtime.
- Encourage increased fluid intake, activity, and dietary fiber intake.
- Auscultate bowel sounds for an increase in intestinal motility.
- Assess for therapeutic and nontherapeutic effects.

Table 22.5 **Antiflatulent**		
Mechanism of Action	**Examples**	**Nontherapeutic Effects**
• Causes coalescence of gas bubbles.	• simethicone (Gas-X)	• None known.

Nursing Care
- Assess bowel sounds and extent of abdominal distention before and after administration.
- Administer after meals and at bedtime.
- Shake liquid preparations well.
- Teach the patient to avoid gas-forming liquids and foods, such as carbonated beverages, beans, and cabbage.
- Assess for therapeutic effects.

CASE STUDY: Putting It All Together

A nurse is admitting a middle-aged adult man to the hospital with a diagnosis of dehydration due to increasing GI distress and diarrhea. The patient was recently discharged from the hospital after being treated with antibiotics for a mild superficial skin infection involving the suture line following a total knee replacement. The patient tells the nurse, "Within a few days after discharge from the hospital, I got diarrhea and I thought it was due to something I ate. I took Lomotil for a few days, but it didn't help, so I went to my doctor. Now I am being put in the hospital for IV fluids and tests to find out what's causing the diarrhea." The nurse reviews the patient's clinical record for the admission history and physical assessment and the primary health-care provider's orders and then obtains the patient's vital signs.

Patient's Clinical Record

Admission History and Physical Assessment

Patient stated, "I have been having loose bowel movements for about a week and then they became watery and increased to 4 to 5 times a day. When I got severe abdominal cramps, I finally went to my doctor."
Reports 3-lb weight loss in the past few days.
Reports thirst and fatigue.
Abdominal distention present.
Stool greenish in color and malodorous.
Perianal irritation and excoriation.
Flat neck veins.

Primary Health-Care Provider's Orders

Contact precautions.
CBC.
Basic metabolic panel and magnesium and phosphorous levels.
Test stools for culture and sensitivity, ova and parasites, and *Clostridium difficile*.
Guaiac stool for occult blood × 3.
Vital signs and BP every 4 hours.
I&O.
Daily weight.
NPO.
OOB in room as tolerated.
IVF: D$_5$ 0.45% Sodium Chloride 125 mL/hour.
Flagyl 500 mg, every 8 hours, IVPB, infuse over 60 minutes.

Vital Signs

Pulse: 98 beats/minute, regular rhythm, thready.
Temperature: 101.2°F, orally
Respirations: 20 breaths/minute.
Blood pressure: 108/68 mm Hg.

CASE STUDY: Putting It All Together *cont'd*

_____ **Case Study Questions** _____

A. Identify at least five additional indicators of GI distress the nurse should monitor that are not included in the scenario.

1. _____

2. _____

3. _____

4. _____

5. _____

B. Identify at least six clinical indicators of dehydration, a complication of diarrhea, the nurse should assess that are not included in the scenario.

1. _____

2. _____

3. _____

4. _____

5. _____

6. _____

C. After interviewing the patient and completing a physical assessment, what is the most likely precipitating factor causing the patient's diarrhea and why?

_____

D. Which order written by the primary health-care provider should the nurse implement first and why?

_____

E. Identify at least ten nursing interventions that are associated with caring for this patient with diarrhea caused by the presence of *C. difficile.*

1. _____

2. _____

3. _____

4. _____

5. _____

6. _____

7. _____

8. _____

9. _____

10. _____

REVIEW QUESTIONS

1. A nurse is caring for a patient who has an order for a fleet enema to be self-administered at home the morning of ambulatory surgery. What is important for the nurse to teach the patient about this enema?
   1. "Insert the tube 6 inches into the rectum to ensure it is beyond the internal rectal sphincter."
   2. "Retain the enema solution as long as possible to promote evacuation."
   3. "Lay on the right side as the solution is administered for best results."
   4. "Warm it in the microwave for 1 minute to promote comfort."

2. A patient comes to the clinic reporting abdominal bloating. The primary health-care provider identifies that the patient has slowed intestinal peristalsis. What should the nurse encourage the patient to do to minimize abdominal bloating. **Select all that apply.**
   1. _____ Eat a high-fiber diet.
   2. _____ Increase fluid intake.
   3. _____ Use laxatives sparingly.
   4. _____ Drink prune juice every morning.
   5. _____ Raise the head of the bed 30° when sleeping.

3. A patient is scheduled for an esophagogastroduodenoscopy. Which is **most** important to discuss when teaching the patient about this procedure?
   1. Inform the patient that mild bloating and flatulence is common after the test.
   2. Teach that a scope will be inserted via the nose and into the stomach and duodenum.
   3. Instruct the patient to call the primary health-care provider if vomiting blood occurs after the procedure.
   4. Explain that drinking a small amount of water after awakening from the anesthesia is considered acceptable.

4. A nurse is caring for a patient who was admitted to the hospital and is scheduled for surgery in the morning due to a partial intestinal obstruction secondary to an intestinal mass. For which clinical indicator **most** associated with an intestinal obstruction should the nurse assess the patient?
   1. Light-brown stool
   2. Mucus in the stool
   3. Ribbon shaped stool
   4. Pungent odor to the stool

5. A nurse is to administer a premixed hypertonic disposable enema. The nurse verifies the primary health-care provider's order and performs all nursing interventions necessary before actually administering the enema. Place the remaining steps of the procedure in the order in which they should be implemented.
   1. Don clean gloves.
   2. Drape the patient with the top sheet so that only the buttocks are exposed.
   3. Position the patient in the left side-lying position with the right leg flexed.
   4. Remove the enema tip from the patient's rectum while holding the container in the rolled up position.
   5. Squeeze the enema container, maintaining slow, steady pressure from the bottom while rolling it up until all fluid is delivered.
   6. Insert the prelubricated enema tip beyond the internal sphincter slowly while directing the enema tip toward the umbilicus.
   Answer: _____

6. A patient reports a long-term problem with constipation. What should the nurse instruct the patient to do to help minimize this problem?
   1. "Include more bananas in your diet."
   2. "Drink a minimum of one quart of fluid a day."
   3. "Hold your breath when bearing down to have a bowel movement."
   4. "Attempt to have a bowel movement after drinking a warm liquid in the morning."

7. A nurse is caring for a patient who was admitted to the hospital with upper gastrointestinal bleeding. For which clinical indicator associated with gastrointestinal bleeding should the nurse assess the patient?
   1. Pale, clay-colored stool
   2. Yellow, greenish stool
   3. Hard, dry brown stool
   4. Black, tarry stool

8. A patient reports frequent episodes of constipation. Which should the nurse teach the patient to do to help relieve this problem? **Select all that apply.**
   1. _____ Use a prepackaged 4 oz enema once a week.
   2. _____ Drink at least 2 quarts of fluid every day.
   3. _____ Exercise at least 15 minutes every day.
   4. _____ Eat fresh vegetables two times a day.
   5. _____ Take a laxative three times a week.

9. A nurse is caring for a patient receiving diphenoxylate HCl with atropine sulfate (Lomotil). Which is **most** important for the nurse to include when teaching the patient about nontherapeutic effects of this medication?
   1. Monitor the pulse for a slow heart rate.
   2. Suck on hard candy when experiencing a dry mouth.
   3. Report abdominal cramps to the primary healthcare provider immediately.
   4. Avoid engaging in hazardous activity until the response to the medication is known.

10. A nurse identifies that a patient may have perceived constipation. What specific question related to perceived constipation should the nurse ask the patient?
    1. "How often do you take a laxative?"
    2. "What is the consistency of your stools?"
    3. "Do you have a sensation of rectal fullness?"
    4. "When was the last time you had a bowel movement?"

11. Which independent nursing actions are associated with caring for a patient with diarrhea? **Select all that apply.**
    1. _____ Suggesting eating the banana from the breakfast tray
    2. _____ Providing perineal care after each defecation
    3. _____ Monitoring the patient's hematocrit level
    4. _____ Administering intravenous fluids
    5. _____ Administering an antidiarrheal

12. A nurse is caring for a patient who just had surgery 6 hours ago to remove a portion of the intestine and the surgical creation of a stoma. Which action is important when caring for this patient?
    1. Assess the color of the stoma.
    2. Explain that bowel function will return in 24 hours.
    3. Wait until the collection bag is full before it is emptied.
    4. Clean the peristomal area with half-normal saline solution and peroxide.

13. A nurse is caring for a patient who has an order for a stool specimen. What should the nurse do when collecting this specimen?
    1. Wear sterile gloves to maintain sterility of the specimen.
    2. Send it to the laboratory promptly to avoid a degraded specimen.
    3. Flush the toilet first so that the water is clean and free from debris.
    4. Collect several inches of formed feces to ensure an adequate sample.

14. A nurse is caring for an older adult who was admitted to the hospital from the emergency department for rehydration therapy. The nurse reviews the patient's clinical record and interviews the patient.

Patient's Clinical Record

Patient Interview

An older adult female stated that she fainted in the yard while gardening and a neighbor called 911 for an ambulance, which took her to the emergency department. She said that she has been following all of her doctor's orders, but she has been taking milk of magnesia daily because she likes having a bowel movement every day. She shared that her stools have been very loose lately, but she would rather have them lose than to be constipated and bloated. She stated that she is very lonely because she has no family living nearby and does not drive anymore, so she watches a lot of television and works in her garden. She said that she just got up too quickly after weeding and that was why she fainted.

Laboratory Results

Hb: 16.8 g/dL.
Hct: 47%.
Creatinine: 1.3 mg/dL.
BUN: 46 mg/dL.
Potassium: 3.4 mEq/L.
Sodium: 147 mEq/L.

Medication Reconciliation Form (medications taken at home)

Centrum Silver vitamin daily.
Calcium 600 mg twice a day.
MOM 2 tablespoons at bedtime daily.
Advil 400 mg every 6 hours when needed for joint pain, not to exceed 1,600 mg daily.

Which nursing intervention is the **most** important for this patient regarding self-health management after discharge?
1. Discuss the patient's reason for taking a cathartic daily.
2. Schedule monthly checkups with the primary healthcare provider.
3. Have a social worker assist the patient with transportation to the local senior center for socialization.
4. Teach the need to change position slowly to allow time for the body to adjust to the change in position.

15. A nurse is caring for a patient who is constipated. Which food is **most** appropriate for the nurse to teach the patient to eat?
    1. Celery
    2. Grapefruit
    3. Bran cereal
    4. Sunflower seeds

16. A nurse is caring for a patient who is scheduled for a lower GI series. What information about this test should the nurse include in a discussion with the patient?
    1. "You will have to implement a bowel prep at home the night before and the morning of the test."
    2. "You will have chalky white colored stool for 1 to 2 days after the test."
    3. "You will remain in the supine position for the duration of the test."
    4. "You will drink 8 ounces of barium just before the test."

17. The attached graphics illustrate bowel diversions with the stoma site and intestinal structures removed. Which intestinal diversion should the nurse anticipate will have the most formed stool?
    1. A
    2. B
    3. C
    4. D

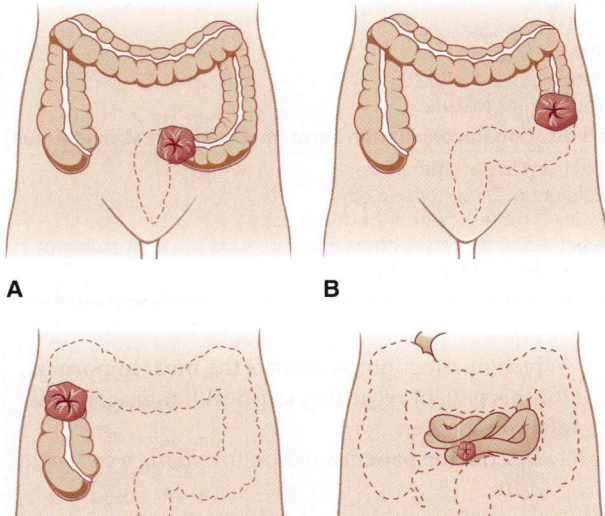

A   B

C   D

18. A nurse is teaching a patient about the best foods to eat to avoid constipation. Which vegetable selected by the patient from the hospital menu indicates that the teaching was effective?
    1. Carrots
    2. Spinach
    3. Zucchini
    4. Cabbage

19. A nurse is teaching a patient with diarrhea about foods that should be avoided. Which foods eliminated from the diet by the patient indicates that the teaching was effective? **Select all that apply.**
    1. _____ Graham crackers
    2. _____ Chicken breast
    3. _____ Kidney beans
    4. _____ Scallops
    5. _____ Yogurt

20. A nurse is teaching a patient about foods to eat when constipated. Which food selected by the patient from a list of foods indicates that the teaching was effective?
    1. Peas
    2. Apples
    3. Cherries
    4. Asparagus

21. A nurse is caring for a patient with a colostomy who has a two-piece ostomy appliance. Which is important for the nurse to do when caring for this patient?
    1. Tuck some gauze into the stoma after cleaning it until the new faceplate and bag is applied.
    2. Cut an opening in the faceplate so that it is at least ½ inch away from around the stoma.
    3. Empty the bag from the bottom, avoiding disconnecting the bag from the faceplate.
    4. Change the faceplate of the appliance every 3 to 5 days or when necessary.

22. A nurse working in a nursing home identifies that a patient may have a fecal impaction. Which clinical manifestation is **most** specific to this problem?
    1. Passage of a small amount of brown liquid from the rectum
    2. Lack of a bowel movement for several days
    3. Distension of the abdomen
    4. Feeling of rectal fullness

23. A nurse is teaching a patient with diarrhea about what foods to select from a menu. Which foods selected by the patient indicate that the teaching was effective? **Select all that apply.**
    1. _____ Shrimp
    2. _____ Chickpeas
    3. _____ Rye bread
    4. _____ Milk shake
    5. _____ Cottage cheese

24. A primary health-care provider orders a tap-water enema. The patient says, "How does this type of enema work?" Which rationale should the nurse include in words the patient will understand when answering the patient's question?
    1. Water causes excessive interstitial fluid loss.
    2. Instilled water stimulates a bowel movement.
    3. Surface tension of water is reduced by soapsuds.
    4. Hypertonic nature of the water irritates the intestinal mucosa.

25. The nurse is caring for a patient who is constipated. The primary health-care provider prescribes bisacodyl (Dulcolax) 15 mg PO h.s. Dulcolax is supplied in 5 mg tablets. How many tablets should the nurse administer? Record your answer using a whole number.
    Answer: _____ tablets

26. A parent brings a child to the clinic because the child has been reporting rectal itching during the night. The primary health-care provider explains a specimen must be obtained so that the standard test for pinworms can be performed. What should the nurse instruct the parent to do?
    1. Wash the anal area and then attempt to collect the specimen.
    2. Insert a cotton-tipped swab into the anus and smear the specimen on a slide.
    3. Pick up any worms found around the anus at night and put them in a sterile container.
    4. Press clear scotch tape to the area around the anus first thing in the morning and place it on a slide.

27. A nurse is caring for a patient adjusting to a colostomy in the descending colon. The patient is concerned about eating foods that may cause a blockage. What foods should the nurse teach the patient to avoid? **Select all that apply.**
    1. _____ Cranberry juice
    2. _____ Green beans
    3. _____ Fresh pears
    4. _____ Popcorn
    5. _____ Rice

28. A nurse is teaching a patient what to expect regarding a colonoscopy. What information is **most** important to include in this discussion with the patient?
    1. "You can expect flatus after the test because air is inflated into the bowel during the test."
    2. "Report abdominal pain, fever, chills, or bleeding to the primary health-care provider."
    3. "Avoid high-fiber food for a week if a polyp or biopsy is taken during the procedure."
    4. "Do not lift anything for a week if a polyp or biopsy is taken during the procedure."

29. A nurse is caring for a patient who has an episode of diarrhea with frothy, odorous stool, containing an excessive amount of fat. Which word should the nurse use when documenting this type of stool?
    1. Chyme
    2. Melena
    3. Meconium
    4. Steatorrhea

30. Which dependent nursing interventions are associated with caring for a patient who is constipated? **Select all that apply.**
    1. _____ Administering Colace 100 mg twice a day
    2. _____ Assisting the patient with ambulation 3 times a day
    3. _____ Encouraging the intake of prunes from the meal tray
    4. _____ Encouraging the patient to turn from side to side in bed
    5. _____ Responding immediately to the patient's urge to defecate

31. A patient self-administers a bowel prep consisting of sodium phosphate (Fleet Phospho-Soda), bisacodyl (Dulcolax), and an enema the night before a colonoscopy. For what serious adverse effect should the nurse assess the patient?
    1. Deficient fluid volume
    2. Intestinal cramping
    3. Hyponatremia
    4. Diarrhea

32. A nurse is teaching a patient how to test stool for the presence of occult blood. Which is important to teach the patient about this test to achieve accurate results?
    1. Collect the specimen in the morning several days in a row.
    2. Apply a thick layer of feces on the designated window of the test packet.
    3. Avoid taking nonsteroidal anti-inflammatory medications before the test.
    4. Read the result as positive if a red color develops in response to the reagent.

33. A patient reports not having a bowel movement for several days. Place the nurse's actions in order of priority.
    1. Obtain an order for an enema.
    2. Request a prescription for a laxative.
    3. Encourage the patient to drink more fluids.
    4. Ask the patient when the last bowel movement occurred.
    5. Explore with the patient how much fiber is being consumed in the diet.
    Answer: _____

34. A patient has multiple fixation devices for fractures of the extremities because of trauma experienced in a motor vehicle collision. The primary health-care provider orders bedrest, regular diet, and morphine sulfate 10 mg every 4 hours prn for moderate pain. What action by the nurse can help limit a common side effect of this medication?
    1. Prolong the times between the administrations of pain medication.
    2. Explain why ingesting yogurt daily is helpful.
    3. Teach the patient to increase dietary fiber.
    4. Place the patient on oxygen therapy.

35. A nurse is caring for a patient with a nasogastric tube to intermittent wall suction. What should the nurse do to ensure that it is functioning effectively?
    1. Verify that the tubing is intact and patent.
    2. Position the patient below the level of the collection bottle.
    3. Elevate the head of the patient's bed to a semi-Fowler position.
    4. Ensure that the collection bottle is attached to a humidification adaptor.

1. ANSWER: 2.
Rationales:
1. The tube is inserted only 3 to 4 inches to clear the internal rectal sphincter.
2. A fleet enema is a hypertonic solution that draws fluid out of interstitial spaces via osmosis, filling the colon with fluid. This causes distention, which stimulates peristalsis, initiating the defecation reflex.
3. The left, not right, lateral or Sims' position allows solution to flow by gravity along the natural curve of the sigmoid.
4. An enema solution should never be warmed in a microwave. The water may become too hot and cause damage to the intestinal mucosa.
TEST-TAKING TIP: Identify the clang association. The word *enema* in the stem and in option 2 is a clang association. Examine option 2 carefully.
Content Area: Gastrointestinal System
Integrated Processes: Teaching/Learning; Nursing Process: Implementation
Client Need: Physiological Integrity; Reduction of Risk Potential
Cognitive Level: Application

2. ANSWER: 1, 2, 4.
Rationales:
1. High-fiber foods increase bulk in fecal material, thereby facilitating intestinal peristalsis; bulkier feces increase pressure against the intestinal wall, which moves feces more rapidly through the colon. Instruct the patient to increase fluid intake when ingesting high-fiber foods to prevent a bowel obstruction.
2. Two thousand to 3,000 mL of fluid daily provides enough fluid to be reabsorbed in the large intestine as well as promote a looser stool. Fluid in the colon mixes with the feces, increasing bulk; the increase in bulk stimulates intestinal peristalsis.
3. The use of laxatives, even sparingly, should be avoided because they weaken the bowel's usual response to pressure against the walls of the bowel.
4. Prune juice is high in fiber and is recommended to increase intestinal peristalsis.
5. Elevating the head of the bed 30° when sleeping helps reduce the risk of gastric reflux; it does not increase intestinal peristalsis.
Content Area: Gastrointestinal System
Integrated Processes: Teaching/Learning; Nursing Process: Implementation
Client Need: Physiological Integrity; Basic Care and Comfort
Cognitive Level: Application

3. ANSWER: 3.
Rationales:
1. Although the patient should be informed that mild bloating and flatulence is common after the procedure, it is not as important as another option.
2. This is incorrect information. The scope is introduced via the mouth, not the nose.
3. If the patient is vomiting blood; has epigastric, substernal or shoulder pain; has black, tarry stools; or a fever, the gastrointestinal tract may have been perforated during the procedure. Immediate medical attention is necessary to treat this complication.
4. The patient should not eat or drink until after the gag reflex and the ability to swallow return.
TEST-TAKING TIP: Identify the word in the stem that sets a priority. The word *most* in the stem sets a priority.
Content Area: Gastrointestinal System
Integrated Processes: Teaching/Learning; Nursing Process: Implementation
Client Need: Physiological Integrity; Reduction of Risk Potential
Cognitive Level: Application

4. ANSWER: 3.
Rationales:
1. Light-brown stool is associated with malabsorption, a diet high in milk, or a diet low in meat, not intestinal obstruction.
2. Mucus in the stool is associated with intestinal inflammation, not obstruction.
3. An intestinal obstruction blocks off part of the lumen of the intestine, causing stool to be ribbon shaped.
4. Pungent odor to stool generally indicates a gastrointestinal infection.
TEST-TAKING TIP: Identify the word in the stem that sets a priority. The word *most* in the stem sets a priority.
Content Area: Gastrointestinal System
Integrated Processes: Nursing Process: Assessment
Client Need: Physiological Integrity; Physiological Adaptation
Cognitive Level: Application

5. ANSWER: 3, 2, 1, 6, 5, 4.
Rationales:
3. Positioning the patient in the left side-lying position facilitates the flow of solution by gravity into the sigmoid and descending colons. Flexing the right leg allows exposure of the anus.
2. Draping the patient supports privacy and dignity.
1. Donning clean gloves protects the nurse from the patient's body fluids.
6. Slow insertion of the enema tip helps prevent sphincter spasm and inserting it beyond the internal sphincter helps minimize outflow of enema solution while it is being instilled. Directing the enema tip toward the umbilicus follows the normal contour of the rectum.
5. Squeezing the container from the bottom and rolling it up toward the tip while maintaining steady pressure prevents fluid from being suctioned back into the container.
4. Removing the container while firmly holding the container in the rolled up position prevents fluid from being suctioned back into the container.
Content Area: Gastrointestinal System
Integrated Processes: Nursing Process: Planning
Client Need: Physiological Integrity; Basic Care and Comfort
Cognitive Level: Analysis

6. ANSWER: 4.
Rationales:
1. Bananas should be avoided because they promote constipation.

2. A minimum of 2 to 3 quarts of fluid should be ingested to promote a soft stool.

3. Bearing down while holding the breath (Valsalva maneuver) should be avoided because it places a strain on the heart and can precipitate a cardiac dysrhythmia.

4. **Warm fluid or food entering an empty stomach precipitates the gastrocolic reflex, which precipitates intestinal peristalsis. Intestinal peristalsis moves fecal material toward the rectum where it can be evacuated.**

Content Area: Gastrointestinal System
Integrated Processes: Teaching/Learning; Nursing Process: Implementation
Client Need: Physiological Integrity; Basic Care and Comfort
Cognitive Level: Application

7. **ANSWER: 4.**
Rationales:

1. Pale, clay-colored stool indicates a lack of bile, generally due to biliary obstruction. Also, it is associated with barium used for intestinal diagnostic tests.

2. Yellow, greenish stool is associated with intestinal infection, such as *C. difficile.*

3. Hard, dry, brown stool indicates decreased intestinal motility (constipation).

4. **Black, tarry stool indicates digested blood emanating from the upper gastrointestinal tract. Stool darkened by blood pigments is call melena.**

Content Area: Gastrointestinal System
Integrated Processes: Nursing Process: Assessment
Client Need: Physiological Integrity; Physiological Adaptation
Cognitive Level: Application

8. **ANSWER: 2, 3, 4.**
Rationales:

1. The consistent use of enemas is contraindicated. Frequent use of enemas will precipitate a reliance on this method to evacuate the bowel.

2. **Two liters of fluid will provide enough fluid to meet metabolic needs and enough fluid to promote a softer stool.**

3. **Exercise promotes intestinal peristalsis, which helps propel fecal material toward the rectum.**

4. **Vegetables contain fiber, which creates a larger fecal mass as well as promotes intestinal peristalsis.**

5. The consistent use of laxatives is contraindicated. Excessive laxative use will precipitate a reliance on this method to evacuate the bowel.

Content Area: Gastrointestinal System
Integrated Processes: Teaching/Learning; Nursing Process: Implementation
Client Need: Physiological Integrity; Basic Care and Comfort
Cognitive Level: Application

9. **ANSWER: 4.**
Rationales:

1. Tachycardia, not bradycardia, is a nontherapeutic response to this medication

2. Sucking on hard candy will stimulate salivation to moisten a dry mouth, which is a manageable side effect associated with this medication.

3. Abdominal cramps are not a side effect of this medication. Abdominal cramps are a side effect of enteric bacterial replacement therapy (*lactobacillus acidophilus* [Bacid]), not diphenoxylate HCl with atropine sulfate.

4. **Diphenoxylate is a synthetic narcotic that can cause sedation, drowsiness, dizziness, lethargy, and weakness. Hazardous activities should be avoided until the patient's response to the medication is evaluated.**

TEST-TAKING TIP: Identify the word in the stem that sets a priority. The word *most* in the stem sets a priority. Identify the word in the stem that indicates negative polarity. The word *nontherapeutic* indicates negative polarity.

Content Area: Gastrointestinal System
Integrated Processes: Teaching/Learning; Nursing Process: Planning
Client Need: Physiological Integrity; Pharmacological and Parenteral Therapies
Cognitive Level: Application

10. **ANSWER: 1.**
Rationales:

1. **"How often do you take a laxative?" is a question that should be asked of patients suspected of having perceived constipation because these individuals frequently self-prescribe the daily use of laxatives, suppositories, or enemas to ensure a bowel movement every day.**

2. "What is the consistency of your stools?" is a question that should be asked of all patients with constipation; it is not specific to perceived constipation.

3. "Do you have a sensation of rectal fullness?" is a question that should be asked of all patients with constipation; it is not specific to perceived constipation.

4. "When was the last time you had a bowel movement?" is a question that should be asked of all patients with constipation; it is not specific to perceived constipation.

Content Area: Gastrointestinal System
Integrated Processes: Communication/Documentation; Nursing Process: Assessment
Client Need: Physiological Integrity; Basic Care and Comfort
Cognitive Level: Analysis

11. **ANSWER: 1, 2, 3.**
Rationales:

1. Although providing a diet is based on an order by a primary health-care provider and therefore a dependent function of the nurse, suggesting a food within the diet that is best for a patient with diarrhea is associated with patient teaching. Patient teaching is an independent function of the nurse.

2. Providing for hygiene needs of a patient is an independent function of the nurse and does not require an order from a primary health-care provider.

3. Monitoring the results of laboratory tests is an independent function of the nurse that does not require an order from the primary health-care provider. When a person has diarrhea the hematocrit level generally is elevated due to hypovolemia. A nurse should notify the primary health-care provider if a level is outside the expected range.

4. Administering intravenous fluids requires an order from a primary health-care provider and, therefore, is a dependent function of the nurse.

5. Administering an antidiarrheal requires a prescription from a primary health-care provider and, therefore, is a dependent function of the nurse.
Content Area: Gastrointestinal System
Integrated Processes: Teaching/Learning; Nursing Process: Implementation
Client Need: Physiological Integrity; Basic Care and Comfort
Cognitive Level: Application

12. **ANSWER: 1.**
Rationales:
1. A stoma should be deep pink/brick red, shiny, and moist. This indicates that the stoma is receiving adequate circulation. If the stoma is pale, purple, or black it indicates ischemia; this should be reported to the primary health-care provider immediately.
2. Bowel motility returns 3 to 6 days, not 24 hours, after bowel diversion surgery.
3. The bag should be emptied when it is half full to avoid the weight of the bag from pulling the appliance away from the surface of the skin. This can cause unnecessary stress and strain on surrounding tissue as well as cause leakage under the seal of the appliance.
4. The peristomal area should be cleaned with gentle soap and warm water. Peroxide is a bleach and oxidizing agent that is caustic to skin and mucosal tissue.
TEST-TAKING TIP: Identify the clang association. The word *stoma* in the stem and in option 1 is a clang association.
Content Area: Gastrointestinal System
Integrated Processes: Nursing Process: Evaluation
Client Need: Physiological Integrity; Basic Care and Comfort
Cognitive Level: Application

13. **ANSWER: 2.**
Rationales:
1. Clean, not sterile, gloves should be worn when collecting a stool specimen to protect the caregiver from the patient's blood or body fluids.
2. A stool specimen should be transported to the laboratory promptly because bacteriological changes may alter test results if testing is delayed.
3. The patient should be encouraged to defecate into a clean, dry bedpan and should be taught not to contaminate the stool specimen with urine, water, or toilet paper, which may alter test results.
4. Only 1 inch of formed stool or 15 to 30 mL of liquid stool is necessary to complete commonly ordered tests on stool.
TEST-TAKING TIP: Identify the clang associations. The word *specimen* in the stem and in options 1 and 2 are clang associations.
Content Area: Gastrointestinal System
Integrated Processes: Nursing Process: Implementation
Client Need: Physiological Integrity; Reduction of Risk Potential
Cognitive Level: Application

14. **ANSWER: 1.**
Rationales:
1. The patient is experiencing perceived constipation and believes she needs to take milk of magnesia to ensure a daily bowel movement. This practice most likely caused the
patient to become dehydrated. Hypovolemia most likely precipitated the "fainting" episode. All of the laboratory results indicate dehydration. The Hb of 16.8 g/dL is higher than the expected range of 12 to 16 g/dL for an older adult female. This is because the total blood volume is decreased with dehydration, but the red blood cell count remains the same. The Hct of 47 percent is higher than the expected range of 34 to 46 percent for an older adult female. This is because the total blood volume is decreased with dehydration, but the red blood cell count remains the same. A creatinine of 1.3 mg/dL is higher than the expected range of 0.5 to 1.2 mg/dL, indicating dehydration secondary to hemoconcentration. A BUN of 46 mg/dL is higher than the expected range of 8 to 21 mg/dL, indicating dehydration secondary to hemoconcentration. The potassium level of 3.4 mEq/L is lower than the expected range of 3.5 to 5.0 mEq/L for an older adult. This occurs when a patient abuses laxatives, causing potassium wasting. The sodium level of 147 mEq/L is higher than the expected range of 135 to 145 mEq/L for an older adult. This occurs with diarrhea because water is lost in excess of the loss of sodium.
2. This intervention will not prevent this event from occurring again in the future. The underlying cause of the patient's fainting must be identified.
3. Although the patient's psychosocial integrity is important, it is not the priority. The underlying cause of the patient's fainting must be identified.
4. Although this teaching is important for safety reasons, it is not the priority. The underlying cause of the patient's fainting must be identified.
TEST-TAKING TIP: Identify the word in the stem that sets a priority. The word *most* in the stem sets a priority. Identify the unique option. Option 1 is unique because it is the only option that attempts to collect more information from the patient.
Content Area: Gastrointestinal System
Integrated Processes: Communication/Documentation; Nursing Process: Assessment
Client Need: Health Promotion and Maintenance
Cognitive Level: Analysis

15. **ANSWER: 3.**
Rationales:
1. One stalk of celery has 1.1 g of fiber, which is significantly less than the amount of fiber in the correct answer.
2. One-half of a medium-size grapefruit has 3.1 g of fiber, which is significantly less than the amount of fiber in the correct answer.
3. One cup of bran cereal has 19.9 g of fiber. This food has the highest amount of fiber from among the foods in the options presented.
4. One-quarter cup of sunflower seeds has 3 g of fiber, which is significantly less than the amount of fiber in the correct answer.
TEST-TAKING TIP: Identify the word in the stem that sets a priority. The word *most* in the stem sets a priority.
Content Area: Gastrointestinal System
Integrated Processes: Teaching/Learning; Nursing Process: Implementation
Client Need: Physiological Integrity; Basic Care and Comfort
Cognitive Level: Analysis

16. ANSWER: 2.

Rationales:

1. A bowel prep for a lower GI series (barium enema) generally involves a clear liquid diet for 24 hours before the test and then NPO for the 8 hours before the test.

2. Stool will be chalky white for 24 to 48 hours after the test. After the barium is completely evacuated, stool returns to its characteristic brown color.

3. The patient starts on the left side, then moves to the back, and then prone during the test; the fluoroscope follows the progress of the barium and x-rays are taken.

4. The patient does not drink barium. Barium is instilled rectally via a rectal tube.

Content Area: Gastrointestinal System

Integrated Processes: Teaching/Learning; Nursing Process: Implementation

Client Need: Physiological Integrity; Reduction of Risk Potential

Cognitive Level: Application

17. ANSWER: 1.

Rationales:

1. This stoma is in the sigmoid colon. The fecal matter (effluent) has passed through most of the large intestine. Fluid within the effluent is reabsorbed in the large intestine, leaving a formed to solid fecal matter.

2. This stoma is in the descending colon. Some fluid in the fecal matter has been reabsorbed in the large intestine. The consistency of fecal matter will be soft to formed.

3. This stoma is in the ascending colon. The fecal matter has not passed through enough of the large intestine for fluid to be reabsorbed. The fecal matter will have a liquid consistency.

4. This stoma is in the ileum of the small intestine (ileostomy). The fecal matter has not yet reached the large intestine where fluid within the fecal matter is reabsorbed; therefore, the fecal matter will have a liquid consistency.

Content Area: Gastrointestinal System

Integrated Processes: Nursing Process: Evaluation

Client Need: Physiological Integrity; Physiological Adaptation

Cognitive Level: Analysis

18. ANSWER: 2.

Rationales:

1. One-half cup cooked carrots has 3.4 g of fiber; this is about half the fiber of the vegetable that is the correct answer.

2. One-half cup cooked spinach has 7 g of fiber; this is twice as much fiber as the vegetables in the options that are distractors.

3. One-half cup cooked zucchini has 3 g of fiber; this is less than half the fiber of the vegetable that is the correct answer.

4. Two-thirds cup cooked cabbage has 3 g of fiber; this is less than half the fiber of the vegetable that is the correct answer.

Content Area: Gastrointestinal System

Integrated Processes: Teaching/Learning; Nursing Process: Evaluation

Client Need: Physiological Integrity; Basic Care and Comfort

Cognitive Level: Analysis

19. ANSWER: 1, 3.

Rationales:

1. Three graham crackers contain 3.1 g of fiber and should be avoided when experiencing diarrhea; fiber provides bulk that probably will prolong the diarrhea.

2. Chicken breasts contain a small amount of fiber.

3. One-half cup of cooked kidney beans contain 9.7 g of fiber and should be avoided when experiencing diarrhea; fiber provides bulk that is likely to prolong the diarrhea.

4. Scallops contain no fiber.

5. Yogurt contains no fiber.

TEST-TAKING TIP: Identify the words in the stem that indicate negative polarity. The words *avoid* and *eliminated* in the stem indicate negative polarity.

Content Area: Gastrointestinal System

Integrated Processes: Teaching/Learning; Nursing Process: Evaluation

Client Need: Physiological Integrity; Basic Care and Comfort

Cognitive Level: Application

20. ANSWER: 1.

Rationales:

1. One-half cup of cooked peas has 6.7 g of fiber; this food contains the greatest amount of fiber of the foods presented in the options.

2. One small apple has 3 g of fiber; this food contains less fiber than the food that is the correct answer.

3. Ten cherries have 1.2 g of fiber; this food contains less fiber than the food that is the correct answer.

4. One-half cup of cooked asparagus has 1.7 g of fiber; this food contains less fiber than the food that is the correct answer.

Content Area: Gastrointestinal System

Integrated Processes: Teaching/Learning; Nursing Process: Evaluation

Client Need: Physiological Integrity; Basic Care and Comfort

Cognitive Level: Analysis

21. ANSWER: 4.

Rationales:

1. The nurse can lay a 4 × 4 gauze over, not tucked into, the stoma to help absorb any leaking effluent; this will help keep the skin clean and dry. Tucking gauze into the stoma may damage the mucous membranes and should be avoided.

2. A ½-inch distance from the flange edge to the stoma is too wide a distance; it will permit digestive enzymes to contact too much peristomal skin. The flange opening should be no more than ⅛-inch to ¼-inch clearance around the stoma. This distance does not infringe on the stoma and yet protects as much skin as possible around the stoma from digestive enzymes contained in stool.

3. The advantage of a two-piece ostomy appliance is that the bag can be disconnected, the area and bag cleansed, and the bag replaced without having to remove the faceplate. The bag is not emptied from the bottom. Using a two-piece ostomy appliance reduces the risk of skin injury caused by repeated removal and application of a bag directly to the skin.

4. A faceplate changed every 3 to 5 days ensures adherence of the faceplate to the skin. The adhesive backing

may loosen from the skin beyond 3 to 5 days, allowing leakage underneath the faceplate, resulting in skin excoriation.

TEST-TAKING TIP: Identify the clang association. The word *appliance* in the stem and in option 4 is a clang association. More often than not, the option with the clang association is the correct answer. Examine option 4 carefully.

Content Area: Gastrointestinal System
Integrated Processes: Nursing Process: Implementation
Client Need: Physiological Integrity; Physiological Adaptation
Cognitive Level: Application

22. **ANSWER: 1.**
Rationales:
1. Intestinal peristalsis increases behind a fecal impaction in an attempt to move the fecal mass toward the rectum. As pressure builds behind the impaction, fluid moves around the mass toward the rectum, resulting in the passage of brown liquid.
2. Although there is a lack of a bowel movement with a fecal impaction, this occurs also with constipation without a fecal impaction.
3. Although abdominal distension occurs with a fecal impaction, this occurs also with constipation without a fecal impaction.
4. The patient may not have a feeling of rectal fullness with a fecal impaction; this depends on where the impaction is located.

TEST-TAKING TIP: Identify the word in the stem that sets a priority. The word *most* in the stem sets a priority.

Content Area: Gastrointestinal System
Integrated Processes: Nursing Process: Assessment
Client Need: Physiological Integrity; Basic Care and Comfort
Cognitive Level: Application

23. **ANSWER: 1, 4, 5.**
Rationales:
1. Shrimp contains no fiber.
2. One-half cup of cooked chickpeas contains 6 g of fiber and should be avoided when experiencing diarrhea. Chickpeas will provide bulk that may prolong the diarrhea.
3. Two slices of rye bread contain approximately 5.8 g of fiber and should be avoided when experiencing diarrhea. Rye bread will provide bulk that may prolong the diarrhea.
4. A milk shake contains no fiber.
5. Cottage cheese contains no fiber.

Content Area: Gastrointestinal System
Integrated Processes: Teaching/Learning; Nursing Process: Evaluation
Client Need: Physiological Integrity; Basic Care and Comfort
Cognitive Level: Application

24. **ANSWER: 2.**
Rationales:
1. Tap water is hypotonic, which can cause water intoxication and fluid and electrolyte imbalance, not excessive interstitial fluid loss. In addition, this is medical terminology that may not be understood.
2. The large volume of instilled tap water distends the colon, which, in turn, stimulates peristalsis; it also softens feces. This terminology should be understood.

3. Soap is not added to a tap-water enema. Soapsuds enemas work by irritating the mucosa and distending the colon, which, in turn, stimulates peristalsis. In addition, this is medical terminology that may not be understood.
4. A tap-water enema is hypotonic, not hypertonic. In addition, this is medical terminology that may not be understood.

Content Area: Gastrointestinal System
Integrated Processes: Communication/Documentation; Nursing Process: Implementation
Client Need: Physiological Integrity; Basic Care and Comfort
Cognitive Level: Application

25. **ANSWER: 3.**
Rationale:
Solve the problem by using the formula for ratio and proportion.

$$\frac{\text{Desire 15 mg}}{\text{Have 5 mg}} \times \frac{\text{x tablet}}{\text{1 tablet}}$$

$$5x = 15 \times 1$$
$$5x = 15$$
$$x = 15 \div 5$$
$$x = 3 \text{ tablets}$$

Content Area: Gastrointestinal System
Integrated Processes: Nursing Process: Planning
Client Need: Physiological Integrity; Pharmacological and Parenteral Therapies
Cognitive Level: Application

26. **ANSWER: 4.**
Rationales:
1. Washing the anal area before collecting the specimen will wash away the pinworm eggs deposited on the skin around the anus.
2. This is unsafe. Inserting a cotton-tipped swab into the anus and rectum places the patient at risk for injury to the intestinal mucosa.
3. The eggs of pinworms, not the actual worms, are collected in the tape test for pinworms; the tape test for pinworms does not require sterile technique.
4. Collecting the specimen upon awakening and before toileting and bathing, using a piece of clear scotch tape pressed against the anus and then applied to a slide, is the standard test for pinworm eggs deposited on the perianal skin surface during the night.

TEST-TAKING TIP: Identify the options that are opposites. Options 3 and 4 are opposites. Option 3 describes steps that are implemented immediately upon awakening and option 4 describes actions that are implemented at night. More often than not, the correct answer is one of the opposites. Examine options 3 and 4 carefully.

Content Area: Gastrointestinal System
Integrated Processes: Teaching/Learning; Nursing Process: Implementation
Client Need: Physiological Integrity; Reduction of Risk Potential
Cognitive Level: Application

27. ANSWER: 2, 3, 4, 5.
Rationales:
1. Cranberry juice is not associated with a blockage of the intestines after a colostomy. Cranberry juice is a beverage that may help control gas or odor.
2. Green beans are considered a "stringy" food that has the potential to cause an intestinal obstruction after a colostomy and, therefore, should be avoided. However, if the beans are cut into tiny pieces and chewed thoroughly, a patient may tolerate green beans without experiencing an obstruction.
3. Fresh pears should be avoided because their tough skin is associated with blockage of the intestines after a colostomy. However, if the skin is removed, the inside of the pear is cut into tiny pieces, and the fruit is chewed thoroughly, a patient may tolerate a pear without experiencing an obstruction.
4. Popcorn should be avoided because it produces a large amount of undigested fiber and could cause a blockage of the intestine after a colostomy.
5. Rice is stripped of its fiber when processed and is a starchy food associated with alleviating diarrhea. Because it is low in fiber, it can reduce transit time of stool through the intestines, allowing more time for fluid absorption and harder and dryer stool. Excessively hard, dry stool can cause an intestinal obstruction.
TEST-TAKING TIP: Identify the word in the stem that indicates negative polarity. The word *avoid* in the stem indicates negative polarity. The question is asking, "Which foods should *not be eaten* because they can cause an intestinal blockage?"
Content Area: Gastrointestinal System
Integrated Processes: Teaching/Learning; Nursing Process: Implementation
Client Need: Physiological Integrity; Basic Care and Comfort
Cognitive Level: Application

28. ANSWER: 2.
Rationales:
1. Although you want to teach the patient to expect an increase in flatus after the procedure, it is not the priority.
2. These signs and symptoms may indicate bowel perforation, hemorrhage, or infection and should be reported immediately to the primary health-care provider.
3. High-fiber food should be avoided for 48 hours, not for a week, after the procedure if a polyp was excised or biopsy was taken during the procedure. High-fiber food has roughage which can injure the site of the polyp or biopsy, causing bleeding.
4. The patient can lift light items but not heavy items for a week after the procedure if a polyp was excised or biopsy was taken during the procedure. This reduces the risk of bleeding at the site of the polyp or biopsy.
TEST-TAKING TIP: Identify the option with a specific determiner. Option 4 contains the word *anything* which is a specific determiner.
Content Area: Gastrointestinal System
Integrated Processes: Teaching/Learning; Nursing Process: Implementation
Client Need: Physiological Integrity; Reduction of Risk Potential
Cognitive Level: Application

29. ANSWER: 4.
Rationales:
1. Chyme is the matter produced by gastric digestion of food.
2. Melena is dark, tarry stool caused by digested blood.
3. Meconium is the term used to describe the initial stool passed by an infant. It is greenish black in color and generally occurs during the first two to three days after birth.
4. Steatorrhea is frothy, odorous stool with an excessive amount of fat; this is associated with malabsorption syndromes.
Content Area: Gastrointestinal System
Integrated Processes: Communication/Documentation; Nursing Process: Implementation
Client Need: Safe and Effective Care Environment; Management of Care
Cognitive Level: Knowledge

30. ANSWER: 1, 2.
Rationales:
1. Administering a medication requires a prescription from a primary health-care provider and is a dependent function of the nurse.
2. A patient's activity level is ordered by a primary health-care provider. Providing for a patient's activity, such as ambulating, sitting in a chair, or remaining in bed, is a dependent function of the nurse.
3. Although providing a diet is based on an order by a primary health-care provider and therefore a dependent function of the nurse, suggesting which foods on the tray that are best for a patient with constipation is associated with patient teaching. Patient teaching is an independent function of the nurse.
4. Implementing some measures to prevent complications of immobility, such as having a patient turn from side to side, does not require an order from a primary health-care provider and therefore is an independent function of the nurse. Movement promotes intestinal peristalsis.
5. Assisting a patient with toileting is an independent function of the nurse. Responding to the urge to defecate helps prevent constipation because the longer feces remains in the large intestine, the more water is reabsorbed, resulting in hard stools.
Content Area: Gastrointestinal System
Integrated Processes: Nursing Process: Implementation
Client Need: Physiological Integrity; Basic Care and Comfort
Cognitive Level: Analysis

31. ANSWER: 3.
Rationales:
1. Although this regimen may cause a fluid volume deficit, it is not as serious a consequence as another option presented. Fluids can be taken up to 8 hours before the test and intravenous fluids are administered during the test.
2. Although abdominal cramps may result from the cleansing regimen, it will not precipitate a life-threatening condition.
3. Sodium phosphate (Fleet Phospho-Soda) is a saline osmotic that draws water into the intestinal lumen. Bisacodyl (Dulcolax) is an intestinal stimulant that also expands intestinal fluid volume. These medications act

together to pull sodium into the intestinal lumen where it is excreted, resulting in a decreased serum sodium level (hyponatremia). Sodium is essential in the functioning of the sodium-potassium pump, which is essential for muscle contraction. Hyponatremia can interfere with the contraction of the heart, resulting in dysrhythmias that can be life threatening.

4. This bowel cleansing regimen will result in stools that will be liquid in consistency. This is the purpose of the regimen; an empty bowel allows for inspection of the intestinal mucosa without being impeded by feces.

TEST-TAKING TIP: Identify the obscure clang association. The words *sodium* in the stem and *hypernatremia* in option 2 is an obscure clang association.

Content Area: Gastrointestinal System
Integrated Processes: Nursing Process: Evaluation
Client Need: Physiological Integrity; Pharmacological and Parenteral Therapies
Cognitive Level: Application

32. **ANSWER: 3.**
Rationales:
1. Specimens do not need to be collected in the morning. A patient may not have a bowel movement every day. Specimens are collected from three consecutive bowel movements.
2. A thin layer of stool is all that is necessary to achieve an accurate result.
3. **Nonsteroidal anti-inflammatory medications and aspirin should be avoided before testing for occult blood because these medications can cause false-positive results.**
4. A blue, not red, color in reaction to the reagent indicates the presence of occult blood.

TEST-TAKING TIP: Identify the clang association. The word *test* in the stem and in options 2 and 3 are clang associations. Examine these options carefully.

Content Area: Gastrointestinal System
Integrated Processes: Teaching/Learning; Nursing Process: Implementation
Client Need: Physiological Integrity; Reduction of Risk Potential
Cognitive Level: Application

33. **ANSWER: 4, 5, 3, 2, 1.**
Rationales:
4. **Clarifying exactly when the patient had the last bowel movement should be the first intervention to determine if the patient is constipated. Some patients believe that they are constipated if they do not have a bowel movement every day or every other day.**
5. After constipation is confirmed, other issues related to constipation (e.g., amount of fiber and fluid in the diet and the amount of exercise) can be explored.
3. After constipation has been confirmed and other data collected, the nurse can make recommendations to help resolve the problem. Constipation is a human response

that nurses are legally permitted to treat. Adequate fluid intake promotes a soft stool.
2. A laxative should not be prescribed until other less invasive interventions are attempted.
1. Obtaining an order for an enema should be the last intervention to be performed in the list above. Less invasive interventions should be attempted first.

Content Area: Gastrointestinal System
Integrated Processes: Communication/Documentation; Nursing Process: Planning
Client Need: Physiological Integrity; Basic Care and Comfort
Cognitive Level: Analysis

34. **ANSWER: 3.**
Rationales:
1. Prolonging the time between opiate administrations will decrease constipation but will reduced its pain control abilities. Pain must be treated effectively and interventions implemented to cope with the potential side effects.
2. This is not as important an intervention when compared to the information in another option. Yogurt may help constipation, but it is more effective when administering antibiotics to maintain the normal intestinal flora.
3. **An opioid will decrease peristalsis; therefore, a high-fiber diet is most effective in preventing constipation because it increases the bulk in the intestine, increasing peristalsis.**
4. This is unnecessary. The administration of oxygen will not prevent respiratory depression associated with the administration of morphine sulfate. If respiratory depression occurs, oxygen may be administered to increase oxygen to body cells.

Content Area: Gastrointestinal System
Integrated Processes: Teaching/Learning; Nursing Process: Implementation
Client Need: Physiological Integrity; Pharmacological and Parenteral Therapies
Cognitive Level: Application

35. **ANSWER: 1.**
Rationales:
1. **For a nasogastric tube to function effectively, the tubing must be connected appropriately, intact, and patent to allow drainage to flow to the collection container.**
2. Wall suction establishes negative pressure, which facilitates the flow of fluid from the patient to the collection container; it does not rely on gravity.
3. Wall suction works by establishing negative pressure. The position of the patient is irrelevant.
4. Humidification is associated with the administration of oxygen, not removal of fluid from the stomach via a nasogastric tube to intermittent wall suction.

Content Area: Gastrointestinal System
Integrated Processes: Nursing Process: Implementation
Client Need: Physiological Integrity; Reduction of Risk Potential
Cognitive Level: Application

Pain, Comfort, Rest, and Sleep

Bruxism—Repetitive clenching and grinding of teeth that last 4 to 5 seconds, usually occurring during stage II nonrapid eye movement sleep.

Dyssomnias—Sleep disorders related to abnormal physiological mechanisms that regulate sleep and wakefulness.

Insomnia—Inability to fall asleep, remain asleep, or go back to sleep, resulting in an inadequate quantity or quality of sleep.

Narcolepsy—Sudden uncontrollable urge to sleep during the day, lasting seconds to 30 minutes.

Parasomnias—Disorders characterized by patterns of abnormal behaviors that intrude on sleep or occur at the threshold between waking and sleeping.

Pain—An unpleasant emotional or sensory experience initiated by potential or actual tissue damage.

Restless leg syndrome—Uncontrollable movements of the legs when resting or just before onset of sleep.

Sleep apnea—Periodic interruption of breathing when sleeping that lasts from 10 seconds to 2 minutes and occurs 50 to 600 times a night.

Sleep deprivation—Situation in which a person experiences extended periods of time without sustained, natural, recurring states of unconsciousness.

Somnambulism (sleepwalking)—Episodic walking around while asleep with minimal awareness of surroundings.

I. Concepts Related to Pain

Pain, which is commonly referred to as the "fifth vital sign," is an unpleasant emotional or sensory experience initiated by potential or actual tissue damage. It is a subjective experience and, therefore, its presence and characteristics are whatever the patient says they are. Nurses must understand the factors that influence pain, the proper method for performing a comprehensive assessment of pain, and independent and dependent nursing interventions that can help to relieve patients' pain.

A. Types
   1. Nociceptive.
      a. Results from stimulation of pain receptors at the site of trauma, ischemia, or inflammation.
      b. Involves visceral pain (i.e., from internal organs) and somatic pain (i.e., from skin, connective tissue, muscles, and bones).
      c. Commonly described as aching, pounding, dull, or gnawing.

   2. Neuropathic.
      a. Results from repeated transmission of pain signals from a site of injury that affected nerve cells.
      b. Associated with chronic problems, such as phantom limb sensation, brain attack, and diabetes.
      c. Commonly described as burning, numbness, or "pins and needles."

B. Pain Threshold
   1. Smallest stimulus that is needed to establish a perception of pain within a person.
   2. Varies from person to person but usually does not vary within a person.

C. Pain Tolerance
   1. Maximal amount of pain a person is willing to endure before seeking relief.
   2. Varies from person to person and within a person, depending on the situation.

A Painful Stimulus and the Perception of Pain:

Pain-sensitive nociceptors are found in the skin, subcutaneous tissue, walls of arteries, joints, and many internal organs. When a mechanical, thermal, or chemical stress damages tissues, the tissues release biochemical mediators (e.g., bradykinin, histamine, and prostaglandins) that activate nociceptors in adjacent tissue. This activation converts the noxious stimulus into an electrical stimulus (transduction). Peripheral nerves then carry the pain message to the dorsal horn of the spinal cord and then via the spinothalamic tracts of the spinal cord to the brain stem and thalamus (transmission). Finally, the pain message travels from the thalamus to the brain, where the pain message is perceived (perception). It involves the somatosensory cortex, where physical sensations are perceived and interpreted; the limbic system, which is involved in emotional reactions to the pain message; and the frontal cortex, which is involved with the affective expression of pain. These physiological processes involved in pain perception are known as *nociception.*

D. Factors That Influence Pain Perception
   1. Emotions.
      a. Influenced by previous pain experiences.
      b. Common emotions that may increase pain perception include anxiety, fear, anger, depression, helplessness, and hopelessness.
   2. Fatigue: Decreases a person's coping abilities, which increases pain intensity.
   3. Ethnic and cultural values.
      a. Behavior and beliefs related to pain are commonly learned through interaction with members of the family and social groups; however, people are individuals and may not reflect the values of their ethnic or cultural group.
      b. May influence communication of pain, such as demonstrative or silent endurance, extent of family involvement, and intensity of pain willing to be tolerated before seeking relief.
   4. Extent of physical and emotional support.
      a. Supportive family, friends, and health team members may help to decrease perception of and increase tolerance to pain.
      b. Lack of empathy may increase intensity of pain.
   5. Environment.
      a. A strange environment, such as a hospital or long-term care facility, has noises, odors, lights, and activity that can increase anxiety, which may increase pain intensity.
      b. A familiar environment, such as one's home and bed, may decrease the intensity of pain.
   6. Spirituality or religious beliefs.
      a. Pain and suffering may be perceived as penance for one's wrongdoings or an avenue to salvation.
      b. Prayers and religious rituals may offer comfort and hope.
   7. Multiplicity of stressors: Intensity of pain increases as the number of issues impacting on an individual's ability to adapt increase.
   8. Developmental level: Age and experiential background influence pain perception and physical and behavioral responses to pain (Table 23.1).

Table 23.1 Developmental Variations Related to Pain and Nursing Care

Developmental Level	Perception of Pain and Pain-Related Behaviors	Nursing Interventions
Infants	• Preterm infants: May have a greater sensitivity to pain. • Newborns: Have the same sensitivity to pain as infants and older children. • Are unable to convey characteristics of pain, such as location, intensity, and description. • Respond by increased physical activity, pulling away, resisting stimuli, quivering chin, and crying.	• Encourage mother to hold the infant to provide comfort. • Encourage skin-to-skin contact against the chest of the mother (kangaroo care) for newborns. • Use a sucrose pacifier. • Play comforting auditory stimuli, such as soft music or heartbeat.
Toddlers and Preschoolers	• Perceive pain as a threat to safety and security. • May consider pain as punishment. • Begin to have the ability to point to location of pain and describe intensity and characteristics. • Toddlers: Respond by crying, screaming, behavioral regression, and difficulty being comforted. • Preschoolers: Responds by a low frustration level, crying, struggling against restraint, and verbal and physical aggressiveness.	• Encourage the parents to remain with the child. • Be honest about the possibility of and acknowledge the presence of pain or discomfort. • Hold to provide comfort. • Use distractions. • Correct misconceptions about pain.

Table 23.1 Developmental Variations Related to Pain and Nursing Care—cont'd

Developmental Level	Perception of Pain and Pain-Related Behaviors	Nursing Interventions
School-Aged Children	• Able to convey characteristics of pain, such as location, intensity, and description. • Understand simple explanations for pain. • May regress to an earlier stage of development as a coping mechanism.	• Provide emotional support. • Role play what will happen when a therapeutic painful procedure is performed and what it will feel like.
Adolescents	• Desire to appear brave in front of others, especially peers. • May be slow to admit the presence of pain.	• Encourage expression of feelings. • Allay fears and anxiety. • Provide privacy during painful procedures.
Adults	• May ignore pain as a result of the desire to be strong, fear of the cause of the pain, or beliefs associated with analgesic use.	• Encourage expression of feelings. • Explore beliefs and correct myths. • Encourage independence as indicated.
Older Adults	• May accept pain as part of aging, which it is not; pain in older adults is related to health problems. • May have decreased sensitivity to painful stimuli. • May ignore pain because fear of treatment, lifestyle changes, or fear of becoming dependent.	

E. Nursing Care of Patients Who Are In Pain

🛑 1. Accept the patient's perception of pain because it is a subjective symptom that is what the patient says it is.

🛑 2. Be nonjudgmental; do not impose own attitudes, beliefs, or expectations onto a patient.

3. Assess characteristics of pain.
   a. Onset.
      (1) Ask, "When did the pain start?"
      (2) Abrupt or gradual onset.
   b. Location.
      (1) Ask, "Where do you feel the pain?"
      (2) Identify the origin and location of pain (Table 23.2 and Fig. 23.1).
      (3) Use anatomical landmarks.
   c. Quality.
      (1) Ask, "What does the pain feel like?" and "Is this pain different than the pain that you have been experiencing all along?"
      (2) Possible descriptions include burning, stabbing, throbbing, crushing, pressure, sharp, dull, and achy.
      (3) Do not give the patient suggestions.

Table 23.2 Origin of Pain

Type	Location	Examples
Superficial or Cutaneous	• Skin or subcutaneous tissue.	• Superficial cut.
Visceral	• Deep internal pain receptors.	• Abdominal organ cancer. • Labor pain.
Somatic	• Ligaments, tendons, blood vessels, and bones.	• Arthritis. • Bone cancer.
Radiating	• Arises in one site and extends to another.	• Sciatic pain from lumbar vertebrae. • Pain associated with lymphatic streaking.
Referred	• Arises in one site but is felt in a distant site (See Figure 23.1).	• Heart ischemia felt as pain in jaw. • Appendicitis causing pain at McBurney's point (halfway between the umbilicus and right anterior iliac crest).
Phantom	• Perceived as arising from a site that was surgically removed.	• Sensations or pain in a limb that was amputated.
Psychogenic	• Perception of pain without a physical cause.	• Any site perceived by the patient.

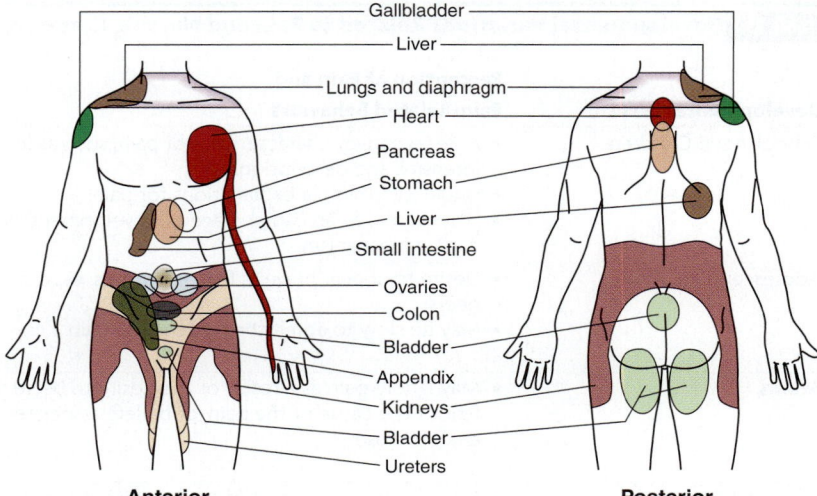

Fig 23.1 Sites of referred pain. (From Burton and Ludwig [2011]. *Fundamentals of nursing care: Concepts, connections & skills.* Philadelphia: F. A. Davis, with permission.)

(4) Is helpful in diagnosing illness because there are commonalities in perceptions of pain, such as with myocardial infarction (crushing); intestinal infections (cramping); urinary tract infection (burning); and arthritis (aching).
d. Intensity.
  (1) Ask, "How severe is the pain?"
  (2) Use an objective scale to provide objectivity and consistency in assessments.
    (a) For individuals aged 12 years and older, use a numerical pain scale (Fig. 23.2).
    (b) For children of different ages, use the Wong-Baker FACES Pain Sale (Fig. 23.3).
    (c) For infants and children from birth to 3 years, cognitively impaired patients, and those who are unable to use other scales, use the FLACC Pain Scale (Fig. 23.4).
e. Duration.
  (1) Ask "How long does the pain last?"
  (2) Seconds, minutes, hours, or days.
  (3) Identify characteristic associated with acute versus chronic pain (Table 23.3.)
f. Pattern.
  (1) Ask, "Is there a pattern to the pain?"
  (2) Continuous or intermittent, frequency, predictable occurrences, and time of day it occurs.

g. Precipitating factors.
  (1) Ask, "What initiates or increases the pain?"
  (2) Can be helpful in diagnosing the cause and/or location of pain.
    (a) Bending, lifting, and coughing: Vertebral pain.
    (b) Lying flat: Heartburn.
    (c) Valsalva maneuver: Hemorrhoids.
    (d) Deep breaths: Pancreatitis.
h. Relieving factors.
  (1) Ask, "What helps to diminish or eliminate the pain?"
  (2) Examples may include immobility, repositioning, eating or eliminating specific foods, analgesics, application of heat or cold, and repetitive behaviors, such as rocking, rubbing, and pacing.
i. Behavioral effects.
  (1) Identify what behavioral indicators of pain are being exhibited.
  (2) Vocalizations, such as moaning, grunting, and crying; body movements, such as restlessness, muscle tension, wringing the hands, guarding and holding or rubbing a part of the body; social interactions, such as withdrawal, avoiding conversation, and reduced attention span; facial expressions, such as wrinkled forehead, tightly closed eyes, grimacing, clenched teeth, and open mouth associated with crying.
4. Validate the patient's pain.
5. Provide emotional support and answer questions the patient has to relieve anxiety and fears.
6. Use distraction techniques, such as soft music, television, conversation, and play appropriate to the patient's developmental level.

No pain	Mild pain		Moderate pain		Severe pain		Worst pain
0	1 2	3	4 5	6	7 8	9	10

Fig 23.2 Numerical pain scale 0 to 10. (From Ward and Hisley [2009]. *Maternal-child nursing care, enhanced revised reprint.* Philadelphia: F. A. Davis, with permission.)

Wong-Baker FACES® Pain Rating Scale

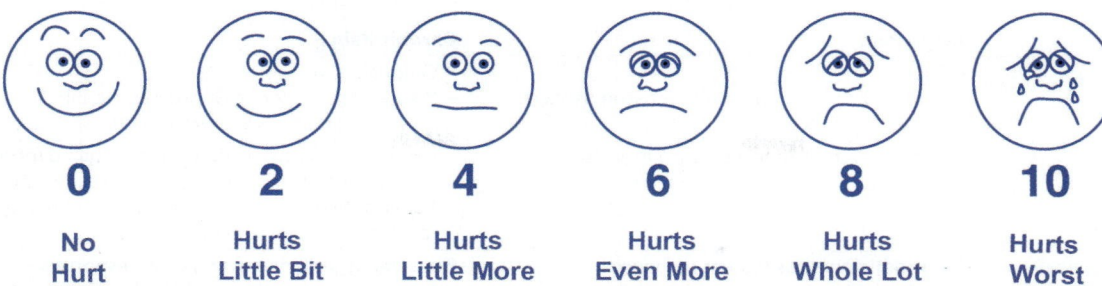

0	2	4	6	8	10
No Hurt	**Hurts Little Bit**	**Hurts Little More**	**Hurts Even More**	**Hurts Whole Lot**	**Hurts Worst**

Fig 23.3 Wong-Baker FACES pain rating scale. (From Hockenberry, M. J. and Wilson, D. [2009]. *Wong's essentials of pediatric nursing,* ed. 8. St. Louis, MO: Mosby. Used with permission.)

FLACC Behavioral Scale

Categories	Scoring		
	0	1	2
Face	No particular expression or smile	Occasional grimace or frown, withdrawn, disinterested	Frequent to constant frown, clenched jaw, quivering chin
Legs	Normal position or relaxed	Uneasy, restless, tense	Kicking, or legs drawn up
Activity	Lying quietly, normal position, moves easily	Squirming, shifting back and forth, tense	Arched, rigid, or jerking
Cry	No cry (awake or asleep)	Moans or whimpers, occasional complaint	Crying steadily, screams or sobs, frequent complaints
Consolability	Content, relaxed	Reassured by occasional touching, hugging, or being talked to, distractible	Difficult to console or comfort

Each of the 5 categories—(F) Face; (L) Legs; (A) Activity; (C) Cry; (C) Consolability—is scored from 0-2, which results in a total score between 0 and 10.

Fig 23.4 FLACC behavioral scale. (© 2002 The Regents of the University of Michigan. All Rights Reserved.)

7. Alter irritating stimuli, such as by limiting noise in the environment, closing curtains or doors, dimming environmental lights, and adjusting room temperature.
8. Teach the patient to use relaxation techniques, such as diaphragmatic breathing, guided imagery, and progressive muscle relaxation.
9. Provide cutaneous stimulation, such as back rubs, warm or cold applications, and transcutaneous electrical nerve stimulation (TENS), that uses the gate-control theory of pain to limit pain; with the exception of a back rub, these interventions require an order.
10. Ensure that the Five Rights of Medication Administration are met.
    a. Right drug: The World Health Organization (WHO) three-step analgesic ladder (Fig. 23.5). Although the ladder focuses on pain associated with cancer, it can be applied to pain from any cause.
       (1) Nonopioids: acetaminophen (Tylenol); NSAIDs, such as aspirin and ibuprofen (Advil, Motrin, Aleve). (See Table 23.6.)
       (2) Opioids: codeine, hydrocodone (Hycodan), oxycodone (OxyContin), hydromorphone (Dilaudid), and fentanyl (Duragesic). (See Table 23.7.)

Table 23.3 Comparison of Acute and Chronic Pain

	Acute Pain	Chronic Pain
Onset	• Rapid. • Related to potential or actual tissue damage.	• Gradual. • Related to a lingering or progressive illness. • May be related to no current tissue damage.
Duration	• Short length of time; usually 6 months or less. • Continuous, diminishes, and resolves.	• Long length of time; usually more than 6 months. • Continuous, recurring (exacerbations and remissions). • Relief difficult to achieve and never permanently resolves (intractable pain).
Patient's Physical Responses	Autonomic nervous system responses • Tachycardia. • Hyperpnea. • Hypertension. • Diaphoresis. • Dilated pupils. • Pressured speech.	Parasympathetic nervous system responses • Decreased pulse rate and blood pressure. • Variable breathing patterns. • Constricted pupils. • Slow, monotonous speech.
Patient's Behavioral Responses	• Restlessness. • Anxiety. • Guarding. • Groaning, wincing, or crying. • Grimacing. • Patient usually reports presence of pain.	• Usual or apathetic facial expression. • Resting or sleeping. • Attempting to focus on distracting activities. • Patient usually does not report presence of pain unless asked.
Psychological Impact	• Briefly impacts physical and emotional energy, but patient is usually able to cope knowing it will eventually end.	• Depletes physical and emotional resources because of no anticipated end. • May be permanently disabling, resulting in interruption in activities of daily living, employment, interpersonal relationships, and so on.
Response to Interventions	• Relief may occur in response to nursing interventions, such as repositioning, back rub, imagery, and distraction, if pain is mild. • Relief usually occurs due to health-care provider orders, such as medications and application of heat or cold.	• Often unresponsive to conventional interventions; relief may be difficult to achieve (intractable pain). • Requires multiple modalities. • Complementary and alternative modalities commonly used, such as acupuncture, therapeutic touch, imagery, yoga, hypnosis, and biofeedback.

(3) Adjuvant analgesics.

(a) Medications given to manage mild pain or concurrently with nonopioid or opioid analgesics to limit escalating doses of the nonopioid or opioid medication.

MAKING THE CONNECTION

Gate-Control Theory of Pain and Effectiveness of Cutaneous Stimulation Therapy:

The gate-control theory of pain claims that the transmission of pain impulses to the central nervous system is modulated by large A-delta fibers and small C fibers. These fibers terminate in the substantia gelatinosa of the dorsal horn cells of the spinal cord. Stimulation of the small C fibers opens the pain gate, enhancing the transmission and perception of pain. Stimulation of the large A-delta fibers through touch, vibration, and thermal stimuli cause the pain gate to close, diminishing the transmission and perception of pain. The large A-delta fibers are stimulated by cutaneous stimulation therapy, such as application of heat or cold, massage, and TENS.

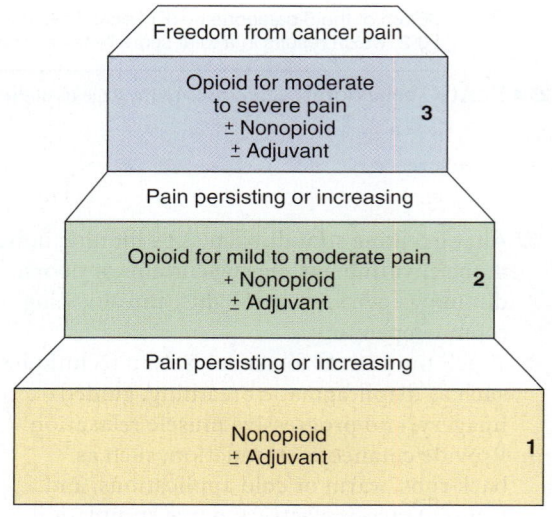

PAIN

Fig 23.5 The WHO's pain relief ladder. (Reprinted with permission from the World Health Organization [2012]. *The WHO's pain relief ladder.* Retrieved November 7, 2012, from www.who.int/cancer/palliative/painladder/en/.)

(b) Examples include anticonvulsants, antidepressants, psychostimulants, muscle relaxants, neuroleptics, and corticosteroids.

b. Right dose.

(1) Computed by weight for infants and children.

(2) Lower doses given to older adults due to decreased metabolism and elimination.

(3) Higher doses may be given for intractable pain.

c. Right route: Although analgesics can be given by any route, the intravenous route provides the most rapid relief from pain, and the transdermal route provides the most prolonged relief from pain.

d. Right time.

(1) Administer at time prescribed to maintain a continuous therapeutic blood level.

🛑 (2) Administer prn medications before pain becomes too intense because doing so helps them to be more effective than when they are administered when the pain is at the high end of a pain scale.

11. Maintain patient-controlled analgesia (PCA) to eliminate highs and lows in the intensity of pain and manage pain at a consistent level that is tolerable.

a. Teach the patient that the pump will deliver a basic dose (basal dose) of analgesic periodically and that compressing the trigger will deliver an extra dose as needed up to a certain point ("lockout"). A lockout prevents the delivery of excessive doses when the trigger is pushed prematurely (Fig. 23.6).

b. Ensure that the flow rate is set at the ordered rate.

c. Monitor the catheter insertion site, such as the peripheral vein or epidural space (Fig. 23.7), for integrity of the line; ensure that the catheter and tubing are not compressed or dislodged.

d. Monitor the number of times the patient uses the trigger in an attempt to relieve pain; excessive attempts to administer a bolus dose may occur when the basal rate is inadequate.

12. Correct misconceptions regarding tolerance as well as physical and psychological dependence.

13. Consult with the primary health-care provider regarding measures to prevent constipation, such as adequate dietary fiber intake, intake of 2 to 3 L of fluid daily, out-of-bed activities, and a stool softener if the patient is receiving an opioid.

🛑 14. Evaluate the patient's response to interventions, such as the extent of pain relief; decrease in vital signs,

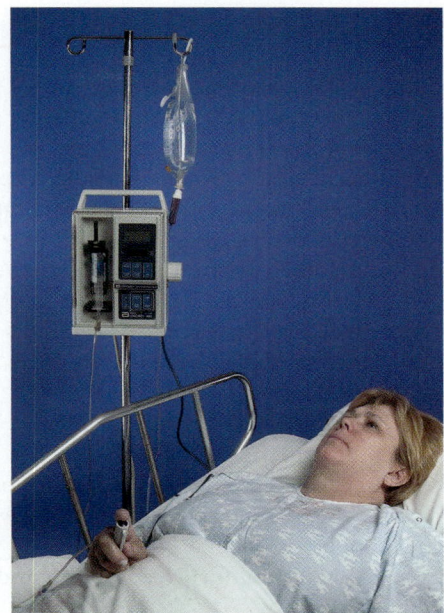

Fig 23.6 Patient-controlled analgesia. (From Wilkinson and Treas [2011]. *Fundamentals of nursing*, Vol. 2, 2nd ed. Philadelphia: F. A. Davis, with permission.)

particularly respirations; and presence of constipation if an opioid is given.

🛑 15. Notify the primary health-care provider if pain is not relieved or the respiratory rate is 10 or less breaths/minute; modify the plan as ordered.

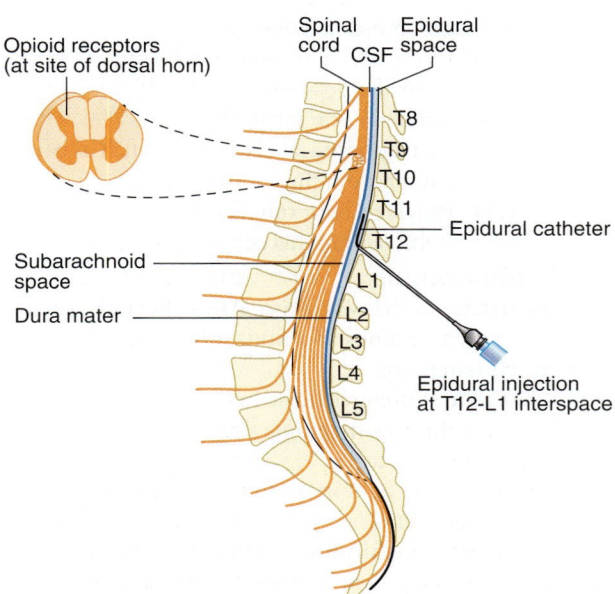

Fig 23.7 Placement of an epidural needle and catheter. (From Wilkinson and Treas [2011]. *Fundamentals of nursing*, Vol. 1, 2nd ed. Philadelphia: F. A. Davis, with permission.)

II. Concepts Related to Comfort

Comfort is more complex than just achieving a state of relief from discomfort or pain. It involves being at ease, content, and rising above discomforts when they cannot be lessened. Comfort exists when an individual expriences a feeling of well-being and a sense of being strengthened. Although comfort measures are defined by and are unique to an individual, some common nursing interventions provide comfort related to physical, environment, socio-cultural, and psychospiritual contexts. Patients expect nurses to help them achieve comfort and nurses should meet these expectations.

A. Dimensions of Comfort (Kolcaba [1994])
  1. Relief: Discomfort or pain is lessened.
  2. Ease: Absence of discomforts and feeling content.
  3. Transcendence: Rising above discomforts when they cannot be lessened.

B. Contexts in Which Comfort Needs Occur and Related Nursing Care
  1. Physical.
     a. Relates to homeostasis, bodily sensations, and basic physiological needs.
     b. Nursing care.
        (1) Administer prescribed medications.
        (2) Assist the patient to maintain regular bowel functioning.
        (3) Assist the patient to maintain regular urinary elimination.
        (4) Monitor and maintain fluid and electrolyte balance.
        (5) Ensure adequate oxygenation.
        (6) Provide hygiene, such as bathing, grooming, and oral care.
        (7) Ensure clean, smooth, dry linens.
        (8) Turn and position the patient.
        (9) Maintain skin integrity.
        (10) Manage physical discomforts such as pain, nausea, vomiting, and dyspnea.
        (11) Provide a back rub (See the section "Back Rub," later in this chapter, page 729).
  2. Environmental.
     a. Relates to that which is outside the body, such as surroundings, location, and ambiance.
     b. Nursing care.
        (1) Limit noxious noise in the environment.
        (2) Adjust room temperature to the patient's preference.
        (3) Modify light in room to the patient's preference.
        (4) Arrange furniture so that the patient has a window view if desired and possible.
        (5) Transport the patient to other surroundings if desired and able, such as to a lounge on the unit, coffee shop, or outside patio.
        (6) Provide environmental stimuli desired by the patient, such as music.
  3. Sociocultural.
     a. Relates to family and societal interpersonal relationships, family traditions, rituals, and cultural customs.
     b. Nursing care.
        🛑 (1) Be nonjudgmental and provide an attitude of caring.
        (2) Ensure continuity of care, such as sharing a written plan of care, assigning consistent caregivers, and performing thorough change of shift reports.
        (3) Provide the patient with information and teaching; include family members when appropriate.
        (4) Enhance support of family and friends by encouraging staying with the patient, involving family in direct care if desired by the patient, and ensuring liberal visiting hours if desired and beneficial to the patient.
        (5) Support cultural customs, such as involving the person who is viewed as the decision maker in the family, supporting the ability to wear culturally appropriate clothing or head coverings, and assigning a specific gender nurse, depending on the patient's culture.

DID YOU KNOW?

People often learn how to respond to pain based on interactions with family members and the culture in which they are raised. For example, in stoical cultures, people avoid demonstrating behavioral responses to or verbalizations of pain because their culture values bravery. Cultural groups generally associated with a stoical response to pain include European American, Native American, Irish, and Filipino cultures. People of Japanese heritage often bear pain without outward expressions as a matter of family honor and may have taboos against use of opioids for relief of pain. People who respond to pain in an outspoken manner may have been raised in a cultural where moaning, crying, and responding loudly to pain is common and acceptable. Cultural groups generally associated with an outspoken response to pain include Italian, Puerto Rican, and Jewish cultures. Although certain patterns of responses to pain are associated with certain cultural groups, the nurse must avoid expecting people of a particular heritage to respond in a manner related to their cultural group. Although nurses should strive to provide culturally competent care, the nurse must avoid stereotyping patients. Pain is a multidimensional experience and each patient should be cared for as a unique person with individual needs.

4. Psychospiritual.
   a. Relates to personal awareness of self, self-esteem, personal meanings in one's life, sexuality, and a relationship to a higher being or force.

   🛑 (1) View each patient as a unique individual.

   (2) Use communication techniques, especially active listening.
   (3) Support self-esteem, such as by treating the patient with respect, providing for privacy, ensuring confidentiality, and meeting patient needs as they arise.
   (4) Promote independence, such as involving the patient in planning and providing choices.
   (5) Increase relaxation to relieve anxiety, such as by encouraging activities, such as imagery, progressive muscle relaxation, and breathing techniques.
   (6) Provide emotional support and instill hope.
   (7) Accommodate the patient's desired religious practices, such as by contacting a spiritual advisor and arranging for distribution of Holy Communion or religious sacraments.

III. Concepts Related to Rest and Sleep

Rest and sleep are universal needs of all humans and are essential for physiological and psychological health. The amount of rest and sleep required by healthy individuals may vary, but all individuals with health problems usually require an increased need for rest and sleep (restorative sleep). Nurses must understand the basic concepts related to rest and sleep, particularly sleep cycles, to provide appropriate nursing care to patients.

A. Rest
1. Is a state when the body's physical and emotional energy expenditure is limited.
2. While resting, the individual is calm, relaxed, alert, and at ease physically and emotionally.
3. Promotes relaxation, conserves energy, and reduces physical and emotional stress; after an episode, the individual should feel refreshed.
4. May involve activities viewed by the individual as relaxing, such as praying, listening to music, watching television, reading, and engaging in needlework.
5. Although beneficial, rest is not as restorative as sleep because it does not filter external stimuli by altering the level of consciousness.

B. Sleep
1. Is a cyclical physiological process characterized by decreased perception and motor activity.
2. While sleeping, the individual exhibits minimal physical activity; has varied levels of consciousness; lacks awareness of the environment but responds selectively to external stimuli; and has varied physiological responses, depending on the stage of sleep.
3. Conserves energy, prevents fatigue, allows physiological processes (e.g., such as metabolism, vital signs) to slow down, and promotes physiological functioning, such as by boosting the immune system, stimulating protein synthesis for tissue repair, and increasing red blood cell production; after an episode of sleep, an individual should feel refreshed, rejuvenated, and satisfied with the amount of sleep achieved.
4. Promotes emotional functioning, such as by restoring balance among parts of the nervous system and reducing brain activity in areas that control emotions, decision making, and interpersonal communication.
5. Basic need required of all humans; amount needed varies by age and other individual factors, such as lifestyle, environment, and illness.
   (1) Newborns: Need 16 to 20 hours a day.
   (2) Adults: May need only 7 to 8 hours a day.
6. Sleep states/cycles.
   a. Sleep is preceded by a 10 to 30 minute period when an individual begins to feel sleepy.
   b. Sleep involves two stages: Nonrapid eye movement (NREM), which has four phases, and rapid eye movement (REM) (Table 23.4 and Table 23.5).
   c. Once asleep occurs, an individual usually has four or five complete sleep cycles per night, lasting 90 to 100 minutes each; with successive cycles, NREM stage I is excluded, NREM stages 3 and 4 shorten, and the REM stage lengthens (Fig. 23.8).
   d. Amount of time in each cycle varies over the life span; infants and children spend more time in stages 3 and 4 than older adults do.
7. Nursing care to promote effective sleep.
   a. Teach patients that sleep hygiene involves activities that control all behavioral and environmental factors that precede sleep or interfere with sleep.
   b. Teach the patient specific sleep hygiene practices.
      (1) Identify personal activity and sleep patterns.
      (2) Engage participation in activity and exercise during the day to reduce stress and deplete energy.
      (3) Avoid daytime naps unless they are less than 30-minute naps (power naps) to prevent insomnia at night.
      (4) Avoid physical exertion for 1 to 2 hours before bedtime to limit stimulation before attempting sleep.

Table 23.4 Comparison of NREM and REM Sleep

Characteristic	NREM Sleep	REM Sleep
Additional Name	• Slow-wave sleep because of the presence of delta waves.	• Paradoxical sleep because of high brain activity with decreased muscle tension.
Physiological Contribution	• Contributes to body tissue restoration. • Biological functions slow, protein synthesis increases, and growth hormone is released, promoting cellular and functional repair. • Parasympathetic nervous system dominates.	• Contributes to cognitive and emotional restoration. • Cerebral blood flow changes, cortical activity increases, and epinephrine is released, promoting filtering of stored information about the day's activities, memory storage, and learning. • Less restful than NREM sleep.
Eye Movements	• No eye movements or slow rolling movements.	• Periodic episodes of rapid eye movements.
Vital Signs	• Temperature, pulse, respirations, and blood pressure progressively decrease during stages 1 through 4.	• Pulse, respirations, and blood pressure increase and fluctuate.
Muscle Tone	• Muscles relax. • Occasionally, the whole body twitches.	• Skeletal muscles become immobile.

Clinical Manifestations of Deprivation	• Precipitate physiological deficiencies.
	  • Fatigue.
	  • Lethargy.
	  • Restlessness.
	  • Delayed wound healing.
	  • Immunosuppression.
	  • Increased sensitivity to pain.
	  • Tremors.
		• Precipitate cognitive, emotional, and behavioral changes.
		  • Anxiety.
		  • Irritability.
		  • Confusion.
		  • Apathy.
		  • Inability to concentrate.
		  • Combativeness.
		  • Disorientation.
		  • Delusions.
		  • Hallucinations.
		  • Paranoia.

Table 23.5 Stages of Sleep

Stage	Characteristics
NREM Stage 1 • Time between wakefulness and sleep. • 5 to 10 minutes long. • 5% of total sleep.	• Light sleep, easy to awaken. • Relaxed but aware of surroundings. • Regular, deep breathing. • Eyes may open and close slowly.
NREM Stage 2 • 10 to 15 minutes long. • 50% of total sleep.	• Light sleep, easy to awaken. • Muscles are relaxed. • Vital signs slightly decreased. • Eyes closed with almost no movement.
NREM Stage 3 • 5 to 15 minutes long. • 8% of total sleep.	• Deep sleep, difficult to awaken. • Muscles are more relaxed. • Vital signs decreased. • Snoring may occur. • Eyes closed with almost no movement.
NREM Stage 4 • 20 to 50 minutes long. • 11% of total sleep.	• Deepest sleep, difficult to awaken. • Confused when awakened. • Muscles are very relaxed. • Eyes closed with almost no movement.
REM, also called Stage 5 • 5 to 30 minutes long. • 25% of total sleep.	• Paradoxical sleep. • Reacts normally when awakened. • Large muscle inactivity; small muscles may twitch, deep-tendon reflexes are depressed. • Vital signs increase; pulse may be rapid and irregular, periods of apnea may occur. • Dreaming may occur.

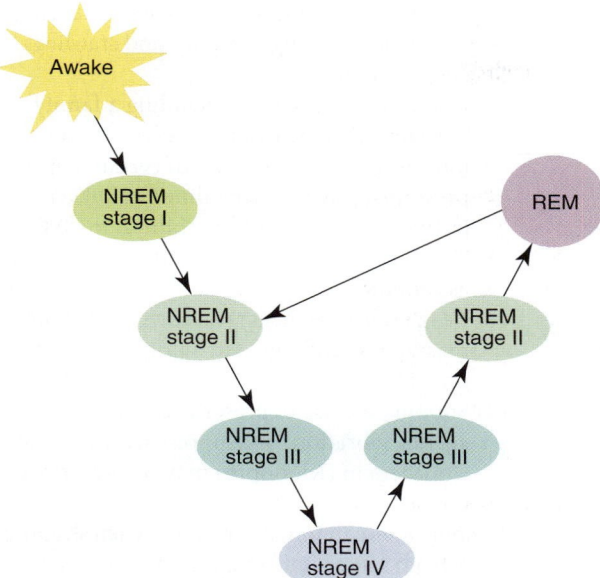

Fig 23.8 The normal adult sleep cycle. From Wilkinson and Treas (2011). *Fundamentals of nursing,* Vol. 1, 2nd ed. Philadelphia: F. A. Davis, with permission.

(5) Avoid heavy and spicy meals for 2 to 3 hours before bedtime to reduce the risk of gastrointestinal (GI) distress and esophageal reflux.

(6) Avoid nicotine and caffeine-containing foods and beverages, such as coffee, tea, colas, and chocolate, for 4 hours before bedtime to limit the stimulating effects of these products (half-life of nicotine is 1 to 2 hours).

(7) Avoid alcohol for 4 hours before bedtime to limit the need to void during the night because of alcohol's diuretic effect and to limit early awakening.

(8) Consume products containing sleep-promoting constituents: Small snack of carbohydrates and protein, such as cheese and crackers; carbohydrates limit the sensation of hunger while protein reduces the sugar boost of the carbohydrate.

(9) Establish a daily bedtime routine, such as reading, taking a warm bath, listening to music, performing specific hygiene practices, and choosing a consistent time to go to bed and arise.

(10) Control the environment, such as by turning off lights, limiting environmental noise, setting a preferred environmental temperature, and using "white noise," such as sounds of rain drops or wind, to limit stimuli that may delay or interrupt sleep.

(11) Perform relaxation techniques, such as imagery, diaphragmatic breathing, and progressive muscle relaxation, to reduce muscle tension and promote relaxation.

(12) Get out of bed if not asleep within 30 minutes and return to bed when sleepy to establish an expectation that sleep should follow when in bed; use the bed only for sleeping and sexual activity.

(13) Avoid consistent use of medication for sleep to prevent physical or emotional dependence.

IV. Sleep Deprivation

Sleep deprivation refers to a situation in which a person experiences extended periods of time without sustained, natural, recurring states of unconsciousness. It results from deprivation of REM sleep, NREM sleep, or both. Nurses should understand the problems associated with sleep deprivation, the clinical manifestations of sleep deprivation, and the nursing care that can promote sleep.

A. Problems Associated With Sleep Deprivation
1. Conditions that interfere with the ability to go to sleep, remain asleep, or return to sleep, such as insomnia, restless leg syndrome, and sleep apnea.
2. Illnesses that interfere with sleeping, such as fever, pain, and dyspnea.
3. Situations impacting the sleep-wake cycle, such as rapid change in time zones (jet lag), rotating shift work, multiple interruptions by health-care providers during sleep, and environmental lights and noise that interfere with sleeping (**ICU psychosis**).

B. Physiological Manifestations of Sleep Deprivation
1. Drooping eyelids (ptosis).
2. Slowed response time.
3. Depressed reflexes.
4. Decreased fine motor skills.
5. Slowed reasoning and judgment.
6. Decreased auditory and visual alertness.
7. Cardiac dysrhythmias.

C. Psychological Manifestations of Sleep Deprivation
1. Excessive sleepiness.
2. Irritability, agitation, and hyperactivity.
3. Decreased motivation, apathy, and withdrawal.
4. Increased sensitivity to pain.
5. Confusion and disorientation.

D. Nursing Care for Patients Experiencing Sleep Deprivation
1. Identify physiological and psychological manifestations of sleep deprivation.
2. Identify causes of sleep deprivation and eliminate them if possible.
   a. Dim lights and limit noise in a hospital unit.
   b. Group patient care to limit interruptions.

c. Administer prescribed medications to reduce pain and promote sleep.

d. Perform specific interventions for dyssomnias.

3. Institute or teach the patient and significant others sleep hygiene practices.

V. Sleep Disorders and Related Nursing Care

The most common disorders that impact sleep are classified as dyssomnias or parasomnias. There are commonalities of nursing care to promote sleep in patients with these sleep disorders. However, each sleep disorder has unique characteristics that require specific nursing interventions. Nurses should be knowledgeable about these sleep disorders and their specific treatments as well as have a comprehensive repertoire of strategies to assist patients to improve their ability to achieve restorative sleep.

A. **Commonalities of Nursing Care for Patients With Sleep Disorders**
   1. Assess patients at risk for sleep disorders.
   2. Validate the patient's and significant other's frustration and anxiety regarding the problem and physical and emotional consequences.
   3. Have the patient keep a sleep/activity/dietary diary.
   4. Teach sleep hygiene practices.
   5. Encourage specific interventions appropriate for the disorder.
   6. Document assessments, nursing interventions, and patient responses.

B. **Dyssomnias:** Sleep Disorders Related to Abnormal Physiological Mechanisms That Regulate Sleep and Wakefulness
   1. **Insomnia.**
      a. Inability to fall asleep, remain asleep, or go back to sleep, resulting in an insufficient quantity or quality of sleep.
      b. May be transient (lasting less than a month) or chronic (lasting longer than a month).
      c. Characterized by awakening without feeling refreshed and excessive daytime sleepiness.
      d. Specific nursing care.
         (1) Assess for risk factors, including female gender, advanced age, anxiety, substance abuse, caffeine intake, inadequate sleep hygiene, and use of medications, such as amphetamines, bronchodilators, decongestants, and beta-adrenergic blockers.
         (2) Support the use of short-term prescribed sedatives-hypnotics to help prevent chronic insomnia.
   2. **Restless leg syndrome.**
      a. Uncontrollable movements of the legs when resting or just before onset of sleep.
      b. Caused by a central nervous system (CNS) disorder.
      c. Characterized by unpleasant sensations in the legs, such as tingling, itching, creeping, and crawling.
      d. Specific nursing care.
         (1) Assess for risk factors, including a family member with the disorder, advanced age, low levels of iron, and use of certain antidepressants, , such as sertraline (Zoloft), a selective serotonin reuptake inhibitor (SSRI).
         (2) Teach the patient to avoid stimulants, such as caffeine.
         (3) Teach self-care measures, such as walking, massage, stretching, and application of heat or cold.
         (4) Support the use of prescribed neuroleptic agents, vibration, or acupressure; note that clonazepam (Klonopin) may be prescribed.
   3. **Sleep apnea.**
      a. Periodic interruption of breathing when sleeping.
      b. Lasts from 10 seconds to 2 minutes and may occur 50 to 600 times a night.
      c. Types.
         (1) **Obstructive sleep apnea** (OSA).
            (a) Caused by airway obstruction due to tongue, tonsils, adenoids, deviated septum, or collapse of soft palate.
            (b) Characterized by struggling to breathe with snoring, gasping, and snorting sounds; patient usually is not aware of awakening.
            (c) Treatment directed at cause.
         (2) **Central sleep apnea** (CSA).
            (a) Caused by dysfunction of central respiratory control.
            (b) Attempts to breathe cease; patient usually is aware of awakening.
            (c) Presently has no effective treatment.
      d. Characterized by excessive daytime sleepiness, fatigue, morning headache, irritability, and difficulty concentrating.
      e. Causes physiological problems if untreated, such as dysrhythmias, hypertension, heart failure, brain attack, and impotence.
      f. Causes emotional problems if untreated, such as mood swings, personality changes, and depression.
      g. Specific nursing care.
         (1) Assess for risk factors, including male gender, age older than 40, and overweight; enlarged tonsils; deviated septum; and associated physical and emotional conditions.
         (2) Obtain the sleeping partner's report about the patient's behavior when sleeping, such as snoring, snorting, and gasps, alternating with periods of silence and flailing of the arms and legs during apneic episodes.

(3) Encourage diagnostic testing, such as electrocardiography, arterial oxygen saturation, electroencephalography, and oral and nasal air flow while sleeping.

(4) Specific nursing care for patients with obstructive sleep apnea.

🛑 (a) Encourage consistent nighttime use of continuous positive airway pressure (CPAP) to maintain an open airway if ordered.

(b) Encourage weight loss and avoidance of alcohol and smoking, if applicable.

(c) Provide perioperative care for procedures, such as tonsillectomy, repair of deviated septum, or laser removal of excess tissue of the platelet and pharynx.

4. **Narcolepsy.**
   a. Sudden uncontrollable urge to sleep during the day, lasting seconds to 30 minutes.
   b. Thought to be caused by a genetic defect of the CNS in which REM sleep cannot be controlled.
   c. Characterized by slurred speech, abrupt bilateral loss of muscle tone (**cataplexy**), and abruptly falling asleep (**sleep attack, sleep episode**).
   d. Associated with patient reports of sleeping well at night; weakness of the knees or inability to move during onset of sleep attack or when waking up (**sleep paralysis**); vivid, bizarre dreams while falling asleep that last 1 to 15 minutes; and awakening from sleep episodes refreshed.
   e. Specific nursing care.
      (1) Assess for risk factors, including onset between 15 and 30 years of age and a family member with the disorder.
      (2) Determine whether the patient sleeps well at night to distinguish between narcolepsy and sleep deprivation; sleep attacks caused by sleep deprivation resolve with sufficient sleep.
      (3) Teach avoidance of shift work, which usually is not tolerated, and passive activities, such as watching television or reading that precipitate sleep.
      (4) Encourage several naps a day at consistent times to decrease sleepiness.

🛑 (5) Recommend avoidance of activities that may result in injury during a sleep attack, such as driving a car and using machinery.

      (6) Encourage intake of prescribed medications, including CNS stimulants, such as amphetamines, methylphenidate (Ritalin), or modafinil (Provigil), and antidepressants, such as monoamine inhibitors and serotonergics.

C. **Parasomnias:** Disorders Characterized by Patterns of Abnormal Behaviors That Intrude on Sleep or Occur at the Threshold Between Waking and Sleeping

1. **Bruxism.**
   a. Repetitive clenching and grinding of teeth; episode lasts 4 to 5 seconds.
   b. Occurs usually during stage II NREM sleep.
   c. May erode tooth enamel, loosen teeth, and cause jaw pain.
   d. May become a habit after the initial cause resolves.
   e. Specific nursing care.
      (1) Assess for risk factors, including increased stress, abnormal bite, and GI disturbances.
      (2) Encourage use of relaxation techniques as part of the bed time routine.
      (3) Encourage the use of a prescribed mouth guard over the teeth when sleeping.

2. **Sleepwalking (somnambulism).**
   a. Episodic walking around while asleep with minimal awareness of surroundings; episode lasts 3 minutes or longer.
   b. Occurs during stage III or IV NREM sleep, 1 to 2 hours after falling asleep.
   c. Patients may have glassy eyes, look through other people as if they do not exist, or perform activities, such as making coffee or dusting furniture.
   d. Patients report no awareness or memory of the episode.
   e. Specific nursing care.
      (1) Assess for risk factors: More common in children but can occur in adults.

🛑 (2) Encourage the use of safety devices, such as bed and house alarms that alert others when the person exits the bed or leaves the house; lock doors to stairs.

3. **Nightmare disorder.**
   a. Repeated episodes of frightening dreams that result in awakening; patients commonly report that the dreams jeopardize their personal safety.
   b. Occurs during REM sleep and may occur every 90 to 110 minutes.
   c. Characterized by increased vital signs, diaphoresis, and difficulty falling back to sleep for fear of having another nightmare.
   d. Specific nursing care.
      (1) Assess for risk factors.
         (a) Occurs most commonly in children 3 to 5 years of age but can occur in older children and adults.
         (b) Is associated with stress; traumatic events; anxiety; guilt; insecurity; depression; fever; medication use, such as stimulants, antidepressants, and antihypertensives; and emotional problems,

such as post-traumatic stress disorder, borderline personality, and dissociative disorder.

(2) Encourage the patient to engage in activities to limit stress, such as daily exercise, relaxation techniques, yoga, and self-hypnosis.

(3) Support taking or discontinuing medications as prescribed.

(4) Teach significant others to provide emotional support.

4. **Sleep terrors (night terrors).**

a. Repeated episodes of abrupt awakening along with a panicky scream.

b. Occurs during stage IV NREM sleep and lasts from 10 to 30 minutes.

c. Characterized by crying or screaming in fear, thrashing about, and resisting attempts at consolation; appearing awake but not being awake; being difficult to awaken; and reporting no awareness or memory of the episode.

d. Specific nursing care.

(1) Assess for risk factors: Most common in children.

(2) Teach significant others that attempts to hold or comfort may be resisted.

🛑 (3) Remain physically close to provide emotional support and maintain safety.

5. **Nocturnal enuresis (bed wetting).**

a. Repeated episodes of involuntary urination when sleeping after toilet training is well established.

b. Occurs when arousing from stages III and IV NREM sleep, 1 to 2 hours after falling asleep.

c. Patient may or may not awaken during the episode.

d. Has multifactorial causes, including hormonal, bladder, and sleep problems; genetics; and medical conditions, such as small bladder, diabetes mellitus, and urinary tract infection.

e. May limit social activities, such as sleepovers and camp; precipitate social exclusion by peers; or cause anger and frustration in significant others.

f. Specific nursing care.

(1) Assess for patients at risk: More common in males than in females; patients with a family member who has or had the disorder; and patients with developmental delays or medical problems associated with the disorder.

(2) Teach the patient to reduce the volume of urine in the bladder at night by limiting fluid intake after 6 p.m. and voiding before going to bed and to decrease bladder irritability by eliminating caffeine in the diet.

(3) Support the use of behavior modification strategies.

(a) Rewards for waking up dry.

(b) Positive imagery, such as thinking about waking up dry.

(c) Use of a bedwetting alarm if ordered; an alarm is activated when the sleeper begins to wet the bed which awakens the sleeper who should attempt to stop the urinary stream and use a toilet to void; its use is controversial.

🛑 (4) Teach parents to be nonjudgmental when episodes occur and have a nonchalant demeanor when changing soiled linens and bed clothes.

🛑 (5) Teach the patient about the disorder and provide emotional support to increase self-esteem and limit embarrassment, shame, and guilt.

VI. Strategies to Decrease Pain and Promote Comfort, Rest, and Sleep

Specific interventions can be used to decrease mild to moderate pain and promote comfort, rest, and sleep by closing the gate for painful stimuli and using emotions and the conscious mind to interfere with the interpretation and perception of pain. The gate-control theory of pain is involved with relaxation techniques that stimulate cutaneous tissues (e.g., back rub). Positive thoughts and emotions (e.g., guided imagery) stimulate the release of endorphins that also are thought to have an effect on closing the gate to painful stimuli. In addition, techniques that require the mind to focus on issues other than the pain (e.g., distraction, progressive muscle relaxation, and breathing techniques) help to interfere with the interpretation and perception of pain because the brain can process only a certain amount of information at one time. These techniques are included within the role of the nurse and do not require a primary health-care provider's order.

A. Guided Imagery

1. Use of auditory suggestions, from a nurse or from an internal dialog, that have the patient picture in the mind places or situations that stimulate emotions that promote relaxation.

2. Nursing care.

a. Have the patient assume a position of comfort with the eyes closed; maintain a quiet environment.

b. Speak in a soft, slow manner.

c. Make suggestions that use a variety of senses in relation to the image selected by the patient, such as, "Hear the waves lapping on the shore," "Smell the roses in the garden," "Savor the taste of the food you are eating," and "Feel the wind blowing through your hair."

B. Distraction
1. Focusing on something else other than the pain.
2. Nursing care.
   a. Carry on a conversation with the patient.
   b. Suggest the use of distraction techniques.
      (1) Visual: Reading, watching television.
      (2) Tactile: Taking a warm bath, petting an animal, cuddling with a significant other.
      (3) Auditory: Listening to music or books on tape, an infant listening to a heartbeat or soothing whispering from a parent.
      (4) Intellectual: Completing crossword or Sudoku puzzles, playing card games alone, such as solitaire, or playing more complex games with another person.

C. Breathing Techniques
1. Inhalation and exhalation of air to maximize lung expansion or require the mind to focus on the pattern of breathing rather than discomfort or pain.
2. May be as simple as diaphragmatic breathing, which utilizes the diaphragm, rather than thoracic muscles, to achieve maximal expansion of the lungs on inhalation and promote muscle relaxation.
3. May involve complex patterns that alternate depths and rates of breaths to distract a person from an uncomfortable or painful experience; can be used by a woman during labor and birth.
4. Nursing care related to diaphragmatic breathing.
   a. Have the patient assume a position of comfort with the hands positioned over the upper abdomen; maintain a quiet environment.
   b. Instruction for the patient.
      (1) Inhale slowly through the nose while counting to the number 4; the patient should first feel the abdomen expand and then the chest.
      (2) Hold the breath at the height of inhalation while counting to the number 4.
      (3) Exhale gently and smoothly while counting to the number 8; the patient should feel the abdomen move toward the middle of the body.
      (4) Repeat steps 1 through 4.

D. Progressive Muscle Relaxation
1. Tensing and relaxing muscles in the body in a sequential pattern to reduce muscle tension and engage the mind in an activity.
2. Nursing care.
   a. Have the patient assume a position of comfort with the eyes closed; maintain a quiet environment.
   b. Encourage the patient to engage in diaphragmatic breathing throughout the procedure.
   c. Begin the sequence of tensing and relaxing muscles with the facial muscles and progress toward the toes.
   d. Instruct the patient to breathe in through the nose while tensing a group of muscles; hold the tension for 15 seconds and then relax the muscles while breathing out.
   e. Instruct the patient to rest for several seconds and then progress to another group of muscles.

E. Back Rub
1. Therapeutic effects.
   a. Relieves muscle tension.
   b. Promotes physical and emotional relaxation.
   c. Facilitates induction of sleep.
   d. Limits transmission of pain impulses via the gate-control theory of pain.
   e. Increases circulation to the skin (friction causes heat that promotes dilation of capillaries).
2. Contraindications.
   a. Personal preference not to receive a back rub; always ask a patient's desire for and permission to perform a back rub.
   b. Rib fractures and vertebral disorders.
   c. Impaired skin integrity, such as burns, pressure ulcers, and open wounds.
   d. Within 48 hours of an acute neurological (e.g., brain attack) or cardiac (e.g., myocardial infarction, cardiac surgery) problem; patient may not tolerate the stimulation of a back rub.
3. Types of back rub strokes.
   a. Effleurage: Long, smooth strokes with gentle pressure that slide over the skin from the small of the back to the shoulders; promotes relaxation and circulation to the skin.
   b. Friction: Continuous, small, circular movements on either side of the vertebrae from the shoulders to the small of the back and then from the small of the back to the shoulders; promotes circulation to the skin.
   c. Pétrissage: Kneading of the skin and muscles; promotes circulation to the skin and reduces muscle stiffness and spasms.
   d. Tapotement: Gentle, rhythmic tapping over tense muscles; reduces muscle tension.
   e. Feathering: Long, soft, fingertip strokes from the shoulders to the small of the back.
4. Nursing care.
   a. Identify whether the patient has any contraindications to a back rub to prevent injury.
   b. Assess the patient's desire for a back rub.
   c. Wash hands to limit the transfer of microorganisms.
   d. Raise the bed to a working height and lower the side rails to prevent reaching and straining of own back and legs.

e. Close the door, pull the curtain, and drape the patient, exposing just the back, to provide privacy and emotional comfort.

f. Place the patient in a side-lying or prone position.

g. Warm the lotion to promote comfort and dilation of the capillaries.

h. Place the lotion on own hands first to prevent startling the patient.

i. Massage using a variety of strokes for 3 to 5 minutes ending with feathering; variety provides several therapeutic effects.

j. Reposition the patient and cover with bed linen.

k. Document the back rub and the patient's response in the patient's clinical record.

VII. Medications That Limit Pain and Promote Rest and Sleep

Many independent and dependent nursing interventions may be inadequate to relieve patients' discomfort or pain. Medications, such as nonopioid analgesics or opioid (narcotic) analgesics, may be prescribed by primary health-care providers to relieve pain. Likewise, sleep hygiene strategies may be inadequate in assisting patients to achieve restorative sleep. Patients may self-prescribe over-the-counter medications, such as antihistamines, dietary supplements, and herbs, and primary health-care providers may prescribe anxiolytics, sedatives, and hypnotics to promote sleep. Nurses should know the mechanisms of action, therapeutic and nontherapeutic effects, and nursing care related to the common medications that are specifically designed to address patient needs in relation to pain, comfort, rest, and sleep.

A. **Nonopioid Analgesics:** Inhibit Prostaglandins Involved in Pain (Table 23.6)

B. **Opioid (Narcotic) Analgesics:** Decrease Transmission of Pain Impulses by Combining With Opioid Receptors in the CNS (Table 23.7)

C. **Anxiolytics, Sedatives, and Hypnotics:** Reduce Anxiety and Promote Rest and Sleep (Table 23.8)

D. **Over-the-Counter (OTC) Products Used to Promote Sleep**
   1. Types of products.
      a. Antihistamines: diphenhydramine (Benadryl).
      b. Dietary supplements: melatonin.
      c. Herbs: kava, valerian, chamomile, passion flower, and lemon balm.

Table 23.6 Nonopioid Analgesics

Examples	Nontherapeutic Effects
acetaminophen (Tylenol)	• Hepatic toxicity.
Nonsalicylate NSAID ibuprofen (Advil, Motrin) naproxen (Aleve, Naprosyn)	• Rash. • Tinnitus. • Flu-like syndrome.
Salicylate NSAID acetylsalicylic acid (aspirin, Ecotrin)	• Agitation. • Hyperventilation. • Lethargy. • Confusion. • Diarrhea. • Bleeding. **Toxicity** • Diaphoresis. • Tinnitus (eighth cranial nerve damage).

Nursing Care
- Assess level of pain.
- Encourage the patient to take the medication with 8 oz of water; sit up 15 to 30 minutes after ingestion, and take the medication with food, except for naproxen and ibuprofen.
- Monitor for nontherapeutic effects.
- Monitor for GI bleeding, such as anemia and melena.
- Encourage the patient to avoid alcohol and over-the-counter (OTC) medications.
- Acetaminophen: Encourage the patient not to exceed 4g in 24 hours because an overdose may cause liver damage.
- Salicylates.
  - Monitor serum salicylate levels.
  - Warn the patient to avoid toxicity by not exceeding the recommended 24-hour dose.
  - Withhold 1 week before invasive procedures to decrease the risk of bleeding.
  - Understand that salicylates are contraindicated in pregnant women, lactating women, and children younger than 2 years of age (associated with Reye's syndrome).

Table 23.7 Opioid (Narcotic) Analgesics

Examples	Nontherapeutic Effects
codeine fentanyl (Duragesic): 72-hour transdermal patch for chronic/intractable pain hydrocodone (Hycodan) hydromorphone (Dilaudid) methadone HCl (Dolophine) morphine (MS Contin, Roxanol): For intractable pain, myocardial infarction, pulmonary edema oxycodone (OxyContin)	• Decreased respiratory rate. • Drowsiness, sedation, confusion. • Hypotension. • Constipation. • Nausea and vomiting. • Pruritus. • Fentanyl: Dry mouth, diaphoresis, weakness.

Opioid/Nonopioid Analgesic Combinations

propoxyphene napsylate and acetaminophen (Darvocet-N)

hydrocodone and acetaminophen (Vicodin)

oxycodone and acetaminophen (Percocet)

codeine phosphate and acetaminophen (Tylenol with codeine 1, 2, 3, or 4)

Nursing Care
- Assess level of pain using a pain rating scale before and after administration (See Fig. 23.2, 23.3, and 23.4, pages 718–719).
- Administer before pain is severe; regularly scheduled doses maintain therapeutic blood levels, which increase effectiveness.
- Administer combinations of analgesics cautiously; combined effect is greater than when each is given independently (synergistic).
- Administer additional prescribed medication for breakthrough pain; common with continuous infusion or sustained release medications or intractable pain.
- Encourage coughing and deep breathing every 2 hours to prevent pooling of respiratory secretions.
- Encourage increased fluids, dietary fiber, and exercise to limit constipation; administer stool softeners or laxatives if prescribed.
- Provide for safety, such as by teaching the patient to avoid hazardous activities and to change positions slowly.
- Teach the patient how to self-administer medication via various routes.
- Monitor pain relief, vital signs, hypotension, drowsiness, confusion, constipation, nausea, and vomiting.
- Monitor for severe respiratory depression; if rate is less than 10 per minute, hold the next dose and notify the primary health-care provider.
- Assess for signs of a decreased physiological response (tolerance); usually requires an increase in dose to achieve effectiveness.
- Assess for signs of physical or emotional reliance on the medication to maintain its effect (dependence); formerly called habituation or addiction.
- Keep naloxone (Narcan) readily available for toxicity or overdose.

Table 23.8 Anxiolytics, Sedatives, and Hypnotics

Types	Examples	Nontherapeutic Effects
Benzodiazepines • Increase action of gamma-aminobutyric acid (GABA) inhibitory neurotransmitter.	**Short acting** alprazolam (Xanax) midazolam (Versed) **Medium acting** lorazepam (Ativan) **Long acting** chlordiazepoxide (Librium) clonazepam (Klonopin) diazepam (Valium)	• Decreased mental alertness. • Decreased blood pressure. • Drowsiness. • Dizziness. • Headache. • Nausea and vomiting. • Paradoxical reactions, such as euphoria and excitement.
Nonbarbiturates • All have CNS depressant effects but variable action depending on the medication.	buspirone (BuSpar) hydroxyzine (Atarax, Vistaril) zaleplon (Sonata) zolpidem (Ambien)	

Nursing Care
- Assess sleep patterns.
- Teach the patient sleep hygiene practices to promote effectiveness of medication.
- Encourage avoidance of products that potentiate effects, such as alcohol, or diminish effects, such as caffeine.
- Teach the patient to provide for personal safety because of decreased mental alertness.
- Discontinue the medication slowly to prevent withdrawal; use longer than 2 weeks may lead to dependence.
- Assess therapeutic effectiveness and for signs of dependence.

2. Nursing care.
   a. Advise the patient that self-medicating with OTC products can be dangerous.
      (1) Products may potentiate, diminish, or interact with other medications being taken. (See Table 15.2 "Common Herbal Supplements and Related Nursing Care" in Chapter 15 "Pharmacology.")
      (2) Products may be habit forming, promoting physical or emotional dependence.
      (3) Products such as dietary supplements and herbs are not regulated by the U.S. Food and Drug Administration.
   b. Encourage the patient to discuss the desire to use these products with the primary health-care provider.

CASE STUDY: Putting it All Together

A nurse is caring for an older man who is being admitted to the hospital for pain management due to progressive metastatic disease. The nurse interviews the patient, completes a pain assessment, and reviews the admitting primary health-care provider's orders.

▮ Patient's Clinical Record

Patient Interview

Patient states that the pain was significantly reduced after surgery 1 year ago to remove as much of a malignant tumor as the surgeon was able to remove. He said that the pain was initially manageable. However, for the last 7 months, the pain has progressively increased in intensity to where now it is "unbearable." Reports constant fatigue. Verbalized that he "feels helpless" because nothing seems to help and stated, "I am so angry that this is happening to me. I was careful about what I ate and lived a healthy lifestyle. I can't take much more of this, and I am afraid of what is going to happen next. I lost my wife 4 months ago because she was hit by a drunk driver and I had to move into my daughter's house because I could no longer take care of myself." He said his family is great and they are always there for him but that he feels like a burden. He shared that his daughter has three small children and the house is always noisy and busy, so it is hard to rest. He went on to say, "Sometimes I think that this suffering is what has to happen because of the things that I did during the Vietnam War that I regret. It was a terrible time in my life."

Pain Assessment

- Pain level before coming to the hospital was "11" on a scale of 0 to 10 and now, 2 hours later, after the first dose of morphine 6 mg, is a level 6.
- The patient stated, "The pain is sharp and piercing and is concentrated all around my belly," as he rubbed his hand in a circular motion over the surface of the abdomen.
- Guarding his abdomen with his hands.
- Makes facial grimaces, clenches the teeth, and tightly closes the eyes when making slight changes in position.

Vital Signs

Temperature:	99.6°F
Pulse:	120 beats/minute
Respirations:	24 breaths/minute, shallow
Blood pressure:	165/92 mm Hg

Primary Health-Care Provider's Orders

Morphine sulfate 6 mg Sub-Q every 4 hours prn for severe pain.
Percocet 2.5 mg/300mg: 1 tablet PO every 6 hours prn for mild pain and 2 tablets PO every 6 hours prn for moderate pain.
Tylenol 500 mg capsule: 1 capsule PO every 4 hours prn for mild pain or PO every 4 hours prn for temp over 101°F.
Colace 100 mg PO every 12 hours.
Senokot 2 tablets PO h.s. prn for constipation.
OOB to chair with assistance.
Regular diet.
Vital signs every 8 hours.
Psychiatry consult for depression.
Oncology consult.
Palliative medicine consult.

Case Study Questions

A. What information collected by the nurse are factors that influence this patient's pain experience?

1. _____
2. _____
3. _____

CASE STUDY: Putting it All Together   *cont'd*

—— **Case Study Questions** ——

4. _____

5. _____

6. _____

7. _____

8. _____

9. _____

B. Identify at least 5 additional questions that the nurse should ask the patient to arrive at a more complete pain assessment.

1. _____

2. _____

3. _____

4. _____

5. _____

C. Identify at least 15 independent nursing interventions that the nurse should implement to address this patient's pain and comfort needs.

1. _____

2. _____

3. _____

4. _____

5. _____

6. _____

7. _____

8. _____

9. _____

10. _____

11. _____

12. _____

13. _____

14. _____

15. _____

D. Identify 5 dependent nursing interventions that the nurse should implement that address this patient's pain and comfort needs.

1. _____

2. _____

3. _____

4. _____

5. _____

REVIEW QUESTIONS

1. A nurse is caring for a patient who was diagnosed with obstructive sleep apnea. Which should the nurse encourage the patient to do because it is **most** effective in supporting restful sleep?
   1. Maintain a side-lying position when going to bed.
   2. Employ breathing exercises for relaxation before bedtime.
   3. Use an ordered positive pressure device when going to sleep.
   4. Position several pillows under the head when retiring at night.

2. A patient with a history of inflammation of the gall-bladder (cholecystitis) comes to the urgent care center with acute pain in the upper right quadrant of the abdomen. The patient states, "We went out for dinner last night and I ate spare ribs, macaroni and cheese, and ice cream. I really overdid it." Where should the nurse anticipate that the patient will report referred pain associated with inflammation of the gallbladder?
   1. A
   2. B
   3. C
   4. D

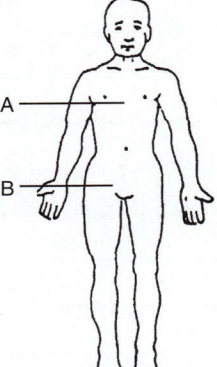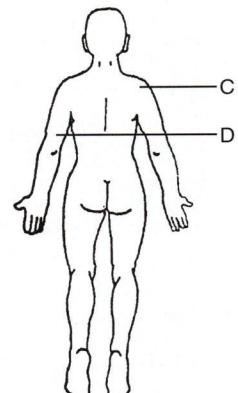

3. A patient on a medical unit tells a nurse, "My heart hurts." What is the nurse's **most** appropriate response?
   1. Say, "Your heart hurts."
   2. Alert the rapid response team.
   3. Obtain the patient's vital signs.
   4. State, "Please be more specific about how it hurts."

4. A nurse is caring for a school-aged child who is to have a bone marrow biopsy. Although a local anesthetic will be used during the biopsy, it may be frightening and uncomfortable for the child. What should the nurse say that will **best** help the child tolerate the procedure?
   1. "Let's practice what will happen during the procedure."
   2. "Do you have any questions about the procedure that you would like to ask?"
   3. "You need to be strong during the procedure and before you know it will be over."
   4. "Would you like me to play a disk with your favorite songs during the procedure?"

5. A nurse is caring for a patient who is reporting pain in the jaw as a result of cardiac ischemia. What word should the nurse use to describe this pain when writing progress notes?
   1. Cutaneous
   2. Radiating
   3. Referred
   4. Visceral

6. An older adult with rheumatoid arthritis comes to the clinic during an exacerbation of the disease. Which patient responses are associated with chronic pain? **Select all that apply.**
   1. _____ Pressured speech
   2. _____ Constricted pupils
   3. _____ Increased heart rate
   4. _____ Increased respiratory rate
   5. _____ Decreased blood pressure

7. A nurse is assessing the presence of pain in a variety of patients. Which patient condition may precipitate phantom pain?
   1. Vertebral stenosis causing sciatica
   2. Above the knee amputation
   3. Myocardial infarction
   4. Acute appendicitis

8. A nurse is caring for a postoperative patient who is receiving patient-controlled analgesia to control postoperative pain. Which concept about patient-controlled analgesia is **most** important for the nurse to convey to the patient?
   1. A basal dose will deliver a basic dose of analgesic periodically.
   2. Excessive doses are locked out if a triggered dose is premature.
   3. Pain medication should be administered before pain becomes intense.
   4. An extra dose of medication is delivered when the trigger is compressed.

9. A nurse is caring for a patient who reports feeling tense and "up tight." The nurse decides to administer a back rub. Which back rub stroke is **most** effective in producing relaxation and circulation to the skin?
   1. Friction
   2. Pétrissage
   3. Effleurage
   4. Feathering

10. A toddler must undergo a painful dressing change. How can the nurse **best** provide emotional support for this child?
    1. Hold the child.
    2. Provide a sucrose pacifier.
    3. Encourage the child to cry.
    4. Obtain a prescription for an opioid.

11. A nurse is assessing a patient with acute pain. What clinical indicators should the nurse expect the patient to exhibit? **Select all that apply.**
    1. _____ Anxiety about the pain
    2. _____ Apathetic facial expression
    3. _____ Relief after taking an analgesic
    4. _____ Grimacing when the pain is intense
    5. _____ Actual tissue damage that caused the pain

12. A nurse plans to administer a back rub to a patient. What should the nurse do **first** before administering the back rub?
    1. Wash the hands.
    2. Warm the lotion.
    3. Pull the curtain for privacy.
    4. Identify any contraindications.

13. Which is unique to sleep versus rest?
    1. Prevents fatigue
    2. Slows vital signs
    3. Conserves energy
    4. Reduces perception

14. A nurse identifies that a patient has been awakening frequently during the night and comes to the conclusion that the patient is experiencing REM sleep deprivation. Which clinical manifestations identified by the nurse supports this conclusion?
    1. Fatigue and lethargy
    2. Irritability and confusion
    3. Tremors and increased sensitivity to pain
    4. Immunosuppression and delayed wound healing

15. Which statement indicates that the patient is experiencing narcolepsy?
    1. "I grind my teeth at night to the point that my jaw is sore in the morning."
    2. "My family says that I snore so loud that I keep everyone awake at night."
    3. "I unexpectedly fall asleep for several minutes in the middle of the day at work."
    4. "My mother says that I walk around in my sleep at night, but I don't remember anything."

16. A nurse has implemented interventions to promote rest and sleep in a postoperative patient. What assessment **best** indicates that the patient probably is sleeping rather than just resting?
    1. Eyes are closed.
    2. Appears physically at ease.
    3. Arms are resting at the side of the body.
    4. Lacks a response to environmental noises.

17. A nurse is caring for a patient whose primary health-care provider prescribes a medication that will provide a palliative reaction. Which patient response indicates that the medication is effective?
    1. The patient has not become pregnant.
    2. The patient's pain has subsided to a tolerable level.
    3. The patient no longer has clinical manifestations of an infection.
    4. The patient's blood glucose level has returned to the normal range.

18. A patient is explaining the pain that is felt in the lower legs as a result of impairment of nervous tissue secondary to diabetes. What words generally expressed by patients to describe this type of neuropathic pain should the nurse expect the patient to use? **Select all that apply.**
    1. _____ Pins and needles
    2. _____ Numbness
    3. _____ Pounding
    4. _____ Burning
    5. _____ Aching

19. A nurse is caring for an adolescent who is scheduled for a painful dressing change after a burn injury caused by "cooking" an illicit medication. Which statement by the nurse is **most** helpful?
    1. "This may cause you some pain, so it is alright if you cry."
    2. "We are going to pull the curtain around your bed for privacy."
    3. "If you experience any pain, it is not because we are trying to punish you."
    4. "I know that you want to be brave, so we will do this as quickly as possible."

20. A nurse asks a patient, "What does the pain feel like?" What characteristic of pain is the nurse assessing?
    1. Quality
    2. Intensity
    3. Behavioral effects
    4. Precipitating factors

21. Which nursing intervention is **most** important when providing nursing care to a patient experiencing pain?
    1. Validate the presence of pain.
    2. Encourage breathing exercises.
    3. Employ a distraction technique.
    4. Teach muscle relaxation techniques.

22. A nurse is assessing a patient with chronic pain. What clinical indicators should the nurse expect the patient to exhibit? **Select all that apply.**
    1. _____ Gradual onset
    2. _____ Dilated pupils
    3. _____ Pressured speech
    4. _____ Recurrent in nature
    5. _____ Variable breathing patterns

23. A nurse is caring for a patient who reports difficulty sleeping for several weeks. What should the nurse encourage the patient to do that will facilitate sleeping?
    1. Drink a small glass of alcohol to relax.
    2. Avoid consuming milk at bedtime.
    3. Read in bed to induce drowsiness.
    4. Establish a daily bedtime routine.

24. Which nursing intervention is related to providing psychospiritual comfort to a hospitalized patient?
    1. Arrange furniture so patients have a view from their rooms.
    2. Respect each patient as a unique individual.
    3. Provide for basic physiological needs.
    4. Ensure continuity of care.

25. A nurse awakens a patient who is sleeping to implement a required nursing intervention. The nurse identifies that the patient is in the deepest stage of sleep and is difficult to awaken. Which stage of sleep is the patient experiencing?
    1. REM sleep stage 5
    2. NREM sleep stage 1
    3. NREM sleep stage 2
    4. NREM sleep stage 4

26. A nurse is caring for a patient who reports having difficulty going to sleep and staying asleep at night. What should the nurse encourage the patient to do? **Select all that apply.**
    1. _____ Limit naps to 1 hour at a time during the day.
    2. _____ Avoid products with nicotine 2 hours before bedtime.
    3. _____ Engage in vigorous exercise 1 to 2 hours before bedtime.
    4. _____ Avoid caffeine containing food and liquids 4 hours before bedtime.
    5. _____ Eat a small snack of carbohydrates and protein, such as cheese and crackers, just before going to bed.

27. A nurse is caring for an older adult who just had alprazolam (Xanax) prescribed for anxiety that has been interrupting sleep. What nursing action is **most** important at this time when caring for this patient?
    1. Institute fall precautions.
    2. Assess for elevated blood pressure.
    3. Monitor the patient for clinical indicators of dependence.
    4. Discontinue immediately if the patient experiences drowsiness.

28. A nurse is caring for a patient receiving an opioid after abdominal surgery. Which nursing intervention is **most** important for the nurse to implement?
    1. Administer before pain is severe.
    2. Encourage coughing and deep breathing.
    3. Assess for signs and symptoms of tolerance.
    4. Monitor for a respiratory rate less than 10 breaths/minute.

29. A nurse is caring for a patient in the intensive care unit who has been exhibiting clinical indicators of sleep deprivation. What is the best intervention to assist this patient to sleep?
    1. Group care into blocks of time.
    2. Encourage napping during the day.
    3. Implement the patient's bedtime ritual.
    4. Provide a back rub at the patient's bedtime.

30. A nurse is caring for an older adult male who was admitted to the hospital with an exacerbation of rheumatoid arthritis. The nurse interviewed the patient, performed a physical assessment, and reviewed the patient's clinical record.

Patient's Clinical Record

Patient Interview

Patient states that his wife of 52 years died 3 months ago after a sudden heart attack. He said that she took care of him and that he had to put his house up for sale and move to a nursing home because he could not take care of himself. He shared that finances are tight and that he could not afford to pay for a private room. He currently shares a room with another man who snores a lot at night, making it difficult for him to sleep. He said that he is able to take a few naps during the day. He is estranged from his son, an only child, because they quarreled over the details of his wife's burial and the sale of the house.

Patient Assessment

Patient is rubbing his knees with the palms of his hands and says that they hurt on a level 3 all the time, even with pain medication. He said that when his wife was alive he was able to deal with the pain but since she passed away he has experienced more pain in his knees. The knees appear slightly swollen, erythema is present, and they are warm to the touch. Temperature is 100.2°F, pulse is 78 beats/minute, respirations are 14 breaths/minute, blood pressure is 110/60 mm Hg. IV fluids running as ordered; IV site is clean, dry, and intact.

Primary Health-Care Provider's Orders

Regular diet.
Activity as tolerated.
Physical therapy consult.
CBC with differential, basic metabolic panel, rheumatoid factor, antinuclear antibody, sedimentation rate, C-reactive protein.
Celecoxib (Celebrex) 200 mg PO daily.
Solu-Cortef 60 mg IVPB every 12 hours.
Oxycodone/acetaminophen (Percocet) 5 mg/325 mg, 1 tablet for moderate joint pain and 2 tablets for severe joint pain, every 4 hours prn
Hydromorphone (Dilaudid) 2 mg Sub-Q every 4 hours, prn for severe joint pain.
Colace 100 mg PO twice daily.

Based on the data collected, what statement is **most** likely related to this patient's situation?
1. Lack of sleep because of noise made by a roommate has made him irritable.
2. The multiplicity of stresses may have reduced the patient's tolerance to pain.
3. The dose of the patient's pain medication should be increased to provide pain relief.
4. He is experiencing respiratory depression due to excessive amounts of pain medication.

31. A nurse is caring for a patient who reports restless leg syndrome. What nursing intervention should help reduce unpleasant sensations related to this sleep disorder?
1. Wrapping the patient's legs with ace bandages snugly before sleeping
2. Teaching the patient how to perform stretching exercises of the legs
3. Encouraging the patient to drink warm tea before bedtime
4. Assisting the patient to implement a weight loss program

32. A nurse plans to provide for a patient's comfort in relation to a psychospiritual need. Which nursing action is an appropriate intervention?
1. Administering a prescribed analgesic
2. Using effective communication skills
3. Dimming the lights in the room at night
4. Encouraging a parent to stay with a hospitalized child

33. A nurse is caring for a patient whose primary health-care provider has prescribed hydromorphone (Dilaudid) 1.5 mg Sub-Q every 4 hours prn for moderate pain. Dilaudid is available in 1 mg per mL. How many mL should the nurse administer? Record you answer using one decimal place.
Answer: _____ mL

34. A nurse is teaching a patient about the acetaminophen prescribed by the primary health-care provider. Which information is important to include in this discussion?
1. Avoid hazardous activities.
2. Take it on an empty stomach.
3. Do not exceed the ordered dose.
4. Use a stool softener when taking this medication.

35. A nurse is caring for an adult who is recovering from abdominal surgery and is receiving an opioid Sub-Q every 6 hours prn for incisional pain. Place the following statements in sequence according to the nursing process.
1. Evaluate the effectiveness of the opioid.
2. The patient will verbalize that the pain level is tolerable.
3. Pain is a level 8 on a pain scale of 0 to 10, with 10 being the most severe pain.
4. Administer the opioid according to the primary health-care provider's prescription.
5. Acute pain related to tissue trauma and reflex muscle spasms secondary to surgery.
Answer: _____

REVIEW ANSWERS

1. ANSWER: 3.
Rationales:
1. Positioning may not help to keep the tongue, tonsils, adenoids, or soft palette from obstructing the airway. An action in another option is the most effective intervention in maintaining a patent airway, thereby providing for more restful sleep.
2. Breathing exercises will not help to minimize airway obstruction when sleeping. The patient does not need to be more relaxed to sleep. The patient needs the airway to be patent.
3. **A continuous positive airway pressure (CPAP) machine has either a mask worn over the nose or prongs positioned in the nostrils. It increases the amount of air entering the respiratory tract through continuous positive airway pressure. CPAP also helps prevent airway collapse during exhalation.**
4. Several pillows under the head may cause flexion of the head, further obstructing the airway. Pillows placed under the shoulders and head may help to maintain an open airway.
TEST-TAKING TIP: Identify the word in the stem that sets a priority. The word *most* in the stem sets a priority. Identify the clang association. The word *sleep* in the stem and in option 3 is a clang association. Examine option 3 carefully.
Content Area: Pain, Comfort, Rest, and Sleep
Integrated Processes: Teaching/Learning; Nursing Process: Implementation
Client Need: Physiological Integrity; Basic Care and Comfort
Cognitive Level: Application

2. ANSWER: 3.
Rationales:
1. Pain that radiates to the sternal area of the chest usually originates in the stomach.
2. Pain that radiates to the right groin area usually originates in the appendix, kidneys, or ureters.
3. **An inflamed gallbladder may irritate the diaphragm. The diaphragm is innervated by spinal nerves C3, 4, and 5 that travel from the shoulder area so that pain is referred along the nerve fibers to the C3, 4, and 5 dermatomes in the shoulder.**
4. Pain that radiates to the left arm usually originates in the heart.
Content Area: Pain, Comfort, Rest, and Sleep
Integrated Processes: Nursing Process: Assessment
Client Need: Physiological Integrity; Basic Care and Comfort
Cognitive Level: Analysis

3. ANSWER: 4.
Rationales:
1. An open-ended question in a potential emergency situation may not gather pertinent information.
2. Alerting the rapid response team is premature at this time.
3. Although obtaining the patient's vital signs is an appropriate intervention and should be done eventually, it is premature at this time.
4. **This response gathers more specific information from the patient. The location, intensity, and characteristics of the pain should be assessed first.**
TEST-TAKING TIP: Identify the word in the stem that sets a priority. The word *most* in the stem sets a priority. Identify

options with a clang association. Options 1 and 4 include the word *hurts,* which also appears in the stem and is a clang association. Consider these options carefully.
Content Area: Pain, Comfort, Rest, and Sleep
Integrated Processes: Communication/Documentation; Nursing Process: Assessment
Client Need: Physiological Integrity; Basic Care and Comfort
Cognitive Level: Application

4. ANSWER: 1.
Rationales:
1. **Role playing enables the child to learn what will happen; it provides an opportunity for the nurse to allay the child's fears and for the child to ask questions and receive answers in a nonthreatening environment. The procedure should be less frightening and threatening when a school-aged child knows what to expect.**
2. This statement is not as good as a response presented in another option. The school-aged child may not know what to ask about the procedure.
3. This statement denies the child's feelings.
4. Although this may be done, it is not the best intervention presented in the options.
TEST-TAKING TIP: Identify the word in the stem that sets a priority. The word *best* in the stem sets a priority. Identify the statement that denies the feelings of the child. Option 3 denies the feelings that a school-aged child would most likely have regarding an unfamiliar and potentially uncomfortable procedure.
Content Area: Pain, Comfort, Rest, and Sleep
Integrated Processes: Communication/Documentation; Nursing Process: Implementation
Client Need: Physiological Integrity; Reduction of Risk Potential
Cognitive Level: Application

5. ANSWER: 3.
Rationales:
1. Cutaneous pain is associated with superficial cuts of the skin or subcutaneous tissue.
2. Radiating pain is when pain arises in one site and extends to another site. For example, sciatic pain from the lumbar vertebrae or pain associated with lymphatic streaking.
3. **When heart ischemia is felt as pain in the jaw, it is identified as referred pain. Referred pain occurs when pain arises in one site but is felt in a distant site.**
4. Visceral pain occurs when deep internal pain receptors are stimulated, such as during labor or in response to cancer of the abdominal organs.
Content Area: Pain, Comfort, Rest, and Sleep
Integrated Processes: Communication/Documentation; Nursing Process: Assessment
Client Need: Safe and Effective Care Environment; Management of Care
Cognitive Level: Knowledge

6. ANSWER: 2, 5.
Rationales:
1. Pressured speech occurs with acute pain because it tends to accompany a crisis. A slow monotonous speech pattern is associated with chronic pain because chronic pain is debilitating, depleting physical and emotional

resources; patients may become apathetic, stoical, or resigned to the pain.

2. Constriction of the pupils occurs with chronic pain because of the action of the parasympathetic nervous system. Dilation of the pupils occurs with acute pain because of the action of the sympathetic nervous system.

3. An increased heart rate occurs with acute pain because of the action of the sympathetic nervous system. A decreased heart rate occurs with chronic pain because of the action of the parasympathetic nervous system.

4. An increase in the respiratory rate (tachypnea) occurs with acute pain because of the action of the sympathetic nervous system. The breathing rate may slow with chronic pain because of the action of the parasympathetic nervous system.

5. A decreased blood pressure occurs with chronic pain because of the action of the parasympathetic nervous system. An increase in blood pressure is associated with acute pain because of the action of the sympathetic nervous system.

Content Area: Pain, Comfort, Rest, and Sleep
Integrated Processes: Nursing Process: Assessment
Client Need: Physiological Integrity; Basic Care and Comfort
Cognitive Level: Analysis

7. ANSWER: 2.
Rationales:
1. Direct extension of pain from one area (vertebrae) to another (sciatic nerve) is called radiating pain.
2. Phantom sensation/pain is discomfort arising from a site that has been surgically removed. The discomfort is perceived as being in the part of the body that no longer exists.
3. A myocardial infarction is associated with referred pain; if feels as if the pain is originating in areas such as the jaw, left arm, or center of back.
4. Acute appendicitis may precipitate pain at McBurney's point, a site halfway between the umbilicus and the right anterior iliac crest. This is an example of referred pain.

Content Area: Pain, Comfort, Rest, and Sleep
Integrated Processes: Nursing Process: Analysis
Client Need: Physiological Integrity; Basic Care and Comfort
Cognitive Level: Application

8. ANSWER: 3.
Rationales:
1. Although this concept is important, it is not as important as the concept in another option.
2. Although this concept is important, it is not as important as the concept in another option.
3. This is an important concept for the patient to understand because a patient may wait until pain is excessively intense before activating the trigger for an interim dose. Research demonstrates that medicating a patient for pain before it becomes intense avoids the highs and lows of pain levels and maintains a tolerable consistent level, which is more effective in controlling pain, requiring less medication overall.
4. An extra dose of medication is delivered only when the trigger is activated after the lockout time has expired and not before.

TEST-TAKING TIP: Identify the word in the stem that sets a priority. The word *most* in the stem sets a priority. Identify the option with a clang association. The word *pain* in the stem and in option 3 is a clang association. Examine option 3 carefully.
Content Area: Pain, Comfort, Rest, and Sleep
Integrated Processes: Teaching/Learning; Nursing Process: Implementation
Client Need: Physiological Integrity; Pharmacological and Parenteral Therapies
Cognitive Level: Application

9. ANSWER: 3.
Rationales:
1. Friction, employing continuous, small, circular movements on either side of vertebrae from the shoulders to the small of the back and then from the small of the back to the shoulders, promotes circulation. It generally does not produce relaxation.
2. Pétrissage, kneading of skin and shoulder muscles, promotes circulation. It generally does not promote relaxation.
3. Effleurage, long, smooth strokes with gentle pressure that slide over skin from the small of the back to the shoulders, promotes relaxation and circulation to the skin.
4. Feathering, long, soft, finger-tip strokes from shoulders to the small of the back, promotes relaxation. It generally does not increase circulation.

TEST-TAKING TIP: Identify the word in the stem that sets a priority. The word *most* in the stem sets a priority.
Content Area: Pain, Comfort, Rest, and Sleep
Integrated Processes: Nursing Process: Implementation
Client Need: Physiological Integrity; Basic Care and Comfort
Cognitive Level: Application

10. ANSWER: 1.
Rationales:
1. Toddlers perceive pain as a threat to their safety and security. Holding the toddler provides comfort and emotional support.
2. The use of a sucrose pacifier is more appropriate for infants rather than toddlers.
3. Toddlers should be permitted to cope with discomfort in their own way. Although they may cry, they also may respond by struggling against the provider of care or use physical or verbal aggression.
4. This may be unnecessary. Other nonprescription interventions should be attempted first. If a medication is prescribed, opioids would be used as a last resort after other analgesics.

TEST-TAKING TIP: Identify the word in the stem that sets a priority. The word *best* in the stem sets a priority. Identify the options with clang associations. Options 1 and 3 and the stem contain the word *child*, which are clang associations. Examine these two options carefully. More often than not, an option with a clang association is the correct answer.
Content Area: Pain, Comfort, Rest, and Sleep
Integrated Processes: Caring; Nursing Process: Implementation
Client Need: Physiological Integrity; Basic Care and Comfort
Cognitive Level: Application

11. **ANSWER: 1, 3, 4, 5.**

Rationales:

1. Acute pain usually has an abrupt onset, may be severe, and requires a diagnostic workup to determine its cause; these factors increase anxiety.

2. An apathetic facial expression often is associated with chronic pain because chronic pain is debilitating, depleting physical and emotional resources; apathy and resignation are common responses to chronic pain.

3. Acute pain usually responds to the administration of analgesics, whereas chronic pain may not. Chronic pain may require multiple modalities to relieve pain.

4. Behavioral responses (e.g., grimacing, wincing, groaning, crying) often occur with acute pain because it is related to a new situation. People with chronic pain due to a life-long condition reach a point where they become apathetic, resigned, or develop other coping mechanisms than overt signs of pain.

5. Acute pain is always related to body tissue changes. Chronic pain may not be related to tissue damage.

TEST-TAKING TIP: Identify the options that are opposites. Options 2 and 4 are opposites. One or the other should be eliminated; rarely are both opposite options correct answers in this type of question.

Content Area: Pain, Comfort, Rest, and Sleep
Integrated Processes: Nursing Process: Assessment
Client Need: Physiological Integrity; Basic Care and Comfort
Cognitive Level: Analysis

12. **ANSWER: 4.**

Rationales:

1. Washing the hands is not the first thing that the nurse should do before administering a back rub.

2. Warming the lotion is not the first thing that the nurse should do before administering a back rub.

3. Pulling the curtain for privacy is not the first thing that the nurse should do before administering a back rub.

4. The stimulation of a back rub may not be tolerated by some patients. A back rub is contraindicated when a patient has certain conditions, such as impaired skin integrity (e.g., pressure ulcer, burn, or open wound), rib fractures, or a vertebral disorder or within 48 hours of experiencing the onset of an acute neurological or cardiac problem.

TEST-TAKING TIP: Identify the word in the stem that sets a priority. The word *first* in the stem sets a priority. Identify the option that is unique. Option 4 is unique. It is the only option that involves assessment.

Content Area: Pain, Comfort, Rest, and Sleep
Integrated Processes: Nursing Process: Planning
Client Need: Physiological Integrity; Basic Care and Comfort
Cognitive Level: Application

13. **ANSWER: 4.**

Rationales:

1. Sleep and rest both prevent fatigue.

2. Sleep and rest both slow vital signs.

3. Sleep and rest both conserve energy.

4. Reduced perception occurs with sleep but not with rest, because the patient is unconscious.

TEST-TAKING TIP: Identify the equally plausible options. Options 1 and 3 are equally plausible. One is no better than the other. Eliminate both from further consideration.

Content Area: Pain, Comfort, Rest, and Sleep
Integrated Processes: Nursing Process: Evaluation
Client Need: Physiological Integrity; Basic Care and Comfort
Cognitive Level: Application

14. **ANSWER: 2.**

Rationales:

1. NREM sleep deficiency precipitates physiological deficiencies, such as fatigue and lethargy.

2. REM sleep deficiency precipitates cognitive, emotional, and behavioral changes that include irritability and confusion. Also, the person may experience anxiety, apathy, an inability to concentrate, combativeness, disorientation, delusions, hallucinations, and/or paranoia.

3. NREM sleep deficiency precipitates physiological deficiencies, such as tremors and increased sensitivity to pain.

4. NREM sleep deficiency precipitates physiological deficiencies, such as immunosuppression and delayed wound healing.

TEST-TAKING TIP: Identify the option that is unique. Option 2 is unique. Options 1, 3, and 4 are related to physiological deficiencies, whereas option 2 is related to an impairment of cognitive function. Examine option 2 carefully.

Content Area: Pain, Comfort, Rest, and Sleep
Integrated Processes: Nursing Process: Assessment
Client Need: Physiological Integrity; Basic Care and Comfort
Cognitive Level: Application

15. **ANSWER: 3.**

Rationales:

1. Grinding the teeth while sleeping is bruxism. It may include repetitive clenching of teeth; it can erode tooth enamel, loosen teeth, and cause pain in the jaw.

2. Snoring is a clinical indicator of obstructive sleep apnea, not narcolepsy.

3. Abruptly falling asleep unexpectedly is a clinical indicator of narcolepsy. Additional clinical indicators include slurred speech and abrupt bilateral loss of muscle tone (cataplexy). The patient may report weakness of the knees and/or inability to move during the onset of a sleep attack or when waking up (sleep paralysis) and vivid or bizarre dreams while falling asleep.

4. Episodic walking around while asleep with minimal awareness of the environment is sleepwalking (somnambulism), not narcolepsy.

Content Area: Pain, Comfort, Rest, and Sleep
Integrated Processes: Communication/Documentation; Nursing Process: Assessment
Client Need: Physiological Integrity; Basic Care and Comfort
Cognitive Level: Application

16. **ANSWER: 4.**

Rationales:

1. When the eyes are closed, the individual may be resting or sleeping. The patient may have the eyes closed when engaged in such activities as praying and imagery.

2. Appearing physically at ease with a reduction in muscle tension can occur with both rest and sleep.

3. A patient may keep the arms at the side of the body when either resting or sleeping.

4. A patient will experience altered levels of consciousness when sleeping, with a lack of response to insignificant environmental noises. A patient at rest will be alert and have no altered level of consciousness.

TEST-TAKING TIP: Identify the word in the stem that sets a priority. The word *best* in the stem sets a priority. Identify the options that are equally plausible. Options 1, 2, and 3 are equally plausible because they are all related to body position.

Content Area: Pain, Comfort, Rest, and Sleep
Integrated Processes: Nursing Process: Evaluation
Client Need: Physiological Integrity; Basic Care and Comfort
Cognitive Level: Application

17. **ANSWER: 2.**
    Rationales:
    1. This outcome is associated with contraceptive therapy, not palliative therapy. Contraceptive therapy prevents a pregnancy.
    2. This outcome describes palliative care, whereby the illness is not cured, but relief of signs and symptoms make the illness more tolerable.
    3. This outcome describes curative care, not palliative care. Curative care completely resolves an illness.
    4. This outcome is associated with health maintenance or substitutive medication therapy, whereby a medication is administered to support normal body function (e.g., regular insulin [Novolin R] for diabetes).

    Content Area: Pain, Comfort, Rest, and Sleep
    Integrated Processes: Nursing Process: Evaluation
    Client Need: Physiological Integrity; Pharmacological and Parenteral Therapies
    Cognitive Level: Application

18. **ANSWER: 1, 2, 4.**
    Rationales:
    1. The feeling of pins and needles generally is associated with neuropathic pain. Neuropathic pain is caused by nerve fibers that are damaged or dysfunctional, which can occur in either the peripheral or central nervous system.
    2. Numbness generally is associated with neuropathic pain.
    3. Pain described as pounding generally results from stimulation of pain receptors at the site of trauma, ischemia, or inflammation. Also, it is associated with pain from internal organs and pain from skin, connective tissue, muscles, and bones.
    4. A burning sensation generally is associated with neuropathic pain.
    5. An aching sensation generally results from stimulation of pain receptors at the site of trauma, ischemia, or inflammation. Also, it is associated with pain from internal organs and pain from skin, connective tissue, muscles, and bones.

    Content Area: Pain, Comfort, Rest, and Sleep
    Integrated Processes: Communication/Documentation; Nursing Process: Assessment
    Client Need: Physiological Integrity; Basic Care and Comfort
    Cognitive Level: Application

19. **ANSWER: 1.**
    Rationales:
    1. Adolescents generally want to appear brave in front of others, especially peers. This statement is patient centered because it gives the adolescent permission to cry when confronted with pain.
    2. Although pulling the curtain addresses the privacy needs of an adolescent, it is not as important as a statement presented in another option.
    3. Although this may be verbalized, it is not as important as a statement presented in another option. Toddlers, not adolescents, may consider pain as punishment.
    4. This is not a patient-centered statement. This statement places the nurse's beliefs onto the patient as well as presents an expected patient response that may be unrealistic.

    TEST-TAKING TIP: Identify the word in the stem that sets a priority. The word *most* in the stem sets a priority.

    Content Area: Pain, Comfort, Rest, and Sleep
    Integrated Processes: Caring, Communication/Documentation; Nursing Process: Implementation
    Client Need: Physiological Integrity; Basic Care and Comfort
    Cognitive Level: Application

20. **ANSWER: 1.**
    Rationales:
    1. This question is assessing the quality of the pain. Descriptions generally include such words as burning, stabbing, throbbing, crushing, pressure, sharp, dull, achy, and so on.
    2. A question that assesses intensity is, "How severe is your pain on a scale of 0 to 10?" A numerical scale provides objective and consistent assessment of pain intensity.
    3. The question does not assess behavioral responses to pain. Observing moaning, grunting, crying, increased muscle tension, hand wringing, guarding, holding or rubbing a part of the body, and so on are examples of observed behaviors associated with a painful experience.
    4. A question that assesses precipitating factors is, "What initiates or increases the pain?" Participating factors may include such actions as bending, lifting, coughing, eating, or breathing deeply.

    Content Area: Pain, Comfort, Rest, and Sleep
    Integrated Processes: Communication/Documentation; Nursing Process: Assessment
    Client Need: Physiological Integrity; Basic Care and Comfort
    Cognitive Level: Application

21. **ANSWER: 1.**
    Rationales:
    1. It is essential that patients know that nurses believe that they are experiencing pain and that the pain is real.
    2. Although breathing exercises may reduce the patient's pain, they are not as important as another option.
    3. Although a distraction technique may reduce the patient's pain, it is not as important as another option.
    4. Although muscle relaxation techniques may reduce the patient's pain, they are not as important as another option.

    TEST-TAKING TIP: Identify the word in the stem that sets a priority. The word *most* in the stem sets a priority. Identify the clang association. The word *pain* in the stem and in option 1 is a clang association. Identify equally plausible options. Options 2, 3, and 4 are strategies to manage pain. Option 1 is the only option that acknowledges the patient's painful experience. Option 1 reflects nursing care that is patient centered.

Content Area: Pain, Comfort, Rest, and Sleep
Integrated Processes: Communication/Documentation; Nursing Process: Implementation
Client Need: Psychosocial Integrity
Cognitive Level: Application

22. ANSWER: 1, 4, 5.
Rationales:
1. **A gradual onset is associated with chronic pain. A quick onset is associated with acute pain.**
2. Constricted pupils are related to stimulation of the parasympathetic nervous system associated with chronic pain. Dilated pupils are related to stimulation of the sympathetic nervous system associated with acute pain.
3. Pressured speech is related to stimulation of the sympathetic nervous system associated with acute pain. Slow, monotonous speech is associated with chronic pain in response to stimulation of the parasympathetic nervous system.
4. **Recurring pain is associated with remissions and exacerbations, which are related to chronic pain. Chronic pain is related to a time frame longer than 6 months.**
5. **Variable breathing patterns are associated with chronic pain in response to stimulation of the parasympathetic nervous system. Hyperpnea is related to acute pain in response to stimulation of the sympathetic nervous system.**

Content Area: Pain, Comfort, Rest, and Sleep
Integrated Processes: Nursing Process: Assessment
Client Need: Physiological Integrity; Basic Care and Comfort
Cognitive Level: Analysis

23. ANSWER: 4.
Rationales:
1. Alcohol should be avoided because it contributes to early awakening. Also, it has a diuretic effect, which may cause nocturia that will interrupt sleeping.
2. Milk at bedtime may be encouraged, not avoided. L-tryptophan in milk converts to melatonin, which maintains the body's circadian rhythms and promotes sleep.
3. The bed should only be used for sleeping and sexual activity. A person should get out of bed if not asleep within 30 minutes and return to bed when sleepy. This trains the body and mind to associate a bed with sleeping.
4. **Rituals and routines promote comfort and relaxation and should be encouraged because they promote sleep.**
TEST-TAKING TIP: Identify the unique option. Option 4 is unique because it is a general comment that incorporates numerous sleep promoting techniques (e.g., every night drink a glass of milk, take a shower, brush the teeth, read a book, perform a muscle relaxation technique, and then turn out the lights). Options 1, 2, and 3 identify just one specific intervention.

Content Area: Pain, Comfort, Rest, and Sleep
Integrated Processes: Teaching/Learning; Nursing Process: Implementation
Client Need: Physiological Integrity; Basic Care and Comfort
Cognitive Level: Application

24. ANSWER: 2.
Rationales:
1. Although arranging furniture so patients have a view from their rooms is a caring intervention, it is unrelated to psychospiritual comfort.
2. **No two people are alike. Viewing each patient as a unique individual is basic to all interactions with a patient. The nurse should view each patient as a distinct individual with personal distinguishing characteristics and plan and implement nursing care accordingly.**
3. Although providing for a patient's basic physiological needs is important, it is related to providing physical comfort, not psychospiritual comfort.
4. Although providing for continuity of care is important, it is unrelated to psychospiritual comfort.

Content Area: Pain, Comfort, Rest, and Sleep
Integrated Processes: Caring; Nursing Process: Implementation
Client Need: Psychosocial Integrity
Cognitive Level: Application

25. ANSWER: 4.
Rationales:
1. Reacting normally when awakened and paradoxical sleep is associated with REM sleep stage 5.
2. Light sleep and easy to awaken is associated with NREM sleep stage 1.
3. Light sleep and easy to awaken is associated with NREM sleep stage 2.
4. **Deep sleep and difficulty awakening is associated with NREM sleep stage 4.**

Content Area: Pain, Comfort, Rest, and Sleep
Integrated Processes: Nursing Process: Assessment
Client Need: Physiological Integrity; Basic Care and Comfort
Cognitive Level: Comprehension

26. ANSWER: 2, 4, 5.
Rationales:
1. Daytime naps should be avoided unless they are less than 30 minutes. Excessive napping contributes to insomnia at night.
2. **Nicotine is stimulating. The half-life of nicotine is 1 to 2 hours.**
3. Physical exertion should be avoided 1 to 2 hours before bedtime because it is too stimulating.
4. **Caffeine is stimulating and should be avoided 4 hours before bedtime.**
5. **Carbohydrates limit the sensation of hunger, which provides for comfort; protein reduces the sugar boost of the carbohydrates.**

Content Area: Pain, Comfort, Rest, and Sleep
Integrated Processes: Teaching/Learning; Nursing Process: Implementation
Client Need: Physiological Integrity; Basic Care and Comfort
Cognitive Level: Application

27. ANSWER: 1.
Rationales:
1. **An increase in falls is associated with older adults receiving Xanax. Xanax, a benzodiazepine, depresses the central nervous system, which may cause impaired coordination, drowsiness, fatigue, confusion, and tremors.**

2. The blood pressure decreases, not increases, in response to Xanax because it may cause central nervous system depression.

3. This is not the priority at this time. Receiving Xanax longer than 2 weeks may lead to dependence.

4. Xanax should be discontinued slowly, not immediately, to prevent signs and symptoms of withdrawal.

TEST-TAKING TIP: Identify the word in the stem that sets a priority. The word *most* in the stem sets a priority.

Content Area: Pain, Comfort, Rest, and Sleep
Integrated Processes: Nursing Process: Implementation
Client Need: Physiological Integrity; Pharmacological and Parenteral Therapies
Cognitive Level: Application

28. ANSWER: 4.

Rationales:

1. Although this should be done, it is not the priority. Usually, relief from pain is achieved more readily when an analgesic is administered before the pain becomes severe.

2. Although this should be done to prevent hypostatic pneumonia, it is not the priority.

3. Although this should be done because tolerance can occur with an opioid, it is not the priority.

4. Opioids depress respirations. If a patient experiences a respiratory rate of less than 10 breaths per minute, hold the next dose and notify the primary health-care provider about the status of the patient. The dose of the opioid should be reduced or a prescription for a different medication may be necessary.

TEST-TAKING TIP: Identify the word in the stem that sets a priority. The word *most* in the stem sets a priority. Identify the unique option. Option 4 is unique because it is the only option with a number.

Content Area: Pain, Comfort, Rest, and Sleep
Integrated Processes: Nursing Process: Evaluation
Client Need: Physiological Integrity; Pharmacological and Parenteral Therapies
Cognitive Level: Application

29. ANSWER: 1.

Rationales:

1. Frequent awakenings to implement nursing care generally are the underlying cause of sleep deprivation in critical care environments. Clustering nursing care provides blocks of uninterrupted periods of time in which the patient can attempt to sleep.

2. Although napping can provide additional sleep, it is not as effective as an action presented in another option.

3. Although supporting a bedtime ritual may help a patient fall asleep, it does not support uninterrupted sleep.

4. Although a back rub may relax a patient, this intervention does not address the most common cause of sleep deprivation in an intensive care unit.

Content Area: Pain, Comfort, Rest, and Sleep
Integrated Processes: Nursing Process: Implementation
Client Need: Physiological Integrity; Basic Care and Comfort
Cognitive Level: Application

30. ANSWER: 2.

Rationales:

1. There is no evidence in the patient interview that indicates that the patient is irritable.

2. Multiplicity of stress can overwhelm a patient physically and emotionally, reducing a patient's pain threshold.

3. A pain level of 3 is within the realm of pain that a person should be able to tolerate. The patient's respirations are 14 breaths/minute. A larger or more frequent dose of an opioid will depress the central nervous system, causing respiratory depression and should be avoided. In addition, opioids can precipitate constipation, hypotension, drowsiness, and confusion.

4. The expected range of respirations for an adult is 12 to 20 breaths/minute. If the respirations are less than 10 breaths/minute, the next dose of the opioid should be held and the primary health-care provider notified. The opioid dose may need to be adjusted or the medication changed. In extreme situations, the antidote naloxone (Narcan) may be required.

TEST-TAKING TIP: Identify the word in the stem that sets a priority. The word *most* in the stem sets a priority.

Content Area: Pain, Comfort, Rest, and Sleep
Integrated Processes: Nursing Process: Analysis
Client Need: Physiological Integrity; Pharmacological and Parenteral Therapies
Cognitive Level: Analysis

31. ANSWER: 2.

Rationales:

1. Wrapping the legs with ace bandages is not associated with reducing unpleasant sensations of restless leg syndrome.

2. Stretching exercises of the leg muscles often provide some relief of the unpleasant tingling, itching, creeping, and crawling sensations associated with restless leg syndrome.

3. Tea contains caffeine, which is a stimulant, and should be avoided in patients with restless leg syndrome.

4. Excessive weight is associated with sleep apnea, not restless leg syndrome.

TEST-TAKING TIP: Identify the clang associations. The word *leg* in the stem and in options 1 and 2 are clang associations. Examine options 1 and 2 carefully.

Content Area: Pain, Comfort, Rest, and Sleep
Integrated Processes: Teaching/Learning; Nursing Process: Implementation
Client Need: Physiological Integrity; Basic Care and Comfort
Cognitive Level: Application

32. ANSWER: 2.

Rationales:

1. Administering an analgesic relieves pain, which is related to a physical, not psychospiritual need.

2. Using effective communication skills, including active listening, addresses psychospiritual needs.

3. Dimming lights in the room at night limits a noxious stimulus, which is related to an environmental, not psychospiritual, need.

4. A parent staying with a hospitalized child addresses the sociocultural, not psychospiritual, needs of both child and parent.

Content Area: Pain, Comfort, Rest, and Sleep
Integrated Processes: Caring; Communication/
Documentation; Nursing Process: Planning
Client Need: Physiological Integrity; Basic Care and
Comfort
Cognitive Level: Analysis

33. ANSWER: 1.5.
Rationale:
Solve the problem by using the formula for ratio and proportion.

$$\frac{\text{Desire 1.5 mg}}{\text{Have 1 mg}} = \frac{x \text{ mL}}{1 \text{ mL}}$$

$$1x = 1.5 \times 1$$
$$1x = 1.5$$
$$x = 1.5 \div 1$$
$$x = 1.5 \text{ mL}$$

Content Area: Pain, Comfort, Rest, and Sleep
Integrated Processes: Nursing Process: Planning
Client Need: Physiological Integrity; Pharmacological and
Parenteral Therapies
Cognitive Level: Application

34. ANSWER: 3.
Rationales:
1. Avoiding hazardous activities is unnecessary. Acetaminophen does not depress the central nervous system.
2. Acetaminophen should be taken with food because it can cause gastrointestinal irritation and bleeding.
3. Intake of greater than 4 g of acetaminophen in 24 hours may cause liver damage.
4. Constipation is not related to the intake of acetaminophen.

Content Area: Pain, Comfort, Rest, and Sleep
Integrated Processes: Teaching/Learning; Nursing Process:
Implementation
Client Need: Physiological Integrity; Pharmacological and
Parenteral Therapies
Cognitive Level: Application

35. ANSWER: 3, 5, 2, 4, 1.
Rationales:
3. The first step in the nursing process is assessment. The patient's pain is a level 8.
5. The second step in the nursing process is identifying the problem. The problem is that the patient is experiencing acute pain related to tissue trauma and reflex muscle spasms secondary to surgery.
2. The third step in the nursing process is planning. Planning includes identifying the expected outcome and planned interventions.
4. The fourth step of the nursing process is implementation. Administering the opioid according to the primary health-care provider's prescription is an action that should achieve the expected outcome.
1. The fifth and last step of the nursing process is evaluation. Evaluating the effectiveness of the administered opioid requires the nurse to reassess the patient's pain to ensure that the expected outcome was achieved.

Content Area: Pain, Comfort, Rest, and Sleep
Integrated Processes: Nursing Process: Planning
Client Need: Physiological Integrity; Pharmacological and
Parenteral Therapies
Cognitive Level: Analysis

Chapter 24

Perioperative Nursing

KEY TERMS

Abdominal distention (tympanites)—Excessive flatus within the intestines.

Ablative surgery—Surgical removal of a body part, pathway, or function.

Atelectasis—Collapsed or airless alveoli due to inadequate lung expansion.

Conscious sedation—Administration of an intravenous agent to produce a depressed level of consciousness that allows a patient to follow directions but to feel little or no pain.

Cosmetic surgery—Surgery to improve appearance.

Curative surgery—Surgical excision or repair of a diseased organ to reestablish function.

Dehiscence—Separation of one or more layers of a surgical abdominal wound before healing.

Diagnostic and explorative surgery—Surgery to validate a diagnosis.

Elective surgery—Surgery that is advised, but life is not imminently threatened.

Emergency surgery—Immediate surgery necessary to preserve life and/or function.

Epidural anesthesia—Agent injected via a catheter into the epidural space to relieve pain while the patient is awake and aware of surroundings.

Evisceration—Spilling of abdominal contents from a surgical abdominal wound as a result of dehiscence.

Hemorrhage—Uncontrolled internal or external bleeding.

Hemovac drain—Drainage tube placed in the body near an operative site and attached to a round collapsible reservoir with springs that, when compressed, establishes low negative pressure, which pulls drainage into the device.

Hypovolemia—Insufficient circulating blood volume.

Hypovolemic shock—Severe insufficient circulating blood volume due to loss of 30 percent or 1,500 mL or more of circulating blood volume.

Hypoxemia—Inadequate oxygen in the blood.

Jackson-Pratt drain—Thin tube placed in the body near an operative site and connected to a self-suction bulb that is compressed to establish low negative pressure, which pulls drainage into the bulb.

Laparoscopic surgery—Minimally invasive surgery using a thin lighted tube (laparoscope) and other instruments inserted through small incisions, allowing the surgical field to be visualized on a video monitor connected to the scope.

Local anesthesia—Agent injected into a specific area that reduces sensation while the patient remains awake and aware of surroundings.

Malignant hyperthermia—Rapid increase in heart and respiratory rates, progressing to hyperthermia, dysrhythmias, and respiratory and metabolic acidosis precipitated by anesthesia in patients with a rare autosomal dominant trait.

Nasogastric (NG) tube—Tube inserted through the nose, down the esophagus, and into the stomach that is generally used to remove gastric contents (gastric decompression) postoperatively when attached to suction.

Negative pressure wound therapy—Treatment in which an occlusive dressing on a wound is attached via tubing to a machine that produces negative pressure, which removes exudate to limit edema and promote granulation.

Nerve block—Agent injected into and around a nerve or group of nerves (plexus) to reduce sensation while the patient is awake and aware of surroundings.

Palliative surgery—Surgery to reduce symptoms without curing.

Patient-controlled analgesia—Device that administers an intravenous analgesic at an hourly dose to manage pain at a consistent, tolerable level and allows the patient to compress a trigger to deliver an extra dose as needed; however, a "lockout" prevents excessive doses when the trigger is pushed prematurely.

Continued

KEY TERMS—cont'd

Penrose drain—Soft, flat tube placed in the body near an operative site to drain blood, pus, tissue, and debris into a gauze dressing via gravity and capillary action.

Postoperative ileus (paralytic ileus, adynamic ileus)—Cessation of intestinal peristalsis characterized by lack of forward movement of intestinal contents.

Pulmonary embolus—A thrombus that travels via venous circulation to the lung, obstructing a pulmonary artery.

Reconstructive (restorative) surgery—Surgery to restore function or appearance.

Regional anesthesia—Agent that causes loss of sensation in a specific area while allowing the patient to remain conscious.

Robotic surgery—Surgery involving the use of mechanical arms to hold surgical instruments that are controlled by a surgeon sitting at a console.

Safety "time out" check—Safety measure performed at various times before surgery to verify the patient's name, surgical procedure, and surgical site.

Spinal anesthesia—Agent injected via a lumbar puncture into the cerebrospinal fluid in the subarachnoid space to block movement and sensation below the level of the injection.

Telesurgery—Robotic surgery implemented remotely, in which the surgeon's console is located in one location and is connected to the surgical system at the patient's location.

Topical anesthetic—Agent applied directly to the surface of the skin or mucous membranes to reduce sensation in the area where it is applied.

T-tube—Tube placed in the common bile duct to maintain patency of the duct and drain bile into a small collection bag via gravity.

Transplant surgery—Replacement of a diseased body part.

Urgent surgery—Surgery necessary within 24 hours of diagnosis.

Urinary retention—Inability to empty the bladder completely, resulting in excessive urine accumulation.

I. Introduction

Perioperative nursing includes the care that is delivered by nurses to patients during the preoperative, intraoperative, and postoperative phases of the surgical experience. Nurses must understand that surgery is an invasive procedure that has various purposes, degrees of urgency, and levels of risk and can be performed in a variety of settings. In addition, numerous personal risk factors can affect a patient's surgical outcome. Nurses must identify the presence of these risk factors and implement appropriate nursing care during each of the phases of the surgical experience to meet the individual needs of patients.

A. Purposes of Surgery
1. **Ablative:** Surgical removal of a body part, pathway, or function (e.g., appendectomy, colectomy, amputation, and obliteration of ectopic foci in the heart).
2. **Cosmetic:** Surgery to improve appearance (e.g., liposuction, facelift, and rhinoplasty).
3. **Curative:** Surgical excision or repair of a diseased organ to reestablish function (e.g., complete removal of a cancerous tumor and repair of an aortic aneurysm).
4. **Diagnostic and explorative:** Surgery to validate a diagnosis (e.g., cardiac catheterization, biopsy of a mass, and identification of a cause of gastrointestinal [GI] bleeding).
5. **Palliative:** Surgery to reduce symptoms without curing (e.g., resection of a nerve root or partial removal of a mass) to provide for comfort.
6. **Reconstructive and restorative:** Surgery to restore function or appearance (e.g., repair of a torn ligament, internal fixation of a fracture, or cleft lip repair).
7. **Transplant:** Replacement of a diseased body part (e.g., kidney, heart, or lung transplant or joint replacement).

B. Degree of Urgency
1. **Elective.**
   a. When surgery is advised but the patient's life is not imminently threatened.
   b. Allows for patient preparation.
   c. Associated with low morbidity and mortality.
   d. Examples: Cataract extraction, knee replacement, and breast reduction.
2. **Urgent.**
   a. When surgery is necessary within 24 hours of diagnosis.
   b. Allows for some patient preparation.
   c. Reduces the risk of complications that can occur with a delay.
   d. Examples: Open reduction internal fixation of a fracture, coronary artery bypass, and removal of a cancerous tumor.
3. **Emergency.**
   a. When immediate surgery is necessary to preserve life and/or function.
   b. Limits time for history taking and patient preparation.

c. Associated with increased morbidity and mortality due to concurrent conditions.

d. Examples: Subdural hematoma, hemorrhaging, and traumatic amputation.

C. Level of Risk of Surgery

1. Major.

a. Involves a high degree of risk.

b. Associated with prolonged and/or complicated surgical procedures, blood loss, total or partial removal of a structure or organ, open abdominal or thoracic surgery, and potential postoperative complications.

c. Examples: Cardiac surgery, removal of a kidney (nephrectomy), removal of a section of the large intestine (colectomy), and organ transplantation.

2. Minor.

a. Involves a low degree of risk.

b. Associated with few potential complications.

c. Generally performed on an outpatient basis.

d. Examples: Hernia repair, arthroscopy, and cataract extraction.

D. Factors Affecting Surgical Risk

1. Age.

a. Older adults.

(1) Decreased physiological reserves, such as decreased cardiac output, cough reflex, immunity, vital capacity, subcutaneous tissue, blood oxygenation, glomerular filtration rate, and basal metabolic rate.

(2) Increased comorbidities, such as heart disease, obstructive lung disease, diabetes, and peripheral vascular disease.

(3) Increased calcium and cholesterol deposits within small arteries that increase the risk of hypertension, fluid and electrolyte imbalances, and shock when blood loss occurs.

b. Infants and children.

(1) Immature immune, renal, cardiovascular, and biliary systems.

(2) Limited ability to regulate body temperature due to underdeveloped shivering reflex.

(3) Limited response to anesthesia that causes vasodilation and heat loss.

(4) Increased psychological and physiological stress because of an inability to understand what is happening and separation from parents.

(5) Limited circulating blood volume, which increases the risk of hypovolemic shock and fluid and electrolyte imbalances, such as fluid volume deficit or excess.

2. Medical history.

a. Cardiovascular disease, such as hypertension, heart failure, and myocardial infarction, affects the ability to maintain cardiac efficiency.

b. Kidney dysfunction, such as acute or chronic kidney disease, reduces the ability to excrete medications and regulate fluid and electrolyte balance.

c. Lung diseases, such as asthma, emphysema, and bronchitis, decrease pulmonary function and increase the risk of postoperative pneumonia and atelectasis.

d. Neurologic disorders, such as spinal cord injury, are associated with vasomotor instability; people with seizure disorders commonly have an increased number of seizures during the perioperative period.

e. Liver disease, such as cirrhosis, increases the risk of hemorrhage because of an inability to make prothrombin and increases the risk of toxic reactions to medications and anesthesia because of an inability to detoxify these agents.

f. Coagulation disorders can contribute to hemorrhage due to delayed clotting mechanisms or risk of brain attack and intravascular clotting due to hypercoagulation.

g. Diabetes mellitus increases the risk of infection and delayed wound healing because of a reduced ability to metabolize carbohydrates, proteins, and fat.

h. Current acute infections challenge physiological and energy reserves, increasing the potential for postoperative complications; upper respiratory infections increase the risk of pneumonia and atelectasis, particularly with general anesthesia.

i. A decreased immune system, such as from cancer and its treatments (e.g., radiation, chemotherapy); bone marrow alterations; immunosuppressives to prevent organ transplant rejection; and steroids to reduce inflammatory disorders, places the patient at risk for postoperative infection and delayed wound healing.

j. Allergies and intolerances can cause uncomfortable—and life threatening—integumentary and respiratory system reactions.

(1) Some patients are allergic to prescription and nonprescription drugs, tape, latex, soaps, ointments, and solutions, such as povidone-iodine, which is used in surgical skin preparation.

(2) Some patients are allergic to iodine; iodine-based dyes are used in many diagnostic procedures.

3. Medications.

a. Anticoagulants: Prolong blood coagulation time, causing bleeding.

b. Antidepressants: Interact with anesthetics and may decrease blood pressure.

c. Antidysrhythmics: Impair cardiac conduction during anesthesia.

d. Antihypertensives: May interact with anesthetic agents, causing hypotension, bradycardia, and reduced circulation.

e. Corticosteroids: Impair wound healing and suppress immunity.

f. Diuretics: May alter fluid and electrolyte balance, precipitating fluid volume deficit, hyponatremia, and hypokalemia.

g. Tranquilizers: May interact with anesthetic agents, causing respiratory depression.

4. Herbal products.
   a. Ephedra (to lose weight): Increases the risk of dysrhythmias.
   b. Feverfew (to limit migraine headaches): Increases the risk of bleeding.
   c. Ginkgo biloba (to increase memory): Affects platelet activity and increases the risk of postoperative bleeding.
   d. Ginseng (to increase energy and immunity): Affects platelet activity and increases the risk of postoperative bleeding; may also increase hypoglycemia with insulin administration when a perioperative patient has diabetes.
   e. Kava (to promote relaxation): Intensifies the effects of sedatives.
   f. Vitamin E (to increase immunity): In high doses, may increase the risk of bleeding.

5. Tobacco smoking.
   a. Increases respiratory complications because anesthesia is a respiratory irritant that stimulates the production of secretions.
   b. Nicotine constricts blood vessels.

6. Illegal drug use: May increase tolerance to anesthetics and analgesics, requiring higher doses to obtain a therapeutic effect.

7. Alcohol abuse.
   a. Alcohol potentiates the action of analgesics and anesthetic agents.
   b. Associated malnutrition delays wound healing.
   c. Associated liver disease and portal hypertension increase the risk of complications, such as hemorrhage.
   d. Withdrawal begins 24 hours after alcohol deprivation.

8. Nutritional status.
   a. Inadequate nutrition increases the risk of infection and delays wound healing.
   b. Increased protein, zinc, and vitamins C and A intake support wound healing.
   c. Daily requirement of 1,500 kcal is needed to maintain basic metabolic needs; because the metabolic rate increases during wound healing, this amount may have to be increased.

9. Obesity.
   a. Presence of comorbidities associated with obesity, such as sleep apnea, hypertension, coronary artery disease, and diabetes mellitus, may increase the risk of perioperative complications.
   b. Obesity decreases postoperative ventilation due to thoracic and abdominal weight impinging on the expansion of the thoracic cavity during inhalation, which may result in respiratory and cardiac postoperative complications.
   c. Fragility of adipose tissue and limited circulation in adipose tissue are associated with increased wound complications, such as delayed wound healing, separation of the wound edges (**dehiscence**), protrusion of the abdominal viscera through the incision (**evisceration**), and wound infection.

10. Fluid and electrolyte balance.
    a. Surgical trauma increases blood glucose and breaks down protein, resulting in a negative nitrogen balance, which impairs wound healing and increases the risk of infection.
    b. Adrenocortical stress response causes sodium and water retention and hypokalemia, which increases the risk of dysrhythmias.

11. Mental status: Impaired cognitive function, such as dementia, delirium, mental retardation, developmental delays, mental illness, confusion, and disorientation, may interfere with the ability to understand teaching or give consent.

12. Emotional health.
    a. Anxiety and a feeling of unease are common reactions.
    b. Patients may express emotions via angry, argumentative, demanding, or overly critical behaviors.

13. Extent of the incision: The larger the incision, the more trauma to body tissues.

DID YOU KNOW?

Historically, all surgery was performed through open incisions. Minimally invasive surgery was introduced with the advent of **laparoscopic surgery**. In laparoscopic surgery, a thin, lighted tube (laparoscope) and other instruments are inserted through small incisions, allowing the surgical field to be visualized by the surgeon on a video monitor connected to the scope. The laparoscopic approach causes less tissue trauma, thereby reducing the length of recovery. Laparoscopic surgery moved to a more complex level with the invention of **robotic surgery**. Robotic systems hold surgical instruments that, when moved by a surgeon sitting at a console, are more deliberate and precise than the human hand. Initially, these consoles were in close proximity to the patient;

however, in 1996, robotic **telesurgery** was introduced in which a computerized interface transmitted the surgical field over the Internet to a console at a great distance from the patient. The continued growth in technology and miniaturization of instruments is predicted to result in robotic devices so small that they will be inserted into the body and directed to the surgical site, where they can be manipulated by the surgeon via computer commands. This technology is not so far-fetched when one notes that it required only several years between the first laparoscopic cholecystectomy in 1986 for this technique to become the industry standard in the early 1990s for such surgeries as appendectomy, cholecystectomy, hysterectomy, and hernia and joint repair.

E. Surgical Settings
1. Health-care provider's offices.
   a. Allow procedures to be performed at the time of an office visit.
   b. Are convenient for patients and primary health-care providers.
   c. Examples: Biopsy, minor plastic surgery, and dermal procedures.
2. Ambulatory surgery centers.
   a. Allow patients to be admitted for surgery in the morning and to be discharged later that day when stable.
   b. Used for surgeries that have minimal risk.
   c. Allow surgeries to be minimally disruptive to a patient's usual routine.
   d. Allow the diagnostic surgical workup to be done on an outpatient basis.
   e. Typically have 23-hour admission, which allows monitoring for complications and pain control after surgery.
   f. Examples: Hernia repair, lumpectomy, laparoscopic cholecystectomy, angioplasty, tonsillectomy, and arthroscopy.
3. Hospital-based settings.
   a. Allow patients to be admitted to the hospital before surgery to perform diagnostic tests and/or correct problems (e.g., fluid and electrolyte imbalances) that may negatively impact the patient's status during the perioperative period.
   b. Allow patients to remain in the hospital after major surgery that requires continued medical and nursing care.
   c. Allow patients admitted for same-day surgery (ambulatory surgery) to be admitted to the hospital after surgery if their status is unstable or a complication occurs.
   d. Examples: Joint replacement, gastric bypass, and emergency exploratory surgery.

F. Anesthesia
1. **General.**
   a. Loss of sensation and consciousness.
   b. Agent administered via IV or inhalation.
   c. Used for major surgery.
   d. Advantages.
      (1) Leaves patient unconscious and motionless, with muscles relaxed.
      (2) Allows dose to be adjusted to age, physical condition, and length of procedure.
   e. Disadvantages.
      (1) Depresses the respiratory system, including cough and gag reflexes, increasing the risk of pneumonia and atelectasis.
      (2) Depresses the circulatory system, increasing the risk of thrombophlebitis.
      (3) Causes postoperative throat discomfort when an endotracheal tube is used.
      (4) Can lead to life-threatening complications, such as brain attack, malignant hyperthermia, and cardiac arrest.
   f. Stages.
      (1) Stage I: Beginning anesthesia, drowsiness, dizziness, and depressed pain sensation.
      (2) Stage II: Excitement, spasmodic muscles, irregular breathing, intact swallowing reflexes, and possible vomiting.
      (3) Stage III: Regular, rhythmic breathing; depressed reflexes and vital functions; relaxed skeletal muscles; constricted pupils; absent eyelid reflexes; and patient readiness for surgery.
      (4) Stage IV: Complete respiratory depression; rapid, thready pulse.
2. **Conscious sedation.**
   a. Produces a depressed level of consciousness that allows the patient to follow directions, but causes the patient little or no pain and usually prevents the patient from remembering the proceedings of the procedure.
   b. Involves IV administration of sedatives and/or analgesic medications.
   c. Used for minor surgery and uncomfortable or painful diagnostic procedures.
   d. Advantages.
      (1) Allows for quick reversal of effects.
      (2) Allows the patient to be able to respond to commands and be aroused easily by touch or speech.
      (3) Allows the patient to retain protective airway reflexes and spontaneous ventilation; vital signs usually remain stable.
   e. Disadvantages.
      (1) May cause discomfort in some patients and some patients experience awareness of the procedure.

(2) Requires patient safety to be maintained during recovery (e.g., vital signs monitored every 15 minutes until fully awake and stable; patient cannot drive after the procedure).

f. Uses.

(1) Endoscopies, such as colonoscopy and bronchoscopy.

(2) Cosmetic surgery.

3. **Regional anesthesia.**

a. Causes loss of sensation in a specific area while the patient remains conscious.

b. Given via a catheter.

c. Types.

(1) **Spinal.**

(a) Agent injected via a lumbar puncture into the cerebrospinal fluid in the subarachnoid space (Fig. 24.1).

(b) Blocks movement and sensation below the level of the injection.

(c) Advantages: Usually does not cause respiratory depression; allows the patient to be awake and aware of surroundings.

(d) Disadvantages: May cause hypotension, urinary retention, nausea and vomiting, and/or headache from leakage of cerebrospinal fluid; agent may migrate upward in spinal cord, depressing respirations and heart rate.

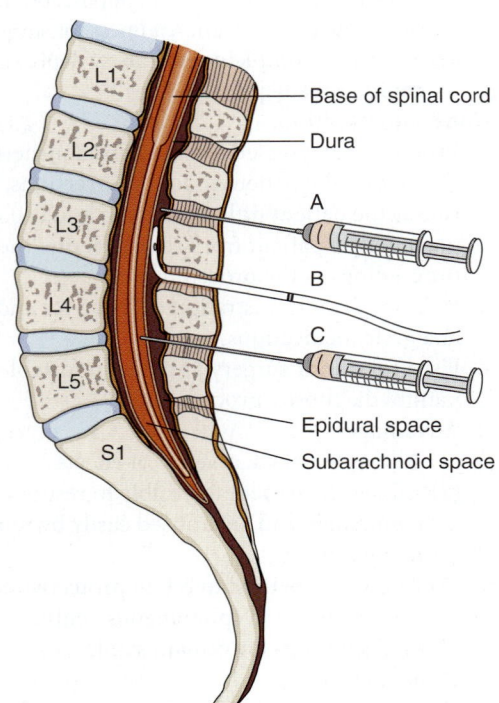

Fig 24.1 Spinal and epidural anesthesia. (From Williams & Hopper [2011]. *Understanding medical surgical nursing,* 4th ed. Philadelphia: F. A. Davis, with permission.)

(e) Uses: Surgical procedures in the lower abdomen, pelvis, or extremities.

(2) **Epidural.**

(a) Agent injected via a catheter into the epidural space (see Fig. 24.1); the catheter can be left in place and taped along the patient's back and over the shoulder for easy access.

(b) Advantages: Depth of anesthesia is less than general and ability to move is maintained; patient is awake and aware of surroundings; is safer than a spinal because it does not enter the subarachnoid space.

(c) Disadvantages: Dose is higher than a spinal; if accidentally injected too deeply, hypotension and respiratory paralysis requiring mechanical ventilation may occur.

(d) Uses: Pain, postoperative analgesia, and cesarean and vaginal births.

(3) **Local.**

(a) Agent injected into a specific area.

(b) Advantages: Allows the patient to be awake and aware of surroundings; has no systemic effects.

(c) Disadvantages: May cause local skin reactions, such as itching and rash.

(d) Uses: Minor procedures, such as suturing a laceration and biopsy.

(4) **Nerve block.**

(a) Injected into and around a nerve or group of nerves (**plexus**).

(b) Advantages: Allows the patient to be awake and aware of surroundings; usually has no systemic effects.

(c) Disadvantages: Has the potential for systemic absorption.

(d) Uses: Anesthetize the facial nerves, brachial plexus, and perineum for repair of an episiotomy.

(5) **Topical.**

(a) Agent is applied directly to the surface of the skin or mucous membranes.

(b) Advantages: Allows agents to be promptly absorbed and act quickly.

(c) Disadvantages: Requires an applicator or gloved hand to prevent exposure of the agent to the caregiver.

(d) Uses: Reduce cutaneous neuropathic pain; limits pain of an injection.

G. Phases of Perioperative Nursing Care

1. Preoperative: Nursing care that is administered before the patient has surgery.

2. Intraoperative: Nursing care that is administered when the patient is in the surgical suite.

3. Postoperative: Nursing care that is administered after the patient has surgery.

II. Preoperative Nursing Care

The preoperative period begins when the patient and primary health-care provider agree that surgery is necessary or desired and ends when the patient is transferred to the surgical suite. The reengineering of the health-care system, resulting in same-day surgery that negates the need for overnight hospital stays (e.g., outpatient surgery, ambulatory surgery) and earlier discharge after hospitalization for surgery, has dramatically changed the role of nurses during this phase. During the preoperative period, nurses are still responsible for collecting patient information, helping with identification of health problems and risk factors that may impact surgery, preparing patients physically just prior to surgery, and participating in obtaining signatures for consents for surgery. However, the teaching role of the nurse has become most significant because the majority of patients are now responsible for their own care before and after a surgical experience. Preoperative teaching decreases patient concerns, prepares patients for the surgical experience, and limits the risk of postoperative complications.

A. Collect Patient Information
1. Collect data from all sources, including the patient, significant other, family members, medical record, and health team members.
2. Collect a health history.
3. Collect a spiritual and cultural history.
4. Perform a physical assessment.
5. Perform a mental and emotional assessment. Notify the primary health-care provider if a patient expresses feelings of impending doom because this finding may herald the potential for an increase in mortality.
6. Identify factors that affect surgical risk, such as age-related issues and allergies, such as latex allergy (Box 24.1).
7. Assess knowledge of surgery and perioperative care.
8. Assess past coping strategies and available support systems.

Box 24.1 Latex Allergy—Nursing Care

- Identify patients at risk, such as those with a history of multiple surgeries or medical procedures and health-care workers. *Note:* Latex allergy commonly is caused by excessive exposure to latex.
- Schedule latex-intolerant patients for the first surgery of the day so that the operating room has not been exposed to latex from a prior surgical procedure.
- Ensure a latex-free environment, such as by using percutaneous, mucosal, parenteral, and inhalation latex-free supplies.
- Identify latex allergy responses in an anesthetized patient, such as flushing, urticaria, facial swelling, bronchospasm, hypotension, and anaphylaxis.

B. Obtain Legal Consent
1. Describe the consent procedure to the patient.
   a. The primary health-care provider explains the type of surgery, options, risks, and benefits.
   b. Information should be provided in language and vocabulary that the patient can understand.
   c. The consent form documents the patient's understanding and confirms that surgery was not coerced; consent protects both the patient and medical/surgical staff.
   d. The patient has the right to refuse or withdraw consent at any time.
2. Ensure that the patient meets the requirements to legally give consent.
   a. Age 18 years or older or emancipated minor (e.g., married, a parent who is younger than 18 years old).
   b. Alert; nonsedated.
   c. Mentally competent (e.g., no signs or symptoms of confusion, dementia, or delirium).
   d. Family member, conservator, or legal guardian for a patient who is younger than age 18 years, unconscious, or mentally or emotionally incompetent.
3. Obtain informed consent.
   a. Reinforce the health-care provider's information if necessary.
   b. Obtain the patient's signature on the consent form.
   c. Sign the consent form as a witness. *Note:* The nurse's signature only verifies that the consent form is signed by the person who legally can give consent.
   d. Ensure that the consent form is in the patient's clinical record.
   e. Notify the primary health-care provider if the criteria for consent are not met—for example, the patient lacks understanding, is emotionally or mentally incompetent, or is not alert; surgery is delayed until the primary health-care provider addresses concerns.
4. Document.
   a. Document all nurse-patient and nurse-primary health-care provider conversations and notifications in the clinical record.
   b. Document all nursing care provided and the patient's responses.

C. Review Common Preoperative Screening Results
1. Arrange for preoperative testing.
   a. Complete blood count: Indicates the oxygen-carrying capacity of the blood and the status of immune function.
   b. Urinalysis: Detects abnormal components, such as protein or glucose, or signs of infection, such as presence of casts or cloudy urine.

c. Chest x-ray: Assesses pulmonary status and the size of the heart.

d. Electrocardiogram: Identifies cardiac disease or dysrhythmias; usually for patients age 40 and older.

e. Blood urea nitrogen: Assesses kidney function.

f. Fasting blood glucose: Detects the possibility of diabetes mellitus.

g. Platelet count and partial thromboplastin time: Assess clotting ability and identify the risk of hemorrhage.

h. Type and crossmatch blood: Prepare for possible blood transfusion.

i. Electrolyte panel: Provides data about fluid and electrolyte status.

j. Serum total protein and albumin: Assess nutritional status.

k. Pregnancy test: Detects pregnancy; implemented for all females of childbearing age.

2. Ensure that the test results are in the patient's clinical record.

3. Report abnormal results to the primary health-care provider.

D. Implement Bowel Preparation

1. Teach the necessity of bowel preparation, which generally is done only for GI procedures to avoid the risk of contaminating the operative site.

2. Teach specific preparations, such as a low-residue diet for several days followed by medications, such as GoLYTELY and/or enemas, the day before and/or day of surgery.

3. Assess for clinical indicators of fluid volume deficit, hyponatremia, and hypokalemia.

4. Teach that bowel function may take 24 to 72 hours to return after GI surgery.

E. Administer or Hold Medications

1. Administer routine medications as prescribed. *Note:* Many medications are held the day of surgery.

DID YOU KNOW?

Some medications that patients routinely take should be adjusted or discontinued before surgery. For example:

• Anticoagulants, such as clopidogrel (Plavix) and warfarin (Coumadin), increase bleeding and usually are discontinued 2 to 10 days before surgery.

• Aspirin and NSAIDs, such as ibuprofen (Advil, Motrin), increase bleeding time and usually are discontinued 5 to 10 days before surgery.

• Insulin doses must be adjusted according to the patient's response to stress and the amount of glucose in intravenous solutions administered during and after surgery.

2. Administer medications when notified to do so by the health team in the surgical suite ("on call"), usually because the medication's onset and duration of action are synchronized with other drugs, anesthesia, and the surgical procedure.

3. Administer medications as prescribed.

a. Antibiotics.

(1) Limit microorganisms that can cause an infection.

(a) May be given to prevent bacterial endocarditis in the presence of a history of rheumatic, congenital, or valvular disease.

(b) Required with "dirty" wounds, such as traumatic injury, perforated thoracic or abdominal cavity, and devitalized tissue.

(c) Recommended with surgery that requires entry into the genitourinary, GI, or biliary tract and with neck dissections.

(2) Usually administered 1 hour before surgery.

(3) Examples: cefazolin (Ancef) and clindamycin (Cleocin).

b. Anticholinergics.

(1) Dry oral and respiratory secretions and help prevent laryngospasm, airway irritability, and risk of aspiration.

(2) Usually administered just before the patient is transferred to the surgical suite.

(3) Examples: scopolamine (Hyoscine) and atropine (Atropisol).

c. Antiemetics.

(1) Reduce the risk of postoperative nausea and vomiting.

(2) Usually administered just before the patient is transferred to the surgical suite.

(3) Examples: ondansetron (Zofran) and famotidine (Pepcid).

d. Anxiolytics, sedatives, and hypnotics.

(1) Ease anxiety, relax skeletal muscles, and facilitate anesthesia induction.

(2) Usually administered just before the patient is transferred to the surgical suite.

(3) Examples: temazepam (Restoril), alprazolam (Xanax), and midazolam (Versed).

e. Antisecretories.

(1) Decrease gastric fluid volume and acidity.

(2) Usually administered just before the patient is transferred to the surgical suite.

(3) Examples: cimetidine (Tagamet), ranitidine (Zantac), omeprazole (Prilosec), and pantoprazole (Protonics).

f. Opioid analgesics.

(1) Provide sedation and decrease the amount of anesthetic needed.

(2) Usually administered just before the patient is transferred to the surgical suite.

(3) Examples: fentanyl (Sublimaze) and morphine (Duramorph).

g. Anticoagulants.

(1) Intravenously administered heparin must be held for 4 hours before surgery.

(2) Subcutaneously administered heparin or low-molecular-weight heparin must be held for 12 hours before surgery.

(3) Warfarin (Coumadin) must be held for a prescribed amount of time as indicated by the primary health-care provider; international normalized ratio (INR) must be stabilized before surgery.

4. Document medications administered and the patient's response; notify the primary health-care provider if a drug has to be held (e.g., antihypertensive when a patient's blood pressure is below indicated parameters).

F. Maintain Nothing-By-Mouth (NPO) Status

1. Dietary restrictions may be necessary preoperatively because general anesthesia decreases GI motility and may cause vomiting.

2. Teach about the length of time of NPO before surgery.

   a. Varies based on the type of surgery, patient's status, and health-care provider's preference.

   b. Teach the patient about specific restrictions, such as 2 hours between clear fluids and surgery, 6 hours between full liquids or light breakfast and surgery, and 8 hours between a regular meal and surgery, as ordered.

G. Detach Removable Items and Indicate the Presence of Implanted Devices

1. Document the presence of a pacemaker, implanted defibrillator, implanted infusion ports, or any implanted metal, such as screws and plates.

2. Remove any nail polish, makeup, false eyelashes, and hairpieces.

3. Remove all prosthetic and metal items, such as artificial limbs, hearing aids, dentures, prosthetic eyes, contact lenses, eyeglasses, jewelry, and hair pins and clips.

H. Implement Skin Preparation

1. Teach the patient to wash, scrub, or shower the surgical area with antibacterial solution the night before and/or day of surgery as ordered. *Note:* Final skin preparation occurs during the intraoperative phase.

2. Remove hair as ordered. *Note:* Hair removal is rarely performed because abrasions and nicks increase the risk of infection. Hair removal is done in the preoperative holding area with clippers, which are less likely to cause injury.

DID YOU KNOW?

Removal of hair (e.g., mustache, beard, and hair on head) before a procedure or surgery requires the patient's written consent.

I. Implement Urinary Preparation

1. Instruct the patient to void just before being transported to the surgical suite.

2. Insert an indwelling urinary catheter if ordered to ensure an empty bladder, reduce the risk of injury during pelvic surgery, and allow for hourly monitoring of urinary output.

J. Implement Safety Protocols

1. Raise the side rails on a patient's bed immediately after administering preoperative medications that depress the central nervous system.

2. Raise the side rails and secure patient straps when a patient is on a stretcher being transported to the surgical suite.

3. Complete a preoperative checklist (Fig. 24.2).

4. Complete a surgical safety check list (Box 24.2).

K. Provide Preoperative Teaching Regarding Postoperative Nursing Care (See the section "Postoperative Nursing Care" later in this chapter, page 756.)

L. Document All Nursing Assessments, Interventions, and Patient Responses

III. Intraoperative Nursing Care

The intraoperative period begins when the patient is admitted to the surgical suite and ends when the patient is transferred to the postanesthesia care unit (PACU). Nurses working in a surgical suite engage in common activities, such as maintaining patient safety, maintaining an aseptic environment, preventing postoperative complications, and working as patient advocates; however, they also are responsible for specific activities unique to their roles, such as circulating nurse or scrub nurse.

A. Scrub Nurse Responsibilities

1. Can be a registered nurse (RN), licensed practical nurse (LPN), or certified assistive personnel (e.g., surgical technologist, surgical first assistant).

2. Works within and maintains the integrity of the sterile field.

   a. Prepares sterilized equipment and field for the procedure.

   b. Scrubs the surgical site with antimicrobial solution (e.g., povidone-iodine [Betadine]) after the patient is anesthetized.

   c. Assists with draping the patient with sterile drapes ensuring that site markings are in view.

PRE-OP SURGICAL CHECKLIST

Patient _____ Surgeon _____
　　　　Last name　　　　First name　　　　　　　Last name　　　　First name

Patient Identification Number _____ Date of Surgery _____ Time of Surgery _____

- -

Date	RN Initial	**Patient Information**
____	_____	ID band on
____	_____	Allergy band on
____	_____	Allergies: _____
____	_____	Advanced directives completed (specify): _____

Medical Information

| ____ | _____ | History and physical completed |
| ____ | _____ | Laboratory studies completed |

RBC _____ HgB _____ HCT _____ WBC _____ Platelets _____
Potassium _____ Urinalysis _____
Pregnancy test: Serum _____ Urine _____
PT _____ PTT _____ Bleeding time _____
Type and screen _____ Crossmatch _____ - _____ units

| ____ | _____ | ECG completed: Yes _____ No _____ |
| ____ | _____ | Chest x-ray completed: Yes _____ No _____ |

Surgical Information

____	_____	Procedure to be performed: _____
____	_____	Site identified by surgeon with X and initials
____	_____	Consent signed
____	_____	Preoperative teaching performed (specify): _____
____	_____	OR prep completed (specify): _____

Day of Surgery

____	_____	Next of kin (specify): _____ Location of family (specify): _____
____	_____	NPO as ordered (specify): _____
____	_____	Hospital gown, head and foot coverings on
____	_____	Jewelry removed—disposition (specify): _____
____	_____	Dentures/bridges, prosthesis, contact lenses, eyeglasses, and hearing aids removed—disposition (specify): _____
____	_____	Hair pins, makeup, nail polish, and one acrylic nail removed
____	_____	Antiembolism stockings on: Yes _____ No _____
____	_____	IV access in place: Yes _____ No _____

Prior to Transfer to Surgical Suite

____	_____	Preoperative medications given (specify): _____
____	_____	Side rails up
____	_____	Voided: Yes _____ No _____ Retention catheter in place: Yes _____ No _____
____	_____	Vital signs: T_____ P_____ R_____ BP_____

- -

Time-Out Safety Check

Patient identification (specify) _____

Procedure to be performed (specify) _____

Site of procedure (specify) _____

Comments:

Verified by: 1. Name (print) _____ Signature _____ Date/Time: _____

Verified by: 2. Name (print) _____ Signature _____ Date/Time: _____

Fig 24.2 Pre-op surgical check list.

- "Time out" checks are implemented to avoid wrong-person, wrong-procedure, and wrong-site surgical errors.
- Time out checks are completed verbally, with the patient if possible, in front of health team professionals who are responsible for the patient's care.
- Time out checks are completed at specific times, such as on admission, before transfer to the surgical suite from the unit; on admission to the surgical holding area, before anesthesia induction; and before the surgeon makes the surgical incision.
- A time out surgical safety check involves three steps.
  1. Verify the name of the patient: Ask the patient his or her name and date of birth; check the arm band for the patient's name, date of birth, and hospital number; use the arm-band bar code to verify this information if the patient's arm band has a bar code.
  2. Verify the procedure: Verbalize the name of the surgery or procedure.
  3. Verify the surgical site: Identify the location of the site; verify that the surgical site is clearly marked according to policy, such as with the word *yes*, and that the mark is visible after the patient is draped for surgery. Also, verify that the mark includes the initials of the patient and the surgeon. The surgeon should mark the site before surgery, preferably the day before surgery, when the patient is awake and aware.

---

    d. Hands instruments, gauze sponges, and other items to the surgeon as needed.

🛑 e. Counts all sponges, sharps, and instruments with the circulating nurse before incision closure.

3. Maintains the integrity of the operating room environment.
   a. Returns instruments for cleaning and sterilization after the procedure.
   b. Ensures cleaning of the operating room for the next procedure.

🛑 4. Protects health team members from exposure to blood and other body fluids.

    a. Uses face shields or goggles to protect mucous membranes.

    b. Changes gloves if worn for a prolonged period because of possible leakage.

    c. Changes masks when moist from breath because they are less effective.

    d. Uses vigilance and caution with sharps.

B. Circulating Nurse Responsibilities
1. Must be an RN.
2. Provides emotional support to the patient.
3. Checks all equipment for malfunctions before surgery, including ensuring proper grounding of electrical equipment.

🛑 4. Provides for patient safety.

    a. Ensures that the preoperative checklist is completed.

    b. Participates in the "time out" surgical safety check before the surgeon makes the first incision.

    c. Ensures that the patient is grounded because cautery devices and laser tools can cause burns.

5. Positions the patient for the surgical procedure.
   a. Positions the patient with input from members of the surgical team (e.g., using wedges, table attachments) to provide adequate access to the surgical site.
   b. Supports skin, neuromuscular, circulatory, and respiratory integrity by using special devices, such as mattresses, pads, and/or foam padding, to support functional alignment and protect bony prominences.
6. Collaborates with members of the surgical team to ensure that anesthesia and monitoring equipment are strategically placed.
7. Provides supplies, equipment, and medications.
8. Monitors the sterile field.

🛑 9. Monitors intake and output (I&O) and blood loss.

🛑 10. Counts all gauze sponges, sharps, and instruments with the scrub nurse before incision closure.

11. Handles and initiates transport of specimens.
12. Assists the anesthesiologist with safe transfer of the patient to the PACU.
13. Gives a nursing report to the nurse receiving the patient in the PACU.
    a. General information: Name, age, procedure, and names of the surgeon and the health team member who provided anesthesia.

MAKING THE CONNECTION

Surgical Sponge Counts and Patient Safety

A surgical sponge retained in the body after a surgical incision is closed can cause many problems. Not only can it lead to infection, but it also requires additional surgery for its removal and is considered professional malpractice. Historically, two nurses are responsible for counting the number of sponges before and after surgery to detect discrepancies that can help to identify retained sponges. Today, however, new technology provides other ways to double-check a sponge count by identifying whether a sponge is still in the wound and where it is located. For example, radiofrequency identification technology enables an operating room nurse to scan a patient's surgical wound to identify the presence of a chip-embedded sponge. Activation of the scanner when it is held over the patient's surgical wound alerts the nurse that a surgical sponge is still in the wound. In addition, some sponges have bar codes that are scanned before and after surgery to help account for the presence of all sponges after incision closure.

b. Patient history: Information such as allergies if present; concurrent health problems.

c. Intraoperative management: Information such as type and duration of anesthesia, medications administered, problems addressed, estimated blood loss, and fluid and blood administered.

d. Patient status: Information such as location and condition of incision and dressing, presence and location of tubes and drains, amount and type of oxygen administration, method and amount of pain management, and patient's condition, including oxygen saturation, urine output, and vital signs, especially respiratory status.

C. Nursing Care to Prevent or Manage Intraoperative Complications

1. **Hypoxemia.**
   a. Aspiration of secretions or vomitus due to loss of cough reflex secondary to anesthesia; also caused by positioning that allows the pressure of abdominal organs to impinge on the diaphragm, limiting lung expansion.
   b. Nursing care.
      (1) Ensure the patient is in a position that allows for lung expansion.
      (2) Monitor pulse oximetry.
      (3) Support the anesthesiologist, who is responsible for monitoring vital signs and tissue perfusion.

2. **Hypothermia.**
   a. Increased risk of heat loss due to exposure of body and internal organs to cool operating room temperature; body heat lost by radiation, convection, evaporation, and conduction.
   b. Nursing care.
      (1) Cover all nonsurgical areas with warm blankets.
      (2) Provide head and feet covering.
      (3) Provide IV and blood-warming machines.

3. **Malignant hyperthermia.**
   a. Rapid increase in heart and respiratory rates, progressing to hyperthermia, dysrhythmias, and respiratory and metabolic acidosis; precipitated by anesthesia in patients with a rare autosomal dominant trait.
   b. Nursing care.
      (1) Administer dantrolene (Dantrium) as prescribed to slow metabolism.
      (2) Provide 100 percent oxygen.
      (3) Maintain hypothermia blanket or ice packs.
      (4) Administer cold IV fluids.

4. **Paresthesia.**
   a. Numbness, prickly, stinging, or burning feeling related to nerve injury.

b. Nursing care.
   (1) Perform routine peripheral vascular assessments.
   (2) Ensure functional alignment when the patient is positioned for surgery.
   (3) Use a special mattress, pads, or foam padding.
   (4) Alter the patient's position during prolonged surgery.

5. **Pressure ulcers.**
   a. Damage to skin or underlying tissue due to capillary tissue compression secondary to immobility.
   b. Nursing care.
      (1) Perform routine peripheral vascular assessments.
      (2) Ensure functional alignment when the patient is positioned for surgery.
      (3) Use a special mattress, pads, or foam padding.
      (4) Alter the patient's position during prolonged surgery.

6. **Hemorrhage, hypovolemia, and hypovolemic shock.**
   a. Insufficient circulating blood volume due to internal or external bleeding, fluid loss, or inadequate fluid intake.
   b. Nursing care.
      (1) Monitor I&O, including output from suction devices used to keep operative areas free from fluids.
      (2) Administer an IV fluid bolus as ordered to increase circulatory volume.
      (3) Administer blood products as ordered.
         (a) Whole blood to correct loss of blood volume.
         (b) Packed red blood cells to correct anemia and improve oxygenation.
      (4) Administer ordered IV colloidal products, such as albumin, hetastarch, and dextran, to treat hypovolemic shock.

IV. Postoperative Nursing Care

The postoperative period begins when the patient is admitted to the PACU and ends when the patient has healed from surgery. Although nurses caring for patients immediately after surgery are concerned about total patient care, the priority of care focuses on supporting patients during their recovery from anesthesia and maintaining airway, breathing, and circulation after the trauma of surgery. After patients are stable and are returned to a surgical unit or are being prepared for discharge home, the focus of nursing care shifts to meeting individual patient needs. These needs include caring for tubes, drains, and wounds;

managing pain; maintaining a balance among activity, rest, and sleep; maintaining fluid and nutritional intake; and promoting fecal and urinary elimination. These needs are met directly by nurses or nurses reinforce the preoperative teaching so that patients can perform competent self-care in the home.

A. Give Report to the Nurse Receiving the Patient in the PACU or Surgical Unit
1. General information: Age, procedure, name of health-care provider, and responsible caregiver; verify the identity of the patient using two indicators.
2. Patient history: Information such as allergies and acute and chronic health problems.
3. Intraoperative and PACU management: Type and duration of anesthesia, medications used, problems addressed, estimated blood loss, fluid and blood administration, urine output, and patient responses.
4. Current physical, emotional, and mental status of the patient.
   a. Use a scoring system to objectively measure patient status during the PACU stay (Fig. 24.3).
   b. Determine when the clinical criteria for discharge from the PACU are met.
      (1) Stable vital signs.
      (2) Presence of spontaneous respiration and effective ventilatory functioning.
      (3) Easy arousal.
      (4) Absence of complications.

(5) Aldrete score of 8 to 10; transfer the patient to the intensive care unit (ICU) if a score of 8 to 10 is not achieved within 4 hours postoperatively.

B. Maintain the Patient's Respiratory Functioning (Includes Preventing Complications of Atelectasis, Pneumonia, and Pulmonary Embolus)
1. Assessments.
   a. Rate and rhythm of respirations; determine whether respirations are more than 10 and less than 30 breaths/minute.
   b. Depth of respirations and use of accessory muscles.
   c. Breath sounds.
   d. Presence of artificial airway.
   e. Presence of gag and cough reflexes.
   f. Amount and characteristics of sputum; productive or nonproductive cough.
   g. Type and flow of oxygen delivery system.
   h. Pulse oximetry.
   i. Clinical indicators of atelectasis, pneumonia, and pulmonary embolus.
2. Nursing care.
   a. Maintain the patient's airway and suction it, if necessary. (See Table 19.7, "Types of Artificial Airways" in Chapter 19, for specific nursing care.)
   b. Administer oxygen as ordered. (See Table 19.6 "Oxygen Delivery Systems" in Chapter 19, for specific nursing care.)

Aldrete Score			On Admission to PCAU	5 Min	15 Min	30 Min	45 Min	60 Min	At Discharge
Able to move 4 extremities voluntarily or on command	= 2	Activity							
Able to move 2 extremities voluntarily or on command	= 1								
Able to move 0 extremities voluntarily or on command	= 0								
Able to deep breathe and cough freely	= 2	Respiration							
Dyspnea or limited breathing	= 1								
Apneic	= 0								
BP ± 20% of Pre-anesthetic level	= 2	Circulation							
BP ± 20%–50% of Pre-anesthetic level	= 1								
BP ± 50% of Pre-anesthetic level	= 0								
Fully awake	= 2	Consciousness							
Arousable on calling	= 1								
Not responding	= 0								
Able to maintain O_2 saturation >92% on room air	= 2	O_2 saturation							
Needs O_2 inhalation to maintain O_2 saturation >90%	= 1								
O_2 saturation <90% even with O_2 supplement	= 0								
		TOTAL							

Fig 24.3 Aldrete score. (From Aldrete, J. A. [1995]. Reprinted from *Journal of Clinical Anesthesia*, Vol. 7/Issue 1, Post-anesthesia recovery score revisited, pp. 89–91, with permission from Elsevier.)

c. Position the patient on the side unless contraindicated and maintain functional alignment to allow secretions to exit the mouth and promote a patent airway.

d. Remove the airway or endotracheal tube when the gag reflex returns to prevent vomiting; usually done in the PACU.

e. Promote lung expansion to prevent atelectasis and pneumonia.
   (1) Elevate the head of the bed.
   (2) Encourage coughing and deep breathing; teach the patient to splint an abdominal incision with a pillow or the hands to limit pain and increase the depth of inhalations.
   (3) Encourage the use of an incentive spirometer 10 times every hour when awake (Fig. 24.4A and Fig. 24.4B).
   (4) Encourage in-bed activity or progressive ambulation if permitted.

f. Notify the rapid response team and primary health-care provider if the patient's oxygen saturation is less than acceptable compared per agency policy or the surgeon's preset parameters (e.g., less than 92 percent) or if the patient exhibits clinical indicators of atelectasis, pneumonia, or pulmonary embolus.

3. Postoperative respiratory complications.
   a. **Atelectasis:** Collapsed or airless alveoli due to inadequate lung expansion.
      (1) Assessments.
         (a) Dyspnea, tachypnea, and pleural pain.
         (b) Reduced or absent breath sounds and crackles.
         (c) Tachycardia.
         (d) Decreased oxygen saturation.
         (e) Anxiety.
         (f) Diaphoresis.
      (2) Nursing care.
         (a) Promote lung expansion.
         (b) Administer humidified oxygen as ordered.
         (c) Monitor for clinical indicators of progression to pneumonia.
   b. **Pneumonia:** Inflammation of the lungs caused by a microorganism.
      (1) Assessments.
         (a) Dyspnea, tachypnea, and chest pain.
         (b) Decreased breath sounds, crackles, and wheezes.
         (c) Blood-tinged and/or purulent sputum; cough that usually is productive.
         (d) Increased temperature.
         (e) Decreased oxygen saturation.
         (f) Increased white blood cell count.
         (g) Infiltrates on chest x-ray examination.
         (h) Identification of causative microorganism on culture of sputum.
      (2) Nursing care.
         (a) Promote lung expansion.
         (b) Suction the airway to maintain patency if necessary.
         🛑 (c) Maintain droplet transmission-based precautions if required.
         (d) Administer humidified oxygen as ordered.
         (e) Balance rest and activity.
         (f) Teach pursed-lip breathing to facilitate exhalation.
         (g) Increase oral and/or IV fluid intake as ordered to liquefy respiratory secretions.
         (h) Teach the patient to dispose of tissues contaminated with sputum into a bag impervious to fluid; provide frequent oral hygiene.
         (i) Administer prescribed medications, such as antibiotics, mucolytics, and bronchodilators.
         (j) Provide chest physiotherapy if ordered.

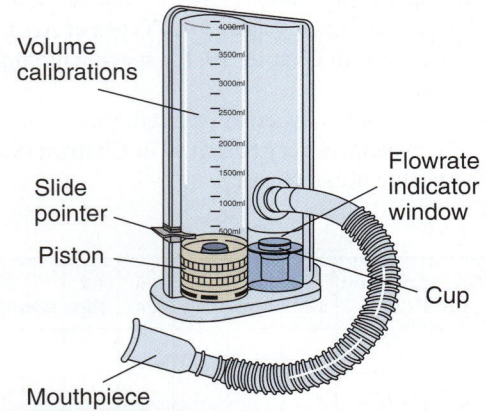

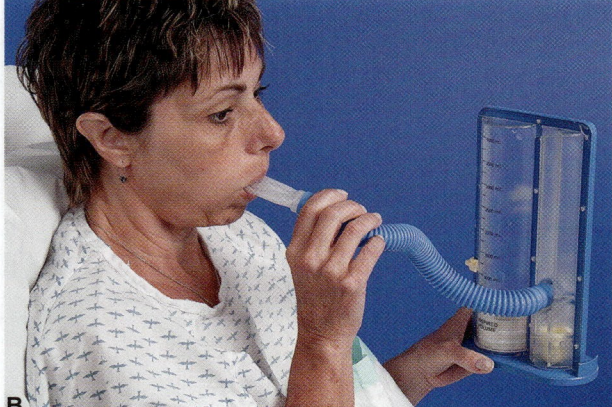

Fig 24.4 Incentive spirometry. (A) Voldyne volumetric deep-breathing exerciser. (B) Patient using an incentive spirometer. (From Williams & Hopper [2011]. *Understanding medical surgical nursing,* 4th ed. Philadelphia: F. A. Davis, with permission.)

c. **Pulmonary embolus:** Obstruction of a pulmonary artery caused by a blood clot (thrombus) that originated in a lower extremity and traveled to the lung.

  (1) Assessments.

    (a) Sudden chest pain, frequently unilateral.

    (b) Shortness of breath (dyspnea).

    (c) Absent breath sounds in affected area of lung.

    (d) Blood-tinged sputum (hemoptysis).

    (e) Tachycardia; decreased blood pressure.

    (f) Cyanosis.

  (2) Nursing care.

    (a) Maintain bed rest.

    (b) Elevate the head of the bed.

    (c) Provide humidified oxygen.

    🛑 (d) Notify the rapid response team and the primary-health care provider immediately.

    (e) Administer prescribed fibrinolytic therapy if ordered.

    (f) Administer analgesics and anticoagulants (e.g., heparin progressing to warfarin [Coumadin]) as prescribed.

    (g) Prepare the patient for insertion of an inferior vena cava filter if ordered.

    (h) Assess the patient's lower extremities for clinical indicators of thrombophlebitis.

C. Maintain the Patient's Circulatory Functioning (Includes Preventing Complications of Thrombophlebitis, Hemorrhage, and Hypovolemic Shock)

1. Assessments.

  a. Continuous cardiac monitoring while in the PACU; heart rate and rhythm and blood pressure routinely after discharge from the PACU based on the patient's status or agency protocol.

  b. Skin color (e.g., pink, dusky, blotchy, cyanotic).

  c. I&O, including blood loss via incision, wound drains, and tubes.

  d. Hourly urine as ordered if a urinary retention catheter is present; expect hourly output to be more than 30 mL.

  e. Neurovascular status of the extremities, such as pedal pulse, capillary refill, color, temperature, movement, and sensation.

  f. Clinical indicators of thrombophlebitis, hemorrhage, and hypovolemic shock.

2. Nursing care.

  a. Promote venous return to prevent venous stasis, thrombophlebitis, and pulmonary embolus.

    (1) Maintain the use of a venous compression device or antiembolism stockings if ordered (Fig. 24.5a and Fig. 24.5b).

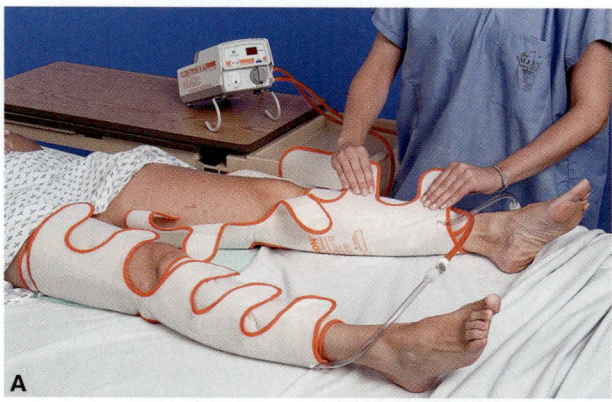

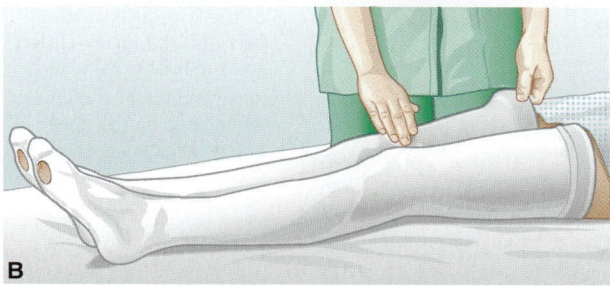

Fig 24.5 Lower extremity compression devices. (A) Sequential compression device. (B) Antiembolism stockings. (From Wilkinson and Treas [2011]. *Fundamentals of nursing,* Vol. 1, 2nd ed. Philadelphia: F. A. Davis, with permission.)

    (2) Teach the patient to avoid crossing the legs, placing pillows behind the knees, and positioning the bed in the contour position ("gatching" the bed) to prevent popliteal pressure; avoid keeping the legs dependent to prevent venous stasis; avoid massaging the legs to prevent a thrombus from becoming an embolus.

    (3) Encourage the patient to perform ankle and leg exercises (Box 24.3).

    (4) Administer prescribed prophylactic anticoagulants, such as low-molecular-weight heparin (e.g., dalteparin [Fragmin], enoxaparin [Lovenox]).

  b. Encourage oral fluid intake if permitted; administer IV fluids as ordered.

  c. Notify the primary health-care provider if hourly urine output is less than 30 mL/hour.

  🛑 d. Notify the rapid response team and primary health-care provider if the patient exhibits clinical indicators of thrombophlebitis, hemorrhage, or hypovolemic shock.

3. Postoperative circulatory complications.

  a. **Thrombophlebitis:** Inflammation of a vein with formation of a blood clot (thrombus) due to injury to a vein, external pressure behind

Box 24.3 Postoperative Leg Exercises

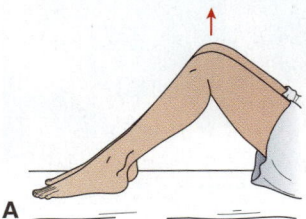

- Flex the knee while sliding the foot on the mattress toward the buttocks.

A

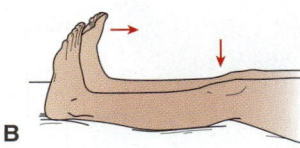

- Extend the knee while sliding the foot on the mattress away from the buttocks; press the back of the knee against the bed with the leg extended and the foot dorsiflexed.

B

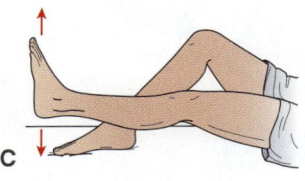

- Raise and lower the leg while keeping the knee extended.

C

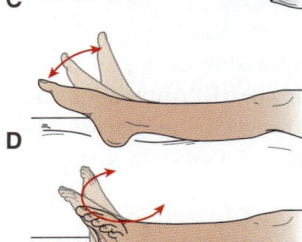

- Keep the knee extended while flexing the foot toward the abdomen (dorsiflexion) and then away from the abdomen (plantar flexion).
- Rotate the ankle while maintaining the foot in dorsiflexion.

D

E

the knees, or venous pooling secondary to immobility.

(1) Assessments.

(a) Discomfort or pain, such as burning, achiness, or cramping in an extremity, usually the calf of a lower extremity.

🛑 (b) Pain on dorsiflexion of a foot (Homan sign); this sign should never be elicited intentionally because doing so can dislodge a thrombus, causing a pulmonary embolus.

(c) Erythema, edema, and warmth in the affected area.

(d) Bilateral measurements of calf and thigh circumferences.

(2) Nursing care.

🛑 (a) Institute bed rest immediately.

(b) Elevate the affected extremity on a pillow.

(c) Notify the primary health-care provider.

(d) Encourage oral fluid intake and IV fluids as ordered.

(e) Apply warm soaks to the affected area if ordered.

(f) Administer anticoagulants as prescribed, usually IV heparin, progressing to warfarin (Coumadin).

(g) Prepare the patient for insertion of an inferior vena cava filter if ordered.

(h) Administer prescribed medications, such as antibiotics and analgesics, as ordered.

b. **Hemorrhage and hypovolemic shock:** Hemorrhage—excessive loss of blood from the circulatory system that is difficult to control; hypovolemic shock—severe blood and fluid loss (class III and class IV hemorrhage) that make the heart unable to pump enough blood to the body.

(1) Assessments.

(a) Internal or external bleeding; blood emanating from a wound, drain, or tube or into a body cavity; arterial blood—bright red blood characterized by spurts; venous blood—dark red blood characterized by a continuous flow.

(b) Class I hemorrhage (up to 15 percent blood loss; 750 mL): No change in vital signs, pale skin, and slight anxiety.

(c) Class II hemorrhage (15 to 30 percent blood loss; 750 to 1500 mL): Tachycardia; tachypnea; increased diastolic blood pressure; narrowed pulse pressure; restlessness; anxiety; pale, cool, clammy skin; confusion; prolonged capillary refill; and urine output 20 to 30 mL/hour.

(d) Class III hemorrhage (30 to 40 percent blood loss; 1,500 to 2,000 mL): Systolic blood pressure 100 mm Hg or less; tachycardia more than 120 beats/minute; tachypnea more than 30 breaths/minute; cool, pale, clammy skin; confusion; agitation; prolonged capillary refill; and urine output 20 mL or less/hour.

(e) Class IV hemorrhage (more than 40 percent blood loss; more than 2000 mL): Systolic blood pressure less than 70 mm Hg; tachycardia more than 140 beats/minute; pronounced tachypnea; extremely pale, sweaty, cool skin; absent capillary refill; negligible urine output; and moribund.

(2) Nursing care.

(a) Apply direct pressure to the site of bleeding.

(b) Reinforce the dressing over the wound.

(c) Ensure that the venous access device is #18 gauge to allow for fluid and blood resuscitation.

🛑(d) Notify the rapid response team and primary health-care provider.

   (e) Administer IV fluids as ordered; usually normal saline or lactated Ringer's solution given at a rate to maintain permissive hypotension so that clotting factors are not excessively diluted.

   (f) Administer blood and blood products as ordered, usually whole blood or fresh frozen plasma.

   (g) Maintain the airway if compromised; administer oxygen.

   (h) Administer prescribed inotrope therapy (e.g., dopamine, noradrenaline).

   (i) Prepare the patient for surgery to repair the site of bleeding.

D. Maintain Safety When the Patient's Central Nervous System is Depressed

1. Assessments.
   a. Level of consciousness (LOC).
   b. Orientation to time, place, and person.
   c. Ability to follow commands.
   d. Movement of the extremities.
2. Nursing care.
   a. Ensure that the patient's airway remains patent.
   b. Provide for patient safety, such as by keeping side rails up, maintaining the integrity of all catheters and monitoring lines, and assisting with ambulation.
   c. Call the patient by name.
   d. Reorient the patient to time, place, and person.

E. Manage the Patient's Pain and Support Comfort

1. Assessments.
   a. Pain location, intensity, quality, onset, duration, nonverbal clues, and aggravating and relieving factors.
   b. Use an objective pain scale to assess pain intensity, such as a numeric pain scale, the Wong-Baker FACES pain scale, or the FLACC pain scale. (See Fig. 23.2, Fig. 23.3, and Fig. 23.4 in Chapter 23.)
   c. Patient responses to interventions, especially 20 minutes after administration of an analgesic; respiratory status after administration of medications that depress the central nervous system.
2. Nursing care.
   a. Validate and accept the patient's description of pain because pain is a subjective experience.
   b. Provide for pain relief before pain becomes severe.
   c. Progress from least invasive independent nursing interventions to dependent nursing interventions.

   d. Institute independent nursing interventions to reduce pain and promote comfort.
   (1) Place the patient in a position of comfort if not contraindicated; support the body in functional alignment.
   (2) Suggest distractions, such as music, television, and reading.
   (3) Use relaxation techniques, such as warm blankets, back rub, imagery, and progressive muscle relaxation.
   (4) Organize care so that the patient has uninterrupted periods of rest and sleep.
   (5) Maintain an environment conducive to rest and sleep, such as by limiting noise, lowering lights, and setting a comfortable environmental temperature.

   e. Institute dependent nursing interventions to reduce pain and promote comfort.
   (1) Implement thermal therapy (e.g., heat or cold) as ordered.
      (a) Heat dilates blood vessels and relaxes muscles.
      (b) Cold anesthetizes nerve endings and constricts blood vessels, limiting edema.
   (2) Administer prescribed analgesics to reduce pain and anxiolytics, sedatives, and hypnotics to reduce anxiety and promote rest and sleep. (See the section "Medications That Limit Pain and Promote Rest and Sleep" in Chapter 23, page 730.)
      (a) Medications can be administered by a nurse via the oral, Sub-Q, IM, IV, or transdermal routes.
      (b) Medications can be controlled by a patient via the intravenous or epidural route (patient-controlled analgesia [PCA]). (For specific nursing care see Chapter 23, page 721.)
   (3) Administer an antiemetic to limit nausea and vomiting. (See Table 18.8, "Antiemetics," Chapter 18.)

F. Maintain the Patient's Position and Promote Activity

1. Assessments.
   a. Intolerance to positioning, such as reports of discomfort or pain.
   b. Intolerance to activity, such as shortness of breath, respirations more than 24 breaths/minute, or heart rate more than 95 beats/minute after 3 minutes of rest.
   c. Skin over bony prominences for clinical indicators of pressure.
   d. Clinical indicators of orthostatic hypotension when moving to an upright position.

2. Nursing care.
   a. Position according to the patient's needs and/or primary health-care provider's order.
      (1) Semiconscious or lethargic patient: Place in a side-lying position with the head slightly elevated to allow secretions to drain from the mouth.
      (2) After spinal anesthesia: Keep flat for 8 to 12 hours to avoid a headache associated with cerebrospinal fluid leakage.
      (3) After surgery that causes edema in an extremity (e.g., mastectomy or internal fixation of a fracture): Elevate the extremity higher than the heart to promote venous drainage and reduce edema via gravity.
      (4) After head and neck surgery (e.g., craniotomy, radical neck dissection, and rhinoplasty): Keep the head of the bed elevated to limit cerebral and tissue edema.
      (5) After spinal surgery: Keep flat and roll the entire body as one unit (**logrolling**) when turning to maintain functional alignment of the spine.
      (6) After open reduction and internal fixation (ORIF) of a hip fracture: Use an abduction pillow if ordered and avoid hip flexion and internal and external rotation of involved leg to prevent femoral head dislocation (Fig. 24.6).
      (7) After total joint replacement (hip, knee or elbow): Use a continuous passive motion (CPM) machine if ordered (Fig. 24.7 and Box 24.4).
   b. Change the patient's position at least every 2 hours.
   c. Assist with or provide range-of-motion exercises.
   d. Encourage in-bed activities, such as turning from side to side, if permitted.
   e. Assist with and encourage being out of bed and ambulating if ordered.
G. Maintain the Patient's Urinary Elimination (Includes Complication of Urinary Retention)
   1. Assessments.
      a. Amount and characteristics of urine, such as color, clarity, and odor.
      b. Urge to void, hesitancy, and frequency.
      c. Patency of urinary retention catheter, if present.
      d. Clinical indicators of urinary retention.
   2. Nursing Care.
      a. Document the time and amount of the first voiding.
      b. Promote urination.
         (1) Provide privacy and assist the patient to the usual position for elimination, such as transfer to toilet, commode, or bedpan,

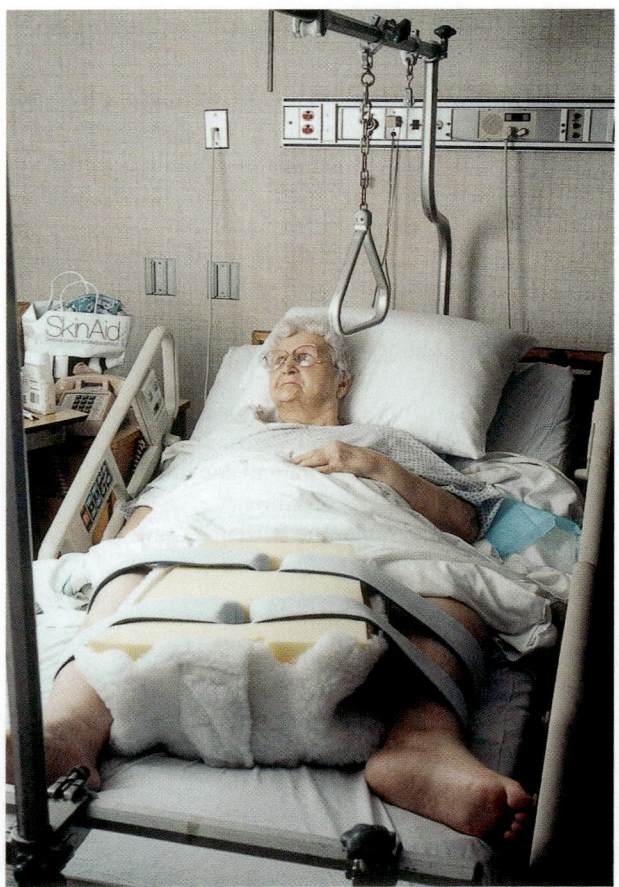

Fig 24.6 Abduction pillow. (From Burton and Ludwig [2011]. *Fundamentals of nursing care: Concepts, connections & skills.* Philadelphia: F. A. Davis, with permission.)

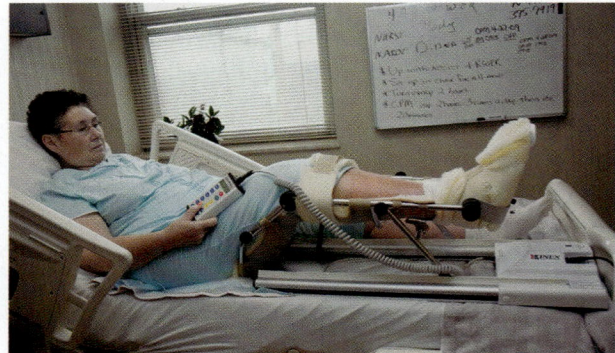

Fig 24.7 Continuous passive motion machine. (From Burton and Ludwig [2011]. *Fundamentals of nursing care: Concepts, connections & skills.* Philadelphia: F. A. Davis, with permission.)

with the head of the bed elevated if not contraindicated.
(2) Stimulate voiding, such as by putting a warm washcloth on the perineum, placing the patient's hands in warm water, or running a faucet.

<table>
<tr><td>

Box 24.4 Continuous Passive Motion Machine— Nursing Care

- Position sheepskin on the platform, especially at the gluteal fold, where there is a risk of pressure.
- Position the patient's extremity on the platform so that the knee/elbow is centered over the break in the platform.
- Ensure that the extremity is in alignment with the patient's hips/torso or shoulder.
- Set the degree of flexion, speed, and time on and off the machine as ordered; speed and degree of flexion increase as recovery progresses.
- Position the controller within easy reach of the patient so that the patient can shut off the machine if unable to tolerate the procedure.
- Assess the patient's skin, and provide skin care when the patient's extremity is removed from the device.
- Evaluate and document the patient's response to continuous passive motion.

</td></tr>
</table>

c. Provide nursing care associated with a variety of urinary catheters (Table 24.1).

🛑 d. Notify the primary health-care provider if the patient does not void within 8 hours after surgery because a straight catheter or urinary retention catheter will be necessary to empty the bladder.

3. **Urinary retention:** Inability to empty the bladder completely, resulting in excessive urine accumulation

due to decreased bladder tone related to anesthetics, analgesics, manipulation during surgery, or pelvic inflammation.

a. Assessments.
  (1) Inability to void despite urge to void.
  (2) Dribbling of urine, urinating small amounts frequently (**overflow incontinence**).
  (3) Suprapubic distension and discomfort.
  (4) Urine output less than intake; output less than 500 mL/24 hours (**oliguria**).
  (5) Restlessness.
b. Nursing care.
  (1) Empty bladder with a single-lumen catheter as ordered.
  (2) Insert and maintain a urinary retention catheter as ordered.
  (3) Administer oral and IV fluids as ordered.
  (4) Promote urination after a urinary catheter is removed; notify the primary health-care provider if the patient does not void within 8 hours.

H. Maintain the Patient's Fluid and Electrolyte Balance (Includes Complication of Hypovolemia)
1. Assessments.
  a. I&O.
  b. Daily weight.
  c. Clinical indicators of electrolyte imbalances (See Table 21.1, "Common Electrolyte Imbalances," in Chapter 21).

Table 24.1 Types of Urinary Catheters—Nursing Care

Catheter Types	Nursing Care
Single-lumen (straight) catheter Single-lumen tube inserted through the urethra one time and then removed. **Double-lumen (indwelling, retention) catheter** Double-lumen tube placed through the urethra and left in place; one lumen allows for inflation of the balloon and the other drains urine. **Triple-lumen catheter** Triple-lumen tube inserted through the urethra or suprapubic area into the bladder; one lumen for inflation of balloon, the second for instillation of a genitourinary irrigant, and third for drainage of urine and the irrigant; used for continuous bladder irrigation (CBI). **Suprapubic catheter** Double-lumen tube surgically placed through the lower abdomen into the bladder and left in place; one lumen allows for inflation of the balloon and the other drains urine.	**Commonalities of nursing care** • Ensure gravity flow by placing the collection bag and tubing below the level of the bladder and preventing dependent loops by curling excess tubing on the bed. • Secure the tubing to the patient's anterior thigh and lower abdomen in males to limit tension on the tubing and prevent the patient from lying on the tubing. • Assess the amount and characteristics of urine; note that hourly amount reflects the glomerular filtration rate; notify the primary health-care provider if output is equal to or less than 30 mL/hour. • Maintain patient safety when ambulating with a urinary catheter; hold catheter tubing so that the patient does not step on it. • Teach the patient about self-care regarding management of a urinary catheter. **Specific nursing care related to a suprapubic catheter** • See Suprapubic Tube under "Urinary Diversions" in Chapter 20, page 627. **Specific nursing care related to continuous bladder irrigation (CBI) through a triple-lumen catheter** • See "Bladder Irrigation" in Chapter 20, page 628.

For illustrations of urinary catheters and the procedure for securing a catheter to a patient's thigh, see Chapter 20 "Urinary Elimination."

d. Clinical indicators of hypervolemia and hypovolemia (See the sections "Fluid Volume Deficit," page 652, and "Fluid Volume Excess," page 653, in Chapter 21).

2. Nursing care.
   a. Administer IV fluids and electrolytes as ordered.
   b. Notify the primary health-care provider if electrolyte imbalances, fluid volume excess, or fluid volume deficit occur.

3. **Hypovolemia:** Decreased blood volume, specifically a decrease in the volume of blood plasma.
   a. Assessments.
      (1) Decreased blood pressure; orthostatic hypotension.
      (2) Thirst; dry mucous membranes.
      (3) Loss of skin elasticity; flushed, dry skin.
      (4) Weight loss.
      (5) Decreased urine output.
      (6) Weak, thready pulse.
      (7) Atonic muscles; weakness; lethargy.
      (8) Mental confusion.
   b. Nursing care.
      (1) Encourage oral fluid intake and administer IV fluids as ordered.
      (2) Provide for safety, particularly in relation to orthostatic hypotension and mental confusion.
      (3) Provide frequent oral hygiene and skin care.

I. Maintain the Patient's Nutritional Status (Includes Preventing Complications of Nausea and Vomiting)

1. Assessments.
   a. Verify dietary order.
   b. Presence of gag and swallowing reflexes.
   c. Presence and quality of bowel sounds; dietary intake usually resumes after intestinal peristalsis returns, which can be verified by bowel sounds and the passing of flatus.
   d. I&O.
   e. Amount of food ingested.

2. Nursing care.
   a. Maintain NPO status until a diet is ordered.
      (1) Remove the water pitcher from the bedside.
      (2) Teach the patient about the restrictions.
   b. Provide meticulous mouth care.
   c. Maintain an aesthetically pleasant environment, such as avoiding odors by uncovering the meal tray before entering the room to dissipate food odors, using an air freshener, and storing the bedpan and urinal.
   d. Initiate the ordered diet, which varies depending on the type of surgery and the organs involved.
      (1) Begin usually with ice chips and then progress to clear liquids, to full liquids, to soft, to regular as tolerated.

(2) Advance the diet to the next level if the patient has no nausea, vomiting, or other signs of GI distress if progression is left to the nurse's judgment.

🛑 e. Encourage intake of foods high in protein and vitamin C to promote wound healing, if permitted.

   f. Assist weak patients with meals; obtain an order for between meal supplements if a patient's intake is inadequate.

3. **Nausea and vomiting: Nausea**—unpleasant wave-like sensation in the throat, epigastrium, or abdomen; **vomiting**—ejection of stomach contents from the mouth in response to pain, anxiety, decreased intestinal peristalsis, or administration of oral intake before return of peristalsis after receiving anesthesia.
   a. Assessments.
      (1) Precipitating factors such as pain, anxiety, and hypoactive or absent bowel sounds.
      (2) Patient reports feeling nauseated.
      (3) Frequent swallowing.
      (4) Retching or gagging.
      (5) Ejection of gastric contents.
   b. Nursing care.
      (1) Reinstitute NPO status.
      (2) Notify the primary health-care provider because vomiting can precipitate fluid and electrolyte imbalances.
      (3) Administer prescribed antiemetics and antisecretories (See the section "Medications Associated With Nutrition" in Chapter 18, page 552).
      (4) Administer ordered IV fluids and electrolytes.
      (5) Administer total parenteral nutrition if ordered.
      (6) Maintain nasogastric (NG) decompression if an NG tube is inserted (Fig. 24.8). A tube is inserted into a naris, down the esophagus, and into the stomach to remove gastric contents when attached to suction (**gastric decompression**) or remove toxic matter from the stomach through repeated irrigations (**lavage**). For additional information about types of tubes, assessing for placement, characteristics of aspirate, and maintaining tube patency, see the section "Enteral Nutrition" in Chapter 18, page 543.
         (a) Secure the tube to the nose; provide skin care to the nares and frequent mouth care.

🛑 (b) Ensure correct placement of the tube; for example, aspirate gastric contents, auscultate sound of 15 to 30 mL of instilled air entering the stomach.

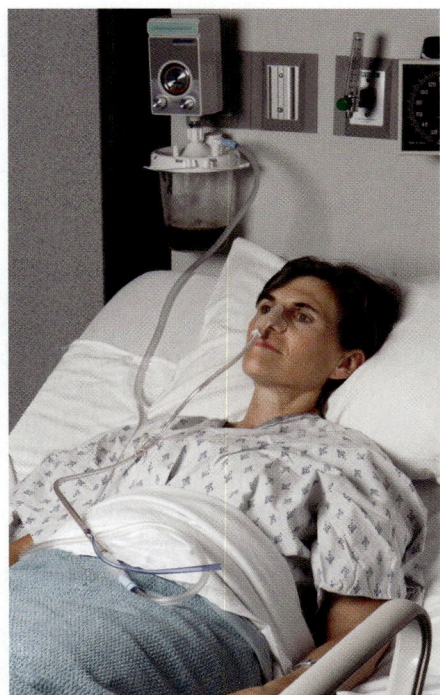

Fig 24.8 Nasogastric tube for gastric decompression. (From Wilkinson and Treas [2011]. *Fundamentals of nursing,* Vol. 2, 2nd ed. Philadelphia: F. A. Davis, with permission.)

   (c) Maintain suction as ordered: Low intermittent suction for a single-lumen tube; low continuous suction for a double-lumen tube with a blue "pigtail."
   (d) Maintain tube patency.
   - Double-lumen tube (e.g., Salem Sump): Keep the blue "pigtail" higher than the drainage catheter; instill 30 mL of air into the blue "pigtail" to ensure patency of air vent tube.
   - Single-lumen tube (e.g., Levin): Instill 30 mL of air into the tube; instill 30 mL of normal saline into the tube after verifying tube placement.
   - Have the patient cough periodically to increase intra-abdominal and intrathoracic pressure that moves tube contents toward the collection container.
   - Instill solution as ordered to dilute gastric contents, usually 30 to 50 mL of normal saline.
   (e) Monitor for clinical indicators of fluid volume deficit and electrolyte imbalances, such as metabolic alkalosis, because hydrochloric acid is part of gastric secretions.

   (f) Empty the collection container, and document the amount and characteristics of output every 8 hours or per agency policy.
J. Maintain the Patient's Intestinal Elimination (Includes Preventing Complications of Abdominal Distention, Constipation, and Postoperative Ileus)
   1. Assessments.
      a. Frequency, amount, and characteristics of stool.
      b. Presence and extent of bowel sounds in all four quadrants of the abdomen.
      c. Contour of the abdomen to identify abdominal distention.
      d. Amount and characteristics of drainage from GI or biliary tubes.
   2. Nursing care.
      a. Document the time and characteristics of the first bowel movement.
      b. Encourage fluids if permitted; administer IV fluids if ordered.
      c. Encourage dietary fiber, if permitted.
      d. Encourage bed exercises and progressive ambulation, if permitted.
      e. Promote defecation.
         (1) Maintain the patient's usual routine for defecation.
         (2) Provide privacy and time to defecate.
         (3) Encourage assumption of a sitting position for defecation if permitted; provide a commode at the bedside if the patient is permitted out of bed but is unable to ambulate safely.
      f. Administer a stool softener, if prescribed.
      g. Care for a tube placed in the common bile duct that exits the abdomen and drains bile into a collection bag via gravity (biliary tube, T-tube); generally anchored with a suture to prevent dislodgement.
         (1) Assess the area around the insertion site for clinical indicators of inflammation or infection.
         (2) Assess the amount and characteristics of drainage; expect 300 to 500 mL in first 24 hours; report output of more than 500 mL; after 4 days, output should be less 200 mL daily; expect color to be green-brown.
         (3) Clean the insertion site and cover the site with a sterile dressing as ordered.
      🛑 h. Notify the primary health-care provider if the patient develops abdominal distension, constipation, or postoperative ileus.

   3. Postoperative intestinal complications.
      a. **Abdominal distention (tympanites):** Excessive flatulence within the intestine, resulting from reduced peristalsis due to manipulation of the

intestines during surgery, anesthesia, opioids, and immobility.

(1) Assessments.

    (a) Enlarged, taut abdomen.

    (b) Abdominal discomfort.

    (c) Hyperactive bowel sounds.

(2) Nursing care.

    (a) Teach the patient to avoid carbonated beverages and foods that produce gas.

    (b) Teach the patient to avoid drinking through a straw to limit swallowing air.

    (c) Administer an antiflatulent as prescribed (See Table 22.5, "Antiflatulents," in Chapter 22).

    (d) Administer a return-flow enema (e.g., Harris drip, Harris flush) as ordered to siphon flatus out of the intestines

    (e) Insert a rectal tube as ordered to facilitate the expulsion of flatus.

b. **Constipation:** No stool or decreased frequency of bowel movements due to reduced peristalsis as a result of manipulation of the intestines during surgery, anesthesia, opioids, and immobility.

(1) Assessments.

    (a) No stool or hard, dry stool.

    (b) Absent or decreased bowel sounds.

    (c) Rectal pressure.

(2) Nursing Care.

    (a) Promote defecation.

    (b) Encourage increased fluid intake if permitted.

    (c) Encourage increased intake of dietary fiber if permitted.

    (d) Encouraged increased ambulation if permitted.

    (e) Administer a laxative or cathartic as prescribed (See Table 22.4, "Laxatives and Cathartics," in Chapter 22).

    (f) Administer an enema as prescribed.

c. **Postoperative ileus (paralytic ileus, adynamic ileus):** Cessation of intestinal peristalsis characterized by a lack of forward movement of intestinal contents; GI secretions continue accumulating in the GI tract; due to anesthesia, opioids, handling of the intestines during surgery, infection, or electrolyte imbalance.

(1) Assessments.

    (a) Absent stool.

    (b) Absent bowel sounds.

    (c) Abdominal distension.

    (d) Abdominal cramps.

    (e) Fecal vomiting.

(2) Nursing care.

    (a) Follow the primary health-care provider's orders concerning conservative interventions (e.g., administer small frequent oral fluids in an attempt to stimulate peristalsis; reinstitute NPO status if the patient vomits; notify primary health-care provider if bowel sounds do not begin within 48 hours).

    (b) Assist with insertion and maintenance of an NG tube for decompression as ordered.

    (c) Assist with insertion and maintenance of a nasoenteric tube as ordered. A long tube with a weighted tip (e.g., Cantor, Miller-Abbott) is inserted via a naris and advanced along the GI tract into the duodenum to remove secretions and gas from the small intestine. Also used for patients with small bowel obstructions; used for 3 to 5 days and if unsuccessful surgery is performed.

      • Position the patient in a semi- to high-Fowler position while the tube is passed through a naris and advanced to the stomach.

      • Turn the patient on the right side to facilitate passage of the tube through the pyloric sphincter into the duodenum.

      • Permit patient to assume position of comfort after tube is in the duodenum.

      • Monitor the markings on the tubing to determine placement.

      • Allow the tube to advance via peristalsis or advance it a specified length (e.g., inch per hour) as ordered.

      • Verify placement of the tube via radiography or a scan as ordered.

      • Secure tube to the naris when the tube has reached the desired site; usually the proximal site of a small bowel obstruction.

    (d) Provide meticulous and frequent oral hygiene and nares care when a GI tube is in place.

    (e) Administer IV fluids and electrolytes, such as potassium, as ordered.

K. Manage the Patient's Operative Site (Includes Preventing Complications of Wound Infection, Dehiscence, and Evisceration)

1. Assessments: For information about assessing a wound, see the section "Assess the Characteristics of the Wound," in Chapter 12, page 308.

2. Nursing care.

  a. Use the principles of surgical asepsis when caring for a patient's wound (See Table 12.3, "Principles of Surgical Asepsis and Related Nursing Care," in Chapter 12).

b. Change a dressing and provide wound care as ordered.

(1) Wash hands, collect all equipment, identify the patient, identify yourself, explain what you are going to do and why, and provide for patient privacy.

(2) Wear clean gloves, remove the soiled dressing, discard the dressing and gloves in a trash container, and discard the dressing in a biohazard container if the dressing is saturated with blood or body fluids.

(3) Wash hands, establish a sterile field with all needed equipment, and don sterile gloves.

(4) Clean the wound using a systematic approach, moving from clean to dirty (Fig. 24.9).

(5) Clean the pins of an external fixation device.

(a) Swipe the base of each pin where it exits from the skin using a circular motion, making one complete revolution with a 4 × 4 gauze pad moistened with normal saline solution.

(b) Repeat using a new wet 4 × 4 gauze pad for each revolution.

(c) Apply a topical antibiotic ointment around each pin if prescribed.

DID YOU KNOW?

External fixation devices are used to stabilize a crushing or splintering bone injury with soft tissue damage. Pins are inserted into the bone and attached to an external metal framework that prevents bone movement. An external fixation device, rather than a cast, prevents pressure on traumatized, edematous soft tissue, permitting soft tissue to heal.

(6) Irrigate the wound as ordered (Fig. 24.10).

(a) Wear personal protective equipment (e.g., gloves, gown, and face shield) to protect yourself from splashing of the patient's blood or body fluid.

(b) Position the patient so that the irrigating solution will flow into an emesis basin.

(c) Hold a piston syringe with irrigating solution 2 inches from the wound surface, just inside the top edge of the wound.

(d) Spray back and forth gently across the inside of the wound and progressively move down the surface of the wound so that the solution and debris move out of the wound via gravity without disrupting granulated tissue in the wound bed.

(e) Refill the syringe and continue the procedure until the entire surface of the wound is cleansed.

(7) Assist a primary health-care provider with mechanical debridement of a wound or im-

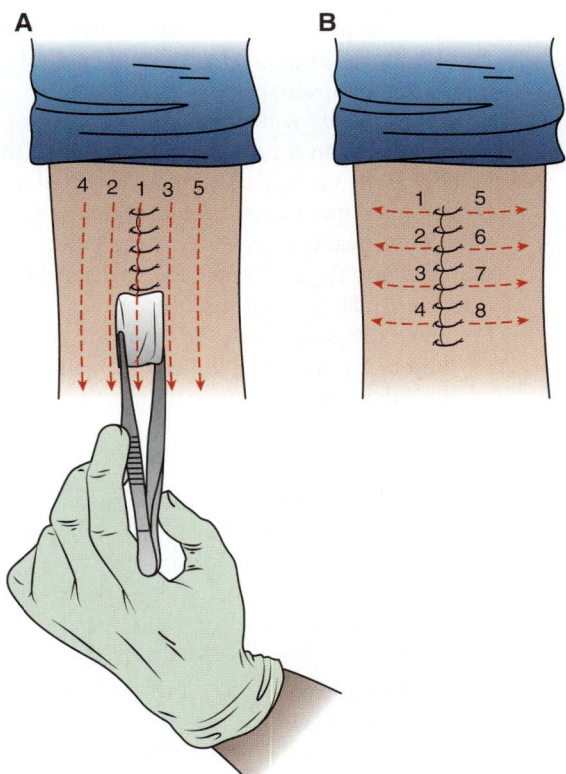

Fig 24.9 Cleaning a wound. Swipe along the line numbered 1 in either illustration A or B first with a 4×4 gauze pad moistened with normal saline solution. Use a new 4×4 gauze pad to swipe along each line numbered 2 through 5 or 2 through 8, depending on the cleansing method used.

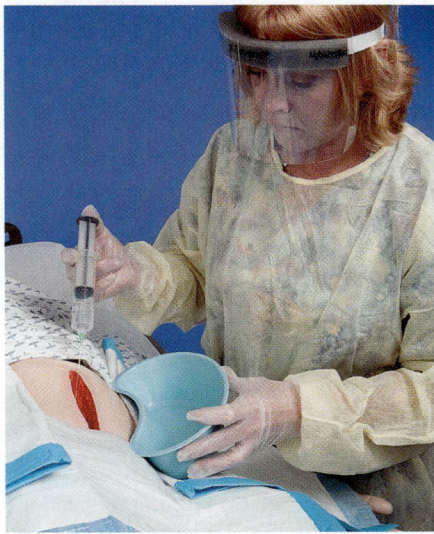

Fig 24.10 Irrigating a wound. (From Burton and Ludwig [2011]. *Fundamentals of nursing care: Concepts, connections & skills.* Philadelphia: F. A. Davis, with permission.)

plement other debridement methods as ordered.

(8) Packing a wound.

(a) Separate the wound edges gently to ensure that the entire wound is accessible so that granulation and healing can occur from the bottom of the wound bed outward.

(b) Open and fluff moistened rolled gauze to increase the surface area for contact with the wound bed (Fig. 24.11a).

(c) Fill the wound completely with the moistened gauze while avoiding the surrounding skin and cover with a dry abdominal pad (Fig. 24.11b).

(9) Secure the dressing.

(a) Use the three-tape method because it uses less tape; protects skin from excessive adhesive, which may impair skin integrity; allows for flexibility of skin; and permits air to circulate under the gauze (Fig. 24.12).

(b) Use the window method of taping to secure the dressing on all sides and contain wound drainage within the gauze window; use for dressings with moist packing (Fig. 24.13).

(c) Use Montgomery straps to secure a dressing that requires frequent changes due to

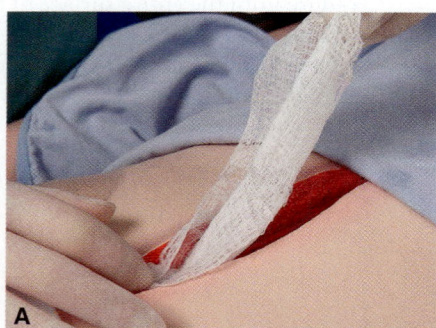

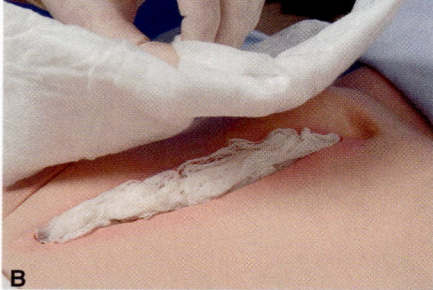

Fig 24.11 Packing a wound. (a) Fluffing moistened gauze. (b) Filling wound with moistened gauze. (From Wilkinson and Treas [2011]. *Fundamentals of nursing*, Vol. 2, 2nd ed. Philadelphia: F. A. Davis, with permission.)

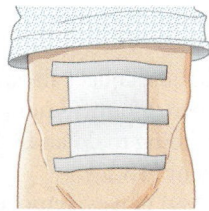

Fig 24.12 Three-tape method for securing a dressing. (From Burton and Ludwig [2011]. *Fundamentals of nursing care: Concepts, connections & skills*. Philadelphia: F. A. Davis, with permission.)

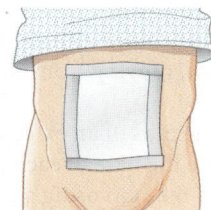

Fig 24.13 Window method for securing a dressing. (Adapted from Burton and Ludwig [2011]. *Fundamentals of nursing care: Concepts, connections & skills*. Philadelphia: F. A. Davis, with permission.)

excessive wound drainage; avoids trauma to the skin caused by constant application and removal of tape (Fig. 24.14).

c. Care for a patient with a **portable wound drainage system:** A catheter is inserted into the body near the operative site and connected to a collection container that is compressed to establish low negative pressure, which pulls drainage into the container (e.g., Jackson-Pratt [Fig. 24.15]; Hemovac [Fig. 24.16]).

(1) Teach the patient that the drain will remove fluid that causes swelling and pain and will limit the potential source of infection.

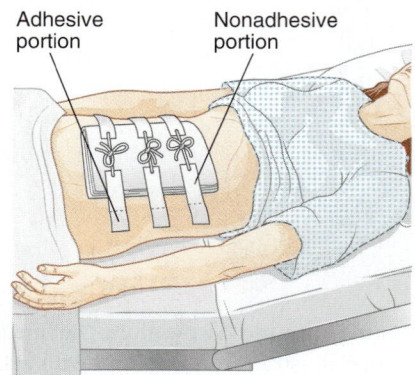

Adhesive portion   Nonadhesive portion

Fig 24.14 Montgomery straps. (From Wilkinson and Treas [2011]. *Fundamentals of nursing*, Vol. 2, 2nd ed. Philadelphia: F. A. Davis, with permission.)

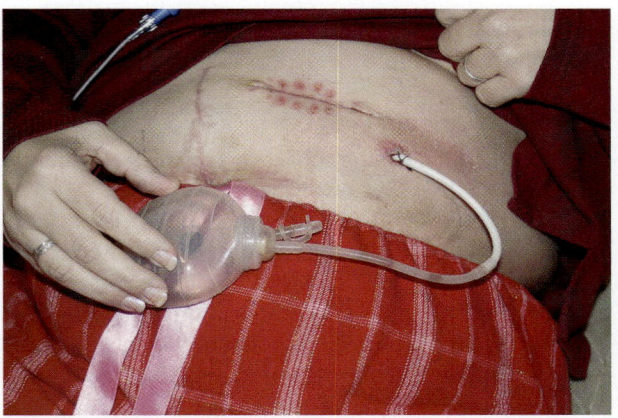

Fig 24.15 Jackson-Pratt drain. (From Wilkinson and Treas [2011]. *Fundamentals of nursing*, Vol. 1, 2nd ed. Philadelphia: F. A. Davis, with permission.)

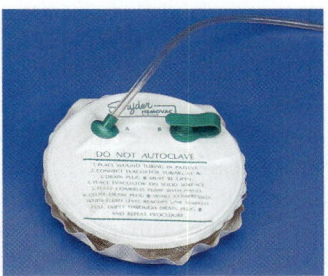

Fig 24.16 Hemovac drain. (From Wilkinson and Treas [2011]. *Fundamentals of nursing*, Vol. 1, 2nd ed. Philadelphia: F. A. Davis, with permission.)

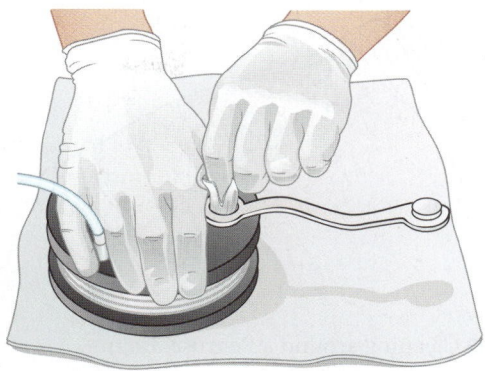

Fig 24.17 Cleaning a Hemovac port. (From Wilkinson and Treas [2011]. *Fundamentals of nursing*, Vol. 2, 2nd ed. Philadelphia: F. A. Davis, with permission.)

(2) Maintain and teach the patient how to care for the drain.

    (a) Maintain the collection container below the insertion site to augment the negative pressure of the system.

    (b) Attach tubing to gown or clothing to prevent tension on the tubing.

    (c) Empty the collection container when half full to prevent weight from pulling on the tubing and to maintain negative pressure; as drainage in the collection container increases, the extent of negative pressure decreases.

    (d) Wear clean gloves when emptying the collection container.

    (e) Empty the collection container by opening the port and draining the contents into a collection container without touching the inside of the port; avoid touching the collection container with the port to maintain sterility.

    (f) Clean the port with an alcohol or a povidone iodine (Betadine) swab before closing (Fig. 24.17).

    (g) Reestablish negative pressure by compressing the collection container, close the port, and release the hand compressing the container.

    (h) Discard drainage in a toilet and flush the toilet twice.

(3) Teach the patient that the drain will be removed when drainage is minimal, generally when the volume is less than 10 mL.

d. Care for a patient with a **Penrose drain:** A soft, flat tube is placed into the body near the operative site; it drains blood, pus, and tissue debris freely via gravity and capillary action into a gauze dressing (Fig. 24.18).

    (1) Ensure that the drain is secured with a sterile safety pin externally to avoid migration into the wound.

    (2) Clean the skin around the insertion site with a 4 × 4 gauze pad moistened with sterile saline solution, using a circular motion, moving outward from the puncture wound (Fig. 24.19).

    (3) Shorten the drain using sterile technique if ordered, such as by pulling the drain out

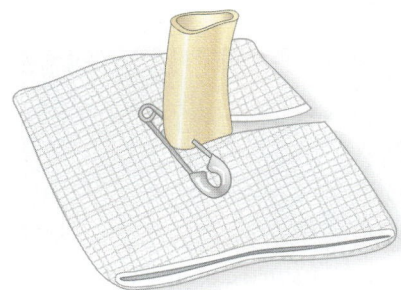

Fig 24.18 Penrose drain. (From Wilkinson and Treas [2011]. *Fundamentals of nursing*, Vol. 2, 2nd ed. Philadelphia: F. A. Davis, with permission.)

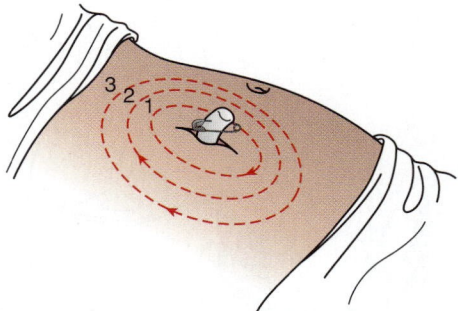

Fig 24.19 Cleaning around a Penrose drain.

6 mm/day, applying an additional pin close to the skin, and then cutting the drain between the pins.

(4) Position the drain between several layers of 4 × 4 gauze pads and cover it with a sterile abdominal pad.

e. Care for a patient with **negative pressure wound therapy:** For example, vacuum-assisted closure (VAC); an occlusive dressing is attached via tubing to a negative pressure machine that removes exudate, thereby reducing edema and promoting granulation (Fig. 24.20).

(1) Ensure that the device is appropriate for the patient's wound—for example, the wound should not have necrotic tissue.

(2) Cut the ordered foam dressing to a size that fills just the wound cavity.

(3) Apply a liquid product around the outside of the wound to protect the skin.

(4) Apply a transparent film that extends 3 to 5 cm (1 to 2 inches) beyond the wound margins.

(5) Cut a 2-cm round hole in the center of the transparent film and attach the suction device with tubing directly over the hole in the transparent film.

(6) Connect the tubing to negative pressure as ordered (continuous or intermittent, 5 to 125 mm Hg).

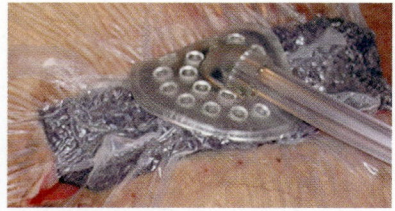

Fig 24.20 Vacuum-assisted closure (VAC). (From Wilkinson and Treas [2011]. *Fundamentals of nursing*, Vol. 2, 2nd ed. Philadelphia: F. A. Davis, with permission.)

(7) Ensure that negative pressure is maintained. *Note*: The film will collapse or wrinkle as pressure is applied and audible leaks can be heard if the film dressing is not secure.

(8) Change the collection container when full or at least once a week.

(9) Observe the site for signs of infection.

(10) Document the amount of drainage, characteristics, and wound assessments.

3. Postoperative wound complications.

a. **Wound infection:** Invasion of an incision by a pathogen that proliferates, resulting in inflammation and purulent drainage.

(1) Assessments.

(a) Local erythema, edema, heat, and pain.

(b) Extent of approximation of wound edges.

(c) Amount and characteristics of purulent exudate, such as color and presence of foul odor.

(d) Increased vital signs.

(e) Increased white blood cell count.

(2) Nursing care.

(a) Institute contact precautions.

(b) Notify the primary health-care provider of clinical indicators of infection.

(c) Obtain a wound specimen for a culture and sensitivity test.

(d) Irrigate and dress the wound as ordered.

(e) Encourage foods high in protein and vitamin C to promote wound healing.

(f) Administer antibiotics as prescribed.

(g) Administer pain medication as prescribed.

(h) Assist with debridement of a wound.

(i) Monitor the incision for clinical indicators of dehiscence and evisceration.

b. **Dehiscence:** Separation of one or more layers of an incision before it heals due to strain on the suture line.

(1) Assessments.

(a) Risk factors including obesity; inadequate nutrition; inadequate circulation; and wound infection; behaviors that use the Valsalva maneuver, such as coughing or bearing down with a bowel movement; abdominal incision 4 to 5 days after surgery while the scar is retracting.

(b) Separation of wound edges so that underlying tissue along an incision is visible (Fig. 24.21).

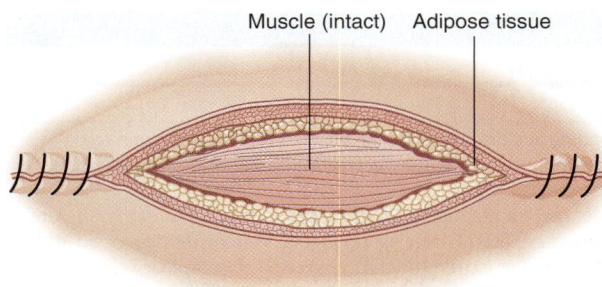

Muscle (intact)   Adipose tissue

Fig 24.21 Dehiscence. (From Burton and Ludwig [2011]. *Fundamentals of nursing care: Concepts, connections & skills.* Philadelphia: F. A. Davis, with permission.)

    (c) Patient reports a "giving way" or "tearing" feeling at the site of the incision.
    (d) Increase in serosanguineous drainage from the incision.
  (2) Nursing care.

🛑 (a) Place patient in the low-Fowler position with knees slightly flexed to limit strain on the suture line.

🛑 (b) Instruct the patient to avoid behaviors such as coughing, holding the breath or bearing down, which will increase tension on the suture line extending the dehiscence to an evisceration.

🛑 (c) Keep the incision covered with a sterile dressing.

🛑 (d) Notify the primary health-care provider immediately.

    (e) Prepare the patient for surgical repair if ordered.

c. **Evisceration:** Spilling of abdominal contents from an abdominal incision as a result of dehiscence.
  (1) Assessments.
    (a) Same risk factors as dehiscence.
    (b) Opening of incision with visible protrusion of internal organs (Fig. 24.22).
  (2) Nursing care.

🛑 (a) Same interventions as dehiscence except cover the incision with a sterile dressing moistened with sterile normal saline.

🛑 (b) Notify the primary health-care provider immediately.

    (c) Change the dressing and perform wound irrigations as ordered.
    (d) Apply and maintain a VAC device if ordered.
    (e) Administer antibiotics if prescribed.
    (f) Prepare the patient for surgical repair if ordered.

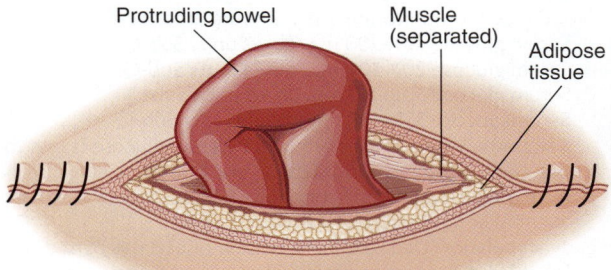

Protruding bowel   Muscle (separated)   Adipose tissue

Fig 24.22 Evisceration. (From Burton and Ludwig [2011]. *Fundamentals of nursing care: Concepts, connections & skills.* Philadelphia: F. A. Davis, with permission.)

CASE STUDY: Putting It All Together

A nurse working on a surgical unit is receiving a patient transferred from the postanesthesia care unit (PCAU) after removal of her uterus via an abdominal incision (abdominal hysterectomy) because of a large benign uterine fibroid. Before surgery, the patient was taking several prescribed medications, including an antiplatelet agent (clopidogrel [Plavix]), a diuretic (hydrochlorothiazide), and an oral hypoglycemic (metformin [Glucophage]). The patient was also taking a self-prescribed over-the-counter herbal supplement (ginseng). The unit nurse received the following report from the nurse in the PACU and reviewed the primary health-care provider's orders.

PACU Transfer Report

- The patient is an obese 74-year-old female with a history of type 2 diabetes mellitus and hypertension. The patient has no history of food or drug allergies. Before surgery, the patient was expressing fear that the mass may be cancerous.
- Under general anesthesia, the patient had an abdominal hysterectomy. Patient experienced one episode of hypotension in the PCAU that immediately responded to an increase in the IVF flow rate. No other untoward anesthesia or surgical events occurred. The surgical procedure required 2 hours of general anesthesia.

Continued

CASE STUDY: Putting It All Together
cont'd

PACU Transfer Report—cont'd

- 500 mL blood loss estimated; two Jackson-Pratt drains #1-30 mL sanguineous drainage and #2-50 mL sanguineous drainage; urinary retention catheter draining 75 mL or more straw colored, sediment-free urine hourly for the past 2 hours while in the PCAU; 100 mL greenish drainage from Salem sump tube (gastric decompression).
- Vital signs are stable: Temperature, 98.8°F (tympanic route); pulse, 80 beats/minute, regular rhythm; respirations, 16 breaths/minute, shallow; oxygen saturation 98% with oxygen via nasal cannula; blood pressure, 110/68 mm Hg; no jugular vein distention or adventitious breath sounds noted; pedal pulses palpable; 1+ dependent edema of lower extremities; skin pink and dry; capillary refill 2 to 3 seconds.
- Patient is able to move from side to side with help; alert when stimulated and capable of summoning help; deep breathing and coughing on request; cough nonproductive.
- Patient in low-Fowler position; sequential venous compression device in place; dressing dry and intact.
- IVF: 0.9% Sodium Chloride 125 mL/hour; site in right median cubital vein dry and intact; no clinical indicators of infiltration or inflammation noted at IV site.
- IV morphine via a PCA pump: Basal rate 1.5 mg/hour; PCA dose 1 mg; lockout interval 12 minutes; maximum dose over 4 hours, 26 mg.
- Patient states that incisional pain is constantly at a level 2, using a numerical scale of 0 to 10, and tolerable.

Postoperative Orders

NG tube (Salem sump tube) to low continuous wall suction.
NPO except ice chips and sips of water with oral medications.
Strict I&O.
IVF: 0.9% Sodium Chloride 125 mL/hour.
CBC, basic metabolic panel daily.
Heparin 5,000 units Sub-Q, every 12 hours.
Blood glucose monitoring every 2 hours times 12 hours then every 6 hours, regular insulin coverage:.
    Serum glucose 150–200 mg/dL—2 units Sub-Q.
    Serum glucose 201–300 mg/dL—4 units Sub-Q.
    Serum glucose 301–350 mg/dL—8 units Sub-Q.
    Serum glucose 351–400 mg/dL—10 units Sub-Q.
    Call primary health-care provider if serum glucose is less than 90 mg/dL or more than 400 mg/dL.
Vital signs, BP, and pulse oximetry every 4 hours.
PCA morphine: Basil rate 1.5 mg/hour; PCA dose 1 mg; lockout interval 12 minutes; maximum dose over 4 hours, 26 mg.
Sequential compression device when in bed.
Early ambulation: Dangle patient on side of bed this p.m.; day 1 postop: Ambulate with assist 25 feet at least 2 times and OOB in a chair for at least 20 minutes times 2; day 3 postop: Ensure patient is OOB (walking frequently and in a chair) at least 6 hours daily; progressively increase walking distance as tolerated.
Urinary retention catheter to gravity; assess hourly output for 4 hours then every shift; notify primary health-care provider if less than 50 mL/hour.

Case Study Questions

A. What is the purpose of this patient's surgery: Ablative, curative, explorative, palliative, or restorative?

_____

B. What degree of surgical urgency is this patient's medical condition: Elective, urgent, or emergency?

_____

C. Is the risk of this patient's surgery considered to be major or minor? Explain why.

_____

  1. _____

  2. _____

  3. _____

  4. _____

  5. _____

CASE STUDY: Putting It All Together   *cont'd*

───────────────────────── **Case Study Questions** ─────────────────────────

D. Identify the clinical criteria required for discharge from the PACU.

1. _____

2. _____

3. _____

4. _____

5. _____

E. Identify at least 10 nursing interventions associated with the patient's Jackson-Pratt drains and explain why they are employed.

1. _____

2. _____

3. _____

4. _____

5. _____

6. _____

7. _____

8. _____

9. _____

10. _____

F. Which postoperative complication is a serious concern in relation to the drugs that the patient was taking before the surgery?

_____

G. For what clinical indicators of stage II hemorrhage (blood loss of 750 to 1,500 mL) should the nurse assess the patient?

1. _____

2. _____

3. _____

4. _____

5. _____

6. _____

7. _____

8. _____

9. _____

10. _____

Continued

CASE STUDY: Putting It All Together   *cont'd*

_____ **Case Study Questions** _____

H. What are the four most common postoperative concerns that require preventive measures that are associated with this patient's obesity and diabetes and why?

1. _____

2. _____

3. _____

4. _____

I. Identify at least 6 nursing interventions that the nurse should employ to reduce the risk of a postoperative wound infection.

1. _____

2. _____

3. _____

4. _____

5. _____

6. _____

J. What nursing interventions should the nurse implement to prevent a postoperative pulmonary embolus and why?

1. _____

2. _____

3. _____

4. _____

5. _____

K. A nurse assesses the patient's blood glucose level and it is 285 mg/dL. What should the nurse do?

_____

REVIEW QUESTIONS

1. A nurse is caring for a postoperative patient who has a history of cigarette smoking. For what complication should the nurse initially monitor the patient?
   1. Airway patency
   2. Dependent edema
   3. Respiratory infection
   4. Pulmonary hemorrhage

2. What should a nurse do when assessing for the presence of dehiscence after a patient had abdominal surgery?
   1. Monitor urine output.
   2. Assess for hypertension.
   3. Palpate around the wound.
   4. Examine the wound edges.

3. Before abdominal surgery, the nurse teaches the patient leg and ankle pumping exercises that are to be done during the postoperative period. What postoperative complication does the nurse explain will be prevented by these exercises?
   1. Atelectasis
   2. Adynamic ileus
   3. Wound infection
   4. Thrombophlebitis

4. A nurse in the postanesthesia care unit is receiving a patient transferred from the operating room. What assessment should the nurse perform **first?**
   1. Vital signs
   2. Urinary output
   3. Airway patency
   4. Wound dressing

5. A nurse is caring for a patient with the wound dressing that appears in the illustration. In what situation should the nurse use this system?

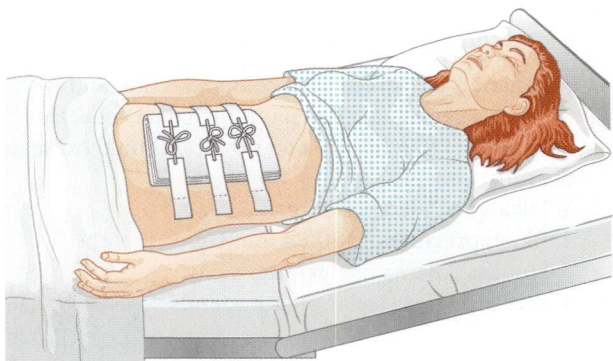

   1. A wound that requires frequent dressing changes
   2. A dressing that should dry out between changes
   3. A wound that has a small amount of drainage
   4. A dressing that the patient will care for

6. A patient goes to the outpatient clinic to be prepared for extensive head and neck surgery for a cancerous tumor of the jaw. Which intervention is the priority?
   1. Initiate discharge planning with a home health agency.
   2. Teach postoperative deep breathing and coughing exercises.
   3. Ensure that the patient has completed a signed consent for the surgery.
   4. Review methods of communicating with the health team after the surgery.

7. A nurse is caring for a patient who had an esophagogastroduodenoscopy two hours ago. The nurse has to attend a meeting and provides information to the nurse accepting responsibility for the patient. What information is **most** important for the relieving nurse to know about this patient?
   1. Vital signs are stable.
   2. Reports a sore throat.
   3. Gag reflex returned 5 minutes ago.
   4. Voided a sufficient quantity 1 hour ago.

8. A primary health-care provider orders the removal of a patient's nasogastric (NG) tube. Place the following steps in the order in which they should be implemented.
   1. Instruct the patient to take a deep breath.
   2. Remove adhesive tape from the patient's nose.
   3. Place a disposable pad across the patient's chest.
   4. Fold the tube on itself and quickly and carefully remove the tube.
   5. Shut off the suction and separate the tube from the suction device.
   Answer: _____

9. A preoperative patient who is wearing a small religious medal around the neck is being prepared for surgery. The patient states, "I never take this medal off because it is very important to me." Which is the appropriate action by the nurse?
   1. Ask the patient to make an exception and give the medal to a family member.
   2. Ensure that the medal is pinned to the linen at the head of the operating room table.
   3. Remove the medal after the patient is under anesthesia and replace it after the surgery.
   4. Explain that patients are not permitted in the operating room with jewelry of any kind.

10. A nurse is providing preoperative teaching for a patient who is scheduled for laparoscopic surgery for removal of the gallbladder (cholecystectomy). Which information is **most** important to teach the patient preoperatively?
    1. Performing ankle pumping exercises
    2. Planning to be out of work for 6 weeks
    3. Avoiding taking drugs that may increase bleeding
    4. Self-administering a hypertonic enema the night before surgery

11. A patient is admitted to the postanesthesia care unit (PCAU) after having a partial gastrectomy. Which nursing interventions should the nurse implement? **Select all that apply.**
    1. _____ Monitor the pulse oximeter.
    2. _____ Auscultate the patient's breath sounds.
    3. _____ Clamp the nasogastric tube intermittently.
    4. _____ Maintain the patient in the dorsal recumbent position.
    5. _____ Push the trigger on the PCA pump when the patient states the presence of pain.

12. A nurse is assessing a patient who is being administered a general anesthetic for abdominal surgery. Which clinical findings indicate that the patient is in stage III of general anesthesia?
    1. Fixed and dilated pupils
    2. Weak respirations and a thready pulse
    3. Absent eyelid reflex and relaxed skeletal muscles
    4. Irregular breathing and involuntary motor movements

13. A nurse in the postanesthesia care unit (PACU) is caring for a patient whose skin becomes cold and clammy; pulse is 112 beats/minute, respirations are 30 breaths/minute, blood pressure is 84/50 mm Hg, and surgical dressing is saturated with blood. Place the following steps in the order in which they should be implemented.
    1. Retake the patient's vital signs.
    2. Activate the rapid response team.
    3. Change the nasal cannula to a face mask.
    4. Place the bed in the Trendelenburg position.
    5. Increase the flow rate of the intravenous solution.
    Answer: _____

14. A patient is transferred from the operating room to the postanesthesia care unit (PACU). What should the PACU nurse assess **first**?
    1. Cardiovascular status
    2. Level of consciousness
    3. Oxygen saturation level
    4. Adequacy of the airway

15. A patient is transferred from the operating room to the postanesthesia care unit (PACU). What should the nurse assess **first** from among the options presented?
    1. Presence of pain
    2. Level of consciousness
    3. Indicators of fluid overload
    4. Patency of a urinary catheter

16. A nurse is caring for a patient wearing the device illustrated in the photograph. What is the expected result that the nurse can anticipate when this patient wears this device? **Select all that apply.**

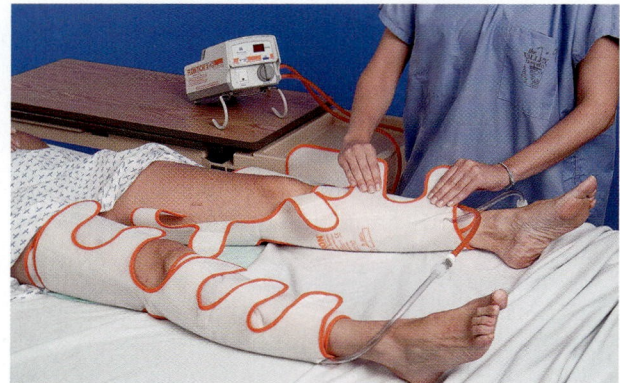

    1. _____ Increased venous return
    2. _____ Minimized muscle atrophy
    3. _____ Reduced lower extremity edema
    4. _____ Increased risk of thrombophlebitis
    5. _____ Reduced lower extremity discomfort

17. A patient is scheduled for a colon resection and is to receive general anesthesia. Which data collected during a nursing history and physical should cause the **most** concern?
    1. History of a latex allergy
    2. Blood pressure of 140/84 mm Hg
    3. Smokes 2 packs of cigarettes a day
    4. Presence of vesicular breath sounds

18. A nurse on a surgical unit is caring for a group of postoperative patients. Which nursing interventions included in the patients' plans of care help reduce the risk of both hypostatic pneumonia and deep vein thrombosis? **Select all that apply.**
    1. _____ Increase fluid intake to 3,000 mL daily.
    2. _____ Encourage coughing and deep breathing.
    3. _____ Ambulate 100 feet in the hall four times daily.
    4. _____ Encourage changing position from side to side when in bed.
    5. _____ Teach how to don compression stockings before getting out of bed in the morning.

19. A nurse in the operating room is caring for a patient who is being anesthetized with general anesthesia. What should the nurse do when the patient is in stage II of anesthesia?
    1. Avoid touching the patient.
    2. Explain that the patient may feel dizzy.
    3. Encourage the patient to take deep breaths.
    4. Begin draping the patient with sterile surgical drapes.

20. A nurse is caring for a patient with a Hemovac. The collection chamber is half filled with drainage and requires emptying. Place the steps in the order in which they should be implemented.
    1. Don clean gloves.
    2. Open the port of the collection chamber.
    3. Press down firmly on the top of the chamber.
    4. Empty the contents into a container for measurement.
    5. Clean the port of the collection chamber with an alcohol wipe.
    6. While the collection chamber is compressed, close the drainage port.
    Answer: _____

21. What is **most** important for the nurse to include in preoperative teaching?
    1. Plan for pain management
    2. Potential complications to be avoided
    3. Risk factors associated with the type of anesthesia
    4. Detailed information related to the type of surgery

22. A nurse is providing preoperative teaching for a patient who is scheduled for surgery in the morning. The primary health-care provider orders antiembolism stockings postoperatively. The patient asks, "Why do I need to wear these ugly stockings?" What information is important for the nurse to include in a response to the patient's question?
    1. Helps prevent muscle atrophy
    2. Supports venous blood return from the legs
    3. Minimizes joint contractures when ambulating
    4. Keeps the legs warm while in the postanesthesia care unit

23. Which nursing action is **most** important when caring for a patient with a portable wound drainage system like the one in the photograph?

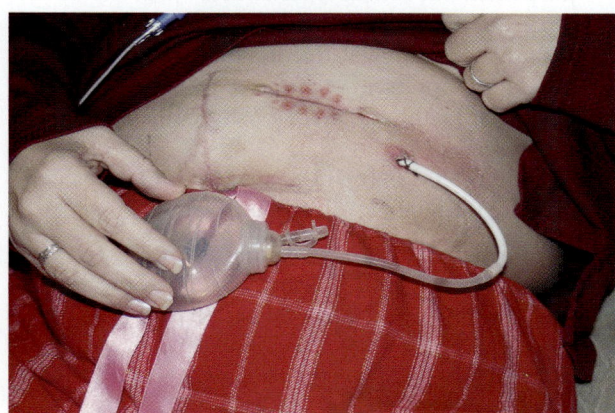

    1. Document the characteristics of the drainage.
    2. Empty the collection container only when it becomes full.
    3. Maintain medical asepsis when emptying the collection container.
    4. Verify that the volume of drainage is consistent with expectations.

24. A nurse is caring for a patient who is obese and is scheduled for abdominal surgery in the morning. Which information is **most** important to include in a preoperative teaching plan for this patient?
    1. How to cough and deep breathe effectively
    2. What to do to prevent a wound infection
    3. What to do to safely ambulate in the hall
    4. How to exit the bed independently

25. A nurse in the PACU is caring for a patient who had debulking surgery for ovarian cancer. The patient's apical pulse is 128 beats/minute, respirations are 22 breaths/minute, blood pressure is 88/60 mm Hg, and two portable wound drainage devices are both half full of sanguineous drainage. What should the nurse do **first**?
    1. Call the surgeon immediately.
    2. Empty the collection containers.
    3. Palpate the abdomen for urinary distention.
    4. Increase the flow rate of the intravenous solution.

26. A nurse is caring for a patient with a Salem sump tube attached to continuous low suction following abdominal surgery. The patient reports feeling nauseated and begins to vomit. The nurse identifies that the patient's abdomen is distended. What should the nurse do **first**?
    1. Ensure the tubing is free from kinks and is not being compressed.
    2. Reposition the patient and instruct the patient to cough.
    3. Administer the prescribed antiemetic to the patient.
    4. Instill the blue pigtail with thirty milliliters of air.

27. Eight hours after surgery, a nurse identifies that a patient has not voided. Which actions by the nurse are appropriate? **Select all that apply.**
    1. _____ Catheterize the patient.
    2. _____ Palpate the patient's bladder for fullness.
    3. _____ Increase the rate of the intravenous fluids.
    4. _____ Encourage the patient to drink more fluids.
    5. _____ Cover the suprapubic area with a warm towel while running water in the sink.

28. A nurse is caring for a patient who just returned from the postanesthesia care unit after abdominal surgery. What should the nurse do **first** when the patient begins to vomit red-colored emesis?
    1. Assist the patient to the lateral position.
    2. Increase the flow rate of the intravenous fluid.
    3. Document the volume of effluent, including its characteristics.
    4. Call the blood bank to deliver a unit of packed red blood cells.

29. A nurse is developing a preoperative plan of care for a patient scheduled for intestinal surgery. The nurse should ensure that the surgeon has prescribed a medication from which drug classification to be administered to the patient preoperatively?
    1. Opioid
    2. Antibiotic
    3. Antiemetic
    4. Thrombolytic

30. A nurse is caring for a patient who recently returned to the surgical unit from the postanesthesia care unit after intestinal surgery. The nurse identifies abdominal distension and the absence of bowel sounds. Which nursing intervention addresses the nurse's main concern?
    1. Inspect proximity of wound edges.
    2. Ensure patency of the nasogastric tube.
    3. Encourage an increase in oral fluid intake.
    4. Assess for clinical indicators of hypovolemia.

31. A nurse is caring for a semiconscious patient in the postanesthesia care unit. The patient begins to try to expel the oropharyngeal airway. What should the nurse do?
    1. Maintain the use of wrist restraints until the patient is fully alert.
    2. Explain to the patient that the airway needs to remain in place.
    3. Remove the airway from the patient's mouth.
    4. Place the patient in the lateral position.

32. Which nursing action is associated with the role of advocate during the intraoperative period? **Select all that apply.**
    1. _____ Providing emotional support
    2. _____ Performing the safety time out check
    3. _____ Providing for patient safety during surgery
    4. _____ Preparing sterile equipment for the procedure
    5. _____ Handing instruments and gauze to the surgeon

33. In which position should the nurse maintain a patient after spinal anesthesia?
    1. Sitting
    2. Supine
    3. Contour
    4. Orthopneic

34. A nurse is caring for a patient 6 hours after surgery to repair a deep 7-inch laceration of an abdominal muscle as a result of a motorcycle accident. In addition, the patient is currently engaged in chemotherapy for stage II lung cancer.

Patient's Clinical Record

Progress Notes 0800

Moderate amount of serosanguineous drainage noted on abdominal dressing. Reinforced with one abdominal pad. IV running at 100 mL/hour via an infusion pump; IV insertion site clean, dry, and intact; no S&S of phlebitis or infiltration. Voided 450 mL of clear, straw-colored urine at 0730.

Vital Signs

Temperature: 100.4°F.
Pulse: 90 beats/minute.
Respirations: 24 breaths/minute and shallow.
Blood pressure: 120/80 mm Hg.
Oxygen saturation: 95%.

Laboratory Results

Hb: 15.5 g/dL.
RBC: 5.6 mm^3.
Platelet count: 200,000 mm^3.
WBC: 2.5 mm^3.
Serum potassium: 4.5 mEq/L.
Serum sodium: 140 mEq/L.

Which is the **most** important concern of the nurse after reviewing the patient's clinical record and interviewing the patient?
1. Hemorrhage
2. Risk for infection
3. Respiratory distress
4. Electrolyte imbalance

35. A nurse is caring for a postoperative patient who had abdominal surgery and who has an impaired immune system because of corticosteroid therapy. Which nursing intervention is essential when caring for this patient?
1. Encourage fluid intake.
2. Institute neutropenic precautions.
3. Suggest ingesting foods high in protein.
4. Maintain medical asepsis when changing the dressing.

36. A nurse is caring for a postoperative patient who is experiencing nausea and vomiting. What is **most** important for the nurse to do?
1. Encourage deep breathing.
2. Maintain ordered NPO status.
3. Use room-deodorizing sprays.
4. Provide frequent oral hygiene.

37. A nurse working in the ambulatory surgical center is admitting a 65-year-old male patient scheduled for elective bowel surgery in 2 hours.

Patient's Clinical Record

Patient Interview

Patient stated that he completed the bowel prep, which included ingesting a clear liquid diet for 2 days, 1.5 oz of Fleet Phospho-Soda at 1 p.m. and 7 p.m. yesterday, and did not eat or drink anything since 12 midnight. He said that he stopped taking his last dose of Plavix yesterday morning but had his vitamins 2 hours ago with a little sip of water.

Vital Signs

Temperature: 99°F.
Pulse: 88 beats/minute, regular.
Respirations: 22 breaths/minute.
Blood pressure: 140/88 mm Hg.

Laboratory Test Results

Hb: 15 g/dL.
RBC: 5.1 mm^3.
Platelets: 280,000 mm^3.
WBC: 6.0 mm^3.

After reviewing the patient's preoperative blood tests, interviewing the patient, and taking the vital signs, what information is **most** important for the nurse to report to the primary health-care provider?
1. Patient's BP is elevated.
2. Patient took a sip of water today.
3. Patient ingested Plavix yesterday.
4. Patient's Hb is lower than the expected range.

38. A nurse is caring for a patient who has an order for wound irrigation. What should the nurse do when implementing this procedure?
1. Use a piston syringe to forcefully cleanse debris from the wound.
2. Spray around the wound, then spray the inside of the wound from top to bottom.
3. Hold a piston syringe four inches from the wound surface when applying the solution.
4. Position the patient so that the irrigating solution will flow from the wound into an emesis basin.

39. A nurse is caring for a patient with an abdominal wound with a vacuum-assisted closure device. What should the nurse do when applying this device?
1. Place the suction apparatus over a hole at the edge of the transparent film.
2. Cut the foam dressing so that it extends 1 inch beyond the wound cavity.
3. Connect the tubing to the positive pressure machine as ordered.
4. Apply the transparent film 2 inches beyond the wound margins.

40. The primary health-care provider orders Versed 2.5 mg IV push for preoperative sedation. It is available in 5 mg/mL. How many milliliters should the nurse prepare to administer?

Answer: _____ mL

REVIEW ANSWERS

1. **ANSWER: 1.**
   Rationales:
   1. **Smoking increases mucus production and destroys the protective action of cilia; a smoker is at risk for ineffective airway clearance.**
   2. Dependent edema is related to heart and peripheral vascular diseases, not smoking.
   3. Although the nurse should monitor the patient for signs of respiratory infection, this is not the priority at this time.
   4. Pulmonary hemorrhage is an unlikely occurrence; it can occur with tissue erosion associated with lung cancer.
   TEST-TAKING TIP: Identify the word in the stem that sets a priority. The word *initially* in the stem sets a priority. Use the principle of the ABCs (Airway, Breathing, and Circulation) when setting a priority. Option 1 is clearly associated with Airway. Options 2 and 4 are associated with Circulation. Option 3 is associated more with Breathing because infection causes inflammation, which can reduce the surface area of the lung, affecting breathing. Although infection can cause obstruction of the airway, in this question, option 1 is more clearly the correct answer.
   Content Area: *Perioperative Nursing*
   Integrated Processes: *Nursing Process: Evaluation*
   Client Need: *Physiological Integrity; Reduction of Risk Potential*
   Cognitive Level: *Application*

2. **ANSWER: 4.**
   Rationales:
   1. Urine output is unrelated to dehiscence.
   2. Hypertension is unrelated to dehiscence.
   3. Palpation assesses for edema and heat; if these signs occur 3 to 6 days postoperatively, infection, not dehiscence, is suspected.
   4. **Dehiscence is a separation of the wound edges at the suture line, which is evidenced by increased drainage and the appearance of underlying tissue. This most frequently occurs 5 to 12 days postoperatively. Dehiscence is precipitated by increased intra-abdominal pressure associated with coughing, vomiting, and distension; obesity is a risk factor.**
   Content Area: *Perioperative Nursing*
   Integrated Processes: *Nursing Process: Evaluation*
   Client Need: *Physiological Integrity; Reduction of Risk Potential*
   Cognitive Level: *Application*

3. **ANSWER: 4.**
   Rationales:
   1. Deep breathing and coughing are the most effective actions to prevent collapse of alveoli (atelectasis).
   2. Early ambulation is the most effective intervention to reduce the likelihood of the absence of peristaltic motility lasting longer than 72 hours (adynamic ileus, postoperative ileus).
   3. Maintaining medical and surgical asepsis will help prevent wound infection.
   4. **Leg and ankle pumping exercises, early ambulation, and the use of antiembolism stockings increase venous return, thereby minimizing venous stasis and thrombophlebitis.**
   Content Area: *Perioperative Nursing*
   Integrated Processes: *Teaching/Learning; Nursing Process: Implementation*
   Client Need: *Physiological Integrity; Reduction of Risk Potential*
   Cognitive Level: *Application*

4. **ANSWER: 3.**
   Rationales:
   1. Although vital signs are important and are associated with Breathing and Circulation, another option has priority.
   2. Although assessing urinary output is important because it assesses glomerular filtration rate and the adequacy of Circulation, it is not associated with Airway or Breathing; another option has priority.
   3. **Airway patency always is the priority because adequate ventilation is essential for life.**
   4. Although assessing the dressing is important to assess for hemorrhage, which is associated with Circulation, it is not the priority.
   TEST-TAKING TIP: Identify the word in the stem that sets a priority. The word *first* in the stem sets a priority. Use the principle of the ABCs (Airway, Breathing, and Circulation) when setting a priority. Option 3 is associated with Airway.
   Content Area: *Perioperative Nursing*
   Integrated Processes: *Nursing Process: Evaluation*
   Client Need: *Physiological Integrity; Reduction of Risk Potential*
   Cognitive Level: *Application*

5. **ANSWER: 1.**
   Rationales:
   1. **Montgomery straps are used when frequent dressing changes are required because of a draining wound. This protects the skin from excessive removal and reapplication of tape that can injure skin. Montgomery straps attach with adhesive to the skin on either side of the wound and the portion that is nonadhesive lays over the dressing and is laced up with gauze strips that hold abdominal pads in place.**
   2. Moist to dry dressings are not advisable because the dry dressing will disrupt new granulated tissue when it is removed. Research demonstrates that a moist wound bed supports the growth of granulated tissue and wound healing.
   3. This type of dressing is not used for wounds with a small amount of drainage. A wound with a small amount of drainage generally is changed only once a day.
   4. Although patients can be taught to change their own dressings, this is not the purpose of this type of dressing.
   TEST-TAKING TIP: Identify the options that are opposites. Option 1, which indicates a wound that requires frequent dressing changes generally because of copious amount of drainage, and option 3, which indicates a wound that has a small amount of drainage, are opposites. Examine options 1 and 3 carefully. More often than not, an option that is an opposite is the correct answer.
   Content Area: *Perioperative Nursing*
   Integrated Processes: *Nursing Process: Planning*
   Client Need: *Physiological Integrity; Physiological Adaptation*
   Cognitive Level: *Analysis*

6. ANSWER: 4.

Rationales:

1. Discharge planning generally is initiated on admission to the hospital when a discharge planner is assigned responsibility for assessing the needs of the patient in preparation for discharge.

2. With extensive head and neck surgery, the patient will have either an endotracheal tube or tracheostomy to facilitate respirations as well as suctioning if necessary to clear the airway.

3. A signed consent generally is obtained when the patient is admitted to the hospital.

4. Establishing a method of communication after head and neck surgery is the priority because the patient will most likely have an endotracheal tube or tracheostomy tube in place. This intervention is important because it meets the emotional and safety needs of the patient when the patient knows how to make needs known to the healthcare team.

TEST-TAKING TIP: Identify the word that sets a priority. The word *priority* indicates that the question is asking what should be done first.

Content Area: Perioperative Nursing

Integrated Processes: Teaching/Learning; Nursing Process: Implementation

Client Need: Physiological Integrity; Reduction of Risk Potential

Cognitive Level: Application

7. ANSWER: 3.

Rationales:

1. Stable vital signs are expected; this indicates that the patient is responding safely after the procedure.

2. A sore throat is expected after this procedure because of irritation of the mucous membranes from the tube inserted into the esophagus.

3. During an esophagogastroduodenoscopy, a local anesthetic is sprayed into a patient's posterior pharynx to lessen the gag reflex. The patient is kept on NPO status until the gag reflex returns. When the gag reflex returns, liquids are permitted; eventually the patient is instructed to eat a light diet during the first 12 to 24 hours.

4. Although assessing urinary output is important because it assesses the glomerular filtration rate and adequacy of <u>C</u>irculation, it is not associated with <u>A</u>irway or <u>B</u>reathing. Voiding urine in a sufficient quantity after the procedure is expected. Urinary retention is not associated with this procedure because conscious sedation, not general anesthesia, is used.

TEST-TAKING TIP: Identify the word in the stem that sets a priority. The word *most* in the stem sets a priority. Use the principle of the ABCs (<u>A</u>irway, <u>B</u>reathing, and <u>C</u>irculation) when establishing a priority. Option 3 is associated with <u>A</u>irway, which is the priority. Option 2 is associated with <u>B</u>reathing. Option 4 indicates that the patient's voiding pattern is of a sufficient quantity. Assessing adequacy of urinary output is associated with <u>C</u>irculation (cardiac output must be maintained to ensure an adequate glomerular flow rate).

Content Area: Perioperative Nursing

Integrated Processes: Communication/Documentation; Nursing Process: Evaluation

Client Need: Safe and Effective Care Environment; Management of Care

Cognitive Level: Application

8. ANSWER: 3, 5, 2, 1, 4.

Rationales:

3. A disposable pad protects the patient from contact with gastric secretions.

5. Shutting off the suction and separating the tube from the suction device prepares for removal of the tube. This is done before removing the tape from the patient's nose.

2. Removal of adhesive tape from the patient's nose allows for unrestricted removal of the tube.

1. Instructing the patient to take a deep breath helps minimize the risk of accidental aspiration of gastric secretions.

4. Folding the tube on itself clamps the tube with the fingers, which helps prevent aspiration of gastric contents exiting from the tube during its withdrawal. Quickly and carefully removing the tube minimizes discomfort and the risk of trauma.

Content Area: Perioperative Nursing

Integrated Processes: Nursing Process: Planning

Client Need: Physiological Integrity; Reduction of Risk Potential

Cognitive Level: Analysis

9. ANSWER: 2.

Rationales:

1. This is not a patient-centered action; it does not meet the spiritual/emotional needs of the patient.

2. A patient cannot wear a metal object in the operating room because of the use of various equipment that conduct electricity. A religious medal can be kept near the patient.

3. A deceptive act violates the trusting relationship that is essential between the patient and nurse.

4. This is not a patient-centered response; it does not meet the spiritual/emotional needs of the patient.

TEST-TAKING TIP: Identify the options that deny the patient's feelings and concerns. Options 1 and 4 deny the patient's feelings and concerns. Eliminate these options from further consideration.

Content Area: Perioperative Nursing

Integrated Processes: Caring; Communication/Documentation; Nursing Process: Implementation

Client Need: Psychosocial Integrity

Cognitive Level: Application

10. ANSWER: 3.

Rationales:

1. Although exercises that increase venous return should be encouraged to reduce the risk of a thrombus and pulmonary emboli, it is not the priority.

2. Generally, patients are advised that they can return to their usual activities within 7 to 10 days, not 6 weeks. People who perform heavy manual labor may require 2 to 4 weeks to recuperate.

3. Medications that can cause bleeding, such as aspirin, clopidogrel (Plavix), and warfarin (Coumadin), increase the risk of postoperative bleeding and should be avoided

before surgery. The primary health-care provider will determine how many days before and after surgery the patient should avoid drugs that increase bleeding time.

4. Generally, an enema the night before this surgery is unnecessary because the bowel is not involved in this surgery.

TEST-TAKING TIP: Identify the word in the stem that sets a priority. The word *most* in the stem sets a priority.

Content Area: Perioperative Nursing
Integrated Processes: Teaching/Learning; Nursing Process: Implementation
Client Need: Physiological Integrity; Reduction of Risk Potential
Cognitive Level: Application

11. **ANSWER: 1, 2.**
   Rationales:
   1. The pulse oximeter informs the nurse about the patient's oxygen saturation. If it decreases below 92 percent, the primary health-care provider should be informed. Generally, patients in the postanesthesia care unit (PACU) receive oxygen until they awaken from anesthesia and the oxygen saturation level is stabilized within the expected range.
   2. Auscultating for breath sounds monitors lung function. Absence of breath sounds indicates a pneumothorax or atelectasis. Adventitious breath sounds, such as rhonchi or crackles, indicate the accumulation of fluid in the lung. Maintaining an airway and providing for adequate oxygenation is a critical role of the nurse in the PACU.
   3. Generally, a NG tube is implemented for decompression of the stomach immediately after surgery. It should be attached to intermittent or continuous suction and should not be clamped without an order. Several days after surgery, a NG tube may be ordered to be clamped intermittently to determine whether gastric emptying is occurring. Once it is determined that gastric emptying is occurring, the NG tube will be removed.
   4. Postoperatively, the head of the bed should be elevated to the low Fowler position after a patient has general anesthesia. Gravity moves the abdominal organs away from the diaphragm, which facilitates respirations and helps prevent aspiration.
   5. Only the patient should activate the trigger on a patient-controlled analgesia pump.

   Content Area: Perioperative Nursing
   Integrated Processes: Nursing Process: Implementation
   Client Need: Physiological Integrity; Physiological Adaptation
   Cognitive Level: Application

12. **ANSWER: 3.**
   Rationales:
   1. Fixed, dilated pupils reflect medullary depression associated with stage IV of anesthesia and indicates that the patient is near death.
   2. Weak respirations and a thready pulse reflect medullary depression associated with stage IV of anesthesia and indicates that the patient is near death.
   3. These clinical findings are associated with stage III of anesthesia; stage III is the appropriate stage for surgical procedures.

4. These clinical findings reflect stage II of anesthesia; often, it is referred to as the *excitement stage.*

Content Area: Perioperative Nursing
Integrated Processes: Nursing Process: Evaluation
Client Need: Physiological Integrity; Reduction of Risk Potential
Cognitive Level: Analysis

13. **ANSWER: 2, 5, 4, 3, 1.**
   Rationales:
   2. The patient's signs and symptoms indicate impending hypovolemic shock. The nurse should mobilize professionals from a variety of health-care disciplines to assist with this emergency.
   5. Increasing the flow rate of the IV will immediately increase the circulating blood volume.
   4. The Trendelenburg position uses the principle of gravity to increase blood return from the legs, which brings more blood to the brain and vital organs. This takes more time to accomplish than increasing the intravenous flow rate but less time than setting up an oxygen delivery system.
   3. Exogenous oxygen will increase the partial pressure of oxygen within the circulatory system. A nasal cannula delivers 24 to 44 percent oxygen depending on the oxygen liter flow while a simple face mask delivers 40 to 60 percent oxygen depending on the oxygen liter flow.
   1. The vital signs should be obtained to determine the patient's response to nursing interventions.

   Content Area: Perioperative Nursing
   Integrated Processes: Nursing Process: Planning
   Client Need: Physiological Integrity; Physiological Adaptation
   Cognitive Level: Analysis

14. **ANSWER: 4.**
   Rationales:
   1. The patient's cardiovascular status should be assessed after airway patency is ensured and respirations are adequate to meet the oxygen needs of the body.
   2. The patient's level of consciousness should be assessed after the patient's airway, breathing, and circulation are assessed.
   3. The patient's oxygen saturation level may be monitored as part of an assessment of the patient's respiratory status. This occurs after the adequacy of the patient's airway is ensured.
   4. The nurse should follow the ABCs of assessing Airway, Breathing, and Circulation, in that order. Maintaining the airway is always the priority to ensure that oxygen can reach the lungs.

   TEST-TAKING TIP: Identify the word in the stem that sets a priority. The word *first* in the stem sets a priority. A nurse should follow the ABCs (Airway, Breathing, and Circulation) as a guide when establishing a priority. Option 4 is associated with airway, which is the priority.

   Content Area: Perioperative Nursing
   Integrated Processes: Nursing Process: Evaluation
   Client Need: Physiological Integrity; Reduction of Risk Potential
   Cognitive Level: Application

15. ANSWER: 3.
Rationales:
1. Although it is important to assess the patient's level of pain, it is not the most important assessment that should be performed among the options presented.
2. Although it is important to assess a patient's level of consciousness, it is not the most important assessment that should be performed among the options presented.
3. **Of the options presented, none refer to airway or breathing. However, assessing a patient for signs of fluid volume excess is associated with circulation. Often, patients are administered a large volume of IV solutions during surgery to ensure that the patient's circulating blood volume is adequate and that the glomerular filtration rate is sufficient to maintain kidney function. The nurse should assess patients for fluid excess or deficit when in the PACU.**
4. Although assessing the patency of a urinary catheter is important, it is not the most important assessment that should be performed among the options presented.
TEST-TAKING TIP: Identify the word in the stem that sets a priority. The word *first* in the stem sets a priority. The nurse should use the ABCs (Airway, Breathing, and Circulation) as a guide when setting a priority. No option refers to Airway or Breathing. Option 3 relates to circulation. Examine option 3 carefully.
Content Area: Perioperative Nursing
Integrated Processes: Nursing Process: Evaluation
Client Need: Physiological Integrity; Reduction of Risk Potential
Cognitive Level: Application

16. ANSWER: 1, 3, 5.
Rationales:
1. **This is a sequential compression device used to prevent deep vein thrombosis by facilitating venous return. It will intermittently inflate chambers and then deflate chambers in the device in a sequential pattern from distal to proximal, thereby promoting venous return.**
2. This device will not minimize muscle atrophy.
3. **This is a sequential compression device used to prevent deep vein thrombosis by facilitating venous return. When lower extremity venous return is promoted, it reduces lower extremity edema.**
4. The risk of thrombophlebitis is reduced, not increased, with a sequential compression device. Venous stasis is a risk factor of thrombophlebitis.
5. **Dependent edema can cause discomfort as fluid collects in the interstitial spaces and dermal tissue becomes taut. This device will promote venous return and limit peripheral edema.**
Content Area: Perioperative Nursing
Integrated Processes: Nursing Process: Evaluation
Client Need: Physiological Integrity; Reduction of Risk Potential
Cognitive Level: Analysis

17. ANSWER: 3.
Rationales:
1. The hospital and operating room can be modified and controlled to ensure a latex-free environment.

2. Slight hypertension may be in response to anxiety associated with the impending surgery. Just before surgery, patients are given medications that reduce anxiety and induce relaxation, which will decrease the blood pressure.
3. **Usually, general anesthesia is administered via a combination of inhalation and the intravenous route. A patient with a history of smoking is at an increased risk for pulmonary complications with general anesthesia. The lungs may be impaired as a result of inhaled toxins associated with smoking. Also, inhaled anesthetic agents are eliminated via the lungs, which may be inefficient because of lung impairment.**
4. Vesicular breath sounds are noiseless breath sounds that are normal and expected.
TEST-TAKING TIP: Identify the word in the stem that sets a priority. The word *most* in the stem sets a priority.
Content Area: Perioperative Nursing
Integrated Processes: Nursing Process: Analysis
Client Need: Physiological Integrity; Reduction of Risk Potential
Cognitive Level: Application

18. ANSWER: 1, 3, 4.
Rationales:
1. **Increasing fluid intake will reduce the viscosity of circulating blood, helping to reduce the risk of a deep vein thrombosis. Also, it reduces the viscosity of respiratory secretions, facilitating expectoration of respiratory secretions; this minimizes pooling of secretions in the lungs, which provides a medium for bacterial growth.**
2. Coughing and deep breathing will facilitate lung expansion and expectoration of secretions, reducing the risk of hypostatic pneumonia; it does not reduce the risk of deep vein thrombosis.
3. **Ambulation requires contraction of muscles of the legs, which increases venous return. Also, it increases the depth of respirations as the body needs more oxygen to meet the needs of muscles. Deep respirations aerate the distal alveoli, preventing the accumulation of fluid. Accumulated fluid precipitates hypostatic pneumonia.**
4. **Changing position from side to side requires the patient to use leg muscles to turn, which increases venous return. It also allows fluid in the lung to move via gravity to dependent sections of the pulmonary system; this in turn facilitates aeration and expansion of alternate lung areas as the patient changes position.**
5. Compression stockings provide external pressure facilitating venous return, thereby reducing the risk of deep vein thrombosis. Compression stockings will not reduce the risk of hypostatic pneumonia.
Content Area: Perioperative Nursing
Integrated Processes: Communication/Documentation; Nursing Process: Planning
Client Need: Physiological Integrity; Reduction of Risk Potential
Cognitive Level: Analysis

19. ANSWER: 1.
Rationales:
1. **Stage II is the stage of excitement. The nurse should avoid stimulating the patient because it can precipitate vomiting and increased activity.**

2. Feeling dizzy and drowsy is associated with stage I of anesthesia.

3. The anesthesiologist, not the nurse, is responsible for implementing anesthesia and giving the patient this direction.

4. Once the patient is in stage III, when the muscles are relaxed, draping the patient for the surgery is implemented.

TEST-TAKING TIP: Identify the unique option. Option 1 is unique because it addresses what should not be done, while the other options address what should be done. Identify the options that are opposites. Options 1 and 4 are opposites. Option 1 indicates not touching the patient and option 4 includes an action that touches the patient.

Content Area: Perioperative Nursing
Integrated Processes: Nursing Process: Implementation
Client Need: Physiological Integrity; Reduction of Risk Potential
Cognitive Level: Application

20. **ANSWER: 1, 2, 4, 3, 5, 6.**
   Rationales:

1. Donning clean gloves protects the nurse from potential contact with drainage from the collection chamber.

2. The port to the collection chamber is opened so that the contents can be emptied into a container for measurement.

4. The content is emptied into a container with marks indicating fluid volume to ensure an accurate measurement of the drainage.

3. Once the collection chamber is empty, the chamber is compressed firmly. This is the first step in reestablishing negative pressure within the portable wound drainage system.

5. Cleansing the port with an alcohol wipe minimizes the introduction of microorganisms that will have direct access to the wound via the Hemovac tubing.

6. The port is closed before compression of the chamber is released. This reestablishes negative pressure. Negative pressure establishes a vacuum and the resulting suction pulls drainage from the wound.

Content Area: Perioperative Nursing
Integrated Processes: Nursing Process: Planning
Client Need: Physiological Integrity; Physiological Adaptation
Cognitive Level: Analysis

21. **ANSWER: 1.**
   Rationales:

1. Most patients anticipate some discomfort/pain after surgery, and this concern should be addressed to decrease anxiety.

2. Teaching should focus on the activities that prevent complications. Stressing potential complications may cause unnecessary anxiety.

3. It is the surgeon's, not the nurse's, responsibility to review the risks and benefits of surgery.

4. It is the surgeon's, not the nurse's, responsibility to discuss the type of surgery that is planned when securing the consent for surgery.

TEST-TAKING TIP: Identify the word in the stem that sets a priority. The word *most* in the stem sets a priority. Identify equally plausible options. Options 2, 3, and 4 are all equally plausible; they all have the potential to raise anxiety.

Identify the unique option. Option 1 is unique because it is the only option that will reduce anxiety that the patient may have about postoperative pain.

Content Area: Perioperative Nursing
Integrated Processes: Teaching/Learning; Nursing Process: Implementation
Client Need: Physiological Integrity; Reduction of Risk Potential
Cognitive Level: Application

22. **ANSWER: 2.**
   Rationales:

1. Only active contraction of muscles will prevent muscle atrophy.

2. Antiembolism stockings are elastic and provide counter pressure supporting muscles in the legs and facilitating venous return to the heart. Avoiding venous stasis helps to minimize the risk of thrombophlebitis.

3. Antiembolism stockings do not prevent contractures; placing joints through their full range of motion several times a day prevents contractures.

4. The purpose of antiembolism stockings is not to keep the legs warm. Blankets may be used to provide warmth if it is considered necessary.

Content Area: Perioperative Nursing
Integrated Processes: Teaching/Learning; Nursing Process: Implementation
Client Need: Physiological Integrity; Reduction of Risk Potential
Cognitive Level: Application

23. **ANSWER: 4.**
   Rationales:

1. Documentation is important, but it is not the priority. Attending to patient needs is the priority.

2. The drainage collection container should be emptied when half full because a full container may place tension on the insertion site. Also, the extent of negative pressure within the device decreases as the container fills with drainage, impeding its effectiveness.

3. Sterile technique, not medical asepsis, is required when emptying the drainage collection container; this minimizes the introduction of pathogens to the wound bed via the container and tubing of the device.

4. This is the most important nursing action of the options presented. The tubing may be clogged or kinked if there is too little drainage. The patient may be hemorrhaging if there is too much drainage. The nurse must respond to both events; the nurse can milk the tubing to relieve a clogged tube or straighten it manually if it is kinked; the nurse should notify the surgeon if the drainage is a larger volume than that which is expected.

TEST-TAKING TIP: Identify the word in the stem that sets a priority. The word *most* in the stem sets a priority. Identify the option with a specific determiner. The word *only* in option 2 is a specific determiner. Rarely is an option with a specific determiner the correct answer. Identify the clang associations. The word *drainage* in the stem and in options 1 and 4 are clang associations. Examine options 1 and 4 carefully.

Content Area: Perioperative Nursing
Integrated Processes: Nursing Process: Evaluation

Client Need: *Physiological Integrity; Physiological Adaptation*
Cognitive Level: *Analysis*

24. **ANSWER: 1.**
Rationales:
1. Individuals who are obese have more adipose tissue in the torso, which can limit the person's ability to take a deep breath, increasing the risk of respiratory complications. Also, intrathoracic pressure increases as the lungs expand on inspiration, causing an increase in intra-abdominal pressure and resulting in abdominal pain. To avoid this painful response, patients may take shallow breaths, thereby increasing the risk of respiratory complications.
2. Although it is important to teach a patient how to prevent a wound infection, it is not the priority at this time.
3. The nurse can teach the patient how to safely ambulate in the hall when assisting the patient to ambulate postoperatively.
4. Although a nurse may teach a patient preoperatively how to exit the bed postoperatively, it is not as important as another option. The nurse has time during the postoperative period to teach the patient how to safely accomplish this activity of daily living.
TEST-TAKING TIP: Identify the word in the stem that sets a priority. The word *most* in the stem sets a priority. Identify equally plausible options. Options 3 and 4 are equally plausible; both are associated with mobility and one option is no better than the other. Identify the unique option. Option 1 is unique because it identifies two, not one, interventions—*cough and deep breathe.*
Content Area: *Perioperative Nursing*
Integrated Processes: *Teaching/Learning; Nursing Process: Planning*
Client Need: *Physiological Integrity; Reduction of Risk Potential*
Cognitive Level: *Application*

25. **ANSWER: 4.**
Rationales:
1. Although this should be done eventually, it is more important that the nurse have more data and institute emergency standing orders.
2. This action is unsafe at this time. Emptying the collection containers will take time, delaying addressing the patient's low blood pressure.
3. This will not correct the low blood pressure. A patient with this type of surgery will have a urinary retention catheter in place and should not experience urinary retention.
4. Increasing the IV flow rate will increase the circulating blood volume, which will help raise the blood pressure; once this is done, the nurse can assess the patient to identify additional data before notifying the surgeon. Nurses in a PACU have standing orders that permit them to increase an IV flow rate if a blood pressure is less than expected during a potential emergency.
TEST-TAKING TIP: Identify the word in the stem that sets a priority. The word *first* in the stem sets a priority.

Content Area: *Perioperative Nursing*
Integrated Processes: *Nursing Process: Implementation*
Client Need: *Physiological Integrity; Reduction of risk Potential*
Cognitive Level: *Application*

26. **ANSWER: 1.**
Rationales:
1. A NG tube must be unobstructed for negative pressure to reach the stomach. The fact that the patient is vomiting and the abdomen is distended indicates that secretions are accumulating in the stomach. The first nursing measure is to ensure that the tube is free from factors that can cause obstruction of the tube, such as kinks in the tubing or compression of the tube.
2. This is the second intervention. Often, repositioning the patient and having the patient cough will alter the pressure in the tubing, alleviating an obstruction.
3. This is unsafe unless placement of the tube is established. An antiemetic will not address the problem of an obstructed NG tube.
4. This action is premature. Once other interventions fail to reestablish the flow of secretions from the tube, 30 mL of air can be added via the blue pigtail. This may clear secretions from the blue tube that are permitting air to enter the stomach and reestablish suction.
TEST-TAKING TIP: Identify the word in the stem that sets a priority. The word *first* sets a priority. Identify the clang association. The word *tube* in the stem and *tubing* in option 1 is a clang association. More often than not, an option with a clang association is the correct answer. Examine option 1 carefully.
Content Area: *Perioperative Nursing*
Integrated Processes: *Nursing Process: Implementation*
Client Need: *Physiological Integrity; Reduction of Risk Potential*
Cognitive Level: *Application*

27. **ANSWERS: 2, 5.**
Rationales:
1. Catheterizing a patient should never be done without an order from the patient's primary health-care provider.
2. **Palpating and percussing the patient's bladder for fullness should be performed first to determine if the patient has urinary retention. If the bladder is not full, the patient may be experiencing kidney dysfunction.**
3. The nurse should never increase the IV flow rate without an order from the patient's primary health-care provider. A standing order would not exist for this situation.
4. Encouraging the patient to drink more fluids should not be done until the cause of the patient's status is confirmed.
5. **Placing a warm towel over the patient's lower abdomen may relax the urinary sphincters and the sound of running water in the patients' sink may psychologically precipitate voiding.**
Content Area: *Perioperative Nursing*
Integrated Processes: *Nursing Process: Implementation*
Client Need: *Physiological Integrity; Physiological Adaptation*
Cognitive Level: *Application*

28. ANSWER: 1.
Rationales:

1. **The initial concern is that the patient may aspirate the vomitus. Turning the patient to the lateral position will facilitate movement of vomitus out of the mouth, thereby reducing the risk of aspiration.**

2. Although this is something the nurse may do after it is determined that the patient has a problem maintaining the blood pressure, it is not the first action that the nurse should implement. A standing order would have to exist for the nurse to implement this action without first notifying the primary health-care provider.

3. Although documenting the amount and characteristics of the emesis is important, it is not the priority at this time.

4. Although this is an action that the nurse may implement if it is determined that the patient is hemorrhaging, it is not the priority at this time. In addition, administering a blood product requires an order from the primary health-care provider.

TEST-TAKING TIP: Identify the word in the stem that sets a priority. The word *first* in the stem sets a priority.
Content Area: Perioperative Nursing
Integrated Processes: Nursing Process: Implementation
Client Need: Physiological Integrity; Physiological Adaptation
Cognitive Level: Application

29. ANSWER: 2.
Rationales:

1. Opioids are prescribed postoperatively, not preoperatively. An opioid is a central nervous system depressant used to manage pain.

2. **An antibiotic generally is prescribed prophylactically preoperatively when a surgeon plans to enter the abdominal cavity, thoracic cavity, GI tract, or biliary tract; surgically repair a traumatic wound (dirty wound); or perform a neck dissection. There is an increased risk of infection associated with these areas of the body.**

3. An antiemetic generally is not administered preoperatively. An antiemetic is prescribed postoperatively to treat nausea and vomiting.

4. An anticoagulant, not a thrombolytic, may be prescribed prophylactically to reduce the risk of thrombophlebitis or a pulmonary embolus. Thrombolytics are prescribed to dissolve clots in blood vessels or venous/arterial catheters after they occur, not before they occur.

Content Area: Perioperative Nursing
Integrated Processes: Communication/Documentation; Nursing Process: Planning
Client Need: Physiological Integrity; Pharmacological and Parenteral Therapies
Cognitive Level: Application

30. ANSWER: 2.
Rationales:

1. Although the nurse may be concerned about an increased risk of dehiscence due to the presence of abdominal distension, another option directly addresses the potential cause of the abdominal distension. The risk of dehiscence will decrease after abdominal distension is reduced. Also, dehiscence is most common 4 to 5 days after surgery, not immediately after surgery.

2. **Identifying whether the tube is patent is the most important intervention. The concern is that the NG tube is not maintaining decompression of the upper GI tract in the presence of a postoperative ileus. A postoperative ileus is a common response to the handling of the bowel during surgery and the effects of anesthesia. The tube may be occluded due to an obstruction within or kink in the tubing.**

3. After bowel surgery, a patient generally is not permitted fluids by mouth until peristalsis returns. Peristalsis is indicated by the presence of bowel sounds.

4. Absent bowel sounds and abdominal distension are not clinical indicators of hypovolemia. Clinical indicators of hypovolemia include decreased blood pressure and urinary output, tachycardia, tachypnea, restlessness, and anxiety.

TEST-TAKING TIP: Identify the word in the stem that sets a priority. The word *main* in the stem sets a priority.
Content Area: Perioperative Nursing
Integrated Processes: Nursing Process: Evaluation
Client Need: Physiological Integrity; Reduction of Risk Potential
Cognitive Level: Analysis

31. ANSWER: 3.
Rationales:

1. Wrist restrains are inappropriate to manage this situation.

2. The patient is semiconscious and probably will not comprehend an explanation at this time. Leaving the airway in place is unsafe.

3. **An attempt to expel the airway indicates that the patient is recovering from the anesthesia and is becoming more alert. As the effects of anesthesia decrease, the gag reflex returns. The use of an oropharyngeal airway in the presence of the gag reflex will cause choking and retching, which may precipitate vomiting. Vomiting should be avoided because it may result in aspiration.**

4. Placing the patient in the lateral position does not address the issue of the patient attempting to expel the airway.

TEST-TAKING TIP: Identify the clang associations. The word *airway* in the stem and in options 2 and 3 are clang associations. Identify the options that are opposites. Options 2 and 3 are opposites. Examine options 2 and 3 carefully.
Content Area: Perioperative Nursing
Integrated Processes: Nursing Process: Evaluation
Client Need: Physiological Integrity; Physiological Adaptation
Cognitive Level: Application

32. ANSWER: 1, 2, 3.
Rationales:

1. **Providing emotional support is an example of the advocate role of the nurse. The nurse functions as an advocate when meeting psychosocial needs.**

2. Performing the safety time out check is an example of the advocate role of the nurse. The nurse functions as an advocate when preventing patient injuries.

3. Maintaining patient safety is an example of the advocate role of the nurse. The nurse functions as an advocate when patient injuries are prevented.

4. This is an example of the caregiver role of the nurse.

5. This is an example of the caregiver role of the nurse.

Content Area: Perioperative Nursing
Integrated Processes: Caring; Communication/Documentation; Nursing Process: Analysis
Client Need: Safe and Effective Care Environment; Management of Care
Cognitive Level: Analysis

33. ANSWER: 2.
Rationales:
1. The sitting position elevates the head of the bed, which can precipitate a postdural puncture headache after spinal anesthesia.

2. A postdural puncture headache can occur as a result of leakage of cerebrospinal fluid when the needle hole in the dura does not close immediately after spinal anesthesia. Cerebrospinal fluid leakage reduces pressure on the spinal cord, resulting in a headache. Positioning a patient in the supine position helps to reduce postdural puncture headaches.

3. The contour position elevates the head of the bed, which can precipitate a postdural puncture headache after spinal anesthesia.

4. The orthopneic position elevates the head of the bed, which can precipitate a postdural puncture headache after spinal anesthesia.

TEST-TAKING TIP: Identify the unique option. Option 2 is unique. It is the only option that positions the patient flat in bed. Options 1, 3, and 4 require the head of the bed to be elevated.

Content Area: Perioperative Nursing
Integrated Processes: Nursing Process: Implementation
Client Need: Physiological Integrity; Physiological Adaptation
Cognitive Level: Application

34. ANSWER: 2.
Rationales:
1. The patient is not hemorrhaging. Serosanguineous drainage is expected. A blood pressure of 120/80 mm Hg is within the expected range of 90 to 120 mm Hg for the systolic blood pressure and 60 to 80 mm Hg for the diastolic blood pressure. If the patient were hemorrhaging, the blood pressure would be lower than the expected range. A hemoglobin level of 15.5 g/dL is within the expected range of 14 to 18 g/dL for an adult male. An RBC count of 5.6 mm³ is within the expected range of 5.0 to 5.80 mm³ for an adult male. If the patient were hemorrhaging, the hemoglobin and RBC count would be lower than the expected range. A platelet count of 200,000 mm³ is within the expected range of 150,000 to 450,000 mm³ for an adult. If the platelet count were lower than the expected range, the patient would be

at risk for hemorrhage. If the drainage changes to sanguineous (abundance of blood), the patient may be hemorrhaging. If the serosanguineous drainage continues to be profuse, the primary health-care provider should be notified because this is an unexpected response that requires further assessment.

2. Infection is a concern because the patient's WBC count is lower than the expected range of 4.5 to 11.0 mm³, which most likely is a complication of the chemotherapy for stage II lung cancer. Also, the patient has a temperature 100.4°F, which is higher than the expected range of approximately 97.5°F to 99.5°F. This may be a response to inflammation associated with trauma and surgery, but it could indicate the presence of infection.

3. The patient is not experiencing respiratory distress. The slightly elevated respirations are most likely a response to the increased temperature. Shallow respirations may be a defensive response to avoid discomfort associated with the abdominal wall trauma when taking a deep breath. Taking a deep breath increases thoracic exertion, which in turn will increase intra-abdominal pressure causing discomfort at the injured site.

4. The patient is not experiencing an electrolyte imbalance. A serum potassium level of 4.5 mEq/L is within the expected range of 3.5 to 5.0 mEq/L, and a serum sodium level of 140 mEq/L is within the expected range of 135 to 145 mEq/L.

TEST-TAKING TIP: Identify the word in the stem that sets a priority. The word *most* in the stem sets a priority. Identify the unique option. Option 2 is unique because it is the only option that involves a "risk for" concern.

Content Area: Perioperative Nursing
Integrated Processes: Nursing Process: Analysis
Client Need: Physiological Integrity; Physiological Adaptation
Cognitive Level: Analysis

35. ANSWER: 2.
Rationales:
1. Although encouraging fluid intake is important to meet fluid requirements and to flush the urinary tract of microorganisms, it is not as essential as another option.

2. Neutropenic precautions protect the patient from pathogens. When a patient has impaired immunity, the white blood cell count is low, which decreases a person's ability to fight infection. The patient is placed in a private room, caregivers and visitors must wear gowns and masks, and strategies, such as wet dusting and mopping; banning of dried, fresh, or potted flowers; a diet of well-cooked food; omission of fresh vegetables and fruit; frequent hand hygiene; meticulous and frequent oral care; and having the patient wear a N95 respirator when being transported for essential reasons, are implemented to protect the patient from pathogens.

3. Although suggesting that the patient ingest high-protein foods facilitates wound healing, it is not as essential as another option.

4. Surgical, not medical, asepsis should be employed when changing a patient's surgical dressings or when emptying drains.

TEST-TAKING TIP: Identify the word in the stem that sets a priority. The word *essential* in the stem sets a priority.
Content Area: Perioperative Nursing
Integrated Processes: Nursing Process: Implementation
Client Need: Safe and Effective Care Environment; Safety and Infection Control
Cognitive Level: Application

36. **ANSWER: 2.**
Rationales:
1. Deep breathing and coughing generally are suggested to minimize the risk of hypostatic pneumonia after anesthesia and surgery.
2. The primary health-care provider ordered that the patient be NPO (nothing-by-mouth). This is the most important intervention of the options ordered. Until the cause of the nausea and vomiting is identified, the patient should be NPO. In addition, drinking and eating may exacerbate nausea and vomiting.
3. Although room-deodorizing sprays may be used to cover up offensive odors, this intervention is not as important as another option.
4. Although frequent oral hygiene should be provided for the patient who is experiencing nausea and vomiting, it is not as important as another option.

TEST-TAKING TIP: Identify the word in the stem that sets a priority. The word *most* in the stem sets a priority. Identify the unique option. Option 2 is unique because it is the only option that involves an intervention ordered by the primary health-care provider. The other actions are all independent nursing interventions.
Content Area: Perioperative Nursing
Integrated Processes: Nursing Process: Implementation
Client Need: Physiological Integrity; Physiological Adaptation
Cognitive Level: Application

37. **ANSWER: 3.**
Rationales:
1. Although the systolic blood pressure is 20 mm Hg above the expected range for a systolic blood pressure (≤120 mm Hg), it is not unusual for a person 65 years of age. In addition, the slight elevation of the systolic pressure most likely is associated with the psychological and physical stress of preparing for bowel surgery.
2. A little sip of water is not critical 2 hours before general anesthesia. This fluid will pass through the stomach in 2 hours and not be a risk factor for aspiration.
3. Plavix is a platelet aggregation inhibitor. It is recommended that Plavix be discontinued 5 to 7 days before surgery because it can cause bleeding and hemorrhage. This is important information that must be reported to the primary health-care provider immediately. Surgery may need to be postponed.
4. A Hb level of 15 g/dL is within the expected range of 14 to 18 g/dL for an adult male.

TEST-TAKING TIP: Identify the word in the stem that sets a priority. The word *most* in the stem sets a priority.
Content Area: Perioperative Nursing
Integrated Processes: Communication/Documentation; Nursing Process: Analysis
Client Need: Physiological Integrity; Pharmacological and Parenteral Therapies
Cognitive Level: Analysis

38. **ANSWER: 4.**
Rationales:
1. A wound should be gently, not forcefully, cleansed so as not to disrupt the granulated tissue in the wound bed.
2. The nurse should spray back and forth across the inside of the wound and progressively move down the surface of the wound. This prevents the introduction of microorganisms surrounding the wound from contaminating the wound.
3. A piston syringe should be held 2, not 4, inches from the surface of the wound. Holding the piston syringe 2 inches away from the wound helps minimize splashing and prevents irrigating solution from contaminating the environment.
4. Positioning the patient so that the irrigating solution flows into an emesis basin uses the principle of gravity to direct the flow of solution and debris away from the wound. Collecting the irrigating solution and debris in an emesis basin protects the environment from contamination.

TEST-TAKING TIP: Identify the clang association. The word *irrigation* in the stem and the word *irrigating* in option 4 is a clang association. Examine option 4 carefully.
Content Area: Perioperative Nursing
Integrated Processes: Nursing Process: Implementation
Client Need: Physiological Integrity; Physiological Adaptation
Cognitive Level: Application

39. **ANSWER: 4.**
Rationales:
1. The suction device and tubing is positioned over a hole at the center, not edge, of the transparent film. This allows for the suction to be maintained over the entire wound, not just one edge.
2. The foam dressing should be contained within the wound, not extended 1 inch over the edge of the wound cavity. This protects the tissue surrounding the wound from becoming macerated.
3. The tubing is connected to negative, not positive, pressure as ordered. Suction can be continuous or intermittent and between 5 to 125 mm Hg.
4. This is the correct way to apply the transparent film of a vacuum-assisted closure device. This ensures that the transparent film has a firm seal around the wound.

TEST-TAKING TIP: Identify the clang associations. The word *wound* in the stem and in options 2 and 4 are clang associations. Examine options 2 and 4 carefully.
Content Area: Perioperative Nursing
Integrated Processes: Nursing Process: Implementation
Client Need: Physiological Integrity; Physiological Adaptation
Cognitive Level: Application

40. ANSWER: 0.5.

Rationale:

Solve the problem by using ratio and proportion.

$$\frac{\text{Desire 2.5 mg}}{\text{Have 5 mg}} = \frac{x \text{ mL}}{1 \text{ mL}}$$

$$5x = 2.5 \times 1$$
$$5x = 2.5$$
$$x = 2.5 \div 5$$
$$x = 0.5 \text{ mL}$$

Content Area: *Perioperative Nursing*
Integrated Processes: *Nursing Process: Planning*
Client Need: *Physiological Integrity; Pharmacological and Parenteral Therapies*
Cognitive Level: *Application*

Comprehensive Final Exam

REVIEW QUESTIONS

1. Which action is associated with a first-level need according to Maslow's hierarchy of needs?
   1. Inviting friends over for a party
   2. Getting a haircut before the holiday season
   3. Locking the car door when alone in the car
   4. Taking a bottle of water along when going for a walk

2. A nurse identifies a 1-cm superficial circular break in the skin over the right trochanter of a patient during an admission assessment. What should the nurse do **first**?
   1. Initiate a turning schedule.
   2. Complete a skin assessment form.
   3. Inform the primary health-care provider of the patient's status.
   4. Start wound care based on the agency's pressure ulcer protocol.

3. Which situation may lead to a legal action for assault?
   1. A nurse threatens a patient with inserting a tube to feed the patient if the patient does not eat all the food on a meal tray.
   2. A nurse administers a medication that the patient has refused by telling the patient that it is different than the refused medication.
   3. A nurse uses a restraint when a patient attempts to leave the hospital before the primary health-care provider writes a discharge order.
   4. A nurse is heard by a patient's relative telling another nurse on an elevator that the patient contracted hepatitis C from IV drug use when, in fact, the patient contracted the disease via a blood transfusion.

4. A nurse is caring for a group of patients who each have an intestinal diversion for fecal matter. The nurse should be concerned about the patient with which ostomy if the fecal matter has a loose consistency?
   1. Ileostomy
   2. Cecostomy
   3. Sigmoid colostomy
   4. Ascending colon colostomy

5. A nurse caring for a newly admitted patient reviews the information in the patient's admission history and performs a chart review.

Patient's Clinical Record

Admission History

An 85-year-old male came to the emergency department reporting urinary frequency and urgency, increased nocturia, and weakness and tiredness. The patient has not been eating well for the last few days but states that he is drinking lots of fluids. Patient states, "Usually when I used to go to the bathroom to urinate, it took a long time to start the stream. Now I barely make it to the bathroom in time." The patient's abdomen is soft and nontender.

Vital Signs Sheet

Temperature: 100.6°F, oral route.
Respirations: 24 breaths/minute, regular.
Pulse: 86, regular.

Urinalysis Results

White blood cell count increased.
Red blood cell count increased.
Glucose negative.
Ketones negative.
Protein negative.
Nitrites positive.

The nurse should assess the patient for which additional human response based on the data collected?
   1. Peripheral edema
   2. Burning on urination
   3. Suprapubic distension
   4. Decreased blood pressure

6. A nurse assesses four patients to determine their hygiene needs. The nurse should anticipate that the patient with which problem will have the greatest difficulty having hygiene needs met by the nurse?
   1. Pain
   2. Dementia
   3. Impaired vision
   4. Limited mobility

7. A patient with the diagnosis of stage 4 pancreatic cancer is consulting with a discharge planner regarding the most appropriate level of care required after palliative surgery. The patient is able to provide self-care but will need pain management. Which setting is **most** appropriate for this patient?
   1. Home hospice care
   2. Rehabilitation facility
   3. Skilled nursing facility
   4. Assistive living apartment

8. A patient comes to the emergency department reporting a sore throat and earaches. The patient has a history of diverticulitis and emphysema with shortness of breath. Which route should the nurse use to obtain this patient's temperature?
   1. Oral
   2. Rectal
   3. Temporal
   4. Tympanic

9. A nurse is teaching a group of patients about diabetes mellitus. Which participant should the nurse anticipate will have the **most** difficulty following a medical regimen associated with a chronic health problem?
   1. Adolescent
   2. Older adult
   3. Young adult
   4. Middle-aged adult

10. A nurse is caring for a middle-aged adult who is deaf. What should the nurse do to facilitate communication?
    1. Talk at a slow rate.
    2. Use shorter phrases.
    3. Overarticulate when speaking.
    4. Stand so his or her face can be easily seen.

11. A patient is frustrated about not being able to perform activities of daily living (ADLs) without help. What should the nurse do to **best** reduce the patient's frustration?
    1. Disregard the patient's behavior.
    2. Offer the patient choices about care.
    3. Distract the patient with an activity.
    4. Assist the patient to recognize personal limitations.

12. A patient comes to the emergency department and reports pain in the hip. Which patient statement **best** reflects chronic pain rather than acute pain?
    1. "Over-the-counter pain killers do not relieve the pain."
    2. "The pain feels like someone stuck me with a knife."
    3. "All of a sudden I started having pain in my hip."
    4. "This pain has been going on for several weeks."

13. What action is unrelated to maintaining airborne precautions for a patient with a diagnosis of suspected primary tuberculosis?
    1. Donning a gown when entering the room
    2. Wearing a N95 respirator when in the room
    3. Maintaining negative air pressure within the room
    4. Having the patient wear a surgical mask when transported outside the room

14. A nurse is to administer eardrops to an adult. The nurse verifies the primary health-care provider's order, washes the hands, and collects the medication, following the three checks and ten rights associated with medication administration. The nurse then dons clean gloves. Place the following steps in the order in which they should be implemented.
    1. Pull the pinna of the ear up and back gently.
    2. Apply slight pressure several times to the tragus of the ear.
    3. Instruct the patient to remain in a side-lying position for 5 to 10 minutes.
    4. Position the patient in a side-lying position with the affected ear facing up.
    5. Hold the dropper one-half inch above the ear canal and instill the drops so that they fall on the side of the ear canal.
    Answer: _____

15. At a nursing organization meeting, the vice president for nursing informs the nurse managers that each patient care unit must engage in one nursing research project a year as part of attaining Magnet status. A nurse manager holds a unit meeting to inform the nursing staff of this new initiative. What nurse manager statement provides the **best** introduction?
    1. "To improve the status of the hospital in the community, we must become involved in nursing research."
    2. "I know that it will require more effort, but you will find it very rewarding to engage in nursing research."
    3. "We have a great opportunity to expand our involvement within our profession by performing nursing research."
    4. "I have just received a new edict from nursing administration that we have to get involved in nursing research."

16. Before going to lunch, a nurse provides information to the nurse accepting responsibility for a patient who returned 2 hours ago after a fiberoptic colonoscopy. Which information is **most** important for the covering nurse to know about this patient?
    1. Gag reflex is present
    2. Reports mild abdominal pain
    3. Passing flatus for the last hour
    4. Dozing intermittently since the procedure

17. Which nursing assessment indicates a period of exacerbation?
1. "Patient was admitted because of a recurrence of clinical manifestations of lymphoma."
2. "Patient reports freedom from left shoulder pain after a cortisone injection for bursitis."
3. "Patient reports long-standing joint pain from rheumatoid arthritis."
4. "Patient status indicates an unexpected response."

18. A patient who abuses alcohol is admitted to the hospital for detoxification. The patient is intoxicated and agitated. The patient's agitation increases and the patient becomes verbally abusive to the nurse. What should the nurse do **next?**
1. Obtain an order for a physical restraint for the patient.
2. Offer emotional support while touching the patient's hand.
3. Stand between the patient and the exit to the room while talking with the patient.
4. Approach the patient's bedside and state that using bad language is unacceptable.

19. Which statement by the nurse **best** helps a patient clarify values regarding a health-care decision that was not supported by the patient's family or primary health-care provider?
1. "There were many possible options. What motivated you to make your decision?"
2. "Your decision was courageous. I give you credit for taking control of your future."
3. "Why did you choose your decision? It was not what your loved ones and doctor preferred."
4. "Your decision would not have been my choice. But everyone has a right to self-determination."

20. A nurse is obtaining a blood specimen for monitoring a blood glucose level by using a lancet. Which action is appropriate when implementing this procedure?
1. Use the first drop of blood that appears at the puncture site.
2. Select an index finger for performing the puncture to acquire a drop of blood.
3. Apply pressure with gauze to the puncture site for a full minute after the procedure.
4. Place the hand in a dependent position before inserting the lancet to obtain the blood specimen.

21. A patient with moderate cognitive impairment who lives in an assisted living facility has been having more difficulty providing self-care over the past year. What intervention is **most** significant to ensure that the patient is receiving adequate nutrition?
1. Feed the patient meals.
2. Weigh the patient weekly.
3. Give the patient a liquid supplement between meals.
4. Provide the patient with opportunities to choose foods that are preferred.

22. A patient is receiving an enteric-coated iron preparation. The patient asks, "Why can't I just chew this pill so it is easier to take?" Which is the **best** response by the nurse?
1. "It has to dissolve slowly in your mouth for best absorption."
2. "If you can stand the taste, you are more than welcome to do that."
3. "If you break the tablet in your mouth, the medication can stain your teeth."
4. "If the tablet coating is damaged, the drug will be deactivated by gastric enzymes."

23. A nurse plans to provide foot care for an older adult. What actions should the nurse include in this procedure? **Select all that apply.**
1. _____ Soak the feet for 30 minutes.
2. _____ Push the cuticles back gently with a washcloth.
3. _____ Dry each foot thoroughly, especially between the toes.
4. _____ Clean under nails with an orangewood stick while a foot is in the water.
5. _____ Soak the feet one at a time in water that has a temperature of 115° to 120°F.

24. A patient who had a brain attack (cerebrovascular accident) is experiencing hemiparesis and fatigue. The nurse plans to progress from passive range-of-motion (ROM) exercises to active ROM exercises as ordered by the primary health-care provider. What should the nurse do to **best** facilitate teaching sessions with this patient?
1. Plan teaching sessions for after lunch.
2. Have another nurse assist with teaching sessions.
3. Conduct patient teaching sessions that are 15 minutes in length.
4. Medicate the patient for pain 30 minutes before a teaching session.

25. A patient is to receive a prescribed drug for the first time at 10 a.m. The laboratory report indicates a newly elevated creatinine level at 6 a.m. Which nursing action is **most** important when caring for this patient?
    1. Assess the patient for clinical manifestations of drug toxicity.
    2. Call the pharmacist to ensure that it is safe to administer the medication.
    3. Hold the medication until repeat test results are within the normal range.
    4. Inform the primary health-care provider of the patient's impaired kidney function.

26. With which patient should the nurse be particularly careful in protecting oneself from potential exposure to the HIV when providing direct physical care?
    1. Patient who is crying
    2. Man who is diaphoretic
    3. Woman who is menstruating
    4. Patient who is incontinent of feces

27. Which skill should the nurse implement **first** when assessing a patient's abdomen?
    1. Palpation
    2. Inspection
    3. Percussion
    4. Auscultation

28. Which should a nurse do when obtaining a patient's peek expiratory flow rate (PEFR)?
    1. Obtain three readings and document the highest reading.
    2. Inform the primary health-care provider if the result is within the green range.
    3. Have the patient always use a rescue medication before performing the procedure.
    4. Instruct the patient to keep the lips sealed around the mouthpiece while forcefully inhaling.

29. Which action is associated with the analysis step of the nursing process?
    1. A nurse takes the vital signs when a patient reports dizziness.
    2. A nurse determines that a patient is at risk for a pressure ulcer because of immobility and edema.
    3. A nurse and patient decide that within two days the patient will learn how to transfer from a bed to a chair safely.
    4. A nurse concludes that further intervention is necessary when the patient does not accurately prepare an insulin injection.

30. A nurse enters the room of a patient who is scheduled to go for surgery within the hour. The nurse observes the patient gazing out the window and that the patient's eyes are filled with tears. The nurse asks, "Are you okay?" The patient responds, "Don't worry. I'll be fine." What is the nurse's **most** appropriate response?
    1. "What are you thinking about?"
    2. "I'll be here if you need to talk."
    3. "Don't you think everything will be alright?"
    4. "When people cry, it usually means something is wrong."

31. Which statement by a patient experiencing insomnia indicates that the nurse must provide further education?
    1. "I enjoy a walk after dinner."
    2. "I always have a snack just before I go to bed."
    3. "I drink a big glass of wine when watching television at night."
    4. "I like to set my bedroom temperature at a cool setting at night."

32. A nurse is providing morning care to a hospitalized patient. Which statement by the nurse is **most** important before leaving the room after providing care?
    1. "Push your call bell if you need anything after I leave."
    2. "Would you like the door to your room closed?"
    3. "Your lunch will be served at around noon."
    4. "Is your room temperature comfortable?"

33. A primary health-care provider orders 1,000 mL of 0.9% NaCl to be administered every 8 hours and an antibiotic to be administered intravenously twice a day. The instructions accompanying the antibiotic indicate that it should be diluted in 100 mL of sterile water. The first dose was administered at 8 p.m. A nurse working the 7 a.m. to 7 p.m. shift the next day continues to implement the primary health-care provider's orders. The antibiotic was administered via a circulatory access device at a different site than the primary infusion. How much intravenous fluid did the patient receive during the 7 a.m. to 7 p.m. shift? Record your answer using a whole number.
    Answer: _____ mL

34. A person who fell down the basement stairs at home is brought to the hospital by the spouse. The patient, who has a psychiatric history, is actively hallucinating and the spouse is upset. The primary health-care provider orders a computed tomography scan with contrast. What should the nurse do?
1. Ask the patient about having an allergy to shellfish.
2. Determine if the patient currently is taking any medications.
3. Obtain an informed consent for the procedure from the spouse.
4. Explain the procedure in detail to limit the anxiety that both are experiencing.

35. Which is **most** effective in helping a patient who has an activity intolerance to shower safely at home?
1. Advise the use of a shower chair.
2. Suggest using a handheld faucet.
3. Encourage the instillation of handrails.
4. Recommend placing a nonskid mat in the shower stall.

36. A primary health-care provider prescribes the proton-pump inhibitor omeprazole (Prilosec). The order states to take 20 mg once a day. Which instruction should the nurse give the patient regarding this medication?
1. "Take the medication several hours before an antacid."
2. "Sprinkle the capsule contents in applesauce."
3. "Take the medication with food."
4. "Swallow the capsule whole."

37. A nurse is teaching a professional athlete with hypertension the reasons for taking all of the prescribed antihypertensive medications, including a diuretic once a day. The patient states, "I take my other drugs, but I have stopped taking the diuretic because there are no toilets near our outside training facilities. What is the nurse's **best** reply?
1. "It must be difficult to be taking all these medications."
2. "It is important that you follow the prescription exactly."
3. "Let's explore a time when it is convenient to take the diuretic."
4. "The other antihypertensives are insufficient without the diuretic."

38. A nurse is caring for patients on a surgical unit. Which patient should the nurse assess **first**?
1. A patient experiencing nausea and vomiting for several hours
2. A patient asking for pain medication for incisional pain on a level 3
3. A patient reporting chest pain 3 days after admission for a fractured pelvis
4. A patient requesting to see the surgeon before signing the consent form for morning surgery

39. A nurse is preparing a medication to be administered to a patient. The nurse identifies that the name of the medication on the unit dose package is not the same as the name on the medication administration record. What should the nurse do?
1. Give it as long as the dose is the same as what is indicated on the prescription.
2. Call the primary health-care provider and ask if the drug provided is the drug prescribed.
3. Ask another nurse on the unit who is more familiar with drugs if it is equivalent to the prescription.
4. Check a drug information resource to determine if the name on the unit dose package is a generic form of the drug.

40. What nursing intervention is **most** important when assisting a patient to eat?
1. Place a bib over the patient's clothes.
2. Engage the patient in conversation when feeding the patient.
3. Open containers, cut meat, and apply condiments to the patient's food.
4. Ask the patient's preference regarding the order of foods and fluids to ingest.

41. A nurse responds to a call light of a patient who had a colon resection 2 days ago for the removal of a cancerous tumor. The patient states, "It feels very wet and funny under my dressing." Which additional information collected by the nurse supports the conclusion that the patient may be experiencing dehiscence?
1. Patient reported throbbing pain at the site of the incision.
2. Patient verbalized, "I just felt a popping sensation at my incision."
3. Patient informed the nurse of voiding excessively during the night.
4. Patient stated, "I feel bloated and will be much better if I have a bowel movement."

42. An 84-year-old man is admitted to a long-term care facility because his daughter can no longer care for him. The nurse reviews the patient's family history and, when the patient is brought to the unit, interviews the patient and performs a physical assessment.

Patient's Clinical Record

Family History

The patient's wife died 10 years ago. Approximately 5 years ago, the patient had a brain attack, resulting in right-sided hemiplegia and expressive aphasia. The patient moved into his daughter's home after discharge from the hospital. The daughter provided almost constant care and supervision of her father. The daughter has 2 children in college and must go to work to earn money to add to her husband's income to pay for tuition.

Physical Assessment

The patient has right hemiplegia and wears a hand and forearm splint on the right arm and a brace on the right leg to manage footdrop. The patient needs assistance with all activities of daily living. The patient usually is continent of urine and feces but occasionally experiences functional urinary incontinence. Transfer from bed to chair or wheelchair is accomplished with a mechanical lift. The ability to chew and swallow solid food safely is intact, but the patient occasionally chokes when drinking liquids.

Patient Interview

The patient has expressive aphasia but was able to write short phrases and use a picture board and gestures to express his needs. The patient was oriented to time, place, and person. He indicated that he understands where he is, but he does not want to be here. The patient was crying and pulled himself to the side of the bed in an attempt to get out of bed. The patient indicated that he is angry with his daughter and will do whatever his daughter wants if he can go back home. The patient banged the bed with his left hand several times and wrote, "WANT TO GO HOME."

Which nursing intervention addresses this patient's *most* important need?
1. Use a product to thicken liquids before giving them to the patient.
2. Maintain splints and braces on extremities at all times.
3. Apply an external urinary drainage device at night.
4. Encourage the patient to explore feelings.

43. A nurse and a nursing assistant are working together caring for a group of patients in a district. Which nursing activity is appropriate for the nurse to assign to the nursing assistant?
1. Turning and repositioning a patient who had spinal surgery
2. Giving a bath and oral care to a patient receiving contact precautions
3. Identifying the signs and symptoms of a patient with a wound infection
4. Assisting a patient to the bathroom the first time after returning from surgery

44. A nurse is teaching the spouse of an immobile patient how to position the patient. What observation indicates to the nurse that the patient was correctly positioned when supine?
1. The patient's heels are placed on a pillow.
2. A pillow is placed between the patient's legs.
3. The patient's hands are turned with the palms facing the ceiling.
4. A trochanter roll is positioned from the patient's hip to the knee bilaterally.

45. A nurse accidentally administers an opioid to a patient. What should the nurse do **first**?
1. Call the nursing supervisor.
2. Administer the antidote immediately.
3. Instruct the patient to drink a glass of water.
4. Contact the patient's primary health-care provider.

46. A nurse is caring for a patient who has an elevated temperature and identifies that the patient's skin is flushed and feels warm. The nurse should assess the patient for which additional clinical manifestation that supports the conclusion that the patient's fever is in the defervescence phase?
1. Pallor
2. Malaise
3. Sweating
4. Shivering

47. A primary nurse is observing a licensed practical nurse (LPN) change a dressing on a patient's abdominal wound. Which action by the LPN requires the primary nurse to interrupt the procedure?
1. Using nonsterile gloves to remove the soiled dressing
2. Removing sterile gloves and applying tape to secure the dressing
3. Touching the sterile irrigating container with the neck of the bottle of normal saline
4. Failing to wash the hands between removing the soiled dressing and donning sterile gloves

48. A 12-year-old child is receiving intravenous patient-controlled analgesia postoperatively. The nurse teaches the child and parents about the trigger connected to the pump and how basal and bolus doses of the analgesic help relieve pain. Later when the child is sleeping, the nurse observes one of the parents pushing the trigger to deliver a bolus dose of medication. What should the nurse do **first**?
1. Review with the parents that the child is still receiving medication even if not pushing the trigger.
2. Tell the parents to stop pushing the trigger when the child is sleeping.
3. Notify the primary health-care provider of the parent's behavior.
4. Increase the dosage of the basal dose.

49. A patient is diagnosed as having herpes simplex type 2, and the primary health-care provider prescribes acyclovir (Zovirax) during outbreaks of lesions. Which statement indicates that the patient understands the nurse's instructions about this medication?
    1. "I should discontinue the medication if I develop dizziness."
    2. "I have to increase fiber in my diet because the medication may cause constipation."
    3. "I must take my pulse before I take this medication because it can raise my heart rate."
    4. "I need to take the medication as soon as I feel tingling in the area where I get the sores."

50. A nurse is caring for a patient who is receiving an anticoagulant. When assisting the patient with hygiene, the patient expresses a desire to shave himself. Which is important for the nurse to teach the patient to do?
    1. Use a safety razor when shaving.
    2. Use an electric razor when shaving.
    3. Apply some aftershave lotion on the skin after shaving.
    4. Wrap the face with a hot towel for a few minutes before shaving.

51. A patient is diagnosed with inflammation of the right lower lobe (RLL) of the lung (pleurisy). The nurse identifies the presence of a pleural friction rub. Where was the stethoscope placed on the patient's chest when the pleural friction rub was heard?
    1. A
    2. B
    3. C
    4. D

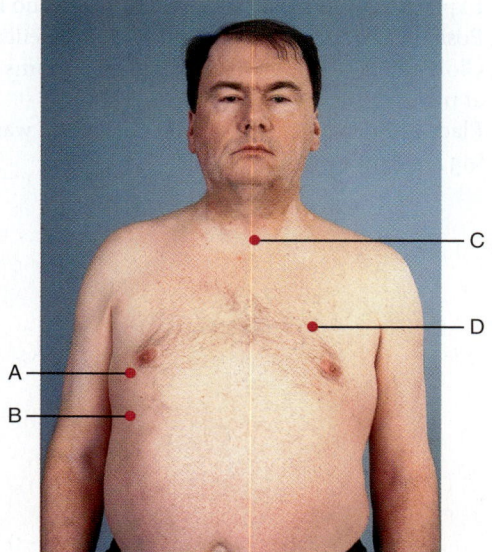

52. A nurse is admitting a patient to an acute care facility. The nurse should explain to the patient that the **most** important member of the health-care team is which person?
    1. Patient
    2. Primary nurse
    3. Nurse manager
    4. Nurse practitioner

53. A primary health-care provider orders a bladder-retraining program for a patient who is incontinent of urine after therapy for bladder cancer. Which nursing intervention promotes a successful bladder-retraining program?
    1. Offer a full-liquid diet.
    2. Follow the scheduled program.
    3. Wash the perineal area every shift.
    4. Maintain a strict record of fluid balance.

54. A nurse is caring for two patients who just had surgery. One patient has a Jackson-Pratt drain and the other patient has a Penrose drain. What nursing intervention is common to both types of drains?
    1. Maintaining negative pressure in the collection device
    2. Emptying the collection device when it is half full
    3. Shortening the drain one inch daily
    4. Assessing color of the drainage

55. A nurse is designing a teaching plan for a patient who speaks a different language. What is a reliable way for the nurse to facilitate patient understanding of the information?
    1. Arrange a telephone translation service to be used during the teaching session.
    2. Have a staff member who is from the same country act as an interpreter.
    3. Provide a pamphlet with pictures to reinforce what is being taught.
    4. Use a translation book that will aid in the conversion of words.

56. A nurse is caring for a patient who tends to become confused. Which information communicated to the patient is the **best** intervention to prevent falls in a hospital setting?
    1. "I am your nurse for today and I will be here for you whenever you call me for help."
    2. "When you finish in the bathroom, activate the call light and I will help you back to your bed."
    3. "When you decide you want to walk around the unit, I would appreciate it if you would use the walker."
    4. "I am going to transfer you to your wheelchair now and move you to an area near the nurses' station."

57. A nurse is assessing the physical status of several patients. Which patient problem should be the nurse's greatest concern?
    1. Tenting of skin
    2. Difficulty breathing
    3. Erythema over the greater trochanter
    4. Body weight inadequate in relation to height

58. A nurse is caring for an obese patient with an abdominal surgical incision that has a separation of wound edges with a large amount of exudate. The primary health-care provider orders a wet to moist dressing with 0.9% NaCl every 6 hours. What is **most** important for the nurse to do when implementing this procedure?
    1. Secure the dressing using Montgomery straps.
    2. Cleanse the wound with half normal saline and peroxide.
    3. Ensure the gauze packing is saturated and dripping with saline.
    4. Dry the wound by patting with gauze from the skin toward the wound.

59. Which action should a nurse implement when administering eye drops to a patient with an eye infection?
    1. Put on sterile gloves.
    2. Pull the upper lid toward the forehead.
    3. Administer drops into the conjunctival sac.
    4. Wipe from the outer toward the inner cantus.

60. Which information should the nurse document under objective data in the patient's clinical record?
    1. Patient statements of always feeling hungry as the reason for excessive eating
    2. Observation of the patient avoiding eye contact when talking with the nurse
    3. Assessment of the presence of bladder spasms after the patient urinates
    4. Reports of epigastric discomfort after meals

61. A nurse observes a patient sitting in bed crying. The nurse enters the room, sits in a chair next to the bed, and states, "You seem upset." The patient says, "I will be fine," but continues to cry. What is the **best** intervention by the nurse?
    1. State, "I will be at the nurses' station if you decide you want to talk."
    2. Say, "It is important that you talk about what is bothering you."
    3. Remain seated in the chair for several minutes
    4. Leave the room so that the patient has privacy

62. A nurse is purchasing toys for children in the child life center. Identify the toys that the nurse purchased that are appropriate for the ages of children progressing from infants to adolescents.
    1. Chess set
    2. Plastic rattles
    3. Decks of cards
    4. Pounding board
    5. Construction set
    Answer: _____

63. A nurse is assessing a postoperative patient's incision. Which clinical manifestation supports the conclusion that the patient may have a wound infection?
    1. Redness
    2. Swelling
    3. Warm to touch
    4. Purulent drainage

64. A nurse is performing range-of-motion exercises for a patient who had a brain attack (cerebrovascular accident) to prevent contractures. How should the nurse move the patient's hip when performing internal rotation?
    1. Position the leg behind the body.
    2. Move the leg laterally across the midline of the body.
    3. Turn the leg and foot pointing away from the other leg.
    4. Rotate the leg and foot pointing inward toward the other leg.

65. A resident in a nursing home wanders during the night and scares other residents by going into their rooms. What is the **most** effective intervention that the nurse should implement to address this situation?
    1. Explain to others that the resident means no harm.
    2. Position a bed alarm on the wandering resident's bed.
    3. Close the doors of the other residents' rooms at night.
    4. Place bolsters against four side rails of the wandering resident's bed.

66. A nurse on the night shift is frustrated with the nurse on the day shift because the day nurse often does not complete patient care, leaving extra work for the night staff. The night nurse tells the nurse manager that intravenous bags are left with less than 100 mL of fluid, urinary collection devices are not emptied, patient teaching has not been performed, and medication drawers do not always contain required medications. What is the nurse manager's **best** response?
    1. "Are there tasks you can delegate to the nursing assistant assigned to work with you?"
    2. "I will arrange a meeting for the three of us so that we can discuss these issues."
    3. "We are team members and we should all extend ourselves to help each other."
    4. "What would you like me to do to help resolve these problems?"

67. A nurse teaches a patient who is lactose intolerant about foods to avoid. Which food eliminated from the diet by the patient indicates an understanding about foods that contain lactose?
    1. Soy milk
    2. Fruit cocktail
    3. Creamed soup
    4. Vegetable juice

68. A nurse must administer a medication through a nasogastric tube that is being used for gastric decompression. What should the nurse do **first**?
    1. Instill an ounce of fluid before the medication is administered.
    2. Use high pressure via a piston syringe while the medication is administered.
    3. Shut off the negative pressure for half an hour after the medication is administered.
    4. Determine accurate placement of the nasogastric tube before the medication is administered.

69. A nurse is caring for a group of patients on a surgical unit. Which clinical finding warrants immediate nursing action?
    1. Mildly active bowel sounds 3 days after a colon resection
    2. Dark pink urine immediately after a transurethral resection of the prostate
    3. Reduced breath sounds on the left side 1 day after a wedge resection of the right lung
    4. Greenish drainage from a nasogastric tube immediately after an abdominal cholecystectomy

70. A nurse is developing a teaching plan for adults who are overweight. What teaching method would be **most** effective to promote behavioral changes?
    1. Online course
    2. Series of lectures
    3. Group instruction
    4. Colorful pamphlets

71. A patient has bilateral wrist restraints because of repeated attempts to pull out tubes. How frequently should the nurse release the restraints, exercise the patient's hands and wrists, and document this activity?
    1. Each hour
    2. Each shift
    3. Every 4 hours
    4. Every 2 hours

72. A nurse is assessing a patient's pain. What question obtains information about whether the patient is experiencing radiating pain?
    1. "Is the intensity of the pain more than 5 on a scale of 0 to 10?"
    2. "Was the onset of pain gradual over a period of time?"
    3. "Did the pain start in 1 area and extend to another?"
    4. "Does the pain tend to come and go?"

73. A patient reports an inability to urinate. What should the nurse do **first** to obtain more information about this problem?
    1. Perform a straight catheterization.
    2. Initiate intake and output monitoring.
    3. Assess the patient's lower abdomen for bladder distension.
    4. Ask the patient about the time and amount of the last voiding.

74. A female patient on bedrest asks the nurse what she can do to prevent her hair from becoming tangled and matted. What should the nurse encourage the patient to avoid?
    1. Conditioning the hair after shampooing
    2. Washing the hair with soap
    3. Placing the hair in braids
    4. Brushing the hair daily

75. A patient is taking furosemide (Lasix) daily because of hypertension. The nurse should teach the patient to consume one or more of which foods daily? **Select all that apply.**
    1. _____ Ten grapes
    2. _____ Five dried figs
    3. _____ One baked potato
    4. _____ Half of a grapefruit
    5. _____ One cup of cooked spinach

76. A person calls the nursing unit of a hospital stating, "I am a lawyer and must speak with a patient on the unit because there is a family emergency." What is the nurse's **most** appropriate intervention?
    1. Bring the patient to the telephone to talk with the lawyer.
    2. Refuse to discuss anything regarding the patient with the lawyer.
    3. Inform the lawyer that the presence of a patient cannot be confirmed or denied.
    4. Take the lawyer's phone number and give it to the patient without revealing that the patient is on the unit.

77. A nurse is caring for a patient who was admitted to the hospital because of a fecal impaction. The nurse identified that inadequate fiber, fluid, and activity contributed to this patient's problem. In addition, which medication that the patient is taking **most** likely contributed to the fecal impaction?
    1. Coumadin
    2. Maalox
    3. Flagyl
    4. Feosol

78. A nurse is caring for an older adult who had a brain attack (cerebrovascular accident) and has a residual problem with chewing and swallowing. What is the greatest risk considering the patient's physical status?
    1. Aspiration
    2. Constipation
    3. Fluid volume deficit
    4. Inadequate nutrition

79. A nurse is assessing a patient with the diagnosis of dehydration. Which assessment should the nurse document on the patient's record to support this diagnosis?
    1. Low urine specific gravity
    2. Bounding radial pulse
    3. Straw-colored urine
    4. Tenting of skin

80. A patient who is a Christian Scientist is admitted to the hospital for medical management and dialysis for renal failure. What intervention is important for the nurse to implement when caring for this patient?
    1. Ensure that pork and pork products are eliminated from the patient's diet.
    2. Position the patient's bed so that the feet are facing toward the entrance to the room.
    3. Encourage expression of feelings regarding the medical management of the patient's problem.
    4. Support the patient's desire to wear an amulet around the neck to chase away evil spirits and support health.

81. A nurse is completing the assessment phase of the nursing process for a group of patients with four different human responses. For which human response did the nurse use the physical examination method of auscultation?
    1. Bruit
    2. Lesion
    3. Ascites
    4. Distention

82. What should the nurse do after administering a gastrostomy tube-feeding formula?
    1. Instill 30 mL of water by gravity into the tube.
    2. Insert 20 mL of air into the tube.
    3. Check the dressing site.
    4. Encourage activity.

83. A primary health-care provider orders total parenteral nutrition for a patient. What should the nurse do when administrating this total parenteral nutrition to the patient?
    1. Remove the solution from the refrigerator 15 minutes before the infusion.
    2. Share the same intravenous tubing set that is being used for medications.
    3. Change the intravenous tubing set every 24 hours.
    4. Assess for placement of the tube in the stomach.

84. A primary health-care provider orders penicillin V potassium 250 mg by mouth every 6 hours for a patient with a staphylococcal infection. The pharmacy provides penicillin V potassium 125 mg per 5 mL. How much solution should the nurse administer? Record your answer using a whole number.
    Answer: _____ mL

85. A nurse is writing progress notes for a variety of patients. Which documentation meets the criteria for a legal record?
    1. Patient tolerated being out of bed in a chair for 1 hour.
    2. Patient urinated 350 mL of clear amber urine at 8 a.m.
    3. Patient received the prn antiemetic at 2 p.m.
    4. Patient reported pain at a level of 5.

86. While assisting a patient to eat, the other patient in the room begins to choke on food and is unable to speak. What should the nurse do **first**?
    1. Initiate the abdominal thrust maneuver.
    2. Instruct the patient to swallow forcefully.
    3. Clap between the patient's scapulae several times.
    4. Wait to see if the patient can cough up the obstruction.

87. A primary health-care provider orders a urinalysis for a patient with an indwelling urinary catheter. Which action is important when collecting a urine specimen from the port of a urinary retention catheter?
    1. Wear sterile gloves to collect the specimen.
    2. Release the clamp after collecting a urine specimen.
    3. Transfer urine to a sterile cup designed for a urine specimen.
    4. Separate the catheter from the tubing to collect the specimen.

88. A nurse is assessing a 78-year-old adult. What changes should the nurse anticipate that the patient will report?
    1. "My short-term memory is better than my long-term memory."
    2. "It takes longer for me to learn something new."
    3. "My level of intelligence has been decreasing."
    4. "I get easily confused."

89. Which nursing intervention should be implemented regardless of the oxygen delivery system being used?
    1. Ensure the oxygen mask is securely placed over the nose and mouth.
    2. Flood the reservoir with oxygen before attaching the mask to the patient.
    3. Set the oxygen flow rate at a minimum of between two and four liters per minute.
    4. Assess the patient's ears and nose for skin trauma to determine if the oxygen devise is too tight.

90. A nurse is transferring a patient from a bed to a chair. Which principle of the mechanics of movement is important for the nurse to employ?
    1. Twist the upper body toward the direction of the move.
    2. Keep arms in a locked position.
    3. Place the feet wide apart.
    4. Bend at the waist.

91. Which nursing action demonstrates the evaluation step of the nursing process?
    1. Identifying a skin lesion during a patient's admission physical examination
    2. Determining activity intolerance after ambulating a patient
    3. Connecting a contributing factor to a problem statement
    4. Formulating an intervention to address a risk factor

92. A nurse enters a patient's room and observes smoke coming out of an air conditioning duct. The nurse transfers the patient into a wheel chair, moves the patient into the corridor, and closes the door to the patient's room while exiting the room. What should the nurse do **next**?
    1. Report the fire.
    2. Attempt to put out the fire.
    3. Close the doors on the unit.
    4. Evacuate all the patients to another unit.

93. A nurse is assessing a patient for signs and symptoms of electrolyte imbalances. What clinical manifestation helps to differentiate hypernatremia from hyponatremia?
    1. Vomiting
    2. Confusion
    3. Increased thirst
    4. Muscle weakness

94. A patient self-administers a bowel prep consisting of sodium phosphate (Fleet Phospho-soda), bisacodyl (Dulcolax), and an enema the night before a colonoscopy. For what serious adverse effect should the nurse assess the patient?
    1. Deficient fluid volume
    2. Intestinal cramping
    3. Hypernatremia
    4. Diarrhea

95. When talking to the school nurse about his decision to drop out of high school and marry his girlfriend who is pregnant, a student says, "I need to do this. It is the right thing to do." What defense mechanism should the nurse determine is being used?
    1. Projection
    2. Suppression
    3. Introspection
    4. Intellectualization

96. A nurse identifies that a patient has inadequate circulation to the right foot as evidenced by prolonged capillary refill, yellow brittle toenails, and an absent pedal pulse. What pulse should the nurse assess **next**?
1. A
2. B
3. C
4. D

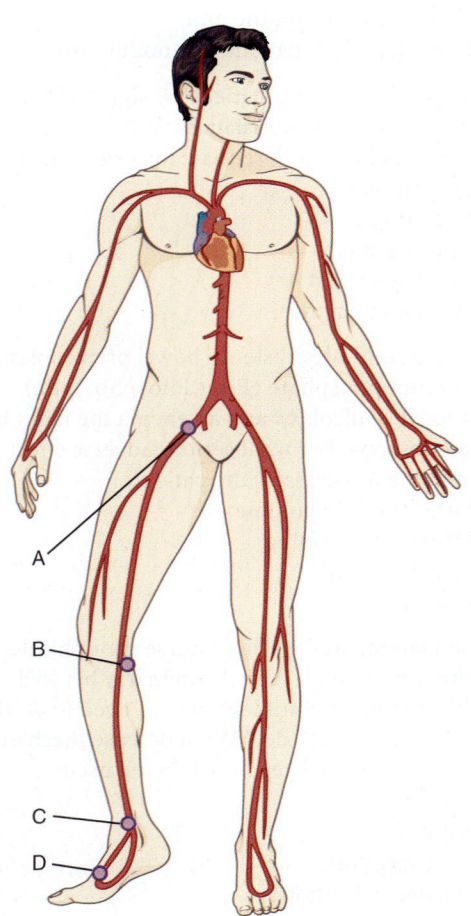

97. A nurse is assessing a patient's urinary status. Which question is appropriate when collecting data about reflex incontinence?
1. "Have you ever had an involuntary loss of urine without sensing the need to void?"
2. "Have you ever had incontinence after a strong sense of urgency to void?"
3. "Do you ever experience urinary dribbling when you sneeze or cough?"
4. "Do you ever experience a weak urinary stream when you pass urine?"

98. A nurse is determining if a prescribed opioid dose is appropriate for a 3-year-old child. What **most** essential information should the nurse gather to assist with this determination?
1. Obtain the child's weight.
2. Take the child's vital signs.
3. Assess the child's level of pain.
4. Explore the child's reaction to previous analgesics.

99. A patient with esophageal reflux has been experiencing heartburn, regurgitation, and a hoarse voice. What should the nurse encourage the patient to do to minimize these signs and symptoms?
1. Eat within one hour before going to bed.
2. Drink a glass of warm water at bedtime.
3. Elevate the head of the bed on blocks.
4. Recline for half an hour after meals.

100. A nurse manager identifies that the number of patient falls on the unit increased by 20 percent in the last 3 months. What should the nurse manager do **next**?
1. Implement a plan of action.
2. Analyze factors precipitating the falls.
3. Choose a solution to address the issue.
4. Explore all possible strategies to prevent future falls.

ANSWERS

1. **ANSWER: 4.**
   Rationales:
   1. Inviting friends over for a party is an example of a third level need, the need for love and belonging.
   2. Getting a haircut before the holiday season is an example of a fourth level need, the need for self-esteem.
   3. Locking car doors when alone in the car is an example of a second level need, the need for safety and security.
   4. Taking a bottle of water along when going for a walk is an example of a first level need, meeting a physiological need.
   Content Area: Theory-Based Nursing Care
   Integrated Processes: Nursing Process: Implementation
   Client Need: Health Promotion and Maintenance
   Cognitive Level: Analysis

2. **ANSWER: 2.**
   Rationales:
   1. This is premature at this time; it will be done eventually.
   2. Assessment is the first step of the nursing process. Risk factors for skin breakdown should be identified first before the nurse can formulate a plan of care.
   3. This is not a life-threatening situation and is not the first action. Notification of the primary health-care provider about the patient's status should be done eventually.
   4. This is an intervention, part of the implementation phase of the nursing process. Other steps of the nursing process must be completed first.
   TEST-TAKING TIP: Identify the word in the stem that sets a priority. The word *first* in the stem sets a priority. Identify the option that is unique. Option 2 is unique because it is an action that is an assessment and the other options are interventions other than assessment.
   Content Area: Mobility
   Integrated Processes: Nursing Process: Assessment
   Client Need: Physiological Integrity; Reduction of Risk Potential
   Cognitive Level: Application

3. **ANSWER: 1.**
   Rationales:
   1. In this scenario, the nurse could be sued for assault. An unjustifiable threat to touch another person is assault.
   2. In this scenario, the nurse could be sued for battery. Patients have a right to refuse treatment. Touching another person without consent, such as administering a medication against the wishes of a patient, is battery.
   3. In this scenario, the nurse could be sued for false imprisonment and battery. The nurse unjustifiably touched and detained the patient without consent.
   4. In this scenario, the nurse could be sued for slander. Spoken words that are untrue and can cause defamation of character are considered slander.
   Content Area: Legal and Ethical Issues
   Integrated Processes: Nursing Process: Evaluation
   Client Need: Safe and Effective Care Environment; Management of Care
   Cognitive Level: Analysis

4. **ANSWER: 3.**
   Rationales:
   1. Liquid fecal effluent from an ileostomy is expected because fluid is absorbed in the transverse and descending colon. An ileostomy is a surgically created opening (stoma) in the small intestine (ileum).
   2. Liquid fecal effluent from a cecostomy is expected because fluid is absorbed in the transverse and descending colon. A cecostomy is a surgically created opening (stoma) in the proximal part of the large intestine.
   3. Stool from a sigmoid colostomy is soft to formed stool. Loose stool should be reported because it indicates diarrhea, which may be due to a gastrointestinal problem that requires medical intervention.
   4. Liquid fecal effluent from an ascending colon colostomy is expected because fluid is absorbed in the transverse and descending colon.
   TEST-TAKING TIP: Identify the key words in the stem that indicate negative polarity. The words *be concerned* are the key words that indicate negative polarity. The question is asking, "Which ostomy *should not produce* loose fecal matter?"
   Content Area: Gastrointestinal System
   Integrated Processes: Nursing Process: Evaluation
   Client Need: Physiological Integrity; Physiological Adaptation
   Cognitive Level: Analysis

5. **ANSWER: 2.**
   Rationales:
   1. There is less concern about assessing for the presence of peripheral edema than another concern. The absence of protein in the urine generally rules out upper urinary system impairment, which could cause fluid volume excess. Also, the patient is not reporting a decrease in urine output.
   2. The clinical indicators of increased vital signs, elevated white and red blood cells, nitrites in the urine, and urinary frequency and urgency support the conclusion that the patient most likely has a urinary tract infection. The slow urinary stream indicates that the patient may have an enlarged prostate gland associated with aging, contributing to urinary stasis. Urinary stasis is a risk factor for a urinary tract infection. A burning sensation on urination is associated with bacteria in the urine that irritates the mucous membranes of the urinary system.
   3. Suprapubic distension is associated with urinary retention. There are no data that indicate the presence of urinary retention, such as anuria, eliminating small amounts of urine frequently (overflow incontinence), or a feeling of fullness in the suprapubic area. Also, assessment revealed that the patient's abdomen was soft and nontender.
   4. The blood pressure increases, not decreases, in response to the increased metabolic rate associated with a fever.
   TEST-TAKING TIP: Identify the clang association. The word *urination* in option 2 and the repetitious use of words associated with the urinary system within the data, such as *urinary frequency, nocturia* (urinating at night), and *to urinate,* are clang associations. Examine option 2 carefully.
   Content Area: Urinary Elimination
   Integrated Processes: Nursing Process: Assessment
   Client Need: Physiological Integrity; Physiological Adaptation
   Cognitive Level: Analysis

6. **ANSWER: 2.**
   Rationales:
   1. A nurse can address a patient's pain control needs before providing care so that interventions can be performed within a tolerable pain level.
   2. **A patient with dementia may have difficulty interpreting environmental stimuli and perceive hygiene care as a threat. This may cause the patient to become frightened or anxious and resist hygiene interventions.**
   3. A patient with impaired vision generally can understand directions regarding the setup of the overbed table with hygiene equipment placed according to the numbers of a clock. Assistance by the nurse may be provided to complete the care.
   4. A patient with impaired mobility generally can participate in hygiene care, even if it is just the ability to make choices regarding preferences. Patients with impaired mobility should be encouraged to participate to their best ability, with the balance of care provided by the nurse.
   TEST-TAKING TIP: Identify the word in the stem that sets a priority. The word *greatest* in the stem sets a priority.
   Content Area: *Hygiene*
   Integrated Processes: *Nursing Process: Analysis*
   Client Need: *Physiological integrity; Basic Care and Comfort*
   Cognitive Level: *Analysis*

7. **ANSWER: 1.**
   Rationales:
   1. **Most people prefer to return home if appropriate supportive care is available. Hospice programs are designed to meet the needs of individuals with less than 6 months to live. Hospice programs approach a patient's needs comprehensively, with an increase in services as a patient's condition requires more constant and varied interventions.**
   2. No data indicate the need for rehabilitation services.
   3. The patient does not need constant services of a skilled nurse.
   4. This requires a major environmental change. This alternative is not capable of meeting this patient's physical and emotional needs when the disease progresses.
   TEST-TAKING TIP: Identify the word in the stem that sets a priority. The word *most* in the stem sets a priority. Identify the word that is clang association. The word *care* is used twice in the stem. The word *care* in option 1 is a clang association. Examine option 1 carefully. More often than not, the option with a clang association is the correct answer.
   Content Area: *Health-Care Delivery*
   Integrated Processes: *Nursing Process: Planning*
   Client Need: *Safe and Effective Care Environment, Management of Care*
   Cognitive Level: *Analysis*

8. **ANSWER: 3.**
   Rationales:
   1. The oral route is contraindicated in a patient with shortness of breath. The patient may become short of breath while the lips are sealed around the probe long enough to obtain a reading.
   2. The rectal route is contraindicated in a patient with anal or large intestine problems. A rectal probe may traumatize the intestinal mucosa and perforate the intestine.

3. **The temporal route will reflect the core body temperature without jeopardizing the patient's physical status.**
4. The tympanic route is contraindicated in a patient with an ear infection because it may traumatize the ear as well as produce an inaccurate measurement due to the presence of inflammation in the ears.
   Content Area: *Physical Assessment*
   Integrated Processes: *Nursing Process: Planning*
   Client Need: *Physiological Integrity; Reduction of Risk Potential*
   Cognitive Level: *Analysis*

9. **ANSWER: 1.**
   Rationales:
   1. **Adolescents have few rigid routines, have busy schedules, and are influenced by peer pressure, which are factors that influence a person's ability to follow a medical regimen. Also, adolescents feel omnipotent, operate most often in the present, and have less ability to appreciate the long-term consequences of inadequate self-care than an older person.**
   2. More often than not, an older adult is capable of recognizing the importance of appropriate self-care when faced with a chronic health condition.
   3. Although a young adult may have some difficulty adjusting to a life-long health problem, a young adult is better able to recognize that appropriate self-care is important than a patient in another option.
   4. More often than not, a middle-aged adult is capable of recognizing the importance of appropriate self-care when faced with a chronic health condition.
   TEST-TAKING TIP: Identify the word in the stem that sets a priority. The word *most* in the stem sets a priority. Identify the option that is unique. Option 1 is unique because it is the only option that contains 1 word and it is the only option that does not contain the word *adult*.
   Content Area: *Nursing Care Across the Life Span*
   Integrated Processes: *Teaching/Learning; Nursing Process: Analysis*
   Client Need: *Health Promotion and Maintenance*
   Cognitive Level: *Analysis*

10. **ANSWER: 4.**
    Rationales:
    1. People should talk at a moderate, not slow, rate when communicating with a person who is deaf. When talking slowly, people tend to overarticulate, which makes it more difficult for the hearing impaired to interpret what is being said.
    2. Longer, not shorter, phrases facilitate understanding. Additional words support a clearer message.
    3. Overarticulation should be avoided because it is harder for a deaf person to understand than when the person speaking articulates normally.
    4. **Standing so that the nurse's face can be seen easily facilitates lip reading. The nurse should gently touch the person and ensure that the person's attention is secured before initiating conversation.**
    TEST-TAKING TIP: Identify the unique option. Options 1, 2, and 3 all present an action that has to do with talking. Option 4 is the only option that does not discuss the process of speaking.

Content Area: Communication and Documentation
Integrated Processes: Communication/Documentation;
Nursing Process: Implementation
Client Need: Psychosocial Integrity
Cognitive Level: Application

11. **ANSWER: 2.**
    Rationales:
    1. All behavior has meaning and requires recognition.
    2. **Offering choices empowers a patient to make decisions. This places a patient in control and supports feelings of independence.**
    3. This action denies the patient's concerns. Patient concerns should be addressed.
    4. Pointing out limitations may intensify the patient's feelings of dependence.
    TEST-TAKING TIP: Identify the word in the stem that sets a priority. The word *best* in the stem sets a priority. Identify the options that deny that patient's feelings. Options 1 and 3 deny the patient's feelings.
    Content Area: Psychosocial and Cultural Support
    Integrated Processes: Caring, Communication/Documentation; Nursing Process: Implementation
    Client Need: Psychosocial Integrity
    Cognitive Level: Application

12. **ANSWER: 1.**
    Rationales:
    1. **Eventually, chronic pain does not respond to the analgesic effect of over-the-counter analgesics when they are used over an extended period of time.**
    2. This characteristic of pain is not a reliable indicator for differentiating acute from chronic pain. Characteristics of the quality of pain (e.g., sharp, throbbing, aching, burning) may be similar for both acute and chronic pain.
    3. Acute pain usually is associated with an abrupt onset. Chronic pain tends to have a gradual onset.
    4. Acute pain is associated with a time frame of 6 months or less. Chronic pain is associated with a long length of time, usually more than 6 months.
    TEST-TAKING TIP: Identify the word in the stem that sets a priority. The word *best* in the stem sets a priority.
    Content Area: Pain, Comfort, Rest, and Sleep
    Integrated Processes: Communication/Documentation; Nursing Process: Assessment
    Client Need: Physiological Integrity; Pharmacological and Parenteral Therapies
    Cognitive Level: Analysis

13. **ANSWER: 1.**
    Rationales:
    1. **Wearing a gown is not necessary to maintain airborne precautions for a patient with a diagnosis of primary tuberculosis. The pathogenic organism is transmitted to others via airborne respiratory secretions. However, a gown is necessary whenever the caregiver has a likelihood of coming into contact with blood, body fluids, excretions, secretions, contaminated items, or nonintact skin.**
    2. A respiratory device (N95 respirator) is necessary to protect a caregiver from the *M. tuberculosis* or *M. bovis* emanating from the patient's respiratory tract.

3. A room with negative air pressure, air change of 6 to 12 air changes per hour, and either discharge of air to the outside or a filtration system for the air in the room is essential to maintain airborne precautions for a patient with a diagnosis of suspected or known tuberculosis.
4. Placing a surgical mask on the patient when being transported for a procedure outside the room is essential to maintaining airborne precautions. This protects others and the environment from contamination from pathogens emanating from the patient's respiratory tract.
TEST-TAKING TIP: Identify the word in the stem that indicates negative polarity. The word *unrelated* indicates negative polarity. The test-taker must identify the intervention that is *not necessary* to maintaining airborne precautions.
Content Area: Infection Control and Wound Care
Integrated Processes: Nursing Process: Implementation
Client Need: Safe and Effective Care Environment; Safety and Infection Control
Cognitive Level: Analysis

14. **ANSWER: 4, 1, 5, 2, 3.**
    Rationales:
    4. **The side-lying position enables medication to flow by gravity into the ear canal.**
    1. **Pulling the pinna of the ear up and backward straightens the ear canal, facilitating distribution of the medication.**
    5. **Holding the dropper one-half inch above the ear canal avoids contamination of the dropper. Directing the flow of medication to the side of the ear canal prevents injury to the tympanic membrane as the drop enters the ear canal.**
    2. **Applying gentle pressure to the tragus of the ear facilitates complete distribution of the medication to all surfaces of the ear canal, which promotes its absorption.**
    3. **Remaining in a side-lying position for 5 to 10 minutes allows for more contact of the medication with the ear canal and tympanic membrane and prevents the medication from exiting the ear.**
    Content Area: Medication Administration
    Integrated Processes: Nursing Process: Planning
    Client Need: Physiological Integrity; Pharmacological and Parenteral Therapies
    Cognitive Level: Analysis

15. **ANSWER: 3.**
    Rationales:
    1. Although this is a true statement, its tone is autocratic. It is not a visionary, charismatic approach.
    2. This statement begins with a negative tone; in addition, it may be false reassurance for some staff members. The nurse manager should accentuate the positive.
    3. **This statement is inspiring and motivating; it creates excitement and relates a new initiative to the role of the nurse.**
    4. An edict is a proclamation, directive, or an order to do something. This approach is autocratic.
    TEST-TAKING TIP: Identify the word in the stem that sets a priority. The word *best* in the stem sets a priority.

Content Area: Leadership and Management
Integrated Processes: Communication/Documentation;
Nursing Process: Implementation
Client Need: Safe and Effective Care Environment;
Management of Care
Cognitive Level: Analysis

16. ANSWER: 2.
Rationales:
1. Generally, conscious sedation, not general anesthesia, is used to sedate a patient for a colonoscopy. Conscious sedation does not cause the loss of the gag reflex.
2. A serious concern after a fiberoptic colonoscopy is bowel perforation. A symptom of bowel perforation is abdominal pain. Although the patient's pain is mild, it needs to be assessed frequently to ensure that it does not intensify. In addition, the nurse should assess for rectal bleeding, abdominal distention, fever, and malaise, which are all associated with bowel perforation after a colonoscopy.
3. Passing flatus is an expected response after a colonoscopy because air is introduced into the intestine to distend the lumen for improved visibility.
4. Dozing intermittently is expected because of the effects of the conscious sedation used during the procedure.
TEST-TAKING TIP: Identify the word in the stem that sets a priority. The word *most* in the stem sets a priority. All the options reflect information that should be communicated, but one is *most* essential.
Content Area: Gastrointestinal System
Integrated Processes: Communication/Documentation;
Nursing Process: Evaluation
Client Need: Safe and Effective Care Environment;
Management of Care
Cognitive Level: Application

17. ANSWER: 1.
Rationales:
1. This statement indicates the concept of exacerbation, a return of signs and symptoms or an increase in the severity of signs and symptoms of a disease.
2. This statement reflects the concept of remission, not exacerbation. Remission refers to a period when symptoms abate or there is an absence of the underlying disease.
3. This statement reflects the concept of chronicity. Chronicity (chronic disease) refers to a disease of long duration or progressive deterioration over a long period of time.
4. This statement reflects the concept of deviation or variance, not exacerbation. Deviation or variance refers to a departure from the norm.
TEST-TAKING TIP: Identify the opposite options. Options 1 and 2 are opposites. Option 1 reflects an increase in clinical manifestations and option 2 reflects a decrease in clinical manifestations.
Content Area: Physical Assessment
Integrated Processes: Nursing Process: Analysis
Client Need: Physiological Integrity; Physiological Adaptation
Cognitive Level: Application

18. ANSWER: 3.
Rationales:
1. Obtaining an order for a restraint is premature. Verbal interactions, one to one observation, or a prescribed sedative are less restrictive measures than a physical restraint.
2. Touching the patient's hand may be viewed as aggressive by the patient and elicit a hostile physical response. A nurse should never touch an agitated, intoxicated patient without the patient's permission.
3. Increasing agitation and verbal abuse may be precursors to physical abuse. The nurse should stand in an area that will provide an escape if the patient attempts physical aggression.
4. This may be viewed as aggressive by the patient and precipitate an altercation. A minimum of three feet should be maintained between the nurse and patient.
TEST-TAKING TIP: Identify the word in the stem that sets a priority. The word *next* in the stem sets a priority. Identify options that are opposites. Options 3 and 4 are opposites. Option 3 positions the nurse at a distance from the patient, while option 4 has the nurse in close proximity to the patient. Consider these options carefully.
Content Area: Safety
Integrated Processes: Communication/Documentation;
Nursing Process: Implementation
Client Need: Safe and Effective Care Environment; Safety and Infection Control
Cognitive Level: Application

19. ANSWER: 1.
Rationales:
1. The response in option 1 is open-ended and noncommittal about the patient's decision. It provides an opportunity for the patient to explore the reasons for the decision.
2. This statement does not provide the patient the opportunity to explore the reasons for the decision. Also, the nurse should not voice personal opinions that could make it difficult for the patient to change the decision in the future.
3. This statement is a challenging statement that puts the patient on the defensive.
4. This statement is judgmental. The second sentence does not invite the patient to explore the reasons for the decision.
TEST-TAKING TIP: Identify the word in the stem that sets a priority. The word *best* in the stem sets a priority. Identify the options that are not patient centered. Options 3 and 4 are judgmental and focus on other people's opinions. These options are not patient centered and can be eliminated.
Content Area: Communication and Documentation
Integrated Processes: Caring, Communication/
Documentation; Nursing Process: Implementation
Client Need: Psychosocial Integrity
Cognitive Level: Analysis

20. ANSWER: 4.
Rationales:
1. The first drop of blood should not be used because it may contain a large volume of serous fluid, which may produce an inaccurate result.

2. The index finger should be avoided because it is reported to be a more painful site than other fingers.
3. Applying 30 seconds of pressure generally is sufficient to stop bleeding from a lancet wound.
4. The hand in the dependent position will increase blood flow to the distal portion of the finger. Squeezing the puncture site should be avoided because it will increase serum and dilute the blood specimen resulting in a false low blood glucose level.
TEST-TAKING TIP: *Identifying clang associations will not help you focus on the correct answer because all options contain a clang association. Options 1 and 2 contain the word blood, option 3 contains the word procedure, and option 4 contains the word lancet.*
Content Area: *Nutrition*
Integrated Processes: *Nursing Process: Implementation*
Client Need: *Physiological Integrity; Reduction of Risk Potential*
Cognitive Level: *Application*

21. **ANSWER: 2.**
Rationales:
1. Feeding the patient will not evaluate the adequacy of the diet; also, the patient should be encouraged to be as independent as possible.
2. Weighing the patient weekly will reflect if the patient is maintaining or losing weight. Maintenance of weight indicates that the patient is receiving adequate nutrition.
3. Although giving a liquid supplement between meals is an appropriate action, it does not evaluate the adequacy of the patient's diet.
4. Encouraging the patient to choose foods that are preferred may be beyond the cognitive ability of the patient, which may increase frustration, anxiety, and agitation. Also, it does not reflect the patient's nutritional status.
TEST-TAKING TIP: *Identify the word in the stem that sets a priority. The word most in the stem sets a priority.*
Content Area: *Nutrition*
Integrated Processes: *Nursing Process: Evaluation*
Client Need: *Physiological Integrity; Reduction of Risk Potential*
Cognitive Level: *Application*

22. **ANSWER: 4.**
Rationales:
1. A lozenge or troche, not an enteric-coated medication, is designed to dissolve slowly in the pocket between the gum and cheek (buccal cavity).
2. The enteric coating is not to protect the mouth from the taste of the medication.
3. The potential to stain the teeth is not the reason why an enteric-coated medication should not be chewed before swallowing.
4. An enteric-coated medication is designed to dissolve in the intestines. This is either because the drug is caustic to the stomach mucosa or because the drug is deactivated by gastric enzymes.
TEST-TAKING TIP: *Identify the word in the stem that sets a priority. The word best in the stem sets a priority. Identify the unique option. Options 1, 2, and 3 are methods that break the surface of the tablet, which will cause the medication to*

become inactivated when in contact with gastric enzymes. *Option 4 is the unique option. It is the only option that states that the tablet must remain intact.*
Content Area: *Medication Administration*
Integrated Processes: *Communication/Documentation, Teaching/Learning; Nursing Process: Implementation*
Client Need: *Physiological Integrity; Pharmacological and Parenteral Therapies*
Cognitive Level: *Application*

23. **ANSWER: 2, 3, 4.**
Rationales:
1. Five to 10 minutes generally is the length of time the nurse should soak a patient's feet. It is enough time to precipitate relaxation and soften debris without excessively removing natural oils that can lead to cracks in the skin.
2. Cuticles should be pushed back gently with a wash cloth; a wash cloth is rough enough to push back the cuticles without causing trauma.
3. Drying the feet thoroughly, especially between the toes, helps prevent maceration of the skin and reduces the risk of a fungal infection.
4. Using the flat side of an orangewood stick to clean under nails while the foot is in the water facilitates removing debris caught under the nail.
5. Although the nurse should soak each foot separately and change water and towels between the feet, the water should be 105°F to 110°F to avoid burning the skin.
Content Area: *Hygiene*
Integrated Processes: *Nursing Process: Planning*
Client Need: *Physiological Integrity; Basic Care and Comfort*
Cognitive Level: *Application*

24. **ANSWER: 3.**
Rationales:
1. Teaching sessions should be conducted early in the morning before the patient becomes fatigued. Fatigue will interfere with learning.
2. Two nurses are unnecessary; one nurse is capable of teaching this patient active range-of-motion exercises.
3. The patient is experiencing fatigue. Teaching sessions should be kept short so that learning can occur before the patient becomes fatigued.
4. There are no data that indicate that the patient is in pain.
TEST-TAKING TIP: *Identify the word in the stem that sets a priority. The word best in the stem sets a priority.*
Content Area: *Teaching and Learning*
Integrated Processes: *Teaching/Learning; Nursing Process: Planning*
Client Need: *Health Promotion and Maintenance*
Cognitive Level: *Application*

25. **ANSWER: 4.**
Rationales:
1. The patient has not yet received the medication.
2. Although the nurse may call the pharmacist for an opinion, it is the nurse's responsibility to intervene in this situation.
3. The laboratory results may never return to the expected (normal) range. Also, this is not within the

scope of nursing practice, except for with a few medications where exact parameters are identified by the primary health-care provider.

4. The primary health-care provider should be informed of the patient's impaired kidney function because the dose of the medication may need to be reduced or the drug cancelled to avoid drug toxicity. Impaired kidney function may interfere with the ability to excrete the drug.

TEST-TAKING TIP: *Identify the word in the stem that sets a priority. The word* most *in the stem sets a priority.*
Content Area: *Pharmacology*
Integrated Processes: *Communication/Documentation; Nursing Process: Implementation*
Client Need: *Safe and Effective Care Environment; Management of Care*
Cognitive Level: *Application*

26. **ANSWER: 3.**
    Rationales:
    1. HIV is not transmitted via tears.
    2. HIV is not transmitted via sweat.
    3. HIV is transmitted via blood and body fluids, such as semen, vaginal secretions, and breast milk. The nurse must use measures associated with standard precautions to protect oneself from exposure to blood and body fluid.
    4. HIV is not transmitted via feces.
    Content Area: *Infection Control and Wound Care*
    Integrated Processes: *Nursing Process: Planning*
    Client Need: *Safe and Effective Care Environment; Safety and Infection Control*
    Cognitive Level: *Application*

27. **ANSWER: 2.**
    Rationales:
    1. Palpating the abdomen first may alter the findings of inspection, auscultation, and percussion.
    2. Inspection should occur before touching the patient. Inspection involves assessing for visual clues of pathology. Options 1, 3, and 4 are all skills that require the nurse to touch the patient's abdomen in some way. The least intrusive assessment method of inspection should be performed first, followed progressively by auscultation, percussion, and palpation.
    3. Percussion should be done after inspection and auscultation.
    4. Auscultation should be done after inspection and before any other hands on assessments are implemented.
    TEST-TAKING TIP: *Identify the word in the stem that sets a priority. The word* first *in the stem sets a priority. Identify the unique option. Option 2 is unique; it is the only option that does not require the nurse to touch the patient. Consider this option carefully.*
    Content Area: *Physical Assessment*
    Integrated Processes: *Nursing Process: Implementation*
    Client Need: *Health Promotion and Maintenance*
    Cognitive Level: *Application*

28. **ANSWER: 1.**
    Rationales:
    1. This ensures greater accuracy when comparing results from day to day.

2. When the result is within the green range, the patient should continue the prescribed maintenance regimen. When the result is in the yellow range the dosage of the maintenance medication may be increased or a rescue medication may be taken as prescribed. When the result is within the red range, immediate use of a prescribed rescue medication should be taken and emergency intervention sought if the condition does not improve.
3. Rescue medication should be taken based on the results of the procedure.
4. The patient should take a deep breath and then forcefully exhale with the lips sealed around the mouth piece.

TEST-TAKING TIP: *Identify the option with a specific determiner. Option 3 contains the word* always, *which is a specific determiner. Generally, an option with a specific determiner is a distractor.*
Content Area: *Oxygenation*
Integrated Processes: *Communication/Documentation; Nursing Process: Implementation*
Client Need: *Physiological Integrity; Reduction of Risk Potential*
Cognitive Level: *Application*

29. **ANSWER: 2.**
    Rationales:
    1. Taking a patient's vital signs in response to a patient's report of dizziness is an example of assessment.
    2. Determining that a patient is at risk for impaired skin integrity because of reduced mobility and edema is associated with the analysis step of the nursing process. Making connections among human responses, contributing factors to illness, disease or injury, and potential negative future developments is part of the analysis step of the nursing process.
    3. Identifying a desired outcome is part of the planning step of the nursing process.
    4. Revising a plan of care in response to a patient not achieving a desired outcome (the ability to accurately prepare an insulin injection) is part of the evaluation step of the nursing process.
    Content Area: *Nursing Process*
    Integrated Processes: *Nursing Process: Analysis*
    Client Need: *Safe and Effective Care Environment; Management of Care*
    Cognitive Level: *Application*

30. **ANSWER: 1.**
    Rationales:
    1. This is a question that offers the patient an opportunity to discuss thoughts, feelings, or concerns with the nurse.
    2. Although this is a supportive statement, it is not the most inviting response.
    3. This is a biased question and may not elicit a true response by the patient.
    4. This is a gross generalization. Nurses should not make assumptions.
    TEST-TAKING TIP: *Identify the word in the stem that sets a priority. The word* most *in the stem sets a priority.*

Content Area: Communication and Documentation
Integrated Processes: Caring, Communication/
Documentation; Nursing Process: Implementation
Client Need: Psychosocial Integrity
Cognitive Level: Application

31. ANSWER: 3.
    Rationales:
    1. Activity performed 2 hours before bedtime will not interfere with sleep and is appropriate. Activity during the day or early evening stimulates physical functioning and increases mental activity.
    2. A snack is appropriate because it prevents hunger and promotes sleep if it contains the amino acid L-tryptophan.
    3. Alcohol shortens sleep onset, but its rapid metabolism causes rebound arousal, resulting in shortened REM sleep. Also, it may cause early morning awakening secondary to a full bladder because alcohol acts as a mild diuretic.
    4. Although excessively cold environmental temperatures will cause frequent awakenings, a cool environmental temperature usually is comfortable for sleeping.
    TEST-TAKING TIP: Identify the word in the stem that sets a priority. The word *must* in the stem sets a priority. Identify the word in the stem that indicates negative priority. The word *further* in the stem indicates negative polarity. The question is asking, "What should the patient with insomnia *not do.*" Identify the option that contains a specific determiner. The word *always* in option 2 is a specific determiner. More often than not, options with specific determiners are distractors and can be eliminated.
    Content Area: Pain, Comfort, Rest, and Sleep
    Integrated Processes: Teaching/Learning; Nursing Process: Evaluation
    Client Need: Physiological Integrity; Basic Care and Comfort
    Cognitive Level: Application

32. ANSWER: 1.
    Rationales:
    1. This is the most important statement because it addresses maintaining the patient's safety and security. This statement tells the patient how to alert the nurse in an emergency or call for any reason that the patient desires assistance.
    2. Although offering choices supports independence, which is important, another statement is more important because it addresses maintaining the patient's safety and security.
    3. Although patients generally want to know when meals are served, another statement is more important because it addresses maintaining the patient's safety and security.
    4. Although the nurse should ensure that the room temperature is comfortable, another statement is more important because it addresses maintaining the patient's safety and security.
    TEST-TAKING TIP: Identify the word in the stem that sets a priority. The word *most* in the stem sets a priority. Identify the clang association. The word *leaving* in the stem and the word *leave* in option 1 is a clang association. Identify equally plausible options. Options 2 and 4 are equally plausible.

plausible. They both have to do with comfort of the environment. Option 2 is no better than option 4. Eliminate both options from further consideration.
Content Area: Safety
Integrated Processes: Communication/Documentation; Nursing Process: Implementation
Client Need: Safe and Effective Care Environment; Safety and Infection Control
Cognitive Level: Application

33. ANSWER: 1,600.
    Rationale:
    To determine the hourly volume of intravenous fluid to be administered, divide 1,000 mL by 8 hours (1,000 ÷ 8 = 125). To identify the total volume of intravenous fluid for a 12-hour period, multiply the hourly rate by 12 hours (125 × 12 = 1,500). During the 7 a.m. to 7 p.m. shift, the antibiotic was administered once at 8 a.m. The total volume of fluid administered intravenously was 1,500 + 100 = 1,600 mL.
    Content Area: Fluid and Electrolyte Balance
    Integrated Processes: Nursing Process: Evaluation
    Client Need: Physiological Integrity; Pharmacological and Parenteral Therapies
    Cognitive Level: Application

34. ANSWER: 3.
    Rationales:
    1. The patient is actively hallucinating and is not a reliable source of information. In addition research has demonstrated that an allergy to shellfish is unrelated to an allergy to the iodine in contrast materials.
    2. Although the nurse should collect information about medications that the patient is taking, it is not the priority in this scenario.
    3. The patient has a psychiatric diagnosis and is actively hallucinating. The patient is incompetent and cannot sign a valid consent. The patient's significant other should be asked to sign the consent.
    4. An involved, detailed explanation may increase anxiety. Significant information should be provided in language that can be understood by the spouse and patient, even if the patient is physiologically or psychologically impaired.
    TEST-TAKING TIP: Identify the option with a clang association. The word *spouse* in the stem and in option 3 is a clang association.
    Content Area: Legal and Ethical Issues
    Integrated Processes: Communication/Documentation; Nursing Process: Implementation
    Client Need: Safe and Effective Care Environment; Management of Care
    Cognitive Level: Application

35. ANSWER: 1.
    Rationales:
    1. A shower chair permits the patient to sit during the procedure. This negates the need to stand on a wet, slippery surface and use excess energy to stand while bathing.
    2. A handheld faucet will increase the risk of a fall because one hand is occupied holding the shower faucet while the

other hand is used for washing; this leaves no hand to hold onto a handrail.

3. Although handrails in a shower stall will contribute to better balance and reduce the risk of a fall, it does not address the patient's activity intolerance.

4. Although a nonskid mat should be used in a shower stall to help prevent a fall, it does not address the patient's activity intolerance.

TEST-TAKING TIP: Identify the word in the stem that sets a priority. The word *most* in the stem sets a priority. Identify the clang associations. The word *shower* in the stem and in options 1 and 4 are clang associations. Examine options with clang associations carefully.

Content Area: Hygiene
Integrated Processes: Teaching/Learning; Nursing Process: Implementation
Client Need: Safe and Effective Care Environment; Safety and Infection Control
Cognitive Level: Application

36. ANSWER: 4.

Rationales:

1. Omeprazole (Prilosec) can be taken concurrently with an antacid; no drug-drug interaction occurs that interferes with absorption of the medication. Ranitidine (Zantac) should be taken 1 to 2 hours before or after an antacid.

2. A capsule of omeprazole (Prilosec) should not be opened, crushed, or chewed. The pellets in the capsule are designed for delayed absorption.

3. Omeprazole (Prilosec) should be given before food is eaten, preferably breakfast.

4. A capsule of omeprazole (Prilosec) should be swallowed whole and should not be opened, crushed, or chewed. The pellets in the capsule are designed for delayed absorption.

TEST-TAKING TIP: Identify the options that are opposites. Options 2 and 4 are opposites. Examine these options carefully because one of the opposite options is commonly the correct answer.

Content Area: Nutrition
Integrated Processes: Communication/Documentation, Teaching/Learning; Nursing Process: Implementation
Client Need: Physiological Integrity; Pharmacological and Parenteral Therapies
Cognitive Level: Application

37. ANSWER: 3.

Rationales:

1. Although this focuses on feelings, it is not the most appropriate nursing statement because the patient is not in denial; the patient is following the rest of the medication regimen.

2. This is a rigid response that denies the patient's concern.

3. The patient is taking the other medications and probably would take the diuretic if there were accessible bathroom facilities. An alternate time of day to take the diuretic should be explored to address the patient's concern and to ensure that all the prescribed medications are taken.

4. Although this may be a true statement, it does not address the patient's concern.

TEST-TAKING TIP: Identify the word in the stem that sets a priority. The word *best* in the stem sets a priority. Identify the option that has a specific determiner. Option 1 contains the word *all*, which is a specific determiner. Most options with a specific determiner are distractors and can be eliminated. Identify the option that denies the patient's concern. Option 2 denies the patient's concern. Identify the options with a clang association. The stem and options 3 and 4 contain the word *diuretic*. Examine options 3 and 4 carefully.

Content Area: Teaching and Learning
Integrated Processes: Communication/Documentation; Nursing Process: Implementation
Client Need: Health Promotion and Maintenance
Cognitive Level: Application

38. ANSWER: 3.

Rationales:

1. The patient has been experiencing nausea and vomiting for several hours. This is not a new event. However, the nurse should be monitoring this patient on a regular basis for electrolyte imbalances and administering an antiemetic if prescribed.

2. Pain on a level of 3 generally is considered tolerable. The patient's pain level should be periodically reassessed.

3. Any patient reporting chest pain should be assessed immediately. The patient may have a pulmonary emboli or myocardial infarction. Both of these events require emergency interventions and the primary health-care provider to be notified immediately.

4. Although this is important for the nurse to explore and resolve, this patient's need is not the priority in this situation.

TEST-TAKING TIP: Identify the word in the stem that sets a priority. The word *first* in the stem sets a priority.

Content Area: Physical Assessment
Integrated Processes: Nursing Process: Assessment
Client Need: Safe and Effective Care Environment; Management of Care
Cognitive Level: Analysis

39. ANSWER: 4.

Rationales:

1. This action is unsafe. Many drugs have similar doses.

2. It is not necessary to call the primary health-care provider. There are other resources that can be accessed to safely manage this concern.

3. This action is unsafe. The other nurse may not provide the nurse administering the drug with accurate information.

4. This is the most appropriate way to verify if the name of the medication on the unit dose package is equivalent to the name of the medication on the medication administration record. A drug usually has only one generic name, but a drug may have many trade names.

TEST-TAKING TIP: Identify the options that contain a clang association. The word *dose* in the stem and in option 1 is a clang association; the words *unit dose package* in the stem and in option 4 is a clang association. Examine options 1 and 4 carefully.

Content Area: Medication Administration
Integrated Processes: Nursing Process: Implementation
Client Need: Physiological Integrity; Pharmacological and Parenteral Therapies
Cognitive Level: Application

40. ANSWER: 4.
Rationales:
1. The term *bib* should be avoided because generally it makes a person feel childlike.
2. This is unsafe. Attempting to speak while chewing or swallowing may result in aspiration.
3. The nurse should not open containers, cut meat, or apply condiments to the patient's food without direction from the patient.
4. Asking about preferences is a patient-centered response; it supports the patient as an individual who is the center of the health team.
TEST-TAKING TIP: Identify the word in the stem that sets a priority. The word *most* in the stem sets a priority Identify the option that is patient centered. Option 4 is a patient-centered option. Identify the options that deny the patient's feelings, needs, and concerns. Options 1, 2, and 3 deny the patient's feelings, needs, and concerns.
Content Area: Nutrition
Integrated Processes: Caring, Communication/ Documentation; Nursing Process: Implementation
Client Need: Physiological Integrity; Basic Care and Comfort
Cognitive Level: Application

41. ANSWER: 2.
Rationales:
1. Throbbing pain at the incision site most likely is associated with the trauma of surgery and the inflammatory process, not dehiscence.
2. Patient's with dehiscence often state that they feel a popping sensation at the site of the incision; it is the release of tension due to the separation of wound edges.
3. This is unrelated to dehiscence. Diuresis is expected because the levels of glucocorticoids and mineralocorticoids increase in response to the stress of surgery return to expected levels after surgery.
4. Feeling bloated is not related to dehiscence; it is related to a postoperative ileus.
Content Area: Perioperative Nursing
Integrated Processes: Communication/Documentation; Nursing Process: Assessment
Client Need: Physiological Integrity; Physiological Adaptation
Cognitive Level: Application

42. ANSWER: 4.
Rationales:
1. Occasional difficulty with swallowing liquids should be managed by giving small amounts of liquid while the patient is in the Fowler position. Direct supervision is essential. Patients should enjoy meals in their usual form until difficulty progresses to a point where it may be unsafe; then a thickening product may be used.
2. Although this is important, it is not the priority. In addition, splints and braces must be removed for hygiene, skin care, and range-of-motion exercises.
3. Although this may be done, it is not the priority. Initially, the nurse should design a bladder retraining program that includes interventions, such as toileting the

patient before going to bed at night and the first thing in the morning, every 2 hours, or 30 minutes before a documented pattern of incontinence. Tubing for a drainage device should be used as a last resort.
4. The patient is experiencing a major change in living arrangements and may be coping with a sense of rejection or punishment. The nurse should stay with the patient and encourage the expression of feelings.
TEST-TAKING TIP: Identify the word in the stem that sets a priority. The word *most* in the stem sets a priority. Identify the option with a specific determiner. Option 2 contains the word *all*, which is a specific determiner.
Content Area: Psychosocial and Cultural Support
Integrated Processes: Caring, Communication/ Documentation; Nursing Process: Planning
Client Need: Health Promotion and Maintenance
Cognitive Level: Analysis

43. ANSWER: 2.
Rationales:
1. A patient with spinal surgery should have assistance with turning and positioning. Nursing knowledge and skill are necessary to maintain alignment of the vertebral column of patients who have had spinal surgery.
2. These activities are within the legal role of unlicensed assistive personnel; the activities are routine ADLs.
3. Assessment is within the legal role of a licensed nurse, not unlicensed assistive personnel.
4. A nurse should assist a postoperative patient to the bathroom the first time after surgery. This provides an opportunity for the nurse to assess the patient's strength and physical ability. In addition, postoperative patients may have IVs, indwelling catheters, etc. that require the nurse's expertise when transferring and ambulating.
Content Area: Leadership and Management
Integrated Processes: Nursing Process: Planning
Client Need: Safe and Effective Care Environment; Management of care
Cognitive Level: Analysis

44. ANSWER: 4.
Rationales:
1. A pillow should be positioned under the patient's calves, not heels, so that the heels are slightly elevated off the surface of the mattress. This reduces pressure on the heels that can cause pressure ulcers.
2. A pillow between the legs is used for the side-lying, not supine, position.
3. This is an awkward position because it places strain on the structures of the arms. Functional alignment of the arms is best achieved with the arms and hands resting on the bed with the palms of the hands facing the side of the body or facing the mattress.
4. A trochanter roll helps to maintain functional alignment by preventing external rotation of the hip.
Content Area: Mobility
Integrated Processes: Teaching/Learning; Nursing Process: Evaluation
Client Need: Physiological Integrity; Basic Care and Comfort
Cognitive Level: Application

45. ANSWER: 4.

Rationales:

1. Informing the nursing supervisor should be done after another more important intervention.

2. This is not within the legal practice of nursing. This is a dependent function of the nurse.

3. This will not safely meet the patient's need at this time.

4. When a medication error is made, the nurse must immediately contact the patient's primary health-care provider, particularly when the medication error may harm or kill the patient.

TEST-TAKING TIP: Identify the word in the stem that sets a priority. The word *first* in the stem sets a priority.

Content Area: *Legal and Ethical*

Integrated Processes: *Communication/Documentation; Nursing Process: Implementation*

Client Need: *Safe and Effective Care Environment; Management of Care*

Cognitive Level: *Application*

46. ANSWER: 3.

Rationales:

1. Pallor occurs in response to vasoconstriction related to the onset, not defervescence, stage of a fever.

2. Malaise, a vague feeling of discomfort, is associated with the course (plateau) phase of a fever. This response occurs because of irritation of cellular function related to the increase in temperature and byproducts of pyrogenic activity.

3. Sweating (diaphoresis) occurs in the defervescence (fever abatement/flush phase) phase of a fever when the cause of the temperature subsides and the set point of the hypothalamic thermostat is reduced. The usual heat loss responses include diaphoresis, warm flushed skin, and decreased shivering as vasodilation occurs during the defervescence stage of a fever.

4. Shivering is a heat production response that occurs during the onset stage of a fever before the new set point of the hypothalamic thermostat adjusts to a higher level.

Content Area: *Physical Assessment*

Integrated Processes: *Nursing Process: Analysis*

Client Need: *Physiological integrity; Reduction in Risk Potential*

Cognitive Level: *Application*

47. ANSWER: 3.

Rationales:

1. Sterile gloves are not necessary to remove a soiled dressing. A nurse wears clean gloves to protect oneself from the patient's body fluids.

2. The outside of the patient's dressing is not considered sterile. A nurse can apply tape to secure the dressing with ungloved hands.

3. A sterile container should not be touched with a bottle of normal saline that is contaminated on the outside. Only sterile objects can touch a sterile field or sterile item for sterility to be maintained. If a sterile object or field is touched by a clean object, it is contaminated and is no longer sterile.

4. This is acceptable practice. To wash the hands at this time requires the nurse to leave the bedside with the wound exposed. If the sterile field was already established, the nurse would have to leave it unattended, which is a violation of a principle of surgical asepsis. If a sterile field is unattended, it is considered contaminated because its sterility cannot be validated when outside the nurse's visual field.

TEST-TAKING TIP: Identify the word in the stem that indicates negative polarity. The word *interrupt* in the stem indicates negative polarity. What action by the LPN is unacceptable? Identify the unique option. Option 3 is the only option that does not contain the word *dressing*, making this option unique. Option 3 is the only option that relates to something other than a dressing.

Content Area: *Infection Control and Wound Care*

Integrated Processes: *Nursing Process: Evaluation*

Client Need: *Safe and Effective Care Environment; Management of Care*

Cognitive Level: *Analysis*

48. ANSWER: 1.

Rationales:

1. The nurse should provide further teaching in an attempt to change the parent's behavior. The parents may stop pushing the trigger if they understand that the child is still receiving an analgesic even when not pushing the trigger.

2. This is an authoritative intervention. A less aggressive approach should be used to change the parent's behavior.

3. This is unnecessary. The nurse should notify the primary health-care provider if the basal and bolus doses are inadequate to control the child's pain.

4. This intervention requires a prescription. This action is a dependent function of the nurse.

TEST-TAKING TIP: Identify the word in the stem that sets a priority. The word *first* in the stem sets a priority. Using the test-taking tip, "Identify the clang associations," will not help in answering this question because each option has a word that is also contained in the stem.

Content Area: *Perioperative Nursing*

Integrated Processes: *Teaching/Learning; Nursing Process: Implementation*

Client Need: *Physiological Integrity; Pharmacological and Parenteral Therapies*

Cognitive Level: *Application*

49. ANSWER: 4.

Rationales:

1. A medication should not be discontinued without collaboration with the primary health-care provider. Safety precautions should be taken if the patient develops dizziness or fatigue.

2. Acyclovir (Zovirax) will not precipitate constipation; it may cause anorexia, nausea, vomiting, and diarrhea.

3. Taking the pulse before the administration of acyclovir (Zovirax) is unnecessary; it does not influence the heart rate.

4. Acyclovir (Zovirax) should be taken at the first indication of an outbreak, such as itching (pruritus), tingling, or pain at the site where lesions develop (usually the perineal area).

Content Area: *Infection Control and Wound Care*

Integrated Processes: *Communication/Documentation, Teaching/Learning; Nursing Process: Evaluation*

Client Need: *Physiological Integrity; Pharmacological and parenteral therapy*

Cognitive Level: *Application*

50. ANSWER: 2.

Rationales:

1. The use of a safety razor is contraindicated when receiving an anticoagulant. Although a safety razor is safer than a straight edge razor, it still has a sharp blade that can cut the skin.

2. An electric razor is designed to trim facial hair with sharp blades safely confined within the shaving surface of the razor. This type razor minimizes the risk of incurring a break in the skin, which may bleed excessively when a person is receiving an anticoagulant.

3. Although aftershave lotion may provide comfort, it does not provide for patient safety.

4. Wrapping the face with a warm, not hot, towel often is done before shaving to soften hair. However, it should be avoided when receiving anticoagulants because this action causes vasodilation. If a break in the skin should occur when shaving, bleeding may be excessive.

TEST-TAKING TIP: Identify equally plausible options. Options 3 and 4 are equally plausible; both are actions that are associated with skin care. One is no better than the other.

Content Area: Hygiene
Integrated Processes: Teaching/Learning; Nursing Process: Implementation
Client Need: Physiological Integrity; Pharmacological and Parenteral Therapy
Cognitive Level: Application

51. ANSWER: 2.

Rationales:

1. Soft, low-pitched, breezy sounds heard in the periphery of the lungs are called vesicular breath sounds; they reflect expected sounds in the tiny airways of the lungs.

2. A low-pitched, grating sound usually during the height of inspiration reflects the sound of inflamed pleura rubbing together. A pleural friction rub is heard at the lateral anterior base of the lung, indicated as RLL in the figure.

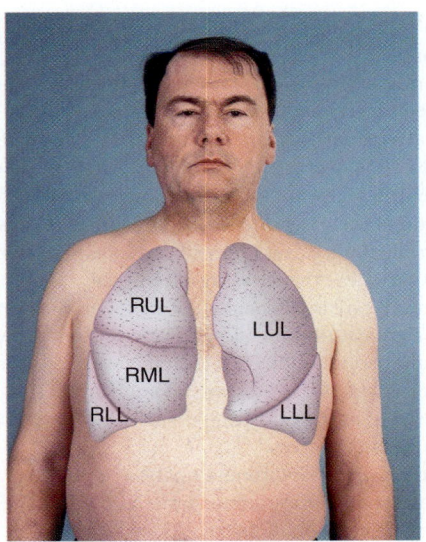

3. Loud, high-pitched, hollow, blowing sounds heard over the trachea anteriorly are called bronchial breath sounds; these sounds are expected breath sounds and do not indicate the presence of pleurisy.

4. Medium-pitched, medium-intensity, blowing sounds heard on inspiration and expiration when the stethoscope is over the major bronchi are called bronchovesicular breath sounds; they are expected breath sounds and are not indicative of pleurisy.

Content Area: Oxygenation
Integrated Processes: Nursing Process: Implementation
Client Need: Physiological Integrity; Physiological Adaptation
Cognitive Level: Analysis

52. ANSWER: 1.

Rationales:

1. The patient is the most important member of the health-care team. All activities of the members of the team focus on the needs of the patient.

2. Although the primary nurse is an important member of the health-care team, the nurse assumes a lesser role compared to the patient.

3. Although the nurse manager is an important member of the health-care team, the nurse manager assumes a lesser role compared to the patient.

4. Although the nurse practitioner is an important member of the health-care team, the nurse practitioner assumes a lesser role compared to the patient.

TEST-TAKING TIP: Identify the word in the stem that sets a priority. The word *most* in the stem sets a priority. Identify the unique option. Option 1 is unique because it is the only option that does not include the word *nurse*.

Content Area: Health-Care Delivery
Integrated Processes: Communication/Documentation; Nursing Process: Implementation
Client Need: Safe and Effective Care Environment; Management of Care
Cognitive Level: Comprehension

53. ANSWER: 2.

Rationales:

1. A balanced diet plus adequate fluid is all that is necessary.

2. Toileting times are purposely scheduled in response to times of fluid intake and the patient's usual elimination pattern; the schedule must be followed exactly to increase success.

3. Washing the perineal area does not contribute to a patient's ability to regain continence.

4. The pattern of voiding, not fluid balance, relative to fluid intake is significant.

TEST-TAKING TIP: Identify the option with a clang association. The word *program* in the stem and option 2 is a clang association.

Content Area: Urinary Elimination
Integrated Processes: Nursing Process: Planning
Client Need: Physiological Integrity; Physiological Adaptation
Cognitive Level: Application

54. ANSWER: 4.
Rationales:
1. Penrose drains function on the principle of gravity and drainage flows directly into a gauze dressing, not a collection device. With a Jackson-Pratt drain, negative pressure is established when the opened collection device is compressed and then closed. The negative pressure establishes gentle suction that pulls drainage from the wound into the collection device. It should be emptied of drainage when half full and negative pressure reestablished to ensure adequacy of the negative pressure.
2. Penrose drains drain directly into a gauze dressing. They do not have a collection chamber.
3. Penrose drains are shortened regularly as healing takes place. Jackson-Pratt drains are not shortened; generally they are removed once drainage decreases to less than 10 mL daily.
4. The color of the drainage of both tubes should be assessed and the results documented.
TEST-TAKING TIP: Identify the clang associations. The word *drain* in the stem and in option 3 and the word *drainage* in option 4 are clang associations. Examine options 3 and 4 carefully.
Content Area: Perioperative Nursing
Integrated Processes: Nursing Process: Evaluation
Client Need: Physiological Integrity; Physiological Adaptation
Cognitive Level: Analysis

55. ANSWER: 1.
Rationales:
1. A telephone translation service employing competent, certified translators ensures that translations will be accurate.
2. Using a staff member to translate a conversation may not ensure accuracy in the translation because the staff member may not be fully competent in the required language. Also, people in different regions of a country may speak a different dialect.
3. Pictures can reinforce learning, but teaching should use the spoken word.
4. A translation book will assist in communicating but cannot guarantee comprehension because the patient may have different interpretation of words.
TEST-TAKING TIP: Identify the option with a clang association. The word *teaching* in the stem and in option 1 is a clang association. Give option 1 careful consideration.
Content Area: Communication and Documentation
Integrated Processes: Communication/Documentation; Nursing Process: Planning
Client Need: Safe and Effective Care Environment; Management of Care
Cognitive Level: Application

56. ANSWER: 4.
Rationales:
1. Although this is something the nurse should instruct the patient to do, this patient is confused at times and cannot be relied upon to call for help when it is needed.
2. A confused patient should not be left unattended in the bathroom; also, the patient may not understand how to use a call light device.

3. A confused patient who needs a walker should not be permitted to walk unattended.
4. This is the best intervention of the options presented to help keep a patient safe from falls. By positioning the patient's wheelchair next to the nurses' station, staff members can continuously supervise a confused patient.
TEST-TAKING TIP: Identify the word in the stem that sets a priority. The word *best* in the stem sets a priority. Identify equally plausible options. Options 1 and 2 are equally plausible. Both options instruct the patient to call for help. Option 1 is no better than option 2.
Content Area: Safety
Integrated Processes: Communication/Documentation; Nursing Process: Implementation
Client Need: Safe and Effective Care Environment; Safety and Infection Control
Cognitive Level: Application

57. ANSWER: 2.
Rationales:
1. Although this reflects dehydration and is an important assessment, it is not the priority among the options presented.
2. Ensuring adequate gas exchange is the priority; inadequate gas exchange is life threatening.
3. Although this reflects a stage I pressure ulcer and is an important assessment, it is not the priority among the options presented.
4. Although this may reflect inadequate nutrition and is an important assessment, it is not the priority among the options presented.
TEST-TAKING TIP: Identify the word in the stem that set a priority. The word *greatest* in the stem sets a priority. Use the ABCs (Airway, Breathing, and Circulation) to identify the priority.
Content Area: Oxygenation
Integrated Processes: Nursing Process: Analysis
Client Need: Safe and Effective Care Environment; Management of Care
Cognitive Level: Analysis

58. ANSWER: 1.
Rationales:
1. Montgomery straps are paired adhesive straps applied several inches on either side of a wound with central sections that can be folded back, allowing access to the primary dressing. On the leading edge of each of the central sections are perforations that allow for a method of securing one side to the other. It is used to secure a primary dressing without having to replace the tape every time the dressing is changed.
2. Wound care is a dependent function of the nurse; half-normal saline solution and peroxide was not ordered. Normal saline solution (0.9% sodium chloride) was ordered because it is isotonic. Research demonstrates that peroxide is caustic to new granulating tissue and counterproductive to the healing process.
3. The gauze packing should not be dripping wet. It should be moist enough to promote granulation of tissue without causing maceration of tissue.

4. Gently wiping away, not toward, the wound avoids contaminating the wound with skin flora. Patting violates surgical asepsis. One 4×4 gauze pad should be used for each swipe from the wound toward the skin.

TEST-TAKING TIP: Identify the word in the stem that sets a priority. The word *most* in the stem sets a priority.
Content Area: Infection Control and Wound Care
Integrated Processes: Nursing Process: Implementation
Client Need: Physiological Integrity; Physiological Adaptation
Cognitive Level: Application

59. **ANSWER: 3.**
Rationales:
1. Clean, not sterile, gloves should be worn to protect the nurse from the patient's body fluids. The patient has an infection and a discharge may be present.
2. The lower lid should be moved by placing a finger just below the lower eyelashes and exerting gentle pressure downward toward the bony prominence of the cheek.
3. Drops should be placed in the conjunctival sac to prevent trauma to the eyeball. The fluid disperses when the eye is closed gently after the insertion of the drops.
4. A new cotton ball for each stroke should be moved from the inner to the outer cantus to prevent debris from entering the lacrimal duct. The eye should be cleansed before the procedure to remove debris and wiped gently after the procedure to remove excess fluid that may have leaked onto the cheek.
Content Area: Medication Administration
Integrated Processes: Nursing Process: Implementation
Client Need: Physiological Integrity; Pharmacological and Parenteral Therapies
Cognitive Level: Application

60. **ANSWER: 2.**
Rationales:
1. Feeling hungry is subjective, not objective, information. Subjective data involve feelings, sensations, and concerns reported by the patient. Subjective data are not observable and can be described only by the patient.
2. Objective data are observable and measurable and can be confirmed by another person though the use of the senses. In this situation, the patient is observed avoiding eye contact when talking with the nurse.
3. Bladder spasms are subjective, not objective, data. They can be reported only by the patient. The patient generally will report feeling abdominal cramping and pain in the lower abdomen when bladder spasms occur.
4. Reports of epigastric discomfort are subjective, not objective, information. Discomfort can be reported only by the patient.
TEST-TAKING TIP: Identify the equally plausible options. Options 1 and 4 are both based on statements by the patient. Option 1 is no better than option 4. Eliminate options 1 and 4.
Content Area: Nursing Process
Integrated Processes: Nursing Process: Assessment
Client Need: Safe and Effective Care Environment; Management of Care
Cognitive Level: Application

61. **ANSWER: 3.**
Rationales:
1. Leaving the patient's room while the patient is in distress without providing an opportunity to emote is inappropriate.
2. Forcing a patient to talk about concerns is inappropriate; nurses must proceed at the patient's pace.
3. Remaining seated in the room with the patient for several minutes allows the patient to gather personal thoughts and not feel abandoned by the nurse.
4. Leaving the room while the patient is upset without giving the patient a chance to verbalize concerns may be viewed by the patient as abandonment.
TEST-TAKING TIP: Identify the word in the stem that sets a priority. The word *best* in the stem sets a priority. Identify opposite options. Options 3 and 4 are opposites. More often than not, one of the options that is an opposite is the correct answer. Examine options 3 and 4 carefully. Identify the equally plausible options. Options 1 and 4 are equally plausible. They both leave the patient when the patient is upset. Eliminate options 1 and 4. Identify the option that denies the patient's feelings. Option 4 denies the patient's feelings.
Content Area: Psychosocial and Cultural Support
Integrated Processes: Caring, Communication/ Documentation; Nursing Process: Implementation
Client Need: Psychosocial Integrity
Cognitive Level: Application

62. **ANSWER: 2, 4, 5, 3, 1.**
Rationales:
2. Infants are developing sensorimotor skills and enjoy the sounds associated with rattles. They become interactive with toys and demonstrate preferences by 3 to 6 months of age.
4. Toddlers are mastering gross and fine motor skills; they enjoy the autonomy of playing with a pounding toy.
5. Preschoolers are developing mastery of fine motor skills. Construction toys allow them to engage in endeavors with purpose and that require skill.
3. School-aged children enjoy associate play and games with increasing complexity.
1. Adolescents develop formal operational thought and are capable of following the rules of complex games.
Content Area: Nursing Care Across the Life Span
Integrated Processes: Nursing Process: Implementation
Client Need: Health Promotion and Maintenance
Cognitive Level: Analysis

63. **ANSWER: 4.**
Rationales:
1. Redness (erythema) indicates the presence of the inflammatory response; the wound may or may not be infected.
2. Swelling (edema) indicates the presence of the inflammatory response; the wound may or may not be infected.
3. A wound that is warm to the touch is a result of an increase in circulation to the area that is indicative of the inflammatory response; the wound may or may not be infected.
4. Thick fluid that appears yellow, green, tan, or brown exiting from a wound is purulent drainage. The drainage

is debris consisting of fluid, cells, or cellular material escaped from blood vessels as a result of an infection.
Content Area: Infection Control and Wound Care
Integrated Processes: Nursing Process: Evaluation
Client Need: Physiological Integrity; Physiological Adaptation
Cognitive Level: Application

64. **ANSWER: 4.**
Rationales:
1. This movement achieves hyperextension.
2. This movement achieves adduction.
3. This movement achieves external rotation.
4. **This movement achieves internal rotation.**
TEST-TAKING TIP: Identify the options that are opposites. Options 3 and 4 are opposites. Examine options 3 and 4 carefully.
Content Area: Mobility
Integrated Processes: Nursing Process: Implementation
Client Need: Physiological Integrity; Basic Care and Comfort
Cognitive Level: Application

65. **ANSWER: 2.**
Rationales:
1. This explanation does not protect the other residents from becoming scared when the wandering resident enters their rooms.
2. **The alarm will ring when the resident exits the bed. When the alarm rings, the nurse can immediately intervene to walk with the resident or engage the resident in a distracting activity. This is the only action among the options offered that effectively protects the other residents.**
3. Some residents may feel isolated if the door is closed. Closing the doors of all residents' rooms at night violates the right of residents to have their doors remain open. Also, a closed door may not stop a wandering resident from entering another resident's room.
4. The wandering resident may climb over a bolster and rail causing a safety concern for the resident. A bolster generally is used to remind a resident to call for assistance when wanting to get of bed, not to keep a resident from climbing out of bed. Four raised side rails are considered a restraint and requires an order from the primary health-care provider.
TEST-TAKING TIP: Identify the word in the stem that sets a priority. The word *most* in the stem sets a priority. Identify the central persons in the question. The other residents are the central persons in the question. The question is asking, "Which intervention is most effective in protecting the other residents from the resident who is wandering at night?" Identify the options that deny residents' feelings, concerns, and rights. Option 1 denies the other residents' feelings and concerns. Delete option 1 from further consideration. Option 3 denies the other residents' rights to have their doors left open at night. Delete option 4 from further consideration.
Content Area: Safety
Integrated Processes: Caring; Nursing Process: Implementation
Client Need: Safe and Effective Care Environment; Safety and Infection Control
Cognitive Level: Application

66. **ANSWER: 2.**
Rationales:
1. This response suggests an intervention before collecting enough information to make an informed decision.
2. **Conflict resolution is best approached by having all the involved people together and discussing the issues. This approach allows each person to explain a personal point of view as well as gain insight into another's point of view. Suggestions from both perspectives will help achieve a win-win resolution.**
3. This response denies the night nurse's concerns.
4. The night nurse's response to this statement may be an action that is inappropriate or impossible to implement. The nurse manager should take the initiative and intervene appropriately from an objective perspective.
TEST-TAKING TIP: Identify the word in the stem that sets a priority. The word *best* in the stem sets a priority. Identify the option that contains a specific determiner. Option 3 contains the word *all*, which is a specific determiner. More often than not, an option that contains a specific determiner is a wrong answer. Identify options that deny the night nurse's concerns. Options 1 and 3 deny the night nurse's concerns.
Content Area: Leadership and Management
Integrated Processes: Caring, Communication/Documentation; Nursing Process: Implementation
Client Need: Safe and Effective Care Environment; Management of Care
Cognitive Level: Analysis

67. **ANSWER: 3.**
Rationales:
1. Soy milk is lactose free and does not have to be avoided when on a lactose-free diet.
2. Fruit cocktail is lactose free and does not have to be avoided when on a lactose-free diet.
3. **Creamed soup has milk, which contains lactose, and should be avoided by a patient following a lactose-free diet.**
4. Vegetable juice is lactose free and does not have to be avoided when on a lactose-free diet.
TEST-TAKING TIP: Identify the words in the stem that indicate negative polarity. The words *avoid* and *eliminated* in the stem indicate negative polarity.
Content Area: Nutrition
Integrated Processes: Teaching/Learning; Nursing Process: Evaluation
Client Need: Physiological Integrity; Basic Care and Comfort
Cognitive Level: Analysis

68. **ANSWER: 4.**
Rationales:
1. This is not the first step of the procedure; however, this should be done before and after administration of a medication to help keep the tube patent.
2. This is not the first step of the procedure. A piston syringe can be used but, the medication should be instilled slowly; gravity flow is preferred.
3. This is not the first step of the procedure. The negative pressure should be shut off immediately before instillation

of the medication and kept off for 30 minutes after medication administration to promote absorption.

4. It is important to identify that the tube is in the stomach. If it inadvertently moved into the esophagus or the trachea, instillation of liquid may be aspirated or flood the respiratory tract, respectively.

TEST-TAKING TIP: Identify the word in the stem that sets a priority. The word *first* in the stem sets a priority. Identify the words that are a clang association. The words *nasogastric tube* in the stem and option 4 is a clang association. Consider option 4 carefully.

Content Area: Medication Administration
Integrated Processes: Nursing Process: Implementation
Client Need: Physiological integrity; Pharmacological and Parenteral Therapies
Cognitive Level: Analysis

69. **ANSWER: 3.**
Rationales:
1. Mildly active bowel sounds 3 days after a colon resection reflects a return of peristalsis, which is expected.
2. Dark pink urine immediately after a transurethral resection of the prostate is expected. If it becomes red or does not become lighter in color several hours after surgery, it may indicate excessive bleeding, which should be reported to the primary health-care provider.
3. The patient has an already reduced surface area for the exchange of oxygen and carbon dioxide as a result of the wedge resection of the right lung. Reduced breath sounds on the nonoperative lung indicate a problem that will further compromise respiratory function. This should be reported to the primary health-care provider immediately.
4. Greenish drainage from a nasogastric tube after an abdominal cholecystectomy is the expected color of gastric secretions.

TEST-TAKING TIP: Identify the word in the stem that sets a priority. The word *immediate* in the stem sets a priority. Use the ABCs (Airway, Breathing, and Circulation) when examining options to establish the priority. No option presents a concern with airway. Option 3 is associated with breathing.

Content Area: Perioperative Nursing
Integrated Processes: Nursing Process: Evaluation
Client Need: Safe and Effective Care Environment; Management of Care
Cognitive Level: Analysis

70. **ANSWER: 3.**
Rationales:
1. An online course is most effective when cognitive learning is required.
2. Lectures are effective for large groups, but interaction among members of the group is not promoted.
3. Overeating has an emotional component. Patients interacting with each other within a group have the opportunity for affective learning that involves changes in feelings, values, attitudes, and beliefs. Also, group members can provide support when designing and maintaining new behaviors.
4. Written materials are effective when cognitive learning is required.

TEST-TAKING TIP: Identify the word in the stem that sets a priority. The word *most* in the stem sets a priority.
Content Area: Teaching and Learning
Integrated Processes: Teaching/Learning; Nursing Process: Planning
Client Need: Health Promotion and Maintenance
Cognitive Level: Application

71. **ANSWER: 4.**
Rationales:
1. Range-of-motion (ROM) exercises every hour are unnecessary unless the patient has an extenuating circumstance, such as a neuromusculoskeletal or peripheral circulation problem.
2. ROM exercises once a shift is too long between releasing restraints and performing ROM and may result in contractures.
3. ROM exercises every 4 hours is too long between releasing restraints and performing ROM and may result in contractures.
4. Every 2 hours is often enough to perform ROM exercises to prevent contractures unless there are extenuating circumstances, such as when a patient has a neuromusculoskeletal or peripheral circulation problem.
Content Area: Safety
Integrated Processes: Communication/Documentation; Nursing Process: Planning
Client Need: Safe and Effective Care Environment; Safety and Infection Control
Cognitive Level: Application

72. **ANSWER: 3.**
Rationales:
1. Rating the intensity of pain on an objective scale assesses the severity of pain.
2. Information about the onset of pain assists in distinguishing the difference between acute and chronic pain, not radiating pain.
3. Pain that extends via direct extension from a point of origin to another close-lying area is known as radiating pain.
4. Pain that comes and goes is known as intermittent pain; it is associated with exacerbations and remissions of an illness.
Content Area: Pain, Comfort, Rest, and Sleep
Integrated Processes: Communication/Documentation; Nursing Process: Assessment
Client Need: Physiological Integrity; Reduction of Risk Potential
Cognitive Level: Application

73. **ANSWER: 4.**
Rationales:
1. A nurse cannot catheterize a patient without an order.
2. Initiating intake and output monitoring is not indicated until further assessment is completed.
3. Physical assessment follows another type of data collection; the data collected will determine how to focus the physical assessment.
4. Before initiating an intervention, the nurse should obtain additional information, such as asking about the time and amount of the last voiding.

TEST-TAKING TIP: Identify the word in the stem that sets a priority. The word *first* in the stem sets a priority. Identify the obscure clang association. The word *urinate* in the stem and *voiding* in option 4 is an obscure clang association. Examine option 4 carefully.
Content Area: Urinary Elimination
Integrated Processes: Communication/Documentation; Nursing Process: Assessment
Client Need: Physiological Integrity; Reduction of Risk Potential
Cognitive Level: Application

74. ANSWER: 2.
Rationales:
1. Conditioners moisturize the hair, which makes the strands supple, preventing tangles.
2. Soap is drying because it removes natural secretions that keep the hair supple. When shampooing is necessary, a gentle moisturizing shampoo should be used.
3. Braids organize the strands of hair, which limits movement of hair into mats and tangles because of friction and pressure.
4. Brushing distributes oils along hair shafts, keeping them supple, preventing tangles and matting.
TEST-TAKING TIP: Identify the word in the stem that indicates negative polarity. The word *avoid* in the stem indicates negative polarity. The question is asking, "What action will promote tangles and matting of hair?"
Content Area: Hygiene
Integrated Processes: Teaching/Learning; Nursing Process: Implementation
Client Need: Physiological Integrity; Basic Care and Comfort
Cognitive Level: Application

75. ANSWER: 2, 3, 5.
Rationales:
1. Ten grapes contain only 116 mg of potassium.
2. Five dried figs contain 712 mg of potassium. Furosemide (Lasix) is not a potassium-sparing diuretic, and a patient may develop hypokalemia unless foods high in potassium are consumed.
3. One baked potato contains 610 mg to 1081 mg of potassium, depending on its size.
4. Half of a grapefruit contains only 165 mg of potassium.
5. One cup of cooked spinach contains 839 mg of potassium.
Content Area: Fluid and Electrolyte Balance
Integrated Processes: Teaching/Learning; Nursing Process: Implementation
Client Need: Physiological Integrity; Basic Care and Comfort
Cognitive Level: Analysis

76. ANSWER: 4.
Rationales:
1. Bringing the patient to talk with the lawyer without written consent from the patient is a breach of Health Insurance Portability and Accountability Act (HIPAA) regulations.
2. Refusing to discuss anything regarding the patient indirectly implies that the patient is on the unit. Also, it does not provide the patient with potentially important information.
3. Although this is correct, it is not the best choice in this scenario because the patient is not given potentially important information.
4. It is against HIPAA regulations to reveal that a patient is on the unit without written consent from the patient. The nurse should take the lawyer's phone number and pass it on to the patient without revealing to the caller that the patient is on the unit. It is important to relay crucial information to the patient without violating HIPAA regulations.
TEST-TAKING TIP: Identify the word in the stem that sets a priority. The word *most* in the stem sets a priority.
Content Area: Legal and Ethical Issues
Integrated Processes: Communication/Documentation; Nursing Process: Implementation
Client Need: Safe and Effective Care Environment; Management of Care
Cognitive Level: Application

77. ANSWER: 4.
Rationales:
1. Side effects of warfarin (Coumadin), an anticoagulant, are bruising, melena, hematuria, epistaxis, bleeding gums, anemia, and thrombocytopenia, not constipation.
2. Magnesium salts in magnesium/aluminum hydroxide (Maalox) may increase peristalsis, causing diarrhea, not constipation.
3. Metronidazole (Flagyl) is an anti-infective; generally, diarrhea, not constipation, is a side effect. It depletes the natural flora in the colon and permits other organisms that do not belong in the colon to grow, causing diarrhea. For example, *Clostridium difficile* causes pseudomembranous colitis, a profuse infectious diarrhea.
4. Constipation is a common side effect of carbonyl iron (Feosol); iron interferes with myoglobin, which helps provide oxygen to muscles, including those associated with the bowel, resulting in decreased bowel motility.
TEST-TAKING TIP: Identify the words in the stem that set a priority. The word *most* in the stem sets a priority.
Content Area: Gastrointestinal System
Integrated Processes: Nursing Process: Analysis
Client Need: Physiological Integrity; Pharmacological and Parenteral Therapies
Cognitive Level: Analysis

78. ANSWER: 1.
Rationales:
1. Difficulty chewing results in food particles that are dangerously large at the time of swallowing and difficulty swallowing may result in secretions, fluids, or solids entering the tracheobronchial tree rather than the esophagus. The patient is at risk for aspiration.
2. Although constipation may occur because the patient may avoid eating foods high in fiber due to the fact that they are difficult to chew, this is not the priority. High-fiber drinks and stool softeners may be ordered to prevent constipation.

3. Fluid volume deficit can be prevented with adequate supervision (e.g., high-Fowler position when drinking small amounts of fluid at a time) and the use of products that thicken the fluid into a gelatin-like consistency.

4. Inadequate nutrition can be prevented by ordering food with an altered consistency (e.g., soft, chopped, puree) along with supplemental nutritional drinks.

TEST-TAKING TIP: Identify the word in the stem that sets a priority. The word *greatest* in the stem sets a priority.
Content Area: Safety
Integrated Processes: Nursing Process: Analysis
Client Need: Safe and Effective Care Environment; Reduction of Risk Potential
Cognitive Level: Application

79. **ANSWER: 4.**
Rationales:
1. A low urine specific gravity reflects diluted urine, which indicates that the patient may have fluid volume excess, not deficit.
2. A bounding pulse indicates an increase in circulating blood volume and is a sign of fluid volume excess, not dehydration.
3. Straw-colored urine indicates that the patient probably is in fluid balance.
4. **Skin turgor refers to expected skin fullness or the ability of the skin and underlying tissue to return to their regular position after being pinched and lifted. When there is decreased skin turgor because of dehydration, the skin remains pinched or "tented" for a longer time after it is released than well-hydrated skin.**
Content Area: Fluid and Electrolyte Balance
Integrated Processes: Communication/Documentation; Nursing Process: Assessment
Client Need: Physiological Integrity; Physiological Adaptation
Cognitive Level: Analysis

80. **ANSWER: 3.**
Rationales:
1. Eating pork and pork products is not prohibited by the Christian Science religion; this is prohibited by observant Jewish and Hindu people.
2. This is not a belief of the Christian Science religion. Observant Jewish people believe that the patient's feet should face toward the exit of a room.
3. **The patient may feel guilty about seeking traditional medical care. Traditional medicine and drugs to treat illness are not accepted by the Christian Science religion. It is believed that illness is caused by ignorance, fear, or sin and that the patient will return to health with prayers and Christian Science treatment.**
4. Amulets to ward off evil spirits are associated with Native American cultures, not the Christian Science religion.

TEST-TAKING TIP: Identify the option that is unique. Option 3 is unique because it is the only option associated with requiring a response from the patient. Identify the option with a clang association. The words *medical management* in the stem and in option 3 is a clang association. Examine option 3 carefully.

Content Area: Psychosocial and Cultural Support
Integrated Processes: Caring; Communication/Documentation; Nursing Process: Implementation
Client Need: Psychosocial Integrity
Cognitive Level: Application

81. **ANSWER: 1.**
Rationales:
1. **A stethoscope can auscultate the abnormality of the venous/arterial system known as a bruit.**
2. A lesion is observed via inspection, not by auscultation.
3. Ascites is assessed by inspection and palpation, not auscultation.
4. Distention of the abdomen is assessed by inspection and palpation, not auscultation.

TEST-TAKING TIP: Identify the equally plausible options. Options 3 and 4 are equally plausible because they both require the assessment techniques of inspection and palpation.
Content Area: Physical Assessment
Integrated Processes: Nursing Process: Assessment
Client Need: Health Promotion and Maintenance
Cognitive Level: Analysis

82. **ANSWER: 1.**
Rationales:
1. **After administration of a tube-feeding formula, instilling 30 mL of water flushes the tube, preventing future blockage from a buildup of formula along the sides of the lumen of the tube.**
2. Inserting 20 mL of air into the tube may be part of the procedure that is done to determine if the tube is in the stomach before a tube feeding is initiated. Aspirating gastric contents is the preferred method of testing placement of a nasogastric tube.
3. Checking the gastrostomy site is not necessarily part of the procedure for administering a gastrostomy tube feeding.
4. Activity is contraindicated immediately after a gastrostomy tube feeding to prevent aspiration. The patient should remain in a sitting or semi-Fowler position for 30 to 60 minutes after a feeding.

TEST-TAKING TIP: Identify options with clang associations. The word *tube* in the stem and in options 1 and 2 are clang associations. Carefully examine option 1 and 2. More often than not, an option with a clang association is the correct answer.
Content Area: Nutrition
Integrated Processes: Nursing Process: Implementation
Client Need: Physiological Integrity; Basic Care and Comfort
Cognitive Level: Application

83. **ANSWER: 3.**
Rationales:
1. The solution should be removed from the refrigerator 1 hour before administration so that it warms to room temperature to prevent pain, venous spasms, and hypothermia. It should never be warmed in a microwave oven or by submerging the bag in warm water.
2. This is unsafe; total parenteral nutrition must be administered via special tubing that has an in-line filter. Also, the

total parenteral nutrition solution and the medication may not be compatible.

3. Total parenteral nutrition intravenous tubing should be changed every 24 hours because the IV filter traps bacteria and particles that may form in the solution tubing.

4. This is unnecessary. Total parenteral nutrition is administered via a vein into the circulatory system, not the stomach. Viability of the intravenous catheter insertion site should be assessed.

Content Area: Nutrition
Integrated Processes: Nursing Process: Implementation
Client Need: Physiological Integrity; Pharmacological and Parenteral Therapies
Cognitive Level: Application

84. ANSWER: 10.
Rationale:
Use ratio and proportion to answer the question.

$$\frac{\text{Desire 250 mg}}{\text{Have 125 mg}} = \frac{\text{x mL}}{\text{5 mL}}$$

$$125x = 250 \times 5$$

$$125x = 1,250$$

$$x = 1,250 \div 125$$

$$x = 10 \text{ mL}$$

Content Area: Medication Administration
Integrated Processes: Nursing Process: Planning
Client Need: Physiological integrity; Pharmacological and Parenteral Therapies
Cognitive Level: Application

85. ANSWER: 2.
Rationales:
1. The word *tolerated* is too general. The nurse should use specific, descriptive terminology to communicate the patient's status after being in the chair.
2. This documentation is specific, descriptive, and has a time frame.
3. The situation indicating the need for a prn medication must be included in the documentation. In addition, the specific drug, dose, route, and patient response should be included.
4. Pain assessment should include location, severity, and characteristics of the pain. The specific pain scale should be referenced (e.g., 5 on a scale of 0 to 10).

Content Area: Communication and Documentation
Integrated Processes: Communication/Documentation; Nursing Process: Evaluation
Client Need: Safe and Effective Care Environment; Management of Care
Cognitive Level: Application

86. ANSWER: 1.
Rationales:
1. The inability to speak indicates a total obstruction. The abdominal thrust maneuver pushes trapped air out of the lungs, forcing out the food causing the obstruction.

2. Attempting to swallow may cause the food to move further down the respiratory passages.
3. Clapping between the scapulae several times may cause aspirated food to lodge deeper in the respiratory passages and is contraindicated.
4. Waiting is unsafe. Letting the patient cough is appropriate if there is a partial obstruction.

TEST-TAKING TIP: Identify the opposite options. Options 1 and 4 are opposites. Identify the unique option. Option 1 is the only option without the word *patient*.

Content Area: Oxygenation
Integrated Processes: Nursing Process: Implementation
Client Need: Physiological Integrity; Physiological Adaptation
Cognitive Level: Application

87. ANSWER: 2.
Rationales:
1. Sterile gloves are not necessary to maintain sterile technique when collecting a urine specimen from a closed urinary catheter and collection set. Clean gloves protect the nurse from the patient's body fluids.
2. A clamp is used to occlude the tubing of a urinary catheter so that fresh urine can collect in the tubing proximal to the clamp. After the specimen is collected from a port proximal to the clamp, the clamp should be released immediately to allow urine to flow out of the bladder via the unobstructed tubing.
3. A sterile specimen cup is not necessary for a urinalysis. However, the use of a sterile specimen cup and maintenance of sterile technique are essential when collecting a sterile urine specimen for a culture and sensitivity examination.
4. Generally, urinary retention catheters are closed systems whereby the catheter, tubing, and collection bag are permanently connected to prevent separation. A closed system reduces the risk of entry of microorganisms, which in turn reduces the risk of a urinary tract infection.

TEST-TAKING TIP: Identify the clang associations. The word *urine* in the stem and in options 2 and 3 are clang associations. Examine options 2 and 3 carefully.

Content Area: Urinary Elimination
Integrated Processes: Nursing Process: Implementation
Client Need: Physiological Integrity; Reduction of Risk Potential
Cognitive Level: Application

88. ANSWER: 2.
Rationales:
1. The opposite is true in older adults; long-term memory is better than short-term memory.
2. Mental acuity slows in older adults and it may take longer to learn something new. Teaching sessions should be short and frequent to allow for repetition and reinforcement.
3. A person's IQ does not change as one ages.
4. People who get easily confused usually have a cognitive disorder (e.g., learning disability, dementia).

Content Area: Nursing Care Across the Life Span

Integrated Processes: Communication/Documentation; *Nursing Process:* Assessment
Client Need: Health Promotion and Maintenance
Cognitive Level: Application

89. **ANSWER: 4.**
Rationales:
1. Not all oxygen delivery systems cover both the nose and mouth. Nasal prongs and a face tent do not cover the nose and mouth.
2. This is not an intervention that is appropriate for all oxygen delivery systems. This is done just with partial-rebreather and nonrebreather masks.
3. Liter flow rates depend on the oxygen flow rate required by the device and the primary health-care provider's order. A simple facemask is set between 5 to 10 L/minute. Nasal prongs are set between 1 to 6 L/minute. Partial-rebreather and nonrebreather masks are set between 6 to 15 L/minute. The liter flow rate for a Venturi mask is set between 4 to 15 L/minute, depending on the size valve used. A face tent is set between 8 to 12 L/minute.
4. All oxygen delivery systems anchor the device around the head with an elastic band or tubing; this can cause pressure, resulting in ischemia and skin breakdown.
Content Area: Oxygenation
Integrated Processes: Nursing Process: Evaluation
Client Need: Physiological Integrity; Physiological Adaptation
Cognitive Level: Analysis

90. **ANSWER: 3.**
Rationales:
1. The nurse's body should remain in functional alignment, not twisted. When the upper body is twisted (torqued), undue stress and strain are placed on muscles, joints, tendons, ligaments, and bones. Twisting the upper body should be avoided to prevent self-injury.
2. The arms should be flexed so that the elbows can act as fulcrums while the arms act as levers.
3. A wide base of support keeps the greatest mass of the body (torso) in the center of gravity, which provides stability.
4. The nurse should bend the knees, not the waist. Bending the knees uses the large muscles of the legs rather than the weaker muscles of the back to assist with a transfer.
Content Area: Mobility
Integrated Processes: Nursing Process: Implementation
Client Need: Safe and Effective Care Environment; Safety and Infection Control
Cognitive Level: Application

91. **ANSWER: 2.**
Rationales:
1. Identifying a skin lesion during an admission physical is associated with the assessment, not evaluation, step of the nursing process.
2. Determining whether a patient has activity intolerance after ambulation is part of the evaluation step of the nursing process. Evaluation is the process whereby the nurse reassesses the patient after nursing care is provided to identify the patient's response (actual out-

come), which is then compared with the goal/expected outcome identified in the plan of care.
3. Connecting a contributing factor to a problem statement is part of the analysis/diagnosis, not evaluation, step of the nursing process.
4. Formulating an intervention to address a risk factor is part of the planning step of the nursing process as a nurse designs a plan of care to meet patient needs.
Content Area: Nursing Process
Integrated Processes: Nursing Process: Evaluation
Client Need: Safe and Effective Care Environment; Management of Care
Cognitive Level: Analysis

92. **ANSWER: 1.**
Rationales:
1. The nurse should report the fire as soon as the safety of the patient in immediate danger is ensured. This guarantees that additional staff members and the fire department are notified to assist in this emergency. Remember the mnemonic RACE: Rescue, Alarm, Confine, and Extinguish.
2. Attempting to put out the fire is premature and unsafe at this time.
3. Closing all the doors on the unit is premature and unsafe at this time.
4. The evacuation of all patients is premature at this time.
TEST-TAKING TIP: Identify the word in the stem that sets a priority. The word *next* in the stem sets a priority. Identify the option with a specific determiner. Option 4 contains the word *all,* which is a specific determiner. More often than not, an option with a specific determiner is a distractor. Although the word *door* in the stem may be interpreted as a clang association with the word *doors* in option 3, they are different in that the *door to the patient's room* is different than the *doors on the unit.* Although a clang association usually helps you to focus on the correct answer, unfortunately in this question it does not.
Content Area: Safety
Integrated Processes: Nursing Process: Implementation
Client Need: Safe and Effective Care Environment, Safety and Infection Control
Cognitive Level: Analysis

93. **ANSWER: 3.**
Rationales:
1. Nausea and vomiting occur with both hypernatremia and hyponatremia because the resting membrane potential of cells is altered with sodium imbalances.
2. Confusion occurs with both hypernatremia and hyponatremia because altered serum sodium levels interfere with cerebral functioning.
3. Dry, sticky mucous membranes and increased thirst are associated with hypernatremia; hypernatremia is often associated with fluid volume deficit. The compensatory mechanism of thirst should increase the intake of fluid to return the elevated serum sodium level to its expected level of 135 to 145 mEq.
4. Sodium is a component of the sodium-potassium pump

that is involved with muscle contraction. An increase or decrease in serum sodium will result in muscle weakness and fatigue.
Content Area: *Fluid and Electrolyte Balance*
Integrated Processes: *Nursing Process: Assessment*
Client Need: *Physiological Integrity, Physiological Adaptation*
Cognitive Level: *Analysis*

94. ANSWER: 3.
Rationales:
1. Although this regimen may cause a fluid volume deficit, it is not as serious a consequence as another option presented. Fluids can be taken up to 8 hours before the test and intravenous fluids are administered during the test.
2. Although abdominal cramps may result from the cleansing regimen, it will not precipitate a life-threatening condition.
3. Sodium phosphate (Fleet Phospho-Soda) is a saline osmotic that draws water into the intestinal lumen. Bisacodyl (Dulcolax) is an intestinal stimulant that also expands intestinal fluid volume. These medications act together to pull sodium into the intestinal lumen where it is excreted, resulting in a decreased serum sodium level (hyponatremia). Sodium is essential in the functioning of the sodium-potassium pump which is essential for muscle contraction. Hyponatremia can interfere with the contraction of the heart, resulting in dysrhythmias that can be life threatening.
4. This bowel-cleansing regimen will result in stools that will be liquid in consistency. This is the purpose of the regimen; an empty bowel allows for inspection of the intestinal mucosa without being impeded by feces.
Content Area: *Gastrointestinal System*
Integrated Processes: *Nursing Process: Evaluation*
Client Need: *Physiological Integrity; Pharmacological and Parenteral Therapies*
Cognitive Level: *Application*

95. ANSWER: 4.
Rationales:
1. No data demonstrate that the student is blaming others (projection).
2. No data demonstrate the intentional dismissing of the event from the mind and opinions.
3. No data demonstrate that the student is concentrating thoughts and emotions on his inner self (introspection).
4. The student is using intellectual reasoning (intellectualization) to avoid confronting the unconscious conflict and the stress of having to cope with his girlfriend's pregnancy.
Content Area: *Psychosocial and Cultural Support*
Integrated Processes: *Communication/Documentation; Nursing Process: Analysis*
Client Need: *Psychosocial Integrity*
Cognitive Level: *Analysis*

96. ANSWER: 3.
Rationales:
1. This site is appropriate for assessing the femoral pulse. This site should be assessed next if palpation of the popliteal pulse reveals an absent pulse or a pulse volume of 1+.
2. This site is appropriate for assessing the popliteal pulse.

This site should be assessed next if palpation of the dorsalis pedis pulse reveals an absent pulse or a pulse volume of 1+.
3. The next proximal pulse should be assessed in an extremity when a distal peripheral pulse is absent or its pulse volume is 1+. The next site is the posterior tibial pulse. The extent of adequacy or inadequacy of circulation to the extremity must be determined.

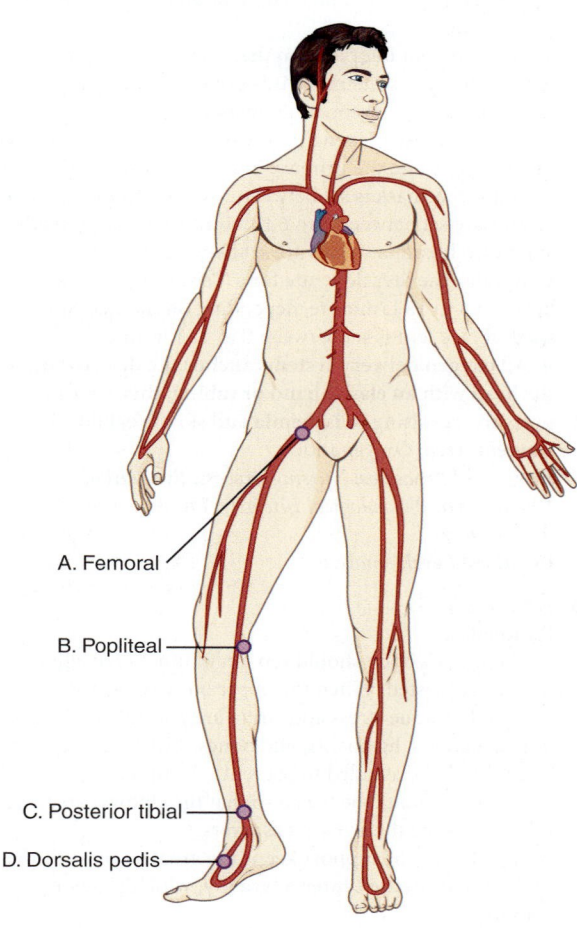

4. This site is appropriate for assessing the dorsalis pedis pulse. The dorsalis pedis pulse is another name for the pedal pulse. The nurse has already identified that the pedal pulse is absent.
Content Area: *Physical Assessment*
Integrated Processes: *Nursing Process: Assessment*
Client Need: *Physiological Integrity; Physiological Adaptation*
Cognitive Level: *Analysis*

97. ANSWER: 1.
Rationales:
1. An involuntary loss of urine without the sensation of the need to void describes reflex incontinence. A relevant factor is spinal cord dysfunction (loss of cerebral awareness or impairment of the reflex arc).
2. Urinary incontinence after a strong sense of urgency to void describes urge incontinence, not reflex incontinence.

Urge incontinence usually is associated with bladder spasms or contractions; also known as an overactive bladder.

3. Experiencing urinary dribbling with increased intra-abdominal pressure (e.g., sneezing, coughing, or lifting with a full bladder) describes stress incontinence, not reflex incontinence. Stress incontinence usually occurs in women who have had numerous pregnancies, a large fetus, or multiple births (e.g., twins, triplets). This also can occur with overflow retention.

4. A weak urinary stream is not associated with reflex incontinence. A weak urinary stream is associated with hyperplasia of the prostate gland or any condition that narrows the diameter of the urethra.

TEST-TAKING TIP: Identify the options that are opposites. Option 1 and option 2 are opposites. More often than not, the correct answer is one of the options that are opposites.

Content Area: Urinary Elimination
Integrated Processes: Communication/Documentation; Nursing Process: Assessment
Client Need: Safe and Effective Care Environment; Reduction of Risk Potential
Cognitive Level: Application

98. ANSWER: 1.
Rationales:

1. **The weight, age, and body surface area of a child must be obtained to individualize a safe, effective analgesic dose specific to the child. The processes of drug absorption, distribution, biotransformation, and excretion, all influenced by age, weight, and body surface area, can alter the safety and effectiveness of a drug.**

2. Although vital signs should be assessed before and after administering an analgesic, this information is not as significant as body weight in determining the appropriate dose of a medication for a child.

3. Although the child's level of pain should be assessed before administering an analgesic, this information does not influence the safe dose for a child.

4. Although this information may influence future doses of analgesics, it is not as essential as another factor.

TEST-TAKING TIP: Identify the word in the stem that sets a priority. The word *most* in the stem sets a priority.

Content Area: Medication Administration
Integrated Processes: Nursing Process: Assessment
Client Need: Physiological Integrity; Pharmacological and Parenteral Therapies
Cognitive Level: Application

99. ANSWER: 3.
Rationales:

1. Food should be avoided 3 hours before bedtime to minimize the risk of regurgitation and aspiration.

2. This is contraindicated in patients with esophageal reflux. Fluids should be avoided 3 hours before bedtime to minimize the risk of regurgitation and aspiration.

3. **Elevating the head of the bed on blocks uses gravity to keep food in the stomach, thereby reducing the risk of regurgitation and aspiration.**

4. The patient should remain in an upright position for at least 1 hour after meals; gravity helps to keep food in the stomach and allows time for food to progress into the jejunum.

TEST-TAKING TIP: Identify the unique option. Option 3 is unique. Options 1, 2, and 3 all relate to something that should be done in relation to food or fluid, while option 3 does not.

Content Area: Nutrition
Integrated Processes: Teaching/Learning; Nursing Process: Implementation
Client Need: Physiological Integrity; Physiological Adaptation
Cognitive Level: Application

100. ANSWER: 2.
Rationales:

1. This action is premature.

2. **The 20 percent increase in the number of falls indicates a need for change. The next step involves identifying the problem. What factors are precipitating the falls?**

3. A variety of strategies should be explored before deciding on a solution.

4. The problem must be identified before potential strategies can be explored.

TEST-TAKING TIP: Identify the word in the stem that sets a priority. The word *next* in the stem sets a priority. Identify options with clang associations. The word *falls* in the stem and in options 2 and 4 are clang associations. Identify the option with a specific determiner. Option 4 contains the word *all,* which is a specific determiner. More often than not, options with specific determiners are distractors, and an option with a clang association is the correct answer.

Content Area: Leadership and Management
Integrated Processes: Nursing Process: Assessment
Client Need: Safe and Effective Care Environment; Management of Care
Cognitive Level: Application

Case Study Answers

Chapter 1

A. 1. Effective breathing promotes the exchange of oxygen and carbon dioxide, which is essential to maintaining life. Air, water, elimination, sleep, activity, sex, and maintenance of body temperature are some of the basic physiological needs necessary for survival. Physiological needs are first level needs according to Maslow's hierarchy of needs.

2. Although fall prevention is important, it is not the patient's priority need. The prevention of falls is related to maintaining patient safety. Safety and security needs are second level needs according to Maslow's hierarchy of needs.

3. Although the patient may have a decreased self-regard, it is not the patient's priority need. Feelings of confidence and self-respect are related to self-esteem needs. Self-esteem needs are fourth level needs according to Maslow's hierarchy of needs.

4. Although the needs to be accepted and loved by another are important, they are not the patient's priority needs. Giving and receiving affection and maintaining positive relationships with significant others and members of the community are related to love and belonging needs, which are third level needs according to Maslow's hierarchy of needs.

B. Data is objective when it can be observed or measured by another person.

1. **Use of accessory muscles of respiration:** People with obstructive lung disease have narrowed airways due to inflammation and mucus and the loss of elastic fibers that cause a lack of expansion and recoil of lung tissue. More effort is required to breathe because of limited airflow. Sinking in of soft tissues adjacent to clavicles and ribs (intercostal, subcostal, and supraclavicular retractions), contraction of the abdominal muscles on exhalation (abdominal breathing), and rising of the shoulders on inhalation (contraction of trapezius muscles) reflect an increased effort to breathe.

2. **Use of pursed lip breathing during exhalation:** The narrowed airways associated with emphysema cause a trapping of air in the alveoli. The alveoli eventually chronically expand, resulting in decreased elastic recoil of the alveoli. On exhalation, the narrowed airways impede the outflow of air, resulting in trapping of air in the alveoli. Exhalation through the mouth with lips positioned to create a small opening (pursed-lip breathing) keeps the alveoli open longer for gas exchange, limits airway constriction, and more efficiently expels trapped air.

3. **Length of exhalation in relation to length of inhalation:** Emphysema is an obstructive airway disorder characterized by difficulty with exhalation. Expanded and weakened alveoli make exhalation difficult because they do not have the ability to move air effectively through the narrowed airways. Exhalation is no longer passive but requires effort. Therefore, it takes longer to move air out of the lungs than into the lungs. In addition, pursed-lip breathing slows the rate of air leaving the lungs, further prolonging exhalation.

4. **Skin color:**
   a. **Pallor, circumoral pallor, or cyanosis, particularly after episodes of intense coughing:** Enlarged alveoli and damaged capillaries in the alveoli impair the exchange of oxygen and carbon dioxide. Changes in skin color indicate a reduction of oxygen to tissues below physiological levels. Mucus and the collapse of respiratory passages precipitate coughing, intensifying the decrease in circulating oxygen levels.
   b. **Yellow or brown discoloration of digits of the hands:** Over time, the nicotine in cigarette smoke causes a superficial discoloration in the skin of the fingers that hold the cigarette.

5. **Presence of clubbing at nail beds of fingers:** Chronic hypoxia results in a proliferation of soft tissue around the terminal phalanges of the fingers.

6. **Extent of respiratory secretions:** The inflammatory process associated with emphysema results in an increase in respiratory secretions. Some of these secretions may be coughed up and expectorated (productive cough) or not (unproductive cough).

7. **Presence of adventitious breath sounds:** Auscultation may reveal loud, coarse, low-pitched sounds heard during inspiration and/or expiration (rhonchi); high-pitched, musical sounds that may be heard throughout inspiration but are more

prominent during expiration (wheezes); and soft, high-pitched, crackling sounds heard at the height of inspiration (crackles). Rhonchi and wheezes are related to narrowed airways due to mucus and inflammation, and crackles are produced by air bubbling through moisture in the alveoli.

8. **Pulse oximetry level:** Pulse oximetry measurement identifies the percentage of arterial oxygen saturation by assessing the percentage of hemoglobin molecules carrying oxygen. The expected value is 95 to 100 percent. A person with chronic hypoxia will have values less than 95 percent.

C. The patient's statement, "The smoking finally got the best of me. I guess I should have stopped smoking when I was diagnosed with emphysema. If I had to do it over, I would do a lot of things differently," indicates that the patient is struggling with Erikson's developmental task of integrity versus despair and tasks related to later maturity in Havighurst's developmental theory. According to Erikson, people 65 years and older are reviewing their life and determining whether their experiences and decisions have been positive or negative. Eventually, they may come to the conclusion that their life accomplishments are acceptable and they develop feelings of self-worth and integrity. On the other hand, if they regret previous actions or decisions, they may develop negative feelings of self-regard and despair. According to Havighurst, tasks that individuals in later maturity are coping with include adjusting to physiological changes of aging and alterations in health. The physiological changes related to aging and emphysema and their impact on quality of life create challenges for the patient.

D. The health belief model proposes that a relationship exists between a person's beliefs and behaviors. The theory stipulates that the likelihood of implementing a healthy action is dependent on several factors.

1. The individual's perceived susceptibility to a disease: The patient in the scenario already has emphysema; it was diagnosed 10 years ago.

2. The individual's perceived severity of the disease: The patient now understands the severity of the disease, as evidenced by the statement: "I have so much phlegm; I cough all the time. I can hardly breathe, and I'm exhausted all the time."

3. The individual's perceived benefits of and perceived barriers to adopting a specific action, as evidenced by the statements, "The smoking finally got the best of me. I guess I should have stopped smoking when I was diagnosed with emphysema. If I had to do it over, I would do a lot of things differently" (benefit) and "I've been smoking since I was 15 years old, but I can't stop" (barrier).

The patient probably did not stop smoking (a major precipitating cause of emphysema) previously because the clinical manifestations of emphysema were tolerable, the pleasures of smoking were more intense than the perceived benefit of stopping smoking, and the patient did not have adequate support systems to make the behavioral change. The patient now is making statements that indicate a readiness for change. However, if the actions are to be implemented and maintained, the patient will require intrapersonal strength, support from significant others, and health-care resources.

Chapter 2

A. Informed consent should be obtained from the infant's mother after the primary health-care provider has given the mother adequate information about the care to be provided. When a patient is an infant, a parent, even if younger than 18 years of age, has the authority to give consent. Because the infant's mother appears dazed and is accompanied by her parent, the nurse must determine whether the mother understands the information surrounding the care to be provided, is giving consent voluntarily, and is alert and has intact cognition. When a person is incapable of participating in the decision-making process (e.g., is an infant or child or has impaired cognition), a surrogate decision maker must be identified. Most states specify the order of priority, such as parents of minors, durable power of attorney for health care, court-appointed guardian, spouse, or partner.

B. 1. This question is inappropriate. It is a probing question that violates the person's rights to privacy. The only purpose this question serves is to satisfy the nurse's curiosity.

2. This question is appropriate. Alcohol crosses the placenta and can negatively impact a fetus, resulting in health problems in the infant during the neonatal period.

3. This question is inappropriate because it is prying into personal information that has no bearing on the present situation. It is a probing question that violates the person's rights to privacy. The mother is the infant's legal guardian. Legally, the father does not have to be involved in the infant's care.

4. This question is appropriate. Many drugs can cross the placenta and negatively impact a fetus, resulting in health problems in the infant during the neonatal period.

5. This question is appropriate. Health problems in a pregnant woman, whether they are related or unrelated to the pregnancy, may negatively impact a fetus, resulting in health problems in the infant during the neonatal period.

6. This question is inappropriate at this time. The mother of the infant appeared dazed, did not make eye contact, and rarely answered the nurse's questions during the initial assessment. The infant's and mother's physical and emotional conditions must be assessed and addressed before future plans can be explored.

C. The nurse intentionally touched the mother in an angry manner when the nurse grabbed the mother's arm and pulled her back to the unit, saying firmly, "Where do you think you are going? Stay here. Your baby needs you!" The nurse's behavior constitutes battery, which occurs when someone touches a person's body or clothing or anything held by or attached to the person in an angry, willful, negligent, or violent manner without consent.

D. The triage nurse made the following statement, "The baby's mother is on drugs. She had no business getting pregnant in the first place." This statement was made without any verifiable data and was made loud enough for other health team members to hear. The nurse could be liable for slander, a form of defamation. Defamation, a quasi-intentional tort, occurs when false, derogatory information is communicated to others that harms a person's reputation, holds the person up to ridicule or contempt, or causes the person to be avoided.

Chapter 3

A. 1. The director of nursing seems to prefer the transformational leadership style. The director has a vision that nurses should be expanding their roles within the profession of nursing and implementing evidence-based practice. The statement made to the nurse managers incorporated the director of nursing's vision concerning these topics; was optimistic and energetic; and attempted to inspire others to be committed to the initiative.

2. The nurse manager of the medical unit seems to prefer the autocratic leadership style. The nurse manager was controlling, did not involve staff members in designing the project, and made decisions for the unit. This autocratic style stifles creativity and ultimately may limit commitment of others to the initiative.

B. 1. The director of nursing seems to prefer theory Y of human relations–oriented management, as evidenced by the director's involvement of the nurse managers in identifying a goal (conducting a research project) and inspiring them to achieve it. The director also gave the nurse managers and staff nurses the autonomy to achieve the goal and ensured that a consultant would be hired to support and assist them in attaining the goal. Approaches that encourage participation and creativity and provide support and appreciation are typical of a person who believes in theory Y management.

2. The nurse manager of the medical unit seems to prefer theory X of human relations–oriented management. An authoritarian approach with strict rules and threats of consequences ("I expect you all to participate in this project and, if you don't, I will have to include that information in your next evaluation.") are typical of a person who believes in theory X management.

C. Examples of resistance.

1. The nurse manager's statements: "I can't believe we are now going to have to do research projects. Don't you think we do enough already?" and "We are going to be conducting a research project on our unit. I am not thrilled about having to do this, but we have no choice." Both of these statements were attempts to influence others to reach a negative attitude regarding the initiative.

2. The nurse manager's statement: "Let's talk with the other nurse managers and see if we can reverse this decision." This statement reflects an attempt to organize resistance.

3. Two nurse mangers did not attend the meeting, stating that they were too busy, and one nurse manager took a day off to avoid the meeting. These avoidance behaviors are forms of passive resistance.

D. 1. **Power of authority:** Both the director of nursing and nurse managers have power by virtue of their positions within the organization.

2. **Power of coercion:** The nurse manager of the medical unit used the power of coercion when threatening staff members with a negative evaluation if they did not participate in the initiative.

3. **Power of expertise:** The director of nursing assured the nurse managers that the budget had enough money to hire a nurse researcher to assist the nurses with their projects.

Chapter 4

A. Immunizations are a form of primary health care. Primary health care focuses on maintaining an optimum level of wellness and implementing interventions to decrease the risk of disease or disability.

B. Complete physical examinations, bone density testing, and mammograms are forms of secondary health care. Secondary health care focuses on early detection and intervention to cure disease and minimize further impairment. Treatment includes acute medical care and surgery.

C. Receiving physical therapy and modifying a home to support a person's independence and safety are associated with tertiary health care. Tertiary health care focuses on rehabilitation, health restoration, and palliative care. It maximizes the ability to accomplish activities of daily living, which supports independence in light of a chronic or irreversible condition.

D. Hospice care focuses on maintaining comfort and quality of life for dying patients and provides emotional support for grieving family members. The location of hospice care varies depending on the patient's condition and the ability of family members to provide care at home. This family has indicated the desire to care for their loved one at home, so services (e.g., direct physical care, management of pain, emotional support, and advocacy within the health-care system) should be made available to assist them with this goal.

Chapter 5

A. Although older adults, immigrants, and homeless migrant workers have characteristics unique to their group, they share common factors that make them all vulnerable populations. These issues include:

1. They tend to be powerless. Older adults are not revered in American society, many immigrants are not citizens and cannot vote, and migrant workers also may be immigrants and do not live in one area to enlist the aid of local social and governmental agencies.

2. They frequently have inadequate financial resources and lack economic status. Older adults may have limited retirement funds or excessive health-care expenses that have exhausted their retirement savings. Immigrants and migrant workers may have a limited ability to speak the English language or lack the education to obtain an adequate-paying job. The inability to obtain a high-paying job is further intensified if the individual is an illegal immigrant because the person does not have a U.S. Permanent Resident Card (green card) that permits nationals of other countries to reside and work in the United States.

3. They may lack access to health care. Lack of access may result from older adults being homebound because of physical disability or the inability to own or drive a car. Immigrants may not understand how to obtain health care in the United States or may be afraid of deportation if the authorities identify that they are illegal immigrants. Migrant workers are constantly moving because the availability of work depends on harvest times or they work in rural areas where health care is sparse.

4. They may engage in unhealthy behaviors. For a variety of reasons, such as physical inability to provide self-care, lack of information, unhealthy cultural practices, or lack of a home environment to meet basic hygienic needs, people may engage in unwholesome behaviors. These behaviors may result in such problems as inadequate nutrition, increased risk of infection, and exposure to abuse, neglect, or violence.

5. They have a higher probability of developing illness (morbidity), less favorable outcomes after receiving care, and have a higher incidence of death (mortality) than other populations because they have a multiplicity of stressors that challenge the health-care delivery system.

B. 1. **Epidemiologist:** The nurse conducted surveillance and monitoring activities and identified that older adults, immigrants, and homeless migrant workers were at-risk populations within the community. Assessment of the community is essential to identify trends in health and risk factors that threaten specific populations within a community. A comprehensive database is the foundation of planning and implementing effective initiatives to help meet the health needs of a community.

2. **Teacher:** The nurse planned or implemented educational programs to increase the knowledge of the members of the community. Knowledge helps to empower people to provide better self-care.

3. **Advocate:** The nurse collaborated with social, religious, and governmental agencies to encourage the provision of services for the identified vulnerable populations. A society has a responsibility to provide help for the physically, emotionally, and financially disadvantaged so that they can eventually become self-sufficient.

4. **Change agent:** The nurse met with governmental representatives to campaign for changes in immigration laws. Vulnerable populations often are powerless and require the assistance of others to help effect change on their behalf.

C. 1. **The nurse collaborated with others.** The nurse collaborated and cooperated with community-based organizations (e.g., social and religious organizations) and the department of social services on behalf of the identified populations to provide appropriate services.

2. **The nurse provided care for individuals across the life span.** The nurse developed educational programs related to prenatal care, child safety, nutrition, weight reduction, and smoking cessation.

3. **The nurse maintained open communication.** The nurse routinely communicated with members of the community and the organizations involved with the delivery of care.

D. Inaccessibility to health care may be due to a lack of financial resources (e.g., no health insurance, low socioeconomic status), social issues (e.g., concern about being identified as an illegal immigrant, embarrassment about a type of illness), or physical inability to be present where health care is provided (e.g., living in a rural area that does not have services, lack of transportation, too frail to travel). To overcome these barriers to health care, nurses should:

1. Provide emotional and culturally sensitive care.
2. Provide dignified, respectful, and nonjudgmental care.
3. Engage patients in the planning process to ensure that they have input and a vested interest in goal achievement.
4. Collaborate with other health-care professionals to ensure that comprehensive care is planned and implemented.
5. Make referrals to appropriate community resources and services.
6. Coordinate home-based care if the patient is unable to leave the home.
7. Bring mobile health-care clinics to the population's specific geographic location.
8. Arrange for transportation and child care to facilitate attendance at appointments.
9. Arrange for telehealth care when appropriate.
10. Arrange for participation in economic support programs, such as food stamps, Medicaid, and the WIC program.

Chapter 6

A. Assessments that meet developmental norms.
1. Turns from abdomen to back and from back to abdomen. *This task is usually achieved by age 6 months.*
2. Holds on to the mother and refuses to go to the nurse. *Fear of strangers is common by age 6 to 8 months.*
3. Reacts to simple commands. *This task occurs by age 9 months.*
4. Enjoys peek-a-boo. *This task occurs by age 7 months.*

Assessments that indicate a developmental delay.
1. Is not sitting. *This task is expected by age 7 months.*
2. Is not crawling or pulling self up. *This task is expected by age 9 months.*
3. Is not using a pincer grasp. *This task is expected by age 9 months.*

B. Data typically associated with toddlers.
1. Sucks thumb while holding a security blanket. *These actions are common toddler behaviors that provide self-comfort.*

2. Is fearful of loud noises. *Fear is a common response of toddlers to loud noises because they may perceive it as a threat.*
3. Is always saying "mine" and "no." *Saying "mine" is associated with an increased concept of ownership and the egocentric nature of toddlers. Saying "no" is related to the need to be independent and is common during toddlerhood.*

Data that raise a cause for concern.
1. Has 14 teeth. *This finding reflects a developmental delay because a toddler should have 20 teeth.*
2. Has made no progress with daytime bladder and bowel control. *Daytime bowel and bladder control should be achieved by age 3 years.*

C. 1. **Cluster:** Climbs stairs using right foot first for each step; hops on two feet. *Most children are able to climb stairs while alternating their feet by age 3 years. Most children are able to hop on one foot by age 4 years.*
   Nursing intervention: Consult with the primary health-care provider to ensure that the child is evaluated by a physical therapist and receives physical therapy. Teach the mother to praise the child's accomplishments and to provide supervision, especially when climbing stairs, to maintain safety.

2. **Cluster:** Needs help with dressing and undressing; is unable to tie shoes. *By age 5 years, children should have the coordination to dress and undress themselves and tie their shoes.*
   Nursing intervention: Consult with the primary health-care provider to ensure that the child is evaluated by an occupational therapist and receives occupational therapy. Teach the mother to praise the child's accomplishments, encourage self-care activities of daily living, encourage choices, and provide toys that require fine motor skills (e.g., threading beads, age-appropriate crafts, and age-appropriate construction sets).

3. **Cluster:** Does not print letters; has a limited vocabulary. *Children who are 5 years old should be able to print a few letters. By age 3 years, children should know 900 words; by age 4 years, children should know 1,500 words; and by age 5 years, children should know 2,100 words.*
   Nursing intervention: Arrange for the child's school district to provide an educational evaluation and receive educational support. Teach the mother to praise the child's progress, work with the child using appropriate activity books that support success, and read to the child.

4. **Cluster:** Is difficult to understand when speaking; has a limited vocabulary. *Children should have totally intelligible speech by age 5 years and should know 2,100 words.*
   Nursing intervention: Consult with the primary health-care provider to ensure that the child is

evaluated by a speech therapist and receives speech therapy. Teach mother to follow-through with speech exercises daily.

D. 1. Demonstrate some simple chair exercises that the grandmother can accomplish several times a day. *These exercises will increase muscle tone and strength.*

2. Teach safety precautions, such as principles associated with using a walker, the need to keep feet wide apart for a wide base of support, and the need to rise slowly. Also suggest removing any scatter rugs from the environment. *These actions will reduce the risk of a fall.*

3. Assess the grandmother for the risk of suicide. *Risk of suicide increases secondary to multiple losses, such as loss of husband and loss of home and friends due to moving into the daughter's home.*

4. Spend some time encouraging the grandmother to reminisce. *Reminiscence is a component of the task of integrity versus despair associated with older adulthood.*

5. Suggest that the daughter give her mother simple chores to do, such as folding laundry or reading to the toddler and 5-year-old. *These activities contribute to a feeling of task accomplishment and contribution to family life, which should support self-esteem.*

6. Assess the patient's perineal area. *This assessment provides information necessary to establish a skin care program to maintain skin integrity.*

Chapter 7

A. 1. The nurse pulled a curtain around the patient's stretcher. *This action provides some privacy and communicates respect.*

2. The nurse made eye contact with the patient. *This action communicates that the nurse's attention is focused on the patient.*

3. The nurse introduced himself and explained what he was going to do. *This action supports the patient's right to know who is providing care and what is going to be done.*

4. The nurse faced the patient at the head of the bed. *Facing a patient enables the patient to see the nurse's face, particularly the lips, which facilitates the reception of verbal messages. In addition, it projects the nurse's voice toward the patient, not away from the patient.*

5. The nurse asked the patient's preference regarding the daughter and grandson staying or leaving the area during the interview. *This action supports the patient's right to make personal decisions regarding confidentiality and demonstrates respect for the patient. Also, the daughter's presence may contribute to the patient's emotional comfort.*

B. 1. The emergency department was filled with noise and commotion. *These can be distracting and interfere with reception of messages.*

2. The stretcher was placed in the alcove of a hallway. *This action does not provide for complete privacy and makes it difficult to communicate due to a noisy, distracting environment.*

3. The grandson was pulling on the bed linen at the foot of the patient's bed. *The grandson's behavior can be distracting.*

4. The nurse was unable to sit at the bedside when conducting the interview because of the hazard of the chair blocking the hallway. *Standing may convey that the nurse is in a rush and not focused on the patient.*

5. The daughter and grandson were at the patient's bedside. *The presence of the daughter and grandson may prevent the patient from being open to discuss information that the patient does not want them to know.*

C. 1. The nurse observed the patient's nonverbal behavior. The nurse identified that the patient was grimacing and rubbing her right hip; breathing in short, shallow breaths; shaking her head from side to side; and closing her eyes before speaking. These behaviors indicate that the patient may be having pain. The nurse should ask appropriate questions in relation to the observations that indicate that the patient may be having pain. *This ensures that the nonverbal behavior is congruent with what the patient verbalizes before concluding that the patient is in pain.*

2. The nurse made a reflective statement: "It must be frustrating to know that you did everything right and still had something like this happen." *Reflection encourages further discussion by focusing on emotional themes and feelings. In addition, it indicates active listening.*

3. The nurse asked direct questions, such as, "What is the intensity of your pain on a scale of 0 to 10?" and "Tell me the location of the pain and what it feels like." *A direct question is used to collect objective information rapidly. In an emergency situation, the nurse wants to quickly obtain information about the location, intensity, and characteristic of the patient's pain.*

4. The nurse asked a clarifying question: "Can you explain in more detail what you mean by 'crazy'?" The patient's message was unclear. *The nurse's response encouraged the patient to elaborate and explain more fully what was meant by the word "crazy."*

5. The nurse touched the patient's arm when the patient began to cry. *Touch communicates caring, concern, and encouragement.*

6. The nurse used the technique of validation by stating, "It's okay to cry. You had a lot happen

to you today." *The first sentence demonstrated acceptance of the patient's crying. The second sentence corroborated that the patient experienced a difficult event.*

D. 1. The nurse used medical jargon when using the word ORIF (which stands for "open-reduction internal fixation"). *Using medical jargon communicates a lack of interest in the patient's understanding of the situation. It also communicates a demeanor of superiority and even arrogance.*

2. The nurse provided false reassurance by saying, "Everything is going to be fine." *False reassurance minimizes the patient's concerns and violates trust.*

3. The nurse demonstrated nonacceptance of the patient's feelings by saying, "Try to be strong and a good role model for your grandson." *This statement could be interpreted as the nurse saying, "Stop your crying. You're being a big baby."*

Chapter 8

A. 1. **Situational.**
   a. Single parent after abandonment by wife.
   b. Hospitalization and rehabilitation that will require prolonged medical treatment.
   c. Children living with neighbors.
   d. On medical leave from his job.

2. **Psychosocial.**
   a. Inability to provide for the daily care of his children.
   b. High cost of hospitalization and rehabilitation.
   c. Fears about how his appearance will affect his relationship with his children and coworkers.
   d. Altered body image and other physiological and physical changes as a result of the initial injury and healing ("I look like a monster").
   e. Potential for altered family dynamics associated with separation from his children.
   f. Financial concerns related to an inability to work, high cost of hospitalization and rehabilitation, and possible inadequate health insurance.

3. **Developmental.**
   a. Stress of raising three children with little help.
   b. Potential inability to be a wage earner and provide for his children.

4. **Microbiological.**
   a. Risk for microbiological stress as a result of multiple open wounds due to the burn injury.
   b. Potential for decreased immune status due to multiplicity of stresses.

5. **Physiological.**
   a. Pain associated with the burn injury and its treatment.
   b. Potential for fluid and electrolyte imbalances related to the consequences of the burn injury.

B. 1. **Stressors:** See answers to question number 1.

2. **Appearance:** Partial-thickness burns (erythema and blanching with pressure) on the neck, hands, and lower arms, involving more than 12 percent of the body, and patches of deep-partial-thickness burns (erythema, moist blebs, and blisters) on the face, chest, and anterior upper arms, involving 5 percent of the body. Singed hair on the forehead and sides of the head, absence of eyebrows and eyelashes, singed nostril hair, and sooty sputum noted.

3. **General attitude:** Openly and willingly shared concerns and feelings. Maintained eye contact most of the time.

4. **Activity and behavior:** Increase in muscle tension, voice tremors when talking, and restlessness, as evidenced by nervously moving about in bed and shaking a lower leg; gestures congruent with expressed feelings, evidenced by shaking his head, shrugging his shoulders, and drawing his hand across his throat as if he were cutting his throat.

5. **Sensory and cognitive status:** Alert and oriented to time, place, and person. Able to recall events surrounding the fire. Appropriately receiving and responding to verbal messages.

6. **Thought processes:** Thought processes were well organized, but talked in a rapid manner when discussing the fire. Content of verbalizations indicated suicide ideation: "Maybe it would be better for the kids if I just killed myself."

7. **Judgment and insight:** Stated, "I have been able to deal with what life has tossed at me because I always want to do right by my kids, but this is more than I can handle. Maybe it would be better for the kids if I just killed myself."

8. **Mood:** Patient's data indicate depression as evidenced by a sad facial expression and tone of voice, the comment "Maybe it would be better if I just killed myself," slumped posture, and avoidance of eye contact at times. Patient data such as increased muscle tension, rapid talking when discussing the event, voice tremors when talking, and restless behavior (e.g., nervously moving about in bed, shaking a lower leg) indicate anxiety.

9. **Affect:** Varied emotional expression based on content of verbalization. Affect was congruent with mood.

10. **Speech:** Talked in a rapid manner when discussing the event, exhibited voice tremors when talking, and at times was hesitant when he became emotional.

11. **Self-concept, self-esteem, and body image:** Said he was able to deal with what life had tossed his way in the past but that this event was more than he could handle; believes that he looks like a

monster; afraid that his face may scare his children and that he may have to get a new job that enables him to stay in the house so that he does not scare others.

12. **Perception:** No altered perception identified.
13. **Impulse control:** No evidence of a lack of impulse control.
14. **Potential for violence:** Risk for suicide as evidenced by the statement, "Maybe it would be better for the kids if I just killed myself."
15. **Family and social systems:** No evidence of family other than children. One neighbor is caring for his three children until other arrangements can be made.
16. **Spiritual status:** No evidence of spiritual status at this time.
17. **Presence of anxiety:** Demonstrating an increase in muscle tension, rapid talking when discussing the event, voice tremors when talking, and restless behavior (e.g., nervously moving about in bed, shaking a lower leg). Several comments indicate that he was worried about finances, anticipation of his children's and coworkers' responses to his appearance, and the need for a change in job in the future.
18. **Use of defense mechanisms:** Used projection when he told his children to "be strong." Used suppression when he said, "This is really going to set me back, but I am not going to worry about that now."

C. The patient's statement, "Maybe it would be better for the kids if I just killed myself," is the most important piece of data. Suicide ideation can progress to actual suicide.

D.
1. Provide constant observation and a safe environment.
2. Identify if the patient's behavior involves giving away possessions or putting affairs in order as precursors to a suicide attempt.
3. Ask the patient whether he has a plan and means to carry out suicide.
4. Encourage writing a no-suicide contract.
5. Focus on strengths rather than weaknesses.
6. Address factors that precipitated the suicide crisis.
7. Encourage exploration of consequences of suicide, such as impact on others if successful, feelings about death, and reasons for living.
8. Assist with problem-solving; help the patient to prioritize problems and focus on one at a time.
9. Help the patient write a list of sources of support, community resources, and ways to ask for help.
10. Accept feelings of worthlessness, helplessness, and powerlessness as real to the patient.

11. Minimize isolation; involve the patient in activities.
12. Assist the patient to identify and replace self-deprecating thoughts with positive thoughts through cognitive restructuring.
13. Avoid false reassurance and overly cheerfulness.
14. Implement measures to support self-esteem.
15. Monitor risk of suicide as depression lifts and energy increases.

Chapter 9

A. The nurse addressed all three learning domains.
1. **Cognitive domain:** During the patient's initial hospitalization, the nurse discussed information about diabetes, made a referral to a nutritionist to provide dietary teaching, and reinforced this teaching at mealtimes. During the counseling center visit, the nurse gave the patient written materials and a CD about diabetes and related self-care activities.
2. **Affective domain:** During hospitalization, the nurse initially gave the patient the opportunity to discuss his shock and disbelief that he had diabetes, and then the nurse met with the patient daily to explore the patient's feelings about having diabetes. During the counseling center visit, the nurse continued to explore the patient's feelings and concerns to identify the etiology of the patient's nonadherence to the medical regimen. The nurse recommended that the patient attend a support group for patients with diabetes.
3. **Psychomotor domain:** Before hospital discharge, the nurse taught the patient how to perform SBGM and self-administer a subcutaneous injection. During the counseling center visit, the nurse reviewed SBGM and self-administration of a subcutaneous injection and had the patient perform return demonstrations.

B.
1. **The patient is a kinesthetic learner.** A kinesthetic learner learns best when processing information by doing. The patient stated, "I learn new things better if I can actually do what I am supposed to do."
2. **The patient has an external locus of control.** A person who has an external locus of control generally is motivated by pressure or rewards outside of the self, not from within. The patient stated, "My wife would kill me if I didn't come this time" and "My wife is on my tail all the time. She doesn't let me out of the house without me taking the insulin."

C.
1. **The patient was in denial.** The patient stated, "I can't believe I have to take insulin. No one in my family who has diabetes has to take insulin," and he failed to adhere to the medical regimen. The

wife stated, "He's had type 2 diabetes for several years, but he didn't take his pills consistently then and he doesn't take his insulin consistently now, never does the fingerstick test, and eats anything he wants."

2. The patient did not attend the first scheduled follow-up visit at the diabetes counseling center. The patient came to the next visit because of coercion by his wife. The patient stated, "My wife would kill me if I didn't come this time."

3. The patient stipulates, "I am not going to give myself insulin at work where everyone can see."

D. 1. **Learning takes place within the learner:** The nurse collected information about what the patient already knew about diabetes so that teaching could move from what was familiar to the unknown. The nurse matched teaching strategies to the patient's learning style (kinesthetic learner) and learning needs (SBGM and self-administration of a subcutaneous injection) when using the teaching strategy of demonstration and return demonstration of self-care skills.

2. **Learning occurs best in an environment that is physically and emotionally conducive to learning:** The nurse addressed the patient's fears and concerns on several occasions before beginning teaching SBGM and self-administration of a subcutaneous injection.

3. **Motivation facilitates learning:** The nurse identified patient behaviors that indicated the patient's lack of readiness to learn (e.g., patient statements indicating denial, failure to attend a counseling appointment, nonadherence to the medical regimen) and explored the patient's feelings and concerns to determine the cause of nonadherence to the medical regimen. The nurse accepted the patient nonjudgmentally and delayed teaching psychomotor skills.

4. **Literacy, language, and communication are essential components of the teaching and learning process:** The nurse in the hospital used repetition of information in the teaching plan to reinforce learning. The nurse met with the patient daily to discuss information about diabetes, explored the patient's feelings about having diabetes, and reviewed the principles of a diabetic diet at mealtimes. During the follow-up counseling visit a nurse again explored the patient's feelings and concerns and reinforced previous teaching. During the visit the nurse demonstrated the procedures for SBGM and self-administration of a subcutaneous injection and had the patient perform return demonstrations. The nurse also gave the patient booklets with illustrations and a CD about these procedures.

E. 1. **One-to-one discussion:** In the hospital, the nurse met with the patient daily and discussed information about diabetes, explored the patient's feelings about having diabetes, and reviewed the diabetic diet at mealtimes. At the subsequent counseling center visit, the nurse primarily provided care in the affective domain by exploring the patient's feelings and concerns and referring the patient to a support group. This patient was attempting to cope emotionally with a chronic health problem with multiple lifestyle changes. One-to-one discussion promotes the nurse-patient relationship, allows the nurse to individualize instruction so that it is patient centered, and provides an opportunity to address identified concerns

2. **Demonstration:** In the hospital and the subsequent counseling center visit, the nurse demonstrated how to perform SBGM and self-administer a subcutaneous injection. The nurse also had the patient perform a return demonstration of these skills. This patient was a kinesthetic learner who learns best when processing information by doing. Demonstration involves hands-on manipulation of equipment with time to practice a skill. During a return demonstration, the nurse can evaluate the patient's performance and intervene immediately if further teaching is required. This approach is especially useful when learning a psychomotor skill.

3. **Support group:** The patient was referred to a support group for individuals with diabetes. The patient was initially having difficulty accepting the diagnosis and adjusting to the medical regimen. A group provides an opportunity for two or more individuals to interact, thereby enhancing learning with the exchange of information. It is particularly effective when addressing issues related to feelings and concerns (affective domain).

F. 1. **Printed materials:** The nurse gave the patient printed materials about diabetes while the patient was in the hospital and provided additional printed materials (e.g., booklets and written instructions with illustrations about self-care procedures) when the patient attended the follow-up counseling session. Written materials support the comprehension of complex concepts and relationships, can be read at the learner's own pace, provide reinforcement of verbal instruction and psychomotor skills, and can be in the patient's first language.

2. **Audiovisual aids:** The nurse gave the patient a CD that included a demonstration of SBGM and self-administration of a subcutaneous injection. Audiovisual aids present information that stimulates both the eyes and ears. A CD can be used to provide new information or reinforce previous learning.

3. **Equipment and models:** The nurse taught SBGM and administration of a subcutaneous injection in the hospital and during the follow-up counseling session. Blood glucose monitoring equipment, a syringe, a vial, and a model of a patient's abdomen were used to learn the skills necessary for self-care. These items stimulate learning because the patient has the opportunity to touch and manipulate actual equipment that will be used in the home. The use of equipment and models is extremely effective when teaching psychomotor skills.

Chapter 10

A. 1. **Inspection**
   a. Skin pale and intact.
   b. Nail beds pale.
   c. Respirations 23 breaths/minute.
   d. Temperature 97.8°F with temporal scanner thermometer.
   e. Clean and well-groomed appearance.
2. **Auscultation.**
   a. Apical pulse rate 95 beats/minute.
   b. Blood pressure 160/86 mm Hg.
   c. Vesicular breath sounds.
   d. Slight expiratory wheeze.
   e. Hyperactive bowel sounds.
3. **Percussion.**
   a. Tympany when the abdomen is percussed.
4. **Palpation.**
   a. Skin dry, warm, and tenting.
   b. Delayed capillary refill.
   c. Slight abdominal distention over suprapubic area.
   d. No lower extremity edema.
B. 1. Patient has felt bloated and uncomfortable in the abdominal area for the past several months.
2. Patient does not feel that he empties the bladder fully after voiding.
3. Patient is afraid that he might become impotent and experience urinary incontinence after the surgery.
4. Patient trusts the urologist.
5. Patient verbalizes that he recognizes that the surgery is necessary.
6. Patient stated, "Having cancer puts a big monkey wrench into my retirement plans. I hope I'll live long enough to do a little traveling."
7. Wife stated, "I don't care if we can't travel. I don't want my husband to die."
C. 1. The patient is the only primary source of data. The patient is the most valuable source of data because the data collected are most recent, unique, and specific to the patient. Only the patient can exhibit clinical indicators and share sensations, feelings, and concerns.

2. The wife is a secondary source of data. A spouse or other family member can provide supplemental information about a patient, such as communicating the patient's likes and dislikes, functioning before and after the occurrence of the health problem, and similarities and differences in the patient's behavior.
3. The primary health-care provider is a secondary source of data. A primary health-care provider provides supplemental information about the patient within the patient's frame of reference.
4. The nurse is a secondary source of data. A nurse provides supplemental information about the patient within the patient's frame of reference.
5. There are no tertiary sources of data in the scenario. Tertiary sources of data include sources such as textbooks, policy and procedure manuals, and commonalities among patients with comparable health problems.

D.
1. Risk for urinary retention related to <u>outlet obstruction</u> secondary to <u>enlarged prostate</u>.
2. Fear of impotence and incontinence related to <u>effects of prostatic surgery</u> secondary to cancer of the prostate.
3. Disturbed sleep pattern related to <u>numerous nighttime awakenings</u> secondary to cancer of the prostate.
4. Situational low self-esteem related to <u>urinary incontinence</u> secondary to <u>urinary urgency</u>.
5. Urge incontinence related to <u>outlet obstruction</u> secondary to <u>an enlarged prostate</u>.

Chapter 11

A. 1. Thermometer to obtain the patient's body temperature.
2. Sphygmomanometer and stethoscope to obtain the patient's blood pressure.
3. Pulse oximetry machine to obtain the patient's oxygen saturation level.
4. Stethoscope to listen to the patient's apical pulse, breath sounds, and bowel sounds.
5. Ophthalmoscope to assess the patient's red eye reflex.
6. Otoscope to assess the patient's external auditory canal.
B. 1. **Inspection:** The nurse observed the movement of the patient's chest or abdomen to determine the rate and depth of respirations and the intercostal, supraclavicular, and trapezius muscles to determine the degree of effort necessary for breathing. The nurse inspected the external auditory canal to determine the presence of cerumen. The nurse inspected the eyes to identify that they were glazed

and had a limited red eye reflex. The nurse also observed the abdomen to determine if it appeared distended.

2. **Auscultation:** The nurse used auscultation to obtain the patient's blood pressure, to listen to the lungs to determine the presence of adventitious breath sounds (e.g., crackles), and to listen to the abdomen to identify the extent of bowel sounds.

3. **Percussion:** The nurse used percussion to identify musical sounds associated with air in the stomach or intestines (tympany).

4. **Palpation:** The nurse used palpation to determine the presence of distension of the abdomen.

C. 1. **Presence and volume of peripheral pulses:** The nurse should assess the peripheral pulses, beginning with the most distal in the extremity and progressing to the most proximal (e.g., begin with the dorsalis pedis, then the posterior tibial, and finally the popliteal). They should be assessed for presence, strong volume (obliterated only with moderate pressure), and symmetry. Absent or weak pulses and asymmetry of pulses indicate impaired arterial circulation.

2. **Length of capillary refill:** Compression of the nail bed or tip of the toe should occlude circulation in the capillary bed, causing the area to appear blanched. Release of compression should result in return of circulation and the color that was present before the compression. This assessment should take less than 3 seconds if cardiac output and circulation to the distal extremity are adequate. If capillary refill takes longer than 3 seconds, further assessment of the cardiovascular system is required.

3. **Color and texture of nails:** The color under nails should be a variation of pink, and the nails should be translucent. If the toenails are thick, yellow, and brittle, the patient might have inadequate circulation to the distal extremity or a fungal infection under the nail.

4. **Color, texture, and temperature of skin:** Inspection should reveal that the skin is similar in color to the rest of the patient's body and its texture is smooth and supple. The skin should be warm to the touch. If the skin is pale, mottled, or red in color, the texture is rough and dry, and the surface temperature is cool to the touch, distal arterial circulation is impaired.

5. **Sensation:** The patient should be able to tell what toes are being touched and distinguish between dull and sharp stimuli (e.g., cotton ball versus end of a paper clip). Impaired sensation indicates peripheral nervous system impairment.

6. **Mobility:** The patient should be able to curl toes downward (flexion), straighten toes (extension),

spread toes apart (abduction), and bring toes together (adduction). If the patient is unable to perform range of motion of the toes, motor function may be impaired.

D. A systematic approach must be used when auscultating for sounds produced by the heart, lungs, and intestines to ensure that all areas of significance are assessed. In addition, an appropriate amount of time should be spent at each location, particularly when sounds are complex, difficult to hear, or infrequent.

Chapter 12

A. The nurse should collect the wound specimen for C&S first, before the first dose of antibiotic is administered.

B. 1. Place the patient in a private room or cohort the patient with another patient who has the same microorganism after the patient's organism is identified and after consultation with infection control personnel.

2. Implement hand hygiene before entering and when leaving the patient's room.

3. Don gloves and a gown after hand hygiene before entering the patient's room.

4. When leaving the room but while still inside the room, untie the ties at the waist, remove gloves, untie ties of the mask and dispose of the mask in an appropriate trash container, and remove the gown by touching only the inside of the gown and place it in an appropriate trash container.

5. Wear other PPE (e.g., mask and face shield) if splashing of body fluids is anticipated.

6. Dedicate patient-care equipment so that microorganisms are not transmitted to others via multiple use.

7. Limit the patient's movement outside of the isolation room to medically necessary purposes. Infected or colonized areas of the body must be contained and covered when the patient is transported outside the room for essential medical purposes. Two people should transport the patient. One person is responsible for touching unclean surfaces, such as elevator buttons, and one person is gowned and gloved ready to care for the patient if necessary.

C. 1. Importance of leaving belongings in the ante room outside the patient's isolation room.

2. Importance of and proper methods for implementing hand hygiene (i.e., use soap and water meticulously for 15 seconds) before entering the room and putting on an isolation gown and gloves.

3. Proper removal of contaminated gloves and gown without contaminating self or the environment.

4. Proper disposal of contaminated gloves and gown without contaminating the environment.

5. Importance of and proper method for implementing hand hygiene after disposing of contaminated gloves and gown and before leaving the patient's room.

D. Yes. Alcohol-based and non-alcohol-based hand sanitizers can be used to reduce the risk of transmission of MRSA when soap and water are not available. However, hand hygiene with soap and water is most effective in preventing the spread of bacterial pathogens.

Chapter 13

A. 1. Impaired mobility associated with left-sided hemiplegia that required a sling on the left arm and a below-the-knee leg brace to prevent foot-drop and facilitate walking increased the patient's risk of a fall.

2. The patient is 72 years old. With age, flexibility, muscle strength, voluntary and autonomic reflexes, and cognitive awareness or ability to manage multiple incoming stimuli decline.

3. Lasix might have caused positional hypotension when the patient suddenly stood at the side of the bed, resulting in syncope and a fall.

4. Scatter rugs are unstable objects that can precipitate a fall.

B. The priority concern is the patient's safety. The patient is confused; she is not aware of the time of day or that she is in a hospital. She is receiving an opioid for pain, which can cause lethargy and reduce cognition and perception. In addition, she is trying to get out of the bed immediately after orthopedic surgery while attached to intravenous tubing and a urinary retention catheter. The scenario provides no evidence that the patient is experiencing hemorrhage. The dressing is dry and intact and vital signs are within expected limits, indicating hemodynamic stability and absence of blood loss. The patient is receiving IV fluids and is voiding a sufficient quantity of urine hourly; therefore, fluid balance is not the priority. The patient rates her pain as a level 3 on a 0-to-10 pain scale, which is considered tolerable; therefore, pain control is not an issue at this time.

C. 1. Ensure that the patient is wearing an identity wrist band.

2. Check on the patient frequently.

3. Orient the patient to the environment frequently.

4. Keep the call bell and personal items within reach.

5. Keep the bed in lowest position with two side rails raised.

6. Keep wheels on moveable objects locked.

7. Inspect all equipment before use.

8. Maintain adequate lighting in the environment for day, evening, and night.

9. Answer the call bell immediately.

D. 1. Apply a wristband that indicates that the patient is at risk for falls.

2. Employ other acceptable indicators to notify nursing staff members that the patient is at risk for falls (e.g., red socks, flower or butterfly insignia on door).

3. Address the patient's risk of falls in the nursing plan of care.

4. Employ nonrestrictive safety measures, such as a bed alarm, position-sensitive ankle alarm, bed bolsters, and wedges for positioning.

5. Document the outcomes of the use of nonrestrictive safety equipment. Only when nonrestrictive measures are ineffective can a nurse seek an order for a restraint.

E. 1. Explain the reason for the restraint to the patient.

2. Ensure that the V opening of the vest is in the front and that the closure is at the back of the restraint.

3. Ensure that there are two fingerbreadths between the patient's body and the vest to ensure that the patient is able to breathe easily.

4. Secure the ties of the vest to the frame of the bed, not the side rails, using a quick-release knot.

5. Check on the patient every 30 minutes to ensure that the patient can breathe easily and that the vest is not too tight.

6. Remove the vest restraint every 2 hours to assess skin integrity; provide for activity, such as range-of-motion; and massage skin surfaces, such as the patient's back and along the lower edge of the vest. Encourage coughing and deep breathing during this time. Reapply the vest, and reposition the patient.

7. Meet hydration, nutrition, elimination, and emotional needs while the patient is restrained.

8. Delegate application and restraint release to unlicensed assistive personnel if necessary, but remember that evaluation of the patient's status and response to the restraint must be implemented by the nurse.

9. Ensure that the primary health-care provider assesses the patient's need for the restraint and renews the order every 24 hours.

10. Discontinue use of the restraint as soon as possible.

Chapter 14

A. 1. Older adults have a decreased rate of medication metabolism and excretion, which increases the risk of drug toxicity.

2. This patient stated that he is forgetful and does not always take his medication every day and also stated that he avoids taking Lasix sometimes because stopping to urinate is inconvenient. Omission of doses does not provide adequate treatment of the patient's medical conditions. Also, a forgetful person may accidentally take a double dose of medication, not remembering that the medication was already taken, leading to drug toxicity.
3. The patient's limited income may prevent the patient from filling his medication prescriptions.

B. 1. Construct a calendar of days and times medications are to be taken.
2. Instruct the patient to place mediations or signs regarding the medications in a prominent place in the home.
3. Teach the patient how to use a divided pill container to minimize the risk of missed doses. If the patient is unsure of having taken daily medications, the patient only has to refer to the divided-dose container to see if the medications are there or have already been ingested.

C. 1. The Lasix 40mg IVPB order does not contain the frequency at which this medication is to be given.
2. The Pepcid 20mg bid order does not contain the route through which this medication is to be given.
3. The Colace 1 tab PO bid order does not contain the milligrams contained in 1 tab.

D. 1. Repeat the order back to the primary health-care provider for confirmation.
2. Have another nurse listen in to the order and countersign the order as well.
3. Ensure that the primary health-care provider countersigns the order within 24 hours.

Chapter 15

A. 1. U.S. Pharmacopoeia.
2. National formulary.
3. U.S. Food and Drug Administration.
4. Physician's Deck Reference (PDR).
5. American Hospital Formulary Service.
6. *Davis's Drug Guide for Nurses.*

B. 1. One trade name medication for cisplatin is Platinol.
2. Cisplatin is classified as an antineoplastic and an alkylating agent.
3. The pregnancy category of cisplatin is D. Category D includes medications that demonstrate evidence of human fetal risk based on research. However, the benefit to a pregnant woman may outweigh the potential risk.

C. 1. Action: Inhibits DNA synthesis by producing cross-linking of parent DNA strands.
2. Therapeutic effect: Death of rapidly replicating cells, particularly malignant ones.

D. The four most serious adverse reactions and side effects of cisplatin, indicated in red print in *Davis's Drug Guide for Nurses,* are
1. Reversible posterior leukoencephalopathy syndrome.
2. Seizures.
3. Leukopenia.
4. Thrombocytopenia.

E. The two most important responses for which the nurse should monitor the patient are bone marrow depression and anaphylaxis (indicated in red under the heading "Nursing Implications" in *Davis's Drug Guide for Nurses*).
1. **Bone marrow depression—Nursing care.**
    a. Assess for bleeding (e.g., bleeding gums, bruising, petechiae, and blood in stools, urine, and emesis).
    b. Avoid giving IM injections and taking rectal temperatures if the patient's platelet count is low (generally lower than $50,000/min^3$).
    c. Apply pressure to venipuncture sites for 10 minutes.
    d. Assess for signs of infection during neutropenia.
    e. Assess for anemia, fatigue, dyspnea, and orthostatic hypotension.
2. **Anaphylaxis—Nursing care.**
    a. Monitor for signs of anaphylaxis (e.g., facial edema, wheezing, dizziness, fainting, tachycardia, and hypotension).
    b. Discontinue the medication and immediately notify the rapid response team; report the episode to the primary health-care provider.
    c. Ensure that epinephrine and resuscitation equipment are readily available.

Chapter 16

A. 1. The purpose of the call bell, its use, and ways to keep it within easy reach.
2. The importance of not using the overbed table as a side rail or for support because it has wheels and is not stationary.
3. The importance of always keeping the bed the in the lowest position to the floor to avoid falls.

B. The nurse must determine whether the patient prefers to have only female caregivers. In the Muslim religion, a Muslim woman cannot be touched by a man other than her husband.

C. 1. Identify the size and shape of the lesion in millimeters.
2. Identify the depth of the lesion.
3. Identify the color of the lesion.
4. Identify the presence of exudate and its color and odor if present.

D. 1. The patient's wound may be infected.
2. The patient may be reluctant to seek assistance with hygiene, grooming, and urine incontinence

because privacy and modesty are a hallmark of the Islamic faith.

3. The patient may limit activity because it may precipitate pain.

4. The patient may be dehydrated. Often, patients who are incontinent of urine do not drink adequate fluid to avoid the frequency of incontinence episodes.

5. The patient's skin may be dry and fragile due to the aging process.

6. The patient's perineal area may be excoriated because of constant exposure to urea on the surface of the skin.

E. 1. Assign a female caregiver to provide patient care if this is the patient's preference.

2. Provide a complete bath less frequently according to a patient's preference to avoid drying the skin.

3. Keep the patient's perineal area clean and dry. Check the patient frequently for incontinence of urine and provide perineal care and dry linens and clothing as necessary.

4. Use mild cleansing products to maintain pH balance of the skin and prevent removal of natural moisturizers and lipids that protect the skin.

5. Use a soft cloth and pat skin surfaces dry to avoid damage by abrasion.

6. Apply a moisturizer or emollient after bathing and at least twice a day to make the skin supple and less dry.

Chapter 17

A. 1. **Ineffective airway clearance:** Maintaining a patent airway is always a priority. A patent airway is necessary to permit exchange of oxygen and carbon dioxide. This patient has a diagnosis of pneumonia and is experiencing thick, yellow secretions and a nonproductive cough. Thick secretions can obstruct the airway, causing a life-threatening situation.

2. **Risk for injury:** The patient is experiencing multiple problems that place him at risk for injury, such as altered mobility due to Parkinson's disease, fatigue related to activity, orthostatic hypotension when changing position, and a history of falls.

3. **Impaired walking:** Walking is the least of the patient's problems at this time. Although impaired walking is a problem evidenced by small, shuffling steps with involuntary accelerations due to the effects of Parkinson's disease, the patient at this time will most likely have an order for bed rest. Bed rest is ordered to minimize exertion. Exertion taxes the respiratory system, which is already compromised by the inflammatory process and thick secretions associated with pneumonia.

B. Propulsive, festinating, or cogwheel gait are all terms used to describe the small, shuffling steps with involuntary accelerations associated with Parkinson's disease.

C. Stage II pressure ulcer.

D. 1. **Increased cardiac workload:** Decreased gravity pressure redistributes blood from the legs to other parts of the body, resulting in an increase in heart rate, stroke volume, and cardiac output. The heart must work harder when a patient is in the supine position than in an erect position.

2. **Thrombus formation:** Venous stasis results from lack of muscle contraction in the legs that promotes venous return. In addition, pressure on blood vessels from bedbound or sitting positions causes intima damage that begins the cascade of clot formation. If a thrombus moves from its place of origin to the lungs, a pulmonary embolus can result.

E. 1. Encourage in-bed exercises to promote muscle contraction and venous return.

2. Encourage the patient to change position every 1 to 2 hours to avoid constant pressure on body parts, helping to prevent damage to venous intima or tissue hypoxia.

3. Encourage fluid intake if not restricted to prevent dehydration and hypercoagulability.

4. Apply ordered venous compression devices to the legs to promote venous return.

5. Teach the patient to avoid the Valsalva maneuver, which causes a surge of blood flow when the held breath is released that can dislodge a thrombus if present.

6. Teach the patient not to massage the legs, which can dislodge a thrombus if present.

F. 1. Assess the patient's status, such as presence of joint stiffness, swelling, or pain; physical ability to perform or assist with exercise; level of motivation; and cognitive ability to follow instructions.

2. Begin each movement with the extremity in functional alignment.

3. Put each joint through the fullest range while moving to the point of resistance.

4. Support each joint distal and proximal to the joint being ranged.

5. Implement range-of-motion slowly, smoothly, and rhythmically; repeat each movement three to five times.

6. Monitor the patient's physical, verbal, and nonverbal responses to interventions.

7. Document interventions, extent of mobility of joints, and the patient's responses.

G. 1. Seek the assistance of another caregiver to move the patient up in bed. *This action shares the stress and strain between two caregivers, decreasing the risk of injury.*

2. Raise the patient's bed to waist level. *This places the bed at a working height, which avoids unnecessary stress and strain on the nurse's joints, ligaments, tendons, muscles, and bones.*

3. Lower the head of the patient's bed when moving the patient up in bed. *This position uses gravity to facilitate moving the patient up toward the head of the bed.*

4. Position a pull sheet under the patient. *Doing so reduces the risk of shearing forces and also causes less strain and stress on the patient than moving the patient up by holding on to the patient's upper body and extremities. Also, it shares the work load between two caregivers.*

5. Position your body so that you are facing the head of the bed before moving the patient. *This position limits stress and strain on the nurse's anatomical structures.*

6. Keep your neck, back, pelvis, and feet in alignment. *Doing so avoids twisting, which stresses anatomical structures.*

7. Spread your feet apart with one foot in front of the other. *Doing so increases stability because the wider the base of support, the more centered is the body mass.*

8. Contract gluteal, abdominal, leg, and arm muscles before the actual move. *This prepares the muscles for action.*

9. Use leg muscles and flex the knees, hips, and ankles when moving the patient up in bed. *Doing so permits the larger muscles of the body to provide the power and decreases strain on back muscles.*

10. Move the patient toward the head of the bed on the count of three. *Doing so coordinates the action of the two caregivers and the patient.*

Chapter 18

A. Nurse's response: Breastfeeding is recommended during the first year of life because it provides the most appropriate nutrients for an infant. It reduces food allergies and intolerances versus cow's milk and is easier to digest. It is convenient, the right temperature, and it is economical. Cow's milk is too concentrated for an infant's kidneys to manage, is a poor source of iron and vitamin C and E, and may cause gastrointestinal bleeding.

B. 1. Teach the mother to provide her toddler with opportunities to explore foods with different textures and tastes.

2. Teach the mother to avoid using food, such as ice cream, to motivate, bribe, or punish because this may cause inappropriate food attitudes.

3. Teach the mother to avoid serving hot dogs and peanut butter because they are associated with an increased risk for choking. In addition, French fries are high in calories, "bad fat" (trans fat, unsaturated fat), and salt and are known to increase cholesterol levels contributing to cardiovascular disease.

C. 1. Spending an excessive amount of time in the bathroom. The adolescent may be engaging in activities such as self-induced vomiting or excessive use of diuretics and laxatives.

2. Gorging followed by self-induced vomiting. Binging and purging are associated with the eating disorder bulimia nervosa.

3. Spending an excessive amount of time exercising. Exercising is an attempt to lose weight.

4. Complaining of a sore throat. A sore throat may indicate mucosal contact with gastric acid during vomiting.

5. Excessive dental caries, enamel erosion, and staining of teeth. These signs may be due to contact with gastric acid during vomiting.

6. Diarrhea. This can result from excessive laxative use.

7. Dehydration. This can result from the excessive use of diuretics and laxatives.

8. Excessive weight loss and muscle wasting. These are signs of malnutrition.

9. Arrested sexual development; amenorrhea. Adequate nutrition and body weight are essential for functioning of the endocrine and reproductive systems.

D. 1. Encourage the grandmother to make an appointment with a dentist for dental care.

2. Encourage the grandmother to chop or puree her food until dental care is implemented.

3. Encourage the intake of foods high in nutritive value to ensure adequate nutritional intake.

4. Encourage between meal snacks that are high in nutritive value to meet caloric needs.

5. Encourage the avoidance of salt when cooking and suggest the use of alternate spices.

6. Provide the grandmother with information about local senior citizens organizations to increase her social life with peers.

E. 1. Teach the mother how to maintain a balanced daily diet to meet nutritional needs of herself and her infant.

2. Encourage the avoidance of alcohol, caffeine, and medications not specifically prescribed by her primary health-care provider because these are transferred via breast milk.

3. Teach the mother to avoid tobacco use because it decreases milk production and is an unhealthy habit.

F. 1. Encourage consultation with a primary health-care provider and a nutritionist to determine a weight reduction diet that is appropriate for a lactating mother.

2. Encourage the mother to use a food diary to help develop insight into eating habits.

3. Help the mother to identify realistic objectives and to review them weekly.

4. Help the mother to understand that healthy eating needs to be an enduring lifestyle change.

5. Explain how to read a food label to identify foods that are high in calories, fat, and carbohydrates that should be reduced when on a weight reduction diet.

6. Teach the mother to avoid food shopping when hungry to reduce the temptation to buy inappropriate comfort foods.

7. Encourage the intake of fresh fruits and vegetables.

8. Encourage incorporation of nutritious morning and afternoon snacks into the meal plan to minimize the desire to graze throughout the day.

9. Encourage the mother to serve food on small plates, take small bites, chew food well, eat slowly and put the fork or spoon down between bites.

10. Encourage participation in an exercise program to increase the resting metabolic rate.

11. Encourage adequate sleep because sleep deprivation negatively affects the hormones leptin and ghrelin that regulate appetite. This may be a challenge with an infant or young child in the household.

12. Encourage participation in a support group, such as Weight Watchers or Overeaters Anonymous, where a person is weighed weekly to evaluate progress and where emotional support is provided.

Chapter 19

A. **Stridor** is a sign of a potential medical emergency that requires immediate medical intervention. It is a harsh, high-pitched breath sound generally heard on inspiration and is associated with a narrowed or obstructed airway, which can be life threatening. A severe allergic reaction to an allergen, such as smoke from a fire, can cause irritation and inflammation of the respiratory tract mucosa, laryngeal spasm, swelling of the tongue, and irritation and edema of the vocal cords. The patient should be assessed frequently for the reoccurrence of stridor because an airway obstruction can be life threatening.

B. 1. **Use of accessory muscles of respiration:** Contraction of the intercostal, abdominal, and trapezius muscles and lifting of the shoulders on inhalation help expand the chest cavity.

2. **Nasal flaring:** Widening of the nares during inhalation decreases airway resistance.

3. **Grunting immediately before exhalation:** A closed glottis at the height of inspiration keeps the alveoli open to enhance gas exchange; the grunt occurs when air is expelled through the larynx.

4. **Pursed-lip breathing:** Exhalation through the mouth with lips positioned to create a small opening prolongs exhalation, keeping alveoli open longer for gas exchange and more efficient expulsion of trapped air.

5. **Barrel chest:** An increased anteroposterior-to-lateral ratio is associated with chronic retention of carbon dioxide. An expected anteroposterior-to-lateral ratio should be 1:2.

6. **Clubbing of the fingers:** Bulbous swelling of the soft tissue of the end of the phalanx of the fingers causes the nail plates to be equal to or greater than 180°.

7. **Presence of sputum and its characteristics:** Sputum color other than clear may indicate a respiratory problem; for example, yellow-green sputum may indicate infection.

8. **Productive or nonproductive cough:** A productive cough indicates the presence of respiratory secretions. A nonproductive cough indicates an inability to raise secretions if secretions are present, which places the patient at risk for impaired gas exchange.

9. **Decreased oxygen saturation level:** A decreased oxygen saturation level indicates the presence of hypoxemia.

C. 1. **Two-pack-a-day smoker with a 20-year history of smoking who experienced secondhand smoke exposure as a child.**
   a. Tobacco smoke contains tars, toxins, and nicotine, which are known to precipitate damage to lung tissue.
   b. Tobacco smoke contains nicotine, which constricts bronchioles.
   c. Tobacco smoke causes mucous membrane inflammation, increases respiratory secretions, breaks down elastin, and decreases the numbers and efficiency of cilia.
   d. Prolonged tobacco use results in chronic bronchitis, smaller diameter of the airways, and loss of alveolar elasticity, leading to emphysema.

2. **Older age.**
   a. As people age, lung compliance and lung elasticity decrease and airway resistance increases, leading to impaired ventilation.
   b. Drier mucus, fewer cilia, a reduced cough efficiency, air trapping in the alveoli, and a decline in immunity in older adults increase the risk of respiratory tract infections.
   c. Other problems, such as gastroesophageal reflux disease (GERD), may result in aspiration, which can precipitate a respiratory infection.

3. **Obesity.**
   a. Excess abdominal adipose tissue limits chest expansion and gas exchange in the alveoli.

b. Obesity increases the risk of sleep apnea due to an increase in neck girth and fat deposits in the upper airway that obstruct the pharynx.

4. **Smoke from the neighborhood fire.**
   a. Smoke is a pulmonary allergen that can precipitate a respiratory hypersensitivity response.

5. **History of asthma.**
   a. Airborne allergens, such as secondhand smoke, can contribute to asthma and other lung diseases, causing a person to experience chronic airway inflammation and sensitivity to various triggers, instigating an allergic reaction.
   b. Smoke from burning wood and tobacco is a common trigger for an allergic reaction for many individuals who have asthma.

D. 1. Factors to assess.
   a. Vital signs, especially for quality, rate, pattern, and depth of respirations; breathing effort; adventitious breath sounds; oxygen saturation; and signs of hypoxemia (tachycardia, restlessness, headache, lethargy, and confusion).
   b. Clinical indicators of atelectasis (e.g., diminished chest excursion, tachycardia, dyspnea, chest pain, reduced breath sounds, crackles, low oxygen saturation).
   c. Skin color for pallor or cyanosis.
   d. Ability to cough effectively.

2. Support the patient in the orthopneic or high-Fowler position.
3. Maintain body alignment for optimal respiratory excursion.
4. Encourage the patient to change position every 2 hours.
5. Encourage the intake of 2 to 3 L of fluid by mouth daily if permitted.
6. Encourage coughing and deep breathing every few hours and use of an incentive spirometer, if permitted.
7. Teach abdominal and pursed-lip breathing techniques.
8. Encourage rest and limit physical activities.
9. Increase activities as tolerated (e.g., progress from passive ROM exercises to active ROM exercises as tolerated).
10. Pace care and schedule rest periods to avoid activity intolerance.
11. Provide for the patient's hygiene and grooming needs and increase the patient's participation in activities of daily living as tolerated.
12. Anticipate needs.
13. Provide emotional support.
14. Teach about ordered medications and the use of a medication delivery device, such as metered-dose inhaler and home nebulizer, as indicated.
15. Refer the patient to a home health agency if oxygen therapy is required at home.

Chapter 20

A. 1. **Age:** Older adults experience a decline in urinary system functioning. They are less able to filter waste and maintain acid-base and fluid and electrolyte balance. They also experience a loss of bladder tone, contributing to urgency, frequency, and incomplete emptying of the bladder. Most importantly, this patient is experiencing an enlarged prostate, which is associated with aging.

2. **Alcohol intake:** Excessive alcohol intake reduces the release of antidiuretic hormone, increasing urine production.

3. **Caffeine intake:** Caffeine increases urine production.

4. **Sodium intake:** Potato chips contain a large amount of sodium, which produces water retention, causing a decrease in urine production.

5. **Smoking history:** Nicotine irritates the detrusor muscle, causing bladder contractions and urinary urgency.

6. **Sedentary lifestyle:** Lack of exercise leads to decreased bladder tone, which can cause incomplete emptying of the bladder when voiding. Stasis of urine in the bladder can contribute to urinary tract infections.

7. **Enlargement of the prostate:** Prostate enlargement can cause a narrowing of the urethra, resulting in incomplete emptying of the bladder and eventual obstruction, causing urinary retention.

8. **Comorbidity of heart disease:** Heart disease can diminish blood flow through the kidneys, reducing GFR.

9. **Sharing a bathroom with others:** Sharing a bathroom may cause a delay in responding to the need to empty the bladder, which can decrease bladder tone and contribute to urinary stasis.

10. **History of urinary tract infections:** An enlarged prostate (an obstructive problem) increases the risk of urinary retention, which leads to the potential for urinary tract infection.

11. **Medications:** Many classifications of drugs can be nephrotoxic or cause urinary retention. The patient is receiving a diuretic, an antihistamine, and an antidepressant, which can cause side effects associated with the urinary system.

B. 1. Presence of small, frequent incontinence episodes.
2. Presence of urinary dribbling.
3. Presence of urgency.
4. Presence of blood in the urine.
5. Decreased daily urine output.

6. Sudden weight gain.

7. Dependent edema.

C. 1. **Hydrochlorothiazide 50 mg PO daily in a.m.:** Diuretics interfere with water reabsorption, causing an increase in urine output.

2. **Loratadine (Claritin) 10 mg PO daily:** Antihistamines have an anticholinergic effect that inhibits involuntary contractions of the bladder, which increases the capacity of the bladder and delays the urge to void; urinary retention is a side effect.

3. **Sertraline (Zoloft) 50 mg PO hour of sleep:** This selective serotonin reuptake inhibitor (SSRI) may cause urinary side effects, such as frequency or urinary retention.

D. **Common principles associated with caring for patients with any type of urinary tube.**

1. Place the collection bag and tubing below the level of the bladder.

2. Curl excess tubing on the bed.

3. Secure the tube to the patient's anterior thigh or abdomen for a male patient.

4. Ensure that the patient is not lying on the tubing and that the tubing is under, not passed through, the side rails.

5. Assess the catheter frequently to ensure tube patency.

6. Ask the patient about the presence or absence of bladder spasms.

7. Administer pain medication as prescribed and needed.

8. Assess the amount and characteristics of urine; assess hourly volumes as ordered to assess GFR, and notify the primary health-care provider if output is equal to or less than 30 mL/hour.

9. Maintain safety when ambulating a patient with a urinary catheter; hold the catheter tubing so that the patient does not step on it and to ensure that it does not drag along the floor.

10. Teach the patient about self-care management of the urinary catheter.

11. Document the patient's status, care provided, and patient responses in the patient's clinical record.

Specific principles when caring for a patient with a triple-lumen urinary catheter for continuous bladder irrigation.

1. Maintain the irrigating solution flow rate as ordered, usually a prescribed amount of flow or to "keep output pink."

2. Increase the irrigating solution flow rate to keep the output free from blood clots.

3. Deduct the volume of irrigating solution from the urinary output to accurately document urine output.

Chapter 21

A. 1. Patient states, "I can't seem to keep anything down."

2. Patient feels weak and dizzy.

3. Patient reports experiencing nausea, vomiting, and diarrhea for 3 days.

4. Patient reports currently taking hydrochlorothiazide (HCTZ).

B. 1. Vital signs that indicate hypovolemia.

2. Tenting over sternum.

3. Sticky, dry oral mucosa, cracked lips.

4. Oliguria and dark amber urine.

5. Weight loss of 5 pounds.

6. Unsteadiness when transferring from chair to bed.

C. Dehydration.

D. 1. **Temperature of 99°F:** A temperature of 99°F may reflect a fever in an older adult because older adults normally have lower core body temperatures due to a decreased metabolic rate and inefficient thermoregulatory mechanisms. In addition, temperature increases because a dehydrated person is less able to cool the body via vaporization due to a decrease in perspiration. Also, an increased temperature is the body's attempt to build a hostile environment that inhibits reproduction of an infectious agent.

2. **Weak, thready pulse of 126 beats/minute with a regular rhythm:** As blood volume decreases, the heart contracts more quickly but less powerfully, causing a rapid, weak, thready pulse.

3. **Blood pressure of 98/64 mm Hg; orthostatic hypotension when mooving from sitting to standing position:** Orthostatic hypotension is caused by hypovolemia associated with dehydration.

4. **Respirations of 26 breaths/minute with a regular rhythm:** Respirations increase in an attempt to increase the amount of oxygen reaching body cells; the need for oxygen increases when the body's metabolic rate increases.

5. **Cracked lips, sticky and dry oral mucosa, and tenting (decreased turgor):** Fluid moves from cells to the interstitial space and then to the vascular system in an attempt to maintain the circulating blood volume.

6. **Fatigue and weakness:** Fatigue and weakness are caused by electrolyte imbalances, such as a low potassium level (hypokalemia) and a high sodium level (hypernatremia).

7. **Unsteadiness when transferring from chair to bed:** Hypotension is associated with hypovolemia, especially when it occurs when a patient moves from a lying down to siting position or from a sitting to standing position. Fluid pools in the lower extremities until the baroreceptors react to the change in position and precipitate vasoconstriction.

8. **Oliguria and concentrated urine:** Oliguria and concentrated urine occur as the body attempts to conserve water; the urine that is excreted is more concentrated (less diluted) due to a higher percentage of waste product to water than when water is not being conserved by the kidneys.

9. **5 pound weight loss in less than 1 week:** One liter of fluid weighs 2.2 pounds. The patient lost over 3.6 L of fluid in less than 1 week. A quick weight loss is related to fluid loss, not a loss of tissue mass.

E. 1. **Elevated serum Na$^+$:** An increased serum sodium level indicates dehydration because the number of sodium ions increases in relation to the amount of the remaining circulating volume (hemoconcentration). Normal serum sodium is 135 to 145 mEq/L.

2. **Elevated blood urea nitrogen:** Elevated blood urea nitrogen levels occur due to hemoconcentration related to dehydration. Normal levels are 8 to 21 mg/dL.

3. **Elevated urine specific gravity:** Increased urine specific gravity levels occur due to concentration of urine as the body attempts to conserve water. Normal range is 1.001 to 1.029.

4. **Elevated serum creatinine:** An increased serum creatinine level is associated with dehydration due to hemoconcentration. Normal range is 0.5 to 1.2 mg/dL.

5. **Elevated hemoglobin:** With dehydration, the total blood volume decreases, but the volume of RBCs remains the same, resulting in hemoconcentration. The normal range is 14 to 18 g/dL in a male; critical levels are 20 g/dL or more.

6. **Elevated hematocrit:** Total blood volume is decreased with dehydration, but the number of RBCs remains the same, resulting in hemoconcentration. Normal hematocrit levels are 40 to 50 percent; critical levels are more than 60 percent.

7. **Decreased serum K$^+$:** A decreased serum potassium level results from gastrointestinal losses due to vomiting and diarrhea as well as losses via the kidneys in response to diuretic therapy. Normal serum potassium levels are 3.5 to 5.0 mEq/L; critical levels are less than 2.5 mEq/L.

F. 1. **Vital signs.**
   a. Assess vital signs every 4 hours and when necessary.

2. **Diagnostic tests.**
   a. Obtain a stool specimen for culture and sensitivity (C&S).
   b. Obtain a urine specimen for C&S and urinalysis.
   c. Obtain blood specimens for CBC and BMP.

3. **Nutrition.**
   a. Maintain NPO status.

4. **Activity.**
   a. Transfer the patient to a chair for 1 hour two times daily.

5. **Hydration.**
   a. Monitor I&O and weight daily.
   b. Assess for nausea and vomiting.
   c. Administer IVF 1,000 mL 0.45% NaCl 20 mEq KCl at 125 mL/hour.

6. **Hygiene.**
   a. Provide frequent mouth care.
   b. Apply a water-soluble lubricant to the lips.
   c. Keep skin and linens clean and dry.
   d. Provide perianal hygiene immediately after an episode of diarrhea.
   e. Apply skin barrier ointment to the perianal area per protocol.
   f. Provide privacy and use room deodorizers.

7. **Prescribed medications.**
   a. Discontinue HCTZ, and explain to the patient the rationale for it being discontinued.
   b. Administer ondansetron (Zofran) 4 mg IVPB every 4 hours prn for nausea.
   c. Tylenol 650 mg every 4 hours prn for temperature more than 101°F.
   d. Ensure that KCl 20 mEq is added to IVF 1,000 mL 0.45% NaCl.

8. **Health teaching.**
   a. Teach about foods high in potassium to include in the diet if a nonpotassium sparing diuretic is prescribed.
   b. Teach the importance of and proper technique for taking blood pressure and weight daily when at home.

G. 1. **Vital signs:** Assess the patient's vital signs to determine whether temperature, pulse, and respirations are decreasing and blood pressure is increasing, indicating a movement toward fluid balance and an appropriate circulating blood volume.

2. **Laboratory results:** Monitor the laboratory results of a complete blood count and BMP to determine the client's fluid volume and electrolyte status in response to the therapeutic regimen. Specific laboratory results should be moving toward the normal range.

3. **Intake and output (I&O):** Monitor I&O to identify a greater intake versus output until dehydration is resolved and then ensure that intake and output remain balanced.

4. **Complications of fluid overload:** Assess for clinical indicators of the complication of fluid overload in response to excessive rehydration therapy, such as bounding pulse; increased blood pressure; increased respirations and pulse; distended neck veins; decreased HCT, Hb level, and BUN levels;

and signs of pulmonary edema with severe fluid overload, such as presence of crackles, dyspnea, and shortness of breath.

Chapter 22

A. 1. Fecal urgency.
2. Hyperactive bowel sounds.
3. Flatus.
4. Anorexia.
5. Nausea and vomiting.
6. Blood in the stool (frank or occult).

B. 1. Decreased tissue turgor.
2. Furrows of the tongue.
3. Flushed, dry skin and mucous membranes.
4. Sunken eyeballs.
5. Hypotension and orthostatic hypotension.
6. Atonic muscles.
7. Mental confusion.
8. Decreased urine output.

C. The patient experienced a wound infection after having surgery for a total knee replacement requiring antibiotic therapy. Antibiotics can suppress the normal GI flora, permitting opportunistic infections to flourish in the bowel. Stool that is malodorous and greenish in color is indicative of *Clostridium difficile* infection. *C. difficile* is a bacterium that causes diarrhea and can extend to a life-threatening inflammation of the colon (pseudomembranous colitis).

D. Stool specimens for C&S, ova and parasites, and *C. difficile* should be collected first. If an antibiotic is implemented before collecting stool specimens, the test results may be inconclusive. Microorganisms might not grow after exposure to an antibiotic or their volume in the specimen may decrease, causing uncertain test results.

E. 1. Factors to assess.
   a. Vital signs and BP every 4 hours.
   b. Daily weight.
   c. Stool for frequency, amount, consistency, color, odor, and other characteristics.
   d. Clinical indicators of fluid volume deficit and electrolyte imbalances.
   e. Perianal area for excoriation.
   f. Bowel sounds.
2. Maintain contact precautions.
3. Monitor I&O.
4. Assist with elimination, provide for privacy, and use air fresheners discretely.
5. Provide perineal care, such as providing for hygiene and using a protective skin barrier or emollient, per policy and procedure.
6. Maintain NPO status and progress the patient's diet as per orders.
7. Increase oral fluid intake gradually once permitted because large amounts can precipitate peristalsis.
8. Administer prescribed metronidazole (Flagyl).
9. Administer D_5 in 0.45% NaCl at 125 mL/hour.
10. Provide health teaching.
   a. Discourage intake of spicy and fatty foods; caffeine; and high-fiber foods until after the acute infection is resolved.
   b. Discourage the intake of hot and cold fluids because they stimulate peristalsis.
   c. Encourage intake of foods high in sodium, such as tomatoes and bullions, and foods high in potassium, such as bananas, oranges, apricots, and potatoes, as the diet is advanced.
   d. Teach the patient to perform perianal skin care after each bowel movement.
11. Evaluate the patient's responses to nursing interventions.
12. Document assessments, interventions, and patient responses in the patient's clinical record.

Chapter 23

A. 1. Malignant tumor physiologically causing visceral pain.
2. Seven-month duration of the pain experience.
3. Emotions, such as feeling helpless and a feeling like a burden.
4. Emotions, such as feelings angry and afraid.
5. Wife killed by a drunk driver 4 months ago.
6. Unfamiliar environment.
7. Noisy and busy environment interfering with rest; constant fatigue.
8. Pain and suffering perceived as penance for wrongdoings during the war.
9. Multiplicity of stressors impacting ability to adapt.

B. 1. "Is there a pattern to the pain?"
2. "What initiates or increases the pain?"
3. "How long does the pain last when it starts?"
4. "What helps to diminish or eliminate the pain?"
5. "Is the pain deep or superficial and does it radiate to other areas of the body?"
6. "Is this pain different than the pain that you have been experiencing all along?"

C. 1. Assess the patient's pain on an ongoing basis.
2. Accept the patient's perception of pain.
3. Be nonjudgmental.
4. Validate the patient's pain.
5. Treat the patient with respect and provide for privacy.
6. Provide opportunities for making choices and being involved in planning care to support independence.

7. Encourage family members to be involved and to provide direct care if desired by the patient and family members.

8. Maintain an attitude of caring that precipitates nursing behaviors, such as responding to needs immediately, ensuring continuity of care, and providing information and teaching that are patient centered.

9. Provide emotional support and answer questions the patient has to relieve anxiety and fears; use interviewing techniques to encourage the patient to verbalize feelings and concerns.

10. Use distraction techniques, such as soft music, television, and conversation.

11. Alter irritating stimuli, such as by limiting noise in the environment, closing curtains or doors, dimming environmental lights, and adjusting room temperature to the patient's preference.

12. Teach relaxation techniques, such as diaphragmatic breathing, guided imagery, and progressive muscle relaxation.

13. Provide physical comfort measures, such as supporting positioning, providing backrubs, providing for hygiene, oxygen, nutrition, and elimination needs.

14. Pace care to minimize fatigue and the risk of activity intolerance.

15. Accommodate the patient's desired religious needs, especially related to his perception that the suffering he is experiencing is penance for past wrongdoings.

16. Teach the patient the need to inform the nurse immediately if the pain level increases, so that appropriate interventions can be implemented before the pain becomes severe.

17. Correct misconceptions regarding drug tolerance as well as physical and psychological dependence.

18. Evaluate the patient's response to nursing intervention, such as the extent of pain relief; decrease in vital signs, particularly respirations; and presence of constipation.

19. Notify the primary health-care provider when an analgesic is ineffective.

20. Document nursing care delivered and the patient's response in the patient's clinical record.

D. 1. Administer morphine sulfate 6 mg Sub-Q every 4 hours prn for severe pain.

2. Administer Percocet 2.5 mg/300mg 1 tablet PO every 6 hours prn for mild pain and 2 tablets PO every 6 hours prn for moderate pain.

3. Administer Tylenol 500 mg 1capsule PO every 4 hours prn for mild pain or PO every 4 hours for temp over 101°F.

4. Administer Colace 100 mg PO every 12 hours.

5. Administer Senokot 2 tablets PO h.s. prn for constipation.

Chapter 24

A. Removal of the uterus, fallopian tubes, and ovaries is curative in its purpose. Excision or repair of a diseased organ via surgery is a therapeutic intervention to achieve a cure.

B. Because this patient is diagnosed with a benign fibroid of the uterus, the patient's surgery is considered to be elective. Elective surgery includes surgical interventions that are advised but are for reasons that do not imminently threaten the patient's life.

C. This surgery is considered major surgery because the incision enters the abdominal cavity and requires the removal of organs and structures. Also, the patient is at risk for postoperative complications because of the patient's age, obesity, and preexisting conditions of diabetes and hypertension.

1. Older adults experience a decrease in physiologic reserves, such as decreased cardiac output, cough reflex, immunity, vital capacity, subcutaneous tissue, blood oxygenation, glomerular filtration rate, and basal metabolic rate.

2. Older adults experience increased calcium and cholesterol deposits within small arteries that increase the risk of hypertension, fluid and electrolyte imbalances, and shock when blood loss occurs.

3. Obesity can decrease postoperative ventilation and cardiac function.

4. Obesity is associated with increased wound complications, such as delayed wound healing, dehiscence (separation of the wound edges), evisceration (protrusion of the abdominal viscera through the incision), and wound infection because adipose tissue contains a limited blood supply.

5. Diabetes mellitus increases the risk of infection and delayed wound healing because of a reduced ability to metabolize carbohydrates, proteins, and fat.

D. 1. Stable vital signs.

2. Presence of spontaneous respirations or effective mechanical ventilator function.

3. Easy arousal.

4. Absence of complications.

5. Aldrete score of 8 to 10.

E. 1. Assign each drainage device a number to ensure that each site is assessed independently. Generally, when drainage volume from a device decreases to less than 10 mL in 24 hours, it is discontinued.

2. Assess the area around the drain insertion sites for clinical indicators of inflammation or infection; this supports early treatment of the problem.

3. Cover the sites with sterile dressings to protect the exit wounds from environmental pathogens.

4. Maintain the collection bulbs below the insertion sites because this uses gravity to move drainage toward the bulbs. This is in addition to the negative pressure within the portable would drainage system.

5. Secure collection blubs in place and attach them to the patient's gown to prevent tension on the tubing.

6. Empty a collection bulb when half full to prevent the weight of a bulb from pulling on the tubing; a less than half-full bulb maintains effective negative pressure. As the volume of drainage in a bulb increases, the extent of negative pressure decreases.

7. Maintain sterility when opening and closing a drainage port to prevent contamination of the port and drain.

8. To empty the bulb open the port and drain the contents into a measuring container without touching the inside of the port; do not touch the measuring container with the port to maintain port sterility and reduce the risk of infection.

9. Clean the port with an alcohol or a povidone iodine (Betadine) swab before closing; doing so helps to reduce pathogens lingering around the port, thereby reducing the risk of infection.

10. Compress the collection bulb, close the port, and release the hand compressing the bulb to reestablish negative pressure.

11. Measure the volume and characteristics of drainage to assess the status of the drainage. Expect drainage to progress from sanguinous to serosanguineous to serous.

12. Discard drainage in the toilet and flush twice and then wash your hands to limit the spread of microorganisms.

13. Document the volume and characteristics of drainage; if more than one device is present, document findings according to the assigned number of the device to ensure the accuracy of the status of each device.

F. Postoperative hemorrhage is a concern because the patient was taking clopidogrel (Plavix), which has antiplatelet activity. In addition, the patient was taking ginseng, which also has antiplatelet activity. Having taken these drugs recently increases the risk of postoperative bleeding.

G.
1. Tachycardia.
2. Tachypnea.
3. Increased diastolic blood pressure.
4. Narrowed pulse pressure.
5. Pale, cool, clammy skin.
6. Prolonged capillary refill.
7. Urine output less than 20 to 30 mL/hour.
8. Restlessness.
9. Anxiety.
10. Confusion.

H.
1. **Pneumonia** is a concern because obesity interferes with a patient's ability to deep breathe, thereby leading to stagnation of respiratory secretions.
2. **Wound infection** is a concern because of the size and depth of the wound required to accomplish the surgery. In addition, the patient's comorbidity of diabetes increases the risk of wound infection because elevated levels of serum glucose support growth of pathogens and because a reduced ability to metabolize carbohydrates, proteins, and fat delays wound healing.
3. **Thromboembolism** is a concern because of venous relaxation that occurs during anesthesia and atherosclerosis associated with diabetes.
4. **Wound dehiscence and evisceration** are a concern with obesity because excessive weight places added stress and strain on the incision and adipose tissue contains a limited blood supply, delaying wound healing. The patient's comorbidity of diabetes additionally contributes to delayed wound healing because of a reduced ability to metabolize carbohydrates, proteins, and fat.

I.
1. Engage in meticulous hand hygiene practices.
2. Change wound dressing as ordered, keeping the wound clean and dry.
3. Maintain sterile technique when changing dressings or when opening and closing drains.
4. Encourage a diet high in protein and vitamin C to promote wound healing as ordered.
5. Encourage fluid intake as ordered.
6. Administer antibiotics prophylactically as prescribed.
7. Ensure that roommates are free from infection.
8. Ensure that the patient's environment is meticulously cleaned.
9. Ensure that family members and visitors understand that they should not visit the patient if they have an infection.

J.
1. Encourage exercises, such as performing flexion and extension of the ankles (ankle pumping) and knees and raising the legs off of the bed, to facilitate venous return, which minimizes venous stasis, thereby reducing the risk of thrombophlebitis. Matter associated with thrombophlebitis can become an embolus that gets carried via the vasculature and lodges in a pulmonary vessel, which is a life-threatening condition.
2. Teach the patient to avoid using pillows behind the knees and raising the lower portion of the bed into the contour position (gatching the bed); this minimizes popliteal pressure and increases venous blood flow, preventing venous stasis.
3. Apply ordered antiembolism stockings or sequential compression devices to facilitate venous return, which minimizes venous stasis, thereby reducing the risk of thrombophlebitis.

4. Provide progressive ambulation as ordered to facilitate venous return, which minimizes venous stasis, thereby reducing the risk of thrombophlebitis. Activity, such as ambulation, increases the depth and rate of respirations as the body attempts to bring more oxygen to muscles. When respirations increase in depth, the lower areas of lungs are aerated, thereby minimizing the risk of stasis of pulmonary secretions.

5. Administer prescribed prophylactic heparin 5,000 units Sub-Q every 12 hours; this interferes with normal coagulation to decrease the risk of thrombus formation.

K. The nurse should verify the prescription for regular insulin coverage and administer the dose based on the patient's blood glucose result. The prescription indicates that a serum glucose level of 201-300 mg/dL requires administration of 4 units of regular insulin via the subcutaneous route. Therefore, the nurse should administer 4 units of regular insulin via the subcutaneous route.

Glossary of English Words Commonly Encountered on Nursing Examinations

Abnormality—Defect, irregularity, anomaly, oddity

Absence—Nonappearance, lack, nonattendance

Abundant—Plentiful, rich, profuse

Accelerate—Go faster, speed up, increase, hasten

Accumulate—Build up, collect, gather

Accurate—Precise, correct, exact

Achievement—Accomplishment, success, reaching, attainment

Acknowledge—Admit, recognize, accept, reply

Activate—Start, turn on, stimulate

Adequate—Sufficient, ample, plenty, enough

Angle—Slant, approach, direction, point of view

Application—Use, treatment, request, claim

Approximately—About, around, in the region of, more or less, roughly speaking

Arrange—Position, place, organize, display

Associated—Linked, related

Attention—Notice, concentration, awareness, thought

Authority—Power, right, influence, clout, expert

Avoid—Keep away from, evade, let alone

Balanced—Stable, neutral, steady, fair, impartial

Barrier—Barricade, blockage, obstruction, obstacle

Best—Most excellent, most important, greatest

Capable—Able, competent, accomplished

Capacity—Ability, capability, aptitude, role, power, size

Central—Middle, mid, innermost, vital

Challenge—Confront, dare, dispute, test, defy, face up to

Characteristic—Trait, feature, attribute, quality, typical

Circular—Round, spherical, globular

Collect—Gather, assemble, amass, accumulate, bring together

Commitment—Promise, vow, dedication, obligation, pledge, assurance

Commonly—Usually, normally, frequently, generally, universally

Compare—Contrast, evaluate, match up to, weigh or judge against

Compartment—Section, part, cubicle, booth, stall

Complex—Difficult, multifaceted, compound, multipart, intricate

Complexity—Difficulty, intricacy, complication

Component—Part, element, factor, section, constituent

Comprehensive—Complete, inclusive, broad, thorough

Conceal—Hide, cover up, obscure, mask, suppress, secrete

Conceptualize—To form an idea

Concern—Worry, anxiety, fear, alarm, distress, unease, trepidation

Concisely—Briefly, in a few words, succinctly

Conclude—Make a judgment based on reason, finish

Confidence—Self-assurance, certainty, poise, self-reliance

Congruent—Matching, fitting, going together well

Consequence—Result, effect, outcome, end result

Constituents—Elements, component, parts that make up a whole

Contain—Hold, enclose, surround, include, control, limit

Continual—Repeated, constant, persistent, recurrent, frequent

Continuous—Constant, incessant, nonstop, unremitting, permanent

Contribute—Be a factor, add, give

Convene—Assemble, call together, summon, organize, arrange

Convenience—Expediency, handiness, ease

Coordinate—Organize, direct, manage, bring together

Create—Make, invent, establish, generate, produce, fashion, build, construct

Creative—Imaginative, original, inspired, inventive, resourceful, productive, innovative

Critical—Serious, grave, significant, dangerous, life threatening

Cue—Signal, reminder, prompt, sign, indication

Curiosity—Inquisitiveness, interest, nosiness, snooping

Damage—Injure, harm, hurt, break, wound

Deduct—Subtract, take away, remove, withhold

Deficient—Lacking, wanting, underprovided, scarce, faulty

Defining—Important, crucial, major, essential, significant, central

Defuse—Resolve, calm, soothe, neutralize, rescue, mollify

Delay—Hold up, wait, hinder, postpone, slow down, hesitate, linger

Demand—Insist, claim, require, command, stipulate, ask

Describe—Explain, tell, express, illustrate, depict, portray

Design—Plan, invent, intend, aim, propose, devise

Desirable—Wanted, pleasing, enviable, popular, sought after, attractive, advantageous

Detail—Feature, aspect, element, factor, facet

Deteriorate—Worsen, decline, weaken

Determine—Decide, conclude, resolve, agree on

Dexterity—Skillfulness, handiness, agility, deftness

Dignity—Self-respect, self-esteem, decorum, formality, poise

Dimension—Aspect, measurement

Diminish—Reduce, lessen, weaken, detract, moderate

Discharge—Release, dismiss, set free

Discontinue—Stop, cease, halt, suspend, terminate, withdraw

Disorder—Complaint, problem, confusion, chaos

Display—Show, exhibit, demonstrate, present, put on view

Dispose—To get rid of, arrange, order, set out

Dissatisfaction—Displeasure, discontent, unhappiness, disappointment

Distinguish—To separate and classify, recognize

Distract—Divert, sidetrack, entertain

Distress—Suffering, trouble, anguish, misery, agony, concern, sorrow

Distribute—Deliver, spread out, hand out, issue, dispense

Disturbed—Troubled, unstable, concerned, worried, distressed, anxious, uneasy

Diversional—Serving to distract

Don—Put on, dress oneself in

Dramatic—Spectacular

Drape—Cover, wrap, dress, swathe

Dysfunction—Abnormal, impaired

Edge—Perimeter, boundary, periphery, brink, border, rim

Effective—Successful, useful, helpful, valuable

Efficient—Not wasteful, effective, competent, resourceful, capable

Elasticity—Stretch, spring, suppleness, flexibility

Eliminate—Get rid of, eradicate, abolish, remove, purge

Embarrass—Make uncomfortable, make self-conscious, humiliate, mortify

Emerge—Appear, come, materialize, become known

Emphasize—Call attention to, accentuate, stress, highlight

Ensure—Make certain, guarantee

Environment—Setting, surroundings, location, atmosphere, milieu, situation

Episode—Event, incident, occurrence, experience

Essential—Necessary, fundamental, vital, important, crucial, critical, indispensable

Etiology—Assigned cause, origin

Exaggerate—Overstate, inflate

Excel—To stand out, shine, surpass, outclass

Excessive—Extreme, too much, unwarranted

Exertion—Intense or prolonged physical effort

Exhibit—Show signs of, reveal, display

Expand—Get bigger, enlarge, spread out, increase, swell, inflate

Expect—Wait for, anticipate, imagine

Expectation—Hope, anticipation, belief, prospect, probability

Experience—Knowledge, skill, occurrence, know-how

Expose—Lay open, leave unprotected, allow to be seen, reveal, disclose, exhibit

External—Outside, exterior, outer

Facilitate—Make easy, make possible, help, assist

Factor—Part, feature, reason, cause, think, issue

Focus—Center, focal point, hub

Fragment—Piece, portion, section, part, splinter, chip

Function—Purpose, role, job, task

Furnish—Supply, provide, give, deliver, equip

Further—Additional, more, extra, added, supplementary

Generalize—To take a broad view, simplify, to make inferences from particulars

Generate—Make, produce, create

Gentle—Mild, calm, tender

Girth—Circumference, bulk, weight

Highest—Uppermost, maximum, peak, main

Hinder—Hold back, delay, hamper, obstruct, impede

Humane—Caring, kind, gentle, compassionate, benevolent, civilized

Ignore—Pay no attention to, disregard, overlook, discount

Imbalance—Unevenness, inequality, disparity

Immediate—Insistent, urgent, direct

Impair—Damage, harm, weaken

Implantation—To put in

Impotent—Powerless, weak, incapable, ineffective, unable

Inadvertent—Unintentional, chance, unplanned, accidental

Include—Comprise, take in, contain

Indicate—Point out, sign of, designate, specify, show

Ineffective—Unproductive, unsuccessful, useless, vain, futile

Inevitable—Predictable, to be expected, unavoidable, foreseeable

Influence—Power, pressure, sway, manipulate, affect, effect

Initiate—Start, begin, open, commence, instigate

Insert—Put in, add, supplement, introduce

Inspect—Look over, check, examine

Inspire—Motivate, energize, encourage, enthuse

Institutionalize—To place in a facility for treatment

Integrate—Put together, mix, add, combine, assimilate

Integrity—Honesty

Interfere—Get in the way, hinder, obstruct, impede, hamper

Interpret—Explain the meaning of, to make understandable

Intervention—Action, activity

Intolerance—Bigotry, prejudice, narrow-mindedness

Involuntary—Instinctive, reflex, unintentional, automatic, uncontrolled

Irreversible—Permanent, irrevocable, irreparable, unalterable

Irritability—Sensitivity to stimuli, fretful, quick excitability

Justify—Explain in accordance with reason

Likely—Probably, possible, expected

Liquefy—To change into or make more fluid

Logical—Using reason

Longevity—Long life

Lowest—Inferior in rank

Maintain—Continue, uphold, preserve, sustain, retain

Majority—The greater part of

Mention—Talk about, refer to, state, cite, declare, point out

Minimal—Least, smallest, nominal, negligible, token

Minimize—Reduce, diminish, lessen, curtail, decrease to smallest possible

Mobilize—Activate, organize, assemble, gather together, rally

Modify—Change, adapt, adjust, revise, alter

Moist—Slightly wet, damp

Multiple—Many, numerous, several, various

Natural—Normal, ordinary, unaffected

Negative—No, harmful, downbeat, pessimistic

Negotiate—Bargain, talk, discuss, consult, cooperate, settle

Notice—Become aware of, see, observe, discern, detect

Notify—Inform, tell, alert, advise, warn, report

Nurture—Care for, raise, rear, foster

Obsess—Preoccupy, consume

Occupy—Live in, inhabit, reside in, engage in

Occurrence—Event, incident, happening

Odorous—Scented, stinking, aromatic

Offensive—Unpleasant, distasteful, nasty, disgusting

Opportunity—Chance, prospect, break

Organize—Put in order, arrange, sort out, categorize, classify

Origin—Source, starting point, cause, beginning, derivation

Pace—Speed

Parameter—Limit, factor, limitation, issue

Participant—Member, contributor, partaker, applicant

Perspective—Viewpoint, view, perception

Position—Place, location, point, spot, situation

Practice—Do, carry out, perform, apply, follow

Precipitate—To cause to happen, to bring on, hasten, abrupt, sudden

Predetermine—Fix or set beforehand

Predictable—Expected, knowable

Preference—Favorite, liking, first choice

Prepare—Get ready, plan, make, train, arrange, organize

Prescribe—Set down, stipulate, order, recommend, impose

Previous—Earlier, prior, before, preceding

Primarily—First, above all, mainly, mostly, largely, principally, predominantly

Primary—First, main, basic, chief, most important, key, prime, major, crucial

Priority—Main concern, giving first attention to, order of importance

Production—Making, creation, construction, assembly

Profuse—A lot of, plentiful, copious, abundant, generous, prolific, bountiful

Prolong—Extend, delay, put off, lengthen, draw out

Promote—Encourage, support, endorse, sponsor

Proportion—Ratio, amount, quantity, part of, percentage, section of

Provide—Give, offer, supply, make available

Rationalize—Explain, reason

Realistic—Practical, sensible, reasonable

Receive—Get, accept, take delivery of, obtain

Recognize—Acknowledge, appreciate, identify, aware of

Recovery—Healing, mending, improvement, recuperation, renewal

Reduce—Decrease, lessen, ease, moderate, diminish

Reestablish—Reinstate, restore, return, bring back

Regard—Consider, look upon, relate to, respect

Regular—Usual, normal, ordinary, standard, expected, conventional

Relative—Comparative, family member

Relevance—Importance of

Reluctant—Unwilling, hesitant, disinclined, indisposed, adverse

Reminisce—To recall and review remembered experiences

Remove—Take away, get rid of, eliminate, eradicate

Reposition—Move, relocate, change position

Require—Need, want, necessitate

Resist—Oppose, defend against, keep from, refuse to go along with, defy

Resolution—Decree, solution, decision, ruling, promise

Resolve—Make up your mind, solve, determine, decide

Response—Reply, answer, reaction, retort

Restore—Reinstate, reestablish, bring back, return to, refurbish

Restrict—Limit, confine, curb, control, contain, hold back, hamper

Retract—Take back, draw in, withdraw, apologize

Reveal—Make known, disclose, divulge, expose, tell, make public

Review—Appraisal, reconsider, evaluation, assessment, examination, analysis

Ritual—Custom, ceremony, formal procedure

Rotate—Turn, go around, spin, swivel

Routine—Usual, habit, custom, practice

Satisfaction—Approval, fulfillment, pleasure, happiness

Satisfy—Please, convince, fulfill, make happy, gratify

Secure—Safe, protected, fixed firmly, sheltered, confident, obtain

Sequential—Chronological, in order of occurrence

Significant—Important, major, considerable, noteworthy, momentous

Slight—Small, slim, minor, unimportant, insignificant, insult, snub

Source—Basis, foundation, starting place, cause

Specific—Exact, particular, detail, explicit, definite

Stable—Steady, even, constant

Statistics—Figures, data, information

Subtract—Take away, deduct

Success—Achievement, victory, accomplishment

Surround—Enclose, encircle, contain

Suspect—Think, believe, suppose, guess, deduce, infer, distrust, doubtful

Sustain—Maintain, carry on, prolong, continue, nourish, suffer

Synonymous—Same as, identical, equal, tantamount

Systemic—Affecting the entire organism

Thorough—Careful, detailed, methodical, systematic, meticulous, comprehensive, exhaustive

Tilt—Tip, slant, slope, lean, angle, incline

Translucent—See-through, transparent, clear

Unique—One and only, sole, exclusive, distinctive

Universal—General, widespread, common, worldwide

Unoccupied—Vacant, not busy, empty

Unrelated—Unconnected, unlinked, distinct, dissimilar, irrelevant

Unresolved—Unsettled, uncertain, unsolved, unclear, in doubt

Utilize—Make use of, employ

Various—Numerous, variety, range of, mixture of, assortment of

Verbalize—Express, voice, speak, articulate

Verify—Confirm, make sure, prove, attest to, validate, substantiate, corroborate, authenticate

Vigorous—Forceful, strong, brisk, energetic

Volume—Quantity, amount, size

Withdraw—Remove, pull out, take out, extract

Bibliography

Chapter 1

American Nurses Association. (1980). *Nursing: A social policy statement.* Kansas City, MO: American Nurses Association.

American Nurses Association. (2004). *Nursing: Scope and standards of practice.* Washington, DC: American Nurses Association.

Anspaugh, D., Hamrick, M., & Rosato, R. (2011). *Wellness: Concepts and applications* (8th ed.). Columbus, OH: McGraw-Hill.

Becker, M. H., & Maiman, L. A. (1975). Sociobehavioral determinants of compliance with health and medical care recommendations. *Medical Care, 13*(1), 10–24.

Dunn, H. L. (1959). High-level wellness for man and society. *American Journal of Public Health and the Nation's Health, 49*(6), 786–792.

Erikson, E. H. (1963). *Childhood and society* (2nd ed.). New York: Norton.

Fowler, J. W. (1981). *Stages of faith: The psychology of human development and the quest for meaning.* New York: Harper & Row.

Gordon, M. (1994). *Nursing diagnosis: Process and application* (3rd ed., p. 70). St. Louis, MO: Mosby.

Havighurst, R. J. (1971). *Developmental tasks and education* (3rd ed.). New York: Longman.

Kohlberg, L. (1968). Moral development. In D. L. Sills (Ed.), *International encyclopedia of social science* (Vol. 18). New York: Macmillan.

Kübler-Ross, E. (1969). *On death and dying.* New York: Macmillan.

Leininger, M. M. (1978). *Transcultural nursing: Concepts, theories, and practices.* New York: Wiley & Sons.

Maslow, A. H. (1970). *Motivation and personality* (2nd ed.). New York: Harper & Row.

Myers, J., Sweeney, T., & Witmer, J. (2000). The wheel of wellness counseling for wellness: A holistic model for treatment planning. *Journal of Counseling & Development, 78*(3), 251–267.

Orem, D. (1991). *Nursing: Concepts of practice* (4th ed., p. 126). St. Louis, MO: Mosby-Year Book.

Piaget, J. (1952). *The origins of intelligence in children.* New York: International University Press.

Rogers, M. E. (1990). Nursing: Science of unitary, irreducible human beings. In E. A. M. Barrett (Ed.), *Visions of Rogers' science-based nursing* (Pub. No. 15-2285). New York: National League for Nursing Press.

Rosenstock, I. M. (1974). Historical origins of the health belief model. In M. H. Becker (Ed.), *The health belief model and personal health behavior.* Thorofare, NJ: Slack.

Roy, C. (2003). *The Roy adaptation model.* Retrieved May 5, 2012, from www.bc.edu/schools/son/faculty/featured/theorist/Roy_Adaptation_Model.html.

Sadock, B., & Sadock, V. (2007). *Kaplan & Sadock's synopsis of psychiatry* (10th ed.). Philadelphia: Lippincott Williams & Wilkins.

Watson, J. (1988). *Nursing: Human science and human care. A theory of nursing* (Pub. No. 15-2236). New York: National League for Nursing Press.

World Health Organization (WHO). (1948). *Preamble to the constitution of the World Health Organization as adopted by the International Health Conference.* New York, 19–22 June 1946; signed on 22 July 1946 by the representatives of 61 States (Official Records of the WHO, no. 2, p. 100) and entered into force on 7 April 1948.

Chapter 2

American Hospital Association. (2003). *The patient care partnership: Understanding expectations, rights and responsibilities.* Retrieved April 15, 2012, from www.aha.org/content/00-10/pcp_english_030730.pdf.

American Nurses Association. (1994). *Position statement: Active euthanasia.* Retrieved June 3, 2012, from www.nursingworld.org/MainMenuCategories/Policy-Advocacy/Positions-and-Resolutions/ANAPosition-Statements/Position-Statements-Alphabetically/prteteuth14450.html.

American Nurses Association. (2001). *The American Nurses Association's Bill of Rights for registered nurses.* Available at http://nursingworld.org/MainMenuCategories/WorkplaceSafety/Work-Environment/NursesBillofRights.

Chapter 3

American Nurses Association. (2009). *ANA Principles for delegation.* Available from www.nursingworld.org/principles.

American Nurses Association & National Council of State Boards of Nursing. (2005). *Joint statement on delegation.* Retrieved April 17, 2012, from www.ncsbn.org/Delegation_joint_statement_NCSBN-ANA.pdf.

American Nurses Credentialing Center. (2012). *ANCC Magnet recognition program.* Retrieved April 25, 2012, from www.nursecredentialing.org/Magnet.aspx.

Bennis, W., Spreitzer, G. M., & Cummings, T. G. (Eds.). (2001). *The future of leadership: Today's top leadership thinkers speak to tomorrow's leaders.* San Francisco: Jossey-Bass.

Hargrove-Huttel, R. A., & Colgrove, K. (2009). *Client management and leadership success: A course review applying critical thinking to test taking.* Philadelphia: F. A. Davis.

Jones, R. P. (Ed.). (2007). *Nursing leadership and management: Theories, processes, and practice.* Philadelphia: F. A. Davis.

Lee, J. A. (1980). *The gold and the garbage in management theories and prescriptions.* Athens, OH: Ohio University Press.

Lewin, K. (1951). *Field theory in social science.* New York: Harper & Row.

Locke, E. A. (1982). The ideas of Frederick Taylor: An evaluation. *Academy of Management Review, 7*(1), 14–24.

McGregor, D. (1960). *The human side of enterprise.* New York: McGraw-Hill.

McNichol, E. (2000). How to be a model leader. *Nursing Standard, 14*(45), 24.

National Council of State Boards of Nursing. (2005). *Working with others: A position paper.* Retrieved April 17, 2012, from www.ncsbn.org/Working_with_Others.pdf.

Porter-O'Grady, T., & Malloch, K. (2011). *Quantum leadership: A textbook of new leadership* (3rd ed.). Boston: Jones & Bartlett.

Tappen, R. M. (2001). *Nursing leadership and management: Concepts and practice* (4th ed.). Philadelphia: F. A. Davis.

Trofino, J. (1995). Transformational leadership in health care. *Nursing Management, 26*(8), 42–47.

Venes, D. (Ed.). (2009). *Taber's cyclopedic medical dictionary* (21st ed.) Philadelphia: F. A. Davis.

White, R. K., & Lippitt, R. (1960). *Autocracy and democracy: An experimental inquiry.* New York: Harper & Row.

Whitehead, D., Weiss, S., & Tappen, R. (2010). *Essentials of nursing leadership and management* (5th ed.). Philadelphia: F. A. Davis.

Chapter 4

American Nurses Association. (2012). *About ANA.* Retrieved April 18, 2012, from www.nursingworld.org/FunctionalMenuCategories/AboutANA.

American Nurses Association. (2012). *What is nursing?* Retrieved April 18, 2012, from www.nursingworld.org/EspeciallyForYou/What-is-Nursing.

Catalano, J. (2012). *Nursing now: Today's issues, tomorrow's trends* (6th ed.). Philadelphia: F. A. Davis.

Hopp, L., & Rittenmyer, L. (2012). *Introduction to evidenced-based practice: A practical guide for nursing.* Philadelphia: F. A. Davis.

International Council of Nurses. (2010). *Definition of nursing.* Retrieved April 18, 2012, from www.icn.ch/definition.htm.

International Council of Nurses. (2011). *Our mission.* Retrieved April 18, 2012, from www.icn.ch/about-icn/icns-mission.

National League for Nursing. (2011). *Mission/Goals/Core Values.* Retrieved April 18, 2012, from www.nln.org/aboutnln/ourmission.htm.

National League for Nursing Accrediting Commission. (2002). *About NLNAC: Mission statement.* Retrieved April 18, 2012, www.nlnac.org/About%20NLNAC/AboutNLNAC.htm#MISSION.

National Student Nurses Association. (n.d.). *About us.* Retrieved April 18, 2012, from www.nsna.org/AboutUs.aspx.

Sigma Theta Tau International (STTI). (2012). *STTI Organizational fact sheet.* Retrieved April 18, 2012, from www.nursingsociety.org/aboutus/mission/Pages/factsheet.aspx.

Chapter 5

Centers for Disease Control and Prevention. (2012). *Minority health: About CDC's Office of Minority Health & Health Equity (OMHHE).* Retrieved April 21, 2012, from www.cdc.gov/minorityhealth/OMHHE.html.

Dawes, D. E. & Weinstock, B. (2011). *Congressional Black Caucus Foundation Health Brain Trust: A practical resource for health equity champions: Policies, grants, programs and publications within the United States Department of Health and Human Services.* Retrieved April 21, 2012, from http://conference.afyainc.com/emhdpolicysummit/resources/Health%20Equity%20Resource%20April%202011.pdf.

Nies, M., & McEwen, M. (2011). *Community/public health nursing: Promoting the health of populations* (5th ed.). St. Louis, MO: Elsevier/Saunders.

Selekman, J. (Ed.). (2006). *School nursing: A comprehensive text.* Philadelphia: F. A. Davis.

Stanhope, M., & Lancaster, J. (2010). *Foundations of nursing in the community: Community-oriented practice* (3rd ed.). St. Louis, MO: Elsevier/Mosby.

Stanhope, M., & Lancaster, J. (2012). *Public health nursing: Population-centered health care in the community* (8th ed.). Maryland Heights, MO: Elsevier/Mosby.

U.S. Department of Health and Human Services. (2012). *About healthy people: Introducing healthy people 2020.* Retrieved April 18, 2012, from www.healthypeople.gov/2020/about/default.aspx.

U.S. Government Accountability Office. (2011). *Improving quality care to vulnerable populations: What needs to be done/key reports.* Retrieved April 21, 2012, from www.gao.gov/highrisk/agency/hhs/improving-care-vulnerable-populations.php.

Watkins, D., & Cousins, J. (Eds.). (2010). *Public health and community nursing: Frameworks for practice* (3rd ed.). Philadelphia: Baillière Tindall/Elsevier.

Chapter 6

Anderson, M. (2011). *Caring for older adults holistically* (5th ed.). Philadelphia: F. A. Davis.

Carlson, D., & Pfadt, E. (2009). *Clinical coach for effective nursing care for older adults.* Philadelphia: F. A. Davis.

Centers for Disease Control and Prevention. (2012). *Basics about childhood obesity.* Retrieved May 8, 2012, from www.cdc.gov/obesity/childhood/basics.html.

Centers for Disease Control and Prevention & National Center for Health Statistics (NCHS). (2009). *Delayed childbearing: More women are having their first child later in life* (NCHS Data Brief No. 21). Retrieved May 8, 2012, from www.cdc.gov/nchs/data/databriefs/db21.pdf.

Chapman, L., & Durham, R. (2010). *Maternal-newborn nursing: The clinical components of nursing care.* Philadelphia: F. A. Davis.

Colyar, M. (2011). *Assessment of the school-age child and adolescent.* Philadelphia: F. A. Davis.

Holloway, B. W., Moredich, C., & Aduddell, K. (2011). *OB/GYN & peds notes: Nurse's clinical pocket guide* (2nd ed.). Philadelphia: F. A. Davis.

Jenny, C. (2011). *Child abuse and neglect: Diagnosis, treatment and evidence.* St. Louis, MO: Saunders/Elsevier.

Lange, J. (2012). *The nurse's role in promoting optimal health of older adults: Thriving in the wisdom years.* Philadelphia: F. A. Davis.

Leifer, G., & Hartston, H. (2004). *Growth and development across the lifespan: A health promotion focus.* St. Louis, MO: Saunders.

Linnard-Palmer, L. (2010). *Peds notes: A nurse's clinical pocket guide.* Philadelphia: F. A. Davis.

Livingston, G., & Cohn, D. (2010). *The new demography of American motherhood.* Retrieved May 9, 2012, from www.pewresearch.org/pubs/1586/changing-demographic-characteristics-american-mothers.

Meiner, S. (2011). *Gerontologic nursing* (4th ed.). St. Louis. MO: Mosby/Elsevier.

Nagtalon-Ramos, K. (2013). *Maternity-newborn nursing care: Best evidence-based practices.* Philadelphia: F. A. Davis.

Ogden, C., Carroll, M., Kit, B., & Flegal, K. (2012). *Prevalence of obesity in the United State, 2009–2010* (NCHS Data Brief, no 82). Hyattsville, MD: National Center for Health Statistics. Retrieved May 8, 2012, from www.cdc.gov/nchs/data/databriefs/db82.pdf.

Polan, E., & Taylor, D. (2011). *Journey across the life span: Human development and health promotion* (4th ed.). Philadelphia: F. A. Davis.

Richardson, V. (2010). *Pediatric success: A course review applying critical thinking skills to test-taking.* Philadelphia: F. A. Davis.

Stanley, M., Blair, K., & Beare, P. (2005). *Gerontological nursing: Promoting successful aging with older adults* (3rd ed.). Philadelphia: F. A. Davis.

Touhy, T., & Jett, K. (2010). *Ebersole and Hess' gerontological nursing & healthy aging* (3rd ed.). St. Louis, MO: Mosby/Elsevier.

U.S. Department of Health and Human Services & Administration on Aging. (2011). *A profile of older Americans: 2011.* Retrieved May 17, 2012, from http://aoa.gov/AoARoot/Aging_Statistics/Profile/2011/docs/2011profile.pdf.

Wold, G. (2012). *Basic geriatric nursing* (5th ed.). St. Louis, MO: Mosby.

Chapter 7

Antai-Otong, D. (2006). *Nurse-client communication: A life span approach.* Burlington, MA: Jones & Bartlett Learning.

Arnold, E., & Boggs, K. (2011). *Interpersonal relationships: Professional communication skills for nurses* (6th ed.). St. Louis, MO: Saunders/Elsevier.

Diefenbeck, C., Paulanka, B., & Phillips, K. (2012). *Interpersonal skills for healthcare professionals—Student version.* Philadelphia: F. A. Davis.

Institute for Healthcare Improvement. (2011). *SBAR technique for communication: A situational briefing model.* Kaiser Permanente of Colorado. Retrieved May 6, 2012, from www.ihi.org/knowledge/Pages/Tools/SBARTechniqueforCommunicationASituationalBriefingModel.aspx.

Institute for Safe Medication Practices (ISMP). (2012). *ISMP's list of error-prone abbreviations, symbols, and dose designations.* Retrieved May 6, 2012, from www.ismp.org/tools/errorproneabbreviations.pdf.

Leonard, M. (2005). *Structured communication—SBAR: Creating a culture of safety* (slides 31–35). Retrieved May 6, 2012, from www.coloradopatientsafety.org/6-Leonard.ppt.

Munoz, C., & Luckman, J. (2005). *Transcultural communication in nursing* (2nd ed.). Clifton Park, NY: Delmar Learning/Thompson Learning.

Riley, J. (2012). *Communication in nursing* (7th ed.). St. Louis, MO: Mosby/Elsevier.

Schuster, P., & Nykolyn, L. (2010). *Communication for nurses: How to prevent harmful events and promote patient safety.* Philadelphia: F. A. Davis.

Sheldon, L. (2009). *Communication for nurses: Talking with patients* (2nd ed.). Sudbury, MA: Jones & Bartlett.

The Joint Commission. (2004). *Facts about the official "Do Not Use" list.* Retrieved July 1, 2012, from www.jointcommission.org/assets/1/18/Do_Not_Use_List.pdf.

Webb, L. (Ed.). (2011). *Nursing: Communication skills in practice.* New York: Oxford University Press.

Chapter 8

A definition of irreversible coma. (1968). *Journal of the American Medical Association, 205*(6), 337–340.

American Psychiatric Association. (2013). *Diagnostic and statistical manual of mental disorders* (5th ed.). Arlington, VA: American Psychiatric Publishing.

Caruso, K. (n.d.). *No-suicide contracts—What they are and how you should use them.* Retrieved June 26, 2012, from www.suicide.org/no-suicide-contracts.html.

Centers for Disease Control and Prevention. (2011). CDC health disparities and inequalities report—United States, 2011. *Morbidity & Mortality Weekly Report, 60*(Suppl.), 1–116. Retrieved July 11, 2012, from www.cdc.gov/mmwr/pdf/other/su6001.pdf.

Centers for Disease Control and Prevention. (2011). *Fact sheet: Tuberculosis in minorities.* Retrieved July 11, 2012, from www.cdc.gov/tb/publications/factsheets/specpop/resources_TB_Minorities.htm.

Centers for Disease Control and Prevention. (2012). *Fact sheets: TB in specific populations.* Retrieved January 10, 2012, from www.cdc.gov/tb/publications/factsheets/specpop.htm.

Coopersmith, S. (1967). *The antecedents of self-esteem.* San Francisco: Freeman Press.

Engel, G. (1964). Grief and grieving. *American Journal of Nursing, 64*(9), 93–98.

Erikson, E. H. (1963). *Childhood and society* (2nd ed.). New York: Norton.

Kaakinen, J., Gedaly-Duff, V., Coehlo, D., & Hanson, S. (2010). *Family health care nursing: Theory, practice, and research* (4th ed.). Philadelphia: F. A. Davis.

Kastenbaum, R. J. (1998). *Death, society, and human experience* (6th ed.). Boston: Allyn and Bacon.

Kübler-Ross, E. (1969). *On death and dying.* New York: Macmillan.

Leininger, M. M., & McFarland, M. R. (2006). *Culture care diversity & universality: A worldwide nursing theory* (2nd ed.). Boston: Jones & Bartlett.

Pew Research Center. (2012). *91.7%—Minorities account for nearly all U.S. population growth.* Retrieved July 11, 2012, from http://pewresearch.org/databank/dailynumbers/?NumberID=1225.

President's Commission for the Study of Ethical Problems in Medicine and Biomedical and Behavioral Research. (1981). *Defining death: A report on the medical, legal, and ethical issues in the determination of death.* Washington, DC: U.S. Government Printing Office.

Purnell, L., & Paulanka, B. (2008). *Transcultural health care: A culturally competent approach* (3rd ed.). Philadelphia: F. A. Davis.

Ray, M. (2010). *Transcultural caring dynamics in nursing and health care.* Philadelphia: F. A. Davis.

Stuart, B., Cherry, C., & Stuart, J. (2011). *Pocket guide to culturally sensitive health care.* Philadelphia: F. A. Davis.

Theobald, D. (n.d.). *Jewish death rituals.* Retrieved June 26, 2012, from http://dying.lovetoknow.com/jewish-death-rituals.

U.S. Census Bureau. (2008). *U.S. population projections: Projections of the population by sex, race, and Hispanic origin in the United States: 2010–2050.* Retrieved January 10, 2012, from www.census.gov/population/www/projections/summarytables.html.

U.S. Department of Health and Human Services & Health Resources and Services Administration. (2010). *The registered nurse population: Initial findings from the 2008 National Sample Survey of Registered Nurses.* Retrieved January 10, 2012, from http://bhpr.hrsa.gov/healthworkforce/rnsurveys/rnsurveyinitial2008.pdf.

Wilkinson, J., & Treas, L. (2011). *Fundamentals of nursing* (2nd ed.). Philadelphia: F. A. Davis.

Wright, L. (2005). *Spirituality, suffering, and illness: Ideas for healing.* Philadelphia: F. A. Davis.

Zerwekh, J. (2006). *Nursing care at the end of life: Palliative care for patients and families.* Philadelphia: F. A. Davis.

Chapter 9

Anderson, A., & Klemm, P. (2008). The Internet: Friend or foe when providing patient education? *Clinical Journal of Oncology Nursing, 12*(1), 55–63.

Bastable, S. (2006). *Essentials of patient education.* Sudbury, MA: Jones & Bartlett.

Bastable, S. (2008). *Nurse as educator: Principles of teaching and learning for nursing practice* (3rd ed.). Sudbury, MA: Jones & Bartlett.

Bietz, J., & Snarponis, J. A. (2006). Strategies for online teaching and learning: Lessons learned. *Nurse Educator, 31*(1), 20–25.

Bradshaw, M., & Lowenstein, A. (Eds.). (2011). *Innovative teaching strategies in nursing and related health professions* (5th ed.). Sudbury, MA: Jones & Bartlett.

Canobbio, M. (2005). *Mosby's handbook of patient teaching* (3rd ed.). St. Louis, MO: Mosby.

Doak, C., Doak, L., & Root, J. (1996). *Teaching patients with low literacy skills* (2nd ed.). Philadelphia: Lippincott Williams & Wilkins.

Dreeben, O. (2010). *Patient education in rehabilitation.* Sudbury, MA: Jones & Bartlett.

Falvo, D. (2011). *Effective patient education: A guide to increased adherence* (4th ed.). Sudbury, MA: Jones & Bartlett.

Hohler, S. (2004). Tips for better patient teaching. *Nursing, 34*(7), 7–8.

Lowenstein, A., Foord-May, L., & Romano, J. (2009). *Teaching strategies for health education and health promotion: Working with patients, families, and communities.* Sudbury, MA: Jones & Bartlett.

Miller, M., & Stoeckel, P. (2011). *Client education: Theory and practice.* Sudbury, MA: Jones & Bartlett.

Piaget, J. (1952). *The origins of intelligence in children.* New York: International University Press.

ProLiteracy. (2011). *The impact of literacy: Basic facts about literacy.* Retrieved July 11, 2012, from www.proliteracy.org/page.aspx?pid=345.

Redman, B. (2007). *The practice of patient education: A case study approach* (10th ed.). St. Louis, MO: Mosby.

Roberts, D. (2004). Advocacy through patient teaching. *MedSurg Nursing, 13*(6), 363, 382.

The Joint Commission. (2012). *Comprehensive accreditation manual for hospitals: The official handbook.* Oakbrook Terrace, IL: The Joint Commission.

Chapter 10

Ackley, B., & Ladwig, G. (2011). *Nursing diagnosis handbook: An evidence-based guide to planning care* (9th ed.). St. Louis, MO: Mosby/Elsevier.

Alfaro-LeFevre, R. (2010). *Applying nursing process: A tool for critical thinking* (7th ed.). Philadelphia: Lippincott Williams & Wilkins.

Bulechek, G. M., Butcher, H. K., Dochterman, J. M., & Wagner, C. (2013). *Nursing interventions classification (NIC)* (6th ed.). St. Louis, MO: Elsevier.

Carpenito-Moyet, L. J. (2006). *Understanding the nursing process: Concept mapping and care planning for students.* Philadelphia: Lippincott Williams & Wilkins.

Doenges, M., & Moorhouse, M. (2013). *Application of nursing process and nursing diagnosis: An interactive text for diagnostic reasoning* (6th ed.). Philadelphia: F. A. Davis.

Gordon, M. (1994). *Nursing diagnosis: Process and application* (3rd ed., p. 70). St. Louis, MO: Mosby.

Gulanick, M., & Myers, J. (2011). *Nursing care plans: Diagnoses, interventions, and outcomes* (7th ed.). St. Louis, MO: Elsevier/Mosby.

Henderson, V. (1964). The nature of nursing. *American Journal of Nursing, 64*(8), 62–68.

Maslow, A. H. (1970). *Motivation and personality* (2nd ed.). New York: Harper & Row.

Moorhead, S., Johnson, M., Maas, M. L., & Swanson, E. (2013). *Nursing outcomes classification (NOC)* (5th ed.). St. Louis, MO: Elsevier.

Murray, M., & Atkinson, L. (2000). *Understanding the nursing process in a changing care environment* (6th ed.). Columbus, OH: McGraw-Hill.

NANDA International. (2011). *Nursing diagnoses: Definitions and classifications 2012–2014.* Hoboken, NJ: Wiley-Blackwell.

University of Iowa, College of Nursing. (n.d.). *Center for nursing classification and clinical effectiveness (CNC).* Retrieved May 24, 2012, from www.nursing.uiowa.edu/center-for-nursing-classification-and-clinical-effectiveness.

University of Iowa, College of Nursing. (n.d.). *CNC—Intervention example (NIC).* Retrieved May 24, 2012, from www.nursing.uiowa.edu/cncce/nic-intervention-example.

University of Iowa, College of Nursing. (n.d.). *CNC Outcome example (NOC).* Retrieved May 24, 2012, from www.nursing.uiowa.edu/cncce/noc-outcome-example.

Wilkinson, J. (2012). *Nursing process and critical thinking* (5th ed.). Upper Saddle River, NJ: Pearson Education.

Chapter 11

Atlanta Medical Center. (n.d.). *What's race got to do with high blood pressure?* Retrieved August 3, 2012, from www.atlantamedcenter.com/en-us/ourservices/communityservices/pages/what%E2%80%99s%20race%20got%20to%20do%20with%20high%20blood%20pressure.aspx.

Centers for Disease Control and Prevention. (2012). *High blood pressure facts.* Retrieved August 3, 2012, from www.cdc.gov/bloodpressure/facts.htm.

D'Amico, D., & Barbarito, C. (2011). *Health & physical assessment in nursing* (2nd ed.). Upper Saddle River, NJ: Pearson Education.

Dillon, P. (2007). *Nursing health assessment: Clinical pocket guide* (2nd ed.). Philadelphia: F. A. Davis.

Fulmer, T. (2007). How to try this, Fulmer SPICES. *American Journal of Nursing, 107*(10), 40–49.

Gordon, M. (2009). *Assess notes: Nursing assessment and diagnostic reasoning.* Philadelphia: F. A. Davis.

Hogstel, M., & Curry, L. (2001). *Practical guide to health assessment through the life span* (3rd ed.). Philadelphia: F. A. Davis.

Hurst, J. (2011). *Anatomy & physiology in a flash! Book & flash cards: An interactive, flash-card approach.* Philadelphia: F. A. Davis.

Iyer, V. N., Mandrekar, J. N., Danielson, R. D., Zubkov, A. Y., Elmer, J. L., & Wijdicks, E. F. (2009). Validity of the FOUR score coma scale in the medical intensive care unit. *Mayo Clinic Proceedings, 84*(8), 694–701. Retrieved June 5, 2012, from www.ncbi.nlm.nih.gov/pmc/articles/PMC2719522.

Jones, S. (2013). *Pocket anatomy and physiology* (2nd ed.). Philadelphia: F. A. Davis.

Lee, A. H. (2005). Why is carcinoma of the breast more frequent in the upper outer quadrant? A case series based on needle core biopsy diagnoses. *Breast, 14*(2), 151–152. Retrieved June 12, 2012, from www.ncbi.nlm.nih.gov/pubmed/15767185.

National Cancer Institute at the National Institutes of Health. (n.d.). *Breast cancer.* Retrieved June 12, 2012, from www.cancer.gov/cancertopics/types/breast.

Perloff, D., Grim, C., Flack, J., Frohlich, E. D., Hill, M., McDonald, M., et al. (1993). Human blood pressure determination by sphygmomanometry. *Circulation, 88*(5 Pt 1), 2460–2470.

Saslow, D., Hannan, J., Osuch, J., Alciati, M. H., Baines, C., Barton, M., et al. (2004). Clinical breast examination: Practical recommendations for optimizing performance and reporting. *CA: A Cancer Journal for Clinicians, 54*(6), 327–344.

Scanlon, V., & Sanders, T. (2011). *Essentials of anatomy and physiology* (6th ed.). Philadelphia: F. A. Davis.

Selye, H. A. (1936). Syndrome produced by diverse nocuous agents. *Nature, 138*(3479), 32. Retrieved June 14, 2012, from www.acutechinternational.com/html/h_selye.html.

Shimek, J. M., Emmanuel, J., Orris, P., & Chartier, Y. (Eds.). (2011). *Replacement of mercury thermometers and sphygmomanometers in health care: Technical guidance.* Retrieved June 1, 2012, from http://whqlibdoc.who.int/publications/2011/9789241548182_eng.pdf.

Teasdale, G., & Jennett, B. (1974). Assessment of coma and impaired consciousness. A practical scale. *Lancet, 2*(7872), 81–84.

Terndrup, T., Allegra, J. A., & Kealey, J. A. (1989). A comparison of oral, rectal, and tympanic membrane-derived temperature changes after ingestion of liquids and smoking. *American Journal of Emergency Medicine, 7*(2), 150 -154.

The World Medical Association, Inc. (2008). *WMA statement on reducing the global burden of mercury.* Retrieved June 1, 2012, from www.mercuryfree-healthcare.org/WMA_Global_Burden_Mercury.pdf.

Tremblay, L. (2011). *What areas of the breast are most lumps found?* Retrieved June 12, 2012, from www.livestrong.com/article/192970-what-areas-of-the-breast-are-most-lumps-found.

U.S. Environmental Protection Agency. (2002). *Eliminating mercury in hospitals: Environmental best practices for health care facilities.* Retrieved June 1, 2012, from www.epa.gov/region9/waste/p2/projects/hospital/mercury.pdf.

U.S. Environmental Protection Agency. (2012). *Mercury: Information for health care providers.* Retrieved June 1, 2012, from www.epa.gov/mercury/healthcare.htm.

Weber, C. (2006). *About.com health: High blood pressure: Ethnicity & high blood pressure.* Retrieved August 3, 2012, from http://highbloodpressure.about.com/od/understandyourrisk/i/ethnic_is_2.htm.

Weber, J., & Kelley, J. (2010). *Health assessment in nursing* (4th ed.). Philadelphia: Lippincott Williams & Wilkins.

Wijkicks, E. F., Bamlet, W. R., Maramattom, B. V., Manno, E. M., & McClelland, R. L. (2005). Validation of a new coma scale: The FOUR score. *Annals of Neurology, 58*(4), 585–593.

Wilson, S., & Giddens, J. (2013). *Health assessment for nursing practice* (5th ed.). St. Louis, MO: Mosby/Elsevier.

Chapter 12

American Nurses Association. (1980). *Nursing: A social policy statement.* Kansas City, MO: American Nurses Association.

Centers for Disease Control and Prevention. (1989). Guidelines for prevention of transmission of human immunodeficiency virus and hepatitis B virus to health-care and public-safety workers: A response to P.L. 100-607, The Health Omnibus Programs Extension Act of 1988. *MMWR Supplements, 38*(S-6), 3–37. Retrieved May 25, 2012, from www.cdc.gov/mmwr/preview/mmwrhtml/00001450.htm.

Centers for Disease Control and Prevention. (2002). Guideline for hand hygiene in health-care settings: Recommendations of the Healthcare Infection Control Practices Advisory Committee and the HICPAC/SHEA/APIC/IDSA Hand Hygiene Task Force. *MMWR Recommendations and Reports, 51*(RR-16), 1–44. Retrieved July 22, 2012, from www.cdc.gov/mmwr/preview/mmwrhtml/rr5116a1.htm.

Centers for Disease Control and Prevention. (2010). *MRSA infections: Precautions to prevent the spread of MRSA in healthcare settings.* Retrieved May 30, 2012, from www.cdc.gov/mrsa/prevent/healthcare/precautions.html.

Centers for Disease Control and Prevention. (2013). Recommended adult immunization schedule—United States, 2013. Retrieved June 22, 2013, from www.cdc.gov/vaccines/schedules/hcp/imz/adult/html.

Centers for Disease Control and Prevention. (2013). *Recommended immunization schedule for persons aged 0 through 18 years—United States, 2013.* Retrieved June 22, 2013, from www.cdc.gov/vaccines/schedules/download/child/0-18years-schedule.pdf.

Centers for Disease Control and Prevention. (2012). *Get smart: Know when antibiotics work.* Retrieved May 24, 2012, from www.cdc.gov/getsmart.

Centers for Disease Control and Prevention. (2012). *Hand hygiene saves lives.* Retrieved May 25, 2012, from www.cdc.gov/Features/HandHygiene.

Centers for Disease Control and Prevention. (2012). *Healthcare-associated infections (HAI) topics.* Retrieved May 24, 2012, from www.cdc.gov/hai.

Centers for Disease Control and Prevention. (2012). *Top CDC recommendations to prevent healthcare-associated infections.* Retrieved May 25, 2012, from www.cdc.gov/HAI/prevent/top-cdc-recs-prevent-hai.html.

Clancy, C. (2010). *Healthcare-associated infections: They can happen to you.* Agency for Healthcare Research and Quality, Rockville, MD. Retrieved May 25, 2012, from www.ahrq.gov/consumer/cc/cc050410.htm.

Clancy, C. (2010). *Simple steps can reduce health care-associated infections.* Agency for Healthcare Research and Quality, Rockville, MD. Retrieved May 24, 2012, from www.ahrq.gov/consumer/cc/cc070108.htm.

Daniels, S. (2007). Protecting patients from harm: Improving hospital care for surgical patients. *Nursing, 37*(8), 36–41.

Holcomb, S. (2008). MRSA infections. *Nursing, 38*(6), 33.

Institute for Healthcare Improvement. (n.d.). *Protecting 5 million lives from harm.* Retrieved May 24, 2012, from www.ihi.org/offerings/Initiatives/PastStrategic-Initiatives/5MillionLivesCampaign/Pages/default.aspx.

Kennamer, M. (2007). *Basic infection control for health care providers* (2nd ed.). Clifton Park, NY: Thomson Delmar Learning.

Liu, C., Bayer, A., Cosgrove, S. E., Daum, R. S., Fridkin, S. K., Gorwitz, R. J., et al. (2011). *Clinical practice guidelines by the Infectious Diseases Society of America for the treatment of methicillin-resistant* Staphylococcus aureus *infections in adults and children.* Retrieved May 30, 2012, from www.idsociety.org/uploadedFiles/IDSA/Guidelines-Patient_Care/PDF_Library/MRSA.pdf.

Mazurek Melnyk, B., & Fineout-Overholt, E. (2011). *Evidence-based practice in nursing and healthcare: A guide to best practice* (2nd ed.). Philadelphia: Wolters Kluwer Health/Lippincott Williams & Wilkins.

Motacki, K., O'Mara, N. B., & Kapoian, T. (Eds.). (2011). *An illustrated guide to infection control.* New York: Springer.

Nursing Diagnosis List. (2011). *Risk for infection nursing diagnosis NIC NOC.* Retrieved May 25, 2012, from www.nursing-diagnosis-list.blogspot.com/2011/10/risk-for-infection-nursng-diagnosis-nic.html.

Perry, C. (2008). *Infection prevention and control.* Hoboken, NJ: Wiley-Blackwell.

Safe Care Campaign. *Preventing health care and community acquired infections.* Retrieved May 28, 2012, from www.safecarecampaign.org/Welcome.html.

San Francisco Department of Public Health. (2005). *Infection control precautions.* Retrieved May 30, 2012, from www.sfcdcp.org/document.html?id=68.

Siegel, J. D., Rhinehart, E., Jackson, M., Chiarello, L., & the Healthcare Infection Control Practices Advisory Committee. (2007). *2007 Guideline for isolation precautions: Preventing transmission of infectious agents in healthcare settings.* Retrieved May 25, 2012, from www.cdc.gov/hicpac/pdf/isolation/Isolation2007.pdf.

U.S. Department of Labor & Occupational Safety and Health Administration. (n.d.). *Bloodborne pathogens and needlestick prevention.* Retrieved May 24, 2012, from www.osha.gov/SLTC/bloodbornepathogens/index.html.

World Health Organization (WHO). (2012). *Global alert and response (GAR): Infection prevention and control in health care.* Retrieved May 23, 2012, from www.who.int/csr/bioriskreduction/infection_control/en/index.html.

World Health Organization (WHO). (2012). *Health topics: Drug resistance.* Retrieved May 23, 2012, from www.who.int/topics/drug_resistance/en.

Yamamoto, L., & Marten, M. (2007). Listen up, MRSA: The bug stops here. *Nursing, 37*(12 Pt 1), 51–55.

Chapter 13

Agency for Healthcare Research and Quality. (n.d.). *Patient safety & medical errors.* Retrieved May 28, 2012, from www.ahrq.gov/qual/patientsafetyix.htm.

Booth, J., & Edwards, A. R. (2011). *Four-point restraint.* Retrieved May 27, 2012, from http://emedicine.medscape.com/article/1941454-overview#a15.

Centers for Disease Control and Prevention. (2009). *10 leading causes of death by age group, United States—2009.* Retrieved June 27, 2012, from www.cdc.gov/Injury/wisqars/pdf/10LCD-Age-Grp-US-2009-a.pdf.

Centers for Disease Control and Prevention. (2010). *CDC falls prevention activities: Research studies.* Retrieved May 29, 2012, from www.cdc.gov/HomeandRecreationalSafety/Falls/FallsPreventionActivity.html.

Centers for Disease Control and Prevention. (2011). *Injury prevention & control: Data & statistics (WISQARTS(tm)).* Retrieved July 24, 2012, from www.cdc.gov/injury/wisqars.

Centers for Disease Control and Prevention. (2012). *Falls among older adults: An overview.* Retrieved May 29, 2012, from www.cdc.gov/HomeandRecreational-Safety/Falls/adultfalls.html.

Centers for Disease Control and Prevention. (2012). *Home & recreational safety: Unintentional drowning: Get the facts.* Retrieved June 27, 2012, from www.cdc.gov/HomeandRecreationalSafety/Water-Safety/waterinjuries-factsheet.html.

Centers for Disease Control and Prevention. (2012). *Leading causes of death.* Retrieved July 22, 2012, from www.cdc.gov/nchs/fastats/lcod.htm.

Giardino, A., DeLago, C., Kersten, H., Matz, P., McGregor, R., Smals, L., & Spector, N. (2007). *Child* safety: A pediatric guide for parents, teachers, nurses and caregivers. St. Louis, MO: STM Learning.

Halm, M. (2009). Hourly rounds: What does the evidence indicate? *American Journal of Critical Care, 18*(6), 581–584. Retrieved May 29, 2012, from http://ajcc.aacnjournals.org/content/18/6/581.full.

Institute for Healthcare Improvement. (2012). *Patient safety.* Retrieved May 28, 2012, from www.ihi.org/explore/patientsafety/pages/default.aspx.

Maslow, A. H. (1970). *Motivation and personality* (2nd ed.). New York: Harper & Row.

Mathias, S. Nayak, U. S., & Isaacs, B. (1986). Balance in elderly patients: The "get-up-and-go" test. *Archives of Physical Medicine and Rehabilitation, 67*(6), 387-389. Retrieved June 25, 2013 from www.ncbi.nlm.nih.gov/pubmed/3487300.

Morse, J. (2009). *Preventing patient falls: Establishing a fall intervention program* (2nd ed.). New York: Springer.

National Highway Traffic Safety Administration. (n.d.). *Is your child in the right car seat?* Retrieved June 19, 2012, from www.nhtsa.gov/Safety/CPS.

National Highway Traffic Safety Administration. (2012). *Motor vehicle traffic crashes are a leading cause of death in US, 2008 & 2009.* Retrieved June 27, 2012, from www-nrd.nhtsa.dot.gov/Pubs/811620.pdf.

National Patient Safety Foundation. (n.d.). *Mission and vision.* Retrieved May 28, 2012, from www.npsf.org/about-us/mission-and-vision.

National Safety Council. (2012). *Child safety seats & boosters.* Retrieved August 3, 2012, from www.nsc.org/safety_road/DriverSafety/Pages/ChildPassengerSafety.aspx.

Nelson, A. (Ed.). (2006). *Safe patient handling and movement: A guide for nurses and other health care providers.* New York: Springer.

Privitera, M. (Ed.). (2011). *Workplace violence in mental and general health settings.* Sudbury, MA: Jones & Bartlett.

Sherwood, G., & Barnsteiner, J. (Eds.). (2012). *Quality and safety in nursing: A competency approach to improving outcomes.* Hoboken, NJ: Wiley & Sons.

The Joint Commission. (2012). *National patient safety goals.* Retrieved May 28, 2012, from www.joint-commission.org/standards_information/npsgs.aspx.

The Leapfrog Group. (n.d.). *The leapfrog safety practices.* Retrieved May 28, 2012, from www.leapfroggroup.org/for_hospitals/leapfrog_hospital_survey_copy/leapfrog_safety_practices.

Tideiksaar, R. (2010). *Falls in older people: Prevention and management* (4th ed.). Baltimore: Health Professions Press.

University of Michigan Health System. (2010). *Gun safety for kids and youth.* Retrieved June 19, 2012, from www.med.umich.edu/yourchild/topics/guns.htm.

U.S. Department of Labor & Occupational Safety and Health Administration. (n.d.). *OSHA law & regulations.* Retrieved May 29, 2012, from www.osha.gov/law-regs.html.

U.S. Department of Labor & Occupational Safety and Health Administration. (n.d.). *Regulations (Standards-29CFR).* Retrieved May 28, 2012, from www.osha.gov/pls/oshaweb/owasrch.search_form?p_doc_type=STANDARDS&p_toc_level=0&p_keyvalue=.

World Health Organization. (2012). *Falls.* Retrieved June 25, 2013, from www.who.int/mediacentre/factsheets/fs344/en.

Chapter 14

Giangrasso, A., & Shrimpton, D. (2012). *Dosage calculations: A multi-method approach.* Upper Saddle River, NJ: Prentice Hall.

Horntvedt, T. (2012). *Calculating dosages safely: A dimensional analysis approach.* Philadelphia: F. A. Davis.

Institute for Safe Medication Practices. (2011). *Throw away your old medicines safely.* Retrieved May 30, 2012, from www.ismp.org/consumers/ThrowAwayMedsSafely.asp.

Institute for Safe Medication Practices. (2012). *ISMP's list of high-alert medications.* Retrieved May 30, 2012, from www.ismp.org/tools/highalertmedications.pdf.

Kee, J., & Marshall, S. (2013). *Clinical calculations* (7th ed.). St. Louis, MO: Saunders/Elsevier.

Lesmeister, M. (2009). *Math basics for the health care professional* (3rd ed.). Upper Saddle River, NJ: Prentice Hall.

Macklin, D., Chernecky, C., & Infortuna, M. H. (2011). *Math for clinical practice* (2nd ed.). Maryland Heights, MO: Mosby/Elsevier.

Morris, D. (2010). *Calculate with confidence* (5th ed.). St. Louis, MO: Mosby/Elsevier.

National Coordinating Council for Medication Error Reporting and Prevention. (2012). *Council recommendations.* Retrieved May 29, 2012, from www.nccmerp.org/councilRecs.html.

Ogden, S., & Fluharty, L. (2012). *Calculation of drug dosages: A work text* (9th ed.). St. Louis. MO: Mosby/Elsevier.

Phillips, L. (2010). *Manual of I.V. therapeutics: Evidence-based practice for infusion therapy* (5th ed.). Philadelphia: F. A. Davis.

Raines, V. (2010). *Davis's basic math review for nurses: With step-by-step solutions.* Philadelphia: F. A. Davis.

Right Diagnosis. (2012). *Chronic illness: Introduction.* Retrieved July 4, 2012, from www.rightdiagnosis.com/c/chronic/intro.htm#whatis.

SMARxT DISPOSAL. (2012). *Responsible medication disposal safeguards lives and protects the environment.* Retrieved May 30, 2012, from www.smarxtdisposal.net.

The Healthy Aging Research Network Writing Group. (2006). Community case study: The prevention research centers healthy aging research network. *Preventing Chronic Disease: Public Health Research, Practice, and Policy, 3*(1), 1–7. Retrieved July 4, 2012, from www.cdc.gov/pcd//issues/2006/jan/pdf/05_0054.pdf.

U.S. Department of Health and Human Services & Agency for Healthcare Research and Quality. (n.d.). *AHRQ's patient safety initiative: Chapter 2. Efforts to reduce medical errors: AHRQ's response to senate committee on appropriations questions.* Retrieved May 30, 2012, from www.ahrq.gov/qual/pscongrpt/psini2.htm.

U.S. Department of Justice, Drug Enforcement Administration, & Office of Diversion Control. (n.d.). *Got drugs: National take-back initiative.* Retrieved May 30, 2012, from www.deadiversion.usdoj.gov/drug_disposal/takeback/index.html.

U.S. Food and Drug Administration. (2011). *Strategies to reduce medication errors: Working to improve medication safety.* Retrieved May 30, 2012, from www.fda.gov/Drugs/ResourcesForYou/Consumers/ucm143553.htm.

Vallerand, A., Sanoski, C., & Deglin, J. (2012). *Davis's Drug Guide for Nurses* (13th ed.). Philadelphia: F. A. Davis.

Chapter 15

Adams, M & Urban, C. (2012). *Pharmacology: Connections to nursing practice* (2nd ed.). Upper Saddle River, NJ: Prentice Hall.

Adams, M. et al. (2010). *Pharmacology for nurses: A pathophysiologic approach* (3rd ed.). Upper Saddle River, NJ: Prentice Hall.

Broyles, B., et al. (2013). *Pharmacological aspects of nursing care* (8th ed.). Clifton Park, NY: Thomson Delmar Learning.

Edmunds, M. (2013). *Introduction to clinical pharmacology* (7th ed.). St. Louis, MO: Mosby.

Hargrove-Huttel, R & Colgrove, K. (2008). *Pharmacology success.* Philadelphia: F. A. Davis.

Kee, J., et al. (2012). *Pharmacology: A nursing process approach* (7th ed.). St. Louis, MO: Saunders.

Lilley, L., et al. (2011). *Pharmacology and the nursing process* (6th ed.). St. Louis, MO: Mosby.

Tomlinson, G., & Ennis, D. (2011),. *Pocket I.V. drugs.* Philadelphia: F. A. Davis.

Ulbricht, C. (2011). *Davis's pocket guide to herbs and supplements.* Philadelphia: F. A. Davis.

U. S. Food and Drug Administration. (April 2012). *Orange book: Approved drug products with therapeutic equivalence evaluations.* Retrieved May 29, 2012, from www.accessdata.fda.gov/scripts/cder/ob/default/cfm.

U.S. Pharmacopeial Convention. (2012). *About us.* Retrieved May 30, 2012, from www.usp.org.

Vallerand, A., & Sanoski, C., & Deglin, J. (2012). *Davis's drug guide for nurses* (13th ed.). Philadelphia: F. A. Davis.

Workman M., et al. (2011). *Understanding pharmacology: Essentials for medication safety.* St. Louis, MO: Saunders.

Chapter 16

Baranoski, S., & Ayello, E. (2012). *Wound care essentials: Practice principles* (3rd ed.). Philadelphia: Lippincott Williams & Wilkins.

Burton, M., & Ludwig, L. (2011). *Fundamentals of nursing care: Concepts, connections and skills.* Philadelphia: F. A. Davis.

Cowdell, F. (2010). Promoting skin health in older people. *Nursing Older People, 22*(10), 21–26.

Cowdell, F. (2011). Older people, personal hygiene, and skin care. *Medsurg Nursing, 20*(5), 235–240.

Dillon, P. (2007). *Nursing health assessment: Clinical pocket guide* (2nd ed.). Philadelphia: F. A. Davis.

Wilkinson, J., & Treas, L. (2011). *Fundamentals of nursing* (2nd ed.). Philadelphia: F. A. Davis.

Williams, L., & Hopper, P. (2011). *Understanding medical surgical nursing* (4th ed.). Philadelphia: F. A. Davis.

Chapter 17

Berman, A., & Snyder, S. (2012). *Kozier and Erb's fundamentals of nursing: Concepts, process, and practice* (9th ed.). Upper Saddle River, NJ: Pearson Education.

Burton, M., & Ludwig, L. (2011). *Fundamentals of nursing care: Concepts, connections and skills.* Philadelphia: F. A. Davis.

Judd, M. (1989). *Mobility: Patient problems and nursing care.* Waltham, MA: Butterworth-Heinemann Medical/Elsevier.

Norton, D. (1962). *The Norton pressure sore risk-assessment scale scoring system.* Retrieved September 3, 2012, from www.rd411.com/wrc/pdf/w0513_norton_presure_sore_risk_assessment_scale_scoring_system.pdf.

Norton, D., McLaren, R., & Exton-Smith, A. (1962/1975). *An investigation of geriatric nursing problems in hospitals.* New York: Churchill Livingstone.

Olson, E., Johnson, B., & Thompson, L. (1990). The hazards of immobility. 1967. *American Journal of Nursing, 90*(3), 43–48.

Wilkinson, J., & Treas, L. (2011). *Fundamentals of nursing* (2nd ed.). Philadelphia: F. A. Davis.

Chapter 18

American Diabetes Association. (2013). *Living with diabetes: Checking your blood glucose level.* Retrieved July7, 2013, from www.diabetes.org/living-with-diabetes/treatment-and-care/blood-glucose-control/checking-your-blood-glucose.html.

BARD Access Systems. (n.d.). *BARD PEG cleaning brush.* Retrieved January 30, 2012, from http://bardaccess.com/feed-peg-brush.php.

Bionix Medical Technologies. (n.d.). *Enteral feeding tube declogger.* Retrieved January 30, 2012, from www.bionixmed.com/MED_Pages/DeClogger.html.

Centers for Disease Control and Prevention & National Center for Health Statistics. (2011). *FastStats: Obesity and overweight.* Retrieved January 30, 2012, from www.cdc.gov./nchs/fastats/overwt.htm.

CORPAK Medsystems. (n.d.). *Clog zapper.* Retrieved January 30, 2012, from www.corpakmedsystems.com/product_main/enteral_main.html#ClogZapper.

Dandeles, L. (n.d.). *What products can be used to unclog feeding tubes?* University of Illinois at Chicago. College of Pharmacy. Drug Information Group. Retrieved January 30, 2012, from http://dig.pharm.uic.edu/faq/Jul10/feedingtube.aspx.

Dudek, S. (2010). *Nutrition essentials for nursing practice* (6th ed.). Philadelphia: Lippincott Williams & Wilkins.

Garcia, J., & Chambers, E. (2010). Managing dysphagia through diet modifications. *American Journal of Nursing, 110*(11), 26–33.

Gedney, L. (2013). *Healthy eating: What is calorie-dense vs. nutrient-dense food?* New York: Demand Media, Retrieved July 7, 2013, from http://healthyeating.sfgate.com/caloriedense-vs-nutrientdense-food-5391.html.

Geissler, C., & Powers, H. (2009). *Fundamentals of human nutrition: For students and practitioners in the health sciences.* New York: Churchill Livingstone/Elsevier.

Grodner, M., Roth, S., & Walkingshaw, B. (2012). *Nutritional foundations and clinical applications: A nursing approach* (5th ed.). St. Louis, MO: Mosby/Elsevier.

Lutz, C., & Przytulski, K. (2004). *Nutri-notes: Nutrition & diet therapy pocket guide.* Philadelphia: F. A. Davis.

Lutz, C., & Przytulski, K. (2010). *Nutrition and diet therapy* (5th ed.). Philadelphia: F. A. Davis.

Metheny, N., Eisenberg, P., & McSweeney, M. (1988). Effect of feeding tube properties and three irrigants in clogging rates. *Nursing Research, 37*(3), 165–169.

Moore, M. (2009). *Mosby's pocket guide to nutritional assessment and care* (6th ed.). St. Louis, MO: Mosby/Elsevier.

National Association of Anorexia Nervosa and Associated Disorders. (2010). *Eating disorders statistics.* Retrieved January 30, 2012, from www.anad.org/get-information/about-eating-disorders/eating-disorders-statistics.

National Osteoporosis Foundation. (n.d.). *Fast Facts.* Retrieved January 30, 2012, from www.nof.org/node/40.

Nix, S. (2009). *Williams' basic nutrition & diet therapy* (13th ed.). St. Louis, MO: Mosby/Elsevier.

Rivero, E. (2009). Elderly women with Dowager's hump may be at higher risk of earlier death. *UCLA Newsroom,* Retrieved July 7, 2013, from http://newsroom.ucla.edu/portal/ucla/hyperkyphosis-may-predict-earlier-92475.aspx.

Schlenker, E., & Roth, S. (2011). *Williams' essentials of nutrition and diet therapy* (10th ed.). St. Louis, MO: Mosby/Elsevier.

Smith, R., & Meyers, S. (2005). 2 devices that unclog feeding tubes. *Modern Medicine.* Retrieved January 30, 2012, from www.modernmedicine.com/modernmedicine/article/articleDetail.jsp?id=142656.

Sorte, J., Daeschel, I., & Amador, C. (2011). *Nutrition, health, and safety for young children: Promoting wellness.* Upper Saddle River, NJ: Pearson.

Stanfield, P., & Hui, Y. (2010). *Nutrition and diet therapy* (5th ed.). Sudbury, MA: Jones & Bartlett.

Takahisa, H. (2011). Glucose monitoring after fruit peeling: Pseudohyperglycemia when neglecting hand washing before fingertip blood sampling, wash your hands with tap water before you check blood glucose level. Published online before print January 32, 2011, doi: 10.2337/dc10-1705, *Diabetes Care,* March 2011 vol.34 no.3 596-597. Retrieved July 7, 2013, from http//care.diabetesjournals.org/content/34/3/596.full?sid=084121aec-dd06-4f4c-a4d-357e6596acd7.

Talbott, S., & Hughes, K. (2007). *Health professional's guide to dietary supplements.* Philadelphia: Lippincott Williams & Wilkins.

U.S. Food and Drug Administration. (2004). *The nutrition facts label—An overview.* Retrieved February 11, 2012, from www.fda.gov/Food/ResourcesForYou/Consumers/NFLPM/ucm274593.htm#twoparts.

U.S. Food and Drug Administration & Center for Nutrition Policy and Promotion. (2011). *10 tips to a great plate.* Retrieved February 11, 2012, from www.choosemyplate.gov/food-groups/downloads/TenTips/DGTipsheet1ChooseMyPlate.pdf.

U.S. Food and Drug Administration & ChooseMyPlate. Gov. (n.d.). *Dietary guidelines.* Retrieved February 11, 2012, from www.choosemyplate.gov/dietary-guidelines.html.

Chapter 19

Auscultation skills: Breath and heart sounds (4th ed.). (2010). Philadelphia: Lippincott Williams & Wilkins.

Berman, A., Snyder, S., & McKinney, D. (2011). *Nursing basics for clinical practice.* Upper Saddle River, NJ: Prentice Hall.

Burton, M., & Ludwig, L. (2011). *Fundamentals of nursing care: Concepts, connections and skills.* Philadelphia: F. A. Davis.

Dillon, P. (2007). *Nursing health assessment: A critical thinking, case studies approach* (2nd ed.). Philadelphia: F. A. Davis.

Dillon, P. (2007). *Nursing health assessment: Clinical pocket guide* (2nd ed.). Philadelphia: F. A. Davis.

Potter, P. A., Perry, A. G., Stockert, P., & Hall, A. (2013). *Fundamentals of nursing* (8th ed.). St. Louis, MO: Mosby/Elsevier.

Sheldon, L. (2008). *Quick look nursing: Oxygenation* (2nd ed.). Sudbury, MA: Jones & Bartlett.

Venes, D. (Ed.). (2009). *Taber's cyclopedic medical dictionary* (21st ed.). Philadelphia: F. A. Davis.

Wilkinson, J., & Treas, L. (2011). *Fundamentals of nursing* (2nd ed.). Philadelphia: F. A. Davis.

Williams, L., & Hopper, P. (2011). *Understanding medical surgical nursing* (4th ed.). Philadelphia: F. A. Davis.

Chapter 20

AllergyExpert.US. Shellfish allergy. Retrieved July 15, 2013, from www.allergyexpert.us/food/shellfishallergy.html.

Boltz, M., Capezuti, E., Fulmer, T., & Zwicker, D. (Eds.). (2012). *Evidence-based geriatric nursing protocols for best practice* (4th ed.). New York: Springer.

Downey, P. (Ed.). (2000). *Introduction to urological nursing.* Philadelphia: Whurr.

Gray, M., & Moore, K. (2009). *Urologic disorders: Adult and pediatric care.* St. Louis, MO: Mosby/Elsevier.

Lynch, D. M. (2004). Cranberry for prevention of urinary tract infections. *American Family Physician, 70*(11), 2175–2177. Retrieved October 18, 2012, from www.aafp.org/afp/2004/1201/p2175.html.

National Kidney Foundation. (2012). *How your kidneys work.* Retrieved October 18, 2012, from www.kidney.org/kidneydisease/howkidneyswrk.cfm.

National Space Biomedical Research Institute. (n.d.). The formation of urine. Retrieved October 18, 2012, from www.nsbri.org/humanphysspace/focus4/ep-urine.html.

Newman, D., & Wein, A. (2009). *Managing and treating urinary incontinence* (2nd ed.). Baltimore: Health Professions Press.

Thiedke, C. C. (2003). Nocturnal enuresis. *American Family Physician, 67*(7), 1499–1506. Retrieved October 18, 2012, from www.aafp.org/afp/2003/0401/p1499.html.

Wang, C., Fang, C., Chen, N., Liu, S., Yu, P., Wu, T., et al. (2012). Cranberry-containing products for prevention of urinary tract infections in susceptible populations. *Archives of Internal Medicine, 172*(13), 988–996. Retrieved October 18, 2012, from http://archinte.jamanetwork.com/article.aspx?articleid=1213845.

Wilkinson, J., & Treas, L. (2011). *Fundamentals of nursing* (2nd ed.). Philadelphia: F. A. Davis.

Chapter 21

Chernecky, C., Macklin, D., & Murphy-Ende, K. (2006). *Saunder's nursing survival guide: Fluids and electrolytes* (2nd ed.). Philadelphia: Saunders/Elsevier.

Hale, A., & Hovey, M. (2012). *Fluid and electrolyte notes: Nurse's clinical pocket guide.* Philadelphia: F. A. Davis.

Hale, A., & Hovey, M. (2013). *Fluid, electrolytes and acid-base imbalances: Need to know content plus practice questions.* Philadelphia: F. A. Davis.

Kee, J., Paulanka, B., & Polek, C. (2010). *Fluids and electrolytes with clinical applications* (8th ed.). Clifton Park, NY: Delmar Cengage Learning.

Kee, J., Paulanka, B., & Polek, C. (2010). *Handbook of fluid, electrolyte and acid-base imbalances* (3rd ed.). Clifton Park, NY: Delmar Cengage Learning.

Metheny, N. (2012). *Fluid & electrolyte balance: Nursing considerations* (5th ed.). Sudbury, MA: Jones & Bartlett Learning.

Phillips, L. (2005). *IV therapy notes: Nurse's clinical pocket guide.* Philadelphia: F. A. Davis.

Phillips, L. (2010). *Manual of I.V. therapeutics: Evidence-based practice for infusion therapy* (5th ed.). Philadelphia: F. A. Davis.

Van Leeuwen, A., Poelhuis-Leth, D., & Bladh, M. (2011). *Davis's comprehensive handbook of laboratory and diagnostic tests with nursing implications* (4th ed.). Philadelphia: F. A. Davis.

Westgard, E. (2011). *Clinical coach for fluid & electrolyte balance.* Philadelphia: F. A. Davis.

Chapter 22

Breckman, B. (2006). *Stoma care and rehabilitation.* St. Louis, MO: Churchill Livingstone/Elsevier.

Burch, J. (Ed.). (2008). *Stoma care.* Hoboken, NJ: Wiley-Blackwell.

Colwell, J., Goldberg, M., & Carmel, J. (2004). *Fecal & urinary diversions: Management principles.* St. Louis, MO: Mosby/Elsevier.

Doughty, D. (2006). *Urinary & fecal incontinence: Current management concepts* (3rd ed.). St. Louis, MO: Mosby/Elsevier.

Meiner, S. (Ed.). (2004). *Care of gastrointestinal problems in the older adult.* New York: Springer.

Ogilvie, J., Hicks, L., & Kalloo, A. (2008). *Johns Hopkins manual of gastrointestinal endoscopic procedures* (2nd ed.). Thorofare, NJ: Slack.

Porrett, T., & McGrath, A. (2005). *Stoma care: Essential clinical skills for nurses.* Malden, MA: Blackwell.

Scanlon, V., & Sanders, T. (2007). *Essentials of anatomy and physiology* (5th ed.). Philadelphia: F. A. Davis.

Chapter 23

Colten, H., & Altevogt, B. (Eds.). (2006). *Sleep disorders and sleep deprivation: An unmet public health problem.* Washington, DC: National Academies Press.

Cranwell-Bruce, L. (2009). PCA delivery systems. *Medsurg Nursing, 18*(2), 127–129, 133.

Gloth, F. M., III (Ed.). (2011). *Handbook of pain relief in older adults: An evidence-based approach* (2nd ed.). New York: Humana Press/Springer Science+Business Media.

Hockenberry, M., & Wilson, D. (2011). *Wong's nursing care of infants and children* (9th ed.). St. Louis, MO: Mosby/Elsevier.

Johnston, N., & Scholler-Jaquish, A. (Eds.). (2007). *Meaning of suffering: Caring practices in the health professions*. Madison, WI: University of Wisconsin Press.

Kolcaba, K. (1994). A theory of holistic comfort for nursing. *Journal of Advanced Nursing, 19*(6), 1178–1184.

Kolcaba, K., & DiMarco, M. (2005). Comfort theory and its application to pediatric nursing. *Pediatric Nursing, 31*(3), 187–194.

Kuebler, K., Heidrich, D., & Esper, P. (2007). *Palliative and end-of-life care: Clinical practice guidelines* (2nd ed.). St. Louis, MO: Saunders/Elsevier.

Macintyre, P., & Schug, S. (2008). *Acute pain management: A practical guide*. St. Louis, MO: Saunders/Elsevier.

Mann, E., & Carr, E. (2006). *Essential clinical skills for nurses: Pain management*. Malden, MA: Blackwell.

Melzack, R., & Wall, P. (1965). Pain mechanisms: A new theory. *Science, 150*(3699), 971–979.

Merkel, S. I., Voepel-Lewis, T., & Malviya, S. (1997). *FLACC Behavioral Pain Assessment Scale*. Retrieved October 18, 2012, from http://wps.prenhall.com/wps/.media/objects/3103/3178396/tools/flacc.pdf.

Morgan, K., & Closs, S. J. (2000). *Sleep management in nursing practice: An evidence-based guide*. Philadelphia: Churchill Livingstone/Elsevier.

Oakes, L. (2011). *Compact clinical guide to infant and child pain management: An evidence-based approach for nurses*. New York: Springer.

Pantley, E. (2005). *The no-cry sleep solution for toddlers and preschoolers: Gentle ways to stop bedtime battles and improve your child's sleep*. New York: McGraw-Hill.

Pasero, C., & McCaffery, M. (2011). *Pain assessment and pharmacologic management*. St. Louis, MO: Mosby/Elsevier.

Quinlan-Colwell, A., & D'Arcy, Y. (2012). *Compact clinical guide to geriatric pain management: An evidence-based approach for nurses*. New York: Springer.

Redeker, N., & McEnany. G. (2011). *Sleep disorders and sleep promotion in nursing practice*. New York: Springer.

U.S. Department of Health and Human Services. (2012). *Sleep disorders* (NOOK Book). Retrieved October 18, 2012, from http://barnesandnoble.com/w/sleep-disorders-us-department-of-health-and-human-services/1111392902?ean=2940014748117.

Chapter 24

Aldrete, J. A. (1995). Post-anesthesia recovery score revisited. *Journal of Clinical Anesthesia, 7*(1), 89–91.

Aldrete, J. A., & Kroulik, D. (1970). A postanesthetic recovery score. *Anesthesia and Analgesia, 49*(6), 924–934.

Browne, N., Flanigan, L., McComiskey, C., & Pieper, P. (2013). *Nursing care of the pediatric surgical patient* (3rd ed.). Burlington, MA: Jones & Bartlett Learning.

Cabanas, J., Manning, J., & Cairns, C. (2011). Fluid and blood resuscitation. In J. Tintinalli, J. S. Stapczynski, D. Cline, O. J. Ma, R. Cydulka, & G. Meckler (Eds.), *Tintinalli's emergency medicine: A comprehensive study guide* (7th ed., pp. 172–176). New York: McGraw-Hill.

Cox. F. (2009). *Handbook of perioperative pain management*. Hoboken, NJ: Blackwell Publishing.

Girard-Powell, V. (Ed.). (2010). *Pain, analgesia and anesthesia, an issue of perioperative nursing clinics*. St. Louis, MO: Saunders/Elsevier.

Goldman, M. (2008). *Pocket guide to the operating room* (3rd ed.). Philadelphia: F. A. Davis.

Hopper, P., & Williams, L. (Eds.). (2011). *Study guide for understanding medical surgical nursing* (4th ed.). Philadelphia: F. A. Davis.

Kost, M., & Odom-Forren, J. (n.d.). *Caring for the postanesthesia patient*. Retrieved October 18, 2012, from http://ce.nurse.com/ce115-60/caring-for-the-postanesthesia-patient/coursepage.

Litwack, K. (2009). *Clinical coach for effective perioperative nursing care*. Philadelphia: F. A. Davis.

Mishra, R. (2011). *History of minimal access surgery*. Retrieved October 18, 2012, from www.laparoscopy-hospital.com/history_of_laparoscopy.htm.

Pudner, R. (Ed.). (2010). *Nursing the surgical patient* (3rd ed.). Philadelphia: Baillière Tindall-Elsevier.

Shippee-Rice, R., Fetzer, S., & Long, J. (2012). *Gerioperative nursing care: Principles and practices in surgical care of the older adult*. New York: Springer.

Smeltzer, S., Bare, B., Hinkle, J., & Cheever, K. (2010). *Brunner and Suddarth's textbook of medical surgical nursing* (12th ed.). Philadelphia: Wolters Kluwer Health/Lippincott Williams & Wilkins.

Timmins, F., & McCabe, C. (2009). *Day surgery: Contemporary approaches to nursing care*. Hoboken, NJ: Wiley-Blackwell.

Watson, D. (2011). *Perioperative safety*. St. Louis, MO: Mosby/Elsevier.

Wicker, P., & O'Neill, J. (2010). *Essential clinical skills: Caring for the perioperative patient* (2nd ed.). Hoboken, NJ: Wiley-Blackwell.

Williams, L., & Hopper, P. (2011). *Understanding medical surgical nursing* (4th ed.). Philadelphia: F. A. Davis.

Woodhead, K., & Fudge, L. (2012). *Manual of perioperative care: An essential guide*. Hoboken, NJ: Wiley-Blackwell.

Credits for Figures in Review Questions

Chapter 1, Question 7: From U.S. Department of Health, Education, and Welfare. Public Health Service. National Office of Vital Statistics.

Chapter 7, Question 11: Courtesy of Smith Northview Hospital, Valdosta, GA.

Chapter 9, Question 26: Adapted from Wilkinson and Treas (2011): *Fundamentals of nursing, Vol. 2* (2nd ed.). Philadelphia: F. A. Davis. With permission.

Chapter 11, Questions 3, 21, and 33: Adapted from Wilkinson and Treas (2011). *Fundamentals of nursing,* Vol. 1, 2nd ed. Philadelphia: F. A. Davis, with permission.

Chapter 12, Question 34: From Burton and Ludwig (2011). *Fundamentals of nursing care: Concepts, connections & skills.* Philadelphia: F. A. Davis, with permission.

Chapter 13, Question 43: From Burton and Ludwig (2011). *Fundamentals of nursing care: Concepts, connections & skills.* Philadelphia: F. A. Davis, with permission.

Chapter 14, Questions 2, 13, 17, and 21: From Burton and Ludwig (2011). *Fundamentals of nursing care: Concepts, connections & skills.* Philadelphia: F. A. Davis, with permission.

Chapter 15, Case Study Question B: From Vallerand, Sanoski, & Deglin (2013) *Davis's drug guide for nurses,* 13th ed. Philadelphia: F. A. Davis, with permission.

Chapter 16, Questions 5, 24, and 27: From Wilkinson and Treas (2011). *Fundamentals of nursing,* Vol. 1, 2nd ed. Philadelphia: F. A. Davis Company, with permission.

Chapter 17, Questions 3 and 6: From Burton and Ludwig (2011). *Fundamentals of nursing care: Concepts, connections & skills.* Philadelphia: F. A. Davis Company, with permission.

Question 17: From Wilkinson and Treas (2011). *Fundamentals of nursing,* Vol. 1, 2nd ed. Philadelphia: F. A. Davis Company, with permission.

Chapter 18: Questions 3 and 19: From Wilkinson and Treas (2011). *Fundamentals of nursing,* Vol. 1, 2nd ed. Philadelphia: F. A. Davis Company, with permission.

Chapter 19, Question 7: From Williams & Hopper (2011). *Understanding medical surgical nursing,* 4th ed. Philadelphia: F. A. Davis, with permission.

Question 30: From Burton and Ludwig (2011). *Fundamentals of nursing care: Concepts, connections & skills.* Philadelphia: F. A. Davis Company, with permission.

Chapter 20, Question 14: From Wilkinson and Treas (2011). *Fundamentals of nursing,* Vol. 2, 2nd ed. Philadelphia: F. A. Davis, with permission.

Chapter 21, Question 5: Adapted from Wilkinson and Treas (2011). *Fundamentals of nursing,* Vol. 1, 2nd ed. Philadelphia: F. A. Davis, with permission.

Question 35: From Burton and Ludwig (2011). *Fundamentals of nursing care: Concepts, connections & skills.* Philadelphia: F. A. Davis, with permission.

Chapter 22, Question 17: From Wilkinson and Treas (2011). *Fundamentals of nursing,* Vol. 1, 2nd ed. Philadelphia: F. A. Davis, with permission.

Chapter 23, Question 2: From Burton and Ludwig (2011). *Fundamentals of nursing care: Concepts, connections & skills.* Philadelphia: F. A. Davis Company, with permission.

Chapter 24, Questions 5 and 16: From Burton and Ludwig (2011). *Fundamentals of nursing care: Concepts, connections & skills.* Philadelphia: F. A. Davis Company, with permission.

Question 23: From Wilkinson and Treas (2011). *Fundamentals of nursing,* Vol. 1, 2nd ed. Philadelphia: F. A. Davis Company, with permission.

Final Exam Questions 51 and 96: From Burton and Ludwig (2011). *Fundamentals of nursing care: Concepts, connections & skills.* Philadelphia: F. A. Davis Company, with permission.

Index

Note: Page numbers followed by *b* indicate boxes, *f* indicate figures, and *t* indicate tables.

A

Abbreviations, to avoid, 138, 139*t*
ABCs (Airway, Breathing, and Circulation), 238
Abdomen
  assessment of, 271–272, 272*f*
  injections in, 388*t*
  percussion of, 273*f*
Abdominal breathing, 569, 584, 729
Abdominal distention, 272, 745, 765–766
Abdominal reflex, 265*t*
Abducens nerve, 267*t*
Abduction, 482*t*, 483*t*, 484*t*
Abduction pillow, 762*f*
Ablative surgery, 745, 746
Absorption, 419, 687
Abuse
  mandated reporting of, 88
  medication, 422–423
  signs of, 88*b*
  victims of, 87–88
Acceptance, 159, 167*t*
Accessory muscles of respiration, 569, 574
Accessory reflex, 269*t*
Accountability, 45, 47
Accreditation, 27
ACEIs (Angiotensin-converting enzyme
  inhibitors), 667*t*
Acetaminophen (Tylenol), 730*t*, 731*t*
Acetylsalicylic acid, 730*t*
Achilles reflex, 266*t*
Acid-base balance, 658–659, 659*f*
Acid-base imbalances, 659, 660*t*–661*t*
Acidosis
  metabolic, 660*t*
  respiratory, 490, 660*t*
Acids, 659
Acquired-active immunity, 298
Acquired-passive immunity, 298
Active immunity, 295, 296
Active transport, 649, 651, 651*f*
Activities of daily living (ADLs), 222, 450
Activity therapist, 67
Acute care hospitals, 65
Acute infections, 747
Acute pain, 257, 720*t*
ADA (American Diabetes Association) diet, 532
Adaptation, 3, 4, 10, 155, 242*t*
Adaptation model, 5
Adaptive capacity, 3, 4
Addiction, 423
Adduction, 482*t*, 483*t*, 484*t*
ADH (Antidiuretic hormone), 651
ADLs (Activities of daily living), 222, 450
Administrative law, 19, 20
Admission nursing assessment, 137
Adolescence, 10, 107
Adolescents
  development of
    cognitive, 107
    language, 107
    physical, 107
    psychosocial, 107, 158

hygiene and, 448
nursing care for, 108
nutrition and, 524*t*
pain perception in, 717*t*
physical assessment of, 239
play in, 107, 108
reaction to illness, hospitalization, and pain,
  107–108
respiratory functioning and, 573
safety issues for, 333
Adults
  See also Middle-life adults; Older adults;
    Young adults
  development of
    cognitive, 110
    physical, 109
    psychosocial, 109
  nursing care for, 110
  nutrition and, 524*t*
  pain perception in, 717*t*
  physical assessment of, 239
  pulse of, 251
  reaction to illness, hospitalization, and
    pain, 110
  safety issues for, 333
Advance health-care directives, 26, 31
Adverse drug effects related to aging, 113*t*
Adverse effect of medications, 415, 417
Advertising, food, 520
Advice giving, 133*t*
Advocate, nurse as, 84
Adynamic ileus, 688, 746, 766
Aerobic exercise, 480*t*
Aerosol, 361, 369
Affect, 155, 161
Affective domain, 191, 192, 192*t*
African Americans, 170, 171*t*, 257
Age
  See also Aging; Developmental
    considerations
  blood pressure and, 257
  metabolic rate and, 243–244
  patient safety and, 332–333
  pharmacokinetics and, 421
  pulse and, 251
  surgical risk and, 747
  wound healing and, 306
Agency policies, 415
Aggression, 155, 165
Aggressive patients, 165–166
Aging
  See also Older adults
  integumentary system and, 448–449, 448*f*
  polypharmacy and, 367
  problems associated with, 113*t*
  self-concept and, 158
Aging population, 82
AHA (American Hospital Association), 258, 338
Air quality, 573
Airborne transmission, 300, 302*t*
Airway obstructions, 587–588, 588*t*
Airway resistance, 571

Airways, 570
ALARA ("As Low as Reasonably Achievable"),
  338
Alarm reaction, 242*t*
Alaska Natives, 170
Albumin, 528*t*, 752
Alcohol abuse, 113*t*, 748
Alcohol consumption, 170, 257, 520, 573
Aldrete score, 757, 757*f*
Alert, 264
Alginate dressing, 310*t*
Alkalosis
  metabolic, 660*t*
  respiratory, 661*t*
Allergens, 337, 573
Allergic reactions to medications, 415, 418, 418*b*
Allergy
  defined, 331, 337
  food, 532
  latex, 337, 751
  nursing care for, 337
  surgical risk and, 747
Alpha cells, 687
Altitude, 573
Alveolar-capillary membrane, 572
Alveoli, 570
Ambulatory surgery settings, 749
American Association of Colleges of Nursing, 27
American culture, 169
American Diabetes Association (ADA) diet, 532
American Hospital Association (AHA), 258, 338
American Indians, 170, 173*t*
American Nurses Association (ANA), 5, 415
  activities of, 68
  on assisted suicide, 32
  certification by, 27
  Code of Ethics for Nursing, 29, 30, 30*b*
  definition of nursing by, 68
  on delegation, 48
  on euthanasia, 32
  mission of, 68
  Nurse's Bill of Rights, 27
  safety guidelines of, 338
  Standards of Nursing Practice, 29
American Nurses Association Credentialing
  Center (ANCC), 46
Americans with Disabilities Act, 25
Amino acids
  essential, 515, 516
  nonessential, 515, 516
Aminoglycosides, 311*t*
Amish, 171*t*
Ampule, 361, 383, 383*f*
Amylase, 516
ANA. *See* American Nurses Association (ANA)
Anabolism, 477, 493, 685, 687
Anal canal, 374
Anal stage, 10, 101
Analgesia, 269
Analgesics, 720–721, 730, 730*t*, 731*t*, 752–753
Analysis, 213, 217–219
Anaphylaxis, 331, 337